原著作者 Contributors

Christopher G. Azzoli, MD
Visiting Assistant Professor, Department of Medicine
Harvard Medical School
Massachusetts General Hospital
Boston, MA, USA

Sonia L. Betancourt Cuellar, MD
Department of Diagnostic Radiology
The University of Texas MD Anderson Cancer Center
Houston, TX, USA

Shanda H. Blackmon, MD, MPH, FACS
Associate Professor, Houston Methodist Hospital, Weill Cornell Medical College of Cornell University, Houston, TX, USA
Clinical Assistant Professor, The University of Texas MD Anderson Cancer Center
Houston, TX, USA

Lauren Averett Byers, MD, MS
Assistant Professor, Department of Thoracic/Head and Neck Medical Oncology
The University of Texas MD Anderson Cancer Center
Houston, TX, USA

David P. Carbone, MD, PhD
Thoracic Oncology Center
James Comprehensive Cancer Center
Ohio State University Medical Center
Houston, TX, USA

Tina Cascone, MD, PhD
Resident Physician
Department of Medicine, Division of Medical Education
Barnes-Jewish Hospital/Washington University School of Medicine in St. Louis
St. Louis, MO, USA

Joe Y. Chang, MD, MS, PhD
Professor
Clinical Section Chief, Department of Radiation Oncology
Director of Stereotactic Radiotherapy Program
The University of Texas MD Anderson Cancer Center
Houston, TX, USA

Caleb T. Chu, MD, MPH
The University of Texas MD Anderson Cancer Center
Houston, TX, USA

James D. Cox, MD
Professor, Department of Radiation Oncology
The University of Texas MD Anderson Cancer Center
Houston, TX, USA

Millie Das, MD
Clinical Assistant Professor, Division of Oncology
Stanford University/Stanford Cancer Institute
Stanford, CA, USA
Staff Oncologist
VA Palo Alto Heath Care System
Palo Alto, CA, USA

Patricia M. de Groot, MD
Assistant Professor, Department of Diagnostic Radiology
The University of Texas MD Anderson Cancer Center
Houston, TX, USA

Steven M. Dubinett, MD
Chief of Pulmonary and Critical Care Medicine
Professor of Medicine and Pathology
Director of UCLA Lung Cancer Research Program
Division of Pulmonary and Critical Care Medicine
University of California at Los Angeles
Los Angeles, CA, USA

George A. Eapen, MD
Associate Professor, Department of Pulmonary Medicine

The University of Texas MD Anderson Cancer Center
Houston, TX, USA

Jeremy J. Erasmus, MD
Professor, Department of Diagnostic Radiology
The University of Texas MD Anderson Cancer Center
Houston, TX, USA

Renata Ferrarotto, MD
Department of Thoracic/Head and Neck Medical Oncology
The University of Texas MD Anderson Cancer Center
Houston, TX, USA

Justin Gainor, MD
Clinical Fellow, Hematology/Oncology
Dana Farber Cancer Institute/Massachusetts General Hospital
Boston, Massachusetts, USA

Amol J. Ghia, MD
Assistant Professor, Department of Radiation Oncology
The University of Texas MD Anderson Cancer Center
Houston, TX, USA

Kathryn A. Gold, MD
Assistant Professor, Department of Thoracic/Head and Neck Medical Oncology
The University of Texas MD Anderson Cancer Center
Houston, TX, USA

Daniel Gomez, MD
Assistant Professor, Department of Radiation Oncology
The University of Texas MD Anderson Cancer Center
Houston, TX, USA

Peter Hammerman, MD, PhD
Assistant Professor of Medicine, Harvard Medical School, Boston, MA, USA
Department of Medical Oncology, Dana-Farber Cancer Institute, Boston, MA, USA

Broad Institute of Harvard and MIT, Cambridge, MA, USA

Mohamed Hassanein, PhD
Research Assistant Professor of Medicine
Division of Allergy, Pulmonary and Critical Care Medicine
Vanderbilt University Medical Center
Nashville, TN, USA

John V. Heymach, MD, PhD
Chair, Department of Thoracic/Head and Neck Medical Oncology
The University of Texas MD Anderson Cancer Center
Houston, TX, USA

Waun Ki Hong, MD, DMSc (Hon)
American Cancer Society Professor
Samsung Distinguished University Chair in Cancer Medicine
Professor and Head, Division of Cancer Medicine
Professor, Department of Thoracic/Head and Neck Medical Oncology
The University of Texas MD Anderson Cancer Center
Houston, TX, USA

Karen Suchanek Hudmon, DrPH, MS, RPh
Associate Head for Operations, Department of Pharmacy Practice
Professor of Pharmacy
Purdue University
Indianapolis, IN, USA

Marcin Imielinski, MD, PhD
Broad Institute of Harvard and MIT, Cambridge, MA, USA
Department of Pathology, Massachusetts General Hospital
Boston, MA, USA

Puneeth lyengar, MD, PhD
Assistant Professor, Department of Radiation Oncology

University of Texas Southwestern, Medical Center
Dallas, TX, USA

David Mark Jablons, MD
Professor and Chief Thoracic Surgery, UCSF Department of Surgery
Nan T. McEvoy Distinguished Professor of Thoracic Surgical Oncology
Ada Distinguished Professor of Thoracic Oncology
Program Leader Thoracic Oncology
UCSF Helen Diller Family Comprehensive Cancer Center
University of California
San Francisco, CA, USA

Rachel Jen, MD, FRCPC
Respiratory Division
Department of Medicine
University of British Columbia
Vancouver, British Columbia, Canada

Humam Kadara, PhD
Assistant Professor, Department of Translational Molecular Pathology
Division of Pathology and Laboratory Medicine
The University of Texas MD Anderson Cancer Center
Houston, TX, USA

Shaf Keshavjee, MD, MSc, FRCSC, FACS
Surgeon in Chief, UHN
James Wallace McCutcheon Chair in Surgery
Professor, Division of Thoracic Surgery & Institute of Biomaterials and Biomedical Engineering
University of Toronto
Toronto, ON, Canada

Edward S. Kim, MD
Chair, Solid Tumor Oncology and Investigational Therapeutics
Donald S. Kim Distinguished Chair for Cancer Research
Levine Cancer Institute
Carolinas HealthCare System
Charlotte, NC, USA

Lucia Kim, MD, PhD
Associate Professor, Department of Pathology
Inha University School of Medicine
Incheon, South Korea

Min P. Kim, MD
Assistant Professor
Weill Cornell Medical College
Department of Surgery
Division of Thoracic Surgery
Houston Methodist Hospital
Houston, TX, USA

Ritsuko U. Komaki, MD, FACR, FASTRO
Professor, Department of Radiation Oncology
Gloria Lupton Tennison Distinguished Endowed Professor in Lung Cancer Research
The University of Texas MD Anderson Cancer Center
Houston, TX, USA

Johannes R. Kratz, MD
Resident, Department of Surgery
Massachusetts General Hospital
Boston, MA, USA

Stephen Lam, MD, FRCPC
Professor of Medicine
University of British Columbia
Chair, Lung Tumour Group
BC Cancer Agency
Vancouver, BC, Canada

Donald R. Lazarus, MD
Interventional Pulmonology Fellow
Department of Pulmonary Medicine
The University of Texas MD Anderson Cancer Center
Houston, TX, USA

J. Jack Lee, PhD, MS
Professor, Department of Biostatistics
The University of Texas MD Anderson Cancer Center
Houston, TX, USA

Jay M. Lee, MD
Chief, Division of Thoracic Surgery
Associate Professor of Surgery
UCLA Lung Cancer Research Program
Jonsson Comprehensive Cancer Center
David Geffen School of Medicine at UCLA
Los Angeles, CA, USA

Zhongxing Liao, MD
Professor and Clinical Director, Department of Radiation Oncology
The University of Texas MD Anderson Cancer Center
Houston, TX, USA

Jie Lin, PhD
Department of Epidemiology
The University of Texas MD Anderson Cancer Center
Houston, TX, USA

Steven H. Lin, MD, PhD
Assistant Professor, Department of Radiation Oncology
The University of Texas MD Anderson Cancer Center
Houston, TX, USA

Geoffrey Liu, MD, FRCPC
Associate Professor
Princess Margaret Hospital/Ontario Cancer Institute;
Department of Medicine, Medical Biophysics, and Epidemiology
University of Toronto
Toronto, ON, Canada

Paolo Macchiarini, MD, PhD
Professor of Regenerative Surgery, Director of Advanced Center of Translational Regenerative Medicine, Director of European Airway Institute and Senior Consultant of Division Ear, Nose and Throat (CLINTEC)
Karolinska University Hospital
Stockholm, Sweden

Edith M. Marom, MD
Professor, Department of Diagnostic Radiology
The University of Texas MD Anderson Cancer Center
Houston, TX, USA

Erminia Massarelli, MD, PhD, MS
Assistant Professor
Department of Thoracic Head and Neck Medical Oncology
The University of Texas MD Anderson Cancer Center
Houston, TX, USA

Matthew Meyerson, MD, PhD
Department of Medical Oncology, Dana-Farber Cancer Institute, Boston, MA, USA
Broad Institute of Harvard and MIT, Cambridge, MA, USA
Department of Pathology, Brigham and Women's Hospital
Boston, MA, USA

Kathryn F. Mileham, MD
Solid Tumor Oncology
Levine Cancer Institute
Carolinas Health Care System
Charlotte, NC, USA

Reginald F. Munden, MD, DMD, MBA
Professor and Chair, Department of Radiology
The Houston Methodist Hospital
Houston, TX, USA

Vassiliki A. Papadimitrakopoulou, MD
Professor, Department of Thoracic/Head and Neck Medical Oncology
The University of Texas MD Anderson Cancer Center
Houston, TX, USA

Mauricio Pipkin, MD
Thoracic Surgery Clinical Fellow
UHN
University of Toronto
Toronto, ON, Canada

Katherine M.W. Pisters, MD
Professor, Department of Thoracic/Head and Neck Medical Oncology
The University of Texas MD Anderson Cancer Center
Houston, TX, USA

Alexander V. Prokhorov, MD, PhD
Professor, Department of Behavioral Science
The University of Texas MD Anderson Cancer Center
Houston, TX, USA

Xia Pu, PhD
Department of Epidemiology
The University of Texas MD Anderson Cancer Center
Houston, TX, USA

David C. Rice, MB, BCh, BAO, FRCSI
Professor of Surgery
Department of Thoracic and Cardiovascular Surgery
The University of Texas MD Anderson Cancer Center
Houston, TX, USA

Kenneth E. Rosenzweig, MD
Chairman and Professor, Department of Radiation Oncology
Icahn School of Medicine at Mount Sinai
New York, NY, USA

Jack A. Roth MD, FACS
Professor and Bud Johnson Clinical Distinguished Chair
Department of Thoracic and Cardiovascular Surgery
Professor of Molecular and Cellular Oncology
Director, W.M. Keck Center of Innovative Cancer Therapies
Chief, Section of Thoracic Molecular Oncology
The University of Texas MD Anderson Cancer Center
Houston, TX, USA

Pierre Saintigny, MD, PhD
Assistant Professor, Department of Thoracic/Head and Neck Medical Oncology
The University of Texas MD Anderson Cancer Center
Houston, TX, USA

Francesco Sammartino, MD
General Surgeon, Department of General and Mininvasive Surgery
San Giovanni di Dio Hospital
Orbetello, Italy

Sherven Sharma, PhD
Professor, Division of Pulmonary and Critical Care Medicine
Department of Medicine
UCLA Lung Cancer Research Program
David Geffen School of Medicine at UCLA
West Los Angeles VA
Los Angeles, CA, USA

Alice Shaw, MD, PhD
Assistant Professor, Department of Medicine, Harvard Medical School
Massachusetts General Hospital
Boston, MA, USA

George R. Simon, MD, FACP, FCCP
Professor of Medicine and Oncology
Section Chief: Translational Research
Department of Thoracic/Head & Neck Medical Oncology
The University of Texas MD Anderson Cancer Center
Houston, TX, USA

Heath D. Skinner, MD, PhD
Assistant Professor, Department of Radiation Oncology
The University of Texas MD Anderson Cancer Center
Houston, TX, USA

Matthew A. Steliga, MD
Associate Professor of Surgery
Division of Thoracic Surgery
University of Arkansas
Little Rock, AR, USA

Sonal Sura, MD
Radiation Oncologist, Queen Hospital Center
Icahn School of Medicine at Mount Sinai
New York, NY, USA

Roman Thomas, MD
Department of Translational Genomics
Center of Integrated Oncology Köln-Bonn
University of Köln
Köln, Germany

Robert D. Timmerman, MD
Professor, Departments of Radiation Oncology and Neurosurgery
University of Texas Southwestern, Medical Center
Dallas, TX, USA

William Travis, MD
Attending Thoracic Pathologist, Department of Pathology
Memorial Sloan-Kettering Cancer Center
New York, NY, USA

Anne S. Tsao, MD
Associate Professor
Director, Mesothelioma Program
Director, Thoracic Chemo-Radiation Program
Department of Thoracic/Head and Neck Medical Oncology
The University of Texas MD Anderson Cancer Center
Houston, TX, USA

Ming-Sound Tsao, MD, FRCPC
Thoracic Pathologist and Professor
University Health Network, Princess Margaret Cancer Centre
Department of Laboratory Medicine and Pathobiology
University of Toronto
Toronto, ON, Canada

Heather Wakelee, MD
Assistant Professor of Medicine, Division of Oncology
Stanford University/Stanford Cancer Institute
Stanford, CA, USA

Howard West, MD
Medical Director, Thoracic Oncology Program
Swedish Cancer Institute
Seattle, WA, USA

William N. William Jr, MD
Assistant Professor
Chief, Head and Neck Section
Department of Thoracic/Head and Neck Medical Oncology
The University of Texas MD Anderson Cancer Center
Houston, TX, USA

Ignacio I. Wistuba, MD
Professor and Chair, Department of Translational Molecular Pathology
Anderson Clinical Faculty Chair for Cancer Treatment and Research
Division of Pathology and Laboratory Medicine
University of Texas MD Anderson Cancer Center
Houston, TX, USA

Xifeng Wu, MD, PhD, MS
Chair and Professor, Department of Epidemiology
Director, Center for Translational and Public Health Genomics
Betty B. Marcus Chair in Cancer Prevention
University of Texas MD Anderson Cancer Center
Houston, TX, USA

译者序
Preface

目前肺癌已成为人类健康的主要"杀手"之一。从小范围来看，肺癌不仅会吞噬掉患者健康的身体，还会导致患者家庭经济状况的骤然恶化和幸福指数直线下降；从大范围来看，随着肺癌发病率的逐年升高，其治疗所面临的沉重经济压力对一个国家、乃至整个社会都会产生巨大的影响。因此，肺癌的预防和治疗不仅是医学界的重大难题，也是政府所关注的重大社会问题。

近年来科学技术迅猛发展，人们对肺癌的认识逐步深入，不仅可以在分子水平揭示肺癌的"真实面目"，而且逐渐实现了肺癌的精准医疗和个体化治疗，在此基础上，与肺癌相关的各类研究成果、文献和著作层出不穷。

由 Jack A. Roth、Waun Ki Hong 和 Ritsuko U. Komaki 主编的《肺癌》第 4 版作为一部权威而系统的专著在众多肺癌相关图书中脱颖而出。本书基于肺癌领域中最新的研究成果，阐述了肺癌最新的诊断和治疗方法，自 1998 年首版发行以来，以新颖性和实用性广受读者欢迎。《肺癌》第 4 版邀请了 80 余位肺癌防治领域的国际顶级专家撰写，全书共分为 38 个章节，涉及吸烟的预防与戒烟、肺癌的易感性和风险评估模型、分子及基因学分析、病理学、影像学、手术及放化疗等治疗方法以及最新研究和前沿临床试验等肺癌相关知识，几乎涵盖了肺癌领域的各个方面，同时也介绍了近年刚刚出现的肺癌诊断和治疗新方法。

应世界图书出版西安有限公司马可为副总编的邀请，由我负责翻译本书，本人深感荣幸。随着翻译工作的逐步开展，我越来越体会到本书的丰富内涵和科技精髓。遂耗费大量精力，联合多位中青年肺癌专业骨干医生，合力呈出本译著，希望可以帮助肿瘤从业者尤其是肺癌专业人员汲取到最新和最先进的肺癌科研成果，开创诊疗新思路，进一步推动我国肿瘤学事业的发展。

译者虽为本书竭尽全力，然因水平所限，书中难免出现翻译不妥甚至错误之处，敬请读者不吝指正。

叶 欣

2018 年 10 月 14 日

主译简介

叶　欣，山东省立医院肿瘤科主任，主任医师，教授，硕士研究生导师。现任中国抗癌协会肿瘤微创专业委员会肺癌微创治疗分会主任委员，中国抗癌协会肿瘤微创治疗专业委员会常委，国家肿瘤微创创新技术联盟肺癌专业委员会主任委员，中国医师协会肿瘤消融专家组肺部肿瘤组组长，中国医师协会介入分会肿瘤消融专业委员会副主任委员，中国临床肿瘤学会（CSCO）肿瘤消融治疗专家委员会副主任委员，中国医师协会微无创肿瘤专业委员会副主任委员，中国研究型医院肿瘤介入专业委员会副主任委员，海峡两岸医药促进会肿瘤微创专业委员会主任委员，山东省医学会综合介入分会副主任委员，山东省抗癌协会临床肿瘤协作分会主任委员，山东省医师协会综合介入分会消融专业委员会主任委员。任 Journal of Cancer Research and Therapeutics 的中国主编。以第一作者或通讯作者发表SCI论文50余篇，累积影响因子超过100。

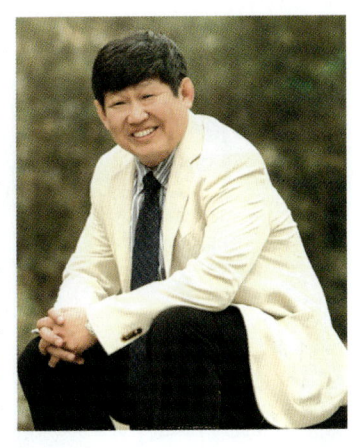

李宝生，山东省肿瘤医院副院长，博士生导师，研究员。现任中国医师协会放射肿瘤治疗医师分会第一届委员会候任主任委员，中华医学会放射肿瘤治疗学分会副主任委员，中国抗癌协会理事会常委理事，中国抗癌协会放射肿瘤治疗学分会副主任委员，山东省医师协会肿瘤放射治疗医师分会主任委员。受聘为《中华放射肿瘤学杂志》、《中华放射医学与防护杂志》、《国际肿瘤学》编委，《中华肿瘤防治杂志》副主编等。作为负责人承担国家重点研发计划子课题1项，国家自然科学基金重点项目1项，面上项目3项；承担省科技攻关项目4项，省自然科学基金重点项目1项。以第一作者或通讯作者发表SCI论文87篇，累积影响因子超过200。作为第一发明人，获得国家发明专利5项。

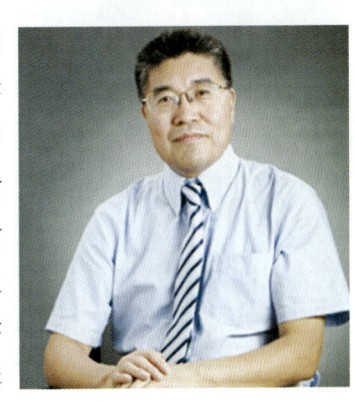

主译简介

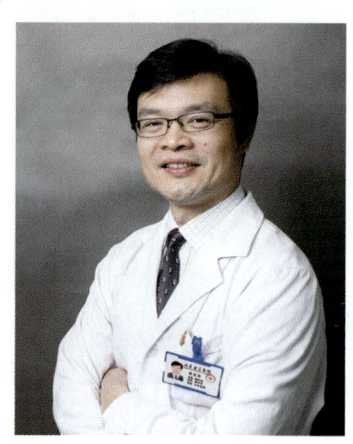

彭忠民，山东省立医院东院区胸外科主任，主任医师，外科学博士，肿瘤学博士后。山东大学教授，博士生导师，二级教授。山东省突出贡献中青年专家。现任中国抗癌协会肺癌分会微创综合治疗委员会常务委员，中国胸外科肺癌联盟山东分盟副主任委员，山东省中青年联盟主任委员，中国胸外科肺癌联盟肺部结节诊治中心主任，中国抗癌协会肺癌专业委员会委员，山东省抗癌协会肺癌专业委员会副主任委员。任《中国肺癌杂志》编委，并主编《胸部微创外科学》、《实用胸部肿瘤外科学》、《胸外科并发症学》及《外科原则》，参编著作10余部。在 Clinical Lung Cancer 等国内外重要期刊上发表论文50余篇。

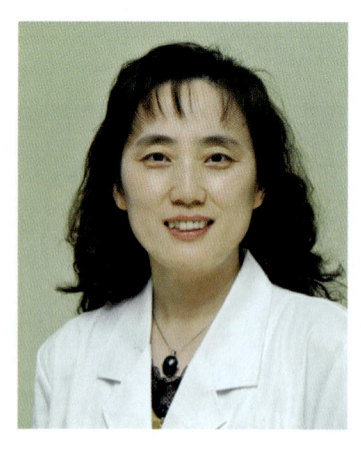

杨　霞，山东省立医院肿瘤研究治疗中心副主任医师。山东大学医学院内科学博士。现任中国抗癌协会微创治疗委员会肺癌微创与综合治疗分会秘书长，中国抗癌协会微创治疗青年委员会委员，中国抗癌协会微创治疗委员会肿瘤急症分会委员，山东省医学会姑息医学分会委员，山东省医师协会肿瘤消融亚专业委员会副主任委员，山东省医师协会综合/肿瘤介入分会副主任委员，山东省抗癌协会肿瘤临床协作分会秘书长，山东省医师协会普外多学科综合治疗专业委员会常委，山东生物医学工程学会生物定向治疗专业委员会常委。

原著序
Preface

在《肺癌》第 1 版出版 20 周年后，第 4 版又与广大读者见面了。过去的 20 年见证了肺癌研究及治疗领域的诸多进展。这些进展集中体现在我们对肺癌发生发展的分子机制理解得更加深刻，针对特异性肺癌驱动基因的靶向药物更加丰富，预测疾病预后及治疗疗效的生物标志物研究更加成熟，手术及放疗技术的革新更加多样，以及对原发及继发肺恶性肿瘤的预防更加有效。

本书的特点之一是为临床医生尽可能简明地总结了肺癌研究领域的主要进展。作者力图在这些最新进展的背景下为读者展示肺癌预防、诊断及治疗方面的最高水平。同时我们还邀请了一批年轻专家进入编委会。在这里我们诚挚地欢迎这些肺癌基础、转化及临床研究的创新者、领导者。

我们需要再次强调，本书中介绍的相关进展仍需要转化医学研究及严格的临床试验验证，但我们坚信肺癌的研究进展将进一步加快，而肺癌引起的死亡将逐渐减少。

郑重声明

未经出版商书面许可授权，禁止将本书内容复制，全部或部分上传至检索系统，以及以电子版、复印、照相复印、录音或其他任何形式传播。

本书的内容旨在进一步促进科学研究、理解和讨论，并不应为特定患者推荐或推广特定的诊断、治疗方法。出版商、作者、译者没有就本书内容的精确性和完整性作任何保证，并且明确否认任何负责任的保证，例如针对特定目的健康和疗效保证。针对正在进行的研究、设备升级、仪器更新换代、政府法规的变化、设备和用药等信息的不断完善，有读者要求审查和评估其包含的详尽信息例如每种药物、设备和装置的各种信息，并希望对部分问题提供详细的指示、警告和预防措施，对于这种情况读者应适当咨询专家。任何组织或网站在本书中被引用时，并不意味着作者或出版商认可该组织或网站提供或建议的任何信息。读者还应意识到，本书所列的互联网网站在著书和阅读时可能发生变化甚至消失，本作品的任何推广声明，不为其提供任何担保。无论是出版商还是作者，都不对由此产生的任何损害负责。

目 录
Contents

第1章　吸烟的预防与戒烟 ……………………………………………………………………… /1
第2章　肺癌的易感性和风险评估模型 ………………………………………………………… /21
第3章　肺癌的分子分析 ………………………………………………………………………… /41
第4章　人类肺癌体细胞基因组的改变 ………………………………………………………… /56
第5章　血清蛋白标志物 ………………………………………………………………………… /74
第6章　肺癌癌前病变的分子生物学 …………………………………………………………… /88
第7章　肺癌癌前病变的检测和治疗 …………………………………………………………… /102
第8章　肺腺癌病理学 …………………………………………………………………………… /114
第9章　多灶性细支气管肺泡癌的治疗 ………………………………………………………… /126
第10章　放射学检查与肺癌筛查 ………………………………………………………………… /140
第11章　肺癌影像学 ……………………………………………………………………………… /152
第12章　纵隔淋巴结分期 ………………………………………………………………………… /160
第13章　孤立性肺结节的处理 …………………………………………………………………… /169
第14章　肺癌的微创手术治疗 …………………………………………………………………… /176
第15章　肺癌扩大切除术 ………………………………………………………………………… /185
第16章　肺癌的支气管镜干预 …………………………………………………………………… /197
第17章　原发性气管肿瘤 ………………………………………………………………………… /208
第18章　肺癌手术后的辅助化疗 ………………………………………………………………… /216
第19章　可手术非小细胞肺癌的新辅助化疗 …………………………………………………… /226
第20章　图像引导的放射治疗 …………………………………………………………………… /242
第21章　立体定向放射治疗在肺癌中的应用 …………………………………………………… /252
第22章　质子治疗 ………………………………………………………………………………… /266
第23章　非小细胞肺癌的放化联合治疗 ………………………………………………………… /277
第24章　基于剂量提升与非常规分割的个体化放疗在非小细胞肺癌中的应用 ……………… /297
第25章　分子靶向治疗与肺癌个体化放疗 ……………………………………………………… /306
第26章　EGFR 酪氨酸激酶抑制剂与单克隆抗体：相关临床试验回顾 ……………………… /319

第 27 章	非小细胞肺癌中表皮生长因子受体耐药机制	/332
第 28 章	EGFR 抑制剂的预测性肿瘤生物标志物	/343
第 29 章	肺癌的免疫治疗	/359
第 30 章	非小细胞肺癌治疗中的新型及新兴药物	/367
第 31 章	转移性肺癌的新临床试验设计	/380
第 32 章	非小细胞肺癌临床试验的新统计学模型	/387
第 33 章	肿瘤的微环境、血管生成及靶向治疗	/400
第 34 章	转移性非小细胞肺癌的抗肿瘤血管生成药物	/418
第 35 章	靶向淋巴瘤激酶（ALK）重排	/430
第 36 章	存在 BRAF 突变的非小细胞肺癌	/443
第 37 章	肺癌预后及预测的生物标志物特征	/449
第 38 章	肺癌脑转移	/455

第 1 章
吸烟的预防与戒烟

Alexander V. Prokhorov[1], *Karen Suchanek Hudmon*[2]
1. Department of Behavioral Science, The University of Texas MD Anderson Cancer Center, Houston, TX, USA
2. Department of Pharmacy Practice, Purdue University, Indianapolis, IN, USA

概 述

烟草的使用已经被公认为世界范围内疾病和死亡率增加的主要诱发因素，而吸烟是肺癌发生的主要危险因素[1]。目前已经掌握了许多导致开始吸烟和产生尼古丁依赖的生物学行为原因的相关知识，预防和戒烟是有效控制吸烟的两个关键措施。2012 年美国卫生总署的报告（Surgeon General's Report，SGR）显示，预防青少年和年轻人使用烟草尤为重要[2]。自 20 世纪 90 年代中期以来，青少年吸烟率急剧下降的趋势已经趋于停滞，与此同时，同年龄段群体中无烟烟草的使用率日益升高[2]。各种措施的实施对预防吸烟产生了积极的影响，包括政策的变更和教育[3]。无论年龄、性别、种族或健康状况如何，戒烟都能为每个人带来广泛的健康受益[4]。最新的戒烟治疗方法包括行为咨询结合一种或多种美国食品药品监督管理局（Food and Drug Administration，FDA）批准的有助于戒烟的药物。美国公共卫生署的《治疗烟草使用和依赖临床实践指引》提出戒烟的 5 个步骤，即询问烟草使用情况、劝告戒烟、评估戒烟的准备状态、协助戒烟和安排随访[5]。向吸烟人员系统地提供有效的戒烟资源，如戒烟热线，是目前行之有效且最具有前景的方法，应鼓励医务工作者对遇到的每位吸烟者进行短暂的干预[5]。

引 言

2011 年，美国约有 19% 的成年吸烟者[6]，2012 年，17% 的高中生每 30d 至少吸一根烟[7]。然而 50 年前，前美国卫生总署的 C. Everett Koop 指出，吸烟是"我们社会上主要的、单一的、可以避免的死亡原因，而且是我们这个时代最重要的公共卫生问题"[8]。吸烟每年导致近 44.3 万人死亡，其中二手烟导致的死亡人数超过 4.9 万人[9]。吸烟也给经济带来了巨大的影响：因吸烟每年产生超过 750 亿美元的医疗费用和因过早死亡导致价值超过 810 亿美元的生产力丧失[10]。虽然公众常将吸烟与癌症危险性升高联系起来，但其对健康的负面影响更加广泛。2004 年美国卫生总署在吸烟对健康影响的报告中提供了引人注目的吸烟对人体有害的证据，并总结出吸烟几乎损害身体的每一个器官[11]（表 1.1）。2000 年，美国有 860 万人患约 1 270 万种由吸烟引起的疾病[12]。有足够的证据表明停止吸烟可带来即时和长期的健康受益，包括降低癌症的累积风险，这一结论在高龄者和已确诊癌症者中也得到了证实[13]。

对青少年开始吸烟的初级预防至关重要，但该重要性却往往被健康专家所低估。事实上，99% 的吸烟者首次使用烟草发生在 26 岁前[2]，所以几乎所有的烟草使用都始于童年或青少年期。虽然青少年的烟草使用率自 20 世纪 90 年代开始有了大幅度下降，但近几年这一令人欣慰的趋势似乎止步不前，尤其是无烟烟草的使用率[7]。青少年的烟草使用不仅仅是一种社会现象，近期发展起来的对尼古丁的生理性依赖阻碍了许多青少年戒掉烟草制品，因此，约有 80% 的青少年吸烟者成年后仍会吸烟[2]。美国每年会新增 100 多万烟草使用者。美国疾病控制与预防中心主任 Thomas R. Frieden 博士在 2012 年的美国卫生总署的报告前言中指出，预防青少年群体吸烟和无烟烟草的使用对终止烟草的流行至关重要[2]。

表 1.1　吸烟的危害（2004 年 USDHHS SGR 报告）

癌症	急性骨髓性白血病
	膀胱
	宫颈
	食管
	胃
	肾
	喉
	肺
	口腔和咽
	胰腺
心血管疾病	腹主动脉瘤
	冠心病（心绞痛、缺血性心脏病、心肌梗死、猝死）
	脑血管疾病（短暂性脑缺血发作、脑卒中）
	外周动脉疾病
肺疾病	急性呼吸道疾病
	－肺炎
	慢性呼吸道疾病
	－慢性阻塞性肺疾病
	－呼吸道症状（咳嗽、咳痰、哮鸣、呼吸困难）
	－难治性哮喘
	－母亲吸烟导致婴儿肺功能下降
生殖影响	妇女生殖能力下降
	妊娠和妊娠结局
	－胎膜早破
	－前置胎盘
	－胎盘早剥
	－早产
	－低体重儿
	婴儿死亡率（婴儿猝死综合征）
其他影响	白内障
	骨质疏松症（妇女绝经后骨硬度下降，增加髋骨骨折风险）
	牙周炎
	消化性溃疡（感染幽门螺杆菌患者）
	外科结果
	－伤口不易愈合
	－呼吸系统并发症

USDHHS：The U. S. Department of Health and Human Services，美国卫生和公共服务部
来源：参考文献 11

吸烟与肺癌

在美国，约 85% 的肺癌患者吸烟或有吸烟史[14]。肺癌对许多患者来说都是致命的，在 21 世纪初预估每年超过 130 万人死于肺癌[15]。在美国，不论性别，肺癌是导致癌症相关死亡的主要原因，预计每年有 174 470 例新诊断病例和 162 460 例死亡病例[16-17]。每年死于肺癌的病例数超过死于乳腺癌、大肠癌和前列腺癌病例数的总和[18]。近年来医疗技术的发展使早期诊断肺癌成为可能，而手术治疗、放射治疗、影像学和化疗的发展提高了治疗效果。然而，治疗技术的进步并未改善肺癌患者 30 年间的总生存率。应用现有的治疗手段仅可以治愈 12%～15% 的肺癌[19]。肺癌的预后主要取决于早发现和及时的、转移前的治疗[20]。肺癌的预防是根除这种致命疾病最好的方法[21]。吸烟在肺癌死亡率中的因果关系已经在许多纵向研究中得到了明确的证实，其中有一项研究持续长达 50 年[15]。被直接吸入或作为二手烟吸入的烟草烟雾中含有约 4 000 种化合物，其中 69 种物质已被证实可以致癌[22]。烟草刺激和致癌物质可损害肺细胞，随着时间的推移，受损的细胞可能发生癌变。吸烟者的肺功能水平低于非吸烟者[23-24]，戒烟明显可以降低肺癌发生的累积危险度[25-26]。

吸烟和肺癌的因果关系得到了生物医学史上最全面的论证[27]。20 世纪 50 年代初 Richard Doll[28] 的研究中首次发现了二者的关系，与同时代的其他流行病学家相比，他的创造性研究成果改变了疾病预防的新局面，在世界范围内挽救了数百万人的生命。美国卫生总署发表的两篇相距 40 年（1964 年和 2004 年）、具有里程碑意义的报告中，进一步证明了吸烟和癌症之间密切的关系。吸烟者比不吸烟者发生肺癌的风险高 15～30 倍，超过 90% 的肺癌由吸烟引起[29]。开始吸烟的年龄越小、吸烟的数量越多和吸烟的年数越长，则发生肺癌的风险越高[30]。吸烟史调查结果显示易感性也与肺癌的发生有关[31]。

二手烟雾与肺癌

虽然已经证实主动吸烟是肺癌主要的可预防

原因，但二手烟雾中也含有与吸烟者所吸入烟雾中相同的致癌物质[22,32]。因此，自1986年美国卫生总署的报告中指出二手烟雾对非吸烟者和吸烟者可以致癌后，这个问题已经引起了关注。虽然评估随暴露地点（例如工作场所、家中）而改变，但2006年美国卫生总署的报告中显示调查估计40%的美国非吸烟人群暴露于二手烟雾中[33]。在美国，估计每年有超过3 000例非吸烟肺癌患者因二手烟雾死亡[33]。根据Glantz及其同事的报道，平均有8例死于吸烟相关疾病的吸烟者时，就有1例非吸烟者因暴露于二手烟雾而死亡[34]。

自1986年以来，2006年美国卫生总署的《被动吸烟的健康后果》报告中发表了大量的研究结果，报告中根据这些证据得出的结论与之前的报告相一致：暴露于二手烟雾中会增加肺癌的发生风险。超过50个非吸烟者在家中和（或）工作场所接触香烟烟雾的流行病学研究显示，肺癌风险增加与接触二手烟雾有关[33]。这意味着在首次确定二手烟雾是终身非吸烟者发生肺癌的原因20年后，又增加了新的支持戒烟和减少接触二手烟雾的证据。因此，消除在家中、工作场所和其他公共场所的二手烟雾对降低非吸烟者的肺癌发生风险非常重要[33]。

肺癌患者的吸烟状况

由于吸烟可导致较高的并发症发生率和死亡率，因此癌症患者烟草的使用成为一个严重的健康问题[35]。有证据显示诊断癌症后继续吸烟对治疗效果[36-37]、总生存率[38]、发生第二原发癌的风险[39-40]存在明确的不良影响，且增加了治疗相关并发症的发生率和严重性，如对心肺功能的影响、增加感染率、伤口愈合差、导致黏膜炎和口干燥症等[41]。

尽管有强有力的证据表明吸烟在癌症发生中起重要作用，但许多癌症患者仍在继续吸烟[42-43]。具体来讲，约1/3的在诊断癌症前吸烟的患者在诊断后仍继续吸烟，并且仅有30%的患者接受手术治疗后停止吸烟[44]。据估计，超过50%曾经吸烟的肺癌患者接受手术后仍继续吸烟[45]。因此，在吸烟相关的恶性肿瘤患者中，诊断时和诊断后吸烟史的相似性很高[46]。

吸烟患者被诊断为肺癌后，如果戒烟可能面临巨大的挑战，并受一系列心理因素的影响[47]。Schnoll和其同事的报道显示头颈部恶性肿瘤和肺癌患者继续吸烟主要与以下因素有关：缺乏戒烟准备，家中亲属吸烟，诊断和治疗间隔延长，尼古丁依赖性较大，自制力和危险意识较低，支持者较少而反对戒烟者较多，宿命论观念较重，情绪压抑等。肺癌患者应被劝告戒烟，但确诊后有些患者可能觉得不能从戒烟中获益[48]。戒烟应是一个特别受关注的贯穿诊断、治疗和生存延续的问题。应利用癌症诊断的"宣教时机"，作为"教育时间"鼓励患者、其家庭成员及关系密切者戒烟[43]。

烟草类型

吸食烟草

在美国，香烟是近几十年来被使用最广泛的烟草类型，然而近几年来，吸香烟人数在多数人口亚群中稳定下降[6]。自2002年以来，美国之前吸烟者的数量超过了现时吸烟者数量[49]。2011年，19%（4 380万）的美国成年人是现时吸烟者，其中77.8%（3 410万）的人每天吸烟，22.2%（970万）的人有时吸烟[6]。吸烟人群在各人群中的变化非常大（表1.2）。据报道，男性（21.5%）比女性（16.5%）现时吸烟人数多，亚洲裔或西班牙裔吸烟率最低（分别为9.9%和12.9%），而美洲印第安人或阿拉斯加本地人最多（31.5%）。另外，美国各地区成人吸烟率变化较大，西部15.0%，中西部21.8%[6]。2012年发表的"未来监测"报告显示，17%的高中生在过去30d内吸过烟[7]。2011年全国青少年烟草调查数据显示，12.9%的高中男生使用无烟烟草，15.7%吸雪茄，这些数据值得关注，因为近90%吸烟者的开始吸烟年龄为18岁之前[50]。

在美国，其他类型的可燃烟草包括雪茄、烟斗烟和比迪烟（bidis）。雪茄是烟叶或其他含有烟草的物质卷成的[51]。过去的10年，雪茄越来越受大众的欢迎[50]。这种现象的可能解释是某一部分

表1.2 18岁以上特定人群当前吸烟率[a]——2011年美国全国健康访问调查

分类	特征	男 ($n=14\,811$)	女 ($n=18\,203$)	合计 ($n=33\,014$)
年龄组（岁）	18~24	21.3%	16.4%	18.9%
	25~44	24.5%	19.7%	22.1%
	45~64	24.4%	18.5%	21.4%
	≥65	8.9%	7.1%	7.9%
种族[b]	白人	22.5%	18.8%	20.6%
	黑人	24.2%	15.5%	19.4%
	非西班牙裔	17.0%	8.6%	12.9%
	美洲印第安人或阿拉斯加本土人	34.4%	29.1%	31.5%
	亚洲裔[c]	29.7%	5.5%	9.9%
教育程度[d]	0~12岁（无文凭）	30.5%	25.1%	25.5%
	普通教育[e]	47.5%	45.2%	45.3%
	高中毕业	27.9%	23.8%	23.8%
	大专毕业	21.4%	17.5%	19.3%
	学院（无学位）	25.2%	20.0%	22.3%
	本科	9.8%	8.7%	9.3%
	研究生	5.2%	4.8%	5.0%
贫困水平[f]	贫困线或以上	20.2%	15.6%	20.6%
	以下	33.6%	25.7%	29.9%
	未知	19.4%	11.4%	18.4%
合计		21.6%	16.5%	19.0%

a：报告显示一个人一生中至少吸100支香烟，且在访问时仍每天吸烟或有时吸烟；86位受访者因吸烟状况不详被排除。b：61位受访者因种族类型不详或为多种族被排除。除非另有说明，否则所有的种族均为非西班牙裔，而西班牙裔可为任何种族。c：排除本土夏威夷居民或其他太平洋地区居民。d：年龄≥25岁，排除173位教育程度不详者。e：普通教育证书。f：根据美国2010年人口统计局贫困线得出。来源：参考文献52

吸烟者由香烟转换为雪茄以及青少年在尝试吸雪茄[50]。1998年，约5%的成年人在过去1个月至少吸1根雪茄[53]。在美国出售的雪茄中尼古丁含量为每支5.9~335.2mg[54]，而香烟中的总尼古丁含量范围较窄，为每支7.2~13.4mg[55]。因此一支大雪茄中含有与一整包香烟相当量的烟草，能够释放足够的尼古丁建立和维持机体的依赖性[56]。

在过去的50年吸烟斗烟的人数稳定下降[57]，只有不足1%的美国人使用烟斗烟[57]。在美国吸比迪烟的人数近年来有所增加，比迪烟是从东南亚进口的手卷褐色香烟，用天杜叶卷成[58]，外表和大麻烟卷有几分相似，能对某些人群产生吸引力。比迪烟有多种香味（例如巧克力、香草、橘皮、草莓、樱桃、芒果等），尤其吸引年轻吸烟者。在对美国的15个州近64 000人的调查中发现，年轻人（18~24岁）曾经使用比迪烟的概率超过16.5%，且现时使用率高于成年人（>25岁），为1.4%。在社会人口特征方面，男性、非洲裔美国人和同时吸香烟者最常使用比迪烟[59]。虽然表面上比迪烟的烟草含量比标准香烟少，但比迪烟可使吸烟者接触到相当数量的有害化合物。一项采用吸烟机装置的研究发现，与传统香烟相比，比迪烟释放3倍的一氧化碳和尼古丁及近5倍的焦油[60]。

无烟烟草

无烟烟草产品通常被称为"唾液烟草",放入口中通过颊黏膜吸收尼古丁。唾液烟草包括嚼用烟草和鼻烟。嚼用烟草含有松散叶、烟草块和绞合成分,被咀嚼后放在颊部或下唇。鼻烟通常以散在的颗粒或香袋(类似茶袋)的形式出现,稠度更高,通常放在口中不必咀嚼。在美国多数鼻烟制品类型为湿性鼻烟,使用时将一小撮鼻烟放在颊和牙龈之间30min或更长时间。相比之下,使用方法为鼻子嗅和吸入的干鼻烟的使用者较少[61]。

2004年,约有3.0% 12岁或以上的美国人在过去的1个月使用唾液烟草。男性使用率(5.8%)高于女性(0.3%)[62]。在18~25岁人群中唾液烟草的使用率最高,美国印第安人、阿拉斯加本地人、南方各州的居民和乡村居民中使用率也相当高[63]。从20世纪80年代中期以来嚼用烟草消耗量出现下降,相反,在2005年鼻烟消耗量较前一年增加了约5%[63],原因可能是由于吸烟者在禁止吸烟的地方和场合使用鼻烟代替香烟。

虽然美国的香烟消费在持续下降,但无烟烟草产品的流行和消费却在增长[64]。近期的一份报告显示,2005至2011年,湿鼻烟产品的销售量增长了65.6%,有袋湿鼻烟和加香湿鼻烟的销售量分别增长了333.8%和72.1%,分别占湿鼻烟产品总体增长率的28.0%和59.4%。加香鼻烟和打折鼻烟的销售增加了对青少年的吸引力和使用量[64],提示应实施强有力的预防措施处理这些烟草制品。

烟草市场的近期发展状况

近10年来,烟草行业增加了大量潜在的有害产品种类,该行业正广泛推广新型低危害卷烟产品(potentially reduced-exposure tobacco products, PREPs)。这些产品通常被市场推广为"传统香烟的替代品",意味着它们有可能比传统烟草形式(即香烟)带来的危害少,或者减少了在PREP使用中人们与有毒物质的接触。这些PREPs包括改进的烟草香烟(如Omni和Advance)、类香烟产品(如Accord和Eclipse)以及无烟烟草产品(如Ariva和Exalt)[65]。

烟草能以小袋加香烟草(骆驼牌和万宝路鼻烟)的形式口服,其锭剂包括压缩低亚硝酸烟草粉(Ariva和Stonewall)或细粒度烟草可溶物及添加剂(骆驼球、骆驼条和骆驼棒),常以禁止吸烟区的烟草替代品形式在市场上推广。无烟烟草产品减少了吸烟者对燃烧相关有害物质的接触,吸烟者的既用香烟品牌并没有发生改变。研究表明,对典型吸烟者来说,非易燃PREP的使用不能提供足够的尼古丁抑制戒烟症状,所以吸烟者不太可能戒烟[66]。总体来说,还没有足够的证据证明此类产品的危害作用[67],但是,显而易见的是所有此类含尼古丁的产品都有潜在的危害性,因此,它们对吸引年轻人吸烟和尼古丁终身依赖方面具有危险性。

水烟袋(aka waterpipe, shisha, narghile, qalyan等)的使用引发了公共卫生中心对健康的担忧,使用这种烟具,烟草烟雾会通过特殊容器中的水被吸入。水烟袋正在美国迅速普及,尤其是在年轻人中[68-74]。例如,在大学生中水烟袋使用率仅次于传统香烟[75]。重要的是,很多水烟袋使用者相信这种吸烟方式比香烟安全[76]。研究表明,使用水烟袋的危害并不亚于香烟,也可能导致众所周知的吸烟相关疾病,并会因尼古丁上瘾妨碍成功戒烟[77]。

电子烟是另一种在美国迅速普及且不受管制的尼古丁传输方式。电子烟用电池做电源,包含尼古丁、各种香料及其他化学物质,外表看起来酷似传统香烟。点燃后电子烟会将化学物质转变成一种烟雾,使用者以一种类似吸普通烟的方式吸入这种烟雾。实验分析已经发现,电子烟中含有毒物质如二甘醇(防冻剂中使用)和致癌物(包括亚硝胺)[78]。此类产品尤其令人关注的问题是它对痴迷科技的现代青年的吸引力[79],年轻的电子烟使用者可能会发展成尼古丁上瘾,并在以后的生活中转向传统香烟。

使用烟草的原因

开始吸烟

在美国,开始吸烟的时间通常是青春期。从20世纪90年代中期到2004年,过去1个月的吸烟率在八年级下降了56%,十年级下降了47%,十二年级下降了32%[80]。但是,近年来这种下降趋势已经减慢[80]，如果没有医务工作者在预防烟草开始使用和帮助年轻吸烟者戒烟方面稳定、系统地努力，这种下降趋势可能无法维持。

一系列社会人口、行为、个人和环境因素作为青少年尝试和开始吸烟的潜在预测指标已被纳入研究，例如，青少年吸烟率与父母的社会经济状况和自己的学习成绩呈负相关[81]。其他被确定的青少年吸烟的预测因素包括：社会影响和规范的信念，负性情感与吸烟有关结果的期望，抵制能力（自我效率），其他冒险行为的吸引、身处电影院中的吸烟环境和吸烟的朋友[82-87]。

虽然许多确定开始吸烟预测因素的研究取得了成功，但只有少数研究提出在青少年中开展戒烟的成功方法，在2005年的研究中发现超过50%的吸烟学生在过去1年试图戒烟但失败[88]。这些结果证明烟草成瘾性强，强调在青少年中推广戒烟需要更有效的方法。

预防吸烟

几十年的研究表明，只有全面协同努力才有可能成功预防青少年群体使用烟草。2012年的美国卫生总署的报告中提出："协调性、多元化的干预，包括大众媒体宣传活动、税收增加所致相关物品价格升高、以学校为本的政策以及全国或社区内禁止吸烟的政策和规范，对减少青少年和青壮年群体吸烟的开始、流行和强度非常有效[2]。"事实上，成功预防烟草的使用需要大家齐心协力，而且，医务工作者是多元化系统中的关键群体。

医务工作者可以多种方式参与青少年吸烟的预防。首先，医疗实践中应定期采取措施预防烟草的使用。询问烟草的使用情况、建议戒烟或不要开始使用，并借助以证据为基础的材料和资源协助培养一种无烟生活方式，这些应当成为患者护理中不可或缺的组成部分。与儿童或青少年的父母通力合作为儿童的成长环境排除所有的二手烟非常重要，一项在社会经济地位明显较低的墨西哥裔美国人社区开展的研究表明，人们对二手烟及与其相关的健康后果知之甚少[89]。一系列的文化影响、印刷材料有效地增加了这方面的知识[89]，并且有效消除了墨西哥裔美国人家庭中的二手烟。除了直接提升健康的努力，这些杜绝措施也可能有助于预防儿童和青少年开始吸烟。

年轻人似乎对拨打戒烟电话的反应并不积极[90]，所以为该群体寻找合适的替代方法非常重要，可以考虑为该群体提供网络资源[91]。医务工作者需要熟知现代技术来帮助青少年做出正确的决定以避免开始使用烟草，这些资源的介绍应当被融入医疗实践。而且，作为在社区备受尊敬的人，医务工作者在其医疗工作中能够对预防青少年烟草的使用产生影响。所开展的活动中成效较高的可能是向学校推荐预防吸烟程序，尽管以学校为本的预防烟草使用[92]教育程序备受争议，但这些程序也是减少青少年烟草使用的系统、综合性措施中不可或缺的一部分。我们必须意识到，儿童、青少年和青壮年皆为特殊群体，他们有特殊的需求，只是经常未被满足或重视。

国际公认的预防青少年吸烟的专家Brian Flay博士的一篇以学校为基础的综述中对几项长期有效的学校本位程序的关键特征进行了概述[93]。他认为如果做到以下几点，学校本位程序将会发挥长期且重要的实际效用：①长期坚持举办15个或更多的教育讲座包括高中讲座；②采用社会影响模式和交互传递方式；③规范组成部分、不吸烟承诺、不吸烟意向，对拒绝吸烟的训练和练习以及其他生活技能；④请同龄人担任某些职位。Flay博士断定，这些程序会让初次吸烟行为减少25%~30%。学校本位程序与社区程序结合可明显降低青少年高中毕业前的初次吸烟行为(35%~40%)。

关于本分析，我们还想补充一点，即学校本位方案要求具有较高的文化灵敏度，以适应美国多元文化中青少年人群的需求。方案制订者应注意目标人群的一般文化水平，并特别留意其健康知识水平。后一概念尤为重要，因为青少年文化水平越低，开始吸烟和终生尼古丁依赖的风险就越高。最后，极为重要的一点是，应认识到我们生活在科技时代，因此，应采用由互联网传输的交互式多媒体程序，因为社交网络（Facebook、Twitter、YouTube等）的应用在青少年群体中非常流行，智能手机程序和应用软件也是如此，对于预防吸烟程序的吸引力、有效性和可持续性具有必要性和标准性。我们根据多项前述原则[91,94-95]，开发了自己有证可循的青少年双语（英语和西班牙语）预防吸烟和戒烟程序，即ASPIRE（A Smoking Prevention InteRactive Experience，预防吸烟互动体验：www.mdanderson.org/aspire）。目前已推广至美国 29 个州，不断收到所参与社区的积极反馈。例如，近 15 000 例学生参与者中，有 92% 了解到了烟草的新知识，83% 表示受该程序的影响他们决定不使用烟草，91% 对烟草的作用有了更深入的了解，而且 77% 表示他们会将 ASPIRE 推荐给亲朋好友。

尼古丁的成瘾性

尼古丁是烟草中的成瘾性物质，会迅速进入大脑（10~20s）[96]，并对其产生广泛的药理作用[97-98]。尼古丁刺激神经递质的释放，引起药理反应，例如愉悦感和奖赏感（多巴胺）、兴奋性（乙酰胆碱、去甲肾上腺素）、认识能力增强（乙酰胆碱）、学习和记忆力增强（谷氨酸）、情绪调节或食欲抑制（5-羟色安）和减轻焦虑或紧张（3-内啡肽和 GABA 即 γ-氨基丁酸）[99]。进入大脑后，大剂量尼古丁激活多巴胺反馈通路——在脑组织中诱导愉悦感觉和刺激释放多巴胺。

在缺乏尼古丁时，依赖尼古丁的戒断患者会表现出由轻到重的症状反应。虽然戒断症状不是戒烟的唯一结果，但大多数戒烟者都经历过戒断反应和对暂停戒烟的渴望过程[100]，因此"旧病复发"非常普遍[101]。一般大部分的戒断症状出现在戒烟后 1~2d，高峰期出现在第 1 周内，在 2~4 周内症状逐渐减轻[100]。对许多吸烟者来说，所谓的尼古丁镇静作用通常与戒断作用减轻有关，而不是尼古丁的直接作用。这种快速剂量反应加上尼古丁半衰期较短（约 2h），成为烟草使用者频繁、反复使用烟草而成瘾的基础。烟草使用者可熟练地调节一天中尼古丁的水平以避免戒断症状，维持愉悦感和兴奋性，调节情绪。戒断症状包括易怒、挫折感、气愤、焦虑、注意力难以集中、焦虑不安、急躁、情绪低落、沮丧、失眠、动作障碍、食欲增加或体重增加以及对香烟的渴望[100]。

开始吸食烟草、使用及依赖性被假设源于许多因素（包括药理、遗传、社会、环境、学习或条件因素）[98]，这些因素部分为全家人共有，如环境、遗传方面。对家庭的研究一致表明与非吸烟的家庭成员相比，家中有吸烟者的家庭成员更有可能成为吸烟者。然而，除了共同的遗传易感性外，还应考虑到环境因素对于助长烟草使用的重要性——同一个家庭中的兄弟姐妹共同受到许多相同的环境因素影响，并有相同的基因。烟草的使用和成瘾与诸多因素有关，因此，烟草管制倡议（例如社区基层的努力）和戒烟咨询服务（此类服务面向个体）更有必要向多方面发展[102]。

戒烟的益处

1990 年和 2004 年美国卫生总署发表的关于吸烟对健康影响的报告中，总结了大量有关戒烟的明显的健康益处[11,103]。在戒烟后不久（2 周至 3 个月）可立即出现肺功能和循环改善；戒烟 1~9 个月，肺上皮纤毛功能恢复，开始时患者可能由于肺清除过量的黏液和烟草颗粒出现咳嗽增多，但几个月内，戒烟所带来的肺功能改善便可检测出来。随着时间的推移，患者出现咳嗽、鼻窦阻塞、疲劳、气促减轻和肺部感染风险下降。戒烟 1 年后，冠状动脑粥样硬化性心脏病（简称冠心病）的风险比继续吸烟者减少一半；5~15 年后，脑卒中的风险降低到接近终身无吸烟者的发病率；戒烟 10 年后，个人死于肺癌的概率约为继续吸烟者的一半，此外，发生口腔、喉、咽、食管、膀胱、肾或胰腺癌的风险下降；最后，戒烟 15 年后，冠心病的发病率降低到与不吸烟者相近的数值。戒烟能直接使男性和女性死于肺癌的累积危险度明显下降。

越来越多的证据提示，在诊断癌症后继续吸烟可产生诸多不良影响。吸烟会降低治疗总有效率，引起并发症，加重治疗副作用，增加第二种原发性肿瘤的风险和降低总生存率。因此，戒烟是各类癌症治疗过程中的必要措施——不单纯限于肺癌[42]。

戒烟干预

有效和及时的戒烟干预能明显降低吸烟相关疾病的发生风险，认识烟草使用的复杂性是对戒烟和预防吸烟进行有效干预和临床试验必要的第一步。

医务人员处于帮助患者戒烟的独特位置，在介入戒烟帮助和为患者提供健康相关建议的问题上有很大的影响力。如今，在科学团体中医生作为戒烟治疗的提供者受到了最大的关注。虽然药剂师和护士较少被关注，但他们也在独特的位置服务于公众并帮助患者改变行为或补充其他医疗服务者的工作。

医务工作者对29项研究进行了meta分析,他们估计与没有接受内科医生戒烟治疗的吸烟者相比,接受内科临床医生或非内科临床医生治疗的吸烟者在戒烟5个月或5个月以上后分别增加了2.2倍和1.7倍的戒烟可能性[101]。为了协助临床医生和其他医务工作者提供戒烟治疗,美国公共卫生署出版了《烟草使用和依赖治疗的临床实践指南》[101],该《指南》以系统回顾和科学文献分析为基础,为医务工作者提供一系列戒烟治疗的建议和策略,并强调了医务工作者系统确定烟草使用者并对每一例使用烟草的患者提供简单治疗的重要性。最有效的戒烟方法是行为咨询和药物治疗,可以单一使用,最好联合使用[101]。各种行为和药物戒烟策略的有效性如表1.3所示。

表1.3 烟草使用和依赖的治疗效果

治疗方法	估计比值比[a] (95% CI)	估计戒烟率[b] (95% CI)
行为干预		
劝告戒烟		
没有劝告戒烟	1.0	7.9%
内科医生劝告戒烟	1.3 (1.1, 1.6)	10.2% (8.5, 12.0)
临床干预		
没有向临床医生咨询	1.0	10.2%
向非内科医生咨询	1.7 (1.3, 2.1)	15.8% (12.8, 18.8)
向内科医生咨询	2.2 (1.5, 3.2)	19.9% (13.7, 26.2)
戒烟咨询形式		
没有形式	1.0	10.8%
自助咨询	1.2 (1.0, 1.3)	12.3% (10.9, 13.6)
主动电话咨询[c]	1.2 (1.1, 1.4)	13.1% (11.4, 14.8)
团队咨询	1.3 (1.1, 1.6)	13.9% (11.6, 16.1)
单独咨询	1.7 (1.4, 2.0)	16.8% (14.7, 19.1)
药物治疗干预		
安慰剂	1.0	13.8%
一线药物	2.0 (1.8, 2.2)	24.2% (22.2, 26.4)
安非他酮	1.5 (1.2, 1.7)	19.0% (16.5, 21.9)
尼古丁口香糖(6~14周)	2.1 (1.5, 2.9)	24.8% (19.1, 31.6)
尼古丁吸入剂	2.0 (1.4, 2.8)	24.2[d]%
尼古丁锭剂(2mg)	1.9 (1.7, 2.2)	23.4% (21.3, 25.8)
尼古丁贴(6~14周)	2.3 (1.7, 3.0)	26.7% (21.5, 32.7)
尼古丁鼻喷剂(2mg/d)	3.1 (2.5, 3.8)	33.2% (28.9, 37.8)
二线药物[e]		
可乐定	2.1 (1.2, 3.7)	25.0% (15.7, 37.3)
去甲替林	1.8 (1.3, 2.6)	22.5% (16.8, 29.4)
联合治疗		
贴剂(>14周)+任意量的尼古丁(口香糖或鼻喷剂)	3.6 (2.5, 5.2)	36.5% (28.6, 45.3)
尼古丁贴+安非他酮	2.5 (1.9, 3.4)	28.9% (23.5, 35.1)
尼古丁贴+去甲替林	2.3 (1.3, 4.2)	27.3% (17.2, 40.4)
尼古丁贴+尼古丁吸入剂	2.2 (1.2, 3.6)	25.8% (17.4, 36.5)

a:评估与对照群体的相关性;b:特定治疗方法的戒烟百分比;c:在吸烟者最初请求或传真戒烟程序之后,临床医生将拨打电话联系并询问患者,之后通过戒烟热线回复来电并进行电话随访;d:一项合格的随机临床试验,在2008版《临床实践指南》中,95% CI未进行报道;e:未经美国FDA批准的戒烟援助;美国公共卫生署《指南》中推荐的治疗烟草使用和依赖的二线药物。

获准引自参考文献108。版权1999—2014加州大学董事会。版权所有。来源:参考文献101

行为咨询

单独行为干预或与药物治疗相结合在整个戒烟治疗中起关键作用[101]。这种干预包括多种方法，从自助资料到个人认知行为疗法，使个人能够更有效地认识到吸烟的高风险，开展可选择的应对策略，管理压力，提高解决问题的能力和增加社会支持。《临床实践指南》列出了临床医生帮助患者戒烟时可应用的 5 步框架：①系统地确定所有烟草使用者；②坚定地劝告所有烟草使用者戒烟；③评估戒烟的准备状况；④协助患者戒烟；⑤安排随访联系方式。这些步骤被称为"5A"：即询问（Ask）、劝告（Advise）、评估（Assess）、协助（Assist）和安排（Arrange）。由于戒烟者存在再次吸烟的可能性，医务工作者必须为患者提供简单的预防再次吸烟的措施。预防再次吸烟应能够增强患者戒烟的决心、重温戒烟的益处和协助患者解决由戒烟带来的问题。在时间不足或缺乏专家提供更全面的咨询的情况下，建议临床医生（最低限度地）询问患者有关烟草的使用情况、劝告戒烟和为这些患者介绍其他戒烟资源，例如免费的戒烟热线。

戒烟热线提供戒烟电话咨询服务，且通常可免费呼叫。近年来，戒烟热线发展迅速，为那些因地理位置不便、经济能力较差或没有保险的患者提供了全面的行为干预。在临床试验中已经证实，对于一些通过戒烟热线发起的咨询，电话咨询服务至少会在促进戒烟方面发挥有效作用[101,104]，并且还表明此类试验结果已在现实生活中发挥了成效[105]。与仅采用药物治疗相比，戒烟热线咨询辅助药物治疗会显著提高戒烟率[106]。在某些国家，临床医生会代表患者向戒烟热线提交一份传真指引表，该表会提供一项戒烟热线顾问可以直接联系患者的程序。研究证明，患者完成所有随访项目的成功率可达 30%。然而，绝大多数内科医生对戒烟热线服务并不熟悉，而且临床医生的指引也比较少——但是即使是最繁忙的临床医生都可以通过询问患者的烟草使用情况、劝告吸烟患者戒烟以及向准备戒烟的患者推荐戒烟热线以寻求更全面的咨询等方式发挥重要作用（询问—劝告—推荐）[107]。

临床医生也应尝试了解并熟悉与戒烟相关的本地社区资源，例如可采用当地医院或诊所提供的群体戒烟计划。对于一些患者，基于互联网的戒烟计划可能更受欢迎，例如"www.quttnet.com"就是一个戒烟者可以在达成戒烟目标的过程中相互分享经验和彼此提供支持的线上社区。目前，患者有更多的获得援助的渠道可供选择，临床医生应该建议患者尽可能多地利用这些服务以获得长期戒烟成功。

作者团队最近开发了一款基于 iOS 系统设计的免费应用 Quit Med Kit©，可以协助医疗工作者为尼古丁依赖患者提供咨询和治疗服务。该程序是根据《临床实践指南》开发的，为尼古丁依赖患者提供当前最先进的行为咨询和药物治疗方法。Quit Med Kit© 可在苹果音乐线上商店获取，适配 iPhone、触控式 iPod 及 iPad，要求 iOS 4.3 以上版本，在 iPhone 5 上效果最佳。

戒烟的药物治疗

根据《临床实践指南》[101]，除特殊情况外，应对所有试图戒烟者鼓励使用一种或多种有效的戒烟治疗药物。100 多项随机研究结果均支持这个建议，这些研究结果表明，与接受安慰剂的吸烟者相比，药物治疗的患者约有 2 倍的可能性维持长期（>5 个月）戒烟（表 1.3）[101,108]。虽然药物治疗价格昂贵且不是每个患者治疗计划中必须的部分，但它是所有戒烟方法中成功率最高、已知最有效的方法，特别是与行为咨询相结合时[101]。

目前，美国有 7 种 FDA 批准用于戒烟的药物上市：5 种尼古丁替代治疗（nicotine replacement therapy，NRT）剂型（尼古丁口香糖、尼古丁锭剂、透皮尼古丁贴片、尼古丁喷雾剂和尼古丁口腔气雾剂），缓释安非他酮和伐伦克林酒石酸盐。每种药物的处方信息见表 1.4。更多药品相关信息请参阅生产商的处方。

表 1.4 美国 FDA 批准的戒烟药物

	尼古丁替代治疗（NRT）剂型					安非他酮缓释剂	伐尼克兰（Varenicline）
	口香糖	锭剂	透皮贴剂	鼻喷剂	口腔吸入剂		
产品	Nicorette[1]，通用类 非处方药 2mg, 4mg 原味、肉桂、水果、薄荷、橙味	Nicorette 含片[1]，Nicotte 迷你含片[1] 通用类 非处方药 2mg, 4mg 樱桃、薄荷	NikoDerm CQ[1]，通用类 非处方药（NikoDerm CQ，通用类） 处方药（通用类） 7mg, 14mg, 21mg（24h 释放）	Nikotrol NS[2] 处方药 定量喷射 0.5mg 尼古丁在 50μL 尼古丁水溶液中	Nikotrol 吸入器[2] 处方药 10mg 药芯释放 4mg 可吸入尼古丁蒸气	安非他酮（Zyban）[1]，通用类处方药 150mg 缓释片	畅沛[2] 处方药 0.5mg, 1mg 片剂
注意事项	• 近期（≤2 周）心肌梗死 • 潜在的严重心律失常 • 严重或恶化的心绞痛 • 颞下颌关节病 • 怀孕[3] 和母乳喂养 • 青少年（<18 岁）	• 近期（≤2 周）心肌梗死 • 潜在的严重心律失常 • 严重或恶化的心绞痛 • 怀孕[3] 和母乳喂养 • 青少年（<18 岁）	• 近期（≤2 周）心肌梗死 • 潜在的严重心律失常 • 严重或恶化的心绞痛 • 怀孕[3]（D 类）和母乳喂养 • 青少年（<18 岁）	• 近期（≤2 周）心肌梗死 • 潜在的严重心律失常 • 严重或恶化的心绞痛 • 潜在慢性鼻窦炎症、鼻息肉、鼻窦炎 • 严重的反应性呼吸道疾病 • 怀孕[3]（D 类）和母乳喂养 • 青少年（<18 岁）	• 近期（≤2 周）心肌梗死 • 潜在的严重心律失常 • 严重或恶化的心绞痛 • 支气管痉挛性疾病 • 怀孕[3]（C 类）和母乳喂养 • 青少年（<18 岁）	• 与其他药物或在已知可降低癫痫发作阈值的条件下同步的医疗 • 严重肝硬化 • 怀孕[3]（C 类）和母乳喂养 • 青少年（<18 岁） **禁忌证：** • 癫痫 • 同时使用其他安非他酮药物（如 Wellbutrin） • 目前或之前诊断出暴食症或神经性食欲缺乏 • 突然中断使用酒精或镇静剂（或苯二氮䓬类药物） • 至少提前 14d 停用 MAO 抑制剂治疗 **警示：** • 黑色警示框中警示的神经精神症状[4]	• 严重肾脏疾病（剂量必须调整） • 怀孕[3]（C 类）和母乳喂养 • 青少年（<18 岁） **警示：** • 黑色警示框中警示的神经精神症状[4] • 现有心血管疾病患者的不良心血管事件

(续表1.4)

	尼古丁替代治疗(NRT)剂型					安非他酮缓释剂	伐尼克兰(Vareni-cline)
	口香糖	锭剂	透皮贴剂	鼻喷剂	口腔吸入剂		
剂量	第一支香烟醒后≤30min:4mg 第一支香烟醒后>30min:2mg 1~6周: 每1~2h 1片 7~9周: 每2~4h 1片 10~12周: 每4~8h 1片 • 最大量:每天24片 • 缓慢咀嚼 • 放在颊和牙龈感之间出现(辛辣或刺激感消失时:咀嚼15~30次) • 当味道和刺激消失时重新咀嚼 • 重新咀嚼到全部尼古丁释放直到味道或刺消感不再出现,通常30min) • 放在口腔不同位置 • 使用前15min 或使用期间不进食 • 持续时间:12周以上	第一支香烟醒后≤30min:4mg 第一支香烟醒后>30min:2mg 1~6周: 每1~2h 1剂 7~9周: 每2~4h 1剂 10~12周: 每4~8h 1剂 • 最大量:每天20剂(标准10min) • 可以缓慢溶解 • 尼古丁释放可以产生热和刺痛感 • 不要咀嚼和吞服 • 有时在口腔不同位置转动 • 使用前15min 和使用时不进食 • 持续时间:12周	每天>10支香烟: 21mg/d,共4周(通用类) 共6周(NikoDerm CQ) 14mg/d,共2周 7mg/d,共2周 每天≤10支香烟: 14mg/d,共6周 7mg/d,共2周 • 如果患者出现睡眠干扰可以贴16h(除睡眠时) • 持续时间: 8~10周	每小时1~2剂(每天8~40剂) 每剂=2次(每鼻孔1次)每次喷鼻释放0.5mg尼古丁到鼻黏膜 • 最大量 每小时5剂或每小时40剂 • 为达到最好的效果,开始到使用时至少每天8剂 • 喷鼻时不应吸入或吞咽 • 疗程: 3~6个月	个体剂量每天6~16包,开始时至少每2h 1包 • 连续吸入20min可达到最好效果 • 开始时至少每天6包 • 主动吸入20min后药芯尼古丁用尽 • 吸入喉咙后部或短气喷出 • 不要像吸烟一样入肺中,而像点烟斗一样吸入 • 打开药芯,维持24h • 使用前15min 和使用时不进食 • 疗程:3~6个月	150mg,共3d,上午口服,之后增至150mg/d • 不要超过300mg/d • 开始治疗后1~2周设定戒烟时间 • 剂量间歇至少8h • 避免睡觉时使用减少失眠 • 不需要将剂量减小 • 能与NRT安全使用 • 疗程7~12周,选择性患者维持至6个月	第1~3天: 上午0.5mg/d 口服 第4~7天: 0.5mg/d 口服 第2~12周:1mg/d 口服 • 患者必须在戒烟前1周开始治疗,即患者可以先接受治疗,然后在治疗8~35d内戒烟 • 饭后饮1杯水冲服 • 不需要减少剂量 • 严重肾病患者必须的剂量调整 • 疗程12周,特殊患者加用12周

(续表 1.4)

	尼古丁替代治疗（NRT）剂型					安非他酮缓释剂	伐尼克兰（Varenicline）
	口香糖	锭剂	透皮贴剂	鼻喷剂	口腔吸入剂		
不良反应	• 口腔或下巴疼痛 • 呃逆 • 消化不良 • 睡液过多 • 与不正常咀嚼有关的副作用： －头痛 －恶心或呕吐 －咽喉和口腔刺激感	• 恶心 • 呃逆 • 咳嗽 • 烧灼感 • 头痛 • 胀气 • 失眠	• 局部皮肤反应（红斑、瘙痒、烧灼） • 头痛 • 睡眠干扰（失眠，异常逼真的梦）；与夜间吸入尼古丁有关	• 鼻和（或）咽部刺激（发热、燥热或烧灼感） • 鼻炎 • 撕裂 • 喷嚏 • 咳嗽 • 头痛	• 口和（或）咽部刺激 • 咳嗽 • 头痛 • 鼻炎 • 消化不良 • 呃逆	• 失眠 • 口干 • 神经过敏或注意力不集中 • 皮疹 • 便秘 • 癫痫（风险 0.1%） • 神经精神症状（罕见，参见注意事项）	• 恶心 • 睡眠干扰（失眠，异常或逼真的梦） • 便秘 • 胃肠胀气 • 呕吐 • 神经精神症状（罕见，参见注意事项）
优点	• 可满足口感 • 可延缓体重增加 • 易于使用和隐藏 • 可调节剂量处理戒断症状 • 提供多种口味	• 可满足口感 • 可延缓体重增加 • 易于使用和隐藏 • 可调节剂量处理戒断症状 • 提供多种口味	• 维持稳定的尼古丁水平 24h 以上 • 易于使用，隐蔽 • 每天 1 次剂量使依从性问题发生较少	• 可调节剂量，快速处理戒断症状	• 患者可调节剂量，处理戒断症状 • 模仿手-口吸烟模式（也可视为缺点）	• 容易使用；口服剂型与依从性较低问题有关 • 可延缓体重增加 • 可以与 NRT 同时使用 • 对抑郁患者有益	• 容易使用：口服剂型与依从性较低问题有关 • 为其他治疗失败的患者提供一种新的治疗方式
缺点	• 需要经常加量才能满足需求 • 牙齿疾病患者很难使用 • 必须使用给当的咀嚼技巧以减少不良反应 • 咀嚼口香糖可能不被社会认可	• 需要经常加量才能满足需求 • 令人不适的胃肠道副作用（恶心、呃逆、烧灼感）	• 不能根据实际戒断症状调节剂量 • 可能出现过敏反应 • 有皮肤问题时不能使用	• 需要经常加量才能满足需求 • 鼻和咽喉刺激可能令人焦虑 • 必须用药 5min 后才能驾驶或操作重型机械 • 有慢性鼻疾病或严重反应性气管炎患者不能使用	• 需要经常加量才能满足需求 • 鼻和咽喉刺激可能令人焦虑 • 不能存放在很热或很冷的地方 • 有支气管痉挛病史者慎用	• 癫痫发作风险升高 • 严重的禁忌证和注意事项阻碍了一些患者的使用（见注意事项） • 监测患者潜在的神经症状[4]（见注意事项）	• 在 1/3 患者中诱发恶心 • 监测患者潜在的神经症状（见注意事项）

(续表1.4)

	尼古丁替代治疗（NRT）剂型				安非他酮缓释剂	伐尼克兰（Varenicline）
	口香糖	锭剂	透皮贴剂	鼻喷剂	口腔吸入剂		
每日花费[5]	2mg 或 4mg：$1.89～$5.48(9片)	2mg 或 4mg:$3.05～$4.38(9片)	$1.52～$3.40(1贴)	$4.12(8剂)	$7.35(6个药芯)	$2.38～$6.22(2片)	$5.96～$6.50(2片)

1. 由葛兰素史克公司注册
2. 由美国辉瑞制药公司注册
3. 《美国临床实践指南》中指出基础安全有效性和理论性的不足，应该鼓励吸烟孕妇不采用药物戒烟，向吸烟孕妇提供超出最小戒烟范围的行为咨询干预
4. 2009年7月，美国FDA要求所有包含安非他酮和伐尼克兰产品的药方信息必须采用黑色警示框警示有出现严重神经症状的风险，如行为改变，敌对倾向，躁动，情绪低落，自杀意念与行为和自杀未遂等，临床医生应对告患者停止服用伐尼克兰产品或盐酸安非他酮缓释片，如果出现临床躁动、情绪低落和任何其他戒烟不典型的行为变化或被自杀想法所困扰，临床医生应联系医务人员。如果因神经症状停止治疗，应监视患者直到症状消失
5. 批发价格来自2012年9月汤姆森路透公司的《药物在线红皮书》

MAO：单胺氧化酶；NRT：尼古丁替代治疗；OTC：非处方药；Rx：处方药
更完整的信息请参考厂家药品说明书
参考文献108。版权1999—2014 加州大学董事会。版权所有

尼古丁替代治疗（NRT）

在临床试验中，患者使用尼古丁替代治疗（Nicotine replacement therapy NRT）产品比使用安慰剂的戒烟成功率高[101]。NRT产品的主要作用机制被认为是刺激大脑腹侧盖膜区的尼古丁受体，导致大脑中伏隔核释放多巴胺。使用NRT的目的是减轻躯体和心理戒断症状，是吸烟者在完全放弃尼古丁之前集中注意于戒烟的行为和心理状况。NRT的主要优点是不必接触烟草和吸烟中发现的致癌物质及其他有毒化合物，且NRT提供的尼古丁作用比通过香烟提供的更为缓慢，因此可以消除通过吸烟获得的具有即刻强化效果的尼古丁（图1.1）。

由于各种不同尼古丁替代产品的剂型（口香糖、锭剂、透皮贴剂、吸入剂、喷鼻剂）的功效相似[101]，患者可根据个人偏好选择。除了每天1次的尼古丁贴片，其他所有尼古丁替代产品的剂型都需要频繁给药以维持所需的尼古丁浓度，缓解戒断效应。为了尽可能地提高成功率，建议患者遵守临床医生推荐的每一次给药，在整个治疗过程中持续坚持推荐的生活习惯。尼古丁替代疗法没有特殊的禁忌证，但是由于尼古丁刺激交感神经系统，并导致心率加快、心肌收缩力增加及血压升高，所以伴有严重心律失常、潜在严重或加重的心绞痛或近期发生过心肌梗死（2周内）的患者应慎用尼古丁替代产品[101]。由于服用推荐剂量的尼古丁替代产品的尼古丁血药浓度通常低于通过吸烟得到的浓度，所以大部分专家认为与继续吸烟的风险相比，伴有心血管系统疾病的患者应用尼古丁替代疗法的风险非常小[112]。

安非他酮缓释剂

安非他酮缓释剂初始是作为一种非典型抗抑郁药上市的，其作用机制被认为是通过抑制中枢神经系统再吸收多巴胺和肾上腺素[101]，以及作为一种尼古丁胆碱受体拮抗剂而促进戒烟[113]。这种神经化学作用被认为能调节多巴胺反馈通路，减少患者对尼古丁的需求和戒断症状[101]。

因为癫痫发作是安非他酮的一种剂量相关毒性反应，这种药物禁用于癫痫患者和同时使用其他安非他酮药物的患者（Wellbutrin、Wellbutrin SR和Wellbutrin XL）。由于会增加癫痫发作的风险，安非他酮也禁用于厌食症或暴食症以及突然中断使用酒精和镇静剂的患者。禁止同时使用安非他酮和单胺氧化酶（monoamine oxidase，MAO）抑制剂，必须在停用单胺氧化酶抑制剂至少14d后再开始使用安非他酮治疗[114]。应用推荐剂量为300mg/d的安非他酮缓释剂治疗无既往癫痫病史患者的抑郁症，癫痫的发病率为0.1%（1/1 000）。因此，对于有癫痫既往病史、颅骨创伤的患者、接受已知可降低癫痫发作阈值治疗的患者及有潜在严重肝硬化的患者，应慎用安非他酮。

2009年7月，美国FDA下令所有含安非他酮的药品说明书中须含有强调严重神经精神病事件风险的黑色警示框，这包括但不限于抑郁症、自杀意念、自杀企图及自杀。所有正在接受安非他酮治疗的患者都必须观察其神经精神症状，包括行为的变化、敌意、躁动、抑郁情绪及自杀相关事件，后者又包括意念、行为及自杀企图。一旦发生躁动、敌意、情绪低落、思维或行动变化异于正常反应，或者产生自杀意念或自杀行为，应建议患者停止服用安非他酮并与医务工作者取得联系，同时提供持续监控及支持性护理直至症状消失[114]。

伐尼克兰（Varenicline）

作为一种 $\alpha_4\beta_2$ 尼古丁乙酰胆碱受体[115-116]部

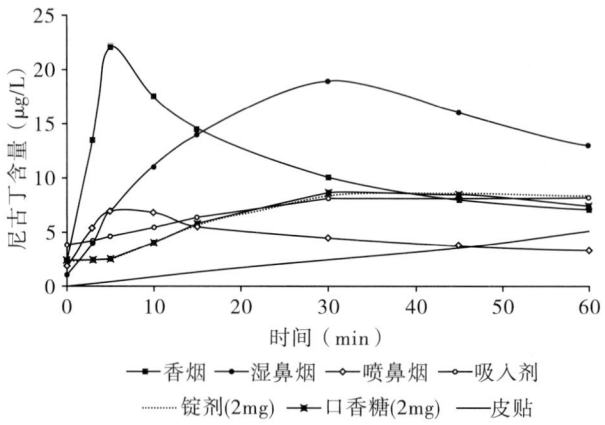

图1.1 各种剂型尼古丁产品的血药浓度
来源：获准引自参考文献108，版权© 1999—2014加州大学董事会。版权所有。血浆尼古丁浓度曲线源于参考文献109~111

分选择性拮抗剂，伐尼克兰被认为具有在受体部位竞争性抑制尼古丁结合以及持续、低水平拮抗作用的效果。这种部分拮抗作用，诱导适度的受体激活，引起多巴胺水平升高，从而减轻尼古丁戒断症状。此外，通过在中枢神经系统竞争性地阻止尼古丁与尼古丁乙酰胆碱受体的结合，伐尼克兰抑制在吸入烟草烟雾后多巴胺的大量释放，这种效应可以减少吸烟的强化效应和奖赏效应，从而有效预防再次吸烟[116]。

与安非他酮类似，2009年美国FDA规定伐尼克兰的药品说明书中须含有强调严重神经精神病事件风险的黑色警示框，这包括但不限于抑郁症、自杀意念、自杀企图及自杀。所有正在接受伐尼克兰治疗的患者都必须观察其神经精神症状，包括行为的变化、敌意、躁动、抑郁情绪及自杀相关事件，后者又包括意念、行为及自杀企图。一旦发生躁动、敌意、情绪低落、思维或行动变化异于正常反应，或者产生自杀意念或自杀行为，应建议患者停止服用伐尼克兰并与医务工作者取得联系[117]。

最近，伐尼克兰的商品标签中增加了一项针对明确有心血管系统疾病患者的警示（预警）。具体内容为：一旦发生新的或恶化的心血管症状，患者必须告知医务工作者；一旦发现心肌梗死或脑卒中的信号或症状，必须立即寻求医疗护理。尽管一项包含15个临床试验（包括一个有明确心血管疾病的患者中进行的试验）的meta分析表明心血管事件整体上罕见，但是在使用伐尼克兰治疗的患者中常被报道，并且这些心血管事件主要发生在明确有心血管疾病的患者中。然而，在临床试验和meta分析中，全因和心血管疾病死亡率在伐尼克兰治疗的患者中反而较低[117]。

联合治疗

当服用戒烟药物使患者戒烟成功的可能性加倍时，需要提高长期戒烟率。根据来自8项临床试验的数据，2008版《临床实践指南》[101]推荐临床医生应考虑将药物联合治疗作为对有戒烟意图患者的一线治疗方法。联合治疗方法通常包括一个长效剂型（例如尼古丁贴）和一个短效剂型（例如口香糖、锭剂、吸入剂、鼻喷剂），这种联合治疗方法的应用正在日益增多。长效剂型有助于阻止严重戒断症状的出现，短效剂型用于控制情境性生理欲望。此外，双尼古丁替代疗法的最佳组合、剂量及持续时间尚不清楚。

妊娠期用药

《临床实践指南》[101]声明，由于缺乏药效证据及对潜在安全性的考虑，应鼓励吸烟的孕妇不通过药物戒烟。

动物实验数据表明，尼古丁对胎儿的发育有害。美国FDA将尼古丁替代疗法的处方剂归入怀孕D类制剂，安非他酮和伐尼克兰被划分为怀孕C类制剂。相应地，制造商推荐仅在对胎儿的潜在益处大于潜在风险的情况下，可在孕期应用该制剂[114,117]。

总　结

烟草使用在人群中仍然很普遍且表现为一个特殊的公共卫生问题。烟草是肺癌发生的主要原因，同时也可导致其他脏器的恶性肿瘤和许多其他疾病。在过去的几十年间，已积累了大量有关吸烟行为方面的理论。青少年中开始吸烟的易感因素的研究可以为开展可行、有效的预防吸烟活动提供重要线索。掌握导致发生尼古丁依赖的生物学行为原因的知识有助于为吸烟者提供更有效的治疗。在美国公共卫生署的《烟草使用和依赖治疗的临床实践指南》中描述了"5A"步骤（即询问烟草的使用情况、劝告戒烟、评估戒烟的准备状态、协助戒烟和安排随访），鼓励医务工作者每遇到一例吸烟患者至少要完成一次简单的干预措施（即询问—劝告—介绍）。

（杨霞　叶欣译）

参考文献

[1] American Cancer Society Cancer Facts and Figures. Atlanta, GA: American Cancer Society, 2014.

[2] US Department of Health and Human Services Preventing Tobacco Use Among Youth and Young Adults: A Report of the Surgeon General. US Department of Health and Human

Services, Centers for Disease Control and Prevention, National Center for Chronic Disease Prevention and Health Promotion, Office on Smoking And Health. Atlanta, GA, 2012.

[3] Pierce JP, White VM Emery SL What public health strategies are needed to reduce smoking initiation? Tob Control, 2012, 21 (2): 258-264.

[4] CDG (2008) Cigarette smoking among adults and trends in smoking cessation-United States. MMWR (Morbidity and Mortality Weekly Report), 2008, 58 (44): 1227-1232.

[5] A Clinical Practice Guideline for Treating Tobacco Use and Dependence: 2008 update. A US Public Health Service report. Am J Prev Med, 2008, 35 (2): 158-176.

[6] CDC (2012) Current cigarette smoking among adults-United States. MMWR. 2011, 61 (44): 889-894.

[7] Johnston LD, O'Malley PM, Bachman JG, et al. Decline in teen smoking continues into 2012. University of Michigan, Ann Arbor MI, 2012.

[8] US Department of Health, Education and Welfare. Smoking and Health: Report of the Advisory Committee to the Surgeon General of the Public Health Service. US Department of Health, Education, and Welfare. Public Health Service. Center for Disease Control PHS Publication No. 1103. Washington, DC, 1964.

[9] CDC Smoking-attributable mortality, years of potential life lost, and productivity losses-United States, 2000—2004. MMWR, 2008, 57 (45): 1226-1228.

[10] CDC Annual smoking-attributable mortality, years of potential life lost, and economic costs-United States, 1995—1999. MMWR, 2002, 51 (14): 300-303.

[11] US Department of Health and Human Services. The Health Consequences of Smoking: A Report of the Surgeon General. US Department of Health and Human Services Centers for Disease Control and Prevention National Center for Chronic Disease Prevention and Health Promotion. Office cm Smoking and Health, 2004.

[12] CDG. Cigarette smoking-attributable morbidity-United States. MMWR, 2003, 52 (35): 842-844.

[13] Wingo PA, Ries LA, Giovino GA, et al. Annual report to the nation on the status of cancer, 1973—1996, with a special section on lung cancer and tobacco smoking. J Natl Cancer Inst, 1999, 91 (S): 675-690.

[14] Peto R, Lopez AD, Boreham J, et al. Mortality from smoking worldwide. Br Med Bull, 1996, 52 (1): 12-21.

[15] Doll R, Peto R. Boreham J, et al. Mortality from cancer in relation to smoking: 50 years observations on British doctors. Br J Cancer, 2005, 92 (3): 426-429.

[16] Yoder LH. Lung cancer epidemiology. Medsurg Nurs, 2006, 15 (3): quiz 5.

[17] Jemal A, Siegel R, Ward E, et al. Cancer statistics. CA Cancer J Clin, 2006, 56 (2): 106-130.

[18] Spiro SG, Silvestri GA. One: hundred years of lung cancer. Am J Respir Crit Care Med, 2005, 172 (5): 523-529.

[19] Knop C. Lung cancer//Cancer Nursing: Principles and Practice, Yarbro CH, Frogge MH//Goodman M, eds. Jones and Barlett. Boston: MA, 2005.

[20] Pastorino U. Early detection of lung cancer. Them atic Review Series, 2006, 73: 5-13.

[21] Rutten LF, Hesse BW, Moser RP, et al. Public perceptions of cancer prevention, screening, and survival: comparison with state of-science: evidence for colon skin and lung cancer. J Cancer Educ, 2009, 24 (1) 40-48.

[22] IARC. Tobacco smoke and involuntary smoking. IARC Monographs on the Evaluation of Carcinogenic Risks to Humans. International Agency for Research on Cancer. 2004, 83.

[23] Anthonisen NR, Connett JE, Murray RP, et al. Smoking and lung function of lung health study participants after 11years. Am J Respir Crit Care Med, 2002, 166 (5): 675-679.

[24] Kamholz SL. Pulmonary and cardiovascular consequences of smoking. Clin Occup Environ Med, 2006, 5 (1): 157-157, x.

[25] Piric K, Peto R, Reeves GK, et al. The 21st century hazards of smoking and benefits of stopping: a prospective study of one million women in the UK. Lancet, 2013, 381 (9861): 133-141.

[26] Agudo A, Bonet C, Travier N, et al. Impact of cigarette smoking on cancer risk in die European prospective investigation into cancer and nutrition study. J Clin Oncol, 2012, 30 (36): 4550-4557,

[27] Lee PN, Forty BA, Coombs KJ. Systematic review with meta-analysis of the epidemiological evidence in the 1900s relating smoking to lung cancer. BMC Cancer 2012, 12: 385.

[28] Doll R, Hill AB. Smoking and carcinoma of the lung; preliminary report. Br Med J, 1950, 2 (4682): 739-748.

[29] Centers for Disease Control and Prevention. Division of

Cancer Prevention and Control. Lung Cancer Risk Faction. Atlanta, GA, 2012. Available at: http://www.cdc.gov/cancer/lung_ inl: o/risk_ factors.htm. Accessed February 20, 2014.

[30] Samet JM, Avila-Tang E, Boffetta P, et al. Lung cancer in never smokers: clinical epidemiology and environmental risk factors. Clin Cancer Res, 2009, 15 (18): 5626-5645.

[31] Alberg AJ, Nonemaker J. Who is at high risk for lung cancer? Population-level and individual-level perspectives. Semin Respir Crit Care Med, 2008, 29 (3): 223-232.

[32] Thomas JL, Guo H, Carmella SG, et al. Metabolites of a tobacco-specific lung carcinogen in children exposed to secondhand or thirdhand tobacco smoke in their homes. Cancer Epidemiol Biomarkers Prev, 2011, 20 (6): 1213-1221.

[33] US Department of Health and Human Services. The Health Consequences of Involuntary Exposure to Tobacco Smoke: A Report of the Surgeon General. US Department of Health and Human Services Centers for Disease Control and Prevention, Coordinating Center for Health Promotion National Center for Chronic Disease Prevention and Health Promotion Office on Smoking and Health, 2006.

[34] Glantz S, Parmley W. Passive smoking and heart disease: epidemiology, physiology and biochemistry. Circulation, 1991, 83 (1): 1-12.

[35] Cox L, Patten C, Ebbert J, et al. Tobacco use outcomes among patients with lung cancer treated for nicotine dependence. J Clin Oncol, 2002, 20: 3461-3469.

[36] van der Bol JM, Mathijssen RH, Loos WJ, et al. Cigarette smoking and irinotecan treatment: pharmacokinetic interaction and effects on neutropenia. J Clin Oncol, 2005, 25 (19): 2719-2726.

[37] Kanai M, Morita S, Matsumoto S, et al. A history of smoking is inversely correlated with the incidence of gemcitabine-induced neutropenia. Ann Oncol, 2009, 20 (8): 1397-1401.

[38] Parsons A, Daley A, Begh R, et al. Influence of smoking cessation after diagnosis of early stage lung cancelr on prognosis: systematic review of observational studies with meta-analysis. BMJ, 2010, 340: b5569.

[39] Underwood JM, Townsend JS, Tat E, et al. Persistent cigarette smoking and other tobacco use after a tobacco-related cancer diagnosis. J Cancer Surviv, 2012, 6 (3): 333-344.

[40] Underwood JM, Rim SH, Fairley TL, et al. Cervical cancer survivors at increascd risk of subsequent tobacco-related malignancies, United States 1992—2008. Cancer Causes Control, 2012, 23 (7): 9-16.

[41] Vander Ark W, DiNardo LJ, Oliver D. Factors affecting smoking cessation in patients with head and neck cancer. Laryngoscope, 1997, 107: 888-892.

[42] Cataldo JK, Dubey S, Prochaska JJ. Smoking cessation an integral part of lung cancer treatment. Oncology, 2010, 78 (5-6): 289-301.

[43] Gritz ER, Fingeret MC, Vidrine DJ, et al. Successes and failures of the teachable moment-smoking cessation in cancer patients. Cancer, 2006, 106 (1): 17-27.

[44] Garces YI, Yang P, Parkinson J, et al. The relationship between cigarette smoking and quality of life after lung cancer diagnosis. Chest, 2004, 126 (6): 1733-1741.

[45] Cooley ME, Sarna L, Kotlernan J, et al. Smoking cessation is challenging even for patients recovering from lung cancer surgery with curative intent. Lung Cancer, 2009, 66 (2): 218-225.

[46] Theadom A, Cropley M. Effects of preoperative smoking cassation on the incidence and risk of intra-operative and postoperative complications in adult smokers: a systematic review. Tob Control, 2006, 15 (5): 352-358.

[47] Berg CJ, Carpenter MJ, Jardin B, et al. Harm reduction and cessation efforts and interest in cessation resources among survivors of smoking-related cancers. J Cancer Surviv, 2013, 7 (1): 44-54.

[48] Schnoll R, Malstrom M, James C, et al. Correlates of tobacco use among smokers and recent quitters diagnosed with cancer. Patient Educ Conus, 2002, 46: 137-145.

[49] CDC. Quitting smoking among adults. MMWR, 2011, 60 (44): 1513-1519.

[50] CDC. Current tobacco use among middle and high school students-United States. MMWR, 2011, 61 (31): 581-585.

[51] Baker F, Ainsworth SR, Dye JT, et al. Health risks associated with cigar smoking. Jama, 2000, 284 (6): 735-740.

[52] CDC. Current cigarette smoking among adults-United States. MMWR, 2012, 61 (44) 889-894.

[53] CDC. State-specific prevalence of current cigarette and cigar smoking among adults-United States. MMWR, 48 (45): 1034-1039.

[54] Henningfield JE, Fant R, Radzius A, et al. Nicotine concentration, smoke pH and whole tobacco aqueous pH of some cigar brands and types popular in the US. Nico-

tine Tob Res, 1999, 1 (2): 163-168.

[55] Kozlowski LT, Mehta N, Sweeney C, et al. Filter ventilation and nicotine content of tobacco in cigarettes from Canada the United Kingdom, and the United States. Tob Control, 1998, 7 (4): 369.

[56] Henningfield JE, Hariharan MM, Kozlowski LT. Nicotine content and health risks of cigars. JAMA, 1996, 276: 1857-1858.

[57] Nelson DE, Davis RM, Chrismon JH, et al. Pipe smoking in the United States, 1965—1991: prevalence and attributable mortality. Prev Med, 1996, 25: 91-99.

[58] CDC. Bidi use among urban youth-Massachusetts, March-April 1999. MMWR, 1999, 48 (36): 796-799.

[59] Delnevo C, Pevzner E, Hrywna M, et al. Bidi cigarette use among young adults in 15 states. Prev Med, 2004, 39 (1): 207-211.

[60] Rickert WS. Determination of yields of "tar", nicotine and carbon monoxide from bidi cigarettes: final report. Ontario, Canada: Labstat International, 1999.

[61] Hudmon KS, Kilfoy BA, Prokhorov AV. The epidemiology of tobacco use and dependence. Crit Care Nurs Clin North Am, 2006, 18 (1): 1-11, xi.

[62] Substance Abuse and Mental Health Services Administration, Office of Applied Studies. The NSDUH Report: Smokeless Tobacco Use, Initiation, and Relationship to Cigarette Smoking: 2002 to 2007. Rockville MD, 2009.

[63] US Department of Agriculture Tobacco Out-look Report (TBS-258), 2005. Available from: http://usda01.library.cornell.edu/usda/ers/TBS/2000s/2005/TBS-04-15-2005.pdf. Accessed February 20, 2014.

[64] Delnevo CD, Wackowski OA, Giovenco DP, et al. Examining Market trends in the United States smokeless tobacco use: 2005—2011. Tob Control, 2014, 23 (2): 107-112.

[65] Pederson LL, Nelson DE. Literature review Lind summary of perceptions, attitudes, beliefs, and marketing of potentially reduced exposure products: communication implications. Nicotine Tob Res, 2007, 9 (5): 525-534.

[66] Blank MD, Eissenberg T. Evaluating oral non-combustiblepotential reduced-exposure products for smokers. Nicotine Tob Res, 2010, 12 (4): 336-343.

[67] Parascandola M, Augustson E, O'Connell ME, et al. Consumer awareness and attitudes related to new potential reduced-exposure tobacco product brands. Nicotine Tob Res, 2009, 11 (7): SS6-95.

[68] AmericanLung Association. An emerging deadly trend: Waterpipe tobacco use. Washington, DC: American Lung Association, 2007. Available from: http://wvvw.lung.org/stop-smoking/tobacco-control-advocacy/reports-resources/tobacco-policy-trend-reports/. Accessed February 20, 2014.

[69] Cobb C, Ward KD, Maziak W, et al. Waterpipe tobacco smoking: an emerging health crisis in the United States. Am J Health Behav, 2010, 34 (3): 275-285.

[70] Eissenberg T, Ward KD, Smith-Simone S, et al. Waterpipe tobacco smoking on a U.S, College campus: prevalence and correlates. J Adolescent Health, 2008, 42 (5): 526-529.

[71] Grekin ER, Ayna D. Argileh use among college students in the United States: an emerging trend. J Stud Alcohol Drugs, 2008, 69 (3): 472-475.

[72] Smith SY, Curbow B, Stillman FA. Harm perception of nicotine products in college freshmen. Nicotine Tob Res, 2007, 9 (9): 977-982.

[73] Martinasek MP, McDermott RJ, Martini L. Waterpipe (hookah) tobacco smoking among youth. Curr Probl Pediatr Adolesc Health Care, 2011, 41 (2): 34-57.

[74] Primack B, Shensa A, Kim KH, et al. Waterpipe smoking among US university students. Nicotine Tob Res, 2013, 15 (1): 29-35.

[75] Sutfin EL, McCoy TP, Reboussin BA, et al. Prevalence and correlates of waterpipe tobacco smoking by college students in North Carolina. Drug Alcohol Depend, 2011, 115 (1-2): 131-136.

[76] Primack BA, Shensa A, Kim KH, et al. Waterpipe smoking among U.S. university students. Nicotine Tob Res, 2013, 15 (1): 29-35.

[77] Maziak W. Thewaterpipe: An emerging global risk for cancer. Cancer Epidemiol, 2013, 37 (1): 1-4.

[78] Food and Drug Administration. Electronic cigarettes, 2009. Available from: http://www.fda.gov/Safety/MedWatch/SafciyInformation/SafetyAlertsforHumanMedical-Products/ucm173327.htm. Accessed February 20, 2014.

[79] Pearson JL, Richardson A, Niaura RS, et al. e-Cigarette awareness use, and harm perceptions in US adults. Am J Public Health, 2012, 102 (9): 1758-1766.

[80] Johnston LD, O'Malley PM, Bachman JG, et al. Decline in teen smoking appeals to be nearing its end. University of Michigan News and Information Services: Ann Arbor MI, 2005. Available from: http: " www.monitoringthefuture.org/data/05data.html#2005data-cigs. Accessed February 20, 2014.

[81] US Department of Health and Human Services. Preventing

Tobacco Use Among Young People: A Report of the Surgeon General, Atlanta, GA, US Department of Health and Human Services, Public Health Service Centers for Disease Control and Prevention, National Center for Chronic Disease Prevention and Health Promotion Office on Smoking and Health, 1994.

[82] Biglan A, Duncan TE, Ary DV, et al. Peer and parental influences on adolescent tobacco use. J Behav Med, 1995, l8 (4): 315-330.

[83] Glitz E. R, Prokhorov AV, Hudmon KS, et al. Predictors of susceptibility to smoking and ever smoking: a longitudinal study in a triethnic sample of adolescents. Nicotine Tob Res, 2003, 5 (4): 493-506.

[84] Hansen WB. Pilot test results comparing the All Stars program with seventh grade D. A. R. E,: program integrity and mediating variable analysis. Subst Use Misuse, 1996, 31 (10): 1359-1377.

[85] MacKinnon DP. Analysts of mediating variables in prevention and intervention research. NIDA Res Monogr, 1994, 139: 127-153.

[86] Sargent J. Smoking in movies: Impact on adolescent smoking. Adoles Med Clin, 2005, 16 (2): 345-370.

[87] Wahlgren DR, Hovell MF, Slymen DJ, et al. Predictors of tobacco use initiation in adolescents: A two-year prospective study and theoretical discussion. Tob Control, 1997, 6 (2): 95-103.

[88] CDC. Youth risk behavior surveillance, United States. MMWR, 2006, 55 (SS-55): 1-108.

[89] Prokhorov AV, Hudmon KS, Marani SK, et al. Eliminating second-hand smoke from Mexican-American households: outcomes from Project Clean Air-Safe Air (CASA). Addict Behav, 2013, 38 (1): 1485-1492.

[90] Cuny SJ, Emery S, Sporer AK, et al. A national survey of tobacco cessation programs for youths. Am J Public Health, 2007, 97 (1): 171-177.

[91] Prokhorov AV, Kelder SH, Shegog R, et al. Impact of A Smoking PreventionInteractive Experience (ASPIRE), an interactive, multimedia smoking prevention and cessation curriculum for culturally diverse high-school students. Nicotine Tob Res, 2008, 10 (9): 1477-1485.

[92] Joffe A, McNeely C, Colantuoni E, et al. Evaluation of school-based smoking-cessation interventions for self-described adolescent smokers. Pediatrics, 2009, 124 (2): e187-194.

[93] Flay BR. The promise of long-term effectiveness of school-based smoking prevention programs: a critical review of reviews. Tob Induc Dis, 2009, 5 (1): 7.

[94] Prokhorov AV, Kelder SH, Conroy JL, et al. Project ASPIRE: An interactive multimedia smoking prevention and cessation curriculum for culturally diverse high school students. Subst Use Misuse, 2010, 45 (6): 983-1006.

[95] Prokhorov AV, Marani SK, Calabro KS, et al. Theory- and technology-driven educational curricula addressing tobacco use. Procedia-Social and Behavioral Sciences, 2012, 46: 4504-4507.

[96] Benowitz NL, Hukkanen J, Jacob P, et al. Nicotine chemistry, metabolism, kinetics and biomarkers. Handb Exp Pharmacol, 2009, 192: 29-60.

[97] Benowitz NL. Neurobiology of nicotine addiction: implications for smoking cessation treatment. Am Med, 2008, 121 (4 Suppl 1): S3-10.

[98] Benowitz NL. Nicotine addiction. N Engl J Med, 2010, 362 (24): 2295-2303.

[99] Benowitz NL. Clinical pharmacology of nicotine: implications for understanding preventing, and treating tobacco addiction. Clin Pharmacol Ther, 2008, 83 (4): 531-541.

[100] Hughes JR. Effects of abstinence from tobacco: valid symptoms and time course. Nicotine Tob Res, 2007, 9 (3): 315-327.

[101] Fiore MC, Jaen CR, Baker TB. Treating Tobacco Use and Dependence: 2008 Update. Clinical Practice Guideline, Rockville, MD: US Department of Health and HumanServices. Public Health Service, 2008.

[102] CDC. Best Practices for Comprehensive Tobacco Control Programs-2007 Notional Center for Chronic Disease Prevention and Health Promotion, Office on Smoking and Health. Atlanta, GA, 2007.

[103] US Department of Health and Human Services. The Health Benefits of Smoking Cessation. A Report of the Surgeon General. US Department of Health and Human Services, Public Health Service, Office on Smoking and Health, Rockville, Maryland, DHHS Publication No. (CDC) 90-8416, 1990.

[104] Stead LF, Perera R, Lancaster T. A systematic review of interventions for smokers who contact quitlines. Tob Control, 2007, 16 Suppl 1: i3-8.

[105] Zhu S, Melcer T, Sun J, et al. Smoking cessation with and without assistance: a population-based analysis. Am J Prev Med, 2000, 18 (4): 305-311.

[106] Smith SS, Keller PA, Kobinsky KH, et al. Enhancing

tobacco quitline effectiveness: Identifying a superior pharmacotherapy adjuvant. Nicotine Tob Res, 2013, 15 (3): 718 -728.

[107] Bonniot Saucedo C, Schroeder SA. Simplicity sells: Making smoking cessation easier. Am J Prev Med, 2010, 38 (3 Suppl): S393 -396.

[108] Rx for Change: Clinician-Assisted Tobacco Cessation. San Francisco, CA: University of California San Francisco, 1999—2014.

[109] Choi JH, Dresler CM, Norton MR, et al. pharmacokinetics of a nicotine polacrilex lozenge. Nicotine Tob Res, 2003, 5 (5): 635 -644.

[110] Schneider NG, Olmstead RE, Franzon MA, et al. The nicotine inhaler: clinicalpharmacokinetics and comparison with other nicotine treatments. Clin pharmacokinet, 2001, 40 (9): 661 -684.

[111] Fant RV, Owen LL, Henningfield JE. Nicotine: replacement therapy. Prim Care, 1999, 26 (3): 633 -652.

[112] Benowitz NL. Pharmacology of nicotine: addiction, smoking-induced disease, and therapeutics. Annu Rev Pharmacol Toxicol, 2009, 49: 57 -71.

[113] Slemmer JE, Martin BR, Damaj MI. Bupropion is a nicotinic antagonist. J Pharmacol Exp Ther, 2000, 295: 321 -327.

[114] GlaxoSmithKlinc, Inc. Zyban package insert. Research Triangle Park, NC, 2012.

[115] Coe JW, Brooks PR, Vetelino MG, et al. Vareniclinc: an alpha4beta2 nicotinic receptor partial agonist for smoking cessation. J Med Chem, 2005, 48 (10): 3474 -3477.

[116] Foulds J. The neurobiological basis for partial agonist treatment of nicotine dependence: vareniclinc. Int J Clin Pract, 2006, 60 (5): 571 -576.

[117] Pfizer, Inc. Chantix Package Insert. New York, NY, 2012.

第2章
肺癌的易感性和风险评估模型

Xifeng Wu, Xia Pu, Jie Lin
Department of Epidemiology, The University of Texas MD Anderson Cancer Center, Houston, TX, USA

引言

从20世纪初开始,全球的肺癌发病率迅速升高。尽管在过去的20年间美国男性肺癌的新发病例数稳步下降,但肺癌仍然是癌症死亡的首要原因[1]。据估计,2013年美国有228 190例新增肺癌病例,与此同时,有159 480人因肺癌死亡,分别占美国男性、女性癌症总死亡人数的28%和26%[1]。尽管吸烟是导致肺癌发病最主要的原因,但肺癌家族史、各种慢性呼吸系统疾病以及环境烟雾等多种因素也会增加个体罹患肺癌的风险。由于仅有一部分吸烟者会最终发展为肺癌,因此宿主的易感性可能也是一种危险因素[2-5]。肿瘤的发生是一个多步骤的过程,因此探索出增加肺癌发生风险的因素可以指导我们鉴别出高危人群,进而使这部分人群通过靶向筛选和其他的干预措施获益。接下来的内容我们总结了关于肺癌分子流行病学的最新进展。

流行病学危险因素

吸烟是肺癌发病最主要的危险因素,一些其他的环境暴露,如石棉、砷、铬、镍、多环芳族化合物、氡、氯乙烯和空气污染等,也与肺癌的发生相关,这在之前的章节中已有论述。本章节我们主要讨论经当前文献证实与肺癌发病相关的一些其他的流行病学因素。

家族史

许多已公布的研究表明,在近亲中肺癌存在家族聚集性[6-12]。此外,许多相关研究证实,一级亲属的肺癌罹患风险会增加1.3~6.0倍[11,13-15]。Matakidou等人对53项肺癌家族史与发病风险相关的研究进行了系统综述和meta分析,发现亲属患有肺癌的个体罹患肺癌的风险显著升高[RR=1.84;95%CI(1.64,2.05)],如果亲属的肺癌发病时间较早,则二者之间的关联会更显著。他们还综合评估了不吸烟者的发病风险,发现了相似的结果[RR=1.51;95%CI(1.11,2.06)],揭示了家族史在不吸烟个体发生肺癌中的作用[15]。另一项研究对国际癌症研究机构(the International Agency for Research on Cancer, IARC)开展的41项多中心病例对照研究进行了meta分析,纳入了2 861例肺癌一级亲属和3 118例健康对照者,亲属患有肺癌的个体罹患肺癌风险提高了1.63倍[95%CI(1.31,2.01)]。如果个体有两个或更多的亲属罹患肺癌,则其发病风险将提高3.60倍[95%CI(1.56,8.31)]。研究者还发现,这种风险在鳞状细胞癌(squamous cell carcinoma, SCC)和大细胞癌等亚型中更加明显[16]。

早期炎性疾病及功能紊乱

慢性阻塞性肺疾病(COPD)

50%~90%的肺癌病例合并有慢性阻塞性肺疾病(chronic obstructive pulmonary disease, COPD)[17],流行病学研究一再表明,COPD是肺癌的高危因素[18-23]。据估计,COPD的存在可将肺癌的发病风险提高4.5倍[21]。无论在美国还是在世界范围内,肺癌和COPD都是发病和死亡的主要原因,而吸烟是他们共同和最主要的致病因素,因此,近年来COPD作为肺癌的伴随疾病获得了越来多的关注。美国国立心肺血液研究所（the National Heart, Lung, and Blood Institute, NHLBI）和美国国家癌症研究所（the National Cancer Institute, NCI）成立工作组并扩大合作范围，聚焦流行病学、遗传学与表观遗传学等方面的高危因素，努力探寻COPD与肺癌的关系，以期能探明它们相同和不同的致病机制。

肺气肿

许多研究已经证实，早期肺气肿病史是罹患肺癌的危险因素。最近一项有关早期肺部疾病和肺癌危险因素的meta分析囊括了20项关于肺气肿和肺癌的数据，研究者发现，肺气肿患者的肺癌发生率将提高2倍[$RR = 2.04$; 95% CI (1.72, 2.41)][24]。另一项包含7 368例行CT扫描患者的meta分析提示，肺气肿会使肺癌罹患风险增加2.11倍[95% CI (1.10, 4.04)]，而且这种风险在肺气肿明显的患者中会更高[$OR = 3.50$; 95% CI (2.71, 4.51)][25]。国际肺癌研究所对24 607例研究组和81 829例对照组患者进行汇总分析发现：肺气肿病史会使个体罹患肺癌的风险增加2.44倍[95% CI (1.64, 3.62)]，而且对于不吸烟的人群，罹患肺癌的风险也会因此提高[26]。

哮喘

在一项meta分析中，排除环境性二手烟的影响后，哮喘是非吸烟者罹患肺癌的显著危险因素，总相对危险度（ralative risk, RR）为1.9 [95% CI (1.4, 2.5)][27]。近期，另一项由国际肺癌研究所发起的包括16个研究项目，涉及585 444人的meta分析指出，在总人群中哮喘与肺癌发病风险密切相关[$RR = 1.28$; 95% CI (1.16, 1.41)]，在鳞状细胞癌亚型中也是如此[$RR = 1.69$; 95% CI (1.26, 2.26)][28]。

花粉症

虽然早期的研究并没有发现花粉症与罹患肺癌风险的关系（Talbot-Smith, et al[29]; Osann, et al[10]），但一项大型对照研究表明，花粉症可能会降低肺癌罹患风险[$OR = 0.58$; 95% CI (0.48, 0.70)][30]。与此研究结果相一致，肺癌、直肠癌、膀胱癌和前列腺癌等恶性肿瘤患者与对照组相比较，有花粉症患者的发病率比较低[31]。这种保护效应可能是通过提高人体的免疫监视功能，从而更好地监测和杀死恶性肿瘤细胞[10,29,31-34]。另外，用于治疗花粉症的抗炎药物也对机体起到了保护作用。

饮食和营养危险因素

饮食摄入的水果和蔬菜

几项队列研究显示，增加蔬菜及水果的摄入量可以降低肺癌的发病风险。欧洲癌症与营养前瞻性调查（European Prospective Investigation into Cancer and Nutrition, EPIC）队列研究通过对478 021例受试者的数据分析发现，当调整了吸烟和其他混杂因素后，水果的高摄入量将使肺癌发病风险降低40%，但蔬菜的摄入却没有这种关系[38]。在一项包括了54 158例参与者的丹麦队列研究中，排除吸烟的影响后，随着植物类食物的摄入增多，肺癌发病率从0.35（0.27, 0.45）增长到0.65（0.45, 0.93）。Neuhouser等对430 281例中的3 206例肺癌患者随访了6～16年，并对8项前瞻性研究进行了汇总分析，发现在摄入总水果量、总水果和蔬菜量、总蔬菜量为消耗量的80%时，与摄入消耗量20%时相比，RR分别是0.77 [95% CI (0.67, 0.87); $P < 0.001$]，0.70 [95% CI (0.69, 0.90); $P = 0.001$]，0.88 [95% CI (0.78, 1.00); $P = 0.12$]。他们总结认为，增加水果和蔬菜的摄入量，主要是水果的摄入量，与肺癌发病率降低有关。一项对日本人群进行的流行病学系统综述表明，水果的摄入能降低肺癌的发病率，但蔬菜的摄入与肺癌发病率的关系尚无确切的数据支持。然而，一项大型前瞻性研究表明，在排除了吸烟等其他因素影响后，水果和蔬菜的摄入与肺癌的发病率并无明显关系。

十字花科植物中有一类具有抑癌作用的非营养化合物——异硫氰酸酯（isothiocyanates, ITCs）。它的一个抑癌机制可能是下调细胞色素P-450生物转化酶的水平并促进其向第Ⅱ期转化[43-44]，ITCs也能诱导凋亡、细胞周期暂停和细胞分化[45]。一些研究表明，十字花科植物的摄入量与肺癌的发病风险呈明显负相关，即使在有敏感突变的肺癌亚组（如GSTM1失活基因组）中依然如此[46-48]。一项关于十字花科植物摄入的meta分析

（18项全十字花科植物摄入研究和11项具体十字花科植物摄入研究）发现，无论在试验组［OR = 0.78；95% CI（0.70，0.88）］还是在对照组［RR = 0.83；95% CI（0.62，1.08）］，十字花科植物的摄入与肺癌的发病率都呈负相关，在GSTM1和GSTT1双突变基因组中，这种关联性则更加明显［OR = 0.41；95% CI（0.26，0.65）；P = 0.01）］[49]。

类胡萝卜素

类胡萝卜素是存在于水果和蔬菜中的红、黄色的脂溶性色素。北美和欧洲通过对399 765例参与者中的3 155例肺癌患者进行7～16年的随访，并对7项早期队列研究汇总分析后，Mannisto等人报道[50]，在控制维生素C、叶酸、其他种类的胡萝卜素、多种维生素的使用和吸烟状况后，只有β隐黄素的摄入与肺癌的发病风险呈负相关［RR = 0.76；95% CI（0.67，0.86）］。ATBC（β胡萝卜素癌症预防研究）[51]是一项囊括了27 084例50～69岁的男性吸烟者的预防研究，通过对其中1 644例肺癌患者的14年随访研究发现，摄入不同营养素标准量的人，患肺癌的风险有不同程度的下降，其中番茄红素下降28%，叶黄素或玉米黄素下降17%，β隐黄素下降15%，总胡萝卜素下降19%，浆液性β胡萝卜素下降16%，浆液性维生素A下降27%。然而，摄入β胡萝卜素、α胡萝卜素和维生素A与肺癌发病率的下降却没有太大关系。在一项有关护士健康和职业健康跟踪随访的汇总分析中，Michaud等认为[52]，只有摄入α胡萝卜素和番茄红素与肺癌危险性的降低有重要关联。通过对各种胡萝卜素总的分析得出，肺癌发病率在那些摄入较高量类胡萝卜素的受试者中降低［RR = 0.68；95% CI（0.49，0.94）］。各种混杂设计的调整不充分，特别是吸烟因素和个体摄入胡萝卜素缺乏多重共线性，可能导致了许多研究得出的结论不一致。最近的一项包括25项前瞻性研究的meta分析表明，类胡萝卜素的摄入量与肺癌发病率呈负相关［RR = 0.79；95% CI（0.71，0.87）］。与此同时，β胡萝卜素的摄入量与肺癌发病率却没有明显关联[53]。

膳食补充β胡萝卜素

流行病学观察研究得出的数据倾向于支持肺癌发病率与β胡萝卜素的摄入量和β胡萝卜素的血清浓度呈负相关，几个大规模随机化学预防试验已经开始对这种假说进行研究。然而，CARET（β胡萝卜素与维生素A药效化试验）和ATBC得出的结果却令人失望[40,51]，通过对当前吸烟者补充β胡萝卜素，肺癌的发病率反而升高了，这与预期的结果和观察到的流行病学证据相反[54-56]。目前争论集中在剂量、试验的持续时间、饮食摄入和补充给药法之间的差异[57]。前期的临床数据为吸烟和β胡萝卜素之间的抵消作用提供了生物学证据。最近的一项包括6个随机对照试验的meta分析表明，补充摄入β胡萝卜素与安慰剂相比RR为1.10，但差异无统计学意义，说明补充摄入β胡萝卜素与肺癌的发病率下降并无关系。

植物雌激素

饮食中的雌激素来源于植物中一些带有弱刺激活性的非类脂醇混合物，据观察，适当增加植物雌激素的摄入量可降低肺癌的发病率[60]。从食物中摄入标准量80%的个体发生肺癌的风险可降低46%［OR = 0.54；95% CI（0.42，0.70）］。针对亚洲人的几项研究表明，他们的饮食中包含大量的雌激素，肺癌的发病率也随着高含量的植物雌激素摄入而降低[61-65]。例如，男性摄入较多量的非发酵豆制品[61]可降低肺癌发病率，与此同时，女性摄入较多量的豆腐食品也可降低小细胞肺癌（small cell lung cancer, SCLC）的发病率。在中国，很多研究都证实了豆制品的摄入可降低肺癌发病率[66-67]。

叶酸

叶酸的缺乏对DNA的甲基化、DNA的合成及修复有不利影响[68-69]，这已被证实与肺部致癌作用有关，然而，观察性研究并没有得出一致的结论[69-72]。在最近的一项关于叶酸和维生素B治疗与癌症发病率和死亡率关系的大型随机试验中，接受叶酸和维生素B治疗的试验组与没有接受治疗的对照组相比，肺癌的发病率显著升高。同样，接受叶酸治疗的试验组与没有接受治疗的试验组相比，叶酸治疗组的肺癌发病率显著提高［HR = 1.59；95% CI（0.92，2.75）］。

遗传易感性

尽管吸烟是肺癌的主要危险因素，但最终仅

有一小部分吸烟者发展为肺癌，这表明遗传因素影响肺癌的易感性。此外，肺癌家族聚集的证据进一步支持肺癌的遗传易感性[73]。因此，肺癌易感基因的发现将有助于理解疾病的发病机制，同时指导个体化治疗和化学预防策略的制订[74]。

肺癌易感基因通常归类为罕见的高风险（OR＞10）、中度风险[OR=（2~5）]或者常见的低风险变异[OR=（1.2~1.5）]。通过对高风险家族（多发肺癌病例的家庭）的连锁分析，我们已确认肺癌的一些高风险基因变异。例如，通过研究52组多发肺癌或喉癌的高风险家庭，6号染色体上的一个潜在的高风险位点q23~25已被确定[75]，后续精细定位已经确定RGS17是一个潜在的高危易感基因[76]。

然而，大多数肺癌易感基因都是中危或低危的。个体易感性可能是由多个中危或低危基因在不同的细胞过程中调控所致，例如致癌物质代谢、DNA修复、细胞周期检查点控制、细胞凋亡、端粒完整性和微环境控制。一些基因相关研究正在检测这些中危或低危基因的变异，通过比较突变组和健康对照组的等位基因，以群体为基础的相关研究通常被用来识别易感基因。单核苷酸多态性（single nucleotide polymorphism，SNP）是癌症相关研究中研究基因变异最常见的形式。有证据显示有功能的单核苷酸多态性对宿主的影响要么是在基因表达方面，要么是在蛋白质的活动方面，这可能会影响肺癌的易感性[77-79]。在过去的几十年间，基因相关研究迅速从候选基因关联研究发展为全基因组关联研究（genome-wide association studies，GWAS），后续部分将着重于这两种研究结果的介绍。

候选基因研究

基于"相同变异相同疾病"假说，候选基因关联研究评估了预期的候选基因突变与致癌风险之间的关系。候选基因研究需要假定驱动基因，这很大程度上取决于对目的基因功能的认知或假设，通常选择的突变都是一些已知的与疾病相关的功能性单核苷酸多态性基因。以此为基础的通路研究是研究候选基因的一个扩展方法，它通过研究整个生物或功能通路中的标记物而增加了基因覆盖面。

大量的分子流行病学研究已经使用候选基因或者通路研究方法对基因突变与肺癌发病风险之间的关系进行了评估。大多数研究都集中在细胞内主要基因的遗传变异过程、主要致癌物质代谢、DNA修复、细胞周期调控途径和一些癌症相关基因如原癌基因或抑癌基因的研究上。然而，很少有研究包含验证阶段，而且除少数外，大多数的研究结果缺乏统一性[74]。

多次报道显示，无效型GSTM1基因会增加肺癌发病风险，原因可能是它可以降低抑癌作用。此外，营养模式和GSTM1基因型之间的相互作用也被不同的研究小组所确认[46-48]。一项包括98项研究的共45 000人参与的meta分析证实了无效性GSTM1基因与肺癌发病风险上升相关[OR=1.22；95% CI（1.14，1.30）]。种族分析发现这种相关性只在亚洲人群中明显[OR=1.38；95% CI（1.38，1.24）][80]。在许多报道中，细胞周期调控的关键位点——CHEK2位点的I157T错义突变是另一个与肺癌发病紧密相关的位点突变，这种突变发生在5%~7%的欧洲中部和北部人群中[81-82]。有趣的是，这个单核苷酸多态性的变异等位基因被发现能增加多种癌症易感性，却可以降低肺癌发病率[81-84]，这种现象的潜在机制还有待阐明。

全基因组关联研究

近年来随着高通量基因分型技术的进步，GWAS已成为一个检测遗传易感位点的强大工具。作为一个替代候选基因的研究方法，GWAS通过扫描人类基因组中数百万个常见的单核苷酸链来进行彻底的全基因组测序[85]。为了获得足够的统计分析能力，GWAS通常需要收入大量人群以进行验证。最近一份关于全基因组单核苷酸多态性分析的报告声称，70%~90%的欧洲人群存在常见变异[86]。然而，尽管人类基因组中常见变异（MAF＞1%）已基本覆盖，但仍有一些罕见变异位点被遗漏了。

与假定驱动候选基因的方法不同，GWAS是发现驱动的基因，它不需要关于疾病的任何前沿知识，因此，GWAS提供了发现那些功能并不明确的小基因位点的机会。近年来，GWAS的方法已经应用在30多个不同的癌症领域并发现了至少

230 个易感基因位点。由于大量的单核苷酸链需要检测，对统计的要求非常严格（$P < 5 \times 10^{-8}$），通常需要多级验证来避免假阳性结果[87]。

第一个肺癌基因组测序结果在 2007 年公布。一个欧洲研究组在一个相对较小的样本人群中使用 Affymetrix 100k SNP 数列进行全基因组扫描，共有 38 个重要的单核苷酸链被确认，但没有 1 个达到当前 GWAS 标准。在接下来的几年中，一些其他团队通过成千上万的病例和对照组进行了大规模的肺癌全基因组测序。此外，所有这些研究均对成千上万的样品进行了验证。重要的是，最早发现的 3 个 GWAS 易感区域都映射到 15q25.1 这个位点，这些发现证明这一区域与肺癌易感性有重要关系，并提供证据证实了 GWAS 可重复检测癌症相关基因的能力。除了 15q25.1，染色体上的变异位点 5p13（89）、6p21（90）和 12p13（91）也被认定与肺癌发病风险相关，这些研究的结果详述如下。

15q25.1

2008 年，3 个独立的研究小组进行了关于欧洲人群肺癌发病风险的全基因组测序：IARC[92]、德克萨斯大学 MD 安德森癌症中心[75]和冰岛 deCODE[93]。*CHRNA*5 的 3 个单核苷酸链（rs10151730、rs8034191 和 rs16969968）被确定与肺癌发病风险显著相关，其 OR 值在 1.30 ~ 1.32。冰岛 deCODE 研究小组进一步发现了 rs1015730 和尼古丁依赖的重要关联。随后，其他几个研究重复验证了在欧洲以及其他种族人群中 rs1015730 与肺癌发病风险的关系[94-97]。

染色体 15q25.1 包含 3 个烟碱乙酰胆碱受体编码基因（*CHRNA*3、*CHRNA*5 和 *CHRNB*4），乙酰胆碱受体在细胞表面参与神经传递，可影响吸烟行为。烟草致癌物比尼古丁更易与乙酰胆碱受体结合，从而通过诱导阳离子进入细胞质而刺激细胞内的信号级联反应[98-99]。因此，这些基因与肺癌易感性[75,92]及尼古丁依赖密切相关[93]。虽然 15q25 单核苷酸链的功能意义是未知的，但这些单核苷酸链可能通过调节宿主基因功能而在肺癌形成过程中发挥重要作用。单核苷酸链 rs16969968 可能就是如此，这是一个错义的单核苷酸链（Asp398Arg），它造成一个氨基酸的变化从而导致了阳离子通道的关闭（例如 Ca^{2+}）。*CHRN* 基因影响肺癌易感性的确切机制尚未完全明确，一些假说提出了 *CHRN* 多态性影响宿主对肺部致癌作用的易感性。由于乙酰胆碱受体对尼古丁的高亲和力和敏感性，并考虑到吸烟在肺癌易感因素中的主导地位，研究者们假设 *CHRN* 基因可以通过诱导一个人吸烟成瘾而增加肺癌的发病风险。除了尼古丁依赖，证据显示 *CHRN* 基因也可增加不吸烟者肺癌的发病风险[75,92,96]。*CHRN* 多态性可能是通过影响支气管上皮细胞的细胞运动导致伤口愈合延迟、持续的组织损伤和炎症，从而为致癌作用和肿瘤进展提供了良好的微环境[74]。吸烟者和非吸烟者乙酰胆碱受体的基因表达模式是不同的[100]。在癌细胞中，*CHRNA*3 的甲基化和基因表达的下调已被确认，这导致更多的细胞凋亡[101]。这些研究为乙酰胆碱受体通路与肺癌易感性之间的联系提供了证据和生物学方面合理的解释[99]。

5p15.33

5 号染色体 p15.33 是被 GWAS 发现的另一个肺癌易感位点[76,89,102]。2008 年，两个研究小组发现 rs401681、rs402710 和 rs2736100 与肺癌发病风险有关；但是，只有 rs401681 达到全基因组的标准[89,102]。2010 年，通过一个国际联合组织的努力，超过 20 000 例样本被重复检验（设计 11 645 例试验组和 14 645 例对照组）。在这项研究中，rs2736100 和 rs402710 都达到了全基因组的标准[103]。

5 号染色体 p15.33，通常称其为 *TERT-CLPTM1L* 位点，包含两个基因编码端粒酶逆转录酶（gelomerase reverse transcriptase，*TERT*）和唇腭裂跨膜蛋白 1 蛋白（Cleft Lip and Palate Transmembrane Protein1 – Like protein，*CLPTM1L*）。除了肺癌，这个区域也是许多其他癌症的易感位点，包括膀胱癌、前列腺癌和宫颈癌[104]。

端粒酶逆转录酶的蛋白质成分复杂，而且在物种间高度保守，它在端粒酶的激活和维护方面发挥着关键作用。端粒酶在干细胞和原始细胞中高度活跃，但在正常细胞中低表达或不表达。癌细胞的特点是通过端粒酶的高表达来克服端粒的磨损。虽然没有明确的证据表明端粒酶的激活导致肺癌，但仍有强有力的证据表明端粒酶逆转录酶在肺癌发展中的作用。人类端粒酶逆转录酶基因在肺癌组织中存在过度表达或突变[105]。许多已知的原癌基因或抑癌基因，如 MYC、RAS 和 p53 均可调节端粒酶的转录。此外，在很多临床试验中，端粒酶亚基化被作为药物靶点来治疗和预防癌症，以期在对正常细胞影响很小的情况下阻止癌细胞的生长[106]。独立 GWAS 研究中的重大发现进一步强调了端粒酶在肺癌中的作用。

CLPTM1L 在其同族 19 号染色体之后被命名[107]，它在癌症中的作用并不像端粒酶那样被深入研究。发现 CLPTM1L 具有致癌作用的第一个证据是其在卵巢癌顺铂耐药细胞株中的过表达[107]。在最近的一份报告中发现 CLPTM1L 在人类肺腺癌组织中高表达，并能阻止肿瘤细胞中基因毒性介导的凋亡[108]。

6p21 和 12p13

6p21 是被 GWAS 确定的第 3 个肺癌易感区域[102,109-110]。一项 meta 分析发现，在 61 个肺癌易感单核苷酸链中，大部分都与 rs3117582 密切相关，其中在鳞状细胞癌中关系最密切[109]。Rs3117582 定位在 BAG6/BAT3 的 5′端，由 BCL2 家族基因编码，与 p53 介导的细胞凋亡有关[111]。动物实验表明这个基因在肺癌发展中起关键作用[112]。另一个单核苷酸链 rs3131379 与 rs3117582 高度相关，定位于 MSH5，编码 DNA 错配修复 MSH5。这个区域也可以影响宿主的 DNA 修复能力，这或许可以解释这个区域与鳞状细胞癌的关系密切，因为鳞状细胞癌与外部致癌物质直接相关[109]。

Shi 等通过一项囊括了 5 355 例肺癌患者和 4 344 例对照组的共约 2 000 条单核苷酸链的通路分析确认 12p13 区域，所有受试者均是欧洲吸烟者。他们发现在 RAD52 上的 rs6489769 是鳞状细胞癌的易感位点，RAD52 同族体基因在 DNA 双链修复和同源重组中是一个关键的基因，因此在生物学上支持这个区域对吸烟患者肺癌的影响[113-114]。在最近的一项大规模 meta 分析中，Timofeeva 等通过对 14 900 例试验组和 29 485 例对照组的全基因组测序分析证实了这个区域在鳞状细胞癌中的重要作用[109]。

种族亚组

肺癌的全基因组测序最初只专注于欧洲人群，近年来由于肺癌的种族差异和遗传特异性，一些研究小组开展了在特定种族或民族亚组的全基因组测序。几种常见的易感位点已在不同种族的人群中被确认，一些种族特定的易感位点也被确认，例如 5p15.33 已在中国的汉族人群中被确认[115]。此外，在非洲裔美国人以及中国人中，一些变异的 CHRNA5 15q25 被发现与肺癌发病率的增加及吸烟行为有关[96,116]。由于之前确认的单核苷酸链（rs1051730、rs8034191 和 rs16969968）是在欧洲人群中被确定的，而在亚洲人群中非常罕见，因此 Wu 等人在这一区域中筛选了中国人群中其他可能的候选单核苷酸链[96]。他们鉴定出 4 种新的达到全基因组标准的单核苷酸链（rs2036534、rs667282、rs12910984 和 rs6495309），这个发现证实了在亚洲人群中该区域对肺癌发病的重要性。然而，并没有相关报道证实该区域与亚洲不吸烟女性的肺癌发病有关，可能是因为这个区域与吸烟行为关系密切[117]。另一个在中国人群中进行的大型全基因组测序分析中，Hu 等人证实 2 个之前在欧洲人群中确认过的易感位点（3q28 和 5p15.33）的关联[118]；此外，他们还发现了 2 个关于亚洲人新的位点（13q12.12 和 22q12.2），这 2 个位点在针对欧洲人口的大型 GWAS 的 meta 分析中并没有重要意义[109]。表 2.1 总结了不同种族人群中的易感位点。

肿瘤组织学

不同的肺癌组织学类型拥有共同和不同的易感位点。Landi 等人报道，5p15 位点只与腺癌亚组关系明显，而与鳞状细胞癌亚组无关[119]。在最近的一项囊括了 14 900 例试验组和 29 485 例对照组的关于欧洲人群的 meta 分析中，调查人员发现了 5p15（TERT：腺癌；CLPTM1L：鳞状细胞癌和大细胞癌）、6p21（BAG6/BAT3：鳞状细胞癌）和 12p13（RAD52：鳞状细胞癌和小细胞癌）的组织特异性，而 15q25 区域在所有组织学类型中都有意义[109]。

不吸烟者

约有 15% 的肺癌患者没有吸烟史[120]。许多假说提出了关于不吸烟肺癌患者的病因学和环境暴露方面的原因，例如二手烟、职业暴露、氡气、烹饪气味、空气污染和病毒感染。然而，很明显，不吸烟肺癌患者与吸烟肺癌患者在分子演变和自然史方面都是不同的,包括表皮生长因子受体(epidermal growth factor receptor, EGFR)基因激活突变的频率增加[121]。最近几年,研究者一直在探索不吸烟患者的遗传易感性。2010年,Li等人进行了第一次尝试,他们通过对377例不吸烟肺癌患者和同等数量的对照组进行2个验证阶段和表达数量性状位点(eQTL)分析,确定了13q31.3基因的2个单核苷酸链为与不吸烟人群肺癌发病风险关联最高的单核苷酸链。此外,这两个单核苷酸链也被确认与 GPC5 基因的表达有关[122]。在随后的一年,韩国人口全基因组测序确定了18p11.22号染色体上的另一个易感位点[73]。然而,这两项研究的结果都没有达到全基因组标准,需要更大的样本量和重复验证来确认这两个位点。最近,Lan等人进行了亚洲不吸烟女性肺癌患者(5 510例患者和4 544例对照组)[117]的全基因组测序,识别了在10q25.2、6q22.2和6p21.32染色体上的3个易感位点。作者也证实了之前报道的5p15.33、3q28和17q24.3均为亚洲人群易感位点[110,115],但15q25单核苷酸链在亚洲人群中却没有意义。

表 2.1 全基因组关联分析确定的易感位点

位点	报道的基因	单核苷酸多态性	人种	参考文献
15q25	psMA4,CHRNA3,CHRNA5,CHRNB4,LOC123688	rs1051730/rs8034191(EUR,AA) rs2036534/rs6495309(EUR,CN) rs16969968/rs6495308(EUR) rs10519203/rs2036527/rs684513/rs1696698(AA) rs667282/rs12910984(CN)	EUR AA* CN	(75,92~94,96,102,109)
sp15.33	TERTICLPTM1L	rs2736100(JPN,AFNS) rs2853677(EUR,JPN) rs10937405/rs4488809(JPN) rs401681(EUR) rs465498(CN)	EUR CN JPN AFNS	(102,109,110,115,117,205)
12p13.33	RAD52	rs6489769(EUR)	EUR	(91,109)
6p21	BAT3IMSH5,HLA-DRA,HLA-DRB5	rs3117582(EUR) rs3817963(JPN) rs2395185(AFNS)	EUR JPN AFNS	(102,109) (110,117)
17q24.3	BPTF	rs7216064(JPN,AFNS)	JPN AFNS	(110,117)
3q28	TP63	rs4488809(CN,AFNS) rs10937405(JPN,AFNS) rs10937405(JPN)	CN JPN AFNS	(110,115,117,205)
13q12.12	MIPEP-TNFRSF19	rs753955(CN)	CN	(115)
22q12.2	MTMR3-HORMAD2-LIF	rs17728461/rs36600(CN)	CN	(115)
9p21	CDKN2A/p16^{INK4},p14^{ARF} CDKN2B/p15^{INK48}	rs1333040(EUR,CN)	EUR CN	(109)
6q22.2p	DCBLD1,ROS1	rs9387478(AFNS)	AFNS	(117)
10q25.2	VTI1A	rs7086803(AFNS)	AFNS	(117)
18p11.22	APCDD1,NAPG,FAM38B	rs11080466/rs11663246(KNS)	KNS*	(73)

*报道的关联没有达到全基因组标准,$P < 5 \times 10^{-8}$
EUR:欧洲人;ASN:亚洲人;AA:非洲裔美国人;CN:中国人;JPN:日本人;AFNS:亚洲不吸烟女性;KNS:韩国不吸烟者

基因易感性评估模型的中间表型分析

DNA 损伤、修复的表型分析

有几种不同的表型分析可以直接或间接地评估外周血淋巴细胞末梢区域（peripheral blood lymphocytes，PBLs）中的 DNA 损伤修复，包括：①某些化学或物理因素诱导的 DNA 损伤修复（例如突变敏感性分析、彗星试验和 DNA 加合物的测定）；②非常规 DNA 合成；③细胞修复损伤报告基因的能力（宿主细胞再激活的分析）；④DNA 修复酶的活性（8-OH-鸟嘌呤修复活性的测量）[123-124]。

突变敏感性

突变敏感性分析是 DNA 修复能力（DNA repair capacity，DRC）的一种间接测量，主要用于体外诱导分化较好的淋巴细胞突变时引起的染色体断裂[125-126]。不同的突变产生不同的 DNA 损伤，并触发专门的 DNA 修复通路。例如，BPDE 是一种烟草致癌物，可以塑造 DNA 加合物并引发核苷酸修复（nucleotide excision repair，NER）；博来霉素是一种断裂剂，可以模仿电离产生氧自由基通过切除修复（base excision repair，BER）和 DNA 单双链断裂修复引起的 DNA 单-双链断裂（DNA single and double-strand breaks，DSB）[127]。Wu 等证实，高浓度的 BPDE 和博来霉素敏感性与肺癌风险的增加没有相关性，这一发现已被其他多项研究证明[2-4,128-129]。

彗星试验

彗星试验是单细胞凝胶电泳分析方法，用于评估个体细胞的 DNA 损伤，它是一种敏感且多功能的高潜能方法[130-131]。彗星试验中的碱性环境（pH>13）可以检测出 DNA 的损伤，如单链损伤、双链损伤和碱性环境中易发生突变的位点[132]。这项试验用一些较普遍的诱导试剂，包括 BPDE、博来霉素和 γ 射线。Wu 等人发现较高剂量的 γ 射线和 BPDE 诱导作用时间最长，是评估 DNA 损伤的参数之一，与肺癌风险的增加有显著关联，分别增加了 2.32 倍和 4.49 倍[133]。Rajaee-Behbahani 等报道，与对照组相比，博来霉素在彗星试验碱性环境中诱导肺癌患者的 DNA 修复率偏低[134]。

DNA 加合物

通过 ^{32}P 标记获得的两项研究结果提示，体外诱导 BPDE 产生 DNA 加合物的水平与肺癌风险明显相关[135-136]，也提示了人体清除这种 BPDE 诱导产生的 DNA 加合物的能力不强，会增加对烟草致癌物暴露的易感性[136]。

宿主细胞再活化试验

宿主细胞再活化试验通过测量在经过 BPDE 处理过的质粒转染未受损的淋巴细胞时应答基因（例如 LUC 基因）的活性来测量 DNA 修复活性[137-139]。单个未经修复的 BPDE 诱导的 DNA 加合物可以阻碍应答基因的转录[140]，被测量的应答基因活性大小可反映出被转染细胞清除质粒中加合物的能力大小。与对照组相比，病例组清除加合物的能力较低，且与肺癌的发病风险增加有关，证明了 DRC 的减少与肺癌风险呈剂量-反应关系[137-139]。

8-OGG 试验

OGG1 基因编码的 8-OGG1 酶主动参与 BER 途径。OGG 活性的大小决定了 OGG 清除 8-过氧化物残余物的能力大小，这种残余物主要来自放射性核素标记合成的 DNA 低聚核苷酸，根据能力的大小可以区别两种 DNA 产物[141]。Paz-Elizur 等人发现，与对照组相比，肺癌患者外周血液中单核细胞 OGG 活性降低，OGG 活性最低的个体与活性最高的个体相比，（non-small cell lung cancer，NSCLC）的易感性升高 [OR=4.8；95% CI（1.5，15.9）][141]。Gackowski 等也报道，正常志愿者血液中的白细胞修复活性较肺癌患者明显升高[142]。

γ-H2AX（磷酸化的 H2AX）

众所周知，DNA 损伤后会出现染色质的改变[143]，在 DNA 双链断裂发生后，H2AX（139 位丝氨酸磷酸化的 H2A 组蛋白变体）在 ATM/ATR/DNA-PK 调解下很快发生磷酸化[144]，进而促进 DSB 的修复并增强 DSB 的信号[145]。通过检测 H2AX 的 C 端肽磷酸化抗体反应引起的免疫荧光聚集，γ-H2AX 细胞分析可以准确敏感地检测出 DNA 双链断裂[146-147]。磷酸化的 H2AX 已经成为广泛应用的生物学标记[148-150]，包括肺癌的研究[151-153]。检测外周血粒细胞的磷酸化 H2AX 的信号并使用 γ 射线照射后，He 等发现在肺癌患者中磷酸化的 H2AX 比例（1.46±0.14）比健康组（1.41±0.12）更高，他们也证实了磷酸化 H2AX 的比例与肺癌发病风险之间的量效关系（$P < 0.001$）[154]。

细胞周期表型分析

两种细胞周期停滞表型分析已被用于评估肺癌风险。通过流式细胞计量，Zhao 等人发现与对照组相比，肺癌患者在 G2 期向 M 期转变过程中有少量的 γ 射线增加，同时细胞凋亡水平进一步下降[155]。而且暴露于这种环境的微量 P53 蛋白水平的改变与 G2/M 延迟转变和染色体断裂有关，提示了肺癌患者细胞周期监测点可能存在缺陷，这与 P53 依赖性 DNA 损伤应答有关。这些发现在 Wu 等进行的一项大规模病例对照研究中进行了详细的阐述，他们报道 γ 射线诱导 S 期和 G2/M 期转变的延迟，可以预测肺癌的易感性[133]。Zheng 等对非裔美国人的研究也得出了类似的结论[156]。

凋亡途径中的表型分析

Zhao 等的报道证实用 TUNEL（Terminal transferase dUTP nick end labeling）方法诱导机体突变物质引起的细胞凋亡能力下降与肺癌风险增加有关[155]。Biros 等[157]报道，含有 p53 Pro72Arg 多态变异等位基因的肺癌患者的白细胞凋亡水平较低，这项发现与 Wu 等[158]得出的结论一致，他证明带有 3 个 p53 多态（第 3 个内含子或第 4 个外显子及第 6 个内含子）野生型等位基因与含有至少 1 个变异的等位基因相比，凋亡指数更高。

肺癌风险和早期检测的新型标志物

炎性生物标志物

一般认为慢性炎症可以促进肺癌的发生，因此，大量研究致力于确认一些新型的且有潜在临床应用价值的炎性标记物[159]。血清 C 反应蛋白（CRP）是已得到广泛认可的慢性炎症标记物，不断有报道指出它与肺癌的发生相关[160-162]。另外，CRP 基因的变异也与不同血液 CRP 水平和肺癌发生相关[160,163]。一些炎性介质［如白细胞介素 6（IL-6）和白细胞介素 8（IL-8）］和其他一些炎性相关分子（如表面活性蛋白 D 和肿瘤坏死因子 α）也与肺癌的发生相关。除 CRP 外的少数炎性标志物在一些独立的研究中已被反复证实。

循环 miRNA

miRNA（microRNA）是一类非编码的小 RNA 分子（18~25 个核苷酸），具有高度的稳定性和组织特异性[168]，它调控人类约 30% 的基因，其在癌症的发生、进展和预后中的作用已被大量研究。正常支气管组织中 miRNAs 的表达方式会因肺癌发生改变[169]，所以 miRNAs 可以用于高患病风险个体化学预防的定量生物标志物[170]。此外，循环 miRNAs 可作为新型肺癌风险评估和早期检测的生物标志物[171-172]，例如在 I 期或 II 期肺癌生物标记研究阶段，Hennessey 等报道，2 个血清 miR-15b 和 miR-27b 组成的 miRNAs 结合物可以将 NSCLC 与对照组相区别[184]。在另一项研究中发现，与对照组相比，I 期肺癌患者血浆中的 miR-155、miR-182 和 miR-197 水平是不同的[173]。Boeri 等发现血浆 miRNA 的含量可以预测肺癌的分期，甚至比从 CT 中得出的临床分期更准确。尽管这些候选的标志物都尚未应用于临床，但这些研究提供了 miRNA 与肺癌的发生和早期检测的一些证据。

循环 DNA 和启动子甲基化

肺癌是一个多步骤的过程，涉及基因变异和表观遗传变异。细胞组分的血液含量与肿瘤细胞的 DNA 脱落有关。血液中无细胞 DNA 是检测这些变化的有效替代标记物，有助于肺癌患者的筛选和早期检测[175]。一项病例对照研究显示，NSCLC 患者的血浆端粒酶逆转录酶的 DNA 含量比对照组高 4 倍[176]。Belinsky 和其同事证实血浆和痰中的无细胞 DNA 启动子的甲基化可以促使肺癌的发生[177]，而且多基因的启动子超甲基化可以在肺癌发生前被检测出来。许多其他的基因变异和表观基因变异在肺癌患者的循环 DNA 中也被证实[179]。然而，由于重复性和质量控制方面的数据较少，所描述的这些方法和结果缺乏一致性。

循环 mRNA 和蛋白质

在肺癌中血浆端粒酶逆转录酶和表皮生长因子受体（EGFR）常过表达，利用定量逆转录聚合酶链反应（reverse-transcription polymerase chain reaction，RTPCR）试验，Miura 等[180]在肺癌患者和对照组分别检测了血清 hTERT 和 EGFR，发现这两个标记物的灵敏度分别为 89% 和 73%，特异度分别为 73% 和 71%，比其他肿瘤标记物［例如癌胚抗原（carcinoembryonic antigen，CEA）］更有效。此外，这些标记物的水平与肿瘤数目和临床分期有关，并预示了未来的复发和转移情况。

CIZ1 基因通过编码细胞周期相互作用因子促使 DNA 开始复制。Higgins 等[181]最近的研究发现，在两组早期肺癌患者血浆中能检测到 Ciz1 蛋白的变异形式，与对照组相比，早期肺癌患者的灵敏度为 95%，特异度超过了 70%。此外，作者表示，使用体外和体内基因的功能作为早期肺癌检测的候选生物标志物非常有前景。

端粒酶长度

端粒是位于染色体末端的帽状结构，有保护 DNA 结构的作用，并且在保证染色体组的完整性和稳定性中起关键作用，端粒变短与恶性肿瘤的发生和发展有关。许多流行病学研究发现，外周血淋巴细胞端粒变短可以促使多种癌症发病率增加，包括肺癌[182-184]；然而，另一项研究却得出了相反的结果[185]。这个矛盾的原因可能是样本大小有差异和试验设计不同，仍需要未来大型前瞻性试验来证实。

肺癌发病风险评估模型

癌症风险预测模型

在总人群中，癌症患病风险是一个连续的范围。因为高风险人群只占总人群的一小部分，实施适当的监控程序并且制订干预策略很大程度上依赖于风险预测的效率。统计模型包含多种风险因素，它是非常具有前景的工具，可以帮助确认高风险个体并有助于制订降低风险的策略。

有不同的试验设计可以用于开发风险模型，但每种设计方案都有各自的优点和局限性[186]。队列研究可以直接得到发病率的基线危险率、竞争风险死亡率和样本人口的相对风险，但局限性是随访时间长和死亡原因数据不确切。病例对照试验是一种有效的方法，可以在相对短的时间内将详细的信息应用于相关变量，但是通常会受到病例对照研究方法的限制，如潜在的回忆偏倚和许多非癌症疾病缺乏全国注册数据。有 3 种统计学标准可用来评价风险评估模型的校准性（可靠性）、辨别力以及准确性[186]。可靠性用来评估风险模型预测亚组人群结局事件发生数量的能力，它可以用统计数据的拟合优度来评估；辨别力是区分这些人是否会发展为患者的能力，通过计算统计数据的一致性或者观查受试者工作特征曲线（recei-ver operating characteristic，ROC）下面积来评估；准确性包括阳性和阴性预测值，反映模型将特定人群分类的能力。然而，由于要考虑治疗方案的获益和危害，用来评估模型表现的统计学标准在临床决策中是受限的。最近提出了两种从临床角度评估风险模型的方法：一种是决策曲线分析，另一种是相关应用曲线分析[187]。应特别指出，相关应用曲线分析可以帮助评估风险预测模型的成本效益[187]。为了量化模型的临床应用价值，需要将危害和获益纳入实用规划中以确定风险阈值。风险阈值是肺癌患病的绝对风险，对于潜在发病人群需要接受筛查。与单一的测试、干预或治疗相比，评估与生活方式改变相关的多级危害和获益较为复杂，这是确认风险阈值的障碍。

在过去的 10 年中，随着分子生物学技术的迅速发展，大量基因组信息受到重视，流行病学已迅速从传统流行病学向综合流行病学研究发展[188]。与传统的调查问卷相比，癌症风险预测模型随着流行病学方法的演变，通过整合其他风险因素获得了更好的模型性能。

肺癌风险预测模型的研究现状

为了对肺癌高危人群进行早期筛查与干预，建立个体化的肺癌风险预测方法（如 CT 检查）越来越受到重视。Colditz 等[189]认为每天吸烟的数量、一级亲属中有肺癌患者、职业暴露、空气污染与肺癌风险有不同程度的关联。这种"以专家意见为基础"的癌症风险指数是迈向肺癌风险评估统计学模型的第一步。

Bach 等[190]利用被调查个体的年龄、性别、石棉接触史和吸烟史来预测肺癌的风险，它是通过来自 5 个 CARET 研究站点的数据分析，然后通过肺癌风险预测模型在第 6 个站点对肺癌发生趋势进行预测，证明了该模型的有效性。这一模型为肺癌风险在吸烟者中的差异提供了强有力的证据，其有效指数高达 0.72，并在吸烟者中得到了认证。α-生育酚、β-胡萝卜素的 ATBC（Alpha-Tocopherol, beta-Carotence Cancer Prevention Study）癌症预防研究项目中的外部验证研究[191]报道，在过去的 10 年中，Bach 模型低估了肺癌的发病率，这归因于对 ATBC 群体监测的加强。由于受到特殊人群（老年重度吸烟患者）的限制，Bach 模型最适用于 50~75 岁的重度吸烟者。

Spitz 等[192]发明了一种分别针对从未吸过烟、以前吸过烟及现时吸烟个体进行肺癌风险评估的模型，所用的数据收集自大型病例对照研究。针对有吸烟史者，除了年龄和吸烟史以外，在模型中还包括他们的家族史、粉尘暴露史和呼吸系统疾病史；对于无吸烟史者，环境二手烟是肺癌家族史以外一项非常重要的预测指标。这一模型的内部有效性和交叉有效性在从未吸过烟、以前吸过烟及现时吸烟人群中的平均吻合度是 0.60，这些模型通过增加吸烟史以外的危险因素扩展了 Bach 模型。然而，这些模型无法解决研究设计的匹配情况和对照组个体年龄、吸烟状况的限制问题。相同的研究小组通过增加 2 个具有 DNA 修复能力的生物标志物扩展了他们的模型，并且声称能够有效改善辨别力[193]。膀胱癌风险预测模型证实，通过整合分子和临床标志物对风险模型带来的改善很小[194]。

利物浦肺癌项目（the Livepool Lung Cancer Project, LLP）模型[195]包括石棉暴露、肺炎、肺癌家族史和发病年龄、既往恶性病史。该模型的曲线下面积统计的调整辨别度为 0.70[195]。与 Bach 和 Spitz 模型相比，LLP 模型是基于较小样本的病例对照设计。LLP 模型被证实在外部同样有效，如欧洲早期肺癌（the European Early Lung Cancer, EUELC）、哈佛病例对照研究和 LLP 以人群为基础的前瞻性队列研究（LLP cohort, LLPC），并且在哈佛和 LLPC 的研究中有着良好的辨别力，在 EUELC 研究中也有中等表现。在决策效用分析中，LLP 分级肺癌风险模型比仅考虑吸烟史和家族史的模型预测效果更好[196]。

Bach、Spitz 和 LLP 模型的局限性在于这些模型并不是从总人群中收集数据。最近公布的从总人群中抽样新建的模型是前列腺癌、肺癌、结肠癌和卵巢癌筛查试验（Prostate, Lung, Colorectal and Ovarian, PLCO）模型[181]，它涉及年龄、教育水平、体重指数、肺癌家族史、慢性阻塞性肺疾病（COPD）、胸部 X 线检查、吸烟状况、每年吸烟量、吸烟时长和戒烟时间（戒烟群体亚组）。该模型是基于超过 70 000 例受试者的 PLCO 前瞻性筛查试验收集的数据，显示了其外部验证的高辨别力和校准性。

欧洲关于肺癌与营养的前瞻性队列研究（the European Prospective Investigation in Cancer, EPIC）是另一个基于总体人群建立的模型[197]，该模型主要通过戒烟者和吸烟者开始吸烟的年龄、吸烟的强度、职业和环境暴露来预测肺癌风险，并确定 GWAS 中的单核苷酸多态性（SNPs）。模型性能评估表明仅考虑吸烟因素时的辨别准确性更好，AUC 为 0.84，结合其他危险因素对 AUC 的改善可以忽略。

如前所述，近期 GWAS 的出现为将遗传变异集成入现有的风险预测模型中提供了可能。然而，截至目前，将 SNPs 增加到风险预测模型中仍面临困难[198-199]。通过增加肺癌全基因组关联分析 SNP 的方法并不能提高模型的预测性[182]。最近 LLP 团队研究比较了 LLP 模型和另一种增强模型的辨别准确性，这种新模型包含了高通量测序识别出来的 SEZ6L SNP（rs663048），此项研究显示 NRI（net reclassification improvements）方法的使用取得了显著的进展[200]，然而对于将基因标记物加入肺癌风险模型的价值仍存在争议。增强的 LLP 模型暗示了包含基因标志物的模型更适用于中度风险的不同个体，这组人群仅使用传统流行病学评估模型进行风险分级通常是模糊不清的。

总的来说，肺癌风险预测模型对改善早期检测的筛查策略有巨大的潜在价值。对重度吸烟人群进行肺癌的 CT 检查可以将肺癌的死亡率降低

20%，但有95%的假阳性率[201]。有必要改进除了吸烟之外的其他风险预测因素，以便确定适合进行CT扫描的人群[203]。整合分子、遗传和其他新的危险因素在接下来的研究中具有很大的价值。

总 结

尽管吸烟是肺癌的主要风险因素，其他流行病学因素和遗传易感基因标志物也已被确定为肺癌潜在的风险指标，但某些环境因素和并发症也增加了肺癌的发病风险，包括各种慢性呼吸系统疾病，如COPD和肺气肿。同样有证据支持饮食和肺癌发病之间的关联，但证据并不确凿。虽然在文献中有大量有关肺癌的候选基因，但这些结果往往不一致且无法重复验证。研究设计方案局限、样本量小、缺乏对混杂因素的控制、选择偏倚和复杂的测试都可能导致不一致的结果。从候选基因和以通路为基础的方法来研究GWAS改变了癌症基因组学的局面，然而，GWAS确认的易感基因位点只能解释不足10%的肺癌风险，因为GWAS只涵盖常见的发生频率较高的基因变异[等位基因频率（minor allele frequency，MAF）>5%]，而没有包括一些具有较大作用的罕见变异（MAF<1%）。鉴于肿瘤是一个多步骤和多因子作用的疾病，从许多用于研究的候选基因中识别出的单个个体变异基因对整个肿瘤风险的影响或许是很小的。多基因模型应发现个体基因位点的影响以及潜在的"基因-基因"和"基因-环境"的相互作用。对结构变异的系统评估有助于对肺癌遗传结构的总体认识，如基因复制数目的变异、插入和缺失、杂合性的缺失（loss of heterozygosity，LOH）和表观遗传学的改变。此外，高功率计算方法可以用来检测遗传因素和环境因素之间的相互作用，这在传统统计学方法中是无法实现的。通过分子和细胞的功能分析可以确定基因型-表型的相关性，也能验证高风险等位基因的生物学意义。由于吸烟和其他环境因素对肺癌的影响，对生活方式因素如吸烟依赖应该进行更深入的研究。此外，新一代高通量测序技术涵盖了整个基因组和外显子组，该技术的应用使全面检测"遗传缺失"成为可能，也能探索肺癌基因组学潜在的复杂性。中间表型生物标志物如DNA修复能力、端粒酶长度和其他表型生物标志物，具有高遗传性和影响肺癌风险的可能性，并有望对风险分层和预测发挥作用。最后，为了提高预测能力并权衡成本效益，这些环境、遗传和表型标志物需要被集成到全面的风险预测模型中，从而改善早期肺癌的筛查和预防策略。

（彭忠民　胡冬鑫　冯　振
李　猛　刘　颖译）

参考文献

[1] Siegel R, Naishadham D, Jemal A. Cancer statistics. CA: A Cancer Journal for Clinicians, 2013, 63: 11-30.

[2] Hsu TC, Spitz MR, Schantz SP. Mutagen sensitivity: a biological marker of cancer susceptibility. Cancer Epidemiology Biomarkers & Prevention. 1991, 1: 83-89.

[3] Spitz MR, Hsu TC, Wu X, et al. Mutagen sensitivity as a biological marker of lung cancer risk in African Americans. Cancer Epidemiology Biomarkers & Prevention, 1995, 4: 99-103.

[4] Wu X, Delclos GL, Anneggers JF, et al. A case-control study of wood dust exposure, mutagen sensitivity, and lung cancer risk. Cancer Epidemiology Biomarkers & Prevention, 1995, 4: 583-588.

[5] Zheng Y-L, Loffredo CA, Yu Z, et al. Bleomycin-induced chromosome breaks as a risk marker for lung cancer: a casecontrol study with population and hospital controls. Carcinogenesis, 2003, 24: 269-274.

[6] Tokuhata GK, Lilienfeld AM. Familial aggregation of lung cancer in humans. J Natl Cancer Inst, 1963, 30: 289-312.

[7] Ooi WL, Elston RC, Chen VW, et al. Increased familial risk for lung cancer. J Natl Cancer Inst, 1986, 76: 217-222.

[8] Samet JM, Humble CG, Pathak DR. Personal and family history of respiratory disease and lung cancer risk. Am Rev Respir Dis, 1986, 134: 466-470.

[9] Shaw GL, Falk RT, Pickle LW, et al. Lung cancer risk associated with cancer in relatives. Journal of Clinical Epidemiology, 1997, 44: 429-437.

[10] Osann KE. Lung cancer in women: The importance of smoking, family history of cancer, and medical history of respiratory disease. Cancer Research, 1991, 51: 4893-4897.

[11] Schwartz AG, Yang P, Swanson GM. Familial risk of

lung cancer among nonsmokers and their relatives. American Journal of Epidemiology, 1996, 144: 554-562.

[12] Mayne ST, Buenconsejo J, Janerich DT. Previous lung disease and risk of lung cancer among men and women nonsmokers. American Journal of Epidemiology, 1999, 149: 13-20.

[13] Bromen K, Pohlabeln H, Jahn I, et al. Aggregation of lung cancer in families: Results from a population-based case-control study in Germany. American Journal of Epidemiology, 2000, 152: 497-505.

[14] Etzel CJ, Amos CI, Spitz MR. Risk for smoking-related cancer among relatives of lung cancer patients. Cancer Res, 2003, 63: 8531-8535.

[15] Matakidou A, Eisen T, Houlston RS. Systematic review of the relationship between family history and lung cancer risk. Br J Cancer, 2005, 93: 825-833.

[16] Lissowska J, Foretova L, Dabek J, et al. Family history and lung cancer risk: International multicenter case-control study in Eastern and Central Europe and meta-analyses. Cancer Causes Control, 2010, 21: 1091-1104.

[17] Adcock IM, Caramori G, Barnes PJ. Chronic obstructive pulmonary disease and lung cancer: New molecular insights. Respiration, 2011, 81: 265-284.

[18] Sin DD, Man SF. Systemic inflammation and mortality in chronic obstructive pulmonary disease. Can J Physiol Pharmacol, 2007, 85: 141-147.

[19] Ben-Zaken Cohen S, Pare PD, Man SF, et al. The growing burden of chronic obstructive pulmonary disease and lung cancer in women: examining sex differences in cigarette smoke metabolism. Am J Respir Crit Care Med, 2007, 176: 113-120.

[20] Mannino DM. Epidemiology and global impact of chronic obstructive pulmonary disease. Semin Respir Crit Care Med, 2005, 26: 204-210.

[21] Punturieri A, Szabo E, Croxton TL, et al. Lung cancer and chronic obstructive pulmonary disease: needs and opportunities for integrated research. J Natl Cancer Inst, 2009, 101: 554-559.

[22] Purdue MP, Gold L, Jarvholm B, et al. Impaired lung function and lung cancer incidence in a cohort of Swedish construction workers. Thorax, 2007, 62: 51-56.

[23] Tockman MS, Anthonisen NR, Wright EC, et al. Airways obstruction and the risk for lung cancer. Ann Intern Med, 1987, 106: 512-518.

[24] Brenner DR, McLaughlin JR, Hung RJ. Previous lung diseases and lung cancer risk: a systematic review and meta-analysis. PLoS One, 2011, 6: e17479.

[25] Smith BM, Pinto L, Ezer N, et al. Emphysema detected on computed tomography and risk of lung cancer: A systematic review and meta-analysis. Lung Cancer, 2012, 77: 58-63.

[26] Brenner DR, Boffetta P, Duell EJ, et al. Previous lung diseases and lung cancer risk: A pooled analysis from the International Lung Cancer Consortium. American Journal of Epidemiology, 2012, 176: 573-585.

[27] Santillan A, Camargo C, Jr., Colditz G. A metaanalysis of asthma and risk of lung cancer (United States). Cancer Causes & Control, 2003, 14: 327-334.

[28] Rosenberger A, Bickeboller H, McCormack V, et al. Asthma and lung cancer risk: a systematic investigation by the International Lung Cancer Consortium. Carcinogenesis, 2012, 33: 587-597.

[29] Talbot-Smith A, Fritschi L, Divitini ML, et al. Allergy, atopy, and cancer: A prospective study of the 1981 Busselton Cohort. American Journal of Epidemiology, 2003, 157: 606-612.

[30] Schabath MB, Delclos GL, Martynowicz MM, et al. Opposing effects of emphysema, hay fever, and select genetic variants on lung cancer risk. American Journal of Epidemiology, 2005, 161: 412-422.

[31] Cockcroft DW, Klein GJ, Donevan RE, et al. Is there a negative correlation between malignancy and respiratory atopy Ann Allergy, 1979, 43: 345-347.

[32] Vena JE, Bona JR, Byers TE, et al. Allergy-related diseases and cancer: An inverse association. American Journal of Epidemiology, 1985, 122: 66-74.

[33] Gabriel R, Dudley BM, Alexander WD. Lung cancer and allergy. Br J Clin Pract, 1972, 26: 202-204.

[34] McDuffie HH. Atopy and primary lung cancer: Histology and sex distribution. CHEST Journal, 1991, 99: 404-407.

[35] Feskanich D, Ziegler RG, Michaud DS, et al. Prospective study of fruit and vegetable consumption and risk of lung cancer among men and women. Journal of the National Cancer Institute, 2000, 92: 1812-1823.

[36] Voorrips LE, Goldbohm RA, van Poppel G, et al. Vegetable and fruit consumption and risks of colon and rectal cancer in a prospective cohort study: The Netherlands Cohort Study on Diet and Cancer. American Journal of Epidemiology, 2000, 152: 1081-1092.

[37] Brennan P, Fortes C, Butler J, et al. A multicenter case-control study of diet and lung cancer among non-smokers.

Cancer Causes & Control, 2000, 11: 49-58.

[38] Miller AB, Altenburg H-P, Bueno-de-Mesquita B, et al. Fruits and vegetables and lung cancer: Findings from the European prospective investigation into cancer and nutrition. International Journal of Cancer, 2004, 108: 269-276.

[39] Skuladottir H, Tjoenneland A, Overvad K, et al. Does insufficient adjustment for smoking explain the preventive effects of fruit and vegetables on lung cancer Lung Cancer, 2004, 45: 1-10.

[40] Neuhouser ML, Patterson RE, Thornquist MD, et al. Fruits and vegetables are associated with lower lung cancer risk only in the placebo arm of the β-Carotene and Retinol Efficacy Trial (CARET). Cancer Epidemiology Biomarkers & Prevention, 2003, 12: 350-358.

[41] Wakai K, Matsuo K, Nagata C, et al. Lung cancer risk and consumption of vegetables and fruit: An evaluation based on a systematic review of epidemiological evidence from Japan. Japanese Journal of Clinical Oncology, 2011, 41: 693-708.

[42] Key TJ. Fruit and vegetables and cancer risk. Br J Cancer, 2011, 104: 6-11.

[43] Zhang Y, Talalay P. Anticarcinogenic activities of organic isothiocyanates: Chemistry and mechanisms. Cancer Research, 1994, 54: 1976s-1981s.

[44] Smith T, Evans K, Lythgoe MF, et al. Dosimetry of pediatric radiopharmaceuticals: uniformity of effective dose and a simple aid for its estimation. Journal of Nuclear Medicine, 1997, 38: 1982-1987.

[45] Thornalley PJ. Isothiocyanates: mechanism of cancer chemopreventive action. Anticancer Drugs, 2002, 13: 331-338.

[46] Brennan P, Hsu CC, Moullan N, et al. Effect of cruciferous vegetables on lung cancer in patients stratified by genetic status: a mendelian randomisation approach. The Lancet, 2005, 366: 1558-1560.

[47] Spitz MR, Duphorne CM, Detry MA, et al. Dietary intake of isothiocyanates: evidence of a joint effect with glutathione s-transferase polymorphisms in lung cancer risk. Cancer Epidemiology Biomarkers & Prevention, 2000, 9: 1017-1020.

[48] Gao C-m, Tajima K, Kuroishi T, et al. Protective effects of raw vegetables and fruit against lung cancer among smokers and ex-smokers: A case-control study in the Tokai area of Japan. Cancer Science, 1993, 84: 594-600.

[49] Lam TK, Gallicchio L, Lindsley K, et al. Cruciferous vegetable consumption and lung cancer risk: A systematic review. Cancer Epidemiology Biomarkers & Prevention, 2009, 18: 184-195.

[50] Männistö S, Smith-Warner SA, Spiegelman D, et al. Dietary carotenoids and risk of lung cancer in a pooled analysis of seven cohort studies. Cancer Epidemiology Biomarkers & Prevention, 2004, 13: 40-48.

[51] Holick CN, Michaud DS, Stolzenberg-Solomon R, et al. Dietary carotenoids, serum β-carotene, and retinol and risk of lung cancer in the alpha-tocopherol, beta-carotene cohort study. American Journal of Epidemiology, 2002, 156: 536-547.

[52] Michaud DS, Feskanich D, Rimm EB, et al. Intake of specific carotenoids and risk of lung cancer in 2 prospective US cohorts. Am J Clin Nutr, 2000, 72: 990-997.

[53] Gallicchio L, Boyd K, Matanoski G, et al. Carotenoids and the risk of developing lung cancer: a systematic review. American Journal of Clinical Nutrition, 2008, 88: 372-383.

[54] The effect of vitamin E and beta carotene on the incidence of lung cancer and other cancers in male smokers. New England Journal of Medicine, 330: 1029-1035.

[55] Hennekens CH, Buring JE, Manson JE, et al. Lack of effect of long-term supplementation with beta carotene on the incidence of malignant neoplasms and cardiovascular disease. New England Journal of Medicine, 1996, 334: 1145-1149.

[56] Omenn GS, Goodman GE, Thornquist MD, et al. Effects of a combination of beta carotene and vitamin A on lung cancer and cardiovascular disease. New England Journal of Medicine, 1996, 334: 1150-1155.

[57] Greenwald P. β-carotene and lung cancer: A lesson for future chemoprevention investigations Journal of the National Cancer Institute, 2003, 95: E1.

[58] Palozza P. Prooxidant actions of carotenoids in biologic systems. Nutrition Reviews, 1998, 56: 257-265.

[59] Touvier M, Kesse E, Clavel-Chapelon F. Dual association of β-carotene with risk of tobacco-related cancers in a cohort of French women. Journal of the National Cancer Institute, 2005, 97: 1338-1344.

[60] Schabath MB, Hernandez L, Wu X, et al. Dietary phytoestrogens and lung cancer risk. JAMA: The Journal of the American Medical Association, 2005, 294: 1493-1504.

[61] Wakai K, Egami I, Kato K, et al. Dietary intake and sources of isoflavones among Japanese. Nutrition and

Cancer, 1999, 33: 139-145.

[62] Swanson CA, Mao BL, Li JY, et al. Dietary determinants of lung-cancer risk: Results from a case-control study in Yunnan province, China. International Journal of Cancer, 1992, 50: 876-880.

[63] Hu J, Johnson KC, Mao Y, et al. A case-control study of diet and lung cancer in Northeast China. International Journal of Cancer, 1997, 71: 924-931.

[64] Koo LC. Dietary habits and lung cancer risk among Chinese females in Hong Kong who never smoked. Nutrition and Cancer, 1988, 11: 155-172.

[65] Seow A, Poh W-T, Teh M, et al. Diet, reproductive factors and lung cancer risk among Chinese women in Singapore: Evidence for a protective effect of soy in nonsmokers. International Journal of Cancer, 2002, 97: 365-371.

[66] Yang G, Shu XO, Chow WH, et al. Soy food intake and risk of lung cancer: evidence from the Shanghai Women's Health Study and a meta-analysis. Am J Epidemiol, 2012, 176: 846-855.

[67] Yang WS, Va P, Wong MY, et al. Soy intake is associated with lower lung cancer risk: results from a meta-analysis of epidemiologic studies. Am J Clin Nutr, 2011, 94: 1575-1583.

[68] Choi S-W, Mason JB. Folate and carcinogenesis: An integrated scheme. Journal of Nutrition, 2000, 130: 129-132.

[69] Bandera E, Freudenheim J, Marshall J, et al. Diet and alcohol consumption and lung cancer risk in the New York State Cohort (United States). Cancer Causes & Control, 1997, 8: 828-840.

[70] Speizer FE, Colditz GA, Hunter DJ, et al. Prospective study of smoking, antioxidant intake, and lung cancer in middle-aged women (USA). Cancer Causes & Control, 1999, 10: 475-482.

[71] Voorrips LE, Goldbohm RA, Brants HAM, et al. A prospective cohort study on antioxidant and folate intake and male lung cancer risk. Cancer Epidemiology Biomarkers & Prevention, 2000, 9: 357-365.

[72] Shen H, Wei Q, Pillow PC, et al. Dietary folate intake and lung cancer risk in former smokers. Cancer Epidemiology Biomarkers & Prevention, 2003, 12: 980-986.

[73] Ahn MJ, Won HH, Lee J, et al. The 18p11.22 locus is associated with never smoker non-small cell lung cancer susceptibility in Korean populations. Hum Genet, 2012, 131: 365-372.

[74] Brennan P, Hainaut P, Boffetta P. Genetics of lung-cancer susceptibility. The Lancet Oncology, 2011, 12: 399-408.

[75] Amos CI, Wu X, Broderick P, et al. Genome-wide association scan of tag SNPs identifies a susceptibility locus for lung cancer at 15q25.1. Nat Genet, 2008, 40: 616-622.

[76] Broderick P, Wang Y, Vijayakrishnan J, et al. Deciphering the impact of common genetic variation on lung cancer risk: a genome-wide association study. Cancer Res, 2009, 69: 6633-6641.

[77] Park JY, Park JM, Jang JS, et al. Caspase 9 promoter polymorphisms and risk of primary lung cancer. Hum Mol Genet, 2006, 15: 1963-1971.

[78] Zhang X, Miao X, Sun T, et al. Functional polymorphisms in cell death pathway genes FAS and FASL contribute to risk of lung cancer. J Med Genet, 2005, 42: 479-484.

[79] Pharoah PD, Dunning AM, Ponder BA, et al. Association studies for finding cancersusceptibility genetic variants. Nat Rev Cancer, 2004, 4: 850-860.

[80] Carlsten C, Sagoo GS, Frodsham AJ, et al. Glutathione S-transferase M1 (GSTM1) polymorphisms and lung cancer: A literature-based systematic HuGE review and meta-analysis. American Journal of Epidemiology, 2008, 167: 759-774.

[81] Brennan P, McKay J, Moore L, et al. Uncommon CHEK2 mis-sense variant and reduced risk of tobacco-related cancers: Case-control study. Human Molecular Genetics, 2007, 16: 1794-1801.

[82] Cybulski C, Masojć B, Oszutowska D, et al. Constitutional CHEK2 mutations are associated with a decreased risk of lung and laryngeal cancers. Carcinogenesis, 2008, 29: 762-765.

[83] Cybulski C, Górski B, Huzarski T, et al. CHEK2 is a multiorgan cancer susceptibility gene. American Journal of Human Genetics, 2004, 75: 1131-1135.

[84] Kilpivaara O, Vahteristo P, Falck J, et al. CHEK2 variant I157T may be associated with increased breast cancer risk. International Journal of Cancer, 2004, 111: 543-547.

[85] Bush WS, Moore JH. Chapter 11: Genome-Wide Association Studies. PLoS Comput Biol, 2012, 8: e1002822.

[86] Zhou K, Pearson ER. Insights from genomewide association studies of drug response. Annu Rev Pharmacol Toxicol, 2013, 53: 299-310.

[87] Pahl R, Schafer H, Muller HH. Optimal multistage designs—a general framework for efficient genome-wide association studies. Biostatistics, 2009, 10: 297-309.

[88] Sugimura H, Tao H, Suzuki M, et al. Genetic susceptibility to lung cancer. Front Biosci (Schol Ed), 2011, 3: 1463-1477.

[89] McKay JD, Hung RJ, Gaborieau V, et al. Lung cancer susceptibility locus at 5p15.33. Nat Genet, 2008, 40: 1404-1406.

[90] Wang Y, Broderick P, Webb E, et al. Common 5p15.33 and 6p21.33 variants influence lung cancer risk. Nat Genet, 2008, 40: 1407-1409.

[91] Shi J, Chatterjee N, Rotunno M, et al. Inherited variation at chromosome 12p13.33 including RAD52 influences squamous cell lung carcinoma risk. Cancer Discovery, 2011, 2: 131-139.

[92] Hung RJ, McKay JD, Gaborieau V, et al. A susceptibility locus for lung cancer maps to nicotinic acetylcholine receptor subunit genes on 15q25. Nature, 2008, 452: 633-637.

[93] Thorgeirsson TE, Geller F, Sulem P, et al. A variant associated with nicotine dependence, lung cancer and peripheral arterial disease. Nature, 2008, 452: 638-642.

[94] Amos CI, Gorlov IP, Dong Q, et al. Nicotinic acetylcholine receptor region on chromosome 15q25 and lung cancer risk among African Americans: a case-control study. J Natl Cancer Inst, 2010, 102: 1199-1205.

[95] Truong T, Hung RJ, Amos CI, et al. Replication of lung cancer susceptibility loci at chromosomes 15q25, 5p15, and 6p21: A pooled analysis from the International Lung Cancer Consortium. J Natl Cancer Inst, 2010, 102: 959-971.

[96] Wu C, Hu Z, Yu D, et al. Genetic variants on chromosome 15q25 associated with lung cancer Risk in Chinese populations. Cancer Research, 2009, 69: 5065-5072.

[97] Shiraishi K, Kohno T, Kunitoh H, et al. Contribution of nicotine acetylcholine receptor polymorphisms to lung cancer risk in a smoking-independent manner in the Japanese. Carcinogenesis, 2009, 30: 65-70.

[98] Grando SA. Cholinergic control of epidermal cohesion. Experimental Dermatology, 2006, 15: 265-282.

[99] Schuller HM. Is cancer triggered by altered signaling of nicotinic acetylcholine receptors? Nat Rev Cancer, 2009, 9: 195-205.

[100] Al-Wadei HAN, Schuller HM. Nicotinic receptor-associated modulation of stimulatory and inhibitory neurotransmitters in NNK-induced adenocarcinoma of the lungs and pancreas. Journal of Pathology, 2009, 218: 437-445.

[101] Paliwal A, Vaissière T, Krais A, et al. Aberrant DNA methylation links cancer susceptibility locus 15q25.1 to apoptotic regulation and lung cancer. Cancer Research, 2010, 70: 2779-2788.

[102] Wang Y, Broderick P, Webb E, et al. Common 5p15.33 and 6p21.33 variants influence lung cancer risk. Nat Genet, 2008, 40: 1407-1409.

[103] Truong T, Hung RJ, Amos CI, et al. Replication of lung cancer susceptibility loci at chromosomes 15q25, 5p15, and 6p21: A pooled analysis from the International Lung Cancer Consortium. Journal of the National Cancer Institute, 2010, 102: 959-971.

[104] Rafnar T, Sulem P, Stacey SN, et al. Sequence variants at the TERT-CLPTM1L locus associate with many cancer types. Nature Genetics, 2009, 41: 221-227.

[105] Fernandez-Garcia I, Ortiz-De-Solorzano C, Montuenga LM. Telomeres and telomerase in lung cancer. Journal of Thoracic Oncology, 2008, 3: 1085-1088.

[106] Chen H, Li Y, Tollefsbol TO. Strategies targeting telomerase inhibition. Molecular Biotechnology, 2009, 41: 194-199.

[107] Yoshiura K-i, Machida J, Daack-Hirsch S, et al. Characterization of a novel gene disrupted by a balanced chromosomal translocation t (2; 19) (q11.2; q13.3) in a family with cleft lip and palate. Genomics, 1998, 54: 231-240.

[108] James MA, WenW, Wang Y, et al. Functional characterization of CLPTM1L as a lung cancer risk candidate gene in the 5p15.33 Locus. PLoS One, 2012, 7: e36116.

[109] Timofeeva MN, Hung RJ, Rafnar T, et al. Influence of common genetic variation on lung cancer risk: metaanalysis of 14 900 cases and 29 485 controls. Human Molecular Genetics, 2012, 21: 4980-4995.

[110] Shiraishi K, Kunitoh H, Daigo Y, et al. A genome-wide association study identifies two new susceptibility loci for lung adenocarcinoma in the Japanese population. Nat Genet, 2012, 44: 900-903.

[111] Sasaki T, Gan EC, Wakeham A, et al. HLA-B-associated transcript 3 (Bat3) /Scythe is essential for p300-mediated acetylation of p53. Genes & Development, 2007, 21: 848-861.

[112] Desmots F, Russell HR, Lee Y, et al. The reaper-bind-

ing protein scythe modulates apoptosis and proliferation during mammalian development. Molecular and Cellular Biology, 2005, 25: 10329-10337.

[113] Mortensen UH, Lisby M, Rothstein R. Rad52. Current Biology, 2009, 19: R676-R677.

[114] Khanna KK, Jackson SP. DNA double-strand breaks: signaling, repair and the cancer connection. Nat Genet, 2001, 27: 247-254.

[115] Hu Z, Wu C, Shi Y, et al. A genome-wide association study identifies two new lung cancer susceptibility loci at 13q12.12 and 22q12.2 in Han Chinese. Nat Genet, 2011, 43: 792-796.

[116] Amos CI, Gorlov IP, Dong Q, et al. Nicotinic acetylcholine receptor region on chromosome 15q25 and lung cancer risk among African Americans: A case-control study. Journal of the National Cancer Institute, 2010, 102: 1199-1205.

[117] Lan Q, Hsiung CA, Matsuo K, et al. Genome-wide association analysis identifies new lung cancer susceptibility loci in never-smoking women in Asia. Nat Genet, 2012, 44: 1330-1335.

[118] Hu L, Wu C, Zhao X, et al. Genome-wide association study of prognosis in advanced non-small cell lung cancer patients receiving platinum-based chemotherapy. Clin Cancer Res, 2012, 18: 5507-5514.

[119] Landi MT, Chatterjee N, Yu K, et al. A genomewide association study of lung cancer identifies a region of chromosome 5p15 associated with risk for adenocarcinoma. American Journal of Human Genetics, 2009, 85: 679-691.

[120] Torok S, Hegedus B, Laszlo V, et al. Lung cancer in never smokers. Future Oncol, 2011, 7: 1195-1211.

[121] Subramanian J, Govindan R. Lung cancer in never smokers: a review. J Clin Oncol, 2007, 25: 561-570.

[122] Li Y, Sheu CC, Ye Y, et al. Genetic variants and risk of lung cancer in never smokers: a genome-wide association study. Lancet Oncol, 2010, 11: 321-330.

[123] Potter JD, Goode E, Morimoto L. AACR Special Conference: The molecular and genetic epidemiology of cancer. Cancer Epidemiol Biomarkers Prev, 2003, 12: 803-805.

[124] Spitz MR, Wei Q, Dong Q, et al. Genetic susceptibility to lung cancer: the role of DNA damage and repair. Cancer Epidemiol Biomarkers Prev, 2003, 12: 689-698.

[125] Hsu TC, Johnston DA, Cherry LM, et al. Sensitivity to genotoxic effects of bleomycin in humans: Possible relationship to environmental carcinogenesis. International Journal of Cancer, 1989, 43: 403-409.

[126] Wu X, Gu J, Amos CI, et al. A parallel study of in vitro sensitivity to benzo (a) pyrene diol epoxide and bleomycin in lung carcinoma cases and controls. Cancer, 1998, 83: 1118-1127.

[127] Burger RM, Peisach J, Band Horwitz S. Mechanism of bleomycin action: In vitro studies. Life Sciences, 1981, 28: 715-727.

[128] Wei Q, Gu J, Cheng L, et al. Benzo (a) pyrene diol epoxide-induced chromosomal aberrations and risk of lung cancer. Cancer Res, 1996, 56: 3975-3979.

[129] Strom SS, Wu S, Sigurdson AJ, et al. Lung cancer, smoking patterns, and mutagen sensitivity in Mexican-Americans. J Natl Cancer Inst Monogr, 1995, 18: 29-33.

[130] Kassie F, Parzefall W, Knasmüller S. Single cell gel electrophoresis assay: a new technique for human biomonitoring studies. Mutation Research/Reviews in Mutation Research, 2000, 463: 13-31.

[131] Tice RR, Agurell E, Anderson D, et al. Single cell gel/comet assay: Guidelines for in vitro and in vivo genetic toxicology testing. Environmental and Molecular Mutagenesis, 2000, 35: 206-221.

[132] Moller P, Knudsen LE, Loft S, et al. The comet assay as a rapid test in biomonitoring occupational exposure to DNA-damaging agents and effect of confounding factors. Cancer Epidemiol Biomarkers Prev, 2000, 9: 1005-1015.

[133] Wu X, Roth JA, Zhao H, et al. Cell cycle checkpoints, DNA damage/repair, and lung cancer risk. Cancer Res, 2005, 65: 349-357.

[134] Rajaee-Behbahani N, Schmezer P, Risch A, et al. Altered DNA repair capacity and bleomycin sensitivity as risk markers for non-small cell lung cancer. International Journal of Cancer, 2001, 95: 86-91.

[135] Li D, Wang M, Cheng L, et al. In vitro induction of benzo (a) pyrene diol epoxide-DNA adducts in peripheral lymphocytes as a susceptibility marker for human lung cancer. Cancer Res, 1996, 56: 3638-3641.

[136] Li D, Firozi PF, Wang LE, et al. Sensitivity to DNA damage induced by benzo (a) pyrene diol epoxide and risk of lung cancer: a case-control analysis. Cancer Res, 2001, 61: 1445-1450.

[137] Shen H, Spitz MR, Qiao Y, et al. Smoking, DNA repair capacity and risk of nonsmall cell lung cancer. In-

ternational Journal of Cancer, 2003, 107: 84 - 88.

[138] Wei Q, Cheng L, Amos CI, et al. Repair of tobacco carcinogeninduced DNA adducts and lung cancer risk: A molecular epidemiologic study. Journal of the National Cancer Institute, 2000, 92: 1764 - 1772.

[139] Wei Q, Cheng L, HongWK, et al. Reduced DNA repair capacity in lung cancer patients. Cancer Res, 1996, 56: 4103 - 4107.

[140] Koch KS, Fletcher RG, Grond MP, et al. Inactivation of plasmid reporter gene expression by one benzo (a) pyrene diol-epoxide DNA adduct in adult rat hepatocytes. Cancer Res, 1993, 53: 2279 - 2286.

[141] Paz-Elizur T, Krupsky M, Blumenstein S, et al. DNA repair activity for oxidative damage and risk of lung cancer. Journal of the National Cancer Institute, 2003, 95: 1312 - 1319.

[142] Gackowski D, Speina E, Zielinska M, et al. Products of oxidative DNA damage and repair as possible biomarkers of susceptibility to lung cancer. Cancer Res, 2003, 63: 4899 - 4902.

[143] Misteli T, Soutoglou E. The emerging role of nuclear architecture in DNA repair and genome maintenance. Nat Rev Mol Cell Biol, 2009, 10: 243 - 254.

[144] Redon C, Pilch D, Rogakou E, et al. Histone H2A variants H2AX and H2AZ. Curr Opin Genet Dev, 2012, 12: 62 - 169.

[145] Huen MS, Chen J. The DNA damage response pathways: at the crossroad of protein modifications. Cell Res, 2008, 18: 8 - 16.

[146] Rothkamm K, Lobrich M. Evidence for a lack of DNA double-strand break repair in human cells exposed to very low x-ray doses. Proc Natl Acad Sci USA, 2003, 100: 5057 - 5062.

[147] Ismail IH, Wadhra TI, Hammarsten O. An optimized method for detecting gamma-H2AX in blood cells reveals a significant interindividual variation in the gamma-H2AX response among humans. Nucleic Acids Research, 2007, 35: e36.

[148] Lobrich M, Rief N, Kuhne M, et al. In vivo formation and repair of DNA double-strand breaks after computed tomography examinations. Proc Natl Acad Sci USA, 2005, 102: 8984 - 8989.

[149] Sedelnikova OA, Horikawa I, Redon C, et al. Delayed kinetics of DNA double-strand break processing in normal and pathological aging. Aging Cell, 2008, 7: 89 - 100.

[150] Redon CE, Nakamura AJ, Zhang YW, et al. Histone gammaH2AX and poly (ADP-ribose) as clinical pharmacodynamic biomarkers. Clin Cancer Res, 2010, 16: 4532 - 4542.

[151] Postel-Vinay S, Vanhecke E, Olaussen KA, et al. The potential of exploiting DNA-repair defects for optimizing lung cancer treatment. Nat Rev Clin Oncol, 2012, 9: 144 - 155.

[152] Gazdar AF. DNA repair and survival in lung cancer-the two faces of Janus. New England Journal of Medicine, 2007, 356: 771 - 773.

[153] Matthaios D, Bouros D, Kakolyris S. H2AX and lung cancer: Is it the Ariadne's thread? DNA Repair, 2013, 12: 90 - 91.

[154] He Y, Gong Y, Lin J, et al. Ionizing radiation-induced γ-H2AX activity in whole blood culture and the risk of lung cancer. Cancer Epidemiology Biomarkers & Prevention, 2013, 22: 443 - 451.

[155] Zhao H, Spitz MR, Tomlinson GE, et al. Gamma-radiation-induced G2 delay, apoptosis, and p53 response as potential susceptibility markers for lung cancer. Cancer Res, 2001, 61: 7819 - 7824.

[156] Zheng Y-L, Loffredo CA, Alberg AJ, et al. Less efficient G2-M checkpoint is associated with an increased risk of lung cancer in African Americans. Cancer Research, 2005, 65: 9566 - 9573.

[157] Biroš E, Kohút A, Biroš I, et al. A link between the p53 germ linepolymorphisms and white blood cells apoptosis in lung cancer patients. Lung Cancer, 2002, 35: 231 - 235.

[158] Wu X, Zhao H, Amos CI, et al. p53 genotypes and haplotypes associated with lung cancer susceptibility and ethnicity. Journal of the National Cancer Institute, 2002, 94: 681 - 690.

[159] Grivennikov SI, Greten FR, Karin M. Immunity, inflammation, and cancer. Cell, 2011, 140: 883 - 899.

[160] Siemes C, Visser LE, Coebergh JW, et al. C-reactive protein levels, variation in the C-reactive protein gene, and cancer risk: the Rotterdam Study. J Clin Oncol, 2006, 24: 5216 - 5222.

[161] Trichopoulos D, Psaltopoulou T, Orfanos P, et al. Plasma C-reactive protein and risk of cancer: a prospective study from Greece. Cancer Epidemiol Biomarkers Prev, 2006, 15: 381 - 384.

[162] Heikkila K, Ebrahim S, Lawlor DA. A systematic review of the association between circulating concentrations

of C reactive protein and cancer. J Epidemiol Community Health, 2007 61: 824-833.

[163] Szalai AJ, Wu J, Lange EM, et al. Single-nucleotide polymorphisms in the C-reactive protein (CRP) gene promoter that affect transcription factor binding, alter transcriptional activity, and associate with differences in baseline serum CRP level. J Mol Med (Berl), 2005, 83: 440-447.

[164] Orditura M, De Vita F, Catalano G, et al. Elevated serum levels of interleukin-8 in advanced non-small cell lung cancer patients: relationship with prognosis. J Interferon Cytokine Res, 2002, 22: 1129-1135.

[165] Yanagawa H, Sone S, Takahashi Y, et al. Serum levels of interleukin 6 in patients with lung cancer. Br J Cancer, 1995, 71: 1095-1098.

[166] Shiels MS, Chaturvedi AK, Katki HA, et al. Circulating markers of interstitial lung disease and subsequent risk of lung cancer. Cancer Epidemiology Biomarkers & Prevention, 2011, 20: 2262-2272.

[167] Il'yasova D, Colbert LH, Harris TB, et al. Circulating levels of inflammatory markers and cancer risk in the health aging and body composition cohort. Cancer Epidemiology Biomarkers & Prevention, 2005, 14: 2413-2418.

[168] Mitchell PS, Parkin RK, Kroh EM, et al. Circulating microRNAs as stable blood-based markers for cancer detection. Proc Natl Acad Sci USA, 2008, 105: 10513-10518.

[169] Mascaux C, Laes JF, Anthoine G, et al. Evolution of microRNA expression during human bronchial squamous carcinogenesis. Eur Respir J, 2009, 33: 352-359.

[170] Mascaux C, Feser WJ, Lewis MT, et al. Endobronchial miRNAs as biomarkers in lung cancer chemoprevention. Cancer Prev Res (Phila), 2012, 12, 100-108.

[171] Bianchi F, Nicassio F, Veronesi G, et al. Circulating microRNAs: next-generation biomarkers for early lung cancer detection. Ecancermedicalscience, 2012, 6: 246.

[172] Hennessey PT, Sanford T, Choudhary A, et al. Serum microRNA biomarkers for detection of non-small cell lung cancer. PLoS One, 2012, 7: e32307.

[173] Zheng D, Haddadin S, Wang Y, et al. Plasma microRNAs as novel biomarkers for early detection of lung cancer. Int J Clin Exp Pathol, 2011, 4: 575-586.

[174] Boeri M, Verri C, Conte D, et al. MicroRNA signatures in tissues and plasma predict development and prognosis of computed tomography detected lung cancer. Proc Natl Acad Sci USA, 2011, 108: 3713-3718.

[175] Pathak AK, Bhutani M, Kumar S, et al. Circulating cell-free DNA in plasma/serum of lung cancer patients as a potential screening and prognostic tool. Clinical Chemistry, 2006, 52: 1833-1842.

[176] Paci M, Maramotti S, Bellesia E, et al. Circulating plasma DNA as diagnostic biomarker in non-small cell lung cancer. Lung Cancer, 2009, 64: 92-97.

[177] Belinsky SA, Klinge DM, Dekker JD, et al. Gene promoter methylation in plasma and sputum increases with lung cancer risk. Clin Cancer Res, 2005, 11: 6505-6511.

[178] Belinsky SA, Liechty KC, Gentry FD, et al. Promoter hypermethylation of multiple genes in sputum precedes lung cancer incidence in a high-risk cohort. Cancer Res, 2006, 66: 3338-3344.

[179] Xue X, Zhu YM, Woll PJ. Circulating DNA and lung cancer. Annals of the New York Academy of Sciences, 2006, 1075: 154-164.

[180] Miura N, Nakamura H, Sato R, et al. Clinical usefulness of serum telomerase reverse transcriptase (hTERT) mRNA and epidermal growth factor receptor (EGFR) mRNA as a novel tumor marker for lung cancer. Cancer Sci, 2006, 97: 1366-1373.

[181] Higgins G, Roper KM, Watson IJ, et al. Variant Ciz1 is a circulating biomarker for early-stage lung cancer. Proc Natl Acad Sci USA, 2012, 109: E3128-3135.

[182] Wu X, Amos CI, Zhu Y, et al. Telomere dysfunction: a potential cancer predisposition factor. J Natl Cancer Inst, 2003, 95: 1211-1218.

[183] Jang JS, Choi YY, Lee WK, et al. Telomere length and the risk of lung cancer. Cancer Sci., 2008, 99: 1385-1389.

[184] Wentzensen IM, Mirabello L, Pfeiffer RM, et al. The association of telomere length and cancer: a meta-analysis. Cancer Epidemiol Biomarkers Prev, 2011, 20: 1238-1250.

[185] Shen M, Cawthon R, Rothman N, et al. A prospective study of telomere length measured by monochrome multiplex quantitative PCR and risk of lung cancer. Lung Cancer, 2011, 73: 133-137.

[186] Freedman AN, Seminara D, Gail MH, et al. Cancer risk prediction models: A workshop on development, evaluation, and application. Journal of the National Cancer Institute, 2005, 97: 715-723.

[187] Baker SG. Putting risk prediction in perspective: relative utility curves. J Natl Cancer Inst, 2009, 101: 1538 – 1542.

[188] Spitz MR, Caporaso NE, Sellers TA. Integrative cancer epidemiology-the next generation. Cancer Discov, 2012, 2: 1087 – 1090.

[189] Colditz GA, Atwood KA, Emmons K, et al. Harvard Report on Cancer Prevention Volume 4: Harvard Cancer Risk Index. Risk Index Working Group, Harvard Center for Cancer Prevention. Cancer Causes Control, 2000, 11: 477 – 488.

[190] Bach PB, Kattan MW, Thornquist MD, et al. Variations in lung cancer risk among smokers. Journal of the National Cancer Institute, 2003, 95: 470 – 478.

[191] Cronin KA, Gail MH, Zou Z, et al. Validation of a model of lung cancer risk prediction among smokers. J Natl Cancer Inst, 2006, 98: 637 – 640.

[192] Spitz MR, Hong WK, Amos CI, et al. A risk model for prediction of lung cancer. Journal of the National Cancer Institute, 2007, 99: 715 – 726.

[193] Spitz MR, Etzel CJ, Dong Q, et al. An expanded risk prediction model for lung cancer. Cancer Prevention Research, 2008, 1: 250 – 254.

[194] Wu X, Lin J, Grossman HB, et al. Projecting individualized probabilities of developing bladder cancer in white individuals. J Clin Oncol, 2007, 25: 4974 – 4981.

[195] Cassidy A, Myles JP, van Tongeren M, et al. The LLP risk model: an individual risk prediction model for lung cancer. Br J Cancer, 2008, 98: 270 – 276.

[196] Raji OY, Duffy SW, Agbaje OF, et al. Predictive accuracy of the Liverpool Lung Project risk model for stratifying patients for computed tomography screening for lung cancer: a case-control and cohort validation study. Ann Intern Med, 2012, 157: 242 – 250.

[197] Hoggart C, Brennan P, Tjonneland A, et al. A risk model for lung cancer incidence. Cancer Prevention Research, 2012, 5: 834 – 846.

[198] Gail MH. Discriminatory accuracy from singlenucleotide polymorphisms in models to predict breast cancer risk. J Natl Cancer Inst, 2008, 100: 1037 – 1041.

[199] Gail MH. Value of adding single-nucleotide polymorphism genotypes to a breast cancer risk model. J Natl Cancer Inst, 2009, 101: 959 – 963.

[200] Raji OY, Agbaje OF, Duffy SW, et al. Incorporation of a genetic factor into an epidemiologic model for prediction of individual risk of lung cancer: the Liverpool Lung Project. Cancer Prev Res (Phila), 2010, 3: 664 – 669.

[201] Bach PB, Mirkin JN, Oliver TK, et al. Benefits and harms of ct screening for lung cancer: A systematic review. JAMA, 2012, 307: 2418 – 2429.

[202] Aberle DR, Adams AM, Berg CD, et al. Reduced lung-cancer mortality with low-dose computed tomographic screening. N Engl J Med, 2011, 365: 395 – 409.

[203] Duffy SW, Raji OY, Agbaje OF, et al. Use of lung cancer risk models in planning research and service programs in CT screening for lung cancer. Expert Rev Anticancer Ther, 2009, 9: 1467 – 1472.

[204] Miki D, Kubo M, Takahashi A, et al. Variation in TP63 is associated with lung adenocarcinoma susceptibility in Japanese and Korean populations. Nat Genet, 2010, 42: 893 – 896.

第3章
肺癌的分子分析

Lauren Averett Byers
Department of Thoracic/Head and Neck Medical Oncology, The University of Texas MD Anderson Cancer Center, Houston, TX, USA

引 言

2001年，两份人类基因组草图的问世标志着分子分析取得了划时代的进步[1-2]。此后，技术的快速发展和生物学的诸多新发现，例如小RNAs（miRNAs）的发现，促进了包括肺癌在内的多种疾病的更多分子信息的阐明。虽然体内蛋白质编码基因多达20 000~25 000种，但是其中仅有部分在细胞内特定时间表达。分子分析研究的核心任务在于明确与肺癌患者相关的活性基因，基因的调控机制，基因对于肿瘤生长、浸润和转移的影响，以及基因特征与特定临床表现（例如治疗的反应性）的相关性。

过去10年间，肺癌的两大进展分别为针对非小细胞肺癌（NSCLC）表皮生长因子受体（EGFR）突变靶点的EGFR抑制剂（厄罗替尼、吉非替尼）和针对棘皮微管相关蛋白样4-间变性淋巴瘤激酶（anaplastic lymphoma kinase，ALK）融合的ALK抑制剂（克唑替尼）[3-7]，均与分子分析直接相关。上述进展促使转移性NSCLCs的治疗由传统肿瘤检测向指导药物选择的异常基因检测转变[8]。ROS1融合和DDR1突变是新确定的可能预测靶向治疗效果的驱动基因[9-10]。目前多项进行中的临床试验正在评估这些基因和其他突变基因对于药物疗效的潜在预测作用。

然而，对于大多数肺癌来说，肿瘤生物学行为相关的驱动基因或驱动通路尚未完全阐明。NSCLCs和小细胞肺癌（SCLC）本身非常复杂，存在大量肿瘤间异质性（例如肿瘤存在多种分子亚型）和肿瘤或患者本身的异质性（例如同一患者体内的肿瘤细胞不同克隆表现出的差异性突变和分子表达谱）。准确测定和分析大量肺癌的DNA、RNA和蛋白（分子表达谱）核心特征有助于更好地理解肺癌的生物学行为，并最终应用于患者治疗的核心方面。分子表达分析的临床应用目标包括：①为患者制订个体化的最佳治疗策略；②发现肿瘤早期诊断或治疗的新型分子标志物；③确定药物靶点。现阶段已存在大量肿瘤相关的分子数据，同样存在分析这些数据且已在临床进行验证的新型工具。这些资源包括主要公共资金援助项目，例如癌症基因分析（the Cancer Genone Atlas, TCGAs）[9-10]，该项目已经完成400例以上肺鳞状细胞癌（简称肺鳞癌）和肺腺癌患者的基因测定。这些资源同样包括个人或研究中心的项目（例如肺癌突变联盟；http://gol-cmc.com）[11-12]。应诸多顶级杂志和美国国立卫生院（the US National Institutes of Health, NIH）的要求，多数分子信息尤其是信使RNA（mRNA）基因表达数据的文章发表后即为公众获得。这些数据可通过如基因表达数据库（Gene Expression Omnibus, GEO）[14]、Oncomine[15]或者cBio癌症基因库[16]等获得。

最后，因为可用于指导患者治疗的突变及其他分子标志物信息不断增长，其他资源必须获得同样的发展才能有效地连接医务人员和患者，而这种连接是基于潜在分子检测结果临床应用的循证医学证据，包括进行中针对具有特定突变或分子标志物患者的临床试验，代表之一就是www.mycancergenome.org网站。该网站由Vanderbilt大学的转化医学专家创建并提供关于特定突变及主要参考文献的信息，同时链接相关临床试验。

分子分析涵盖测定特定样本中数以百计甚至数以千计的特定基因（例如 mRNA、基因组 DNA、蛋白质）表达（图 3.1）。例如研究者可能分析特定肿瘤 DNA 以评估特定基因突变频率，基因拷贝数变化（例如扩增、缺失），或者基因甲基化模式（例如表观遗传学调节）。同样，肺癌中提取的 RNA 也用于分析单一肿瘤中数以千计的 mRNAs 或 miRNA 水平。

采用多种统计工具识别具有特定疾病行为的分子特征或分子分析，并与已收集到的大量患者样本信息进行比较。表达谱和疾病行为的相关性由基于"火车模型"的样本分析得以阐明。该结论随后在另一个新的模型或样本中进行验证，以确定"火车模型"所阐明的相关性在其他独立样本中同样存在[17]。分子分析是一个动态概念，理论上，它可以用于研究和确定任何可分析数据与任一特定变异现象的相关性（例如疾病分子、药物反应性、突变状态），从而为彼此提供可描述性和可信的数据测定。

分子分析工具

分子分析试验可用来研究任何临床变量和任何被分析物的相关性。因此，任何测定单一样本大量差异分子的工具均可用于解决临床问题，部分原因是：①蛋白质在细胞调节过程存在多样性；②蛋白质翻译对 mRNA 转录及转录后修饰具有依赖性；③核心技术的进步，最主要的技术是 DNA 谱（基因组）、RNA 谱（例如基因表达谱）和蛋白质谱（蛋白质组学），这些都推动了对疾病进一步的认识。

基因组学和蛋白质组学是一组具有互补性的研究模型。基因组学目前应用更广泛且发展更为成熟。DNA 和 RNA 互补碱基配对的生物学特性简化了分析过程。蛋白质尤其是自身异质性的存在导致更难进行归类，然而，蛋白质对于病理学行为具有更直接的影响，并且其调节和（或）功能方面的复杂性不能从基因表达水平上阐明。基于以

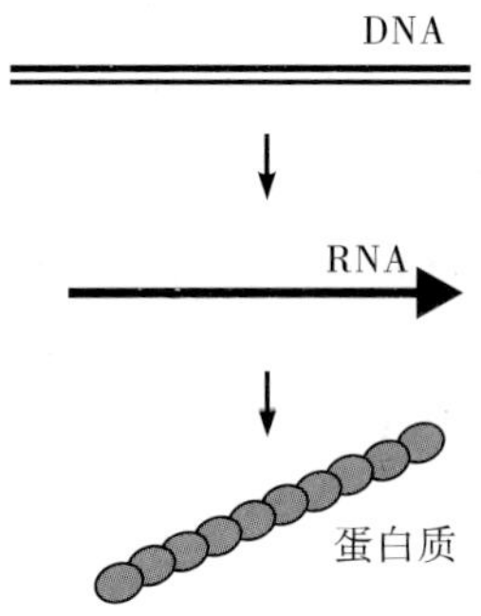

		分子分析举例	平台举例
	DNA	突变	质谱分析（如 Sequenom） 靶向基因测序（如 Ion Torrent） 全基因组测序 全外显子组测序
		拷贝数变异	CGH 分析 SNP 分析 DNA 测序
		单核苷酸多态性（SNP）	SNP 分析
		表观遗传学 （如甲基化、组蛋白修饰等）	DNA 甲基化分析
	RNA	mRNA	mRNA 微阵列（如基因表达数组） RNA 测序
		miRNA, lincRNA	miRNA 分析 RNA 测序
	蛋白质	总蛋白，磷酸化蛋白	反向蛋白质阵列（RPPA） 谱技术（MALDI；质谱）

图 3.1 DNA、RNA 和蛋白质分析的模式。多种基因分析测序平台可分析 DNA、RNA 和蛋白质水平的变化。DNA 突变可以被大量的序列或基因分型技术识别，DNA 的拷贝数变化通常与 DNA 测序分析、CGH 及 SNP 数组共同分析。SNP 数组以及甲基化分析也可以检测 DNA 甲基化的变化。基因表达阵列常用于检测 mRNA 水平的变化。虽然 RNA 测序可以监测 mRNA、miRNA 或 lincRNA 的变化，但是，蛋白质最常应用反相蛋白数组或质谱技术进行分析

CGH：比较基因组杂交；SNP：单核苷酸多态性；miRNA：微小 RNA；lincRNA：大型基因间的非编码 RNA；MALDI：基质辅助激光解析电离

上原因，DNA、RNA 和蛋白质表达的整合分析将成为理解肺癌复杂生物学行为和异质性的核心。

现有测定肿瘤 DNA、RNA 和蛋白质特定特征的技术——通常为泛基因组规模，过去数年中进步快速并将得到更迅速的扩展。在此我们将展示目前正在应用的几个核心平台。

DNA 测序

如前所述，肺癌治疗的巨大进步在于如 EGFR、ALK 等药物驱动性突变的发现。近期许多研究都将 NSCLC 中上述突变及其他突变的频率纳入其中，例如来自肺癌突变联盟（the Lung Cancer Mutation Consortium, LCMC）[18]的研究。随着靶向药物的增长（>800 项研究中），研究终点为对患者肿瘤更大量的潜在活性基因异常进行分析，这些异常包括突变、基因拷贝数变化（例如缺失和扩增）及基因融合。这些特定突变和变异可直接指导患者接受已知标准治疗或入组临床试验。

随着 DNA 测序费用的降低，迫切需要进行更大规模的基因分析。研究和临床中常用的一种方法是对可用于药物选择或其他潜在临床应用的个体肿瘤基因（如 EGFR、KRAS、BRAF）或基因组合（50~400 个基因）进行靶向性测序。既往研究方法侧重于分析热点突变[19]，但是随着相应费用和劳动力成本的快速下降，现阶段许多分子病理实验室转向对整个基因外显子（蛋白质编码区域）进行深度测序。许多学术中心和商业公司（如麻省剑桥的 Foundation 医药和 Oregon Health&Science 大学的 Knight 诊断实验室）正在采用上述方法。

除了对于特定选择的肿瘤基因进行靶向性分析，全外显子测序和全基因组测序也越来越多地用于可能有助于阐明肿瘤行为和（或）潜在治疗靶点的 DNA 变异的研究。随着人类基因组草图在 2001 年首次公布[1-2]，二代测序技术使全基因分析变得更加便捷和经济。2008 年，采用二代测序方法的首个完整人类基因自测序完成[20]。现阶段，大批完整的肺癌基因组已公布[10,12-13]。

全外显子组测序（对应全基因组测序）是一种关注于外显子且相对便宜的高通量测序方法。外显子代表了约 3% 的全部 DNA 内容并且是基因转录为 mRNA 的一部分。相反，全基因组测序提供的是蛋白质编码和非编码区域的全部信息。全基因组测序的优势在于更好地检测基因拷贝数变异和融合基因（如 EML4-ALK、Kif5b/RET）[21-22]，涵盖非编码 DNA 区域［例如 miRNA 和较大融合非编码 RNA（slincRNAs）］，这些在 mRNA 调节、蛋白质表达和肿瘤生物学行为方面至关重要。

然而，与所有新技术一样，DNA 测序目前也存在争议，争议点在于开展、分析和保存海量信息的必要性。因为信息不完整，测序结果解读也很困难，截至目前，哪些 DNA 改变是正常变异以及哪些 DNA 改变与生物学相关尚不明确。例如，尽管多数 DNA 测序结果存在于人类甚至不同物种间，但是单一细胞内人类基因组存在多达 60 亿个碱基对，由于正常个体间的差异，近 2 400 万个碱基对（<1%）存在变异。

最后，即便采用高度准确性的测序技术，也会存在大量假阳性的基因变异（每个基因组高达 6 000 个）[23]。尽管多数全外显子组和全基因组测序仍处于研究阶段，但是随着测序费用的降低、转化周期的缩短及可直接提供结果给患者使测序在不久的将来可迅速应用于临床。从大量"无意"突变环境中识别具有临床意义的突变或变异是分子生物学家、生物信息分析师和内科医生等面临的最大挑战。

其他 DNA 分析，例如单核苷酸多态性（single-nucleotide polymorphism, SNP）、拷贝数评估和甲基化分析可提供更多的基因组信息并在 mRNA 表达水平进行互补（如下所述）[24-29]。比较基因组杂交是一种可快速区分与正常组织类似基因组拷贝数变异的方法。与 mRNA 谱分析类似，该方法可采用基因芯片，也可采用荧光原位杂交方法（fluorescent in situ hybtidization, FISH）分析特定基因扩增，该方法目前主要用于检测乳腺癌组织中 HER2 拷贝数的变化。大量 SNPs 分析可连接遗传表型与人群中特定染色体区域以及肿瘤样本中的异质性，而这种异质性可能与肿瘤的恶性转换和疾病表型相关。

RNA 分析

mRNA 和 miRNA 是分子分析中最常见的两种

RNA。mNRA 由细胞 DNA 中的蛋白质编码基因转录形成，并随后翻译为蛋白质。尽管所有细胞具有完全相同的 DNA，但所有特定细胞仅有 3%～5% 的基因可转录为 mRNA。分子分析中 mRNA 广泛用于分析哪些基因出现或表达于细胞中，这种分析方法也被称作基因表达分析。mRNA 表达在肺癌不同病理类型中（例如 NSCLC 和 SCLC）存在不同的方式，并且可能与药物敏感性相关。

与 mRNA 相同，miRNA 同样可以采用芯片技术进行分析。miRNA 较 mRNA 更短，非编码 RNA（通常 22 个核苷酸）可抑制多种 mRNA 从而调节细胞行为。因为单个 miRNA 可调节多个靶点，所以可作为复杂生物学过程的开关[23,30-31]。肺癌中，miRNA 的差异与生存、NSCLC 类型[32-34]及核心生物学程序例如上皮间叶转化相关[35]。此外，出现了一种被称作 lincRNA 的新型 RNA[36]，这种 RNA 见于全基因组测序。

目前 mRNA 表达水平的测定共有 3 种常用方法，包括：寡核苷酸芯片（微芯片）、转录组测序（也称 RNA 测序）及反转录实时定量聚合酶链反应（reverse-transcription quantitative polymerase chain reaction, RT-PCR）。早期微芯片研究采用固定于芯片上的寡核苷酸探针，这些探针总数不足 10 000[37-38]。微芯片技术的潜力在于浅显易懂，并且微芯片原型在首次合成 3 年后，相关文献于 1991 年在科学杂志上发表[39]。随着兴趣点及应用的快速增加，目前芯片商业化生产明显，并且同一芯片中低聚物探针的数目也显著增加（每个阵列 >1 000 000）。具有里程碑意义的研究是对乳腺癌中分子亚组和具有不同临床特征的淋巴瘤的描述[40-41]。

寡核苷酸阵列（微阵列芯片）是 cDNA 阵列的现代版本，已应用于多种早期高影响力微阵列试验[42-43]。与 cDNA 探针目的基因位于载玻片上不同，寡核苷酸阵列上 20～60bp 的短探针直接合成在每个阵列上。mRNA 随后从目的细胞或组织中分离，反转录为 cDNA，并转录为生物素标记的 cRNA，cRNA 代表了所有表达于试验样本中（如细胞系、肿瘤）的 mRNA，并以互补的方式与阵列和结合探针杂交。为进一步对样本中各 cRNA 定量，探针采用荧光标记，标记有荧光的探针在荧光镜下可发出荧光。阵列上绑定探针的荧光信号强度可定量原始样本的 cRNA（从而定量 mRNA）。

目前常用的商用 mRNA 阵列来自于 Affymetrix（Santa Clara, CA）和 Illumina（San Diego, CA）公司。miRNA 阵列亦有临床应用，该阵列采用类似方法对样本中超过 1 000 种 miRNAs 进行定量。

转录组测序（RNA-Seq）是一种测定肿瘤细胞中 RNA 表达的新方法。该方法采用 RNA 直接测序的方法对 mRNA 表达水平进行定量。除了提供 mRNA 表达水平方面的信息，该方法还具有识别样本中其他基因组特征的潜能，可识别转录中的突变和多态性[44]。

最后，RT-PCR 可用于测定小基因的 RNA 表达（然而，微阵列及 RNA-Seq 方法常规测定所有蛋白质编码基因）。RT-PCR 通常用于具有临床意义的 RNA 表达分析，例如，一种可预测乳腺癌患者复发风险的 RT-PCR 方法，已用于指导临床是否进行辅助化疗。

随着表达阵列快速应用于生物医学研究，顶级同行评审期刊及 NIH（指 NIH 基金资助研究）在最早的研究文章一发表就授权公布实验中的全部表达数据。阵列数据的发布使得提供全部基因表达结果的透明度大大提高（除了重要发现的归纳分析），同样使得数据方便其他研究者用于进行假说检验或验证的独立集。表达矩阵数据可在线 Gene Expression Omnibus（GEO；http://www.ncbi.nlm.nih.gov/gco/）获得，该数据库由 NIH 生物技术信息国家中心负责运行，完全开放[14]。

蛋白质组学

蛋白质组学涵盖蛋白质表达的研究，包括时间和空间分析、翻译后修饰以及与其他分子的关系。肺癌中蛋白质功能通常是失调的，有时这些异常在 RNA 或 DNA 水平表现不出来。例如，蛋白质通常在由影响其活性或功能的关键通路上的 mRNA 翻译后进行修饰（例如磷酸化或分裂）。因此，这些翻译后的修饰需要在蛋白质分析中体现。此外，比较基因及蛋白质数据的研究表明基因和蛋白质水平或许存在重大差异，并且这些在表达水平的差异也存在不同[24-25,45]。

明确肿瘤内特定信号蛋白质的表达和活化特征有助于医生为患者提供最佳治疗。多种重要的分析工具和方法已在蛋白质组学的研究中获得了广泛应用。这些应用包括反向蛋白阵列（reverse phase protein arrays，RPPA）、质谱法（mass spectrometry，MS）、前向蛋白阵列（例如受体酪氨酸激酶阵列）、用于单个蛋白质分析的酶联免疫吸附试验（enzyme-linked immunosorbent assay，ELISA）、用于多种蛋白质分析的磁珠阵列以及循环肿瘤细胞的分析。

抗体微阵列是一种分析蛋白质表达和蛋白质活性非常有效的技术。RPPAs用于分析较小样本时与mRNA微阵列的原理类似：将蛋白溶菌产物固定于特定底物上，通常是载玻片，底物需要在应用前稀释到相同浓度并溶于多种稀释液中，随后载玻片与富含一种或多种已知蛋白质的抗体孵育。RPPAs一次可检测近200种抗体，从而使研究者可同时检测属于同一或互补信号通路或网络中大量蛋白质的变化。荧光或化学发光检测法随后可用来检测相应靶蛋白的表达。因为应用了同时检测磷酸化蛋白及总蛋白的抗体，RPPAs可揭示与蛋白磷酸化水平密切相关的蛋白活性的变化，而这种变化通常对应蛋白质的一种磷酸化形式。与基因分析技术类似，RPPAs同样可用来检测肺癌表型相关蛋白质并且分析样本间的潜在相似性。例如，RPPAs试验最近证明，NSCLC和SCLC蛋白信号通路存在显著差异[46-47]。此外，RPPAs或可促进现实临床矩阵分析的发展，目前已存在应用其他技术验证的预测因子。

RPPAs的敏感性很高，但是也存在缺陷。由于每种抗体结合位点存在细微差异，因此获得适合的RPPA抗体和明确最佳的试验条件存在困难。在采用该方法选择抗体时，需要考虑试验条件从而确定相应抗体。与采用一系列非选择性的蛋白质抗体相比，采用已知生物学行为的细胞信号通路相关蛋白质抗体更容易成功。采用临床组织样本时尤其需要注意这一点。尽管采用细胞、快速冰冻组织或福尔马林固定石蜡包埋组织的溶解产物进行分析时RPPAs的敏感性及可信性更高，但检测磷酸化蛋白时可能存在错误。

MS是一种测定蛋白质分子量的准确方法，也是低浓度下测定蛋白质的敏感方法。MS可与一系列蛋白质分离方法相结合，包括凝胶过滤和电泳法，同样也可以直接用于分析组织或血液中的蛋白质（不需要分离步骤）。质谱仪分离样本中的分子并测定在特定敏感阈值下所有粒子组成电荷（m/z）具体的分子构成含量和比例。样本在真空环境下进行分离，各分离样本的m/z比例可通过不同检测方法的物理学特性进行分离，例如飞行时间（time-of-flight，TOF）、傅里叶转换（fourier-transform，FT）以及磁极等。基质辅助激光解吸电离（matrix-assisted laser desorptionlionization，MALDI）和电喷雾电离（electrospray ionization，ESI）是目前最常用的两种分离方法。这两种方法重要的区别在于，MALDI法通过激光激发涂有机酸结晶层的固体导电板来产生离子，而ESI则是溶液通过具有高度选择性的毛细管小孔进行分离。MALDI可用于对冰冻组织切片或全细胞学的准备，可惜该方法不适用于石蜡包埋标本。多蛋白质谱分析可从多个角度进行冰冻组织切片的分析，从而明确蛋白质的空间结构以及其产物蛋白质的空间定位及分布。因此，MALDI有助于区分场效应或将肿瘤与邻近间质及淋巴细胞区分开。MALDI同样可用于分析生物样本的干滴，例如血液、血清、血浆、胸水、腹水或通过柱状层析分离所得的蛋白碎片，单向或双向凝胶层析提取蛋白质。ESI需要样品溶解并且尤其适用于柱状层析分离时在线分析蛋白质和肽。MALDI试验已用于肺癌患者的样本和血清分析。

近年来，串联质谱分析（MS/MS）已用于混合物中肽的直接测序。质谱第一步将完整的肽离子分开，而后碰撞气体被引入真空环境中，从而使离子断裂，并发生由于碳碳结合或碳氮结合形成多肽支架的特征性断裂离子。这些片段随后由质谱在第二步进行分离和检测。该片段并非完整的蛋白质，需要由例如胰蛋白酶的蛋白酶消化为小肽。对于接受MS/MS分析的各肽，新的质谱分析可测定片段离子的m/z比例并通过与人类蛋白质数据库中预测性的多肽片段结合识别原代离子。这些片段同样适用于翻译后蛋白质的修饰研究。

ELISA是一种常用的检测特定蛋白质的实验室技术，可用于检测细胞因子、趋化因子以及血管形成及生长因子。该试验分析在96孔板上进行，价格低廉。通常96孔板上被覆目标抗体，样本随后滴入小孔中进行孵育，通过比色度变化可识别蛋白质。临床上，ELISA方法可用于分析来自人体的血液或其他体液中的循环蛋白。ELISA的缺点在于单次检测仅能分析单一分泌蛋白。尽管 ELISA 需要的样本量很小（50～100μL），但为了检测一系列蛋白质必须同时进行多次 ELISA 试验。

多种基于磁珠技术的检测与 ELISA 方法类似，可用于分析少量分泌蛋白质，但是，与 ELISA 相比，基于磁珠技术的检测的一大优势在于可最多同时检测 100 种蛋白质。该方法采用聚苯乙烯珠，内部由 2 种不同荧光进行染色，每个荧光具有 10 个不同的荧光强度，从而组成具有 100 个珠的组合。这种分析包含染色珠结合于特定的蛋白质或肽，例如细胞因子或磷酸化蛋白。100 个珠中每个均含有针对特定目标蛋白质的捕获抗体。抗体结合珠允许与样本相互作用并且随后进行检测，微孔上的抗体可与目标蛋白质发生免疫反应。多重分析通过混合珠集与不同连接蛋白质可实现单一样本的多种分析。这一技术也获得了广泛应用，并且效果可与 ELISA 媲美[48-50]。

基于血液标志物的蛋白质分析较其他检测方法具有一个重大优势，即样本取材容易且准备和储存简单，并且在治疗前、治疗中和治疗后均可获得，可识别抗癌治疗的可能获益人群，确定药物剂量并且明确耐药机制。该方法可基于基线特征和治疗过程中标志物的变化分析预测标志物、活性标志物和耐药标志物[51-53]。

识别、分离以及分析循环肿瘤细胞（circulating tumor cells, CTCs）对于肿瘤早期检测、快速监测肿瘤反应以及药物有效性具有一定作用，并最终阐明"转移先导"的特征。转移先导是一种现阶段尚未明确的肿瘤细胞亚组，针对该亚组的新型靶向治疗能有效阻止肿瘤转移[54-55]。然而迄今为止，由于细胞检测技术的限制，无法把基于 CTCs 的检测应用于诊断和治疗[56-57]。目前针对该亚组细胞进行研究的商业化机器名为 Cell Search 分析仪（Veridex 公司），该仪器采用针对连接于磁珠的特异性上皮黏附标志物 EpCAM 的抗体经过多步骤纯化固定细胞，而后在磁场环境下进行细胞分离[58-61]。尽管设计完美，但仅有 50% 的转移患者采用该方法可发现 CTCs，平均数为 1CTC/mL（cut-off 值为每 7.5mL 中有 5 个细胞），最终纯化率为每 1 000 个白细胞中有 1 个 CTC（0.1%）。即便如此，考虑到每 10 亿个血细胞中仅有 1 个 CTC 的现实，这仍是一项重大成果。采用该方法进行 CTCs 的分离和纯化灵敏度较低，尚不足以进行有效的临床动态监测，亦不能进行具体分子分析。因此，CTCs 目前推荐作为通用的预后因子，而不是直接用于监测或指导肿瘤的治疗[62]。

数据统计分析

不同样本在进行分子分析时存在大量有关 mRNA 或蛋白样本的信息。统计学计算可对具有相似表达特征的样本进行汇总分析。当与单一样本的生物学或临床数据例如化疗疗效、转移特性或生存相结合可分析分子与临床特征的相关性。尽管不同分析方法及分子分析定量方面存在差异，但数据分析的方法异常简单。第一步是在分析中去除可信度低的样本或数据变量，并去除表达较少或样本间变异度低的分子变量；而后采用多种分析方法明确具有统计学意义的分子或明确临床特征与测定分子变量的相关性，多数研究采用队列测定的方法明确两者的相关性。一项高度可信的队列可用于定义一系列的预测基因或蛋白质，而后再独立地测定集中明确这一模型的准确性，并且在队列和测定中样本无重叠[17]。

一旦选定样本和基因，就可采用一系列的统计学方法明确肿瘤生物学行为或潜在表型的基因或蛋白质表达。这些方法可简单地分为"管理性"和"非管理性"两大类。非管理性技术采用不包括非基因描述的基因表达数据以明确具有相似基因的亚组。管理性技术涵盖一种或多种临床特征（如病理类型、远处转移与否或临床预后），并且采用基因表达数据明确临床特征与基因表达两者间的相关性。

非管理性集合基于不同亚组可通过其不同表达谱完全区分这一假设进行分析，并且这种集合可呈现出既往尚未阐明的完全不同的生物学行为。聚类分析是一种常用的限定基因集合的方法，该方法可明确两个样本中基因表达的相关性，并且在聚类图中可清晰地显示潜在的类似基因表达。研究者根据聚类结果区分部分特定亚组并明确这些基因组是否与临床特征显著相关。通常采用 Kaplan-Meier 生存曲线分析比较特定亚组与其他组别在总生存时间或无病生存时间方面的区别。亚组中任一成员可通过特定聚类实验中两种肿瘤样本相同或不同的临界值进行区分。一个既定的临界值可区分两组患者，但是不能完全掌握各样本的基因变异。另外一种更加严格的临界值可区分更大样本的亚组，每个亚组包含更多一致性的表达基因，然而，这种方法观察具有统计学差异的基因表达存在困难，因为各组间患者例数更少，而且由于采用多种亚组分析增加了出现错误结论的概率。另一方面，如果新发现的临床特征具有显著统计学差异，相关数据会在前瞻性研究中进一步证实并且可用于指导个体化治疗。

管理性分类计划从两种或多种临床或生物学特征的亚组出发，例如淋巴结阴性与淋巴结阳性、有效与无效或特定突变存在与否，试图明确可预测这些特征的差异基因并对未知样本进行预测。可以采用类似于前文提到的聚类分析方法，但是必须依据目标临床变量限定两种主要聚类。当然，也可以采用统计学分析［例如 t 检验、方差分析（analysis of variance，ANOVA）］明确与目标临床变量相关的个体基因或蛋白质，并且通过对这些特征进行线性加权组合创建可预测未知基因的模型。

重复试验对于研究结果的意义非常重大。当对两组间数以千计的变量进行分析时，少数观察变异会存在假阳性。可采用多种分析方法进行多种比较检验并且预估出可能发现真正观察值的 P 值（或显著水平）。例如，常用的一种方法为 Bonferroni 检验，其中合理的 P 值（通常设定为 $P=0.05$ 意味着两组间无差异时检测出差异的概率为 1/20）由进行分析的变量数目确定。换言之，如果对两组患者间 10 000 个基因的 mRNA 表达进行分析时，P 值小于 0.05/1 000 的差异（等同于 $P=5\times10^{-6}$）认为存在统计学差异。这种方法使假阳性发生率最小化，但是存在将部分低于 P 临界值但存在真正差异的变量剔除的可能。另一种方法是采用 Benjamini-Hochberg 方法设定一个合理的错误发现率（false discovery rate，FDR），并且该值可以进行适当调整[63-64]，该合理 FDR（或者基因概率或假阳性允许的观察值）随后用于确定 P 值。例如，如果 5 000 个基因低于对应于 0.05FDR（或 5%）的特定 P 值，250 个基因可被认为是假阳性。这种方法依据可接受的假阳性率值允许更大的灵活性，而假阳性率值由试验目标及设计决定。

管理性和非管理性技术具有过度使用依据样本来源进行的样本产量模型数据的可能，但是在独立检验时准确率较低。因为即便有显而易见的相关性在对独立样本进行检验时也可能表现为非相关性，因此任何分子分析中结果的验证都是最重要的一步。

目前普遍认为高质量的临床样本难以获取并且收集及储存费用较高，临床数据随访耗费大量人力，因此，充分应用所有可能的样本对于多数规模较小的研究很有必要，并且需设定大样本对于小样本结论及非严格预测模型进行验证。此外，作为预测因子的基因很大程度上取决于研究队列中的患者[65]。交叉验证是一种可实现研究队列最大化并且仍可在大样本研究队列中验证结果的方法[66-67]，这种方法从数据集中划分为单一样本或小部分样本，其他样本用于创建预测模型。这种模型用于模拟创建时保留的样本，并且记录预测目标特征的准确性，然后在更大样本中进行多次验证，将所有保留样本的总准确率作为该模型可能的分类准确率。

验证结果所需样本数最小化的另一种方法为使用既往已发表的作为独立预测因子的基因表达在线数据库，这些数据库前文中已提到。随着技术标准化的快速进步，这种方法的吸引力逐步增加[68-72]，但是不同试验中数据集的有效融合是一个巨大的挑战。获取基因表达分析的方法或许存在显著差别，例如研究中采用不同公司的微阵列芯片，甚至来自于同一公司不同的微阵列生产设备生产的阵列都可能存在差别。甚至采用同一公司的新版芯片获取的关于同一基因的数据可能无法直接与采用早期版本芯片获取的数据进行比较分析。同样，与早期版本相比，新版微阵列含有更多的探针，涵盖更多的基因组分。因此，许多基因或许不能出现于共同的数据集中，并且将基因表达数据从一种转为另一种存在困难。随着外显子阵列的出现，转录数据中寡核苷酸的位置差别会出现不同的测定结果。此外，样本处理和试验流程中的特定差异可能导致基因表达集间的系统性差异。

尽管存在这些挑战，但多数研究表明，单一数据集中发现的相关性可在更大样本独立数据集中得到确认，当试图将过程标准化后，数据间的重复性相当好[68-71,73]。目前微阵列基础上的分析可能获益于各实验室间的标准化，对可控的错误或验证的关注（例如批量工作处理），以及尽管各实验室间存在区别但大数据集及数据融合分析的生物信息学工具不断发展，这些进展不但可对模型进行有效验证而且可进行大规模的 meta 分析以明确大样本数据集分子-临床的相关性，同时确定统计学把握度更高的分子特征。当然，不管队列和验证集的重复性如何，前瞻性临床试验中证实的分子分类中数据结论可明确其临床应用是否与患者的预后相关。

临床应用

大量数据的出现将会使肺癌的治疗在未来 5 年、10 年和 20 年发生巨大变化，而且我们很难想象这种变化的速度。现在，临床中最常用的临床分析也是一种会对临床决策产生即刻影响的方式，是进行肺癌组织 DNA 检测以确定突变或融合方式（通常是已确诊活检组织的福尔马林固定石蜡包埋标本）。同一反应中多种基因同时检测技术的出现使得小组织样本大量基因检测变得可行并且不增加费用。肿瘤基因套餐检测已经在诸多科研机构常规开展，并且由肿瘤学专家集体进行商业化分析。相应的，患者的肿瘤组织同样用于进行特定治疗疗效相关的 mRNA 和蛋白质表达水平分析。尽管多种检测的临床应用前景尚不明确，但是随着分子标志物指导下靶向治疗药物相关临床试验阳性结果的出现，部分检测方法可能会成为标准。除了药物选择相关预测性因子，分子分析可能影响临床决策的几个方面，包括早期检测和诊断、分组和分期以及监测。最后，分子检测技术的进步使得血液、唾液、尿液或者其他微创方式获得的样本分子分析成为可能。非肿瘤组织（例如血液基础上的）生物标志物检测方法的进步使得肿瘤组织较少、不能安全获得肿瘤组织以及不能重复检测（例如疾病进展或出现耐药时）患者的分子检测成为可能。

早期诊断与治疗

在早期诊断和治疗方面，外周血无疑是最易获得并且具有临床应用价值的标本。由于分泌蛋白细胞表达的改变，细胞死亡后直接释放于细胞外液，分裂所致的翻译后修饰及糖基化或宿主对疾病的反应，病理学水平可出现疾病相关的循环分子的变化。如果疾病存在的情况下血液蛋白组分的变化持续产生，那这种变化就有助于疾病的检测和诊断。例如，心肌梗死所致心肌细胞损伤后血液中的肌钙蛋白及其他蛋白可用于诊断心肌梗死并评估预后，虽然这些蛋白质并非自身存在。

肺癌患者生存时间短的原因之一是缺乏有效的早期诊断方法。以往高危人群中多种肺癌筛查方法均未对患者的生存时间产生影响，包括每年胸部 X 线检查、痰脱落细胞学检查以及支气管镜检查。然而，近期的一项大型随机临床试验证实，螺旋 CT 扫描可早期检测具有重度吸烟史高危人群的肺癌，而这种早期检测可延长患者的生存时间[74]。

部分试验预设对入组患者的血液和（或）痰标本进行分子分析，该分析方法可作为影像学研究的一种补充，提供分子标志物以识别肺癌的高危人群并协助进行肺癌的早期诊断，而早期诊断的肺癌易于根治。对于不吸烟的患者来说，这些无创性检测方法尤其重要，因为对于他们来说，肺癌发生率相对较低，但 CT 筛查的获益不足以弥补 CT 筛查中反复暴露于射线所带来的危害。

分子分类及分期

肺癌治疗方法的选择很大程度上依赖于疾病的分期以及组织学类型相关的生物学行为，而分期最有可能预测患者从何种治疗中获益。然而，相同的分期或组织学亚组患者的临床预后亦存在显著差异，部分肺癌患者的恶性程度更高，表现为转移潜能更大、更易出现疾病进展或对化疗产生耐药。阐明预测患者预后及治疗反应的因子有助于识别从强化治疗例如辅助化疗中获益的人群。

迄今为止，病理学方面最重要的内容在于区分 SCLC 与 NSCLC。两者可通过组织学及免疫组化进行区分，且在起源细胞、自然病程及对化疗反应性方面存在显著差异。NSCLC 亚组分类对患者的治疗影响较小，当然也有例外，例如非鳞状细胞癌中 EGFR 突变及 ALK 融合富集，非鳞状细胞癌的治疗中，与吉西他滨化疗相比，培美曲塞化疗有效率更高。但最有可能影响预后的行为特征——侵袭性、转移可能、凋亡耐药、治疗反应性，这些在传统显微镜下并不能进行区分，而这些特征可以决定潜在基因特征，并且揭示那些可能在肺癌治疗中产生巨大影响的分子。

其他肿瘤中的基因分析试验已经证实了部分基因的作用。例如，乳腺癌中采用 mRNA 表达分析已将乳腺癌分为可重复的 5 种基因型，并且对应于预后及治疗反应，其中基底细胞样或者"三阴性"预后最差[75-78]。其他表达研究证实存在可区分女性淋巴结阴性、激素受体阳性乳腺癌接受他莫昔芬治疗时预后的独立基因。临床上，Oncotype DX 分析是一种常用的 21-基因标志物，该标志物采用 RT-PCR 方法进行表达分析并预测最有可能从化疗中获益的人群[79-80]。

探索肺癌中有效预测因子的技术也已成熟。多项研究[24,26-27,46-47,81-94]已经采用与成功的乳腺癌及其他癌症研究相类似的方法识别具有总体相似基因及蛋白质表达谱的亚组。这些研究中入组患者数从 50 例至 200 例以上不等，并且随着商业芯片技术的进步，RNA 探针的数目在近期研究中逐步增多。

Bhattacharjee 等进行的早期研究证实多种临床及组织学类型存在天然基因的相似性[82]。正常肺组织可与肿瘤、NSCLC 与 SCLC 进行区分，腺癌、鳞状细胞癌、大细胞癌可在很大程度上区分为各自亚型。识别不同样本组织类型的差异并非是一种进步，但证实基因分析试验可进行有意义的分类。多项研究证实一种或多种组织学亚组样本存在富集现象[24,83,85,88-90,95-100]，这些结果表明，在主要组织学亚组中可能存在特定基因型亚组，而这些亚组间的生物学行为存在显著差异。近期的多项研究例如 TCGA 进行的肺鳞癌分析等证实了上述可能[11]。

肺癌中的部分特征或分子特征可作为预后预测因子[22,101]，这些可以是单独生物标志物（例如 EGFR 突变与总生存时间延长相关）或标志特征。例如，Beer 等采用微阵列分析方法对 86 例肺腺癌患者进行分析，发现该队列中存在 3 个主要富集区域，其中 1 个与其他预后因子存在显著差异[83]。已有研究报道特定患者人群例如接受辅助化疗者的预后相关特征，并且未来可能用于筛选最有可能从已知治疗中获益的患者[102]。此外，近期研究数据表明，这些分子异常可能与新型药物靶点的表达有关，例如非鳞状细胞癌患者的 DDR2 突变及 FGFR1 变异或 SCLC 患者的 PARP1 基因[10,46,103]。最后，对 mRNA 或蛋白表达水平及 DNA 水平异常的综合分析能提高我们对于潜在分子亚组如 LKB1 及 KRAS 突变的 NSCLC 生物学行为的分析能力，并促进存在常见基因异常患者新型药物治疗的进展[104-105]。

治疗选择

尽管多种化疗方案和（或）靶向治疗在肺癌治疗中具有确切的临床效应，但对于患者个体的疗效差异较大。对特定患者来说，选择最有效的治疗方案是分子分析的核心目标，尤其是考虑到持续治疗相关致死风险及无效治疗相关的机会/费用比等情况。对特定肿瘤进行分子分析以有效预测不同治疗相关临床获益将对患者的治疗产生深远影响。目前最典型的例子是采用 EGFR 突变及 ALK 融合识别最有可能从美国 FDA 批准的口服靶向治疗（分别为厄洛替尼及克唑替尼）获益的患者，已作为转移性 NSCLC 的主要治疗策略在 2012 年收入美国国立综合癌症网络指南。这些预测分子标志物及其在临床中的应用将在后续章节中进一步阐述。

除了 EGFR 及 ALK，发现了肺癌患者中的一系列新型驱动基因，包括 BRAF、PIK3CA、ROS1、RET 及 HER2（图 3.2），这些基因可抑制这些靶点的药物，或许对具有上述分子特征的患者（例如肿瘤中存在上述基因突变、融合或扩增的患者）具有生存获益。然而，因为每个驱动基因仅存在于部分 NSCLC 患者（如 1%~5%），即使是对多数患者具有疗效的药物，如果其活性未在相应分子亚组中进行分析（至少部分），临床试验也可能得出阴性结果。HER2 抑制剂（曲妥珠单抗、拉帕替尼）就存在上述情况，其对 HER2-扩增乳腺癌患者具有确切的临床疗效，并且是临床标准治疗方法，但这些药物的活性在未经选择的乳腺癌患者中缺少临床获益。

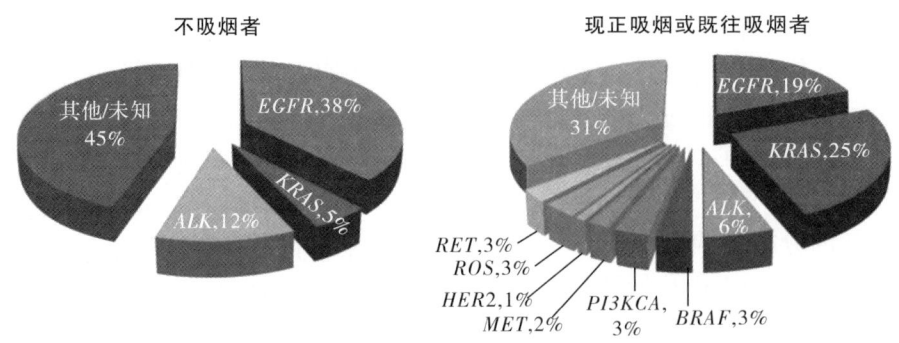

图 3.2 不吸烟者和现时吸烟或既往吸烟肺腺癌患者的不同突变谱。与现时吸烟或既往吸烟肺腺癌患者相比，EGFR 突变和其他靶向突变（如 ALK 融合）更常见于不吸烟者；然而 45% 的不吸烟者未发现驱动性突变。来源：摘自 Paik 等[108]。已获得 John Wiley 和 Sons 的许可

相反，部分无已知驱动性突变的患者仍可从靶向治疗中获益，关于疗效预测的分子标志物假说可能是不准确或不完整的。例如，近期的一项对复发、难治性 NSCLC 患者的研究发现，上皮间叶转化可预测患者正常的 EGFR 对 EGFR 抑制剂（厄罗替尼）的活性[47]。基于上述原因，临床试验设计——精心策划的相关生物标志物研究，对确保我们不会遗漏潜在活性药物或可从这些药物中获益的患者至关重要。标准治疗及临床试验中传统分子检测方法面临的挑战主要是需要足量的肿瘤组织及可获取的组织类型，例如多数活检标本为福尔马林固定石蜡包埋组织标本，尽管对于多数 DNA 分析石蜡标本不是问题，但问题在于石蜡标本用于例如基因表达及蛋白质组学分析等其他类型分析时具有明显的缺陷。此外，多项研究表明，肿瘤会发生分子水平的改变，尤其是治疗有效时。例如 Sequist 等的研究发现 EGFR 突变患者对 EGFR 抑制剂耐药后出现一系列耐药相关组织学或分子改变。重复活检标本证实耐药特征的存在（例如，耐药突变的出现、EGFR 基因 T790M 突变或 EMT 标志物的表达[106-107]）或许对于选择二线或后续治疗具有重要作用。因此，在疾病进展或出现获得性耐药时对患者的肿瘤细胞（或其他标本，例如血液）进行重复分子检测明确目前肿瘤的特征具有重要的临床意义。

总结与未来发展方向

在分析技术实现最大化潜能前仍存在诸多挑战。过去，多数肺癌研究的主要缺陷是所研究患者样本量较小不能得出可信的结论。然而，随着分子标志物数据库的公开、分子分析费用的降低以及对更小组织样本分析技术的进步，这些困难正逐步被克服。随着 DNA 测序及其他高通量平台的应用越来越广泛，分子信息学及计算机辅助工具需要持续改进以有效利用大量数据，在实验室间进行质量控制，并融合不同类型的分子数据（例如蛋白质组学及基因组学研究）。

某种预测性分析方法一旦出现并得到验证，就需要在临床中进行确认，这对于来自于细胞系、动物模型或平台有限的精密技术的相关结论尤其困难。分析一旦进行，将试图通过小样本研究并从潜在低质量的"真实世界"临床样本中获得临床疗效相关数据。对于 mRNA 标志物，实时定量 PCR 高度敏感并在临床中用于测定各基因的表达水平。此外，进行微阵列分析时，该技术同样适用于石蜡包埋组织标本，而不必限定为新鲜冰冻组织。对于高通量平台识别的蛋白标志物，免疫组化及 ELISA 均为快速将这些标志物转化至临床的潜在选择。

尽管存在许多挑战，但分子分析实验已经在肺癌中取得了可喜的成绩并逐步改变着肺癌患者的治疗。早期分子分析实验通过个体化危险分层及优化治疗选择的方式实现了其基本潜能。随着蛋白质组学及基因组学技术与数据分析方法的成熟，分子分析试验无疑会越来越多地应用于试验和患者的治疗中。分子分析中获得的信息及认知水平的提高，以及这些技术的进步必将导致肿瘤生物学的研究及临床肿瘤学的实践发生重大变革。

（危志刚　译）

参考文献

[1] Lander ES, Linton LM, Birren B, et al. Initial sequencing and analysis of the human genome. Nature, 2001, 409 (6822): 860-921.

[2] Venter JC, Adams MD, Myers EW, et al. The sequence of the human genome. Science, 2001, 291 (5507): 1304-1351.

[3] Lynch TJ, Bell DW, Sordella R, et al. Activating mutations in the epidermal growth factor receptor underlying responsiveness of non-small-cell lung cancer to gefitinib. N Engl J Med, 2004, 350 (21): 2129-2139.

[4] Paez JG, Janne PA, Lee JC, et al. EGFR mutations in lung cancer: correlation with clinical response to gefitinib therapy. Science, 2004, 304 (5676): 1497-1500.

[5] Fukuoka M, Yano S, Giaccone G, et al. Multi-institutional randomized phase II trial of gefitinib for previously treated patients with advanced non-small-cell lung cancer (The IDEAL 1 Trial) [corrected]. J Clin Oncol, 2003, 21 (12): 2237-2246.

[6] Inamura K, Takeuchi K, Togashi Y, et al. EML4-ALK lung cancers are characterized by rare other mutations, a TTF-1 cell lineage, an acinar histology, and young onset. Mod Pathol, 2009, 22 (4): 508-515.

[7] Kwak EL, Bang YJ, Camidge DR, et al. Anaplastic lymphoma kinase inhibition in non-small-cell lung cancer. N Engl J Med, 2010, 363 (18): 1693-1703.

[8] National Comprehensive Cancer Network. NCCN Guidelines on Non-Small Cell Lung Cancer V, 2013. www.nccn.org.

[9] Bergethon K, Shaw AT, Ou SH, et al. ROS1 rearrangements define a unique molecular class of lung cancers. J Clin Oncol, 2012, 30 (8): 863-870.

[10] Hammerman PS, Sos ML, Ramos AH, et al. Mutations in the DDR2 kinase gene identify a novel therapeutic target in squamous cell lung cancer. Cancer Discov, 2011, 1 (1): 78-89.

[11] Comprehensive genomic characterization of squamous cell lung cancers. Nature, 489 (7417): 519-525.

[12] Imielinski M, Berger AH, Hammerman PS, et al. Mapping the hallmarks of lung adenocarcinoma with massively parallel sequencing. Cell, 2012, 150 (6): 1107-1120.

[13] Rudin CM, Durinck S, Stawiski EW, et al. Comprehensive genomic analysis identifies SOX2 as a frequently amplified gene in small-cell lung cancer. Nat Genet, 2012, 44 (10): 1111-1116.

[14] NCBI. Gene Expression Omnibus, 2012. Available from: http://www.ncbi.nlm.nih.gov/geo/.

[15] Bioscience C. Oncomine, 2012. Available from: https://www.oncomine.org/resource/login.html.

[16] Cerami E, Gao J, Dogrusoz U, et al. The cBio cancer genomics portal: an open platform for exploring multidimensional cancer genomics data. Cancer Discov, 2012, 2 (5): 401-404.

[17] Ransohoff DF. Rules of evidence for cancer molecular-marker discovery and validation. Nat Rev Cancer, 2004, 4 (4): 309-314.

[18] Kris MG, Johnson BE, Kwiatkowski DG, et al. Identification of driver mutations in tumor specimens from 1 000 patients with lung adenocarcinoma: The NCI's Lung Cancer Mutation Consortium (LCMC). J Clin Oncol, 2011, 29 (suppl): abstr CRA7506.

[19] Thomas RK, Baker AC, Debiasi RM, et al. Hight-hroughput oncogene mutation profiling in human cancer. Nat Genet, 2007, 39 (3): 347-351.

[20] Wheeler DA, Srinivasan M, Egholm M, et al. The complete genome of an individual by massively parallel DNA sequencing. Nature, 2008, 452 (7189): 872-876.

[21] Kohno T, Ichikawa H, Totoki Y, et al. KIF5B-RET fusions in lung adenocarcinoma. Nat Med, 2012, 18 (3): 375-377.

[22] Lipson D, Capelletti M, Yelensky R, et al. Identification of new ALK and RET gene fusions from colorectal and lung cancer biopsies. Nat Med, 2012, 18 (3): 382-384.

[23] Feero WG, Guttmacher AE, Collins FS. Genomic medicine-an updated primer. N Engl J Med, 2010, 362 (21): 2001-2011.

[24] Chen G, Gharib TG, Wang H, et al. Protein profiles associated with survival in lung adenocarcinoma. Proc Natl Acad Sci USA, 2003, 100 (23): 13537-13542.

[25] Chen G, Gharib TG, Huang CC, et al. Discordant protein and mRNA expression in lung adenocarcinomas. Mol Cell Proteomics, 2002, 1 (4): 304-313.

[26] Shibata T, Uryu S, Kokubu A, et al. Genetic classification of lung adenocarcinoma based on array-based comparative genomic hybridization analysis: its association with clinicopathologic features. Clin Cancer Res, 2005, 11 (17): 6177-6185.

[27] Li R, Wang H, Bekele BN, et al. Identification of putative oncogenes in lung adenocarcinoma by a comprehen-

sive functional genomic approach. Oncogene, 2006, 25 (18): 2628-3635.

[28] Massion PP, Kuo WL, Stokoe D, et al. Genomic copy number analysis of non-small cell lung cancer using array comparative genomic hybridization: implications of the phosphatidylinositol 3 - kinase pathway. Cancer Res, 2002, 62 (13): 3636-3640.

[29] Weir BA, Woo MS, Getz G, et al. Characterizing the cancer genome in lung adenocarcinoma. Nature, 2007, 450 (7171): 893-898.

[30] Carthew RW, Sontheimer EJ. Origins and mechanisms of miRNAs and siRNAs. Cell, 2009, 136 (4): 642-655.

[31] Bartels CL, Tsongalis GJ. MicroRNAs: novel biomarkers for human cancer. Clin Chem, 2009, 55 (4): 623-631.

[32] Yanaihara N, Caplen N, Bowman E, et al. Unique microRNA molecular profiles in lung cancer diagnosis and prognosis. Cancer Cell, 2006, 9 (3): 189-198.

[33] Takamizawa J, Konishi H, Yanagisawa K, et al. Reduced expression of the let-7 microRNAs in human lung cancers in association with shortened postoperative survival. Cancer Res, 2004, 64 (11): 3753-3756.

[34] Lebanony D, Benjamin H, Gilad S, et al. Diagnostic assay based on hsa-miR-205 expression distinguishes squamous from nonsquamous non-small-cell lung carcinoma. J Clin Oncol, 2009, 27 (12): 2030-2037.

[35] Gibbons DL, Lin W, Creighton CJ, et al. Contextual extracellular cues promote tumor cell EMT and metastasis by regulating miR-200 family expression. Genes Dev, 2009, 23 (18): 2140-2151.

[36] Birney E, Stamatoyannopoulos JA, Dutta A, et al. Identification and analysis of functional elements in 1% of the human genome by the ENCODE pilot project. Nature, 2007, 447 (7146): 799-816.

[37] Schena M, Shalon D, Davis RW, et al. Quantitative monitoring of gene expression patterns with a complementary DNA microarray. Science, 1995, 270 (5235): 467-470.

[38] Churchill GA. Fundamentals of experimental design for cDNA microarrays. Nat Genet, 2002, 32 (Suppl): 490-495.

[39] Fodor SP, Read JL, Pirrung MC, et al. Light-directed, spatially addressable parallel chemical synthesis. Science, 1991, 251 (4995): 767-773.

[40] van't Veer LJ, Dai H, van de Vijver MJ, et al. Gene expression profiling predicts clinical outcome of breast cancer. Nature, 2002, 415 (6871): 530-536.

[41] Alizadeh AA, Eisen MB, Davis RE, et al. Distinct types of diffuse large B-cell lymphoma identified by gene expression profiling. Nature, 2000, 403 (6769): 503-511.

[42] DeRisi J, Penland L, Brown PO, et al. Use of a cDNA microarray to analyse gene expression patterns in human cancer. Nat Genet, 1996, 14 (4): 457-460.

[43] Wang SM, Rowley JD. A strategy for genome wide gene analysis: integrated procedure for gene identification. Proc Natl Acad Sci USA, 1998, 95 (20): 11909-11914.

[44] Wang Z, Gerstein M, Snyder M. RNA-Seq: a revolutionary tool for transcriptomics. Nat Rev Genet, 2009, 10 (1): 57-63.

[45] Nishizuka S, Charboneau L, Young L, et al. Proteomic profiling of the NCI-60 cancer cell lines using new high density reverse-phase lysate microarrays. Proc Natl Acad Sci USA, 2003, 100 (24): 14229-14234.

[46] Byers LA, Wang J, Nilsson MB, et al. Proteomic profiling identifies dysregulated pathways in small cell lung cancer and novel therapeutic targets including PARP1. Cancer Discov, 2012, 2 (9): 798-811.

[47] Byers LA, Diao L, Wang J, et al. An epithelial-mesenchymal transition gene signature predicts resistance to EGFR and PI3K inhibitors and identifies axl as a therapeutic target for overcoming EGFR Inhibitor resistance. Clin Cancer Res, 2013, 19 (1): 279-290.

[48] Skogstrand K, Thorsen P, Norgaard-Pedersen B, et al. Simultaneous measurement of 25 inflammatory markers and neurotrophins in neonatal dried blood spots by immunoassay with xMAP technology. Clin Chem, 2005, 51 (10): 1854-1866.

[49] Giavedoni LD. Simultaneous detection of multiple cytokines and chemokines from nonhuman primates using luminex technology. J Immunol Methods, 2005, 301 (1-2): 89-101.

[50] Dupont NC, Wang K, Wadhwa PD, et al. Validation and comparison of luminex multiplex cytokine analysis kits with ELISA: Determinations of a panel of nine cytokines in clinical sample culture supernatants. J Reprod Immunol, 2005, 66 (2): 175-191.

[51] Hanrahan EO, Heymach JV. Vascular endothelial growth factor receptor tyrosine kinase inhibitors vandetanib (ZD6474) and AZD2171 in lung cancer. Clin Cancer Res, 2007, 13 (15 Pt 2): s4617-s4622.

[52] Norden-Zfoni A, Desai J, Manola J, et al. Blood-based biomarkers of SU11248 activity and clinical outcome in patients with metastatic imatinib-resistant gastrointestinal stromal tumor. Clin Cancer Res, 2007, 13 (9): 2643-2650.

[53] Nikolinakos PG, Altorki N, Yankelevitz D, et al. Plasma cytokine and angiogenic factor profiling identifies markers associated with tumor shrinkage in early stage non-small cell lung cancer patients treated with pazopanib. Cancer Res, 2010, 70 (6): 2171-2179.

[54] Papadopoulos N, Kinzler KW, Vogelstein B. The role of companion diagnostics in the development and use of mutation-targeted cancer therapies. Nat Biotechnol, 2006, 24 (8): 985-995.

[55] Greenman C, Stephens P, Smith R, et al. Patterns of somatic mutation in human cancer genomes. Nature, 2007, 446 (7132): 153-158.

[56] Allard WJ, Matera J, Miller MC, et al. Tumor cells circulate in the peripheral blood of all major carcinomas but not in healthy subjects or patients with nonmalignant diseases. Clin Cancer Res, 2004, 10 (20): 6897-6904.

[57] Zieglschmid V, Hollmann C, Bocher O. Detection of disseminated tumor cells in peripheral blood. Crit Rev Clin Lab Sci, 2005, 42 (2): 155-196.

[58] Braun S, Marth C. Circulating tumor cells in metastatic breast cancer-toward individualized treatment? N Engl J Med, 2004, 351 (8): 824-826.

[59] Cristofanilli M, Budd GT, Ellis MJ, et al. Circulating tumor cells, disease progression, and survival in metastatic breast cancer. N Engl J Med, 2004, 351 (8): 781-791.

[60] Cristofanilli M, Hayes DF, Budd GT, et al. Circulating tumor cells: a novel prognostic factor for newly diagnosed metastatic breast cancer. J Clin Oncol, 2005, 23 (7): 1420-1430.

[61] Smerage JB, Hayes DF. The measurement and therapeutic implications of circulating tumour cells in breast cancer. Br J Cancer, 2006, 94 (1): 8-12.

[62] Smirnov DA, Zweitzig DR, Foulk BW, et al. Global gene expression profiling of circulating tumor cells. Cancer Res, 2005, 65 (12): 4993-4997.

[63] Storey JD, Tibshirani R. Statistical significance for genomewide studies. Proc Natl Acad Sci USA, 2003, 100 (16): 9440-9445.

[64] Benjamini Y, Hochberg Y. Controlling the false discovery rate: A practical and powerful approach to multiple testing. Journal of the Royal Statistical Society Series B (Methodological), 1995, 57 (1): 289-300.

[65] Michiels S, Koscielny S, Hill C. Prediction of cancer outcome with microarrays: A multiple random validation strategy. Lancet, 2005, 365 (9458): 488-492.

[66] Braga-Neto UM, Dougherty ER. Is crossvalidation valid for small-sample microarray classification? Bioinformatics, 2004, 20 (3): 374-380.

[67] Simon R, Radmacher MD, Dobbin K, et al. Pitfalls in the use of DNA microarray data for diagnostic and prognostic classification. J Natl Cancer Inst, 2003, 95 (1): 14-18.

[68] Canales RD, Luo Y, Willey JC, et al. Evaluation of DNA microarray results with quantitative gene expression platforms. Nat Biotechnol, 2006, 24 (9): 1115-1122.

[69] Guo L, Lobenhofer EK, Wang C, et al. Rat toxicogenomic study reveals analytical consistency across microarray platforms. Nat Biotechnol, 2006, 24 (9): 1162-1169.

[70] Shi L, Reid LH, Jones WD, et al. The MicroArray Quality Control (MAQC) project shows inter- and intraplatform reproducibility of gene expression measurements. Nat Biotechnol, 2006, 24 (9): 1151-1161.

[71] Shippy R, Fulmer-Smentek S, Jensen RV, et al. Using RNA sample titrations to assess microarray platform performance and normalization techniques. Nat Biotechnol, 2006, 24 (9): 1123-1131.

[72] Tong W, Lucas AB, Shippy R, et al. Evaluation of external RNA controls for the assessment of microarray performance. Nat Biotechnol, 2006, 24 (9): 1132-1139.

[73] Dobbin KK, Beer DG, Meyerson M, et al. Interlaboratory comparability study of cancer gene expression analysis using oligonucleotide microarrays. Clin Cancer Res, 2005, 11 (2 Pt 1): 565-572.

[74] Aberle DR, Adams AM, Berg CD, et al. Reduced lung-cancer mortality with low-dose computed tomographic screening. N Engl J Med, 2011, 365 (5): 395-409.

[75] Hu Z, Fan C, Oh DS, et al. The molecular portraits of breast tumors are conserved across microarray platforms. BMC Genomics, 2006, 7: 96.

[76] Perou CM, Sorlie T, Eisen MB, et al. Molecular portraits of human breast tumours. Nature, 2000, 406 (6797): 747-752.

[77] Sorlie T, Perou CM, Tibshirani R, et al. Gene expression patterns of breast carcinomas distinguish tumor subclasses with clinical implications. Proc Natl Acad Sci

[78] Sorlie T, Tibshirani R, Parker J, et al. Repeated observation of breast tumor subtypes in independent gene expression data sets. Proc Natl Acad Sci USA, 2003, 100 (14): 8418-8423.

[79] Paik S, Shak S, Tang G, et al. A multigene assay to predict recurrence of tamoxifen-treated, node-negative breast cancer. N Engl J Med, 2004, 351 (27): 2817-2826.

[80] Paik S, Tang G, Shak S, et al. Gene expression and benefit of chemotherapy in women with node-negative, estrogen receptorpositive breast cancer. J Clin Oncol, 2006, 24 (23): 3726-3734.

[81] Guo L, Ma Y, Ward R, et al. Constructing molecular classifiers for the accurate prognosis of lung adenocarcinoma. Clin Cancer Res, 2006, 12 (11 Pt 1): 3344-3354.

[82] Bhattacharjee A, Richards WG, Staunton J, et al. Classification of human lung carcinomas by mRNA expression profiling reveals distinct adenocarcinoma subclasses. Proc Natl Acad Sci USA, 2001, 98 (24): 13790-13795.

[83] Beer DG, Kardia SL, Huang CC, et al. Gene-expression profiles predict survival of patients with lung adenocarcinoma. Nat Med, 2002, 8 (8): 816-824.

[84] Creighton C, Hanash S, Beer D. Gene expression patterns define pathways correlated with loss of differentiation in lung adenocarcinomas. FEBS Lett, 2003, 540 (1-3): 167-170.

[85] Endoh H, Tomida S, Yatabe Y, et al. Prognostic model of pulmonary adenocarcinoma by expression profiling of eight genes as determined by quantitative real-time reverse transcriptase polymerase chain reaction. J Clin Oncol, 2004, 22 (5): 811-819.

[86] Garber ME, Troyanskaya OG, Schluens K, et al. Diversity of gene expression in adenocarcinoma of the lung. Proc Natl Acad Sci USA, 2001, 98 (24): 13784-13789.

[87] Hayes DN, Monti S, Parmigiani G, et al. Gene expression profiling reveals reproducible human lung adenocarcinoma subtypes in multiple independent patient cohorts. J Clin Oncol, 2006, 24 (31): 5079-5090.

[88] Takeuchi T, Tomida S, Yatabe Y, et al. Expression profiledefined classification of lung adenocarcinoma shows close relationship with underlying major genetic changes and clinicopathologic behaviors. J Clin Oncol, 2006, 24 (11): 1679-1688.

[89] Talbot SG, Estilo C, Maghami E, et al. Gene expression profiling allows distinction between primary and metastatic squamous cell carcinomas in the lung. Cancer Res, 2005, 65 (8): 3063-3071.

[90] Tomida S, Koshikawa K, Yatabe Y, et al. Gene expressionbased, individualized outcome prediction for surgically treated lung cancer patients. Oncogene, 2004, 23 (31): 5360-5370.

[91] Yanagisawa K, Shyr Y, Xu BJ, et al. Proteomic patterns of tumour subsets in non-small-cell lung cancer. Lancet, 2003, 362 (9382): 433-439.

[92] Nanjundan M, Byers LA, Carey MS, et al. Proteomic profiling identifies pathways dysregulated in non-small-cell lung cancer and an inverse association of AMPK and adhesion pathways with recurrence. J Thorac Oncol, 2010, 5 (12): 1894-1904.

[93] Wilkerson MD, Yin X, Walter V, et al. Differential pathogenesis of lung adenocarcinoma subtypes involving sequence mutations, copy number, chromosomal instability, and methylation. PLoS One, 2012, 7 (5): e36530.

[94] Wilkerson MD, Yin X, Hoadley KA, et al. Lung squamous cell carcinoma mRNA expression subtypes are reproducible, clinically important, and correspond to normal cell types. Clin Cancer Res, 2010, 16 (19): 4864-4875.

[95] Blackhall FH, Wigle DA, Jurisica I, et al. Validating the prognostic value of marker genes derived from a non-small cell lung cancer microarray study. Lung Cancer, 2004, 46 (2): 197-204.

[96] Wigle DA, Jurisica I, Radulovich N, et al. Molecular profiling of non-small cell lung cancer and correlation with disease-free survival. Cancer Res, 2002, 62 (11): 3005-3008.

[97] Borczuk AC, Gorenstein L, Walter KL, et al. Non-small-cell lung cancer molecular signatures recapitulate lung developmental pathways. Am J Pathol, 2003, 163 (5): 1949-1960.

[98] Larsen JE, Pavey SJ, Passmore LH, et al. Expression profiling defines a recurrence signature in lung squamous cell carcinoma. Carcinogenesis, 2007, 28 (3): 760-766.

[99] Raponi M, Zhang Y, Yu J, et al. Gene expression signatures for predicting prognosis of squamous cell and adenocarcinomas of the lung. Cancer Res, 2006, 66 (15): 7466-7472.

[100] Yamagata N, Shyr Y, Yanagisawa K, et al. A training-testing approach to the molecular classification of resec-

ted non-small cell lung cancer. Clin Cancer Res, 2003, 9 (13): 4695-4704.

[101] Xie Y, Xiao G, Coombes KR, et al. Robust gene expression signature from formalin-fixed paraffin-embedded samples predicts prognosis of non-small-cell lung cancer patients. Clin Cancer Res, 2011, 17 (17): 5705-5714.

[102] Zhu CQ, Ding K, Strumpf D, et al. Prognostic and predictive gene signature for adjuvant chemotherapy in resected non-small-cell lung cancer. J Clin Oncol, 2010, 28 (29): 4417-4424.

[103] Weiss J, Sos ML, Seidel D, et al. Frequent and focal FGFR1 amplification associates with therapeutically tractable FGFR1 dependency in squamous cell lung cancer. Sci Transl Med, 2010, 2 (62): 62ra93.

[104] Fernandez P, Carretero J, Medina PP, et al. Distinctive gene expression of human lung adenocarcinomas carrying LKB1 mutations. Oncogene, 2004, 23 (29): 5084-5091.

[105] Sanchez-Cespedes M, Parrella P, Esteller M, et al. Inactivation of LKB1/STK11 is a common event in adenocarcinomas of the lung. Cancer, 2002, 62 (13): 3659-3662.

[106] Sequist LV, Waltman BA, Dias-Santagata D, et al. Genotypic and histological evolution of lung cancers acquiring resistance to EGFR inhibitors. Sci Transl Med, 2011, 3 (75): 75ra26.

[107] Zhang Z, Lee JC, Lin L, et al. Activation of the AXL kinase causes resistance to EGFR-targeted therapy in lung cancer. Nat Genet, 2012, 44 (8): 852-860.

[108] Paik PK, Johnson ML, D'Angelo SP, et al. Driver mutations determine survival in smokers and never-smokers with stage IIIB/IV lung adenocarcinomas. Cancer, 2012, 118 (23): 5840-5847.

第4章
人类肺癌体细胞基因组的改变

Marcin Imielinski[1], Peter S. Hammerman[1], Roman Thomas[2], Matthew Meyerson[1]
1. Broad Institute of Harvard and MIT, Cambridge, MA, USA
2. Department of Translational Genomics, Center of Integrated Oncology Köln-Bonn, University of Köln, Köln, Germany

肺癌基因概述

本章节将分别对肺腺癌、肺鳞状细胞癌（简称肺鳞癌）及小细胞肺癌（SCLC）的特异性基因改变进行综述分析。分别讨论肺癌基因组常见的基因特征——尤其是常见的体细胞突变，以及相对少见的家族性或生殖性病因，并识别基因靶向治疗相关的驱动基因。

肺癌的典型特征为罕见的高频体细胞突变（仅见于肿瘤细胞而非生殖源性或其他细胞或组织）、高水平染色体内或染色体间重排，以及常见的染色体水平及区域拷贝数变异[1-5]。与黑色素瘤相同，肺癌同样存在最高频体细胞突变[5-6]——这两种肿瘤类型均具有特征性DNA损伤突变，黑色素瘤表现为紫外线相关损伤，肺癌表现为烟草暴露相关致癌性改变。

此外，肺癌处于肿瘤基因组靶向治疗改革的核心。对于肺腺癌，针对表皮生长因子受体酪氨酸激酶基因EGFR[7-9]和间变性淋巴瘤基因ALK[10-12]的靶向治疗，均证实具有显著临床获益。对于肺鳞癌来说，多种靶向治疗相关基因变异的发现同样为直接靶向治疗提供了良好前景。最后，对于SCLC，综合分析已经识别了一系列的基因改变，但是多数患者靶向治疗的前景尚不明朗。

对于所有类型的肺癌，系统性基因组相关研究均证实已知基因变异，同时也发现了新的基因变异：蛋白激酶信号转导通路、常见TP53突变及非整倍性包括细胞周期和染色体修饰及细胞分裂相关的周期性突变。认识肺癌信号通路上这些改变类型的作用对于靶向治疗的发展和进步至关重要，当了解肺癌相关高频突变负荷时有助于免疫调整治疗的进展。

肺腺癌基因组

肺腺癌是最常见的肺癌类型，并且是人类上皮源性恶性肿瘤基因特征最多的肿瘤之一。近年来，关于肺腺癌体细胞突变特征的研究众多并逐步转向治疗靶点，从而影响患者的治疗选择。

与其他肿瘤类似，对肺癌体细胞变异特征的研究大致可分为3个阶段。第一个阶段来自于细胞遗传学、病毒学以及系谱研究，这些早期研究采用转化、克隆及靶向测序的方法阐明与肺癌发生相关的特定基因变异，包括Ras家族（KRAS、NRAS、HRAS）、TP53、CDKN2A及其他基因突变[13-21]。2001年人类基因组测序的完成[22-23]显著提高了靶向基因分析的可行性，预示着第二个研究阶段的到来，这一阶段包括EGFR治疗敏感性突变[24-26]、ERBB2[27]及BRAF突变[28-30]、ALK融合[31-32]以及STK11[33]与SMARCA4突变[34-35]。

在过去的10年间，高通量分子基因技术的进步，包括微阵列芯片及大规模平行测序的发展，促进了癌症基因的变革[36-40]。该研究的第三个阶段促进了大规模体细胞改变的发展，这些体细胞改变包括肺腺癌肿瘤样本相关的基因表达、拷贝数变异、重排和（或）突变[41-47]。大量关于肺腺癌组织及对应正常组织的大规模平行测序研究包括外显子组、基因组及转录组的开展同样具有重要作用[2-4,48-52]。

基因组关联研究提供了肿瘤病理分类分子特征的概况，并可提供肿瘤逃避假说相关的再发性基因变异。第 3 个阶段的相关发现包括系谱特异性转录因子基因 NKX2-1 的局部扩增[45,47,53-54]、受体酪氨酸激酶基因 RET 及 ROS1 相关的复发融合基因[4,31,55-58]以及既往尚未阐明的肿瘤基因及通路上的基因变异（U2AF1、RBM10、ARID1A、SETD2）。

肺腺癌分子变异谱

肺腺癌分子变异是人类肿瘤中发生最多的，不论是体细胞突变的频率、广泛程度，发生局部拷贝数变异、重排，还是基因表达改变。肺腺癌每个外显子碱基含有 12 个体细胞突变（碱基替换或小插入/缺失）[2-3,50]，26 个区域复发水平臂扩增或缺失（跨度为半个基因组），31 个区域复发性局部拷贝数获得或缺失[47]，以及 98 个可检测重排断裂点。

肺腺癌基因的复杂性决定了区分癌症发生相关变异（如驱动基因）及潜在变异机制的旁路因子（如过路基因）的重要性。事实上，基因活化及灭活的所有已知机制均在肺腺癌中发挥重要作用：肺腺癌基因可能集合异常数目的截断突变（如 NF1）[44]或特定密码子区域周围的特异性突变（如 KRAS G12V）[59]。它们可能通常局部扩增至较高拷贝数（如 NKX2-1）[45,47,53-54]或表现为纯合子删除（如 PTEN）[47,60]，也可能经历复发性基因融合，而这些融合可能保持编码蛋白的关键催化区域（如 ALK）[31-32]。它们可以通过启动子甲基化（如 CDKN2A）、选择性剪切（如 MET）或上调转录因子（如 MYC）的活性实现转录抑制。尽管具有上述改变，但大多数肺腺癌基因异常尤其是 DNA 水平的异常是中性的。泛基因组数据进行统计学分析时必须准确校准以区分肿瘤内中性基因改变及体细胞突变选择[3]。

全球分子分析可将肺腺癌病例进行分组并发现复杂特征来预测患者的预后，这一方法首先在微阵列相关基因表达分析中进行探讨。最早该类分析采用非监测性方法将肺腺癌病例进行分组，并且观察相应分组表现出的不同生存情况及分子病理学特征[41,43,61]。一种复杂的分析方法已将肺腺癌分为 3 种以重复基因表达为基础的类别：支气管、鳞状以及大细胞型[62]。其他研究采用监测性方法进行基因表达基础上的预后分类，其中，Shedden 等采用多盲法回顾性分析 442 例患者以粗略区分基因表达基础上的总生存相关预后因子[46]，该方法针对介导细胞增殖、分化及免疫功能的信号通路上数以百计的基因表达区分侵袭性或惰性肺腺癌。该方法对于联系临床及病理因素有效。

应用以 DNA 变异为基础的特征如点突变已经用于对肺腺癌分组。例如，吸烟者及不吸烟者因具有不同背景特异性突变率，所以通常区分对待。通常，不吸烟者中的肺腺癌比吸烟者具有更高的基因突变率，其中多数出现 CpG 岛区域胞嘧啶去氨基化［C（pG）→T］。相反，重度吸烟者的肿瘤更多存在 C→A 转换，可在 CpG 岛区域内或区域外[2-3]，C→A 被认为来自于烟草摄入的细胞周期蛋白胺碳氢化合物[63]。吸烟者及不吸烟者在驱动性改变特征（后续将讨论）方面存在显著差异，而这些驱动性改变可表现为完全不同的疾病[64]。不吸烟的肺腺癌患者更容易在激酶区域出现 EGFR 及 ERBB2 突变，ALK、RET 及 ROS1 重排，然而吸烟的肺腺癌患者通常存在 KRAS、TP53 及 STK114 突变。

部分信号通路中肺腺癌关键基因变异

临床样本及（多数）癌症试验模型已证实肺腺癌（或其他病理类型）的关键基因变异具有重要作用[36-37,65-67]。该模型包括良性及恶性细胞系，该模型中过表达某一基因的突变形式或敲除该基因，然后进行增殖分析或观察锚定于细胞培养基中独立生长或在裸鼠体内的移植瘤形成情况。这些模型同样包括基因导向性小鼠，这些小鼠中突变基因稳定整合于生殖基因组中并且持续在组织特异性启动子作用下表达及增殖，然后表现为特定行为（例如降低肿瘤潜伏期）。对于多数这些关键变异，连接特定基因改变与细胞内过程例如肿瘤生长、迁移及凋亡的生物化学模型的具体信号通路已经阐明。部分情况下，已发展出了针对肺腺癌相关基因及通路的靶向治疗，其中临床疗效最显著的是针对 EGFR 突变[7-8,68]及 ALK 重排[10-12]的小分子抑制剂。

增殖通路

生长与增殖是细胞内的精密调节过程,该过程中恶性肿瘤持续活化[36-37,65-67]。肺腺癌通过 MAPK 通路、PI3K/mTOR 通路及 c-Myc 的增殖活化该信号通路。这些通路已作为肺腺癌的治疗靶点进行了诸多研究,但仅有部分证实具有临床应用价值[69-71]。

良性肿瘤中 MAPK 通路调节增殖,该过程中受体首先与细胞外配体结合,而后出现受体酪氨酸激酶同源或异源二聚化,最后通过小 G 蛋白 Ras 及 Raf、Mek 及 Erk 丝氨酸及苏氨酸激酶介导级联反应。

北美 10%~20% 的肺腺癌患者(亚洲 30%~50%)存在受体酪氨酸激酶基因 EGFR 激酶区域突变[24-26,72]。主要为 18 外显子 G719A 突变,第 746 位氨基酸近 ELREA 19 外显子缺失突变,20 外显子框移插入,21 外显子 L858R 突变,这些突变位点多数可引起激酶持续活化。靶向于 EGFR 的抑制剂如小分子厄洛替尼及吉非替尼对 EGFR 突变具有确切疗效[24-26],但外显子 20 的插入突变除外[73]。EGFR 区域扩增可与 EGFR 激酶区域突变同时存在;然而,EGFR 扩增与抗 EGFR 治疗相关小分子抑制剂(如厄洛替尼)或抗体相关药物(如西妥昔单抗)的敏感性无关。

在另外 2%~3% 的肺腺癌患者中相应的酪氨酸激酶基因 ERBB2 同样存在细胞外或激酶区域的点突变及框移突变[27,44,74]。尽管初始细胞相关研究证实,突变与抗 Erbb-2 抗体(曲妥珠单抗)或小分子 Erbb2 抑制剂(拉帕替尼、来那替尼、阿法替尼)的疗效具有相关性,但临床证实这些突变与药物作用无关[74-77]。

肺腺癌患者尤其是非吸烟者中有 3%~8% 存在受体酪氨酸激酶基因重排[31-32,48,55-58]。酪氨酸激酶 ALK、RET 及 ROS1 的保留激酶活性的 3′区域存在重排并与 5′端至少 6 个不同基因进行融合,包括 EML4、CCD6 及 KIF5B[31,32,48,55-58]。这些由上述基因 5′端蛋白编码的蛋白以同源二聚化的方式结合并发挥正常细胞功能,从而保证这些融合蛋白产物具有原癌活性。存在 ALK 融合的患者使用 ALK 抑制剂克唑替尼具有显著疗效[11],同样对于存在 ROS1 重排的患者亦有疗效[55]。关于肺癌细胞系存在 RET1 融合的早期研究证实,多种激酶抑制剂包括 RET 特异性小分子凡德他尼具有活性[57]。

吸烟的肺腺癌患者的 MAPK 信号通路活化最常见的机制为 RAS 家族基因第 12、13 及 61 位氨基酸的替代性突变[14,16-17,78-79]。这些突变主要为 KRAS 突变(20%~30%),同样也可以是 NRAS 及 HRAS 突变[<(1%~2%)]。Ras 蛋白在细胞内发生从无活性 GDP 结合形式向活性 GTP 结合形式的转变,后者可通过热点突变的形式持续存在并消除 Ras 的内在 GTP 酶活性。目前临床尚无靶向于 RAS 突变的药物,尽管既往研究采用法尼基转移酶(farnesyltransferase)抑制剂,但近期研究多采用针对下游 Mek 蛋白的小分子抑制剂[80]。

肺腺癌可通过 NF1 无活性突变或缺失方式获得 Ras 持续活性。NF1 编码一种关键 GTP 酶活性蛋白,该蛋白将 Ras 转变为无活性 GDP 结合状态[81]。NF1 缺失及截断突变见于 10%~20% 的肺腺癌患者,以吸烟者最为常见[3,44,49]。

BRAF 编码 MAPK 通路上 Ras 的第一个效应器,在 5%~10% 肺腺癌患者中存在两个热点突变,分别位于 G469 及邻近 V600 区域(V600E)[3,28,30,44,49]。尽管在黑色素瘤中 V600E 突变对于突变特异性 B-raf 抑制剂维罗非尼(vemurafenib)高度敏感,但在肺腺癌中尚未证实 BRAF 突变与维罗非尼具有相关性。尽管活性 MEK 突变(p.K57N)在该病中曾进行过描述(<1%),但另外两个在 MAPK 信号通路上的激酶在肺腺癌中的突变率较低[84]。其他已报道的 MAPK 通路突变包括 MET 接合突变[52,85],Ntrk 基因家族点突变(NTRK1、NTRK2、NTRK3)、PTPN11 点突变[44,52,86]。

受体酪氨酸激酶活化有 PI3K 介导的细胞内二级信号通路[87-88]。该通路依据周围营养环境由一个高度保守的真核机制进行生长控制,并且与 mTOR 通路存在相关性[89]。PIK3CA 编码 110KdPI3K 催化亚基,5%~10% 的肺腺癌患者中存在突变或局部扩增[3,44,49]。多数突变位于外显子 9 及外显子 20 这两个热点区域,可介导持续的激酶活性及第二信使因子 PtdIns(3、4、5)P_3,后者可活化下游信号因子 Akt。

肺腺癌 PI3K 信号通路活化的第二种机制为

Pten 缺失或突变性失活[3,44,47,49]。Pten 是一种液体磷酸酶，可引起 PtdIns（3、4、5）P_3 水解从而逆转 PI3K 引起的反作用性催化。PTEN 缺失或突变性失活见于 2%～8% 的肺腺癌患者。Akt 作为 PI3K 的下游因子，存在少见的 N-末端持续活化性突变，该突变为 E17K，见于不足 1% 的肺腺癌患者[44,49]。Akt 活化的致癌作用可通过 mTOR 进行介导，该活性可通过药物雷帕霉素（rapamycin）及其化学诱导剂进行抑制。PIK3CA 及 PTEN 突变肺腺癌采用针对 PI3K、Akt 或 mTOR 的小分子抑制剂相关临床试验目前正在进行中[90]。

5%～15% 的肺腺癌存在局部或高水平 MYC 扩增[3,47,91]。MYC 编码转录因子 c-Myc 通常与细胞增殖的启动及细胞培养时纤溶酶重组后的生存模式相关[65-66]。已证实 c-Myc 的生物学作用范围更广泛：该基因直接调节高达 15% 的人类基因，目前被认为是一种全面的放大器或转录因子[92]。c-Myc 同样是 MAPK 信号通路的关键下游转录因子之一，尽管 MYC 扩增与 MAPK 通路突变不存在突变互斥[3]。

细胞周期及 TP53 回路

肺腺癌（及人类肿瘤）中最常见的突变基因是 TP53[3,44,49]。TP53 编码一种转录因子，该转录因子可促进 DNA 损伤、缺氧、代谢性应激状态下细胞死亡及细胞周期阻滞[93]。TP53 介导的基因上调同样催化 DNA 修复，促进自噬，阻碍糖酵解，促进有氧呼吸，降低活性需氧物种的水平并促进肝细胞分化。超过 50% 的患者存在 TP53 截断、接合或缺失突变[3,44,49]。TP53 突变缺失肺腺癌通常含有变异蛋白，而这些蛋白可与 TP53 直接结合：7%～10% 的肺腺癌存在 ATM 突变[3,44,49]，该突变编码一种 DNA 损伤感受器和细胞周期监测点激酶，该激酶可通过磷酸化作用活化 TP53；6%～8% 的患者存在 MDM2 的局部或高水平扩增，MDM2 可编码在蛋白连接酶靶向于 TP53 的降解。尽管肺腺癌中 TP53 基因区域直接或间接基因损害的普遍存在使得其成为有吸引力的治疗靶点，但直接针对该通路的药物研究极具挑战性。在 TP53 突变肿瘤中保留 TP53 功能（通过基因重组或原始蛋白构象稳定）或靶向于致死性合成脆弱点（如 G2 检查点废除）无显著临床获益。

细胞周期通路中，TP53 连接作用通常由于体细胞基因改变抑制 Rb 蛋白而出现调节异常，Rb 是一种基因转录抑制因子，可加速 G1 细胞周期的程序[65-67]。RB1 是编码 Rb 的基因，在 3%～4% 的肺腺癌患者中存在突变并且靶点拷贝数缺失见于另外 10%～20% 的患者[3,44,47]。此外，Rb 更多地因 p16/CDKN2A 的基因缺失失活，而 p16/CDKN2A 通过抑制 Rb 磷酸化介导 G1 细胞周期阻滞。CDKN2A 在 10%～30% 的肺腺癌患者中存在缺失或突变性失活，包括 5% 的患者发生截断或缺失突变[3,18-19,44,47]。相反，CDK4、CCND1 及 CCNE1 扩增（10%～20%）[47]促进 Rb 磷酸化并加速 G1 细胞周期进程。研究显示，Rb 同样与来源于 TGF-Beta 通路的上游细胞外生长抑制因子相互作用，2%～4% 的肺腺癌患者中该通路通常由于 SMAD4 突变发生静默[3]。

生存能力回路

肺腺癌中最常见的局部拷贝数改变是 NKX2-1（10%～20%）[45,47,53-54]。定位于染色体 14q13.3 的 NKX2-1（亦称 TITF1），可编码一种转录因子，该转录因子对于位于肺腺泡中的 II 型肺泡上皮细胞至关重要。这些特征表明 NKX2-1 或许是一种线形特异性生存因子。初始细胞系研究表明 NKX2-1 对于表达 NKX2-1 的肺癌细胞系锚定独立生长是必需的，因此推断其具有原癌活性。然而，近期转基因小鼠模型相关研究表明，在特定背景下 NKX2-1 或可表现为肺癌肿瘤抑制基因[94]。

肺腺癌中另外一个活化信号介导氧化应激下的生存。KEAP1 编码一种富含半胱氨酸且具有氧化还原作用的感受器蛋白，该蛋白可与转录因子 NRF2 结合并以其作为靶点进行变换中的降解[95]。氧化应激破坏 KEAP1-NRF2 的结合，导致 NRF2 转位于细胞核并完成压力下生存启动基因的转录，KEAP1 突变常见于肺腺癌中（11%）[3,49,96]，并且推测可能会破坏 KEAP1-NRF2 复合体并促进氧化应激状态下的生存。KEAP1 及 NFE2L2 基因突变更常见于肺鳞癌，详见下文[1,97]。尽管大量证据表明 KEAP1 是肺癌及其他类型肿瘤的一个突变靶点，但 KEAP1 变异的致瘤性尚需在细胞及动物肿

能动性回路

肺腺癌中更常见的序列变异之一为丝氨酸-苏氨酸蛋白激酶11（也称Lkb1）的缺失[33]。靶向于STK11的截断突变及缺失见于15%~35%的肺腺癌患者，并且主要见于吸烟者[3,49]。STK11对于介导细胞代谢、生长及极性的14种结构相关Lkb1依赖性激酶的催化活性必不可少[98]。这些靶点包括AMPK，AMPK是一种多功能蛋白激酶，可通过TP53依赖性通路介导凋亡（细胞去除相关凋亡）从而抑制mTOR及SIK1。NSCLC的KRAS突变小鼠模型证实STK11敲除加速成瘤及转移过程[99]。这些结果表明，STK11缺失同其他基因区域协同在肿瘤形成的多个阶段调节肿瘤浸润、转移及分化过程。

APC通路连接细胞黏附及生长和增殖过程[100]。这一通路通过CTNNB1（编码β-联蛋白）活性突变及APC（结肠腺瘤性息肉病）截断性突变和缺失可作为肺腺癌的靶点。β-联蛋白通常隐于黏附接头内或作为包含APC"破坏复合物"的降解靶点，该复合物通过N-端4个丝氨酸或苏氨酸残基磷酸化发挥作用。近期发现肺腺癌上述残基中存在CTNNB1突变（1%~2%）或APC功能缺失性改变（3%~5%）[3,44,49]。这些改变可保证β-联蛋白转移到核内并且活化转录程序，从而促进浸润、转移及增殖。

表观遗传修饰通路

表观遗传修饰作为一种基因类型，近期发现在肺腺癌及其他肿瘤类型中存在突变[101-102]。10%的肺腺癌存在SMARCA4截断和（或）缺失突变，该基因可编码SWI/SNF复合物（又称为BRG1）的ATP酶亚单位[34-35]。SWI/SNF复合物可促进靶基因的静默及活化，包括信号通路相关基因介导的细胞周期检查点控制、细胞迁移、增殖及胚胎性干细胞程序化。肺癌原癌基因诱发小鼠模型中SMARCA4敲除增加肿瘤的数目及大小[103]。近期已发现肺腺癌存在另外一种SWI/SNF复合物ARID1A（10%）及组蛋白甲基化基因SETD2（13%）的截断或缺失突变[3]。RNA结合蛋白是另外一种基因类别，近期在基因组广泛性体细胞突变分子中作为一种重要突变。U2AF1编码U2剪切体的一个核心部分，并且近期在3%~5%的肺腺癌[3]以及50%以上脊髓发育不良综合征的患者中[104]发现存在特定密码子（p.S34F）的突变。RBM10是一种特征不明显的RNA结合蛋白，在7%的肺腺癌中存在截断性及缺失突变，可作为治疗靶点。RBM10、U2AF1、SETD2及ARID1A变异尚未在细胞系或动物模型中得到证实。此外，这些后生性及衔接性调节因子影响肿瘤发生的生物化学机制尚需进一步完整阐述。

药物敏感性及耐药相关基因

2004年EGFR突变与厄洛替尼敏感相关性的发现标志着肺腺癌进入靶向治疗新时代[24,26,105]。随后2010年ALK融合与克唑替尼敏感性的发现进一步推动了靶向治疗新模式的发展[10-12]。目前进行的探索针对BRAF、HER2、PI3K、AKT、MEK及MET等靶点的临床试验均在特定患者亚组中采用此种治疗模式[106]。

限制肿瘤患者靶向治疗广泛应用的问题主要是耐药性[69]。接受EGFR抑制剂治疗的患者无疑存在显著的生存获益，但是，肿瘤最终出现耐药，通常表现为新型体细胞突变和（或）组织类型改变[107]。约50%的肿瘤患者发生耐药后存在EGFR"闸门"区域p.T790位点转变为甲硫氨酸从而阻止药物结合[108-109]。少数患者发生新型变异，包括MET扩增[110]。有趣的是，部分患者（14%）发生病理性改变并最终转变为SCLC[107]。类似的克唑替尼治疗后ALK基因发生二次突变（p.C1196M、C1156Y）亦有报道，然而ALK/克唑替尼相关的耐药性改变谱尚未完全阐明[111-113]。

上述例子表明，肿瘤分子基因（和靶向治疗）下一步可能涉及基因型的动态改变，换言之，必须考虑数个周期治疗后的基因改变。靶向治疗后新型选择性压力相关的肿瘤基因组可能涉及新型基因改变，并且需要变更治疗药物。未来肺腺癌患者或需要接受动态活检并且接受特殊设计的多种靶向治疗药物以防止发生耐药。作为一种统计及观察科学，未来临床肿瘤基因需要设计动态预测模型以评估体细胞改变与靶向药物治疗的相关性[114]。

种系倾向

目前关于肺癌基因的讨论主要涉及患者生命历程中的体细胞基因变异。截至目前,关于肺癌遗传风险相关的基因调节因子尚未阐明。当前GWAS采用SNP序列对大样本病例对照研究进行分析以明确多种复杂遗传性疾病(包括肿瘤)的共同基因变异[115-116]。

采用GWAS方法对欧洲人群的分析发现,多组独立队列中存在可重复的3个相关富集基因座(15q25.1、5p15.33及6p21.33)。与这些基因座相关的基因包括 CHRNA5、CHRNA3、CHRNB4 (15q25.1)、TERT、CLPTM1L (5p15.33)及 BAT3-MSH5 (6p21.33)[117-122]。15q25.1相关基因编码尼古丁乙酰胆碱受体亚单位,该亚单位表达于神经元及肺泡细胞中并且已知与尼古丁及其变异体结合。既往研究表明,该区域的变异体与尼古丁成瘾相关,但是这些变异对于肿瘤易感性的影响与吸烟行为无关。

采用GWAS方法对东亚人群进行分析发现,除了欧洲人群中发现的易感区域,仍有多个人群特异性风险相关基因座:韩国及日本人中存在3个基因座:3q28(近 TP63)、17q24(近 BPTF)及6p21.3(近 BTNL2),这些似乎有人群特异性[123-124]。中国汉族人中已发现在近13q12.12(仅 MIPEP 及 TNFRSF19)及22q12.2(近 MTMR3、HORMAD2、LIF)区域存在其他基因座[125]。肺癌基因组中最明显的现象之一为东亚不吸烟女性的肺癌发生风险增加,尤其是存在 EGFR 活性突变的患者。欧洲及东亚人的肺癌易感基因的显著差异表明,生殖基因与体细胞基因存在一种复杂的关系,但尚未阐明。

与孟德尔等位基因遗传学不同,GWAS研究发现的常见变异对于预后的预测作用有限,并且多数情况下仅与(并且可能罕见)遗传等位基因相关。对于已知基因座更加详细的描述及基因GWAS的二代基因测序将进一步扩展对肺腺癌种系遗传的认识。

未来发展方向

二代测序及大数据统计时代旨在充分加强对肺腺癌基因的认识。通过对大量临床样本及相应肿瘤样本进行分析,明确少见驱动性变异可进一步提高对疾病的认识。大样本研究中DNA基础上基因变异的相关性及突变互斥现象将提供一条重要的信号通路,从而解决复杂的肿瘤信号通路。亚特兰大肿瘤基因组(the Cancer Genome Atlas,TCGA)开展的大规模甲基化、组蛋白、mRNA及miRNA表达与测序分析研究[1,126-128]有助于明确肺腺癌相关的体细胞基因变异。分子特征与近期修正的肺腺癌组织病理学亚分类相关性分析将提高治疗水平并形成新的生物学视角。在多种新型靶向治疗药物出现的背景下,分子基因变化的纵向分析将对治疗耐药及体细胞演进产生影响。基于种系的二代测序相关研究将进一步明确肺腺癌的遗传易感性。随着新型靶向治疗药物的进展及肿瘤细胞和动物模型中基因变异筛查方法的进步,这些观点将得到进一步完善。

肺鳞癌基因组

肺鳞癌基因变异概述

肺鳞癌是第二种常见的NSCLC类型。肺鳞癌被认为起源于气道近端,由以吸烟为代表的慢性气道损伤所致鳞状上皮化生引起[130]。鳞状上皮通常不存在于成人肺中并且驱动化生的分子事件近期才得到阐明[130-131]。肺鳞癌与其他类型NSCLC可通过形态学及免疫组化分析进行区分,肺鳞癌的典型免疫组化标志为TTF-1阴性及p40/p60阳性。截至目前,尚不明确肺鳞癌与其他类型NSCLC是否具有不同的分子特征。然而,近期多项研究表明,肺鳞癌与肺腺癌及SCLC明显不同,肺鳞癌与头颈部鳞状细胞癌更相似,而非其他类型的肺癌[1]。尽管靶向治疗药物在肺鳞癌中的应用效果明显不及肺腺癌,但随着近年来对肺鳞癌分子特征的深入研究,肺鳞癌的个体化治疗指日可待。

肺鳞癌与其他类型的肺癌相似,与吸烟密切相关。既往对于肺鳞癌患者的研究表明,90%以上的患者为吸烟者[132]。与肺腺癌不同,尚无关于不吸烟肺鳞癌患者的研究,并且尚不明确不吸烟肺鳞癌患者是否具有不同的基因变异。此外，比较不同种族背景的肺鳞癌相关研究尚未公布，并且尚不明确不同种族肺鳞癌患者是否与肺腺癌一样存在分子特征的显著差异。

肺鳞癌具有相当程度的基因组复杂性。TCGA报道，肺鳞癌体细胞突变、拷贝数变化及所有上皮肿瘤类型的基因重排发生率最高[1]。该研究表明，识别肺鳞癌中对肿瘤发展及治疗最重要的变异非常具有挑战性。

基因表达

多个中心关于 NSCLC 队列的分析表明肺鳞癌基因表达谱与肺腺癌显著不同[43,46,61,133]。此外，肺鳞癌可依据基因表达分析分为具有不同生物学及临床特征的亚组，这些亚组表现为正常肺的不同细胞类型及分化程度[134]。近期这些亚组采用 RNA 测序分析的方法进行了复制并且与特定基因变异相关。例如，与其他 3 种表达亚组相比，最常见的表达亚组即"经典型"与染色体 3q23（包括 SOX2、PIK3CA 及 TP63）扩增、NFE3L2 及 KEAP1 突变密切相关，并且 CpG 启动子甲基化程度更高。相反，FGFR 家族受体变异、RB1 及 PTEN 与其他表达类型关系更密切。多项研究表明，基因表达特征与肺鳞癌患者的预后相关，然而，目前独立样本的验证数据显示，基因表达数据预测临床预后仍极具挑战性。

体细胞拷贝数变异

肺鳞癌 SNP 及 aCGH 分析证实与肺腺癌相比，肺鳞癌存在复杂且差异显著的拷贝数特征。与其他组织来源如皮肤及宫颈的鳞状细胞癌相比，肺鳞癌具有同样的基因扩增及缺失区域[42]。肺鳞癌的特征性表现及与肺腺癌具有显著差异的特征在于 3q26、8p11-12 及 7p11 区域扩增，3q26 区域的转录因子 SOX2 在鳞癌分化中具有重要作用，8p11-12 区域包括 FGFR1 及 WHSC1L1，7p11 区域为 EGFR 基因定位点[135-140]。SOX2 及 FGFR1 是肺鳞癌细胞系的核心因子[135-136,140]，并且抗 FGFR1 治疗目前正处于临床试验阶段[141]。肺鳞癌的其他扩增区域包括 PDGFRA、CCND1、MYC、CDK6、BCL2L1、MDM2 及 NFE2L2[1]，其中 CDKN2A 及 PTEN 已获得较为深入的研究[1]。

体细胞突变

早期肺鳞癌 Sanger 测序研究发现，抑癌基因 TP53[21,142] 及原癌基因 NFE2L2 突变普遍存在[97]。此外，集中测序研究发现，肺鳞癌普遍缺乏肺腺癌[14,24-26,59]常见的 EGFR 或 KRAS 突变[143]。对所有酪氨酸激酶更加深入的 Sanger 测序研究发现，3%~4% 的肺鳞癌患者存在 DDR2 激酶突变[144]。已知 DDR2 是多种激酶抑制剂的靶点，并且抗 DDR2 治疗的相关临床试验目前正在进行中。采用 DNA 错配修复技术进行的测序分析发现，肺鳞癌普遍存在 TP53、NFE2L2、KEAP1、BA13、FBXW7、GRMB、MUC16、RUNX1T1、STK11 及 ERBB4 突变，并且其中部分存在统计学证实的突变富集情况[49]。

近期才出现关于肺鳞癌全外显子测序及全基因组测序分析的报道。TCGA 完成了 178 例肺鳞癌患者的全外显子组测序及 19 例肿瘤或正常配对组织的全基因组分析[1]。分析表明，肺鳞癌突变率极高，中位突变率为 8.4/Mb，CpG 岛区域突变率（20.6/Mb）显著高于非 CpG 岛区域，并且存在反义突变的富集，类似现象见于吸烟相关肺腺癌[2-3]及 SCLC[4-5,145]。

与肺腺癌类似，肺鳞癌基因组中大量基因突变仅见于单一或多个病例中，因此，识别具有重要生物学行为的基因非常困难。为解决这一问题，可引入统计学软件对数据集进行分析以识别单一基因特定突变背景下发生的基因突变情况。该分析发现 10 种具有统计学意义且在肿瘤中显著表达的富集突变：TP53、CDKN2A、PTEN、PIK3CA、KEAP1、MLL2、HLA-A、NFE2L2、NOTCH1 及 RB1[1]。其他统计分析发现存在其他突变富集相关基因，包括：FAM123B（WTX）、HRAS、FBXW7、SMARCA4、NF1、SMAD4、EGFR、APC、TSC1、BRAF、TNFAIP3 及 CREBBP。重点在于文献中仅有 2 例患者存在 EGFR L861Q 突变，而无 EGFR L585R 突变或 19 外显子缺失突变。KRAS 突变同样少见。BRAF V600E 突变具有统计学意义，因此该突变是否具有治疗意义值得进一步探讨[1]。

全基因组测序证实肺鳞癌基因高度复杂并且

基因重排率较高，平均每个肿瘤中存在 165 个重排基因，该数量与吸烟的肺腺癌患者接近。尽管发现一定数量抑癌基因（CDKN2A、RB1 及 NF1）等的重排[1]，但由于样本量较小尚未发现激酶区普遍存在的融合基因。

通路变异

肺鳞癌基因组变异表明疾病中存在一系列关键细胞通路的改变。肺鳞癌中最常见的两种突变基因为 NFE2L2 及 KEAP1，编码结合组件并且明确参与对氧化压力细胞反应相关基因转录的调节[96-97,146]。有假说认为 NFE2L2 及 KEAP1 变异是通过持续活化细胞保护转录程序减轻气道细胞慢性暴露于烟草相关致癌剂所致损伤，从而表现出生存优势。然而，肿瘤背景下，该通路的活化可促进肿瘤细胞化疗及放疗耐药的发生[150-155]。在老鼠模型中，突变型 NF2L2、KEAP1 与突变型 KRAS 协同驱动肺癌的发生，表明该通路除调节氧化损伤的细胞反应外还可调节过程[156]。

头颈部及皮肤鳞癌中有关于功能缺失 NOTCH1 突变的报道[157-159]。NOTCH 基因在鳞状化生中具有重要作用，表明鳞状上皮正常活动中的参与基因可能在鳞癌中发生异常调节。NOTCH1 同样是肺鳞癌的功能性缺失突变；肿瘤分化中的其他基因包括 SOX2 及 TP53 同时在鳞癌中存在改变并且多数与 NOTCH 突变互斥[1]。考虑到鳞状上皮细胞在正常人气道中并不存在，或许肺鳞癌发生过程中的鳞状分化相关基因改变必不可少。

除了氧化还原反应及鳞状分化相关基因的异常调节，有丝分裂及促生存激酶同样在肺鳞癌中存在改变。肺鳞癌中最常见的发生改变的激酶通路为 PI3K/AKT 信号通路[1]。TCGA 队列中近一半的肺鳞癌患者存在突变和体细胞拷贝数变化。PI3K/AKT 通路基因最常见的为 PIK3CA 或 PTEN 表达明显上调或下调[1]。其他常见改变的激酶家族为 EGFR 基因，在 10%～20% 的患者中存在 EGFR 拷贝数变化或突变[1]。EGFR 及其他 ERBB 激酶同样经常受到扩增或错误表达的影响，并且这些影响的后果尚未阐明。其他激酶家族同样存在如 DDR2、BRAF 及 JAK 激酶等变异，并且上述变异可能是治疗的重要靶点[1]。

TCGA 在肺鳞癌研究中的重要发现是确定存在 HLA-A 基因的功能性缺失突变[1]，这些变异或可减少肿瘤对于免疫系统的免疫源性多肽并可保证肿瘤脱离一定程度的免疫监测。疾病中常见识别肺鳞癌相关的体细胞基因突变可解释前期临床试验研究中的免疫检查点抑制剂的有效性[160-161]，该抑制剂可保持免疫系统的识别能力并对肿瘤应答。

总之，肺鳞癌存在高度靶向基因改变，表明靶向治疗可能在疾病中发挥重大作用。此外，肺鳞癌具有免疫浸润的疾病特征，提示免疫调节治疗的前景广阔。

SCLC 的基因特征

SCLC 是一种恶性程度极高的肿瘤，属于肺部神经内分泌肿瘤的范畴。除了 SCLC，神经内分泌肿瘤同样包括大细胞神经内分泌癌（large-cell neuroendocrine lung cancer, LCNECs）及临床上的肺部良性肿瘤（含类癌）。SCLC 是最常见的肺神经内分泌肿瘤，约占所有病例的 80%，其次为 12% 的 LCNEC[162]。SCLC 与 LCNEC 共占人类肺癌总病例数的 20%～25%[163]。

既往 SCLC 的分子发现

SCLC 与 LCNEC 存在大量基因变异，这些变异集中于 3p、13q、9p 及 17p，其中小细胞肺癌一定存在 3p 区域基因变异[164-166]。此外，TP53 突变常见于 LCNEC（59%）及 SCLC（71%）[21,167-168]。类癌存在 G:C>T:A 转换或无义突变，而 SCLC 与 LCNEC 存在 G:C>T:A 易位[5]。该现象支持一种结论：吸烟涉及 SCLC 与 LCNEC 的病理形成过程与类癌不同[169]。P16INK4/CyclinD1/Rb 通路的基因改变在神经内分泌癌的细胞周期调控中起决定性作用。RB1 缺失是 SCLC 与 LCNEC 的常见现象之一[18,170-172]，但在类癌中少见[170]。依据癌症中体细胞突变的 COSMIC 数据库（www.sanger.ac.uk/genetics/CPG/cosmic/），SCLC 中最常见的突变位于 TP53（占检测病例的 90%）、RB1（57%）、PTEN（15%）、PIK3CA（10%）及 EGFR（5%）。

传统基因研究中 SCLC 与 LCNEC 最重要的改

变为 TP53 及 RB1 突变。与其他类型的肺癌相比，RB1 缺失在 SCLC 与 LCNEC 中更常见。此外，小鼠模型研究对基因处理发现 TP53 及 KRAS 同时失活可形成腺癌[173]，而小鼠中肺上皮 TP53 及 RB1 缺失可促进 SCLC 的发生[174]。因此，RB1 缺失似乎是 SCLC 病理形成过程的核心因素。越来越多的证据表明其作用不仅限于细胞周期调控，RB1 同样存在于其他影响肿瘤启动及进展的细胞通路中（详见下文）。

SCLC 大规模基因组研究

遗憾的是，由于可获取组织有限，对神经内分泌癌进行综合基因组分析异常困难。SCLC 通常由较小的活检标本证实，不适宜进行综合基因组分析。仅在极少数接受手术切除的肺癌病例中可获得较大组织标本进行深度基因组分析。因此，尽管人群中 SCLC 的发生率较高，但获得足够组织病理进行分析非常困难。

近期，两项研究对 SCLC 进行了综合基因组特征分析[4,145]。研究共对 100 例 SCLC 样本进行了外显子组测序、拷贝数分析及转录组测序，其中最重要的发现之一为较高的背景突变率，高达 7.4 个体细胞突变/Mb。G：C＞T：A 易位为典型烟草相关致癌基因所致，常见于 SCLC 中，从而证实其与重度吸烟的相关性。SCLC 较高的基因突变率使得识别如肺腺癌或肺鳞癌中生物学相关的基因突变变得困难。为了实现该目标，需要对常见突变基因进行统计学分析以获得具有统计学意义的基因突变。该过程对基因大小及特异性基因突变进行过滤，然后明确特定基因是否依然表达，进而分析突变类型是否为抑癌基因（框外插入或缺失、引入终止密码子的突变）或原癌基因（框内插入或缺失），最后明确突变富集是否集中于某一特定基因。当采用这些方法时，研究者发现 TP53 突变及 RN1 突变[4,145]几乎普遍存在。此外，两项研究发现 PTEN 及组蛋白修饰基因的突变，如 EP300 及 MLL2。另外一种组蛋白甲基化转移酶 CREBBP 同样存在于其中一项研究中[4]。CREBBP 与 EP300 突变存在互斥，提示两种基因失活可满足重叠功能。此外，CREBBP 及 EP300 突变在组蛋白甲基化转移酶区域聚集。总之，18% 的 SCLC 患者中存在影响两种基因之一的基因组事件。因此，除了 TP53 及 RB1，两种组蛋白甲基化转移酶基因 CREBBP 及 EP300 是 SCLC 最常见的第 3 种突变。SCLC 中发现的其他基因突变中影响激酶活性的例子可能涉及 PI3K 通路[145]。

对染色体基因拷贝数的具体分析揭示了一种重要的体细胞拷贝数变异（SCNAs）模型[4,145,175]。重点在于，较多染色体改变被发现，而高度局部扩增及缺失较少。这些事件包括导致 3 号染色体短臂缩短的半合子缺失、5p 延长（可能靶向于端粒酶基因 TERT）、RB1（13q）及 TP53（17p）缺失、MYC 家族 3 个成员（MYCL1、MYCN、MYC）的扩增以及 FGFR1（8p）扩增见于约 6% 的患者[4,145]。至少一种 FGFR1 扩增细胞系对于 FGFR 抑制剂高度敏感[140,176]，表明 FGFR1 扩增的 SCLC 可从 FGFR 抑制剂治疗中获益。SOX2 基因在接近 25% 的患者中存在高水平扩增[145]。SOX2 是一种线性转录因子，有研究表明其扩增见于很大一部分肺鳞癌患者[135]。与 SOX2 扩增可能有助于 SCLC 的致癌活性概念类似，两种 SOX2 扩增 SCLC 细胞系在 SOX2 敲除后表现为增殖活性降低[145]。现阶段尚不明确 SCLC 中 3q 扩增是否具有与肺鳞癌相同的生物学行为。

SCLC 基因组改变的生物学特征及临床应用

尽管 SCLC 中发现了数个特征性新型突变，但目前尚无研究详细阐述这些肿瘤类型的临床特征，其类型、扩增概率、早期转移倾向、化疗敏感性及快速复发情况尚不明确。

对化疗高度敏感的可能解释在于 RB1 趋势几乎普遍存在。RB1 部分通过与 E2F1 及其前凋亡靶向基因的相互作用参与 DNA 损伤修复[177]。因此，RB1 缺失可能通过抑制 DNA 损伤修复提高化疗敏感性。近期一项关于 SCLC 的细胞系对于 PARP1 抑制剂高度敏感的研究支持该现象[178]。RAPR1 参与 DNA 损伤修复，并且可作为转录因子 E2F1 的转录共活化因子，而 RB1 抑制 E2F1 的活性。RAPR 抑制剂抑制存在 DNA 损伤反应的 E2F1 靶向基因，因此，这些 SCLC 细胞中存在指向内在 DNA 损伤修复缺陷的大量体细胞突变[4,145]。在大量背景突变存在的情况下，抑制 DNA 双链修复机制（通过 PRAP 自身）及涉及单独碱基替换的损伤修复机制，可能在抑制 SCLC 生长方面具有协同作用。

此外，多项研究表明 SCLC 基因缺陷可影响组蛋白调节基因。但目前尚不明确组蛋白乙酰化转移酶 CREBBP 或 EP300，以及组蛋白甲基化转移酶 MLL 失活会对 SCLC 的肿瘤发生产生何种影响。除了急性组蛋白修饰，有报道发现，这些组蛋白乙酰化转移酶可直接乙酰化其他蛋白，而这些蛋白可能参与保护细胞免于恶性转变的核心过程。相应的，EP300、CREBBP 及 MLL 基因失活可能改变组蛋白乙酰化的模式，从而引起基因表达的显著改变。CBP 及 p300 的首要靶点为组蛋白 H3；乙酰化过程尤其见于赖氨酸残基 K18 及 K27[179]。因为 H3K18 低乙酰化与肿瘤恶性转化相关[180-182]，因此有研究者认为 SCLC 中该组蛋白信号也是 CREBBP 及 EP300 失活的产物。

如前所述，SCLC 中仅有少数潜在变异可作为治疗靶点，其中，FGFR1 扩增或可作为 FGFR1 扩增 SCLC 的治疗靶点[140,176]。此外，PTEN 失活的肿瘤可能对 PI3K、AKT 或 HSP90 抑制剂敏感[176]。另外，存在 EPHA 激酶融合的肿瘤[145]可能接受 EPHA 激酶抑制剂治疗。然而，现阶段存在这些潜在基因变异的临床前模型数量极其有限。此外，目前多数这些基因的分子流行病学特征尚未阐明。因此，这些潜在靶点的临床前验证程度尚需进一步研究。

近期一项研究提供的临床前研究证据表明 SCLC 存在 Hedgehog 信号通路活化[183]，显示 SCLC 模型中小鼠对化疗联合 Hedgehog 信号通路抑制剂 NVP-LDE225 敏感，目前该研究处于 Ⅱ 期临床试验阶段。该现象的具体机制中对 Hedgehog 通路的依赖程度尚不明确。髓母细胞瘤及皮肤基底细胞癌相关研究显示存在引起 Hedgehog 通路活化的体细胞突变[184]，但在 SCLC 中未发现上述突变[4,145]。

总之，近期发现 SCLC 存在多种新型基因组变异，其中部分为高频变异（如 CREBBP、EP300 突变）。这些变异如何诱发 SCLC，以及这些变异与治疗相关通路活性有价相关性，这些问题还需要通过对细胞和小鼠机制的研究进一步阐明。

（危志刚　译）

参考文献

[1] Cancer Genome Atlas Research N. Comprehensive genomic characterization of squamous cell lung cancers. Nature, 2012, 489 (7417): 519 - 525. PubMed PMID: 22960745. Pubmed Central PMCID: 3466113.

[2] Govindan R, Ding L, Griffith M, et al. Genomic landscape of non-small cell lung cancer in smokers and never smokers. Cell. 2012, 150 (6): 1121 - 1134. PubMed PMID: 22980976.

[3] Imielinski M, Berger AH, Hammerman PS, et al. Mapping the hallmarks of lung adenocarcinoma with massively parallel sequencing. Cell, 2012, 150 (6): 1107 - 1120. PubMed PMID: 22980975. Pubmed Central PMCID: 3557932.

[4] Peifer M, Fernandez-Cuesta L, Sos ML, et al. Integrative genome analyses identify key somatic driver mutations of small-cell lung cancer. Nat Genet, 2012, 44 (10): 1104 - 1110. PubMed PMID: 22941188.

[5] Pleasance ED, Stephens PJ, O'Meara S, et al. A small cell lung cancer genome with complex signatures of tobacco exposure. Nature, 2010, 463 (7278): 184 - 190.

[6] Pleasance ED, Cheetham RK, Stephens PJ, et al. A comprehensive catalogue of somatic mutations from a human cancer genome. Nature, 2010, 463 (7278): 191 - 196. PubMed PMID: 20016485.

[7] Mitsudomi T, Morita S, Yatabe Y, et al. Gefitinib versus cisplatin plus docetaxel in patients with non-small cell lung cancer harbouring mutations of the epidermal growth factor receptor (WJTOG3405): an open label, randomised phase 3 trial. Lancet Oncol, 2009, 12. PubMed PMID: 20022809.

[8] Mok TS, Wu YL, Thongprasert S, et al. Gefitinib or carboplatin-paclitaxel in pulmonary adenocarcinoma. N Engl J Med, 2009, 361 (10): 947 - 957. PubMed PMID: 19692680.

[9] Rosell R, Moran T, Queralt C, et al. Screening for epidermal growth factor receptor mutations in lung cancer. N Engl J Med, 2009, 361 (10): 958 - 967. PubMed PMID: 19692684.

[10] Camidge DR, Bang YJ, Kwak EL, et al. Activity and safety of crizotinib in patients with ALK-positive non-small cell lung cancer: updated results from a phase 1 study. Lancet Oncol, 2012, 13 (10): 1011 - 1019. PubMed PMID: 22954507.

[11] Kwak EL, Bang YJ, Camidge DR, et al. Anaplastic lymphomakinase inhibition in non-small-cell lung cancer. N Engl J Med, 2010, 363 (18): 1693-1703. PubMed PMID: 20979469.

[12] Shaw AT, Yeap BY, Solomon BJ, et al. Effect of crizotinib on overall survival in patients with advanced non-small-cell lung cancer harbouring ALK gene rearrangement: a retrospective analysis. Lancet Oncol, 2011, 12 (11): 1004-1112. PubMed PMID: 21933749. Pubmed Central PMCID: 3328296.

[13] Cairns P, Mao L, Merlo A, et al. Rates of p16 (MTS1) mutations in primary tumors with 9p loss. Science, 1994, 265 (5170): 415-417. PubMed PMID: 8023167.

[14] Capon DJ, Seeburg PH, McGrath JP, et al. Activation of Ki-ras2 gene in human colon and lung carcinomas by two different point mutations. Nature, 1983, 304 (5926): 507-513. PubMed PMID: 6308467.

[15] Kamb A, Gruis NA, Weaver-Feldhaus J, et al. A cell cycle regulator potentially involved in genesis of many tumor types. Science, 1994, 264 (5157): 436-440.

[16] McCoy MS, Toole JJ, Cunningham JM, et al. Characterization of a human colon/lung carcinoma oncogene. Nature, 1983, 302 (5903): 79-81. PubMed PMID: 6298638.

[17] Sakaguchi AY, Naylor SL, Shows TB, et al. Human c-Ki-ras2 proto-oncogene on chromosome 12. Science, 1983, 219 (4588): 1081-1083. PubMed PMID: 6823569.

[18] Shapiro GI, Edwards CD, Kobzik L, et al. Reciprocal Rb inactivation and p16INK4 expression in primary lung cancers and cell lines. Cancer Res, 1995, 55 (3): 505-509.

[19] Shapiro GI, Park JE, Edwards CD, et al. Multiple mechanisms of p16INK4A inactivation in non-small cell lung cancer cell lines. Cancer Res, 1995, 55 (24): 6200-6209.

[20] Shiraishi M, Noguchi M, Shimosato Y, et al. Amplification of protooncogenes in surgical specimens of human lung carcinomas. Cancer Res, 1989, 49 (23): 6474-6479. PubMed PMID: 2573414.

[21] Takahashi T, Nau MM, Chiba I, et al. p53: a frequent target for genetic abnormalities in lung cancer. Science, 1989, 246 (4929): 491-494.

[22] Lander ES, Linton LM, Birren B, et al. Initial sequencing and analysis of the human genome. Nature, 2001, 409 (6822): 860-921. PubMed PMID: 11237011.

[23] Venter JC, Adams MD, Myers EW, et al. The sequence of the human genome. Science, 2001, 291 (5507): 1304-1351. PubMed PMID: 11181995.

[24] Lynch TJ, Bell DW, Sordella R, et al. Activating mutations in the epidermal growth factor receptor underlying responsiveness of non-small-cell lung cancer to gefitinib. N Engl J Med, 2004, 350 (21): 2129-2139. PubMed PMID: 15118073.

[25] Paez JG, Janne PA, Lee JC, et al. EGFR mutations in lung cancer: correlation with clinical response to gefitinib therapy. Science, 2004, 304 (5676): 1497-1500. PubMed PMID: 15118125.

[26] Pao W, Miller V, Zakowski M, et al. EGF receptor gene mutations are common in lung cancers from "never smokers" and are associated with sensitivity of tumors to gefitinib and erlotinib. Proc Natl Acad Sci USA, 2004, 101 (36): 13306-13311. PubMed PMID: 15329413.

[27] Stephens P, Hunter C, Bignell G, et al. Lung cancer: intragenic ERBB2 kinase mutations in tumours. Nature, 2004, 431 (7008): 525-526. PubMed PMID: 15457249.

[28] Brose MS, Volpe P, Feldman M, et al. BRAF and RAS mutations in human lung cancer and melanoma. Cancer Res, 2002, 62 (23): 6997-7000. PubMed PMID: 12460918.

[29] Davies H, Bignell GR, Cox C, et al. Mutations of the BRAF gene in human cancer. Nature, 2002, 417 (6892): 949-954. PubMed PMID: 12068308.

[30] Naoki K, Chen TH, Richards WG, et al. Missense mutations of the BRAF gene in human lung adenocarcinoma. Cancer Res, 2002, 62 (23): 7001-7003. PubMed PMID: 12460919.

[31] Rikova K, Guo A, Zeng Q, et al. Global survey of phosphotyrosine signaling identifies oncogenic kinases in lung cancer. Cell, 2007, 131 (6): 1190-1203. PubMed PMID: 18083107.

[32] Soda M, Choi YL, Enomoto M, et al. Identification of the transforming EML4-ALK fusion gene in non-small cell lung cancer. Nature, 2007, 448 (7153): 561-566. PubMed PMID: 17625570.

[33] Sanchez-Cespedes M, Parrella P, Esteller M, et al. Inactivation of LKB1/STK11 is a common event in adenocarcinomas of the lung. Cancer Res, 2002, 62 (13): 3659-3662. PubMed PMID: 12097271.

[34] Medina PP, Carretero J, Fraga MF, et al. Genetic and epigenetic screening for gene alterations of the chromatin-remodeling factor, SMARCA4/BRG1, in lung tumors. Genes Chromosomes Cancer, 2004, 41 (2): 170-

[35] Medina PP, Romero OA, Kohno T, et al. Frequent-BRG1/SMARCA4-inactivating mutations in human lung cancer cell lines. Hum Mutat, 2008, 29 (5): 617-622. PubMed PMID: 18386774.

[36] Futreal PA, Coin L, Marshall M, et al. A census of human cancer genes. Nat Rev Cancer, 2004, 4 (3): 177-183. PubMed PMID: 14993899. Pubmed Central PMCID: 2665285.

[37] Futreal PA, Kasprzyk A, Birney E, et al. Cancer and82 Lung Can-cer genomics. Nature, 2001, 409 (6822): 850-852. PubMed PMID: 11237008.

[38] Meyerson M, Gabriel S, Getz G. Advances in understanding cancer genomes through second generation sequencing. Nat Rev Genet, 2010, 11 (10): 685-696. PubMed PMID: 20847746.

[39] Stratton MR, Campbell PJ, Futreal PA. The cancer genome. Nature, 2009, 458 (7239): 719-724. PubMed PMID: 19360079. Pubmed Central PMCID: 2821689.

[40] Weir B, Zhao X, Meyerson M. Somatic alterations in the human cancer genome. Cancer Cell, 2004, 6 (5): 433-438. PubMed PMID: 15542426.

[41] Beer DG, Kardia SL, Huang CC, et al. Gene-expression profiles predict survival of patients with lung adenocarcinoma. Nat Med, 2002, 7. PubMed PMID: 12118244.

[42] Beroukhim R, Mermel CH, Porter D, et al. The landscape of somatic copy-number alteration across human cancers. Nature, 2010, 463 (7283): 899-905. PubMed PMID: 20164920. Pubmed Central PMCID: 2826709.

[43] Bhattacharjee A, Richards WG, Staunton J, et al. Classification of human lung carcinomas by mRNA expression profiling reveals distinct adenocarcinoma subclasses. Proc Natl Acad Sci USA, 2001, 98 (24): 13790-13795. PubMed PMID: 11707567.

[44] Ding L, Getz G, Wheeler DA, et al. Somatic mutations affect key pathways in lung adenocarcinoma. Nature, 2008, 455 (7216): 1069-1075. PubMed PMID: 18948947.

[45] Kendall J, Liu Q, Bakleh A, et al. Oncogenic cooperation and coamplification of developmental transcription factor genes in lung cancer. Proc Natl Acad Sci USA, 2007, 104 (42): 16663-16668. PubMed PMID: 17925434.

[46] Shedden K, Taylor JM, Enkemann SA, et al. Gene expression-based survival prediction in lung adenocarcinoma: a multi-site, blinded validation study. Nat Med, 2008, 14 (8): 822-827. PubMed PMID: 18641660.

[47] Weir BA, Woo MS, Getz G, et al. Characterizing the cancer genome in lung adenocarcinoma. Nature, 2007, 450 (7171): 893-898. PubMed PMID: 17982442.

[48] Ju YS, Lee WC, Shin JY, et al. A transforming KIF5B and RET gene fusion in lung adenocarcinoma revealed from whole-genome and transcriptome sequencing. Genome Research, 2012, 22 (3): 436-445. PubMed PMID: 22194472. Pubmed Central PMCID: 3290779.

[49] Kan Z, Jaiswal BS, Stinson J, et al. Diverse somatic mutation patterns and pathway alterations in human cancers. Nature, 2010, 466 (7308): 869-873. PubMed PMID: 20668451.

[50] Lee W, Jiang Z, Liu J, et al. The mutation spectrum revealed by paired genome sequences from a lung cancer patient. Nature, 2010, 465 (7297): 473-477. PubMed PMID: 20505728..

[51] Liu J, Lee W, Jiang Z, et al. Genome and transcriptome sequencing of lung cancers reveal diverse mutational and splicing events. Genome Res, 2012, 22 (12): 2315-2327. PubMed PMID: 23033341. Pubmed Central PMCID: 3514662.

[52] Seo JS, Ju YS, Lee WC, et al. The transcriptional landscape and mutational profile of lung adenocarcinoma. Genome Res, 2012, 22 (11): 2109-2119. PubMed PMID: 22975805. Pubmed Central PMCID: 3483540.

[53] Kwei KA, Kim YH, Girard L, et al. Genomic profiling identifies TITF1 as a lineage-specific oncogene amplified in lung cancer. Oncogene, 2008, 27 (25): 3635-3640. PubMed PMID: 18212743.

[54] Tanaka H, Yanagisawa K, Shinjo K, et al. Lineage-specific dependency of lung adenocarcinomas on the lung development regulator TTF-1. Cancer Res, 2007, 67 (13): 6007-6011. PubMed PMID: 17616654.

[55] Bergethon K, Shaw AT, Ou SH, et al. ROS1 rearrangements define a unique molecular class of lung cancers. Journal of Clinical Oncology, 2012, 30 (8): 863-870. PubMed PMID: 22215748. Pubmed Central PMCID: 3295572.

[56] Kohno T, Ichikawa H, Totoki Y, et al. KIF5B-RET fusions in lung adenocarcinoma. Nature Medicine, 2012, 18 (3): 375-377. PubMed PMID: 22327624.

[57] Lipson D, Capelletti M, Yelensky R, et al. Identification of new ALK and RET gene fusions from colorectal and lung cancer Somatic Genome Alterations in Human Lung Cancers 83 biopsies. Nature Medicine, 2012, 18 (3): 382-384. PubMed PMID: 22327622.

[58] Takeuchi K, Soda M, Togashi Y, et al. RET, ROS1 and ALK fusions in lung cancer. Nature Medicine, 2012,

[59] Rodenhuis S, van de Wetering ML, Mooi WJ, et al. Mutational activation of the K-ras oncogene. A possible pathogenetic factor in adenocarcinoma of the lung. N Engl J Med, 1987, 317 (15): 929-935.

[60] Forgacs E, Biesterveld EJ, Sekido Y, et al. Mutation analysis of the PTEN/MMAC1 gene in lung cancer. Oncogene, 1998, 17 (12): 1557-1565.

[61] Garber ME, Troyanskaya OG, Schluens K, et al. Diversity of gene expression in adenocarcinoma of the lung. Proc Natl Acad Sci USA, 2001, 98 (24): 13784-13789. PubMed PMID: 11707590.

[62] Hayes DN, Monti S, Parmigiani G, et al. Gene expression profiling reveals reproducible human lung adenocarcinoma subtypes in multiple independent patient cohorts. J Clin Oncol, 2006, 24 (31): 5079-5090. PubMed PMID: 17075127.

[63] Hainaut P, Olivier M, Pfeifer GP. TP53 mutation spectrum in lung cancers and mutagenic signature of components of tobacco smoke: lessons from the IARC TP53 mutation database. Mutagenesis, 2001, 16 (6): 551-553. PubMed PMID: 11682648.

[64] Sun S, Schiller JH, Gazdar AF. Lung cancer in never smokers—a different disease. Nat Rev Cancer, 2007, 7 (10): 778-790. PubMed PMID: 7882278.

[65] Hanahan D, Weinberg RA. The hallmarks of cancer. Cell, 2000, 100 (1): 57-70. PubMed PMID: 10647931.

[66] Hanahan D, Weinberg RA. Hallmarks of cancer: the next generation. Cell, 2011, 144 (5): 646-674. PubMed PMID: 21376230.

[67] Vogelstein B, Kinzler KW. Cancer genes and the pathways they control. Nat Med, 2004, 10 (8): 789-799. PubMed PMID: 15286780.

[68] Maemondo M, Inoue A, Kobayashi K, et al. Gefitinib or chemotherapy for non-small-cell lung cancer with mutated EGFR. N Engl J Med, 2010, 362 (25): 2380-2388. PubMed PMID: 20573926.

[69] Pao W, Chmielecki J. Rational, biologically based treatment of EGFR-mutant non-small-cell lung cancer. Nat Rev Cancer, 2010, 10 (11): 760-774. PubMed PMID: 20966921. Pubmed Central PMCID: 3072803.

[70] Sebolt-Leopold JS, Herrera R. Targeting the mitogen-activated protein kinase cascade to treat cancer. Nat Rev Cancer, 2004, 4 (12): 937-947. PubMed PMID: 15573115.

[71] Zhang J, Yang PL, Gray NS. Targeting cancer with small molecule kinase inhibitors. Nat Rev Cancer, 2009, 9 (1): 28-39. PubMed PMID: 19104514.

[72] Sharma SV, Bell DW, Settleman J, et al. Epidermal growth factor receptor mutations in lung cancer. Nat Rev Cancer, 2007, 7 (3): 169-181. PubMed PMID: 17318210.

[73] Greulich H, Chen TH, Feng W, et al. Oncogenic transformation by inhibitor-sensitive and resistant EGFR mutants. PLoS Med, 2005, 2 (11): e313. PubMed PMID: 16187797.

[74] Greulich H, Kaplan B, Mertins P, et al. Functional analysis of receptor tyrosine kinase mutations in lung cancer identifies oncogenic extracellular domain mutations of ERBB2. Proc Natl Acad Sci USA, 2012, 109 (36): 14476-14481. PubMed PMID: 22908275. Pubmed Central PMCID: 3437859.

[75] Engelman JA, Zejnullahu K, Gale CM, et al. PF00299804, an irreversible pan-ERBB inhibitor, is effective in lung cancer models with EGFR andERBB2 mutations that are resistant to gefitinib. Cancer Res, 2007, 67 (24): 11924-11932. PubMed PMID: 18089823.

[76] Minami Y, Shimamura T, Shah K, et al. The major lung cancer-derived mutants of ERBB2 are oncogenic andare associated with sensitivity to the irreversible EGFR/ERBB2 inhibitor HKI-272. Oncogene, 2007, 26 (34): 5023-5027. PubMed PMID: 17311002.

[77] Shimamura T, Ji H, Minami Y, et al. Non-small-cell lung cancer and Ba/F3 transformed cells harboring the ERBB2G776insV_ G/C mutation are sensitive to the dual specific epidermal growth factor receptor and ERBB2inhibitor HKI-272. Cancer Res, 2006, 66 (13): 6487-6491. PubMed PMID: 16818618.

[78] Feinberg AP, Vogelstein B, Droller MJ, et al. Mutation affecting the 12th amino acid of the c-Ha-ras oncogene product occurs infrequently in human cancer. Science, 1983, 220 (4602): 1175-1177. PubMed PMID: 6304875.

[79] Shimizu K, Goldfarb M, Suard Y, et al. Three human transforming genes are related to the viral ras oncogenes. Proc Natl Acad Sci USA, 1983, 80 (8): 2112-2116. PubMed PMID: 6572964. Pubmed Central PMCID: 393767.

[80] Greulich H. The genomics of lung adenocarcinoma: opportunities for targeted therapies. Genes & Cancer, 2010, 1 (12): 1200-1210. PubMed PMID: 21779443. Pubmed Central PMCID: 3092285.

[81] Ballester R, Marchuk D, Boguski M, et al. The NF1 lo-

cus encodes a protein functionally related to mammalian GAP and yeast IRA proteins. Cell, 1990, 63 (4): 851-859. PubMed PMID: 2121371.

[82] Chapman PB, Hauschild A, Robert C, et al. Improved survival with vemurafenib in melanoma with BRAF V600Emutation. N Engl J Med, 2011, 364 (26): 2507-2516. PubMed PMID: 21639808. Pubmed Central PMCID: 3549296.

[83] Sosman JA, Kim KB, Schuchter L, et al. Survival in BRAF V600 - mutant advanced melanoma treated with vemurafenib. N Engl J Med, 2012, 366 (8): 707-714. PubMed PMID: 22356324.

[84] Marks JL, Gong Y, Chitale D, et al. Novel MEK1 mutation identified by mutational analysis of epidermal growth factor receptor signaling pathway genes in lung adenocarcinoma. Cancer Res, 2008, 68 (14): 5524-5528. PubMed PMID: 18632602. Pubmed Central PMCID: 2586155.

[85] Kong-Beltran M, Seshagiri S, Zha J, et al. Somatic mutations lead to an oncogenic deletion of met in lung cancer. Cancer Res, 2006, 66 (1): 283-289. PubMed PMID: 16397241.

[86] Bentires-Alj M, Paez JG, David FS, et al. Activating mutations of the noonan syndrome-associated SHP2/PTPN11 genein human solid tumors and adult acute myelogenous leukemia. Cancer Res, 2004, 64 (24): 8816-8820. PubMed PMID: 15604238.

[87] Samuels Y, Wang Z, Bardelli A, et al. High frequency of mutations of the PIK3CA gene in human cancers. Science, 2004, 304 (5670): 554. PubMed PMID: 15016963.

[88] Yamamoto H, Shigematsu H, Nomura M, et al. PIK3CA mutations and copy number gains in human lung cancers. Cancer Res, 2008, 68 (17): 6913-6921. PubMed PMID: 18757405. Pubmed Central PMCID: 2874836.

[89] Shaw RJ, Cantley LC. Ras, PI (3) K and mTOR signalling controls tumour cell growth. Nature, 2006, 441 (7092): 424-430. PubMed PMID: 16724053.

[90] Liu P, Cheng H, Roberts TM, et al. Targeting the phosphoinositide 3 - kinase pathway in cancer. Nature Reviews Drug Discovery, 2009, 8 (8): 627-644. PubMed PMID: 19644473. Pubmed Central PMCID: 3142564.

[91] Little CD, Nau MM, Carney DN, et al. Amplification and expression of the c-myc oncogene in human lung cancer cell lines. Nature, 1983, 306 (5939): 194-196.

[92] Nie Z, Hu G, Wei G, et al. c-Myc is a universal amplifier of expressed genes in lymphocytes and embryonic stem cells. Cell, 2012, 151 (1): 68-79. PubMed PMID: 23021216. Pubmed Central PMCID: 3471363.

[93] Whibley C, Pharoah PD, Hollstein M. p53 polymorphisms: cancer implications. Nat Rev Cancer, 2009, 9 (2): 95-107. PubMed PMID: 19165225.

[94] Winslow MM, Dayton TL, Verhaak RG, et al. Suppression of lung adenocarcinoma progression by Nkx2-1. Nature, 2011, 473 (7345): 101-104. PubMed PMID: 21471965. Pubmed Central PMCID: 3088778.

[95] Sporn MB, Liby KT. NRF2 and cancer: The good, the bad and the importance of context. Nat Rev Cancer, 2012, 12 (8): 564-571. PubMed PMID: 22810811.

[96] Singh A, Misra V, Thimmulappa RK, et al. Dysfunctional KEAP1 - NRF2interaction in non-small-cell lung cancer. PLoS Med, 2006, 3 (10): e420. PubMed PMID: 17020408. Pubmed Central PMCID: 1584412.

[97] Shibata T, Ohta T, Tong KI, et al. Cancer related mutations in NRF2 impair its recognition by Keap1-Cul3 E-3ligase and promote malignancy. Proc Natl Acad Sci USA, 2008, 105 (36): 13568-13573. PubMed PMID: 18757741. Pubmed Central PMCID: 2533230.

[98] Shaw RJ. Tumor suppression by LKB1: SIKness prevents metastasis. Sci Signal, 2009, 2 (86): pe55. PubMed PMID: 19724060.

[99] Ji H, Ramsey MR, Hayes DN, et al. LKB1 modulates lung cancer differentiation and metastasis. Nature, 2007, 448 (7155): 807-810. PubMed PMID: 17676035.

[100] Fodde R, Smits R, Clevers H. APC, signal transduction and genetic instability in colorectal Somatic Genome Alterations in Human cancer. Nat Rev Cancer, 2001, 1 (1): 55-67. PubMed PMID: 11900252.

[101] Baylin SB, Jones PA. A decade of exploring the cancer epigenome-biological and translational implications. Nat Rev Cancer, 2011, 11 (10): 726-734. PubMed PMID: 21941284. Pubmed Central PMCID: 3307543.

[102] Ryan RJ, Bernstein BE. Molecular biology. Genetic events that shape the cancer epigenome. Science, 2012, 336 (6088): 1513-1514. PubMed PMID: 22723401.

[103] Glaros S, Cirrincione GM, Palanca A, et al. Targeted knockout of BRG1 potentiates lung cancer development. Cancer Res, 2008, 68 (10): 3689-3696. PubMed PMID: 18483251.

[104] Yoshida K, Sanada M, Shiraishi Y, et al. Frequent pathway mutations of splicing machinery in myelodysplasia. Nature, 2011, 478 (7367): 64-69. PubMed

PMID: 21909114.

[105] Paez JG, Lin M, Beroukhim R, et al. Genome coverage and sequence fidelity of phi29 polymerase-based multiple strand displacement whole genome amplification. Nucleic Acids Res, 2004, 32 (9): e71. PubMed PMID: 15150323.

[106] Pao W, Girard N. New driver mutations in non-small-cell lung cancer. Lancet Oncol, 2011, 12 (2): 175 - 180. PubMed PMID: 21277552.

[107] Sequist LV, Waltman BA, Dias-Santagata D, et al. Genotypic and histological evolution of lung cancers acquiring resistance to EGFR inhibitors. Science Translational Medicin, 2011, 3 (75): 75ra26. PubMed PMID: 21430269.

[108] Kobayashi S, Boggon TJ, Dayaram T, et al. EGFR mutation and resistance of non-small-cell lung cancer to gefitinib. N Engl J Med, 2005, 352 (8): 786 - 792. PubMed PMID: 15728811.

[109] Pao W, Miller VA, Politi KA, et al. Acquired resistance of lung adenocarcinomas to gefitinib or erlotinib is associated with a second mutation in the EGFR kinase domain. PLoS Med, 2005, 2 (3): e73. PubMed PMID: 15737014.

[110] Engelman JA, Zejnullahu K, Mitsudomi T, et al. MET amplification leads to gefitinib resistance in lung cancer by activating ERBB3 signaling. Science, 2007, 316 (5827): 1039 - 1043. PubMed PMID: 17463250.

[111] Choi YL, Soda M, Yamashita Y, et al. EML4 - ALK mutations inlung cancer that confer resistance to ALK inhibitors. N Engl J Med, 2010, 363 (18): 1734 - 1739. PubMed PMID: 20979473.

[112] Heuckmann JM, Balke-Want H, Malchers F, et al. Differential protein stability and ALK inhibitor sensitivity of EML4-ALKfusion variants. Clin Cancer Res, 2012, 18 (17): 4682 - 4690. PubMed PMID: 22912387.

[113] Tanizaki J, Okamoto I, Okabe T, et al. Activation of HER family signaling as a mechanism of acquired resistance to ALK inhibitors in EML4-ALK-positive non-small cell lung cancer. Clin Cancer Res, 2012, 18 (22): 6219 - 6226. PubMed PMID: 22843788.

[114] Michor F, Liphardt J, Ferrari M, et al. What does physics have to do with cancer Nat Rev Cancer, 2011, 11 (9): 657 - 670. PubMed PMID: 21850037.

[115] Fletcher O, Houlston RS. Architecture of inherited susceptibility to common cancer. NatRev Cancer, 2010, 10 (5): 353 - 361. PubMed PMID: 20414203.

[116] Pharoah PD, Dunning AM, Ponder BA, et al. Association studies for finding cancer susceptibility genetic variants. Nat Rev Cancer, 2004, 4 (11): 850 - 860. PubMed PMID: 15516958.

[117] Amos CI, Pinney SM, Li Y, et al. A susceptibility locus on chromosome 6q greatly increases lung cancer risk among light and never smokers. Cancer Res, 2010, 70 (6): 2359 - 2367. PubMed PMID: 20215501. Pubmed Central PMCID: 2855643.

[118] Amos CI, Wu X, Broderick P, et al. Genome-wide association scan of tag SNPs identifies a susceptibility locus for lung cancer at 15q25.1. Nat Genet, 2008, 40 (5): 616 - 622. PubMed PMID: 18385676. Pubmed Central PMCID: 2713680.

[119] Hung RJ, McKay JD, Gaborieau V, et al. A susceptibility locus for lung cancer maps to nicotinic acetylcholine receptor subunit genes on 15q25. Nature, 2008, 452 (7187): 633 - 637. PubMed PMID: 18385738.

[120] Landi MT, Chatterjee N, Yu K, et al. A genome-wide association study of lung cancer identifies a region of chromosome 5p15 associated with risk for adenocarcinoma. Am J Hum Genet, 2009, 85 (5): 679 - 691. PubMed PMID: 19836008. Pubmed Central PMCID: 2775843.

[121] Liu P, Vikis HG, Wang D, et al. Familial aggregation of common sequence variants on 15q24 - 25.1 in lung cancer. J Natl Cancer Inst, 2008, 100 (18): 1326 - 1330. PubMed PMID: 18780872. Pubmed Central PMCID: 2538550.

[122] Wang Y, Broderick P, Webb E, et al. Common 5p15.33and 6p21.33 variants influence lung cancer risk. Nat Genet, 2008, 40 (12): 1407 - 1409. PubMed PMID: 18978787. Pubmed Central PMCID: 2695928.

[123] Miki D, Kubo M, Takahashi A, et al. Variation in TP63 is associated with lung adenocarcinoma susceptibility in Japanese and Korean populations. Nat Genet, 2010, 42 (10): 893 - 896. PubMed PMID: 20871597.

[124] Yoon KA, Park JH, Han J, et al. A genome-wide association study reveals susceptibility variants for non-small cell lung cancer in the Korean population. Hum Mol Genet, 2010, 19 (24): 4948 - 4954. PubMed PMID: 20876614.

[125] Hu Z, Wu C, Shi Y, et al. A genome-wide association study identifies two new lung cancer susceptibility loci at 13q12.12and 22q12.2 in Han Chinese. Nat Genet, 2011, 43 (8): 792 - 796. PubMed PMID: 21725308.

[126] Cancer Genome Atlas N. Comprehensive molecular por-

traits of human breast tumours. Nature, 2012, 490 (7418): 61 - 70. PubMed PMID: 23000897. Pubmed Central PMCID: 3465532.

[127] Cancer Genome Atlas N. Comprehensive molecular characterization of human colon and rectal cancer. Nature, 2012, 487 (7407): 330 - 337. PubMed PMID: 22810696. Pubmed Central PMCID: 3401966.

[128] Cancer Genome Atlas Research N. Integrated genomic analyses of ovarian carcinoma. Nature, 2011, 474 (7353): 609 - 615. PubMed PMID: 21720365. Pubmed Central PMCID: 3163504.

[129] Travis WD, Brambilla E, Noguchi M, et al. International Association for the Study of Lung Cancer/American Thoracic Society/European Respiratory Society International Multidisciplinary Classification of Lung Adenocarcinoma. J Thorac Oncol, 2011, 6 (2): 244 - 285. PubMed PMID: 21252716.

[130] Rock JR, Onaitis MW, Rawlins EL, et al. Basal cells as stem cells of the mouse trachea and human airway epithelium. ProcNatl Acad Sci USA, 2009, 106 (31): 12771 - 12775. PubMed PMID: 19625615. Pubmed Central PMCID: 2714281.

[131] Guseh JS, Bores SA, Stanger BZ, et al. Notch signaling promotes airway mucous metaplasia and inhibits alveolar development. Development, 2009, 136 (10): 1751 - 1759. PubMed PMID: 19369400. Pubmed Central PMCID: 2673763.

[132] Kenfield SA, Wei EK, Stampfer MJ, et al. Comparison of aspects of smoking among the four histological types of lung cancer. Tobacco Control, 2008, 17 (3): 198 - 204. PubMed PMID: 18390646. Pubmed Central PMCID: 3044470.

[133] Raponi M, Zhang Y, Yu J, et al. Gene expression signatures for predicting prognosis of squamous cell and adenocarcinomas ofthe lung. CancerRes, 2006, 66 (15): 7466 - 7472. PubMedPMID: 16885343.

[134] Wilkerson MD, Yin X, Hoadley KA, et al. Lung squamous cell carcinoma mRNA expression subtypes are reproducible, clinically important, and correspond to normal cell types. Clin Cancer Res, 2010, 16 (19): 4864 - 4875. PubMed PMID: 20643781. Pubmed Central PMCID: 2953768.

[135] Bass AJ, Watanabe H, Mermel CH, et al. SOX2 is an amplified lineage-survival oncogene in lung and esophageal squamous cell carcinomas. Nat Genet, 2009, 41 (11): 1238 - 1242. PubMed PMID: 19801978. Pubmed Central PMCID: 2783775.

[136] Dutt A, Ramos AH, Hammerman PS, et al. Inhibitor-sensitiveFGFR1 amplification in human non-small cell lungcancer. PLoS ONE, 2011, 6 (6): e20351. PubMed PMID: 21666749. Pubmed Central PMCID: 3110189.

[137] Lockwood WW, Chari R, Coe BP, et al. Integrative genomic analyses identify BRF2 as a novel lineage-specific oncogene in lung squamous cell carcinoma. PLoS Med, 2010, 7 (7): e1000315. PubMed PMID: 20668658. Pubmed Central PMCID: 2910599.

[138] Ramos AH, Dutt A, Mermel C, et al. Amplification of chromosomal segment 4q12 in non-small cell lung cancer. Cancer Biology & Therapy, 2009, 8 (21): 2042 - 2050. PubMed PMID: 19755855.

[139] Tonon G, Wong KK, Maulik G, et al. High-resolution genomic profiles of human lung cancer. Proc Natl Acad Sci USA, 2005, 102 (27): 9625 - 9630. PubMed PMID: 15983384. Pubmed Central PMCID: 1160520.

[140] Weiss J, Sos ML, Seidel D, et al. Frequent and focalFGFR1 amplification associates with therapeutically tractable FGFR1 dependency in squamous cell lung cancer. Sci Transl Med, 2010, 2 (62): 62ra93. PubMed PMID: 21160078.

[141] Guagnano V, Kauffmann A, Wohrle S, et al. FGFR genetic alterations predict for sensitivity to NVP-BGJ398, a selective panFGFR inhibitor. Cancer Discov, 2012, 2 (12): 1118 - 1133. PubMed PMID: 23002168.

[142] Chiba I, Takahashi T, Nau MM, et al. Mutations in the p53gene are frequent in primary, resected non-small cell lung cancer. Lung Cancer Study Group. Oncogene, 1990, 5 (10): 1603 - 1610.

[143] Rekhtman N, Paik PK, Arcila ME, et al. Clarifying the spectrum of driver oncogene mutations in biomarker-verified squamous carcinoma of lung: lack of EGFR/KRAS and presence of PIK3CA/AKT1 mutations. Clin Cancer Res, 2012, 18 (4): 1167 - 1176. PubMed PMID: 22228640. Pubmed Central PMCID: 3487403.

[144] Hammerman PS, Sos ML, Ramos AH, et al. Mutations in the DDR2kinase gene identify a novel therapeutic target insquamous cell lung cancer. Cancer Discov, 2011, 1 (1): 78 - 89. PubMed PMID: 22328973. Pubmed Central PMCID: 3274752.

[145] Rudin CM, Durinck S, Stawiski EW, et al. Comprehensive genomic analysis identifies SOX2 as a frequently amplified gene in small-cell lung cancer. Nat Genet, 2012, 44 (10): 1111 - 1116. PubMed PMID: 22941189. Pubmed Central PMCID: 3557461.

[146] Shibata T, Kokubu A, Gotoh M, et al. Genetic alteration of Keap1 confers constitutive Nrf2 activation and resistance to chemotherapy in gallbladder cancer. Gastroenterology, 2008, 135 (4): 1358–1368, 68 e1–4. PubMed PMID: 18692501.

[147] Frohlich DA, McCabe MT, Arnold RS, et al. The role of Nrf2 in increased reactive oxygen species and DNA damage in prostate tumorigenesis. Oncogene, 2008, 27 (31): 4353–4362. PubMed PMID: 18372916.

[148] Itoh K, Mochizuki M, Ishii Y, et al. Transcription factor Nrf2 regulates inflammation by mediating the effect of 15-deoxy-Delta (12, 14) -prostaglandin j (2). Mol Cell Biol, 2004, 24 (1): 36–45. PubMed PMID: 14673141. Pubmed Central PMCID: 303336.

[149] Osburn WO, Wakabayashi N, Misra V, et al. Nrf2 regulates an adaptive response protecting against oxidative damage following diquat-mediated formation of superoxide anion. Archives of Biochemistry and Biophysics, 2006, 454 (1): 7–15. PubMed PMID: 16962985. Pubmed Central PMCID: 1851923.

[150] Kobayashi A, Kang MI, Watai Y, et al. Oxidative and electrophilic stresses activate Nrf2 through inhibition of ubiquitination activity of Keap1. Mol Cell Biol, 2006, 26 (1): 221–229. PubMed PMID: 16354693. Pubmed Central PMCID: 1317630.

[151] Li QK, Singh A, Biswal S, et al. KEAP1 gene mutations and NRF2 activation are common in pulmonary papillary adenocarcinoma. Journal of Human Genetics, 2011, 56 (3): 230–234. PubMed PMID: 21248763. Pubmed Central PMCID: 3268659.

[152] Ohta T, Iijima K, Miyamoto M, et al. Loss of Keap1 function activates Nrf2 and provides advantages for lung cancer cell growth. Cancer Res, 2008, 68 (5): 1303–1309. PubMed PMID: 18316592.

[153] Shibata T, Kokubu A, Saito S, et al. NRF2 mutation confers malignant potential and resistance to chemoradiation therapy in advanced esophageal squamous cancer. Neoplasia, 2011, 13 (9): 864–873. PubMed PMID: 21969819. Pubmed Central PMCID: 3182278.

[154] Singh A, Bodas M, Wakabayashi N, et al. Gain of Nrf2 function in non-small-cell lung cancer cells confers radioresistance. Antioxidants & Redox Signaling, 2010, 13 (11): 1627–1637. PubMedPMID: 20446773. Pubmed Central PMCID: 3541552.

[155] Solis LM, Behrens C, Dong W, et al. Nrf2 and Keap1 abnormalities in non-small cell lung carcinoma and association with clinicopathologic features. Clin Cancer Res, 2010, 16 (14): 3743–3753. PubMed PMID: 20534738. Pubmed Central PMCID: 2920733.

[156] Bauer AK, Cho HY, Miller-Degraff L, et al. Targeted deletion of Nrf2 reduces urethane-induced lung tumor development in mice. PLoS ONE, 2011, 6 (10): e26590. PubMed PMID: 22039513. Pubmed Central PMCID: 3198791.

[157] Agrawal N, Frederick MJ, Pickering CR, et al. Exome sequencing of head and neck squamous cell carcinoma reveals inactivating mutations in NOTCH1. Science, 2011, 333 (6046): 1154–1157. PubMed PMID: 21798897. Pubmed Central PMCID: 3162986.

[158] Stransky N, Egloff AM, Tward AD, et al. The mutational landscape of head and neck squamous cell carcinoma. Science, 2011, 333 (6046): 1157–1160. PubMed PMID: 21798893.

[159] Wang NJ, Sanborn Z, Arnett KL, et al. Loss-of-function mutations in Notch receptors in cutaneous and lung squamous cell carcinoma. Proc Natl Acad Sci USA, 2011, 108 (43): 17761–17766. PubMed PMID: 22006338. Pubmed Central PMCID: 3203814.

[160] Brahmer JR, Tykodi SS, Chow LQ, et al. Safety and activity of antiPD-L1 antibody in patients with advanced cancer. N Engl J Med, 2012, 366 (26): 2455–2465. PubMed PMID: 22658128. Pubmed Central PMCID: 3563263.

[161] Topalian SL, Hodi FS, Brahmer JR, et al. Safety, activity, and immune correlates of anti-PD–1 antibody in cancer. N Engl J Med, 2012, 366 (26): 2443–2454. PubMed PMID: 22658127. Pubmed Central PMCID: 3544539.

[162] Chen LC, Travis WD, Krug LM. Pulmonary neuroendocrine tumors: What (little) do we know? Journal of the National Comprehensive Cancer Network: JNCCN, 2006, 4 (6): 623–630. PubMed PMID: 16813729.

[163] Travis WD. Lung tumours with neuroendocrine differentiation. Eur J Cancer, 2009, 45 Suppl1: 251–266. PubMed PMID: 19775623.

[164] Whang-Peng J, Kao-Shan CS, Lee EC, et al. Specific chromosome defect associated with human small-cell lung cancer; deletion 3p (14–23). Science, 1982, 215 (4529): 181–182.

[165] Naylor SL, Johnson BE, Minna JD, et al. Loss of heterozygosity of chromosome 3p markers in small-cell lung cancer. Nature, 1987, 329 (6138): 451–454.

[166] Mori N, Yokota J, Oshimura M, et al. Concordant deletions of chromosome 3p and loss of heterozygosity for

[166] chromosomes 13 and 17 in small cell lung carcinoma. Cancer Res, 1989, 49 (18): 5130-5135.

[167] Takahashi T, Takahashi T, Suzuki H, et al. The p53 gene is very frequently mutated in small-cell lung cancer with adistinct nucleotide substitution pattern. Oncogene, 1991, 6 (10): 1775-1778.

[168] Sameshima Y, Matsuno Y, Hirohashi S, et al. Alterations of the p53 gene are common and critical events for the maintenance of malignant phenotypes in small-cell lung carcinoma. Oncogene, 1992, 7 (3): 451-457.

[169] Onuki N, Wistuba, II, Travis WD, et al. Genetic changes in the spectrum of neuroendocrine lung tumors. Cancer, 1999, 85 (3): 600-607. PubMed PMID: 10091733.

[170] Beasley MB, Lantuejoul S, Abbondanzo S, et al. The P16/cyclinD1/Rb pathway in neuroendocrine tumors of the lung. Hum Pathol, 2003, 34 (2): 136-142. PubMed PMID: 12612881.

[171] Kelley MJ, Nakagawa K, Steinberg SM, et al. Differential inactivation of CDKN2 and Rb protein in non-small-cell and small-cell lung cancer cell lines. J Natl Cancer Inst, 1995, 87 (10): 756-761.

[172] Yokota J, Akiyama T, Fung YK, et al. Altered expression of the retinoblastoma (RB) gene in small-cell carcinoma of the lung. Oncogene, 1988, 3 (4): 471-475.

[173] Zheng S, El-Naggar AK, Kim ES, et al. A genetic mouse model for metastatic lung can-cer with gender differences in survival. Oncogene, 2007, 26 (48): 6896-6904. PubMed PMID: 17486075.

[174] Meuwissen R, Linn SC, Linnoila RI, et al. Induction of small cell lung cancer by somatic inactivation of both Trp53 and Rb1 in a conditional mouse model. Cancer Cell, 2003, 4 (3): 181-189. PubMed PMID: 14522252.

[175] Voortman J, Lee JH, Killian JK, et al. Array comparative genomic hybridization-based characterization of genetic alterations in pulmonary neuroendocrine tumors. Proc Natl Acad Sci USA, 2010, 107 (29): 13040-13045. PubMed PMID: 20615970. Pubmed Central PMCID: 2919980.

[176] Sos ML, Dietlein F, Peifer M, et al. A framework for identification of actionable cancer genome dependencies in small cell lung cancer. Proc Natl Acad Sci USA, 2012, 109 (42): 17034-17039. PubMed PMID: 23035247. Pubmed Central PMCID: 3479457.

[177] Burkhart DL, Sage J. Cellular mechanisms of tumour suppression by the retinoblastoma gene. Nat Rev Cancer, 2008, 8 (9): 671-682. PubMed PMID: 18650841.

[178] Byers LA, Wang J, Nilsson MB, et al. Proteomic profiling identifies dysregulated pathways in small cell lung cancer and novel therapeutic targets including PARP1. Cancer Discov, 2012, 2 (9): 798-811. PubMed PMID: 22961666. Pubmed Central PMCID: 3567922.

[179] Bedford DC, Brindle PK. Is histone acetylation the most important physiological function for CBP and p300? Aging, 2012, 4 (4): 247-255. PubMed PMID: 22511639. Pubmed Central PMCID: 3371760.

[180] Barber MF, Michishita-Kioi E, Xi Y, et al. SIRT7 links H3K18 deacetylation to maintenance of oncogenic transformation. Nature, 2012, 487 (7405): 114-118. PubMed PMID: 22722849. Pubmed Central PMCID: 3412143.

[181] Ferrari E, Lucca C, Foiani M. A lethal combination for cancer cells: synthetic lethality screenings for drug discovery. Eur J Cancer, 2010, 46 (16): 2889-2895. PubMed PMID: 20724143.

[182] Horwitz GA, Zhang K, McBrian MA, et al. Adenovirus small e1a alters global patterns of histone modification. Science, 2008, 321 (5892): 1084-1085. PubMed PMID: 18719283. Pubmed Central PMCID: 2756290.

[183] Park KS, Martelotto LG, Peifer M, et al. A crucial requirement for Hedgehog signaling in small cell lung cancer. Nat Med, 2011, 17 (11): 1504-1508. PubMed PMID: 21983857. Pubmed Central PMCID: 3380617.

[184] Teglund S, Toftgard R. Hedgehog beyond medulloblastoma and basal cell carcinoma. Biochimica et biophysica acta, 2010, 1805 (2): 181-208. PubMed PMID: 20085802.

第 5 章
血清蛋白标志物

Mohamed Hassanein[1], *David P. Carbone*[2]
1. Division of Allergy, Pulmonary and Critical Care Medicine, Vanderbilt University Medical Center, Nashville, TN, USA
2. James Comprehensive Cancer Center, Ohio State University Medical Center, Columbus, OH, USA

肺癌的自然进展史和生物标志物在临床中的潜在效用

肺癌是一种在病理和分子水平上高度异质性的疾病[1-4]，而吸烟作为一种危险因素与其异质性密切相关。全世界有 10 亿人吸烟，而美国约有 20% 的成年人吸烟，由肺癌引起的死亡人数比乳腺癌、前列腺癌、结肠癌、肝癌、肾癌和黑色素瘤的总死亡人数还要多[5-6]。尽管近年来支气管镜技术、手术以及化疗、靶向治疗、放射治疗得到了快速发展，但改善晚期癌症患者的预后仍面临巨大的挑战。为了更早期地发现癌症，最大限度地提高治愈率，一些非侵入性检查技术正在研究中。包括 X 线、CT 在内的影像学技术，痰细胞学检查以及各种生物样本中的分子标志物检测已证实对肺癌的早期诊断有重要价值[7-8]。尽管这些检查在灵敏度和特异性上各有差异，但仅有胸部 CT 能较小幅度地降低肺癌特异死亡率，这项发现显著提高了寻找新分子标志物用于疾病风险评估及无创诊断的重要性，而这些分子标志物也能最大限度地界定从特异性化学预防或治疗措施中获益的潜在患者群体。这些分子标志物将被反复检测以证实其临床效用及其对目前检查策略的互补价值。

在吸烟人群中，肺癌可被视为是一个长期反复气管损伤与修复的过程，该疾病的反复过程在引起临床重视之前需历经多年，这个相当长的病程（图 5.1）称为窗口期，在此期间进行干预可能会阻止病情进展（如基本的戒烟或化学预防）。尽

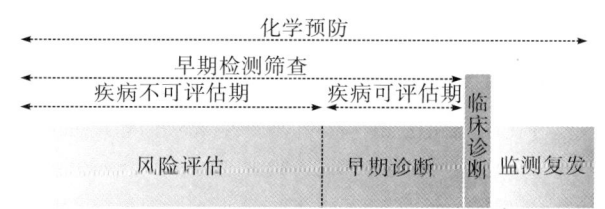

图 5.1 关于肺癌进展期间生物标志物效用的临床因素。此图说明了在 4 个时间窗内包括了 4 个临床因素。在肺癌不可测和诊断前期是风险评估时期；在病程发展和与预防时机相对应的期间，代表了一个长的时间窗。当疾病被检测到但暂无症状时，我们进入早期诊断。另外 2 个临床时期与临床诊断相关，此时疾病可检测，患者表现出症状并可出现复发。这些时间窗与不同的时期相对应，此时不同的生物标志物产生

管只有约 20% 的高危人群发展为肺癌，但其中仍有一些关键且无法解释的问题，包括：哪些人的肿瘤会发展到恶性（哪些人可能从筛选或预防中获益）？当肿瘤进展时，会以怎样的速度发展（即疾病表现为"临床征象"）？以及哪些患者人群能最大限度地从靶向治疗中获益（治疗选择）？为达到这一目标，有关肺癌特定生物标志物的研究正在加强，但尚没有生物标志物可有效或广泛地应用于肺癌的临床诊断[13]。

血液蛋白质组

血液是一种复杂的动态介质，其成分能反映人体不同的生理或病理状态，包括多种癌症的发生。血液蛋白质组分析认为，肿瘤或宿主的组织灌注会对循环中新的或变化的蛋白质或多肽类应答（图 5.2）。由于可无创获得相当数量的样本，所以血液蛋白质组分析是研究人员绝佳的选择。

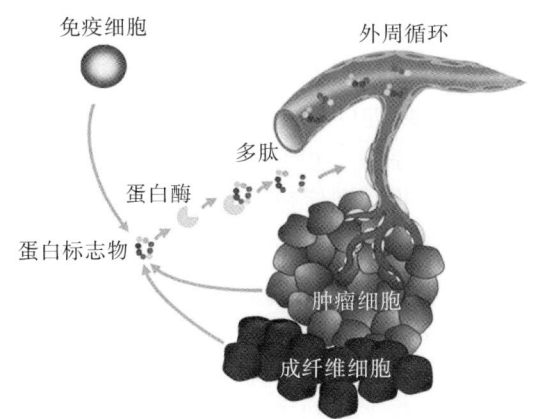

图5.2 血清蛋白质及多肽生物标志物的来源。肿瘤相关蛋白可由肿瘤细胞直接产生，或者由肿瘤微环境中的周边细胞如成纤维细胞或免疫细胞应答致癌物发生宿主反应产生。组织内蛋白水解级联（细胞生态学如基质上皮反应的产物），主要组织相容性复合体（MHC）免疫细胞出现，或凋亡产生的蛋白片段（多肽）被动进入血液循环

血液样本的这些特点有助于早期诊断肺癌、监测病情发展、开发靶向药物、评价疗效及预后。血浆和血清中已知的肿瘤标志物尚不丰富，故选择蛋白质组技术为发现生物标志物提供深入有效的分析就显得尤其重要。最近几篇研究报告已经研究了蛋白质组技术如何解释血浆蛋白质组的复杂性，人类蛋白质组组织也发表了一篇研究人类血清及血浆蛋白质组特点的综合协作研究报告。

蛋白质组发现平台

几种新的分析方法已被用于鉴定新型蛋白和明确其分子结构、功能及其与其他蛋白质、小分子物质间的相互作用。正在将这些理论尽可能地尝试应用于临床，如寻找新的诊断及预测指标和新的治疗靶点。我们在表5.1中总结了大多数普通蛋白质组途径，并会在其他章节进行详细讨论。

发现与确认外周血生物标志物的蛋白质组学研究途径

通过分子生物学技术来明确肿瘤特征的研究在过去的10年中取得了令人瞩目的进展。许多此类进展是建立在我们对肿瘤相关核苷酸异常遗传、转录及翻译水平知识逐步增加的基础上。基因组通过调控其最终功能产物——蛋白质的表达水平、转录后修饰及功能来控制细胞的关键生物学行为。不仅如此，细胞合成的蛋白质数量要远超基因数量，因为蛋白质相较于mRNA的稳定性各有差异，

表5.1 肿瘤生物标志物探测研究的蛋白质组学方法比较

	2-D胶分离	MALDI MS	LC-MS/MS	LC-MRM/MS	蛋白或抗体实验
目的	性能分析，分离及鉴定	性能分析	量表及鉴定	靶向蛋白定量	靶向蛋白检测
蛋白检测及鉴定	蛋白PI及MW，肽谱识别及测序	检测完整蛋白及测序	通过肽序列识别	肽段特异性的MS或MS转换	使用抗体或配体检测
定量	半定量	半定量	半定量	定量，标记参考肽段，无标记技术	不定量
PTM检测	有	无	有	有	有
通量	低	高	高	低	高
再生性	高	高	高	高	高
灵敏度	中	低	高	高	高
深度分析	100~1000蛋白	100~300峰	500~4000蛋白	1~100蛋白	50~500蛋白
缺点	受PI和MW限制，存在多糖和核酸的污染	检测到大量的蛋白，MW限制（2~30kDa），无识别作用	高错误率	完全定量中标记肽段的浪费	抗体的特异性和可获得性。只有已知的蛋白能检测到

2-D：2围；LC：液相色谱法；MALDI MS：基体辅助激光解吸电离质谱法；MRM：多反应检测；MW：分子质量；PI：等电点；PTM：翻译后修饰

并受到例如剪切、融合及翻译后修饰等多种转录后及翻译后调控水平的调节。因此，为加强对肺癌细胞生物学的理解并获得关于该疾病生物学更为完整的分析，尽可能完整地获得癌症细胞蛋白表达谱、翻译后修饰及功能十分关键。因此完整的分析遗传组及转录组学信息能为我们理解疾病本质提供更多的信息。表5.2总结了几篇关于肺癌诊断标志物蛋白质组研究的结果。

诊断性 MALDI-TOF MS 血清分析

在蛋白质组研究中，基质辅助激光解吸飞行时间质谱仪（MALDI-TOF MS）是一项在肿瘤生物学中突飞猛进的技术，主要用于对血清、尿液及组织等多种复杂生物复合物进行高通量分析，具有敏感性适中、特异性较高的特性。这项技术需要一个共结晶矩阵，对激光能量吸收并随后弹出，进入气相电离分子生物，离子的离子源有一个固定的电位差，并在到达检测器的飞行时间之前，与它们的 M/I 成反比（图5.3）。每个离子到达检测器所需要的时间产生一个信号，X 轴代表 M/I 比，Y 轴代表离子强度。由于 MALDI 过程本质上有利于产生单分子离子，因此不论是否进行分馏，均可以分析复杂蛋白混合物[18]。可准确分析分子量从 1kDa 至 100kDa 以上的物质。

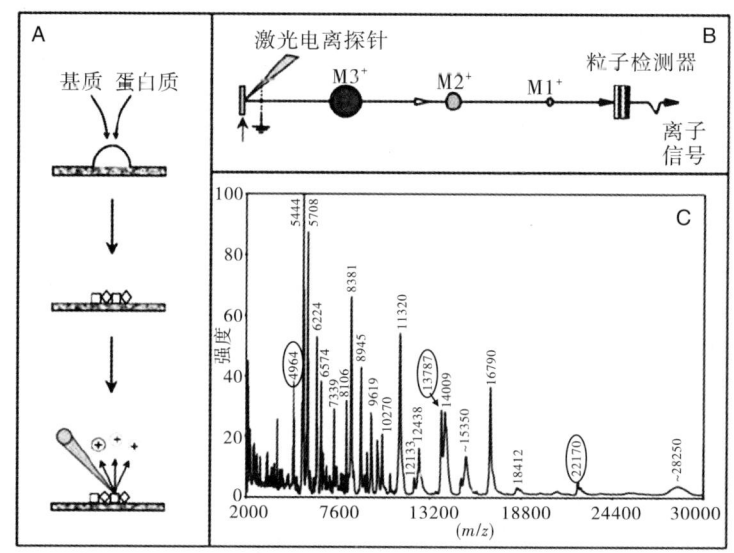

图5.3 MALDI-TOF MS 的原理。A. 待分析分子首先与基质分子以 1~5 000 的比例混合，通过溶剂蒸发，基质－分析物共晶体形成。工具中的离子源，辐射带有简短的激光脉冲开启了解吸电离（desoiption-ionization）事件。B. 新形成的分子离子在恒定电位差下不断加速，给具有相同电荷的例子相同的能量，当离子经过飞行质谱时，依据它们的质量分开。C. MALDI-TOF MS 是在阳离子模式下对复杂的蛋白质混合物进行分离的结果

表5.2 肺癌早期检测过程中血样生物标志物的特性及性质

参考文献	样本	标志物类型	分析	数量	亚型	检测平台	临床前样本	BM Dev 期	测试群	验证群	灵敏度	特异度	AUC
Zhong, 2006[66]	血清	AutoAB	噬菌肽克隆	5	肺癌	ELISA	n/a	II	46	56	91*	91*	99*
Chapman, 2008[72]	血清	AutoAB	p53, cmyc; HER2, NY-ESO-1, CAGE, MUC1, GBU4-5	7	肺癌	ELISA	n/a	I	154	n/a	n/a	n/a	n/a

(续表5.2)

参考文献	样本	标志物类型	分析	数量	亚型	检测平台	临床前样本	BM Dev 期	测试群	验证群	灵敏度	特异性	AUC
Qiu, 2008[84]	血清	AutoAB	膜联蛋白1, 14-3-3θ, LAMR1	3	NSCLC	蛋白实验	170	Ⅲ		170	51	82	73
Wu, 2010[85]	血清	AutoAB	噬菌肽克隆	6	NSCLC	ELISA	n/a	Ⅱ	20	180	92	92	96
Farlow, 2018[86]	血清	AutoAB	IMPDH, PCAM1, 泛素, ANXA1, ANXA2, HSP7Q-9B	6	NSCLC	ELISA	n/a	Ⅱ	196	n/a	94.8	91.1*	96.4*
Boyle, 2010[87]	血清	AutoAB	P53, NY-ESO-1, CAGE, GBU4-5, 膜联蛋白1, SOX2	6	NSCLC	ELISA	n/a	Ⅱ	241	255	32	91	64
Kulpa, 2002[88]	血清	蛋白	CEA, CYFRA21-1, SCC抗原, NSE	4	SCC	ELISA	n/a	Ⅱ		420	20~62	95	71~90
Patz, 2007[21]	血清	蛋白	CEA, RBP4, hTTA, SCCA	4	LC	ELISA	n/a	Ⅱ	100	97	78	75	n/a
Takano, 2009[89]	血清	蛋白	粘连蛋白-4	1	NSCLC	ELISA	n/a	Ⅱ		295	54	98	n/a
Yildiz, 2007[20]	血清	蛋白	MALDI MS 标签	7	NSCLC	MALDI MS	n/a	Ⅱ	185	106	58	85.7	82
Pecot, 2012[90]	血清	蛋白	模型: MALDI M 标签 + 临床和显影数据		肺结节	MALDI MS	n/a	Ⅱ		100	n/a	n/a	72
Diamandis, 2011[91]	血清	蛋白	穿透素-3	1	LC	ELISA	n/a	Ⅰ		426	37~48	80~90	60~74
Ostroff, 2010[92]	血清	适配子	钙黏素-1, CD30配体, 内皮抑素, HSP90a, LRIG3, MIP-4, 多效生长因子, PRKCI, RGM-C, SCF-Sr, sL选择素, YES	6	NSCLC	适配子	n/a	Ⅱ	985	341	89	83	90
Zhong, 2005[67]	胞质	AutoAB	TAA 标签	5	NSCLC	蛋白微阵列	5	Ⅰ	81	n/a	90*	95*	n/a
Taguchi, 2011[93]	胞质	蛋白	EGFR, SFTPB, WFDC2, ANGPTL-3, ANXA1 YWHAQ, Lmr1	7	NSCLC	ELISA	52	Ⅲ		n/a	n/a	n/a	89

AUC: 曲线下面积; *: 只来源于测试群的值; BM Dev Phage: 生物标志物形成时期; n/a: 不可得; LC: 肺癌。来源: 引自 Hassanein 等, 2012[78]

MSLDI-TOF MS 由于具有较高的准确度（远高于任何凝胶系统）、高通量（样品分析只要几秒钟）、所需样品量少（几个细胞就能进行分析）等特点，同时对盐、缓冲液、生物污染物具有耐受性，被广泛用于各种生物样本（例如组织样本、细胞、激光微切割的细胞、血液、血清、尿液）的分析。此外，当其与表面层析技术一起使用时则被称为 SELDI-TOF MS。该方法利用层析柱实验从样本中选择吸附所需要的目的蛋白，而非特异性吸附的蛋白及对电离过程有干扰作用的物质则被洗掉。然后矩阵就被用于蛋白结合实验，SELDI-TOF MS 完成实施。

通过使用峰型作为诊断工具，利用最小的样本量，对血、组织及尿液进行快速的蛋白质组学特性分析已取得了令人鼓舞的结果，然而将其应用于早期临床诊断还有一段距离。MALDI-TOF MS 的一个应用就是检测蛋白和多肽用于诊断肿瘤。在该应用中，MS 峰值表示的是与疾病情况相对应的最典型且丰富的蛋白或片段，但它不易与疾病的发病机制相联系（图 5.4）。目前有几个研究利用 MALDI MS 来研究血清中蛋白或多肽的诊断特性[19-20]。例如，我们之前利用该技术分析血清鉴定出 I 期非小细胞肺癌（NSCLC）诊断中的 7 个蛋白质组学信号标志，且其准确度和灵敏度分别为 78% 和 67.4%[20]。Patz 及其同事也发现了在 NSCLC 和对照组间存在表达差异的 4 种血清蛋白[转铁蛋白、视黄醇结合蛋白（retinol binding protein, RBP）、抗胰蛋白酶和结合珠蛋白][21]。利用该技术，其他研究组也区分出了各种肿瘤与对照组中表达差异的血清蛋白[15]。

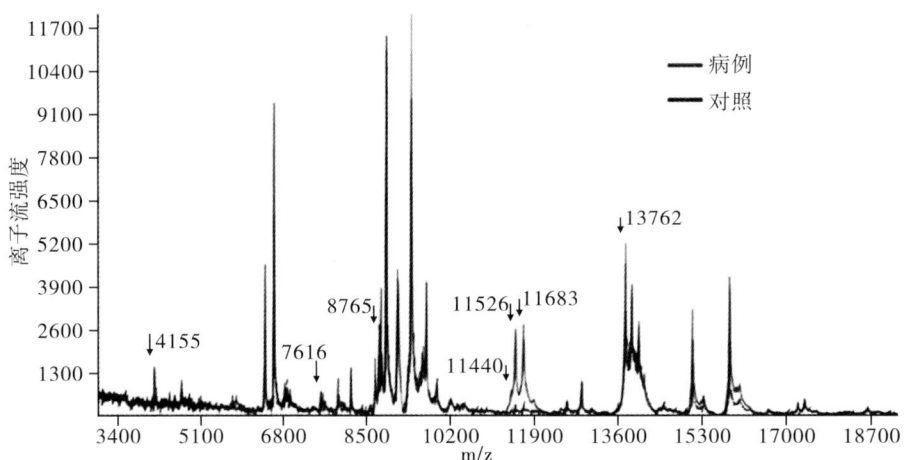

图 5.4（见彩插）　肺癌患者及其对照的 MALDI MS 血清图谱。图中列出了匹配案例（红色，平滑线）和对照（蓝色，点线）的图谱分析的平均强度。箭头代表有差异性的 M/Z 值

Han 等将 253 份血清样本分为测试组（89 例 NSCLC，68 例对照）和验证组（62 例 NSCLC，34 例对照），并应用 SELDI-TOF MS 进行分析[22]。通过测试组中获得的血样蛋白质谱，利用 Biomarker Pattern 软件，建立了包含 3 个不同蛋白质量分类树，且肺癌组和对照组的准确度、灵敏度以及特异度分别为 94%、91% 及 97%。当用验证组进行验证时，其灵敏度、特异度及阳性预测值分别为 89%、90% 及 91%。作者也用电化学发光免疫分析法检测了血清中的 CEA 及 Cyfra21-1 水平，结果显示，无论单独或联合分析，生物标志物的特异度和灵敏度都显著低于 SELDI 蛋白质组学分析（Cyfra21-1 的灵敏度和特异度分别为 42% 和 72%，CEA 的灵敏度和特异度分别为 46% 和 76%）。同样使用该方法对 158 例肺癌患者和 50 例对照进行分析，Yang 等人发现了 5 个信号蛋白质标志物，且其在验证群中的灵敏度和特异度分别为 86.9% 和 80.0%。

尽管 MALDI-TOF MS 和 SELDI-TOF MS 有很强的技术优势，但由于存在分析前及分析过程中的限制，所以制约了该方法在临床领域的广泛使用。分析前的困难与收集及制备样本的多样性有关，这些困难导致了分析的偏倚及可再生性。在分析过程中，对于低丰度及大分子量蛋白，检测是十

分困难的。此外对于单个患者分类，很难形成一个可进行分析的强烈信号。

生物液体的极端复杂性（如血液、血清、胞质）以及特殊蛋白标志物的较低数量都是减少 MS 技术灵敏度的制约因素。事实上，无论是 MALDI MS 还是其他 MS 技术的灵敏度都在 1μg/mL 左右，而血清样本中生物标志物的浓度往往比该值低 1 000 倍。因此，使用 MALDI MS 技术分析新鲜组织或血样虽能得到大量的分离峰，但却不能鉴定出所对应的目的蛋白[15]。

通过 MS 分析血清的直接方法就是通过 1 或 2 围凝胶电泳分离血样，然后切除所需要的被消化的目的条带，用质谱技术进行分析（表 5.1）。Patz 等利用 2 围差异凝胶电泳以及 SELDI-TOF MS 分别识别了表达具有差异的 3 种蛋白［转铁蛋白、视黄醇结合蛋白（RBP）和结合珠蛋白］和 1 种蛋白酶（抗胰蛋白酶）[21]。使用测试血清群［100 例患者（50 例肺癌，50 例对照）］。他们利用上述 4 种蛋白以及之前被鉴定与鳞状细胞癌的相关抗原（CEA）进行了试验。通过使用分类回归树分析（classification and regression tree，CART），他们在肺癌与对照组间，鉴定出 4 种蛋白（CEA、RBP、抗胰蛋白酶和 SCC 抗原），其在测试群中的灵敏度和特异度分别为 89.3% 和 84.7%。当用独立验证群进行验证时，这些标志物的灵敏度和特异度分别为 77.8% 和 75.4%。利用 CART 分析产生的分类方案，患者终端节点类别的差异决定了其患癌风险。对于有 3 种不同终端节点的患者，其测试群和验证群中患癌的可能性分别为 92% 和 90%。但当单独使用时，4 种标志物都不具有诊断价值，只有当它们联合使用时，才对肿瘤诊断及严重程度的评估有临床意义。

治疗反应的血清蛋白质组学

为了界定最能从表皮生长因子受体（EGFR）酪氨酸激酶抑制剂（tyrosine kinase inhibitors，TKIs）治疗中获益的 NSCLC 患者，Taguchi 等[24] 应用 MALDI MS 法对 302 例服用吉非替尼或厄洛替尼的患者治疗前的血清进行分析，其中 139 份样本为测试组（含 3 个队列），163 份样本为验证组（含 2 个独立队列），同时也测试了来自于 158 例未接受 EGFR TKIs 治疗的 NSCLC 患者的血清。基于 EGFR TKIs 治疗后的生存期和疾病进展时间，最终开发出了一个 8 质谱分析信号的算法，该分类算法随后也被用于验证群中。最终，分类算法成功地鉴别出了在 EGFR TKIs 治疗后受益的患者。实际上，在第一队列中，预测的"好"与"差"的各组中间存活时间分别为 207d 和 92d［"好"与"差"的死亡 HR = 0.50；95% CI（0.24，0.78）］。在第二队列中分别为 306d 和 107d［HR = 0.41；95% CI（0.17，0.63）］。该算法的预测值不依赖于与 EGFR TKIs 灵敏度相关的临床因素，如性别、吸烟史以及组织学。此外该算法也鉴别出疗效较好的吸烟者亚组，显示其在预测临床特征显示药物敏感性差的人群中的预测优势。对于未接受化疗或 EGFR TKIs 治疗的患者，算法并不依据患者的生存时间进行分类。该分类也被用于 BR.21 临床试验的样本分析，该试验主要比较不适合化疗的患者行厄洛替尼对比安慰剂作为 2 线或 3 线治疗的疗效[25]，这种分类法充分地预测了厄洛替尼的治疗应答。19 例应答者中 18 例被界定为"好"。蛋白质组学界定为"好"的患者，其生存时间显著优于"差"组（中位生存期为 10.5 个月 vs 6.6 个月），但对照组却无显著差异（中间存活时间为 4 个月 vs 3.4 个月）。近期一项随机前瞻试验验证了该结果的显著性，且另一项肺鳞癌患者大型随机临床试验也正在进行[26]。

使用候选蛋白标志物的另一项研究中，E4599 Ⅱ期/Ⅲ期临床试验评估了两种黏附分子——可溶性细胞间黏附分子（intercellular adhesion molecule，ICAM）和 E - 选择素，以及两种血管生成因子——血管内皮生长因子（vascular endothelial growth factor，VEGF）和碱性成纤维细胞生长因子（Basic fibroblast growth factor，bFGF）的胞质水平的预后及预测价值。该试验中，878 例晚期 NSCLC 患者随机接收卡铂 + 紫杉醇（PC 组）及 PC + 贝伐单抗（BPC 组）治疗。只有 ICAM 表达水平是患者生存期的预后指标，且不论是否联用贝伐单抗均能预测化疗疗效，但 VEGF 水平只能预测贝伐单抗治疗疗效却不能预测生存期[27]。在另一项 33 例早期 NSCLC 患者参与的单臂 Ⅱ 期临床试验中，通过多重检验及 ELISA 测定的 8 种细胞因子及血管生成因子的胞质水平能准确预测帕唑帕尼的应答效果。该药是一种靶向抑制 VEGFR、血小板生长因子受体及 c-kit 的抗血管生成药物[28]。

最近，一种自动化技术被用于同时测量血清肽。在该方法中，多肽被捕获并在基于磁珠格式的反向批处理过程中浓缩，该过程由自动化液体机器人处理，之后是 MALDI-TOF MS 操作。该技术简单并具有规模生产化，也具有较好的可再生性、多维性以及高通量性[29]，但必须在更大的人群及多个研究机构中进行反复验证。

血清蛋白质组复杂度的解决策略

血清蛋白质组中不同浓度、种类的蛋白质，各种蛋白产生的大量多肽，不同的翻译后修饰方式以及个体间不同的亚型，给当前蛋白质组学技术带来了无限的挑战[30-31]。为克服这些困难，多种方法被用于减少其复杂程度，其中一种方法是亲和性移除如白蛋白等最丰富的血清蛋白[32-35]，并检测量较少的蛋白，这些蛋白能提供更多关于肿瘤特异性标志物的相关信息，但却容易被丰富的蛋白所湮没。第二种方法是在 MS 之前利用蛋白质的理化性质对样本进行分离，如分子量、残余电荷以及亲水性[34,36-37]，当然这种分离方法有其局限性，例如需要大量样本、价格昂贵且耗时，以及增加了样品内及样品间变化的风险。

液相色谱－串联质谱法

液相色谱－串联质谱法是从复杂的混合物中分离鉴定目的肽段和蛋白的有力工具。该技术直接偶联液相色谱和 ESI MS，对肿瘤蛋白质分析具有较深远的意义[38]。这种全自动化的工具遵循自下而上的方法（与之相反的是自上而下的方法，在这种方法中，完整的蛋白被电离成碎裂的肽片段）。在自下而上的方法中（也叫猎枪法），蛋白质首先被特异性的蛋白酶消化，所获得的肽段通过 LC 分离，并由 ESI MS 以及 MS/MS 在线分析（图 5.5）[15,39]。在第一个 MS 中，较短的电荷依据 m/z 比例测量，最丰富的肽段被选择用来 MS/MS 分析。所获得的碎片离子依据 m/z 比例进行二次 MS 分析。基于我们对破碎细胞所获得水平的理解以及其准确的分子量，可以准确地推断肽段的序

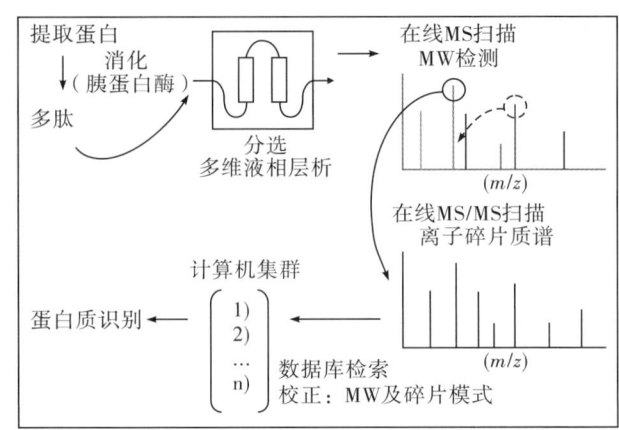

图 5.5 使用 LC-MS/MS 猎枪识别蛋白。蛋白混合物先被胰酶消化，所获得肽段通过多维液相色谱（典型的强阳离子交换后反相分离）在线偶联质谱进行分离。洗脱后，肽段 M/Z 比值第一次确定后，最丰富的肽信号进行再一次或几次 MS/MS 循环直到所有的肽段都从层析柱上洗脱下来为止，对于 MS/MS 中的每一个选择的肽，与之名义质量类似的肽段就从数据库中提取，预测来自硅片的碎片模式。这些模式然后与实验所产生的碎片图谱进行比较得到一个相关数。一个蛋白质的鉴定要依据两个甚至更多已知序列的肽段所获取

列。通过将预测的序列与数据库中具有相同标志质量的序列进行比较，就能识别肽段，并能推导其所构成的蛋白质。然而对于结构极其复杂的蛋白质混合物，通过 MS/MS 进行准确及重复的识别会有难度。此外，高丰度蛋白也可能湮没低丰度蛋白。为克服该缺陷，不同分离方法可与 MS 联合应用，例如分子排阻层析、阴离子交换、强阳离子交换、等电聚焦和反相色谱分析，其中，多维蛋白质鉴定技术结合强阳离子交换和反相柱技术，可以适应猎枪 MS 蛋白质组平台[40-42]。这种方法充分利用了离子交换和反相色谱分离，进行独立数据扫描[3]，能减少总分析时间。通过猎枪蛋白质组结合多维蛋白质鉴定技术分析肺癌患者的胞质，可显示肺腺癌患者中 120 种独立表达的蛋白[46]。

在上述策略中，特异性化学探针也能被用来标记及促进目的肽段的分离。在猎枪法中，经过胰酶消化后，由于每个蛋白含有大量的冗余肽段，分析将变得更复杂。通过靶向包含唯一或稀少氨基酸或翻译后修饰的肽段，如磷酸化或糖基化[47]，我们能减少生物样本的复杂性，分析亚蛋白质组。例如，Zhou 等[48]利用固相从糖蛋白中萃取 N－连

接糖肽的方法，研究出了一种高通量分析血清糖蛋白的技术。通过使用酰肼化学，糖蛋白能结合到固相上，未糖基化的蛋白被胰酶消化除去，N-段糖肽在被识别之前通过肽-N-糖苷酶F释放，并被串联的MS量化[49]。虽然这些策略非常吸引人，但都处于发展早期，需要进行标准化。

使用多反应（LC MRM MS）检测靶向蛋白质组学

多反应检测（多反应检测：分子质量）通过对蛋白质和肽段准确定量从而对候选生物标志物进行验证。在该策略中，需要一个三重四极杆串联质谱[50]，质量选择分为两个阶段：第一个阶段，选择部分有预先设计特定值的容易破碎的前体离子；第二个阶段，将给予假定离子相关的预先鉴定的碎片离子一个光谱。双重过滤器将诱导一个极其特异及敏感的识别。几个前体离子或碎片离子在单一的LC-MS/MS中就能实现特异化，从而使多个蛋白或肽段进行平行定量成为可能。通过在MS2阶段[51]使用iTRAQ（isobaric tags for relative and absolute quantification; covalent linkage to lysines, -NH$_2$ termini）或在MS1阶段使用无标记的方法就能提高定量能力。胞质或血清中的CRP[52]、阿朴脂蛋白A~I[53]、人生长激素[54]和前列腺特异性抗原[55]通过多反应检测都已被测量。

血清蛋白生物标志物的生物分析验证

新的生物标志物被发现以后，接下来的关键步骤就是验证及评估他们在临床相关患者中的预测作用[56]。在生物标志物确定应用于临床之前，必须进行多层次验证[57-58]。这就包括使用不同的技术验证在蛋白质水平是否发生改变，如肺癌的生物学表现是否与早期的检测、化学灵敏度以及生存时间有关。临床验证的这些阶段将评估在相关临床环境中生物标志物的性能，以及它们如何影响临床管理的风险或疾病[59]（见下文"血清生物标志物的临床验证"）。

蛋白标志物的生化方法验证主要是基于免疫学的实验方法。虽然基于免疫学的检测分析已十分真实和可靠，其主要依赖于抗体与靶向分子之间的紧密及特异性的结合。但这些方法也受抗体质量、高劳动强度以及较低通量等因素限制[60]。最近，Kuhn等应用多反应检测从类风湿关节炎患者体内鉴定出一系列血清生物标志物[61]。其他的联合免疫法的特异度、质谱的灵敏度、同位素标准稳定以及抗多肽抗体捕获或SISCAPA的新技术也被研发出来并用于复杂消化物中肽段的量化[62]。在这些方法中，固定在纳米亲和柱上的抗肽抗体对目的肽段进行富集，且同时加入具有相同序列的同位素稳定标记的标准物。从抗肽抗体中洗脱下来后，电喷雾质谱就被用来量化肽段（天然的和标记的）。虽然SISCAPA只能用于序列已知的分析物，但它通过移除MS传递过程中不需要的肽段，提高了灵敏度。通过该技术，肺癌的非血清生物标志物已经得到了验证。未来随着蛋白质分离及检测技术的不断提高，这些技术可能用于验证平台。最近通过NCI/SPORE/EDRN的联合努力，已建立了血液样本库，可用于候选生物标志物的Ⅱ期验证（http://edrn.nci.nih.gov/resources/sample-reference-sets）。

自身循环抗体

肿瘤相关抗原（tumor associated antigens, TAA）是肿瘤细胞中由于各种原因使蛋白发生改变，从而具有免疫原性的蛋白。这些改变方式包括过量表达、突变、错误折叠、截短或降解[63]。通过使用cDNA噬菌体展示文库以及蛋白质微阵列等高通量筛选平台，从几个免疫性疾病及恶性肿瘤患者的血清中已鉴定出大量的TAA靶点[64]。对于肺癌，通过使用抗肿瘤蛋白的患者血清，蛋白基因产物9.5（PGP 9.5）的自身抗体已被证实是一种潜在的肺癌肿瘤相关抗原[65]。有趣的是，通过噬菌体展示文库，可比螺旋CT早5年发现肿瘤患者血清中的TAA。因此，监测具有高肺癌风险个体血清中的自身抗体是进行筛选试验的较好选择。使用这种方法，几组研究人员识别了大量可能是自身抗体靶点的免疫原性肽，例如通过使用T7-cDNA噬菌体展示文库，对NSCLC患者的血清进行筛选，两组团队分别识别了自身抗体所对应的几个免疫反应性多肽[66-68]。使用类似技术，Chen 等从早期肺腺癌患者的血清中识别且验证了包含泛素1在内的其他几种肽段，它们是自身抗体的潜在靶点[69]。此外，最近 Wu 等使用噬菌体展示技术，从 NSCLC 中识别出了6种有差异的肽段克隆，但它们中只有一种蛋白质的身份被确认[70]。然而，大多数已被鉴定的抗原只在小部分患者中产生抗体，其特异度较好，灵敏度偏低。

噬菌体展示技术的另一个缺点是其不能检测翻译后修饰。最近，通过使用液相层析分离肿瘤细胞系的天然蛋白质混合物来研发的多维分离技术克服了上述障碍。该技术可在结肠癌及肺腺癌患者的外周血中识别 C 端水解酶 L3 泛素蛋白的特异性抗体[71]。这些新的肺癌自身抗体的鉴别推动了高灵敏度、可再生性及高通量检测方法的发展。

为测试自身抗体能否用于肺癌的诊断，研究人员应用间接 ELISA 法测试了6种已知肿瘤相关抗原 [p53，NY-ESO-1，cancer-associated antigen (CAGE)，GBU4-5，Annexin 1 and SOX2][72-73]。这些努力获得了一个高可再生性、精密度及线性的方法。通过外周血检测，它能检测出近40%的原发性肺癌。该方法尤其能满足发病及治疗前的早期诊断需求（图5.2）。当然这些试验还需在大样本高危患者中进行进一步的临床研究，在进入临床实践运用前，还需行回顾性和前瞻性验证。

血清生物标志物的临床验证

合理的实验设计是成功获得潜在的生物标志物并应用于临床的关键。验证一种生物标志物能否用于肺癌的诊断或早期筛选，其验证过程应按照 PRoBE 设计在前瞻性纵向队列中使用巢式病例对照研究设计[74]。具体而言，从一个建立好的队列人群中随机抽取试验组和对照组能保证试验组和对照组来自于同一人群，从而为病例对照研究提供可实现性，例如匹配策略，在采样的同时可以考虑使用发病密度，对每一个案例，在同一时间使病例和对照组进行时间的匹配。虽然有匹配优势，但匹配的缺陷在实施之前应仔细斟酌[74-75]。

对于临床应用的生物标志物，评估在不同临床环境及不同人群中生物标志物的一般性是有必要的。在生物标志物发现过程中，包含案例组和对照组的前瞻性队列必须能代表生物标志物将应用的临床靶向人群，因此，队列研究人群必须包含靶向人群各种环境下的个体，如炎症、肉芽肿或良性肿瘤，只有这样，假阳性率才能被最小化，患肺癌的个体才能与未患病的个体区分开。

用于研究生物标志物的生物标本应该在前瞻性队列研究开始、确诊肺癌状态之前就被收集[74]，如果生物标志物随着年龄及疾病的侵袭状态发生改变，生物标本同时应该在多个时间点进行收集[76]，为了能研发一个经济、有效、可临床应用的生物标志物，生物标本须在确诊的肿瘤患者（试验组）和未形成肿瘤的患者（对照组）之间进行评估。重要的是，结果应该明确表述，为了避免偏倚，在试验过程中试验组和对照组的信息应该盲编[74]。为了验证一个生物标志物能否用于肺癌的早期检测，其诊断验证应该在不同、尽可能复杂的人群中进行，而不仅局限于用于测试特异性的肺癌患者[78]。之后，应该以肺癌死亡率作为研究终点，使用筛选试验进行早期诊断验证。

评估一个生物标志物是否能有效应用于临床，需要计算灵敏度和特异度。这个可以利用受试者工作特征曲线（receiver operator characteristic curve，ROC）进行总结[80]。通过 ROC 曲线能测量的其他两个临床相关数据包括阳性预测值（positive predictive value，PPV）和阴性预测值（negative predictive value，NPV），这两个值使用灵敏度和特异度来进行计算。阳性预测值和阴性预测值这两个重要的临床指数分别描述有和无疾病的可能性。阳性预测值和阴性预测值的计算受到疾病的患病率、患者的年龄、人群分布以及疾病状态的影响，因此仅仅只基于人口因素，只对高危人群进行筛选可能会改变筛选试验的结果[81]。因此，对于一个能有效用于临床且可被验证的生物标志物，其验证过程必须在有不同人群特性的多人群中展开，并且每个人群可能对生物标志物的临床应用要求不同。

当前肺癌生物标志物研发及应用的挑战

分子医学在肺癌研究中的一个主要目标就是识别及区分低危和高危人群、良性和恶性肿瘤的生物标志物。最终，这些生物标志物要尽可能转化为无创、简单、可靠，且能用于疾病早期检测的诊断工具。这些努力背后的潜在假设是可以在一些复杂的临床样本，如替代组织和生物液体中，简单准确地检测到肿瘤特异性或高表达的蛋白。旨在识别生物标志物的基因组学和蛋白质组学研究已经发现了大量可能的诊断生物标志物，但很少能达到美国 FDA 批准用于诊断的水平[82]。表 5.2 总结了最近关于血清蛋白生物标志物的相关研究，这些生物标志物的选择要基于两个准则：第一，所提出的标志物或标志物群必须能够定量测量，且其必须要在至少一种临床相关的样本中进行性能测试；第二，报告必须严格遵守上述临床验证指南，报告中的验证群体必须是一个真实的独立人群[83]。

肺癌生物标志物发现及验证的停滞不前受到大量的技术和方法学的限制。在期望和产品之间的阻碍部分是由于当前的检测方法是不可靠或无效的。当前分析方法的限制主要在于很难从极其复杂的物质如胞质和血清中，在很高的背景下，从丰富的分子中（如蛋白质）检测到低丰度的肿瘤生物标志物。在生物液体（如血清）中的低丰度标志物很可能就是肿瘤生物标志物，最终的结果是，很多最好的候选者可能会在发现阶段丢失。

另一个难题就是缺乏高通量的方法去证明和验证已经存在的候选标志物，这一点在蛋白质组学研究中尤其突出。缺乏合适的试剂如抗体，或者合适的方法去验证组织样本中已发现的候选者，同时也没有办法测量其在循环中的浓度，这些都是巨大的挑战。因此，可能很多生物标志物已经被发现，但却还没有得到验证。此外，即使大量的候选生物标志物被编译，也没有标准的方法进行选择。当然，生物标志物数据的可再生性也不强，原因可能是实验设计不佳[74]、模型过度拟合、缺乏交叉验证、低浓度的信号、前瞻性研究太少以及发病率较低等。所有这些因素给生物标志物研究领域带来了巨大挑战。

总结及未来临床价值

各种生物样本的分子分析已经发现了很多相关的候选生物标志物，且这些新鉴定的蛋白质可能有助于肺癌的研究。最近几年，"Omics"资源大量临床样本的高通量分析已获得了大量的数据，其发展速度十分惊人，产生了大量的候选生物标志物。目前已发表的生物标志物没有一个用于临床，也很少能进入Ⅲ期研发。肺癌是一种复杂的异质性疾病，它不仅表现在生化水平（基因、蛋白、代谢），同时也在组织、器官以及人群中表达。我们有必要将目前多个研究平台的结果整合到一个数字化的框架中，只有这样，才能进一步加深我们对该疾病的理解。通过 CT 筛选，基于生物液体的测试可能提高高危人群的筛选，从而能将恶性肿瘤与良性肿瘤区分开，识别出具有侵袭性的患者，这样做才可以降低死亡率，为公共卫生系统减少开支。

随着血清生物标志物不断对致病机制、疾病侵袭等影响的验证，其作用也在不断加强，它将为疾病的早期检测、预后以及治疗和管理提供新的机会。本章我们阐述了血清蛋白质组学技术的最新研究进展，以及其在肺癌中的广泛应用，我们主要强调的是早期检测。蛋白质组学技术的快速发展已经导致了大量蛋白的合成以及肽段的发现，同时我们对它们之间如何作用及特异性翻译后修饰的作用有了更进一步的理解，此外，也解决了它们中的一些生物学功能。

尽管目前还未确定肺癌血清蛋白质组学特性分析以及相关的生物样本的临床价值，它可以突出肺癌与良性病变，以及不同危险因素、分期及组织学类型的病变之间的差异。分子特异性分析将帮助识别高危人群，提供研究致癌机制的机会，帮助患者从特异性靶向治疗中获益。运用系统生物学方法整合不同水平的成果（基因→蛋白→细胞）将为与肿瘤侵袭相关的关键分子的改变提供一个全面的视野。因此，未来系统生物学将加速"Omics"向个人分子医学的发展。

从生物液体如痰、血液或呼出气中研发出特异性、灵敏的诊断性生物标志物，将改善早期检测方法、疾病进展监测、治疗效果以及复发监测。新的蛋白质组学研究平台的使用需要进行验证，并证明其在临床中的应用价值。

（李庆玉　倪　阳　译）

参考文献

[1] Bhattacharjee A, Richards WG, Staunton J, et al. Classification of human lung carcinomas by mRNA expression profiling reveals distinct adenocarcinoma subclasses. Proc Natl Acad Sci USA, 2001, 98 (24): 13790-13795.

[2] Brambilla E, Travis WD, Colby TV, et al. The new World Health Organization classification of lung tumours. European Respiratory Journal, 2001, 18 (6): 1059-1063.

[3] Beer DG, Kardia SL, Huang CC, et al. Gene-expression profiles predict survival of patients with lung adenocarcinoma. Nature Medicine, 2002, 8 (8): SI6-S24.

[4] Garber ME, Troyanskaya OG, Schluens K, et al. Diversity of gene expression in adenocarcinoma of the lung. Proc Natl Acad Sci USA, 2001, 93 (24): 13784-13789.

[5] Siegel R, Naishadham D, Jemal A. Cancer statistics, 2012. CA: A Cancer Journal for Clinicians, 2012, 62 (1):10-29.

[6] Zhu L, Pickle LW, Ghosh K, et al. Predicting US-and state-level cancer counts for the current calendar year: Part II: evaluation of spatiotemporal projection methods for incidence. Cancer, 2012, 118 (4): 1100-1109.

[7] Hoffman PC, Mauer AM, Yokes EE. Lung cancer. Lancet, 2000, 355 (9202): 479-485.

[8] Patz EF, Jr., Caporaso NE, Dubinett SM, et al. National Lung Cancer Screening Trial American College of Radiology Imaging Network Specimen Biorepository originating from the Contemporary Screening for the Detection of Lung Cancer Trial (NLST, ACRIN6654): design, intent, and availability of specimens for validation of lung cancer biomarkers. J Thorac Oncol, 2010, 5 (10): 1502-1506.

[9] Manser RL, Irving LB, Eyrnes G, et al. Screening for lung cancer: a systematic review and meta-analysis of controlled trials. Thorax, 2003, 58 (9): 784-789.

[10] Manser R. Screening for lung cancer: a review. Curr Opin Pulm Med, 2004, 10 (4): 266-271.

[11] Pastorino U. Lung cancer screening. Br J Cancer, 2010, 102 (12): 1681-1686.

[12] National Institute of Health NCIN, NCI Office of Media Relations. Twenty percent fewer lung cancer deaths seen among those who were screened with low-dose spiral CT than with chest X-ray. US NIH New, 2010.

[13] Ludwig JA, Weinstein JN. Biomarkers in cancer staging, prognosis and treatment selection. Nat Rev Cancer, 2005, 5 (11): 845-856.

[14] Anderson L, Hunter CL. Quantitative mass spectrometiic multiple reaction monitoring assays for major plasma proteins. Mol Cell Proteomics, 2006, 5 (4): 573-588.

[15] Ocak S, Chaurand P, Massion PP. Mass speetrometry-based proteomic profiling of lung cancer. Proceedings of the American Thoracic Society, 2009, 6 (2): 159-170.

[16] Addona TA, Abbatiello SE, Schilling B, et al. Multi-site assessment of the precision and reproducibility of multiple reaction monitoring-based measurements of proteins in plasma. Nat Biotechnol, 2009, 27 (7): 633-641.

[17] Gonzalez-Angulo AM, Hennessy BT, Mills GB. Future of personalized medicine in oncology: a systems biology approach. J Clin Oncol, 2010, 28 (16): 2777-2783.

[18] Beavis RC, Chait BT. Rapid, sensitive analysis of protein mixtures by mass spectrometry. Proc Natl Acad Sci USA, 1990, 87 (17): 6873-6877.

[19] Sidransky D, Irizarry R, Caiifano JA, et al. Serum protein MALDI profiling to distinguish upper aerodigestive tract cancer patients from control subjects. J Natl Cancer Inst, 2003, 95 (22): 1711-1717.

[20] Vildiz PB, ShyrY, Rahman JS, et al. Diagnostic accuracy of MALDI mass spectrometric analysis of unfractionated scrum in lung cancer. J Thorac Oncol, 2007, 2 (10): 893-901.

[21] Patz EF, Jr, Campa MJ, Gottlin EB, et al. Panel of serum biomarkers for the diagnosis of lung cancer. J Clin Oncol, 2007, 25 (35): 5578-5583.

[22] Han KQ, Huang G, Gao CF, et al. Identification of lung cancer patients by serum protein profiling using surface-enhanced laser desorption/ionization time-of-flight mass spectrometry. Am J Clin Oncol, 2008, 31 (2): 133-139.

[23] Yang SY, Xiao XY, Zhang WG, et al. Application of serum SELDI proteomic patterns in diagnosis of lung cancer. BMC Cancer, 2005, 5: 83.

[24] Tagucbi F, Solomon B, Gregorc V, et al. Mass spectrometry to classify non-small-cell lung cancer patients for clinical outcome after treatment with epidermal growth factor receptor tyrosine kinase inhibitors: a multicohort cross-institutional study. J Natl Cancer Inst, 2007, 99 (11):838-846.

[25] Carhone DP, Ding K, Roder H, et al. Prognostic arid predictive role of the VeriStrat plasma test in patients with advanced non-small-cell lung cancer treated with erlotinib or placebo in the NCIC Clinical Trials GroupBR. 21 trial.

J Thorac Oncol, 2012, 7 (11): 1653-1660.

[26] Lazzati C, Novello S, Barni S, et al. Randomized proteomic stratified phase Ⅲ study of second-line erlotinib (E) versus chemotherapy (CT) in patients with inoperable non-small cell lung cancer (PROSE). J Clin Oncol, 2013, 31 (suppl): abstr LBA8005.

[27] Dowlati A, Gray R, Sandler AB, et al. Cell adhesion molecules, vascular endothelial growth factor, and basic fibroblast growth factor in patients with non-small cell lung cancer treated with chemotherapy with or without bevacizumab-an Eastern Cooperative Oncology Group Study. CI in Cancer Res, 2008, 14 (5): 1407-1412.

[28] Nikolinakos PG, Altorki N, Vankelevitz D, et al. Plasma cytokine and angiogenic factor profiling identifies markers associated with tumor shrinkage in early-stage non-small cell lung cancer patients treated with pazopanib. Cancer Res, 2010, 70 (6): 2171-2179.

[29] Villanueva J, Philip J, Entenberg D, et al. Serum peptide profiling by magnetic particle-assisted, automated sample processing and MALDI-TOF mass spectrometry. Anal Chem, 2004, 76 (6): 1560-1570.

[30] Anderson NL, Anderson NG. The human plasma proteome: history, character, and diagnostic prospects. Mol Cell Proteomic, 2002, 1 (11): 845-867.

[31] Nedelkov D, Kiernan UA, Niederkofler EE, et al. Investigating diversity in human plasma proteins, Proc Natl Acad Sci USA, 2005, 102 (31): 10 352-10 357.

[32] Pieper R, Gatlin CL, Makusky AJ, et al. The human serum proteome: display of nearly 3700 chromatographically separated protein spots on two-dimensional electrophoresis gels and identification of 325 distinct proteins. Proteomics, 2003, 3 (7): 1345-1364.

[33] Pieper R, Su Q, Gatlin CL, et al. Multi-component immunoaffinity subtraction chromatography: an innovative step towards a comprehensive survey of the human plasma proteome, Proteomics, 2003, 3 (4): 422-432.

[34] Adkins JN, Varnum SM, Auberry KJ, et al. Toward a human blood serum proteome: analysis by multidimensional separation coupled with mass spectrometry. Mol Cell Proteormics, 2002, 1 (12): 947-955.

[35] Liu T, Qian WJ, Chen WN, et al. Improved proteome coverage by using high efficiency cysteinyl peptide enrichment: the human mammary epithelial cell proteome. Proteomics, 2005, 5 (5): 1263-1273.

[36] Shen Y, Jacobs JM, Camp DG, et al. Ultra-high-efficiency strong cation exchange LC/RPLC/MS/MS for high dynamic range characterization of the human plasma proteome. Anal Chem, 2004, 76 (4): 1134-1144.

[37] Tirumalai RS, Chan KC, Prieto DA, et al. Characterization of the low molecular weight human serum proteome. Mol Cell Proteomics, 2003, 2 (10): 1096-1103.

[38] McCormack AL, Schieltz DM, Goodie B, et al. Direct analysis and identification of proteins in mixtures by LC/MS/MS and database searching at the low-femtomole level. Anal Chem, 1997, 69 (4): 767-776.

[39] Ocak S, Sos ML, Thomas RK, et al. High-throughput molecular analysis in lung cancer: insights into biology and potential clinical applications. European Respiratory Journal, 2009, 34 (2): 489-506.

[40] Link AJ, Eng J, Schieltz DM, et al. Direct analysis of protein complexes using mass spectrometry. NatBiotechnol, 1999, 17 (7): 676-682.

[41] Wolters DA, Washburn MP, Yates JR, et al. An automated multidimensional protein identification technology for shotgun proteomics. Anal Chem, 2001, 73 (23): 5683-5690.

[42] Washburn MP, Wolters D, Yates JR. Large-scale analysis of the yeast proteome by multidimensional protein identification technology. NatBiotechnol, 2001, 19 (3): 242-247.

[43] Liebler DC. Shotgun mass spec goes independent. Nat Methods, 2004, 1 (1): 16-17.

[44] Chen EI, Hewel J, Felding-Habermann B, et al. Large scale protein profiling by combination of protein fractionation and multidimensional protein identification technology (Mud PIT), Mol Cell Proteomics, 2006, 5 (1): 53-56.

[45] Jessani N, Niessen S, Wet BQ, et al. A streamlined platform for high-content functional proteomics of primary human specimens. Nat Methods, 2005, 2 (9): 691-697.

[46] Fujii K, Nakano T, Kanazawa M, et al. Clinical-scale high-throughput human plasma proteome analysis: lung adenocarcinoma. Proteomics, 2005, 5 (4): 1150-1159.

[47] Zhang Z, Bast RC, Jr., Yu Y, et al. Three biomarkers identified from serum proteomic analysis for the detection of early stage ovarian cancer. Cancer Res, 2004, 64 (16): 5882-5590.

[48] Zhou Y, Aebersold R, Zhang H. Isolation of N-linked glycopeptides from plasma. Anal Chem, 2007, 79 (35): 5826-5837.

[49] Zhang H, Li XJ, Martin DB, et al. Identification and quantification of N-linked glycoproteins using hydrazide chemistry, stable isotope labeling and mass spectrometry. Nat Biotechnol, 2003, 21 (6): 660-666.

[50] Domon B, Aebersold R. Mass spectrometry arid protein analysis. Science, 2006, 312 (5771): 212-217.

[51] Wolf-Yadlin A, Hautaniemi S, Lauffenburger DA, et al. Multiple reaction monitoring for robust quantitative proteomic analysis of cellular signaling networks. Proc Natl Acad Sci USA, 2007, 104 (14): 5860-5865.

[52] Kulm E, Wu J, Karl J, et al. Quantification of C-reactive protein in the serum of patients with rheumatoid arthritis using multiple reaction monitoring mass spectrometry and relabeled peptide standards. Proteomics, 2004, 4 (4): 1175-1186.

[53] Barr JR, Maggio VL, Patterson DG, et al. Isotope dilution-mass spectrometric quantification of specific proteins: model application with apolipoprotein A-I. Clin Chem, 1996, 42 (10): 1676-1682.

[54] Wu CC, MacCoss MJ. Shotgun proteomics: tools for the analysis of complex biological systems. Curr Opin Mol Ther, 2002, 4 (3): 242-250.

[55] Barnidge DR, Goodmanson MK, Klee GG, et al. Absolute quantification of the model biomarker prostate-specific antigen in scrum by LC-Ms/MS using protein cleavage and isotope dilution mass spectrometry. J Proteome Res, 2004, 3 (3): 644-652.

[56] George SL. Statistical issues in translational cancer research, Clin Cancer Res, 2008, 14 (19): 5954-5958.

[57] Pepe MS, Etzioni R, Feng Z, et al. Phases of biomarker development for early detection of cancer. J Natl Cancer Inst, 2001, 93 (14): 1054-1061.

[58] Srivastava S, Gopal-Srivastava R. Biomarkers in cancer screening: a public health perspective. J Nutr, 2002, 132 (8 Suppl): 2471S-2475S.

[59] Moons KG. Criteria for scientific evaluation of novel markers: a perspective. Clin Chem, 2010, 56 (4): 537-541..

[60] Huang SN, Minassian H, More JD. Application of immunofluorescent staining on paraffin sections improved by trypsin digestion, Lab Invest, 1976, 35 (4): 383-390.

[61] Kuhn E, Wu J, Karl J, et al. Quantification of G-reactive protein in the serum of patients with rheumatoid arthritis using multiple reaction monitoring mass spectrometry and C-13-labeled peptide standards. Proteomics, 2004, 4 (4): 1175-1186.

[62] Anderson NL, Polanski M, Pieper R, et al. The human plasma proteome: a non-redundant list developed by combination of four separate sources. Mol Cell Proteomics, 2004, 3 (4): 311-326.

[63] Caron M, Choquet-Kastylevsky G, Joubert-Garon R. Cancer immunomics using autoantibody signatures for biomarker discovery. Mol Cell Proteomics, 2007, 6 (7): 1115-1122.

[64] Feng Z, Prentice R, Srivastava S. Research issues and strategies for genomic and proteomic biomarker discovery and validation: a statistical perspective. Pharmacogenomics, 2004, 5 (6): 709-719.

[65] Brichory F, Beer D, Lc Naour F, et al. Proteomics-based identification (if protein gene product 9.5asa tumor antigen that induces a humoral immune response in lung cancer. Cancer Res, 2001, 61 (21): 7903-7912.

[66] Zhong L, Coe SP, Stromberg AJ, et al. Profiling tumor-associated antibodies for early detection of non-small cell lung cancer. J Thorac Oncol, 2006, 1 (6): 513-19.

[67] Zhong L, Hidalgo GE, Stromberg AJ, et al. Using protein microarray as a diagnostic assay for non-small cell lung cancer. Am J Respir Crit Care Med, 2005, 172 (10): 1308-1314.

[68] Khattar NH, Coe-Atkinson SP, Stromberg AJ, et al. Lung cancer-associated autoantibodies measured using seven amino acid peptides in a diagnostic blood test for lung cancer. Cancer Biology-Therapy, 2010, 10 (3).

[69] Chen EI, Cociorva D, Norris JL, et al. Optimization of mass spectrometry-compatible surfactants for shotgun proteomics. J Proteome Res, 2007, 6 (7): 2529-2533.

[70] Wu D, Gao Y, Chen L, et al. Anti-tumor effects of a novel chimeric peptide on SI80 and H22 xenografts bearing nude mice. Peptides, 2010, 31 (5): 850-864.

[71] Hanash S. Harnessing immunity for cancer marker discovery. Nat Biotechnol, 2003, 21 (1): 37-38.

[72] Chapman CJ, Murray A, McElveen JE, et al. Autoantibodies in lung cancer: possibilities for early detection and subsequent cure. Thorax, 2003, 63 (3): 223-233.

[73] Murray A, Chapman CJ, Healey G, et al. Technical validation of an autoantibody test for lung cancer. Ann Oncol, 2010, 21 (8): 1687-1693.

[74] Pepe MS, Feng Z, Janes H, et al. Pivotal evaluation of the accuracy of a biomarker used for classification or prediction: standards for study design. J Natl Cancer Inst, 2003, 100 (20): 1432-1438.

[75] Janes H, Pepe MS. Matching in studies of classification accuracy: implications for analysis, efficiency, and assessment of incremental value. Biometrics, 2003, 64 (1): 1-9.

[76] Baker SG, Kramer BS, Srivastava S. Markers for early detection of cancer: Statistical guidelines for nested case-control studies. BMC Med Res Methodol, 2002, 2 (1): 4.

[77] Moons KG, Altman DG, Vergouwe Y, et al. Prognosis and prognostic research: application and impact of prognostic models in clinical practice. BMJ, 2009, 338: b606.

[78] Hassanein M, Callison JC, Callaway-Lane C, et al. The state of molecular biomarkers for the early detection of lung cancer. Cancer Prev Res (Phila), 2012, 5 (8): 992-1006.

[79] Baker SG. Improving the biomarker pipeline to develop arid evaluate cancer screening tests. J Natl Cancer Inst, 2009, 101 (16): 1116-1119.

[80] Taylor JM, Ankerst DP, Andridge RR. Validation of biomarker-based risk prediction models. Clin Cancer Res, 2008, 14 (19): 5977-5983.

[81] Moons KG, Biesheuvel CJ, Grobbee DE. Test research versus diagnostic research. Clin Chem, 2004, 50 (3): 473-476.

[82] Andersen JE, Hansen LL, Mooren FC, et al. Methods and biomarkers for the diagnosis and prognosis of cancer and other diseases: towards personalized medicine. Drug Resist Updat. 2006, 9 (4-5): 193-210.

[83] Brenner DE, Normolle DP. Biomarkers for cancer risk, early detection, and prognosis: the validation conundrum. Cancer Epidemiol Biomarkers Prev, 2007, 16 (10): 1918-1920.

[84] Qiu J, Choi G, Li L, et al. Occurrence of autoantibodies to annexin I, 14-3-3 theta and LAMR 1 in prdiagnostic lung cancer sera. J Clin Oncol, 2003, 26 (31): 5060-5066.

[85] Wu L, ChangW, Zhao J, et al. Development of autoantibody signatures as novel diagnostic biomarkers of non-small cell lung cancer. Clinical Cancer Research, 2010, 16 (14): 3760-3768.

[86] Farlow EC, Patel K, Basil S, et al. Development of a multiplexed tumor-associated autoantibody-baaed blood test for the detection of non-small cell lung cancer. Clin Cancer Res, , 2010, 16 (13): 3452-3462.

[87] Boyle P, Chapman CJ, Holdenrieder S, et al. Clinical validation of an autoantibody test for lung cancer. Ann Oncol, 2011, 22 (2): 383-389.

[88] Kulpa J, Wojcik E, Rein fuss M, et al. Carcinoembryonic antigen, squamous cell carcinoma antigen, CYFRA 21-1, and neuron-specific enolase in squamous cell lung cancer patients. Clin Chem, 2002, 48 (11): 1931-1937.

[89] Takano A, Ishikawa N, Nishino R, et al. Identification of Ncctin-4 oncoprotein as a diagnostic and therapeutic target for lung cancer. Cancer Res, 2009, 69 (16): 6694-6703.

[90] Pecot CV, Li M, Zhang XJ, et al. Added value of a serum proteomic signature in the diagnostic evaluation of lung nodules. Cancer Epidemiol Biomarkers Prev, 2012, 21 (5): 786-792.

[91] Diamandi EP, Goodglick L, Planque C, et al. Pentraxin-3 is a novel biomarker of lung carcinoma. Clinical Cancer Research, 2011, 17 (8): 2395-2399.

[92] Ostroff RM, Bigbee WL, Franklin W, et al. Unlocking biomarker discovery large scale application of aptamer poteomic technology for early detection of lung cancer. PLoS ONE, 2010, 5 (12): el 5003.

[93] Taguchi A. Politi K, Pitteri SJ, et al. Lung cancer signatures in plasma based on proteome profiling of mouse tumor models. Cancer Cell, 2011, 20 (3): 289-299.

[94] Hassanein M, Rahman JS, Chaurand P, et al. Advances in proteomic strategies toward the early detection of lung cancer. Proc Am Thorac Soc, 2011, 8 (2): 183-188.

第 6 章
肺癌癌前病变的分子生物学

Humam Kadara, Ignacio I. Wistuba
Department of Translational Molecular Pathology, Division of Pathology and Laboratory Medicine, The University of Texas MD Anderson Cancer, TX, USA

引 言

从组织病理学和生物学角度看，肺癌是多种相互关联的不同类型肿瘤的高度混杂体[1]，因此可能存在多条癌前病变通路。肺癌包括多种病理类型：小细胞肺癌（SCLC）以及由鳞状细胞癌、腺癌（包含非侵袭性细支气管肺泡癌）、大细胞癌构成的非小细胞肺癌（NSCLC）[2]。肺癌可发生于主支气管（中央型肿瘤）或肺远端的小支气管、终末细支气管、肺泡（周围型肿瘤）等不同位置。鳞癌及SCLC通常发生于中央，而腺癌及大细胞肺癌通常发生于外周[2]。但每种肺癌具体由哪些特定的呼吸道上皮发展而来尚不明确。如同其他上皮来源的恶性肿瘤，肺癌的发生也经历了一系列渐进的病理变化，即癌前病变[3-4]。尽管目前对中央型肺鳞癌的癌前病变连续过程已较为清楚，但对其他类型肺癌的相关过程我们还知之甚少[3-4]。

已有相当多的研究提供了参与肺鳞癌及肺腺癌发病的癌前病变的分子生物学特征信息[5-8]。不仅如此，较早的研究也发现肺癌表现出一种区域癌变现象，即癌细胞或癌组织与相邻的组织学正常的组织会共表达某些异常的分子特征（如异质性丧失）[2,9-10]，并且其中多种分子改变可在组织学正常的吸烟者的呼吸道黏膜中检测到[9-12]。早期筛查出的高危人群为大量吸烟者和既往患上消化道恶性肿瘤者，说明进一步理解区域癌变现象将有助于肺癌的早期诊断[9,13]。值得注意的一点是，经典的识别癌前细胞形态学的方法有较大的局限性。这驱使着研究者们在分子生物学方面开展研究工作，主要包括呼吸道上皮及周边癌前病变细胞的分子和遗传学改变。

相较于有明显症状或临床确诊的肺肿瘤的分子病理学[1-2,14-15]，目前我们对肺癌发生前相关分子事件及癌变的潜在遗传基础了解甚少。因此我们目前的知识不足以判定用于评估肺癌风险的确定性相关分子标志物，以采取针对性的预防或治疗措施和早期发现肺内癌前病变。而且，肺癌癌前病变定义的完善又受制于细胞病变的相对隐蔽性及其在呼吸道内的随机分布性。尽管近期美国肺癌筛检试验（National Lung Screening Trial, NLST）带来了一些振奋人心的研究结果[16]，但由于缺乏早期诊断生物标志物，且在肺癌发生过程中有多条肿瘤相关分子信号通路参与介导，故肺癌的早期诊断和预防仍是一项艰巨的任务。对该领域进行深入研究从而提高对肺癌（包括正常上皮细胞）发展早期阶段的认识将有助于形成有效的早期诊断和预防措施。

在本章中，我们总结了肺癌的分子及组织病理学发病机制，并将讨论肺组织癌变的分子机制研究进展及其与早期诊断和预防的关系。另外，我们还描述了几种主要类型肺癌的癌前病变，并回顾了目前重要组织类型肺癌的早期发病机制和病变进展的定义；总结了区域癌变现象的研究进展，及其对进一步明确肺癌分子发病机制的作用。

肺癌癌前病变的病理机制

在认识到肺癌是发生于呼吸道黏膜一系列渐进的病理变化（肿瘤前或癌前病变）之后[2,5]，国际肺癌研究协会（International Association for the study of Lung Cancer，IASLC）对与肺内侵袭前病变相关的组织学分型列出了 3 种肺癌癌前病变的形态学类型[17]：①鳞状上皮不典型增生与原位癌（carcinoma in situ，CIS）；②非典型腺瘤样增生（atypical adenomatous hyperplasia，AAH）；③弥漫性特发性肺神经内分泌细胞增生（diffuse idiopathic pulmonary neuroendocrine cell hyperplasia，DIPNECH）。尽管在中央型肺鳞癌中可观察到连续的癌前变化，但在大细胞肺癌、肺腺癌及 SCLC 中，这些变化尚不明确[3-4,15]。发生于侵袭性鳞状细胞癌之前的气道病变包括鳞状上皮不典型增生及原位癌（CIS）[3-4]。先于腺癌发生的病变包括外周支气管细胞 AAH 等形态变化[3,18]。而 DIPNECH 被认为是类癌的癌前病变。SCLC 尚无确切的癌前病变。

肺鳞癌的癌前病变

增生、鳞状上皮化生、鳞状上皮不典型增生及原位癌是大气道侵袭性鳞状细胞癌发生前以及发生过程中的一系列病变[2-4,8]（图 6.1）。值得注意的是，正常气管上皮内没有鳞状细胞以及可发生鳞状上皮化生的祖细胞或干细胞。有研究推测，大气道基底细胞暴露于香烟烟雾后会表现出多能性并引起鳞状上皮化生和不典型增生，起到鳞状细胞癌前体的作用。

不典型增生鳞状上皮病变通常分为轻度、中度和重度，但这些病变呈连续性细胞学及组织形态不典型改变，每种分级间常有重叠。轻度鳞状上皮异型增生以组织、细胞的轻度紊乱为特征，中度异型增生表现为更多数量的不规则细胞，重度则是异常细胞及大量多形性细胞的进一步增多。另外，在一类称为伴新生血管的鳞状上皮不典型增生中，基底膜显著增厚且于上皮组织中出现血管出芽，进而引起上皮的乳头状突起[19]。这些病变高度提示，血管生成作为肿瘤标志之一[20]，在早期癌前病变中已发生。CIS 表现为细胞结构的高度混乱，间质浸润的同时基底膜完整。CIS 病灶通常分布在段支气管分叉处，然后延伸至邻近的肺叶支气管及远端的亚段支气管。这些病变通常难以被传统支气管镜或整体检查发现，但肺成像荧光内镜（lung-imaging fluorescent endoscopy，LIFE）等荧光支气管镜可以显著提高鳞状上皮不典型增生及 CIS 的检测敏感性[21]。

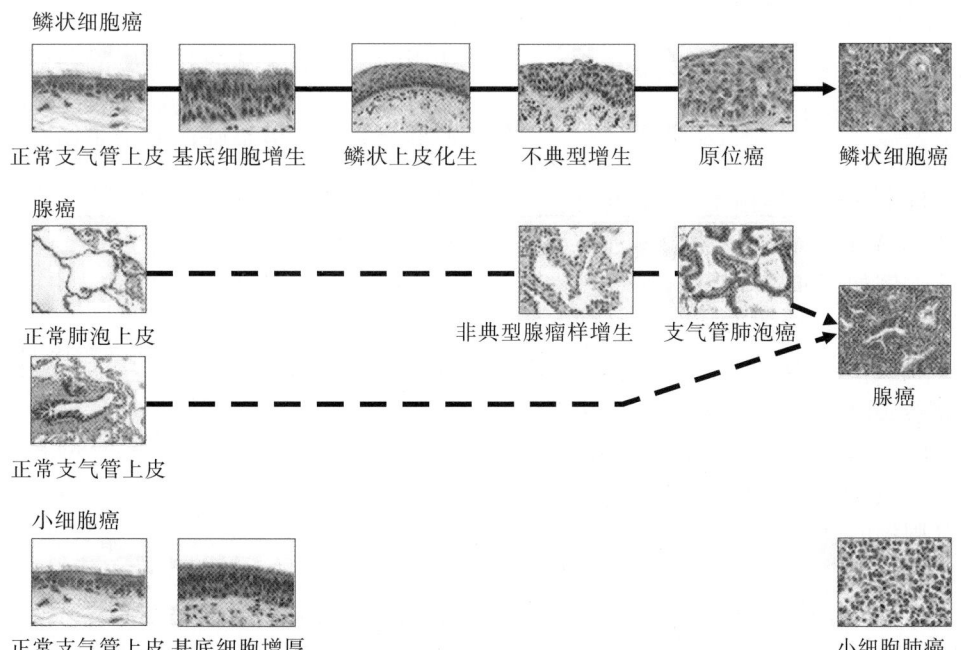

图 6.1（见彩插） 肺癌癌前病变的组织病理学变化总结。肺鳞癌发生发展中癌前病变的次序已被阐述。肺腺癌目前唯一已知的癌前病变是 AAH（非典型腺瘤样增生），其被认为是肺腺癌某一亚型的前驱病变。SCLC 尚未发现明显的癌前病变（经病理组织切片 HE 染色）

肺腺癌的癌前病变

Clara 细胞和 Ⅱ 型肺泡细胞被认为是外周支气管的祖细胞，发生于外周的肺腺癌通常表达该种类型细胞的分子标识[22-24]。AAH 被认为是外周肺腺癌的癌前病变之一[2-3,18]。然而到目前为止，AAH 是侵袭性肺腺癌发展唯一、必然经历的形态学改变，多数肺腺癌的发病机制尚不清楚。分子生物学研究结果支持了 AAH 向以非侵袭性肿瘤细胞伴行肺泡结构为特征的原位肺腺癌发展的过程[4,18]。准确辨别高度不典型 AAH 及细支气管肺泡癌（bronchioalveolar carcinoma，BAC）有时并不容易。值得注意的是，国际肺癌研究协会（International Association for the study of Lung Cancer，IASLC）、美国胸科学会（American Thoracic Society，ATS）、欧洲呼吸学会（European Respiratory society，ERS）在 WHO 2004 标准的基础上进行了修改并提出肺腺癌诊断的新分型标准。新标准建议不再沿用 BAC 概念而改用原位腺癌（adenocarcinoma in situ，AIS），同时用微浸润腺癌（invasive adenocarcinoma，MIA）替代纯贴壁生长或主要为贴壁生长但浸润深度小于 5mm 的小腺癌。重要的是，这两种肺腺癌的临床特征均较为独特，如果接受根治手术，患者的 5 年生存率可达 100%[17]。

依据免疫组化及超微结构特征诊断出的分化表型显示，AAH 起源于外周气道的祖细胞[2,15,22-24]。几乎所有的 AAH 细胞均表达肺泡表面活性蛋白及 Clara 细胞特异性 10-kDd 蛋白。另外，更多证据提示 AAH 可能作为至少一种类型肺腺癌的初期形式，例如，肺癌患者肺内 AAH 检测率较高（9%~20%），而相较于肺鳞癌（11%），肺腺癌的发生率则更高（40%）[25]。且 AAH 在东亚患者中的检出率显著高于欧美患者。在这些研究中，由于 AAH 与 TRU（终末呼吸单元）共表达多个基因，故 AAH 在 TRU 进展为原位腺癌并最终发展为侵袭性肺腺癌的过程中起直接作用[24,26-27]。研究推测 AAH 作为一种癌前病变介导了大多数正常肺泡发展为外周型肺腺癌的肿瘤进展过程。正如接下来我们要讨论的，我们注意到，在不吸烟者中发生的腺癌及肺腺癌邻近区域的细支气管间表达相似的分子异常（如 EGFR 突变），说明肺腺癌不仅起源于肺泡，也有可能起源于支气管上皮及细支气管[28-29]。最近在 Yatabe 及其同事发表的一篇论著中，提出了肺腺癌非线性进展模式[26]。在这种模式中，Yatabe 提出了 TRU 亚型肺腺癌的概念，并假设这种类型的肺癌由 AAH 发展而来。从另一个角度看，某些肺腺癌由 TRU 之外的其他细胞通过未知癌前病变过程演变而来，而我们认为这类细胞仍是支气管上皮细胞[15,28-29]。

神经内分泌肿瘤的癌前病变

如前所述，作为最常见的一种神经内分泌肿瘤，SCLC 的癌前病变尚未明确[2-4]（图 6.1）。然而，一种被称为弥漫性特发性肺神经内分泌细胞增生（DIPNECH）的罕见病变与肺内其他神经内分泌肿瘤、典型及不典型类癌的发展相关[3,30]。DIPNECH 病变包括以肺微小瘤为表现形式的外生增殖。在神经内分泌增殖大于 0.5cm 的类癌中，肿瘤细胞被杂乱分布的肺微小瘤隔离开。

肺癌发病的分子机制

先前的研究已经揭示了肺癌发病中重要的分子机制，主要包括以下几点：①几种主要类型的 NSCLC 发生发展中，多条组织病理学及分子信号通路与其密切相关[2]；②疾病发生发展中起关键作用的细胞谱系基因在肺腺癌与鳞癌中表达存在差异[15]；③尽管肺癌的癌前病变存在场效应现象，但最近的研究提示肺癌至少来源于两种不同的气管（中央和周围型）[9]；④炎症可能是参与肺癌发展以及场效应现象的重要因素[2,10]；⑤肺腺癌中已经明确的吸烟与非吸烟相关通路分别为 KRAS 和 EGFR 癌基因[14,31-38]。

一些研究显示肺癌中存在多种遗传学改变，主要包括多种确定和假定的抑癌基因及癌基因的突变[1,14]。肺癌由组织学正常的支气管上皮细胞发生一系列分子突变而来，并有一定的序列[5,8]。3p 等位基因（多个 3p 位点）缺失继以 9p（$p16^{INK4a}$ 区）缺失是最早的正常组织形态支气管上皮发生基因突变的常见顺序[5-6,39]（表 6.1）。有多个 3p 染色体基因参与肺癌的发病，主要包括 3p24 区的 RARβ，3p14.2 区的 FHIT，3p21.3 区的 RASSF1A、BLU、FUS1、SEMA3B、3p12 区的 ROBO1 也很有可能与肺癌的发病有关[6,40-41]。

表 6.1 肺癌癌前病变的组织病理学及分子异常

异常病变	肺腺癌	肺鳞癌	SCLC
组织病理学			
前驱病变	可能存在	已知	未知
病变	AAH?	鳞状上皮化生及原位癌	正常上皮及化生?
分子			
基因异常	KRAS 突变	TP53 基因杂合性缺失及突变	MYC 过表达
	EGFR 突变	SOX2 扩增	TP53 基因杂合性缺失及突变
基因不稳定性	低	中等	高
频率	13%	10%	68%
杂合性缺失	低	中等	高
频率	10%	54%	90%
染色体区	9p21，17p/TP53	8p21~23，9p21，17p/TP53	5q21，8p21~23，9p21，17p/TP53

LOH：杂合性缺失

端粒酶激酶也是肺癌发病的早期事件之一[42-43]。端粒酶缩短是支气管癌变的早期遗传学异常之一，先前的端粒酶表达及 p53/Rb 基因失活则主要出现在高病变程度的鳞癌癌前病变中[44]。对肺癌患者、目前或既往无吸烟史的肺癌患者进行显微镜下上皮组织精确切割及吸烟损害肺扫描，结果显示在组织学正常及轻度异常的支气管上皮（增生及鳞状上皮化生）以及癌前病变（不典型增生）的支气管上皮中可检测到包括等位基因缺失在内的多种损伤[45]。尽管这些变化常存在于未患肺癌的吸烟者或既往吸烟者中，但在终生不吸烟者中则几乎检测不到这些改变[11-12]。有趣的是，即使在戒烟之后这些克隆变化也持续存在[11]。这些研究发现显示了肺癌发展的多阶段过程。

有必要提到的是，我们不能忽略另一种假设，即分子及遗传学的改变是分子变异的积累，而与肺癌的发病无关。例如，KRAS 突变在 AAH 中较侵袭性肺腺癌的发生率更高[24,26]。相反，我们的研究显示在肺腺癌的进展过程中，支气管或细支气管上皮细胞中发生的 EGFR 突变早于癌基因拷贝数的增加[29]。增进肺癌癌变中的分子病理学有助于明确疾病的自然进展过程（连续或非连续），且目前相关研究指向肺癌的发病机制与渐进的、序列特异性遗传改变及分子遗传学分子异常的积累有关[9]。

肺鳞癌的发病机制

目前肺鳞癌的癌变过程中连续分子生物学异常的模式显示，遗传学异常起始于组织学正常的上皮细胞并且随着组织形态的改变而逐步累加[45]（图 6.2）。

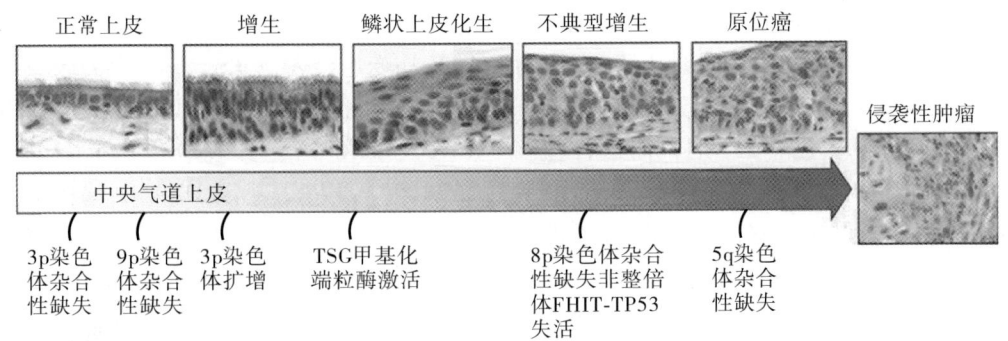

图 6.2（见彩插）　肺鳞癌发病的分子机制。肺鳞癌发病的多步骤中发生一系列分子异常，并可在高危个体中检测到该类异常

不仅如此，吸烟者及肺癌患者呼吸道上皮的分子学改变广泛存在，并在整个支气管树内形成多个病灶，形成区域效应或区域性癌变[5-6,11-12]。重要的是，基因突变常遵循一个次序，以3p染色体上多个位点（3p21，3p14，3p22~24及3p12）和9p21（p16^{INK4a}）缺失为最早可检测的基因改变。随后的突变包括8p21~23、13q14（RB）和17p13（TP53）染色体位点[5-6,39]。p16^{INK4a}甲基化也出现于肺鳞癌癌前病变的早期，其发生频率随组织学进展而逐步提高（鳞状上皮化生中为24%，CIS中为50%）[46]。在肺癌患者的正常或轻度异常的支气管上皮中可用荧光支气管镜检测到由40 000~360 000个细胞构成的克隆或亚克隆集落[45]，除了个别文献报道了有意义的阳性结果[47]，大多数研究发现对肺癌的发病风险评估、早期诊断及化学预防并无太大作用。

如前所述，作为鳞状细胞不典型增生的一个亚类，血管生成性鳞状细胞不典型增生（angiogenic squamous dysplasias，ASDs）主要表现为皮下组织中基底膜增厚和血管出芽并导致上皮细胞乳头状突起[19]。对该类病变的支气管活检显示其微血管密度高于正常黏膜组织，但与其他增生或异常相比无升高现象。因此ASD与血管生成的本质区别在于其毛细血管存在组织结构重建。对病变表面上皮的遗传学分析显示，53%的病变区存在3p染色体杂合性缺失（loss of heterozygosity，LOH），且ASD的增殖能力显著高于正常上皮。约19%的未患癌高危吸烟者的荧光支气管镜检查结果显示有ASD发生[48]，而对16例非吸烟正常对照者的活检则未发现相关病变[19]。该种病变在高危吸烟者中的出现提示支气管癌变的早期阶段可能就已发生微血管异常。在支气管鳞状上皮不典型增生中，应用半定量逆转录PCR及免疫组化均证实血管内皮生长因子（vascular endothelial growth factor，VEGF）及VEGF受体较正常上皮显著升高[49]，提示血管生成出现于癌变早期，而这种概念也促成了靶向抗血管生成化学预防治疗策略的发展。有趣的是，多数调控肺癌，尤其是肺鳞癌细胞生长的信号通路在肺癌癌前病变中也存在异常，这些通路主要有炎症相关多不饱和脂肪酸代谢通路[50]、维甲酸信号通路[51]、Ras[14,18]、EGFR[52]、PI3K/AKT[53]、IGF[54]及mTOR[55]信号通路。因此，针对性调控癌变早期相关通路为设计肺癌靶向预防治疗提供了可能[56]。

最新的分子生物学研究进展也增进了我们对肺癌关键信号通路相关知识的了解。Bass及Hussenet等的研究发现肺鳞癌及食管鳞癌中，3q（3q26.3）区谱系特异性基因SOX2大量扩增，并介导鳞癌的增殖及存活[57-58]。并且，免疫组化显示肺腺癌中SOX2表达完全缺失，但在鳞状细胞癌特别是肺鳞癌中显著升高[59]。另外，也有多项研究强调了该基因对促进肺鳞癌癌变的作用[57,60-61]。McCaughan及其同事随后特异性分析了不同等级及程度的支气管上皮不典型增生中3q拷贝数变化，并发现肺鳞癌中发生的SOX2扩增也表达于高级别支气管不典型增生而非低级别病变中，重要的是，该基因扩增与高级别原位鳞状上皮病变患者的疾病进展相关[62]。这里有必要提到的是，Yuan等的研究发现正常支气管及细支气管结构中表达较高水平的SOX2蛋白[59]。Yuan和McCaughan的研究均显示SOX2参与了早期鳞状细胞癌的癌变过程[59,62]。

肺腺癌的发病机制

肺腺癌中常见的分子异常在AAH中亦有发生，进一步验证了AAH代表真正的癌前病变[22]（图6.3），其中最重要的发现是在多达39%的AAH中可检测到KRAS（12密码子）突变，此突变在肺腺癌中也相对常见[2,63]。其他可在AAH中检测到的分子异常包括Cyclin D1过表达（70%），survivin（48%）及HER2/neu（7%）蛋白[2]。不仅如此，在Wistuba和Gazdar的综述中也提到，部分AAH病变表达3p（18%）、9p（p16^{INK4a}、13%）、9q（53%）、17q和17p（TP53，6%）染色体杂合性缺失[2]。值得注意的是，尽管并非全部，但大多数上述分子变化也频发于肺腺癌。随后的研究发现，AAH病变也会表达TSC基因相关区域杂合性缺失、端粒酶激活、LKB1基因缺失、DICER（小干扰RNA及miRNA重要效应蛋白）过表达以及CDKN2A和PTPRN2基因DNA甲基化等诸多分子特征[2,64-65]。已有多项研究试图全面比较低级别病变（如癌前病变）或原位癌与侵袭性肿瘤间基因表达谱和拷贝数的差异，发现癌基因EGFR的扩增是不同级别腺癌间的主要分子生物学差异，且通常发生于基因突变之后[26]。

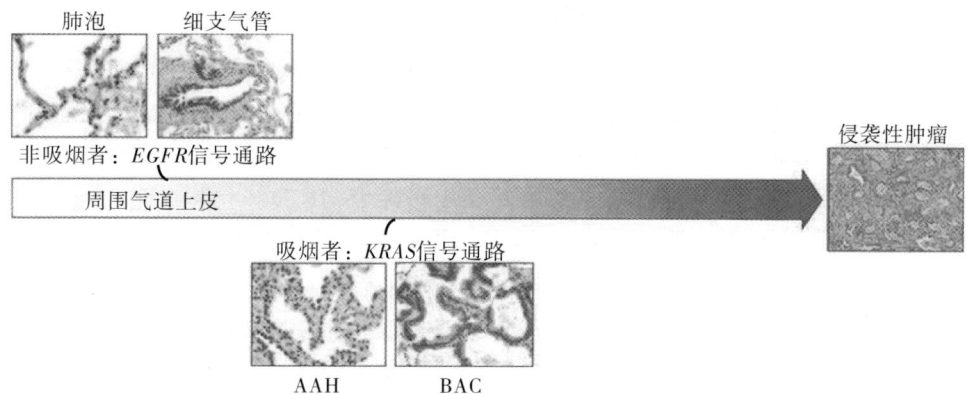

图 6.3（见彩插） 肺腺癌的分子学发病机制。吸烟或不吸烟相关性肺腺癌发展中已知至少发生两种病变

大量证据表明，至少有两条分子信号通路参与了肺癌的发生，分别为吸烟患者中的 KRAS 通路及非吸烟患者中的 EGFR 通路[14,31-38]。EGFR 突变，特别是 19 外显子及 21 外显子 L858R、L861Q 的框内缺失，在不吸烟的东亚女性患者中多见并提示对 EGFR-TKIs 疗效良好[14,33,36-37,66-67]。另一方面，KRAS 突变与吸烟者的肺癌发病密切相关[14,32-35,37]。

绝大多数 AAH 癌前病变和原位肺腺癌与"终末呼吸单元"亚型的腺癌相关，由于这种类型的腺癌高表达 TITF-1 和表面活性蛋白，因此推断该型腺癌与终末呼吸上皮同源[27]。另外，研究显示，97 例 EGFR 突变阳性腺癌表达 TITF-1，且 97 例肿瘤中有 91 例为终末呼吸单元型（TRU 型）[68]，因此假设 EGFR 突变主要或特异性存在于由 AAH 癌前病变发展而来的终末呼吸单元型周围型肺腺癌中[24,27,68]。另外，该假说还提出，EGFR 突变与肺癌 TRU 亚型相关或是肺癌中特异性的 TRU 亚型，另外一部分依据也在于 AAH 病变、原位肺腺癌及侵袭性肺腺癌之间 EGFR 和 KRAS 表达频率存在显著差异[24,26]。EGFR 突变在腺癌进展过程中呈均一表达，而 KRAS 突变率则由 AAH 中的 33% 降至腺癌中的 8%，也说明 KRAS 突变的 AAH 极少进展为腺癌。

EGFR 酪氨酸激酶区突变与肺癌早期癌变相关，可于组织学正常的小支气管上皮及毗邻 EGFR 突变的肺腺癌周边细支气管中检测到[28]。在表达 EGFR 突变的肺腺癌患者中，表观正常的外周呼吸上皮也可以检测到 EGFR 突变[28]，而在肿瘤细胞未发生突变的患者中这种情况则几乎不会发生[28]。这些结果意味着，包括被检查的上皮在内的不同类型细胞可能是 EGFR 突变肺腺癌的起源部位。尽管表达这些突变的细胞尚不明确，但我们的研究结果假设支气管和细支气管上皮内的干细胞或祖细胞含有这些突变。EGFR 突变在所有检测的 40 例 AAH 中仅表达 3 例[68-69]，且在 BAC 中表达缺失[36] 或频率相对低也是一个值得注意的现象。这些早期研究显示，EGFR 突变不仅参与肺泡型肺癌的癌变，而且可能驱动完全不同于终末呼吸及肺泡细胞的支气管上皮细胞发展为外周肺腺癌[2,15,24]。

TITF-1 是主要表达于发育期及成年小鼠终末细支气管及肺周边的一类含有同源结构域的反式激活因子[70-71]。另外，TITF-1 在正常肺组织的分支结构形成中起关键作用[70-72]，并反式激活 SPs-A、SPs-B 和 SPs-C 等表面活性蛋白的表达，随后这些蛋白通常表达于 Clara 细胞并在肺泡 II 型细胞的分化中发挥重要作用[73]。一些研究显示，含有 TITF-1 基因的 14q13.3 染色体区拷贝数及扩增的增加，表明该反式激活因子具有细胞特异性癌基因功能[74-75]。应用 RNA 干扰特异性敲除肺腺癌细胞中的 TITF-1 可导致细胞生长受阻并诱导凋亡，因此可以推断肺腺癌对 TITF-1 癌基因具有特异性遗传依赖[74-76]。但最近一项在 Kras（LSL-G12D/+）、p53（flox/flox）小鼠模型中进行的动物实验却显示 TITF-1 抑制细胞癌变及转移[77]。

SCLC 的发病机制

前面我们提到，SCLC 没有明确的癌前病变（图 6.1）。在一项比较 NSCLC 及 SCLC 患者中间气管上皮分子（部分染色体位点 LOH 及微卫星位点不稳定）差异的研究中，结果显示毗邻 SCLC 的正常或轻度异常支气管上皮遗传学异常显著高于邻近 NSCLC（鳞癌及腺癌）的正常或轻度异常支气管上皮[7]。该结果说明 SCLC 患者支气管上皮发生异常遗传学特征的范围明显广泛。毗邻 SCLC 的表观正常组织发生分子异常的现象也说明 SCLC 可能直接起源于组织学正常或轻度异常的上皮，而不需要通过更复杂的组织序列。动物模型试验显示 SCLC 的驱动因素为 TP53 和 RB 基因失活[78] 及 Hedgehog 信号通路激活[79-80]。最近，SCLC 的整合基因组分析明确了 TP53 及 RB1 失活及组蛋白修饰因子 CREBBP、EP300 及 MLL 的经常性突变，PTEN、SLIT2 及 EPHA7 突变和 FGFR1 扩增[81]。

肺癌发病的区域癌化

Danely Slaughter 早期对口腔癌和口腔癌前病变的研究显示，毗邻肿瘤或癌前病变的正常形态组织会发生一些与肿瘤组织相同的分子异常[82]。Auerbach 等于 1961 年发表的一篇研究报告显示，香烟烟雾能诱导吸烟者肺内支气管上皮发生广泛的组织学改变，癌前病变广泛、多灶性分布于支气管上皮，提示"区域癌化"现象的发生[83]。这种被称为"区域癌化"的现象随后被证实发生于包括肺癌在内的多种恶性肿瘤。一定程度的炎症和炎症相关损害几乎无一例外地存在于吸烟者的中间和外周气道，并可能早于肺癌的发生[2,9]。因此，区域癌化可解释为烟草致癌物的直接作用或者炎症反应的开始。在此背景下，Steiling 等提出并回顾了有关区域癌化起源或吸烟相关受损区的不同理论[10]。

吸烟损伤上皮及肺部区域癌化

肺癌患者及吸烟者支气管上皮往往遍布多发病灶[5-7]。对肺鳞癌患者中表观正常、癌前及恶变上皮的具体分析显示，鳞状细胞癌多阶段癌变的早期即发生了多发、有序的引起杂合性缺失的染色体特异性缺失[5-6]，尤其是 31% 的组织学正常上皮及 42% 轻度异常（增生/化生）组织切片有不止一个检查区域出现等位基因缺失细胞。Nelson 等的研究显示毗邻肺部肿瘤的组织学正常肺组织也会出现 KRAS 突变[84]。此外，也有研究报道了类似的一些肿瘤及邻近组织学正常上皮的表观遗传学及基因甲基化改变特征。Belinsky 等报道，有 44% 的受试肺癌患者在至少一个支气管上皮位点可检测到广泛表达于肺部肿瘤的 p16 基因启动子甲基化[46,85]。并且，吸烟的肺癌患者支气管上皮会发生 p16 及死亡相关蛋白激酶（death associated protein kinase, DAPK）启动子的甲基化，即使在戒烟后仍持续存在，但这种情况却不会发生于不吸烟的肺癌患者[85]。

前述的诸多分子异常也见于已通过手术切除的肺癌患者的癌组织周边正常上皮。未患肿瘤的吸烟者远端组织学正常的支气管上皮内也可检测到多灶性杂合性缺失及微卫星位点异常改变[11-12]。重要的是，这些在无肿瘤的既往吸烟者支气管上皮内检测到的分子异常即使在戒烟多年后仍然存在。另外，对经支气管镜检出的肺癌患者正常或异常肺组织支气管镜刷检获得的 DNA 检测显示有杂合性缺失的表达，且对健侧或患侧肺组织的检测均为阳性[86]。TP53 突变也广泛存在于无肿瘤的吸烟者支气管上皮细胞内[87]。无瘤患者吸烟损伤的肺上皮中也能发现类似的关于启动子甲基化及表观遗传学改变的证据。在重度吸烟者支气管上皮中可检测到包括 RAR-β2、CDH13、APC、p16、RASSFF1A 在内的多种基因突变[88]。并且，有 1/3 的无瘤吸烟者支气管上皮刷检可检测到 p16、GSTP1 和 DAPK 基因的甲基化[89]。Heller 的综述则更为具体地分析了肺癌患者及无瘤吸烟者的基因甲基化情况[90]。

区域癌化的转录组

高通量微阵列分析对研究肺气道的转录组学非常有用。Hackett 等运用支气管刷检测了无瘤吸烟者及不吸烟者中 44 个抗氧化相关基因的表达，发现其中 16 个基因在吸烟者中显著上调[91]。之后，Spira 分析比较了健康无瘤吸烟者及非吸烟者正常外观支气管上皮基因表达的差异[92]。重要的是，既往吸烟者在戒烟数年后仍存在的气道不可逆性改变是其肺癌发病风险升高的病理基础[92-93]。吸烟者与不吸烟者的大气道中 miRNA 表达量也存在差异[94]。尤其是转录组学研究显示大气道支气管上皮内有 80 种基因存在特定表达特征，而这种表达特征则有助于区别无可见肿瘤的吸烟者及吸烟的肺癌患者[95]。最近，Gustafson 等利用重组腺病毒技术在原代人上皮细胞中表达 PI3K 激酶 110α 亚基以获得 PI3K 通路激活[96]。吸烟的肺癌患者中组织学正常的支气管上皮内 PI3K 通路活性显著增强，重要的是，在接受 PI3K 抑制剂——肌醇治疗后，伴不典型增生的高危吸烟者气道中 PI3K 通路活性降低[96]。微列阵及基因表达谱研究方法同样也被用来证实肺癌广泛的区域癌化现象。吸烟者的支气管、鼻腔及口腔上皮常见基因表达改变[97]，另一项研究则显示吸烟能在支气管及鼻腔上皮中引起类似的 119 种基因表达的改变[98]。最近，Beane 等运用下一代 RNA 测序技术比较分析了健康不吸烟者与吸烟者（肿瘤及非肿瘤患者）支气管上皮刷检样本[99]，该研究强调了既往用微列阵法检测显著性不高的基因转录的重要性，说明下一代测序方法（next-generation sequencing，NGS）能为吸烟及肺癌相关的气管区域癌化现象的研究提供新的视野[99]。

区域癌化的划分

Tang 及其同事在表达 EGFR 突变的肺腺癌尤其是不吸烟患者毗邻肿瘤的正常支气管和细支气管内检测研究了 EGFR 突变情况。在 44% 有突变、组织学正常的肺腺癌患者的外周上皮中检测到了 EGFR 突变，但无突变患者则无一例出现这种情况[28]。并且，该研究显示肿瘤内正常上皮 EGFR 突变表达率（43%）显著高于周边正常上皮（24%），提示该突变在呼吸道上皮中的局部区域效应[28]。这些研究显示肺腺癌的区域癌化不同于鳞状细胞癌。

相较于肺鳞癌，周围型肺腺癌患者的中央支气管上皮发生分子异常的频率要低得多[6]，提示在这两种不同类型的病变中，因吸烟引起的基因损伤程度不同。因此，吸烟诱发的肺鳞癌主要表现为中央支气管上皮的吸烟相关性遗传损伤，而肺腺癌则主要表现为周围气道的分子及组织学损伤。尽管某些分子变化（如炎症和信号通路激活）可于整个呼吸道（包括中央和周围支气管）中检测到，其他病变则更频发于中央气道（如杂合性缺失、微卫星重复遗传不稳定性）或周围气道（如 EGFR 突变）[2,9]。这种有趣的现象表明肺腺癌和肺鳞癌中区域性癌化的差异，而该差异也反映了 NSCLC 各个亚型间发病机制的不同（图 6.4，左）[2,9]。

最近，我们在接受手术治疗并随后进行 II 期监测试验（国防部先锋队列）的早期 NSCLC 患者中研究了吸烟损伤相关区域性癌化现象，发现毗邻原发切除肿瘤的气道上皮发生的表达方式改变显著高于肿瘤对侧气道上皮及从基线时点或纳入研究（分别从术后 1 年内）开始 3 年内的区域癌变或损伤[100]。另外，离原发肿瘤距离不同或活检时间点不同，也会引起磷酸化 ERK1/2 及 AKT 激酶免疫组化表达量的显著差异[100]。我们团队最近的研究结果扩展了气道区域性癌化现象的分子定义[100-101]，并对肺癌的预防有重要意义。该研究中描述的表达差异究竟反映了业已形成的不同肿瘤相关通路诱导肿瘤进展的损伤梯度场，还是反映了原发肿瘤对周围区域产生了异化分子作用尚不清楚[9]。未来的研究将从时间和空间分子角度深入探讨早期肺癌患者手术切除后的区域性损伤或

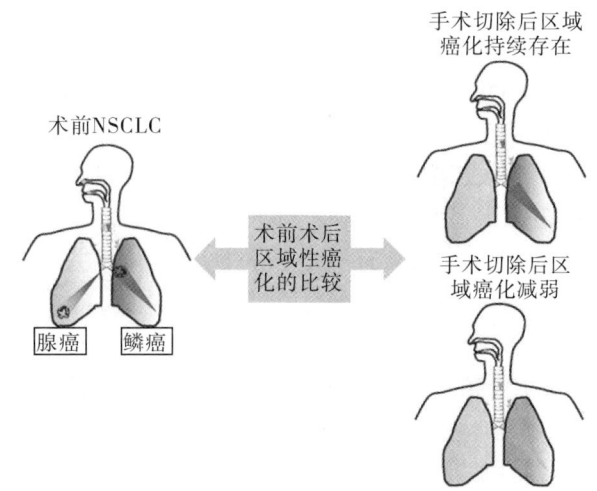

图 6.4（见彩插）　早期 NSCLC 患者中的区域性癌化现象。相较于肺鳞癌，区域性癌化与肺癌的某特定亚型（如肺腺癌）的相关性尚不明确。通过分析肺腺癌（黄色点区）及鳞癌（红色点区）之外多点支气管镜刷检物转录组物来分析局部及远端癌化区域，能为探讨这两种主要病变的分子学发病机制提供线索（左图）。区域性癌化与早期肺癌患者的潜在相关性可通过研究术前及术后分子癌化现象在手术切除后是否持续（右上）或下降（右下）来进行阐明。该类分析将有助于确定肺癌患者术后区域癌化现象与术后复发的相关性。如此，对该效应的分析可能发展为新的预防措施

癌化，这将解答上述疑问并对肺癌的三级预防具有重大意义（图 6.4）[9]。另外，还有一种有趣的假设是尽管部分早期 NSCLC 患者的分子区域性癌化现象在手术后会减弱（图 6.4，右下），但在其他患者中仍持续存在并可能预示疾病的高复发风险（图 6.4，右上）。

炎症和肺癌

对肺部慢性炎症环境与癌症的相关性已有广泛的研究[102]。一些研究发现罹患 COPD 的吸烟者的肺癌发病风险要高于未患 COPD 的吸烟者[102]。在 COPD 患者的肺泡水平，炎细胞引起的细胞外基质降解进而导致蛋白酶释放及抗蛋白酶的氧化失活[103-104]。在传导气道水平，主要表现为气道上皮化生黏液分泌型，基质分子沉积引起的气道壁增厚，间叶细胞增生及纤维化引起的狭窄[103-104]，这些变化同样也出现在未患 COPD 的吸烟者中，但损伤程度较轻[105]。每年累计吸烟 40 包及以上的 COPD 患者的痰脱落细胞检查显示癌前病变不典型增生的发生率更高（24% 重度癌变及原位癌）[106]。女性吸烟者比男性吸烟者的高级别癌前病变发生率低（14% vs 31%），且女性的癌前病变发生率也较低。即使戒烟 10 年以上也不会对癌前病变的发生率产生实质性改变。肺功能与癌前病变的发生有一定相关性，但其相关性在女性中弱于男性[107]。

较多试验显示炎症通过激活包括 NF-κB 通路在内的多条分子信号通路诱发肺部癌变[102]。NSCLC 细胞株中，烟草成分能刺激 NF-κB 相关细胞的活性[108]。并且，NF-κB p65 蛋白在细胞核内的过表达是肺部癌变的早期频发现象，在支气管鳞状上皮不典型增生及外周肺 AAH 病变中发生率较高[109]，但在未患肺癌吸烟者中鳞状上皮不典型增生的发生频率有限[110]。前列腺素类相关通路，尤其是 COX-2，与肺癌的发病有关。COX-2 是一类受生长因子、癌基因、致癌物及肿瘤促进因子——佛波酯等刺激后早期发生应答的基因[111]，在肺腺癌及肺鳞癌中过表达[112]。塞来考昔预防肺癌的临床前及临床试验均显示 PGE2 表达量的降低[113]。免疫组化显示 COX-2 在支气管鳞状上皮不典型增生特别是高等级不典型增生（重度不典型增生及原位癌）中显著高表达[114]。最近的研究提示 COX-2 抑制剂塞来考昔对吸烟者支气管上皮的增殖指数及凋亡平衡具有重要的调控作用[115-117]。

总结与未来展望

肺癌的发生是由多种遗传学、表观遗传学突变以及分子生物学改变的累积造成的。目前肺癌的癌前病变主要有 3 种形态学类型：鳞状上皮不典型增生、AAH 及弥漫性特发性肺神经内分泌细胞增生。然而，这些病变仅是部分肺癌发生发展的原因。目前的模型显示，肺鳞癌中出现了一系列渐进次序的分子及组织病理学变化，而分子改变常起始于组织学正常或轻度异常的支气管上皮。AAH 被认为是肺腺癌亚型的潜在癌前病变，与侵袭性肿瘤表达相似的分子变化。在肺腺癌癌变过程中可检测到至少两条分子信号通路：吸烟相关性 KRAS 通路及非吸烟相关性 EGFR 突变，后者也可在组织学正常的支气管上皮中检测到。肺部肿瘤及相关癌前病变中发生的分子学改变也能在组织学正常的吸烟损伤支气管上皮中检测到。吸烟者及肺癌患者支气管树呼吸道上皮可检测到严重及广泛的分子和组织病理学变化，即区域性癌化现象。相当多的证据显示慢性炎症通过激活多条分子信号通路参与肺癌癌变过程。

NGS 通过全基因组、全外显子组和全转录组技术，在肺癌生物学、诊断、预防和治疗方面具有巨大的潜力[118]。最近，NGS 以及深度测序技术阐明了肺腺癌、肺鳞癌及 SCLC 的基因组特征[81,119-121]。运用目前在肿瘤中的高通量技术研究肺癌癌前病变、上皮内病变、组织学正常的肿瘤旁区域及正常气道上皮将会加深我们对该类疾病生物学机制的理解。

尽管在肺癌生物学研究方面我们做了相当多的努力，但肺癌仍然是全美国乃至世界范围内造成癌症死亡人数最多的疾病。相较于 NSCLC 靶向治疗及个性化治疗的进展，其个体预防尚未取得突破。随着最近 NLST 的振奋人心的结果，这种情况将有望得到改变[16]。肺部气道及区域性癌化微侵袭灶中表达的多种分子标志物及表达分类物可用于筛选最适合行 CT 筛查的高危人群。

对 NSCLC 发病机制中的早期分子事件进行综合分析，无疑将能确定肺癌检测和预防新的重要生物标志物。

(倪 阳 译)

参考文献

[1] Minna JD, Roth JA, Gazdar AF. Focus on lung cancer. Cancer Cell, 2002, 1: 49-52.

[2] Wistuba, II, Gazdar AF. Lung cancer preneoplasia. Annu Rev Pathol, 2006, 1: 331-348.

[3] Colby TV, Wistuba, II, Gazdar A. Precursors to pulmonary neoplasia. Adv Anat Pathol, 1998, 5: 205-215.

[4] Kerr KM. Pulmonary preinvasive neoplasia. J Clin Pathol, 2001, 54: 257-271.

[5] Wistuba, II, Behrens C, Milchgrub S, et al. Sequential molecular abnormalities are involved in the multistage development of squamous cell lung carcinoma. Oncogene, 1999, 18: 643-650.

[6] Wistuba, II, Behrens C, Virmani AK, et al. High resolution chromosome 3p allelotyping of human lung cancer and preneoplastic/preinvasive bronchial epithelium reveals multiple, discontinuous sites of 3p allele loss and three regions of frequent breakpoints. Cancer Res, 2000, 60: 1949-1960.

[7] Wistuba, II, Berry J, Behrens C, et al. Molecular changes in the bronchial epithelium of patients with small cell lung cancer. Clin Cancer Res, 2000, 6: 2604-2610.

[8] Wistuba, II, Mao L, Gazdar AF. Smoking molecular damage in bronchial epithelium. Oncogene, 2002, 21: 7298-7306.

[9] Kadara H, Wistuba, II. Field cancerization in non-small cell lung cancer: implications in disease pathogenesis. Proc Am Thorac Soc, 2012, 9: 38-42.

[10] Steiling K, Ryan J, Brody JS, et al. The field of tissue injury in the lung and airway. Cancer Prev Res (Phila Pa), 2008, 1: 396-403.

[11] Wistuba, II, Lam S, Behrens C, et al. Molecular damage in the bronchial epithelium of current and former smokers. J Natl Cancer Inst, 1997 (89): 1366-1373.

[12] Mao L, Lee JS, Kurie JM, et al. Clonal genetic alterations in the lungs of current and former smokers. J Natl Cancer Inst, 1997, 89: 857-862.

[13] Gold KA, Kim ES, Lee JJ, et al. The BATTLE to personalize lung cancer prevention through reverse migration. Cancer Prev Res (Phila), 2011, 4: 962-972.

[14] Herbst RS, Heymach JV, Lippman SM. Lung cancer. N Engl J Med, 2008, 359: 1367-1380.

[15] Kadara H, Kabbout M, Wistuba, II. Pulmonary adenocarcinoma: a renewed entity in 2011. Respirology, 2012, 17: 50-65.

[16] Aberle DR, Adams AM, Berg CD, et al. Reduced lung-cancer mortality with low-dose computed tomographic screening. N Engl J Med, 2011, 365: 395-409.

[17] Travis WD, Brambilla E, Noguchi M, et al. International Association for the Study of Lung Cancer/American Thoracic Society/European Respiratory Society International Multidisciplinary Classification of Lung Adenocarcinoma. J Thorac Oncol, 2011, 6: 244-285.

[18] Westra WH. Early glandular neoplasia of the lung. Respir Res, 2000, 1: 163-169.

[19] Keith RL, Miller YE, Gemmill RM, et al. Angiogenic squamous dysplasia in bronchi of individuals at high risk for lung cancer. Clin Cancer Res, 2000, 6: 1616-1625.

[20] Hanahan D, Weinberg RA. Hallmarks of cancer: the next generation. Cell, 2011 144: 646-674.

[21] Lam S, MacAulay C, leRiche JC, et al. Detection and localization of early lung cancer by fluorescence bronchoscopy. Cancer, 2000, 89: 2468-2473.

[22] Kitamura H, Kameda Y, Ito T, et al. Atypical adenomatous hyperplasia of the lung. Implications for the pathogenesis of peripheral lung adenocarcinoma. Am J Clin Pathol, 1999, 111: 610-622.

[23] Osanai M, Igarashi T, Yoshida Y. Unique cellular features in atypical adenomatous hyperplasia of the lung: ultrastructural evidence of its cytodifferentiation. Ultrastruct Pathol, 2001, 25: 367-373.

[24] Yatabe Y. *EGFR* mutations and the terminal respiratory unit. Cancer Metastasis Rev, 2010, 29: 23-36.

[25] Chapman AD, Kerr KM. The association between atypical adenomatous hyperplasia and primary lung cancer. Br J Cancer, 2000, 83: 632-636.

[26] Yatabe Y, Borczuk AC, Powell CA. Do all lung adenocarcinomas follow a stepwise progression? Lung Cancer, 2011, 74: 7-11.

[27] Yatabe Y, Mitsudomi T, Takahashi T. TTF-1 expression in pulmonary adenocarcinomas. Am J Surg Pathol, 2002, 26: 767-773.

[28] Tang X, Shigematsu H, Bekele BN, et al. EGFR tyrosine kinase domain mutations are detected in histologically normal respiratory epithelium in lung cancer patients. Cancer Res, 2005, 65: 7568-7572.

[29] Tang X, Varella-Garcia M, Xavier AC, et al. Epidermal growth factor receptor abnormalities in the pathogenesis and progression of lung adenocarcinomas. Cancer Prev Res (Phila Pa), 2008, 1: 192-200.

[30] Armas OA, White DA, Erlandson RA, et al. Diffuse idiopathic pulmonary neuroendocrine cell proliferation presenting as interstitial lung disease. Am J Surg Pathol, 1995, 19: 963-970.

[31] Gazdar AF, Thun MJ. Lung cancer, smoke exposure, and sex. J Clin Oncol, 2007, 25: 469-471.

[32] Le Calvez F, Mukeria A, Hunt JD, et al. TP53 and KRAS mutation load and types in lung cancers in relation to tobacco smoke: distinct patterns in never, former, and current smokers. Cancer Res, 2005, 65: 5076-5083.

[33] Mounawar M, Mukeria A, Le Calvez F, et al. Patterns of EGFR, HER2, TP53, and KRAS mutations of p14arf expression in non small cell lung cancers in relation to smoking history. Cancer Res, 2007, 67: 5667-5672.

[34] Ridanpaa M, Karjalainen A, Anttila S, et al. Husgafvel-pursiainen K. Genetic alterations in p53 and k-ras in lung-cancer in relation to histopathology of the tumor and smoking history of the patient. Int J Oncol, 1994, 5: 1109-1117.

[35] Rodenhuis S, Slebos RJ, Boot AJ, et al. Incidence and possible clinical significance of K-ras oncogene activation in adenocarcinoma of the human lung. Cancer Res, 1988, 48: 5738-5741.

[36] Shigematsu H, Lin L, Takahashi T, et al. Clinical and biological features associated with epidermal growth factor receptor gene mutations in lung cancers. J Natl Cancer Inst, 2005, 97: 339-346.

[37] Tam IY, Chung LP, Suen WS, et al. Distinct epidermal growth factor receptor and KRAS mutation patterns in non-small cell lung cancer patients with different tobacco exposure and clinicopathologic features. Clin Cancer Res, 2006, 12: 1647-1653.

[38] Shigematsu H, Takahashi T, Nomura M, et al. Somatic mutations of the HER2 kinase domain in lung adenocarcinomas. Cancer Res, 2005, 65: 1642-1646.

[39] Wistuba, II, Behrens C, Virmani AK, et al. Allelic losses at chromosome 8p21-23 are early and frequent events in the pathogenesis of lung cancer. Cancer Res, 1999, 59: 1973-1979.

[40] Lerman MI, Minna JD. The 630-kb lung cancer homozygous deletion region on human chromosome 3p21.3: identification and evaluation of the resident candidate tumor suppressor genes. The International Lung Cancer Chromosome 3p21.3 Tumor Suppressor Gene Consortium. Cancer Res, 2000, 60: 6116-6133.

[41] Zochbauer-Muller S, Fong KM, Maitra A, et al. 5'CpG island methylation of the FHIT gene is correlated with loss of gene expression in lung and breast cancer. Cancer Res, 2001, 61: 3581-3585.

[42] Miyazu YM, Miyazawa T, Hiyama K, et al. Telomerase expression in noncancerous bronchial epithelia is a possible marker of early development of lung cancer. Cancer Res, 2005, 65: 9623-9627.

[43] Yashima K, Milchgrub S, Gollahon LS, et al. Telomerase enzyme activity and RNA expression during the multistage pathogenesis of breast carcinoma. Clin Cancer Res, 1998, 4: 229-234.

[44] Lantuejoul S, Soria JC, Morat L, et al. Telomere shortening and telomerase reverse transcriptase expression in preinvasive bronchial lesions. Clin Cancer Res, 2005, 11: 2074-2082.

[45] Park IW, Wistuba, II, Maitra A, et al. Multiple clonal abnormalities in the bronchial epithelium of patients with lung cancer. J Natl Cancer Inst, 1999, 91: 1863-1868.

[46] Belinsky SA, Nikula KJ, Palmisano WA, et al. Aberrant methylation of p16 (INK4a) is an early event in lung cancer and a potential biomarker for early diagnosis. Proc Natl Acad Sci USA, 1999, 95: 11891-11896.

[47] Belinsky SA, Liechty KC, Gentry FD, et al. Promoter hypermethylation of multiple genes in sputum precedes lung cancer incidence in a high-risk cohort. Cancer Res, 2006, 66: 3338-3344.

[48] Hirsch FR, Prindiville SA, Miller YE, et al. Fluorescence versus white-light bronchoscopy for detection of preneoplastic lesions: a randomized study. J Natl Cancer Inst, 2001, 93: 1385-1391.

[49] Merrick DT, Haney J, Petrunich S, et al. Overexpression of vascular endothelial growth factor and its receptors in bronchial dypslasia demonstrated by quantitative RTPCR analysis. Lung Cancer, 2005, 48: 31-45.

[50] Hirsch FR, Lippman SM. Advances in the biology of lung cancer chemoprevention. J Clin Oncol, 2005, 23: 3186-3197.

[51] Khuri FR, Cohen V. Molecularly targeted approaches to the chemoprevention of lung cancer. Clin Cancer Res, 2004, 10: 4249s-4253s.

[52] Merrick DT, Kittelson J, Winterhalder R, et al. Analysis

of c-ErbB1/epidermal growth factor receptor and c-ErbB2/HER-2 expression in bronchial dysplasia: evaluation of potential targets for chemoprevention of lung cancer. Clin Cancer Res, 2006, 12: 2281-2288.

[53] Tsao AS, McDonnell T, Lam S, et al. Increased phospho-AKT (Ser (473)) expression in bronchial dysplasia: implications for lung cancer prevention studies. Cancer Epidemiol Biomarkers Prev. 2003, 12: 660-664.

[54] Lee HY, Moon H, Chun KH, et al. Effects of insulin-like growth factor binding protein-3 and farnesyltransferase inhibitor SCH66336 on Akt expression and apoptosis in nonsmall-cell lung cancer cells. J Natl Cancer Inst, 2004, 96: 1536-1548.

[55] Wislez M, Spencer ML, Izzo JG, et al. Inhibition of mammalian target of rapamycin reverses alveolar epithelial neoplasia induced by oncogenic K-ras. Cancer Res, 2005, 65: 3226-3235.

[56] Abbruzzese JL, Lippman SM. The convergence of cancer prevention and therapy in early-phase clinical drug development. Cancer Cell, 2004, 6: 321-326.

[57] Bass AJ, Watanabe H, Mermel CH, et al. SOX2 is an amplified lineage-survival oncogene in lung and esophageal squamous cell carcinomas. Nat Genet, 2009, 41: 1238-1242.

[58] Hussenet T, Dali S, Exinger J, et al. SOX2 is an oncogene activated by recurrent 3q26.3 amplifications in human lung squamous cell carcinomas. PLoS ONE, 2010, 5: e8960.

[59] Yuan P, Kadara H, Behrens C, et al. Sex determining region YBox 2 (SOX2) is a potential cell-lineage gene highly expressed in the pathogenesis of squamous cell carcinomas of the lung. PLoS ONE, 2010, 5: e9112.

[60] Lu Y, Futtner C, Rock JR, et al. Evidence that SOX2 overexpression is oncogenic in the lung. PLoS ONE, 2010, 5: e11022.

[61] Xiang R, Liao D, Cheng T, et al. Downregulation of transcription factor SOX2 in cancer stem cells suppresses growth and metastasis of lung cancer. Br J Cancer, 2011, 104: 1410-1417.

[62] McCaughan F, Pole JC, Bankier AT, et al. Progressive 3q amplification consistently targets SOX2 in preinvasive squamous lung cancer. Am J Respir Crit Care Med, 2010, 182: 83-91.

[63] Westra WH, Baas IO, Hruban RH, et al. K-ras oncogene activation in atypical alveolar hyperplasias of the human lung. Cancer Res, 1996, 56: 2224-2228.

[64] Chiosea S, Jelezcova E, Chandran U, et al. Overexpression of Dicer in precursor lesions of lung adenocarcinoma. Cancer Res, 2007, 67: 2345-2350.

[65] Selamat SA, Galler JS, Joshi AD, et al. DNA methylation changes in atypical adenomatous hyperplasia, adenocarcinoma in situ, and lung adenocarcinoma. PLoS ONE, 2011, 6: e21443.

[66] Rudin CM, Avila-Tang E, Harris CC, et al. Lung cancer in never smokers: molecular profiles and therapeutic implications. Clin Cancer Res, 2009, 15: 5646-5661.

[67] Sun S, Schiller JH, Gazdar AF. Lung cancer in never smokers-a different disease. Nat Rev Cancer, 2007, 7: 778-790.

[68] Yatabe Y, Kosaka T, Takahashi T, et al. *EGFR* mutation is specific for terminal respiratory unit type adenocarcinoma. Am J Surg Pathol, 2005, 29: 633-639.

[69] Yoshida Y, Shibata T, Kokubu A, et al. Mutations of the epidermal growth factor receptor gene in atypical adenomatous hyperplasia and bronchioloalveolar carcinoma of the lung. Lung Cancer, 2005, 50: 1-8.

[70] Minoo P, Su G, Drum H, et al. Defects in tracheoesophageal and lung morphogenesis in Nkx2.1 (-/-) mouse embryos. Dev Biol, 1999, 209: 60-71.

[71] Yuan B, Li C, Kimura S, et al. Minoo P Inhibition of distal lung morphogenesis in Nkx2.1 (-/-) embryos. Dev Dyn, 2000, 217: 180-190.

[72] Kimura S, Hara Y, Pineau T, et al. The T/ebp null mouse: thyroid-specific enhancer-binding protein is essential for the organogenesis of the thyroid, lung, ventral forebrain, and pituitary. Genes Dev, 1996, 10: 60-69.

[73] Ikeda K, Clark JC, Shaw-White JR, et al. Gene structure and expression of human thyroid transcription factor-1 in respiratory epithelial cells. J Biol Chem, 1995, 270: 8108-8114.

[74] Kwei KA, Kim YH, Girard L, et al. Genomic profiling identifies TITF1 as a lineage-specific oncogene amplified in lung cancer. Oncogene, 2008, 27: 3635-3640.

[75] Weir BA, Woo MS, Getz G, et al. Characterizing the cancer genome in lung adenocarcinoma. Nature, 2007, 450: 893-898.

[76] Tanaka H, Yanagisawa K, Shinjo K, et al. Lineage-specific dependency of lung adenocarcinomas on the lung development regulator TTF-1. Cancer Res, 2007, 67: 6007-6011.

[77] Winslow MM, Dayton TL, Verhaak RG, et al. Suppression of lung adenocarcinoma progression by Nkx2-1.

Nature, 2011, 473: 101-104.

[78] Meuwissen R, Linn SC, Linnoila RI, et al. Induction of small cell lung cancer by somatic inactivation of both Trp53 and Rb1 in a conditional mouse model. Cancer Cell, 2003, 4: 181-189.

[79] Park KS, Martelotto LG, Peifer M, et al. A crucial requirement for Hedgehog signaling in small cell lung cancer. Nat Med, 17: 1504-1508.

[80] Watkins DN, Berman DM, Burkholder SG, et al. Hedgehog signaling within airway epithelial progenitors and in small-cell lung cancer. Nature, 2003, 422: 313-317.

[81] Peifer M, Fernandez-Cuesta L, Sos ML, et al. Integrative genome analyses identify key somatic driver mutations of small-cell lung cancer. Nat Genet, 2012, 44: 1104-1110.

[82] Slaughter DP, Southwick HW, Smejkal W. Field cancerization in oral stratified squamous epithelium; clinical implications of multicentric origin. Cancer, 1953, 6: 963-968.

[83] Auerbach O, Stout AP, Hammond EC, et al. Changes in bronchial epithelium in relation to cigarette smoking and in relation to lung cancer. N Engl J Med, 1961, 265: 253-267.

[84] Nelson MA, Wymer J, Clements N, Jr, et al. Detection of K-ras gene mutations in non-neoplastic lung tissue and lung cancers. Cancer Lett, 1996, 103: 115-121.

[85] Belinsky SA, Palmisano WA, Gilliland FD, et al. Aberrant promoter methylation in bronchial epithelium and sputum from current and former smokers. Cancer Res, 2002, 62: 2370-2377.

[86] Powell CA, Klares S, O'Connor G, et al. Loss of heterozygosity in epithelial cells obtained by bronchial brushing: clinical utility in lung cancer. Clin Cancer Res, 1999, 5: 2025-2034.

[87] Franklin WA, Gazdar AF, Haney J, et al. Widely dispersed p53 mutation in respiratory epithelium. A novel mechanism for field carcinogenesis. J Clin Invest, 1997, 100: 2133-2137.

[88] Zochbauer-Muller S, Lam S, Toyooka S, et al. Aberrant methylation of multiple genes in the upper aerodigestive tract epithelium of heavy smokers. Int J Cancer, 2003, 107: 612-616.

[89] Soria JC, Rodriguez M, Liu DD, et al. Aberrant promoter methylation of multiple genes in bronchial brush samples from former cigarette smokers. Cancer Res, 2002, 62: 351-355.

[90] Heller G, Zielinski CC, Zochbauer-Muller S. Lung cancer: from single-gene methylation to methylome profiling. Cancer Metastasis Rev, 2010, 29: 95-107.

[91] Hackett NR, Heguy A, Harvey BG, et al. Variability of antioxidant-related gene expression in the airway epithelium of cigarette smokers. Am J Respir Cell Mol Biol, 2003, 29: 331-343.

[92] Spira A, Beane J, Shah V, et al. Effects of cigarette smoke on the human airway epithelial cell transcriptome. Proc Natl Acad Sci USA, 2004, 101: 10143-10148.

[93] Beane J, Sebastiani P, Liu G, et al. Reversible and permanent effects of tobacco smoke exposure on airway epithelial gene expression. Genome Biol, 2007, 8: R201.

[94] Schembri F, Sridhar S, Perdomo C, et al. MicroRNAs as modulators of smoking-induced gene expression changes in human airway epithelium. Proc Natl Acad Sci USA, 2009, 106: 2319-2324.

[95] Spira A, Beane JE, Shah V, et al. Airway epithelial gene expression in the diagnostic evaluation of smokers with suspect lung cancer. Nat Med, 2007, 13: 361-366.

[96] Gustafson AM, Soldi R, Anderlind C, et al. Airway PI3K pathway activation is an early and reversible event in lung cancer development. Sci Transl Med, 2010, 2: 26ra5.

[97] Sridhar S, Schembri F, Zeskind J, et al. Smoking-induced gene expression changes in the bronchial airway are reflected in nasal and buccal epithelium. BMC Genomics, 2008, 9: 259.

[98] Zhang X, Sebastiani P, Liu G, et al. Similarities and differences between smoking-related gene expression in nasal and bronchial epithelium. Physiol Genomics, 2010, 41: 1-8.

[99] Beane J, Vick J, Schembri F, et al. Characterizing the impact of smoking and lung cancer on the airway transcriptome using RNA-Seq. Cancer Prev Res (Phila), 2011, 4: 803-817.

[100] Kadara H, Shen L, Fujimoto J, et al. Characterizing the molecular spatial and temporal field of injury in earlystage smoker non-small cell lung cancer patients after definitive surgery by expression profiling. Cancer Prev Res (Phila), 2019, 6: 8-17.

[101] Gomperts BN, Walser TC, Spira A, et al. Enriching the molecular definition of the airway "field of cancerization:" establishing new paradigms for the patient at risk for lung cancer. Cancer Prev Res (Phila), 2013, 6: 4-7.

[102] Anderson GP, Bozinovski S. Acquired somatic mutations in the molecular pathogenesis of COPD. Trends Pharmacol Sci, 2003, 24: 71-76.

[103] Barnes PJ. Chronic obstructive pulmonary disease. N Engl J Med, 2000, 343: 269-280.

[104] Hogg JC. Pathophysiology of airflow limitation in chronic obstructive pulmonary disease. Lancet, 2004, 364: 709-721.

[105] Hida T, Kozaki K, Muramatsu H, et al. Cyclooxygenase-2 inhibitor induces apoptosis and enhances cytotoxicity of various anticancer agents in non-small cell lung cancer cell lines. Clin Cancer Res, 2000, 6: 2006-2011.

[106] Kennedy TC, Proudfoot SP, Franklin WA, et al. Cytopathological analysis of sputum in patients with airflow obstruction and significant smoking histories. Cancer Res, 1996, 56: 4673-4678.

[107] Lam S, leRiche JC, Zheng Y, et al. Sex-related differences in bronchial epithelial changes associated with tobacco smoking. J Natl Cancer Inst, 1999, 91: 691-696.

[108] Tsurutani J, Castillo SS, Brognard J, et al. Tobacco components stimulate Akt-dependent proliferation and NFkappaB-dependent survival in lung cancer cells. Carcinogenesis, 2005, 26: 1182-1195.

[109] Tang X, Liu D, Shishodia S, et al. Nuclear factor-kappaB (NF-kappaB) is frequently expressed in lung cancer and preneoplastic lesions. Cancer, 2006, 107: 2637-2646.

[110] Tichelaar JW, Zhang Y, leRiche JC, et al. Increased staining for phospho-Akt, p65/RELA and cIAP-2 in preneoplastic human bronchial biopsies. BMC Cancer, 2005, 5: 155.

[111] Dannenberg AJ, Altorki NK, Boyle JO, et al. Cyclooxygenase 2: a pharmacological target for the prevention of cancer. Lancet Oncol, 2001, 2: 544-551.

[112] Hasturk S, Kemp B, Kalapurakal SK, et al. Expression of cyclooxygenase-1 and cyclooxygenase-2 in bronchial epithelium and nonsmall cell lung carcinoma. Cancer, 2002, 94: 1023-1031.

[113] Mao JT, Cui X, Reckamp K, et al. Chemoprevention strategies with cyclooxygenase-2 inhibitors for lung cancer. Clin Lung Cancer, 2005, 7: 30-39.

[114] Mascaux C, Martin B, Verdebout JM, et al. COX-2 expression during early lung squamous cell carcinoma oncogenesis. Eur Respir J, 2005, 26: 198-203.

[115] Mao JT, Fishbein MC, Adams B, et al. Celecoxib decreases Ki-67 proliferative index in active smokers. Clin Cancer Res, 2006, 12: 314-320.

[116] Kim ES, Hong WK, Lee JJ, et al. Biological activity of celecoxib in the bronchial epithelium of current and former smokers. Cancer Prev Res (Phila), 2010, 3: 148-159.

[117] Mao JT, Roth MD, Fishbein MC, et al. Lung cancer chemoprevention with celecoxib in former smokers. Cancer Prev Res (Phila), 2011 (4): 984-993.

[118] Meyerson M, Gabriel S, Getz G. Advances in understanding cancer genomes through secondgeneration sequencing. Nat Rev Genet, 2010, 11: 685-696.

[119] Govindan R, Ding L, Griffith M, et al. Genomic landscape of non-small cell lung cancer in smokers and neversmokers. Cell, 2012, 150: 1121-1134.

[120] Hammerman PS, Hayes DN, Wilkerson MD, et al. Comprehensive genomic characterization of squamous cell lung cancers. Nature, 2012, 489: 519-525.

[121] Imielinski M, Berger AH, Hammerman PS, et al. Mapping the hallmarks of lung adenocarcinoma with massively parallel sequencing. Cell, 2012, 150: 1107-1120.

第7章
肺癌癌前病变的检测和治疗

Rachel Jen, Stephen Lam
Department of Medicine, University of British Columbia, Vancouver, British Columbia, Canada

引 言

目前，肺癌确诊患者的 5 年生存率仅有 15% 左右[1]，尽管系统治疗和放化疗的发展对改善患者的生存质量有一定的作用，但总体死亡率仍然居高不下。肺癌生存率与肿瘤的分期相关，流行病学统计结果提示，仅 16% 的肺癌患者病变较局限，其他患者多有局部甚至远处转移[2]。因此，在肿瘤较为局限时对患者进行早期诊断，是改善患者预后的重要措施。

肺部癌前病变的定位有其独特的挑战性。与其他上皮器官不同，肺是一个有复杂通气系统的内部器官，它与外周气体单位的表面积相当于一个网球场的面积。另外，肺癌细胞类型众多，不同类型肺癌可生长于支气管树的不同部位，目前还没有方法可以检测整个支气管树上皮来寻找癌前病变，以及取得组织样本并做出分子学或者病理学诊断。生物光学成像技术的出现，如自发荧光支气管镜检查（autofluoresacence bromchoscopy, AFB）及光学相干层析成像（optical coherence tomography, OCT）都可以用来定位光纤探针可及的癌前病变。多层螺旋 CT 也是检查外周肺野癌前病变的敏感方法，并可指引进一步的活检病理学检查。CT 可以作为虚拟地图，通过导航系统实现对外周肺病变活组织的检查。本章主要讨论上述方法应用的证据支持及未来的研究方向。

中央型肺癌癌前病变检测

生物成像原理

当光线照射气道表面时，光线有可能被吸收、反射、散射或诱发荧光[3]。这种光学原理同样应用于检测正常或者异常支气管组织的结构、分子生物学组成及功能改变。白光支气管镜（white-light bronchoscopy, WLB）检查利用可见光镜面反射、散射吸收宽带的不同反映支气管表面的不同结构，从而区分正常和不正常的支气管表面组织。尽管是最简单的检测技术，仍有接近 40 种原位癌可通过此法检测出来[4]。WLB 检查法利用自发荧光与吸收特性不同的原理，提供支气管组织不同的生物化学合成及代谢信息。大多数内源性荧光基团与组织或细胞代谢有关，胶原和弹力纤维是最重要的荧光基团。荧光基团有关的细胞代谢包括二磷酸吡啶核苷酸（nicotinamide adenine dinu-cleotide, NADH）和黄素类。其他的荧光基团包括芳香族氨基酸（如色氨酸、酪氨酸、苯丙氨酸），多种卟啉类以及脂质素（如蜡样脂、脂褐素）。支气管组织荧光的特性是由荧光基团集聚及分布特性决定的，由它们不同的发射光谱、荧光基团的分布、代谢、组织结构以及不同非荧光发色基团如血红蛋白的分布等因素共同决定[3]。在紫光或蓝光照射下，正常支气管组织发出强烈的绿色荧光。随着支气管上皮从正常发展到不典型增生甚至原位癌及侵袭性病变，绿色荧光会逐渐衰弱而红色荧光逐渐增强[5]。这种变化与黏膜下层的细胞外基质如胶原和弹力蛋白减少及增厚上皮对光的重吸收减少、细胞核增大、细胞密度、分布及微血管密度增加有关[6-7]。血红蛋白的聚集将导致蓝色激发光增加而荧光减少。例如，已发现血管源性鳞状上皮不典型增生导致荧光减少[8]。另外，在癌前病变和恶性细胞中黄素类及还原型辅酶 I 的量是减少的，其他因素如 pH 和氧合作用都有可能改变荧光量[9]。在支气管镜检查法中，最大肿瘤到正常组织的激发波长范围是 400 ~

480nm，峰值是 405nm[5,10]。而正常组织、癌前病变及恶性组织光谱差的不同（500～700nm）为局限性早期支气管肺癌设计自发荧光内镜显像装置奠定了基础[5,11-12]。最近出现的这些装置通常是利用光学特性以及反射和荧光联合显像以提高癌前病变的检测敏感性[12-18]。

自发荧光支气管镜（AFB）检查法

AFB 可以快速、较大范围地检查支气管表面黏膜，并可能发现 WLB 检查难以发现的不明显病变。目前大多数设备使用比光纤支气管镜分辨率更高的电视支气管镜技术，可以在白光与荧光之间快速转换，并能够同时播放检查影像[13,18]。小量的反射光（蓝光、绿光及近红外光）被用来加强影像的彩色对比，并纠正因光学及几何原因，如病变与气管镜距离变化及气管镜与支气管壁成角等导致的成像问题。鉴于成像依赖反射光的不同，病变区域表现为棕红色、红色、紫色或洋红色，而正常黏膜表现为绿色或者浅蓝色[12-18]。

除了多个单中心研究[19]，还有两个随机试验[20-21]及 3 个大型多中心试验[11-12,22]比较了 WLB 及 AFB。这些研究发现，与 WLB 相比，AFB 检查发现气道发育不良、原位癌以及微浸润肿瘤的概率更高。AFB 的灵敏度是 WLB 的两倍，但它的特异度却仅有 60%，远不如 WLB 的 90%。最近的一项 meta 分析显示，AFB 检查发现单一浸润前病变的灵敏度为 85%。与 WLB 检查相比，相对灵敏度为 2.04，95% CI（1.56，11.55）[23]。然而，在发现侵袭性鳞状细胞癌方面，AFB 与 WLB 相比，优势并不明显，特异性尚不如 WLB 检查[23]。

AFB 的特异度偏低与其荧光检测炎症、黏膜腺体增生、吸入损伤假阳性及观察者之间的不同有关。在检查过程中通过定量求红/绿荧光比值，可以将 AFB 的特异度提高至 80%[24]；调节不同光线比率结合肉眼观察，可以改善特异度至 88%。在一项多中心研究中发现，在检查支气管黏膜病变时红绿光比率的变化，导致假阳性率增高。定量显像降低了观察者自身及观察者之间的偏差。某些病例检查时存在自发荧光改变，提示这部分患者的癌症发病率升高。在 AFB 中表现阳性但活检却是发育不良或低级别病理改变的病例，比检查正常的组织更容易有基因改变[25-26]，并可能具有侵袭性。支气管镜检查下多部位病变，似乎是肺癌进展的潜在危险因素。Pasic 等报道，支气管镜检查发现两处或更多处异常的病例，未来 4 年发展为肺癌的概率为 50%，远高于仅一处黏膜异常的患者（8%）[27]。

窄带成像技术（NBI）

在肿瘤进展过程中新生血管形成是肿瘤进展过程中的早期事件，且是重要的影响因素[28]。窄带成像技术（narrow band imaging，NBI），即图像强化内镜，被用于检查浅表微血管形成[29]。这种技术在胃肠内镜检查早期巴特（Barrett）食管中广泛应用[30]，但在常规支气管镜检查中它的地位仍待商榷。NBI 利用符合血红蛋白吸收峰值的波长 415nm（400～430nm）的窄带蓝光及 540nm（530～550nm）的绿光进行成像。蓝光可以显示表浅的毛细血管，绿光则更有穿透力，可以检测黏膜下的较大血管。NBI 降低了其他波长光线的散射，并增强了血管的可视性[31]。NBI 可以改善侵袭前病变的发现率及明确侵袭性肿瘤的分化程度。点状血管及细小的螺旋形血管及不同大小的曲折走形血管都存在发育不良。在原位癌中，存在点状血管、小螺旋或螺旋血管。在具有侵袭性的肺癌组织中小螺旋或螺旋形血管更加明显[31]。一项前瞻性研究比较了 WLB 检查后进行 AFB 检查或 NBI 检查发现上皮间瘤样新生物的准确性[32]。WLB 发现高度不典型增生或原位癌的灵敏度为 18%，特异度为 88%。WLB 检查结合 AFB 检查及 WLB 结合 NBI 检查与单独 WLB 检查相比，相对灵敏度分别为 3.7 和 3.0，差异没有统计学意义。WLB 结合 AFB 与 WLB 结合 NBI 的相对特异度分别为 0.5 和 1.0。WLB 结合 NBI 的特异度相比 WLB 结合 AFB 的更高（$P<0.001$）。

目前对如何比较 NBI 和运用高清晰度图像的 WLB 检查尚不清楚。英国哥伦比亚癌症中心（the British Columbia Cancer Agency，BCCA）发现，从中心型鳞状细胞癌和小细胞癌到周围型腺癌，使用标准成人尺寸（5.8～6mm）支气管镜进行的

AFB 检查结果显示，患者的发病率 10 年来正逐渐降低（图 7.1）。为了更广泛地应用 AFB 及 NBI 技术，将气管镜直径控制在 4mm 以下，活检孔径控制在 2mm 左右将是未来发展趋势。

光学相干层析成像（OCT）

OCT 是一种可以提供细胞、胞外及组织表面以下组织学信息的光学成像技术[33-35]。它类似于超声，但使用的是红外光线。这种光线可以被组织分解或反射，利用光学干涉量度法生成一个一维组织图。通过扫描组织表面的光束，可以呈现二维或三维图像。这种检查方法使用纤维光束探针进行，它们可以到达末端支气管肺泡组织。在清醒状态下用标准支气管镜做组织活检时会形成一些腔隙，探针可通过插入这些腔隙进行检查。轴位和横向的检查方法可依从于成像要求实现 5～30μm 的调整，成像深度为 2～3mm[35]。分辨率及成像深度的结合是检查起源于上皮组织的癌前病变及小气道肿瘤的理想途径。不同于超声，光线不需要液体介质，这都有利于气道成像，且它使用的微弱近红外线相关风险较小。

将正常支气管、原发性肺癌和 7 例肺癌患者的肺叶切除标本中的肺泡 OCT 成像结果与组织病理学结果进行了对比研究。OCT 图像可以显示在肺癌组织中丢失的正常支气管壁结构。在外周肺组织、含气肺泡显示为蜂巢样结构。Lam 等曾对 OCT 作为不典型增生及癌前病变无创检查的效果进行了研究[34]。正常及增生组织在 OCT 检查中表现为黏膜下及高度分散的基底膜上的 1～2 层细胞层。随着上皮从正常组织增生至化生，发展为不同级别的不典型增生及癌前病变，上皮厚度不断增加。上皮厚度的量化测量提示侵袭性肿瘤较原位癌的厚度明显增加（$P=0.004$），而不典型增生较化生及增生明显增厚（$P=0.002$）。细胞核在高度不典型增生及癌前病变中更加明显。基底膜在原位癌中还是完整的，但在浸润癌中基底膜变的不连续[34-35]。鳞癌与腺癌的体积测定不同[36]。而 OCT 检查就可在活检前区分这些特点。

自发性荧光支气管镜的适应证

对痰细胞学异常患者进行评估

痰细胞学检查发现可疑或确诊的恶性肿瘤细胞时需要行进一步检查，通常是气管镜和 CT，这一点没有争议。Sato 等报道，在痰脱落细胞学诊断为鳞状细胞癌且胸片检查结果为阴性的患者中，根据气管镜进行肿瘤定位接受治疗的患者较拒绝治疗患者的预后有明显改善。治疗组的 10 年生存率为 94.9%，而拒绝治疗组为 33.5%[37]。

有数项研究报道，痰细胞学检查结果为重度异型性的患者中大约 45% 在两年内进展为肺癌[38-39]。Johns Hopkins 早期肺癌筛查计划同样发现中度异型性者将来进展为肺癌的风险增加。有 14% 伴中度异型性的参加者进展为肺癌，而不伴异型性的参加者中仅有 3% 进展为肺癌[38]。在伴气道阻塞的高危吸烟和戒烟者的 Colorado SPORE 队列研究中，在校正年龄、性别、累计吸烟量及吸烟状态后，轻度异型性、中度异型性、中度异型性或更差，以及重度异型性或更差者进展为肺癌的相对危险度（RR）分别增加 1.10、1.68、3.18 及 31.4 倍[40]。痰细胞学呈重度异型性或更差者进展为肺癌的风险显著增加，有必要行 WLB + AFB 等有创检查进行进一步诊断。尽管证据没有重度异型性患者那么明显，但中度异型性患者也应行气管镜检查。在一项病例报道中，79 例患者痰细胞学呈中度异型性且胸片检查结果为阴性，

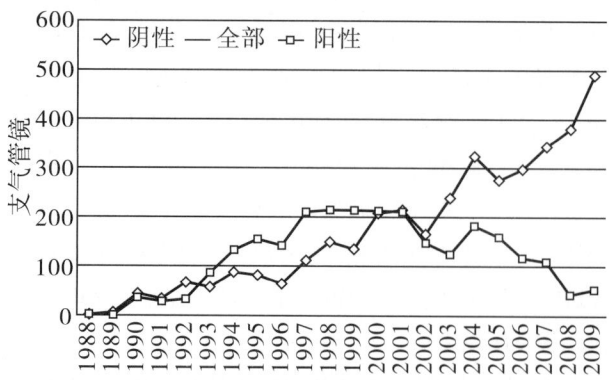

图 7.1（见彩插） 1998—2009 年加入 BCCA 肺部健康研究的重度吸烟者的比例。使用自发荧光支气管镜检查及 5.8mm 的支气管镜活检发现，这些患者存在至少 1 处以上的支气管异型增生，自 2000 年开始，支气管异型增生的发病率稳固下降

气管镜检查发现了 5 例肺癌［RR = 6.3%；95% CI（0.7%，11%）］[41]，其中 2 例为癌前病变，3 例为浸润性病变。气管镜对肿瘤的发现率超过了大便潜血试验阳性时结肠镜对结肠癌的发现率。

对可疑、确诊或既往曾行肺癌完全切除术患者的评估

在拟行根治性手术切除的早期肺癌患者中，AFB 在界定肿瘤的边界及评估多原发病变方面发挥着重要作用[27,41-43]。Ikeda 等对 30 例术前行 AFB 检查进而行手术切除的 NSCLC 患者进行了详细的临床病理学研究，结果发现与 WLB 相比，AFB 对肿瘤边界的界定更加准确且能发现其他部位的异型增生[44]。AFB 在多达 15% 的早期肺癌患者中发现了同时性癌[43-45]。多同时性癌的发现改变了对这些患者的治疗策略。

有报道称，NSCLC 患者成功行根治性切除术后，第二原发（异时性）肿瘤的发生率较高（每年 1%～3%）[46]。在之前患有早期肺鳞癌的患者中，报道的异时性病变的发生率似乎更高，近 30% 的患者在 4 年内发生第二中央型恶性肿瘤[47-48]。术后对行肿瘤完全切除术的 NSCLC 患者应用 WLB 和 AFB 进行随访[27,48-49]。在 25 例患者中，Weigel 等发现 12% 的患者在经过平均 20.5 个月的随访后发展为 3 处中度或重度异型增生，1 例发展为微浸润性癌[48]。Pasic 等发现 28% 的肺癌患者经过 47 个月的中位时间后发展为肺鳞癌[27]。一项对之前患有鳞癌或周围型腺癌的患者发生中央气道为主的异时性病变进行的对比研究结果显示，30% 之前患有鳞癌的患者发生高度异型增生或更严重的病变，而在之前接受手术切除的腺癌患者的发生率仅为 4%[50]。之前接受根治性切除的肺癌患者发生第二原发性肺癌的风险较高，而之前患有肺鳞癌且一般情况良好、没有严重合并症的患者可能会从 AFB 随访中获益。

对早期中央型肺癌患者接受气管内治疗前的评估

当考虑对早期中央型肺癌患者进行根治性气管内治疗时，AFB 在判断病变的范围方面发挥着重要作用。气管内治疗，例如光动力治疗后的完全缓解受病变表面积以及是否所有的边缘均直观的影响[51]。这些因素仅凭 WLB 难以进行准确评估。Sutedja 等对 23 例行腔内治疗的 NSCLC 患者在 WLB 以后又进行了 AFB 检查[52]。由 CT 和 AFB 分别发现 4 例（17%）和 19 例（68%）患者因病变范围太广泛而不适合行腔内治疗。

气管上皮内瘤变的监测

异型增生和原位癌被认为是肺鳞癌的癌前病变，但在纵向研究中这种情况的病例很少，由癌前病变进展为浸润性鳞癌的风险及发病率以及进展或消退的机制尚不明确。一项已发表的综述表明，平均 60% 的重度异型增生自发消退，40% 出现进展或持续存在[53]。对同一部位重复活检实际上在多大程度上移除了病变尚不能估计。癌前病变的自然病程更难以评估，因为除一项研究外[54]，所有的研究都在诊断的同时对治疗进行了干预，或者在 3 个月内原位癌持续存在时对患者反复行支气管镜检查和活检。原位癌在分子水平与重度异型增生不同，并且两者的临床结局也不同。原位癌自发消退率在 13% 以下，而高度异型增生超过 50%[53]。一项针对未经过初始治疗的 16 例患者的 36 处高级别病变（7 例重度异型增生，29 例原位癌）的单中心研究中，9 例患者被诊断出 11 处恶性肿瘤；5 例患者的 6 处高级别病变在经过 4～17 个月的时间后进展为浸润性癌，这 5 例患者中的 3 例虽经过治疗仍然未能治愈[54]。因此，如果放任原位癌进展为浸润癌，局部治疗可能无法治愈[53-54]。对于重度异型增生的患者进行气管镜检查比较合适，而对原位癌应该进行治疗而不能反复做气管镜检查和活检。正如下面将要讨论的，气管内治疗如电烙治疗和冷冻治疗，是一种简单、廉价及安全的治疗方式[55-56]。

基因改变如 3p 染色体杂合性缺失或染色体异倍性，以及宿主因素如肺内抗炎蛋白的炎症负荷和水平影响癌前病变的进展或消退[53,57]。BCCA 的一项研究中，与进展为肺腺癌的患者相比，进展为肺鳞癌的患者有着显著增高的进展率[53]。中度异型增生的恶变率在进展为肺鳞癌者为 30.9%，而在进展为腺癌者为 3.3%（$P = 0.041$），其作用

机制尚未明确。一些病变进展得非常快，在两年内就从增生或化生进展到原位癌或浸润癌[53,58]，这比我们传统认为的10~20年要短很多。在组织病理学分级以外加入细胞核形态或分子分析可以对癌前病变进行更准确的分类及对生物学行为更具有侵袭性的病变进行更好的鉴定。近期 van Boerdonk 等的研究[26]对同一部位的鳞状上皮化生病变进展为原位癌或浸润癌的6例患者与鳞状上皮化生病变未进展的20例患者的基因改变进行了比较，p53，p63及Ki-67免疫组化结果对病变的不同临床结局不具有预测性。在出现进展病例的基线鳞状上皮化生性病变中，其平均拷贝数改变（copy number alteration，CNA）较对照组明显增高（$P<0.01$）。基于 3p26.3~p11.1，3q26.2~29 及 6p25.3~24.3 CNAs 的一个模型在预测癌症进展方面具有97%的准确度。如果这些发现能被验证，将为支持明显低程度病变的患者应用 AFB 进行监测或进行气管内治疗提供证据。

无论在中央气道还是周围肺组织，高度异型增生或原位癌的存在都是肺癌的危险因素[53-54]。对存在这些病变的患者应当考虑应用 AFB 和 CT 进行密切随访。

周围肺组织癌前病变的检测

不典型腺瘤样增生（AAH）被认为是腺癌的侵袭前病变[59-60]。这些病变的直径通常≤7mm，在CT上表现为小的毛玻璃密度影[61-62]。在切除的肺组织中，AAH 的发生率在原发性肺癌患者中估计为9%~21%，在不伴肺癌的患者中为4%~10%[59]。实验室研究证实 AAH 细胞具有 Clara 细胞或Ⅱ型肺泡上皮细胞[63]的超微结构，肺腺癌中存在的多数分子改变在这些病变中也存在，支持 AAH 病变是周围型腺癌癌前病变这一概念。在CT上发现毛玻璃密度影、小的半实性或非钙化结节并非 AAH、原位腺癌、微浸润或浸润性腺癌的特异性表现。这些肺部小结节中的大多数并不是癌前或癌性病变[61-62]。逐渐增大或密度增加的小于1cm 肺结节的诊断需要依靠活检。

对于≤15mm 的病变，CT 引导下经胸细针穿刺或活检的灵敏度为70%~82%[64-65]。经胸细针穿刺活检平均有15%的气胸发生率。大约有6.6%需要胸管引流[66]。一些气管镜活检方法可以在并发症显著降低的同时获得与CT引导经胸肺活检相接近的获益。随着薄层CT和影像重建技术的发展，虚拟支气管镜导航（virtual bronchoscopy navigation，VBN）可以应用计算机生成3D路线图来定位肺部病变。在每个分支点，气管镜检查者通过使实际的支气管镜图像与虚拟的图像相匹配来控制气管镜[67]。Ishida 等的一项随机试验显示，与不使用 VBN 相比，使用 VBN 的诊断获益显著增高（对于<20mm 的病变，为75.9% vs 59.3%）[68]。随着技术的发展和进步，VBN 可以叠加气管镜导航与真实的图像来实时指引所要到达的气管，同样还可以在不能通过气管直接到达病灶的情况下显示出病灶位于气管壁后方的位置和距离[69]。VBN 显著缩短了气管镜检查的时间。

VBN 还可以被用来与一条可操纵的导管配准，这条导管在头端安装有传感器并且可以用类似于全球定位系统的外部电磁装置来追踪气管镜或活检钳。这种方法被称为电磁导航（electromagnetic device similar，EMN）。一旦虚拟图像到达靶病灶，其位置将进一步由径向超声内镜（radial endoscopic ultrasound，R-EBUS）或者荧光气管镜进行确认以使配准误差减到最小[70]。R-EBUS 可以使荧光气管镜定位欠佳的病灶变得更加形象化[71]。一项关于 EMN 的 meta 分析显示其平均诊断率为67%，95% CI（62.6%，71.4%）[72]，在社区中诊断率要低一些。最近的一项关于 EMN 的多中心临床试验显示，其对≤2cm 病灶的灵敏度为50%[73]。各种技术的联合应用可以提高诊断率。随机试验显示对于≤20mm 的病灶，与分别单独应用 R-EBUS 或 EMN 的78%与75%相比，VBN+EMN+R-EBUS 可以使灵敏度提高到90%[74]。最近的一项关于气管镜引导的 meta 分析得出了类似的结果[72]。

有两项小的随机试验对经胸细针穿刺活检与 R-EBUS 气管镜进行了比较，结果显示二者总的诊断率相似[75-76]。气胸及其他并发症的发生率非常低。对 R-EBUS 检查而言，气胸的平均发生率为1%（0~5%）[72,75-76]。

新技术如 OCT[35-36]可以使诊断率进一步提高并可以实时采样，OCT 可以达到微米分辨率或类似小望远镜的可视化，应用光导纤维探头使小至1mm 的气道变得直接可视化。将导航系统与 OCT 相结合可能对肺部小结节能进行更好的定位，对其生长行为进行更好的描述，从而将癌前病变及早期腺癌与良性病变区分开。如图 7.2 所示，基于连续的 CT 扫描对腺癌体积倍增时间进行计算，并未在第一次 CT 扫描时就对肺结节进行活检，这种方法可能是错误的，因为肺结节在进展为浸润癌之前可能表现为 AAH。

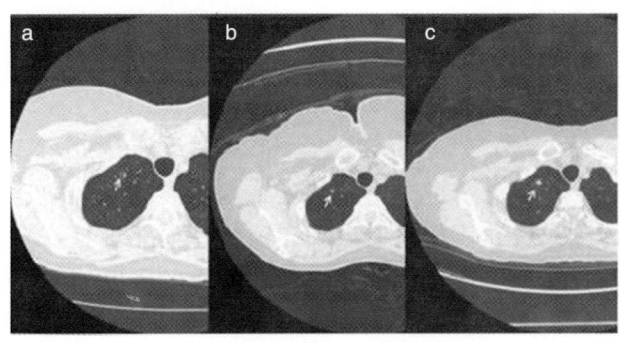

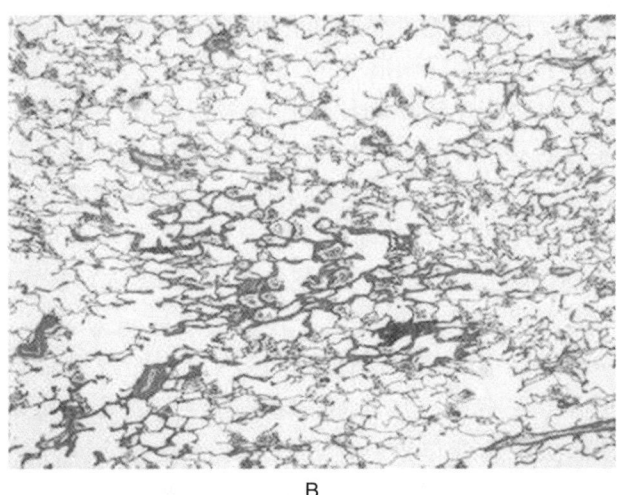

图 7.2（见彩插） A. 连续两年的低剂量螺旋 CT 复查显示右肺上叶（箭头所示）小结节的大小及密度逐渐增加（b、c）。B. 肺楔形切除病理检查示 AAH

侵袭前支气管病变的治疗

手术仍然是治疗原位癌的金标准，其 5 年生存率在 80%~90%[47,78-79]。然而，手术存在严重的局限性，那就是为了达到根治性治疗目的，需要切除大量肺组织。为了达到治愈，高达 30% 的患者需要行双肺叶切除或全肺切除，剩余的 70% 需要行肺叶切除术[47,78-79]。肺段切除仅用于一小部分经过选择的患者。所报道的最佳 5 年存活率超过了 90%[79]。

一些患者由于并发症或肺功能储备有限并不适合手术切除。高达 30% 的中央型肺鳞癌患者会发展为异时性癌并且大约 15% 的患者被发现合并同时性癌[42-43,45,47,78-80]。因此对于不能行支气管内治疗的患者，应考虑用尽可能保留肺组织的局部手术治疗。

在根治性支气管内治疗之前，排除支气管周围肿瘤侵犯、局部浸润或远处转移非常重要。胸部 CT 及 PET 是非常有用的检查方法[81]。CT 已被证实改变了 22%~35% 的考虑行根治性治疗患者的临床策略[81]。不管是 CT 还是 PET 上的阳性淋巴结都必须行进一步研究以排除转移。

支气管内治疗通常不能治愈侵及或超过支气管软骨的病变[81-83]。Konaka 等认为，长度超过 10mm 的扁平病变以及结节样或息肉样肿瘤出现软骨侵犯的风险显著增高[84]。EBUS 已被证明是评价软骨侵犯的有效工具，其评估小的中央型肺鳞癌软骨侵犯的灵敏度和特异度分别为 89% 和 100%[82,85]。此外，EBUS 可以对淋巴结进行采样从而用于分期。经过 WLB 和胸部 CT 检查后认为可以通过支气管内治疗达到根治的肿瘤中，EBUS 改变了 36% 的肿瘤治疗策略[82]。

除了确定肿瘤浸润支气管壁的深度和排除支气管外侵犯以外，在气管镜治疗时，病变的边缘必须可视化并且可以接近。如果可以手术，不符合这些标准的病变应考虑接受根治性手术。AFB 是精确显示病变所有边缘的最好方法[44,52]。

支气管内治疗

尽管没有比较原位癌行手术与支气管内治疗的前瞻性、随机对照研究，但看起来这似乎与早期中央型肺癌患者行支气管内治疗与手术治疗的对比研究结果类似[47,56]。除了保留肺组织及操作风险较低外，支气管内治疗的成本效益较高，与手术切除相比，可节省高达 70% 的费用[56]。

应用广泛并且有详细文献记录的支气管内治疗技术包括光动力学疗法（photodynamic therapy, PDT）、电烙术、氩离子凝固术（argon plasma coagulation, APC）、冷冻疗法、短距离放射疗法以及 Nd-YAG 激光疗法。所有这些技术在用于原位癌病灶时通常使用纤维支气管镜在患者清醒镇静状态下完成，而不是像较大的阻塞性病灶那样需要使用硬质支气管镜完成，其中，PDT 在世界范围内应用最广泛，但是费用较高和皮肤光过敏是其主要的缺点。电烙术或 APC 以及冷冻疗法是较 PDT 更便宜且简单的选择，但是它们的疗效缺乏数据支持。由于穿孔和出血的风险增加，通常认为 Nd-YAG 激光疗法不适用于浅表性原位癌的根治性治疗[86]。

光动力疗法（PDT）

PDT 指静脉注射光敏剂，如在肿瘤组织中比周围组织优先高浓度聚集的光卟啉，24~72h 内药物在特定波长光的作用下活化，发生光化学反应从而破坏肿瘤组织[51,87-88]。与光卟啉相比，新的光敏剂如单-L-天门冬酰氯 e6（他拉泊芬钠，NPe6）的皮肤光过敏时间更短[89-90]。

Kato 等报道的 264 例早期中央型恶性肿瘤患者中，85% 获得完全缓解[91]。随着肿瘤体积的增加，完全缓解率逐渐下降：纵向长度 <10mm 的肿瘤为 94%，10~20mm 的肿瘤为 80%，>20mm 的肿瘤为 44%。来自北美和欧洲的小样本研究所报道的 CR 率为 62%~100%[92-93]。局部复发见于约 12% 的患者[88,91]，且多数发生于 12 个月内[94]，这些多被认为是周围边界或深度可视化不充分导致照射不足所致。为了提高 PDT 的疗效，EBUS、OCT 及 AFB 已经被联合应用以更好地界定病灶的边界[82,91]。

电烙术

支气管镜下电烙术通过探针的直接接触传递高频交流电产生的热能从而破坏组织。电烙术通过一系列工具如钳子、切割环及钝热探头等使组织破坏，并且通过功率、接触表面积及能源持续时间的调整使组织凝固。这是一项花费小且并发症发生率较低的技术。Van Boxem 等的报道显示，13 例患者的 15 处 CT 上正常、≤10mm² 的腔内小病变的完全缓解率为 80%。经过 22 个月的中位随访，未发现残留病变[95]。同一组作者接下来的一项研究纳入了 32 例患者，评估了包括应用电烙术治疗小的腔内、微浸润 IA 期病变（除外原位癌）在内的多种根治性支气管内治疗模式。这些患者中 75% 接受电烙术治疗，超过 95% 的患者达到气管镜下根治。经过 5 年的平均随访，半数患者死亡，但仅有 1 例患者的死亡归因于支气管镜治疗的失败或并发症[80]。

APC 是另外一种相对廉价的非接触型热消融技术[96]。电离的氩气喷出探针，在探针的活动电极与组织之间传导电子。这些在人体组织内遇到高阻抗的电子产生热量，导致表面组织破坏。目前尚缺乏 APC 治疗支气管内原位癌疗效的数据[97]，但从理论上讲，其结果应该与电烙术相似。

冷冻疗法

冷冻疗法是应用一氧化二氮或液氮实现快速冷冻及融化，使组织破坏，这是一项廉价且安全的技术。支气管软骨和细胞外基质的高度耐冷特点使冷冻外科相对安全，没有气道穿孔或狭窄形成的危险[98]。与基于高温技术所导致的蛋白变性不同，保留细胞外基质可以促使不需要的组织消融且不遗留明显瘢痕[99-100]。

对冷冻疗法作为原位癌或微浸润支气管恶性肿瘤的根治性治疗方法的研究尚有限。Deygas 等[100] 报道了 35 例患者的 41 处原位癌或微浸润病变，经过 12 个月的随访，患者未见严重不良反应且 CR 值达到 91%。10 例患者（占 28%）在 12 个月内出现局部复发，总的长期治愈率为 80%。应用支气管内冷冻探针进行冷冻治疗的效果并不十分令人满意，并且操作起来有一定困难，其效果取决于病变位置。最近研制出了喷雾冷冻疗法（spray cryotherapy，SCT），通过内镜导管传送比冷冻探针温度更低的液氮。这种非接触方法便于在更大的范围进行更精确的治疗。已有的应用 SCT 的临床经验主要在大的阻塞性支气管肿瘤[101-102]。短时间且多周期应用 SCT 以及导管的恰当定位对避免由于气体快速膨胀导致的气胸至关重要。

近距离放射疗法

支气管内近距离放射疗法（endobronchial brachytherapy，EBBT）可以进行局部放射，这一过程通过纤维支气管镜将作为放射源（通常是铱^{192}）管道的聚氨酯导管置入气道内肿瘤来实现。这项技术已经被有效地用于阻塞性支气管内肿瘤的姑息治疗，但 EBBT 在治疗原位癌和微浸润肿瘤方面的报道较少。EBBT 独特的优势在于它对侵入支气管软骨的肿瘤的治疗效果较好。最大的系列报道之一来自 Hennequin 等，他们对 106 例 CT 上看不到且厚度 <10mm 的中央型气道肿瘤患者进行了 EBBT 治疗[103]。由于存在禁忌证，这些患者不适合手术或体外放射治疗。EBBT 使 59% 的患者达到了完全组织学缓解。支气管内长度较短的肿瘤以及 CT 上看不到的肿瘤接受 EBBT 治疗后有显著的效果，两项小样本研究观察到的反应率（response，RR）为 83% ~ 85%[104-105]。EBBT 潜在的并发症包括咯血以及辐射导致的支气管炎或支气管狭窄。

支气管内治疗后随访

因为 10% ~ 15% 的患者为了达到治愈目的需要进行二次治疗，所以对最初接受支气管内治疗后患者需要通过重复活检进行仔细的随访[80,92,100]。此外，由于高达 30% 的患者将来会在其他部位发展为异时性疾病，建议在根治性治疗后对患者进行长期随访。随访时通常应行气管镜检查及活检，在初始治疗后 4 ~ 6 周做 1 次，在 1 ~ 2 年内每 3 ~ 6 个月做 1 次，以后每年做 1 次直到满 5 年。尽管没有关于 CT 作用的数据发表，考虑到这些患者发展为异时性疾病的风险较高，CT 随访可能会带来额外的益处。

（于　洋　王　晖　王功朝　彭忠民　译）

参考文献

[1] Siegel R, Naishadham D, Jemal A. Cancer statistics. CA: a Cancer Journal for Clinicians, 2012, 62（1）: 10 - 29.

[2] Surveillance, Epidemiology, and End Results (SEER) Program (www. seer. cancer. gov) SEER* Stat Database: Incidence—SEER 17 Regs Public-Use, Nov 2005 Sub (1973 - 2003 varying). released April 2006, based on the November 2005 submission.

[3] Wagnieres G, McWilliams A, Lam S. Lung cancer imaging with fluorescence endoscopy//Mycek M, Pogue B (eds). Handbook of Biomedical Fluorescence. New York: Marcel Dekker, 2003: 361 - 396.

[4] Woolner L. Pathology of cancer detected cytologically//Atlas of Early Lung Cancer. Tokyo: Igaku-Shoin: National Institutes of Health. US Department of Health and Human Services, 1983: 107 - 213.

[5] Hung J, Lam S, LeRiche JC, et al. Autofluorescence of normal and malignant bronchial tissue. Lasers in Surgery & Medicine, 1991, 11（2）: 99 - 105.

[6] Qu J, MacAulay C, Lam S, et al. Laserinduced fluorescence spectroscopy at endoscopy: tissueoptics, Monte Carlo modeling, and in vivo measurements. Optical Engineering, 1995, 34: 3334 - 3343.

[7] Qu J, Macaulay C, Lam S, et al. Optical properties of normal and carcinomatous bronchial tissue. Appl Opt, 1994: 33（31）: 7397 - 7405.

[8] Keith RL, Miller YE, Gemmill RM, et al. Angiogenic squamous dysplasia in bronchi of individuals at high risk for lung cancer. Clinical Cancer Research, 2000, 6（5）: 1616 - 1625.

[9] Gardner CM, Jacques SL, Welch AJ. Fluorescence spectroscopy of tissue: recovery of intrinsic fluorescence from measured fluorescence. Appl Opt, 1996, 35（10）: 1780 - 1792.

[10] Zellweger M, Grosjean P, Goujon D, et al. In vivo auto fluorescence spectroscopy of human bronchial tissue to optimize the detection and imaging of early cancers. J Biomed Opt, 2001, 6（1）: 41 - 51.

[11] Lam S, Kennedy T, Unger M, et al. Localization of bronchial intraepithelial neoplastic lesions by fluorescence bronchoscopy. Chest, Mar, 1998, 113（3）: 696 - 702.

[12] Edell E, Lam S, Pass H, et al. Detection and localization of intraepithelial neoplasia and invasive carcinoma using fluorescence-reflectance bronchoscopy: an international, multicenter clinical trial. Journal of Thoracic Oncology, 2009, 4（1）: 49 - 54.

[13] Chiyo M, Shibuya K, Hoshino H, et al. Effective detection of bronchial preinvasive lesions by a new autofluorescence imaging bronchovideoscope system. Lung Cancer, 2005, 48（3）: 307 - 313.

[14] Ikeda N, Honda H, Hayashi A, et al. Early detection of bronchial lesions using newly developed videoendoscopy-based autofluorescence bronchoscopy. Lung Cancer, 2006, 52（1）: 21 - 27.

[15] Haussinger K, Stanzel F, Huber RM, et al. Autofluorescence detection of bronchial tumors with the D-Light/AF. Diagnostic & Therapeutic Endoscopy, 1999, 5（2）: 105 - 112.

[16] Goujon D, Zellweger M, Radu A, et al. In vivo autofluorescence imaging of early cancers in the human tracheobronchial tree with a spectrally optimized system. J Biomed Opt, 2003, 8（1）: 17 - 25.

[17] Tercelj M, Zeng H, Petek M, et al. Acquisition of fluo-

rescence and reflectance spectra during routine bronchoscopy examinations using the ClearVu Elite device: pilot study. Lung Cancer, 2005, 50 (1): 35-42.

[18] Lee P, Brokx HA, Postmus PE, et al. Dual digital video-autofluorescence imaging for detection of pre-neoplastic lesions. Lung Cancer, 2007, 58 (1): 44-49.

[19] Lam S. The role of autofluorescence bronchoscopy in diagnosis of early lung cancer//Hirsch F, Bunn PJ, Kato H, et al (eds). IASLC Textbook for Prevention and Detection of Early Lung Cancer. London: Taylor & Francis, 2006: 149-158.

[20] Hirsch FR, Prindiville SA, Miller YE, et al. Fluorescence versus white-light bronchoscopy for detection of preneoplastic lesions: a randomized study. J Natl Cancer Inst, 2001, 93 (18): 1385-1391.

[21] Haussinger K, Becker H, Stanzel F, et al. Autofluorescence bronchoscopy with white light bronchoscopy compared with white light bronchoscopy alone for the detection of precancerous lesions: A European randomized controlled multicentre trial. Thorax, 2005, 60 (6): 496-503.

[22] Ernst A, Simoff M, Mathur P, et al. D-light autofluorescence in the detection of premalignant airway changes: a multicenter trial. Journal of Bronchology, 2005, 12 (3): 133-138.

[23] Sun J, Garfield DH, Lam B, et al. The value of autofluorescence bronchoscopy combined with white light bronchoscopy compared with white light alone in the diagnosis of intraepithelial neoplasia and invasive lung cancer: a meta-analysis. Journal of Thoracic Oncology, 2011, 6 (8): 1336-1344.

[24] Lee P, van den Berg RM, Lam S, et al. Color fluorescence ratio for detection of bronchial dysplasia and carcinoma in situ. Clinical Cancer Research, 2009, 15 (14): 4700-4705.

[25] Helfritzsch H, Junker K, Bartel M, et al. Differentiation of positive autofluorescence bronchoscopy findings by comparative genomic hybridization. Oncol Reports, 2002, 9 (4): 697-701.

[26] van Boerdonk RA, Sutedja TG, Snijders PJ, et al. DNA copy number alterations in endobronchial squamous metaplastic lesions predict lung cancer. American Journal of Respiratory & Critical Care Medicine, Oct 15, 2011, 184 (8): 948-956.

[27] Pasic A, Vonk-Noordegraaf A, Risse EK, et al. Multiple suspicious lesions detected by autofluorescence bronchoscopy predict malignant development in the bronchial mucosa in high risk patients. Lung Cancer, 2003, 41 (3): 295-301.

[28] Gazdar AF, Minna JD. Angiogenesis and the multistage development of lung cancers. Clinical Cancer Research, May, 2000, 6 (5): 1611-1612.

[29] Tajiri H, Niwa H. Proposal for a consensus terminology in endoscopy: How should different endoscopic imaging techniques be grouped and defined? Endoscopy, 2008, 40 (9): 775-778.

[30] Curvers WL, Singh R, Song LM, et al. Endoscopic trimodal imaging for detection of early neoplasia in Barrett's oesophagus: a multi-centre feasibility study using high-resolution endoscopy, autofluorescence imaging and narrow band imaging incorporated in one endoscopy system. Gut, 2008, 57 (2): 167-172.

[31] Shibuya K, Nakajima T, Fujiwara T, et al. Narrow band imaging with high-resolution bronchovideoscopy: a new approach for visualizing angiogenesis in squamous cell carcinoma of the lung. Lung Cancer, 2010, 69 (2): 194-202.

[32] Herth FJ, Eberhardt R, Anantham D, et al. Narrow-band imaging bronchoscopy increases the specificity of bronchoscopic early lung cancer detection. Journal of Thoracic Oncology, 2009, 4 (9): 1060-1065.

[33] Tsuboi M, Hayashi A, Ikeda N, et al. Optical coherence tomography in the diagnosis of bronchial lesions. Lung Cancer, 2005, 49 (3): 387-394.

[34] Lam S, Standish B, Baldwin C, et al. In vivo optical coherence tomography imaging of preinvasive bronchial lesions. Clinical Cancer Research, 2008, 14 (7): 2006-2011.

[35] Ohtani K, Lee A, Lam S. Frontiers in bronchoscopic imaging. Respirology, 2012, 17 (2): 261-269.

[36] Hariri L, Applegate M, Mino-Kenudson M, et al. Volumetric optical frequency domain imaging of pulmonary pathology with precise, correlation to histopathology. Chest, 2013, 143 (1): 64-74.

[37] Sato M, Sakurada A, Sagawa M, et al. Diagnostic results before and after introduction of autofluorescence bronchoscopy in patients suspected of having lung cancer detected by sputum cytology in lung cancer mass screening. Lung Cancer, 2001, 32 (3): 247-253.

[38] Frost JK, Ball WC, Jr, Levin ML, et al. Sputumcytopathology: use and potential in monitoring the workplace environment by screening for biological effects of exposure.

[39] Risse EK, Vooijs GP, van't Hof MA. Diagnostic significance of "severe dysplasia" in sputum cytology. Acta Cytol, 1988, 32 (5): 629-634.

[40] Prindiville SA, Byers T, Hirsch FR, et al. Sputum cytological atypia as a predictor of incident lung cancer in a cohort of heavy smokers with airflow obstruction. Cancer Epidemiology, Biomarkers & Prevention, 2003, 12 (10): 987-93.

[41] Kennedy TC, Franklin WA, Prindiville SA, et al. High prevalence of occult endobronchial malignancy in high risk patients with moderate sputum atypia. Lung Cancer, 2005, 49 (2): 187-191.

[42] Pierard P, Faber J, Hutsebaut J, et al. Synchronous lesions detected by autofluorescence bronchoscopy in patients with high-grade preinvasive lesions and occult invasive squamous cell carcinoma of the proximal airways. Lung Cancer, 2004, 46 (3): 341-347.

[43] van Rens MT, Schramel FM, Elbers JR, et al. The clinical value of lung imaging fluorescence endoscopy for detecting synchronous lung cancer. Lung Cancer, 2001, 32 (1): 13-18.

[44] Ikeda N, Hiyoshi T, Kakihana M, et al. Histopathological evaluation of fluorescence bronchoscopy using resected lungs in cases of lung cancer. Lung Cancer, 2003, 41 (3): 303-309.

[45] Pierard P, Vermylen P, Bosschaerts T, et al. Synchronous roentgenographically occult lung carcinoma in patients with resectable primary lung cancer. Chest, 2000, 117 (3): 779-785.

[46] Johnson BE. Second lung cancers in patients after treatment for an initial lung cancer. J Natl Cancer Inst, 1998, 90 (18): 1335-1345.

[47] Nakamura H, Kawasaki N, Hagiwara M, et al. Early hilar lung cancer-risk for multiple lung cancers and clinical outcome. Lung Cancer, 2001, 33 (1): 51-57.

[48] Weigel TL, Yousem S, Dacic S, et al. Fluorescence bronchoscopic surveillance after curative surgical resection for non-small-cell lung cancer. Annals of Surgical Oncology, 2000, 7 (3): 176-180.

[49] Weigel TL, Kosco PJ, Dacic S, et al. Postoperative fluorescence bronchoscopic surveillance in non-small cell lung cancer patients. Ann Thorac Surg, 2001, 71 (3): 967-970.

[50] Moro-Sibilot D, Fievet F, Jeanmart M, et al. Clinical prognostic indicators of high-grade pre-invasive bronchial lesions. European Respiratory Journal, 2004, 24 (1): 24-29.

[51] Kato H, Okunaka T, Shimatani H. Photodynamic therapy for early stage bronchogenic carcinoma. J Clin Laser Med Surg, 1996, 14 (5): 235-238.

[52] Sutedja TG, Codrington H, Risse EK, et al. Autofluorescence bronchoscopy improves staging of radiographically occult lung cancer and has an impact on therapeutic strategy. Chest, 2001, 120 (4): 1327-1332.

[53] Ishizumi T, McWilliams A, MacAulay C, et al. Natural history of bronchial preinvasive lesions. Cancer & Metastasis Reviews, 2010, 29 (1): 5-14.

[54] Jeremy George P, Banerjee AK, Read CA, et al. Surveillance for the detection of early lung cancer in patients with bronchial dysplasia. Thorax, 2007, 62 (1): 43-50.

[55] Sutedja G, Postmus PE. Bronchoscopic treatment of lung tumors. Lung Cancer, 1994, 11 (1-2): 1-17.

[56] Pasic A, Brokx HA, Vonk Noordegraaf A, et al. Cost-effectiveness of early intervention: Comparison between intraluminal bronchoscopic treatment and surgical resection for T1N0 lung cancer patients. Respiration, 2004, 71 (4): 391-396.

[57] Salaun M, Sesboue R, Moreno-Swirc S, et al. Molecular predictive factors for progression of high-grade preinvasive bronchial lesions. American Journal of Respiratory & Critical Care Medicine, 2008, 177 (8): 880-886.

[58] Breuer RH, Pasic A, Smit EF, et al. The natural course of preneoplastic lesions in bronchial epithelium. Clinical Cancer Research, 2005, 11 (2 Pt 1): 537-543.

[59] Miller RR. Bronchioloalveolar cell adenomas. Am J Surg Pathol, 1990, 14 (10): 904-912.

[60] Travis WD, Brambilla E, Noguchi M, et al. International Association for the Study of Lung Cancer/American Thoracic Society/European Respiratory Society International Multidisciplinary Classification of Lung Adenocarcinoma. Journal of Thoracic Oncology, 2011, 6 (2): 244-285.

[61] Vazquez MF, Flieder DB. Small peripheral glandular lesions detected by screening CT for lung cancer: A diagnostic dilemma for the pathologist. Radiol Clin North Am, 2000, 38 (3): 579-589.

[62] McWilliams AM, Mayo JR, Ahn MI, et al. Lung cancer screening using multislice thin-section computed tomography and autofluorescence bronchoscopy. Journal of

Thoracic Oncology, 2006, 1 (1): 61-68.

[63] Mori M, Kaji M, Tezuka F, et al. Comparative ultrastructural study of atypical adenomatous hyperplasia and adenocarcinoma of the human lung. Ultrastruct Pathol, 1998, 22 (6): 459-466.

[64] Kothary N, Lock L, Sze DY, et al. Computed tomography-guided percutaneous needle biopsy of pulmonary nodules: impact of nodule size on diagnostic accuracy. Clinical Lung Cancer, 2009, 10 (5): 360-363.

[65] Heyer CM, Reichelt S, Peters SA, et al. Computed tomographynavi-gated transthoracic core biopsy of pulmonarylesions: which factors affect diagnostic yield and complication rates? Acad Radiol, 2008, 15 (8): 1017-1026.

[66] Wiener RS, Schwartz LM, Woloshin S, et al. Population-based risk for complications after transthoracic needle lung biopsy of a pulmonary nodule: an analysis of discharge records. Ann Intern Med, 2011, 155 (3): 137-144.

[67] Asano F. Virtual bronchoscopic navigation. Clin Chest Med, 2010, 31 (1): 75-85.

[68] Ishida T, Asano F, Yamazaki K, et al. Virtual bronchoscopic navigation combined with endobronchial ultrasound to diagnose small peripheral pulmonary lesions: a randomized trial. Thorax, 2011, 66 (12): 1072-1077.

[69] Eberhardt R, Kahn N, Gompelmann D, et al., Lung-Point-a new approach to peripheral lesions. Journal of Thoracic Oncology, 2010, 5 (10): 1559-1563.

[70] Becker HD, Herth F, Ernst A, et al. Bronchoscopic biopsy of peripheral lung lesions under electromagnetic guidance: A pilot study. Journal of Bronchology & Interventional Pulmonology, 2005, 12 (1): 9-13.

[71] Herth FJ, Eberhardt R, Becker HD, et al. Endobronchial ultrasound-guided transbronchial lung biopsy in fluoroscopically invisible solitary pulmonary nodules: a prospective trial. Chest, 2006, 129 (1): 147-150.

[72] Wang Memoli J, Nietert P, Silvestri G. Metaanalysis of guided bronchoscopy for the evaluation of the pulmonary nodule. Chest, 2012, 142 (2): 385-393.

[73] Jensen KW, Hsia DW, Seijo LM, et al. Multicenter experience with electromagnetic navigation bronchoscopy for the diagnosis of pulmonary nodules. Journal of Bronchology & Interventional Pulmonology, 2012, 19 (3): 195-199.

[74] Eberhardt R, Anantham D, Ernst A, et al. Multimodality bronchoscopic diagnosis of peripheral lung lesions: A randomized controlled trial. American Journal of Respiratory & Critical Care Medicine, 2007, 176 (1): 36-41.

[75] Steinfort DP, Vincent J, Heinze S, et al. Comparative effectiveness of radial probe endobronchial ultrasound versus CT-guided needle biopsy for evaluation of peripheral pulmonary lesions: a randomized pragmatic trial. Respir Med, 2011, 105 (11): 1704-1711.

[76] Fielding DI, Chia C, Nguyen P, et al. Prospective randomized trial of endobronchial ultrasound-guide sheath versus computed tomography-guided percutaneous core biopsies for peripheral lung lesions. Intern Med J, 2012, 42 (8): 894-900.

[77] Delage A, Godbout K, Martel S, et al. Evaluation of pulmonary nodules using the spyglass direct visualization system combined with radial endobronchial ultrasound: A feasibility study. American Journal of Respiratory and Critical Care Medicine, 185 (1): A1103.

[78] Cortese DA, Pairolero PC, Bergstralh EJ, et al. Roentgenographi-cally occult lung cancer. A ten-year experience. Journal of Thoracic & Cardiovascular Surgery, 1983, 86 (3): 373-380.

[79] Fujimura S, Sakurada A, Sagawa M, et al. A therapeutic approach to roentgenographically occult squamous cell carcinoma of the lung. Cancer, 2000, 89 (11 Suppl): 2445-2448.

[80] Vonk-Noordegraaf A, Postmus PE, Sutedja TG. Bronchoscopic treatment of patients with intraluminal microinvasive radiographically occult lung cancer not eligible for surgical resection: A follow-up study. Lung Cancer, 2003, 39 (1): 49-53.

[81] Sutedja G, Golding RP, Postmus PE. High resolution computed tomography in patients referred for intraluminal bronchoscopic therapy with curative intent. European Respiratory Journal, 1996, 9 (5): 1020-1023.

[82] Miyazu Y, Miyazawa T, Kurimoto N, et al. Endobronchial ultrasonography in the assessment of centrally located early-stage lung cancer before photodynamic therapy. American Journal of Respiratory and Critical Care Medicine, 2002, 165 (6): 832-837.

[83] Kurimoto N, Murayama M, Yoshioka S, et al. Assessment of usefulness of endobronchial ultrasonography in determination of depth of tracheobronchial tumor invasion. Chest, 1999, 115 (6): 1500-1506.

[84] Konaka C, Hirano T, Kato H, et al. Comparison of endoscopic features of early-stage squamous cell lung cancer and histological findings. Br J Cancer, 1999, 80 (9): 1435-1439.

[85] Herth F, Ernst A, Schulz M, et al. Endobronchial ultrasound reliably differentiates between airway infiltration

and compression by tumor. Chest, 2003, 123 (2): 458-462.

[86] Bolliger CT, Sutedja TG, Strausz J, et al. Therapeutic bronchoscopy with immediate effect: laser, electrocautery, argon plasma coagulation and stents. European Respiratory Journal, 2006, 27 (6): 1258-1271.

[87] Lam S. Photodynamic therapy of lung cancer. Semin Oncol, 1994, 21 (6 Suppl 15): 15-19.

[88] Furuse K, Fukuoka M, Kato H, et al. A prospective phase II study on photodynamic therapy with photofrin II for centrally located early-stage lung cancer. The Japan Lung Cancer Photodynamic Therapy Study Group. Journal of Clinical Oncology, 1993, 11 (10): 1852-1857.

[89] Ikeda N, Usuda J, Kato H, et al. New aspects of photodynamic therapy for central type early stage lung cancer. Lasers in Surgery & Medicine, 2011, 43 (7): 749-754.

[90] Kato H, Furukawa K, Sato M, et al. Phase II clinical study of photodynamic therapy using mono-1-aspartyl chlorin e6 and diode laser for early superficial squamous cell carcinoma of the lung. Lung Cancer, 2003, 42 (1): 103-111.

[91] Kato H, Usuda J, Okunaka T, et al. Basic and clinical research on photodynamic therapy at Tokyo Medical University Hospital. Lasers in Surgery & Medicine, 2006, 38 (5): 371-375.

[92] Cortese DA, Edell ES, Kinsey JH. Photodynamic therapy for early stage squamous cell carcinoma of the lung. Mayo Clin Proc, 1997, 72 (7): 595-602.

[93] Moghissi K, Dixon K, Thorpe JA, et al. Photodynamic therapy (PDT) in early central lung cancer: a treatment option for patients ineligible for surgical resection. Thorax, 2007, 62 (5): 391-395.

[94] Furukawa K, Kato H, Konaka C, et al. Locally recurrent central-type early stage lung cancer <1.0 cm in diameter after complete remission by photodynamic therapy. Chest, 2005, 128 (5): 3269-3275.

[95] Van Boxem TJ, Venmans BJ, Schramel FM, et al. Radiographically occult lung cancer treated with fibreoptic bronchoscopic electrocautery: A pilot study of a simple and inexpensive technique. European Respiratory Journal, 1998, 11 (1): 169-172.

[96] Sutedja G, Bolliger C. Endobronchial electrocautery and argon plasma coagulation. Interventional bronchoscopy. Progress in Respiratory Research, 2000, 30: 120-132.

[97] Schuurman B, Postmus PE, Van Mourik JC, et al. Combined use of autofluorescence bronchoscopy and argon plasma coagulation enables less extensive resection of radiographically occult lung cancer. Respiration, 2004, 71 (4): 410-411.

[98] Shepherd JP, Dawber RP. Wound healing and scarring after cryosurgery. Cryobiology, 1984, 21 (2): 157-169.

[99] Vergnon JM, Huber RM, Moghissi K. Place of cryotherapy, brachytherapy and photodynamic therapy in therapeutic bronchoscopy of lung cancers. European Respiratory Journal, 2006, 28 (1): 200-218.

[100] Deygas N, Froudarakis M, Ozenne G, et al. Cryotherapy in early superficial bronchogenic carcinoma. Chest, 2001, 120 (1): 26-31.

[101] Au JT, Carson J, Monette S, et al. Spray cryotherapy is effective for bronchoscopic, endoscopic and open ablation of thoracic tissues. Interactive Cardiovascular & Thoracic Surgery, 2012, 15 (4): 580-584.

[102] Finley DJ, Dycoco J, Sarkar S, et al. Airway spray cryotherapy: Initial outcomes from a multiinstitutional registry. Ann Thorac Surg; 2012, 94 (1): 199-203; Discussion 203-204.

[103] Hennequin C, Bleichner O, Tredaniel J, et al. Long-term results of endobronchial brachytherapy: A curative treatment? Int J Radiat Oncol Biol Phys, 2007, 67 (2): 425-430.

[104] Marsiglia H, Baldeyrou P, Lartigau E, et al. High-dose-rate brachytherapy as sole modality for early-stage endobronchial carcinoma. International Journal of Radiation Oncology Biology Physics, 2000, 47 (3): 665-672.

[105] Perol M, Caliandro R, Pommier P, et al. Curative irradiation of limited endobronchial carcinomas with high-dose rate brachytherapy: Results of a pilot study. Chest, 1997, 111 (5): 1417-1423.

第 8 章
肺腺癌病理学

William D. Travis
Department of Pathology, Memorial Sloan-Kettering Cancer Center, New York, NY, USA

引 言

在大多数国家，腺癌是肺癌最常见的组织学类型之一。据美国癌症协会（the American Cancer Society，ACS）估计，2013 年美国将有 228 190 例新增肺癌患者[1]，同时有 159 480 例肺癌患者死亡（其中 41% 为腺癌）[2]，2013 年美国肺腺癌患者将超过 93 000 例。

肺腺癌的异质性表现在多个方面，如临床影像、病理、手术和分子表型等。即使同一个体的肿瘤，也存在大量的组织学异质性，因此，与预后相关的重要临床分类方法的提出遭遇了很大的挑战。在过去的 10 年间，为了能提出一个国际性多学科分类方法，人们做了大量的努力，基于这些努力，国际肺癌研究协会（ASLC）、美国胸科学会（ATS）和欧洲呼吸学会（ERS）提出了一种新的肺腺癌分类方法，对肺腺癌的诊断产生了重大影响[3-5]。这种方法不仅考虑了切除样本（表 8.1），同时也考虑了小型活检和细胞样本（表 8.2）。本章主要讨论切除样本的分类，同时也将简单介绍小活检和细胞样本的分类。

2011 ATS/ERS 肺腺癌的分类建议有多处较大改动（表 8.1）[3-6]：①不再使用细支气管肺泡癌（BAC）这一术语，主要是因为在当前分类方法下，该肿瘤已分为 5 种不同类型的肿瘤；②新增了原位腺癌（AIS）和微浸润腺癌（MIA）两个概念；③全面组织型分型代替混合型分型这一术语，用以计算肿瘤主要型别的最终分类有 5% 增量的组织模式的百分数；④之前非黏液型 BAC 为主要成分的肿瘤被划分为鳞状上皮腺癌；⑤新增微乳头状生长方式亚型，因其预后差；⑥浸润性黏液型腺癌代替之前的黏液型支气管肺泡癌一词。最后，提出小活检及细胞标本的专业术语和诊断标准，以及晚期腺癌患者的组织样本管理和表皮生长因子突变检测[3-6]。

切除样本的腺癌分类

癌前病变

2011 年新的肺癌分类中，AIS 新增为腺癌的癌前病变（表 8.1）[4]。AAH 与鳞状上皮不典型增生性质相当，AIS 亦相当于鳞状细胞原位癌。

不典型腺瘤样增生（AAH）

AAH 是一种不典型的细胞增殖，类似于 AIS，但其标准低于 AIS[4,7-12]。AAH 常见于肺癌切除样本的肺实质中[13-15]。大多数 AAH 病灶区直径小于 5mm，但表现为多病灶[15-16]。组织学上，AAH 包含一个不典型立方形低柱状细胞沿肺泡壁表面匍匐样生长的病灶增生区，有时也可能有肺泡间隔增厚。

AAH 的鉴别诊断包括非黏液型 AIS、MIA 以及鳞状上皮腺癌[17]，由于 AAH 和鳞屑样腺癌的形态特征相似，因此区分 AAH 和 AIS 比较困难[13-14,18-19]。

原位腺癌（AIS）

AIS 是 IASLC/ATS/ERS 定义的一种新的腺癌类型，其腺性增生直径不超过 3cm，表现为单纯的鳞屑样生长且无浸润性（图 8.1）[4]。大多数情况

表 8.1 切除样本的腺癌组织分类

癌前病变
　AAH
　AIS（单纯的鳞屑样生长且无浸润性）
　　非黏液型，黏液型，混合型
　　非黏液型或黏液型

MIA
　直径≤3cm，鳞屑样生长方式为主且浸润灶≤5mm 的腺癌
　　非黏液型，黏液型，混合型
　　非黏液型或黏液型

浸润性腺癌
　鳞屑样生长方式为主（之前的非黏液型 BAC，浸润灶＞5mm）
　腺泡样为主
　乳头状为主
　微乳头状为主
　实性生长方式为主

浸润性腺癌的变异型
　浸润性黏液型腺癌（之前的黏液型 BAC）
　胶样型腺癌
　胎儿型腺癌
　肠型腺癌

引自 2004 年世界卫生组织（WHO）分类[10]和 2011 年 IASLC/ATS/ERS[11]分类。只强调切除样本的腺癌组织分类

下，肿瘤细胞为非黏液型，主要增殖细胞为 Ⅱ 型肺泡上皮细胞和 Clara 细胞。极少数情况下会出现富含顶端黏蛋白的高柱状上皮杯状细胞黏液型 AIS。对于黏液型 AIS 必须谨慎，应确保病变孤立且受到严格限制，对周围软组织没有粟粒性浸润。AIS 若接受根治性切除手术，5 年生存率可达 100%[20-27]。对于非黏液型 AIS 和孤立整合性黏液型 AIS，其 CT 表现为毛玻璃样结节[4]。

符合 1999 年和 2004 年 WHO 分类标准中 BAC 定义的大多数病变也都符合当前 AIS 的定义[10]。AIS 概念的提出是基于多个孤立性肺腺癌的观察性研究，在这些研究中，肺腺癌都表现为单纯的鳞屑样生长，直径小于 2cm 或 3cm，且接受根治性切除手术后，其生存率为 100%[20-26,28]。尽管大部分已发表的文献都聚焦于非黏液型肿瘤，但 Noguchi 在 1995 年报道的 28 例肿瘤中有 2 例分别是 A 型和 B 型黏液型肿瘤[26]。在 AIS 的新定义中，直径 ＜3cm，且有一个离散的限制边界是非常重要的，不包括粟粒性浸润至周边肺实质和（或）大叶性实变案例，尤其是黏液型 AIS。大部分数据表明，接受根治性切除手术后，5 年生存率为 100% 的肿瘤直径均小于 2cm 或 3cm，很少有直径超过 3cm 的研究报道。但是，关于黏液型 AIS 的研究数据很少[20-26,28]。

微浸润腺癌（MIA）

MIA 定义为直径 ＜3cm、鳞屑样生长方式为主且浸润灶 ＜ 5mm 的腺癌（图 8.2）[4]。直至 IASLC/ATS/ERS 提出新的分类方法，只有少数几个研究支持 MIA 患者的 5 年生存率为 100%[4,27,29]，其中一些研究甚至没有使用相同的标准[30-31]。与 AIS 类似，大多数 MIA 是非黏液型的，当然极少数情况下也会出现黏液型的案例[4]。非黏液型 MIA 在 CT 下表现为毛玻璃样结节样，且其固体成分小于 5mm，但黏液型 MIA 在 CT 下却表现为固体结节[4]。

MIA 的浸润测量需满足以下条件：①浸润的组织亚型［腺泡，乳头状、微乳头状和（或）实性］而不是鳞屑样；②肿瘤细胞浸润肌纤维母细胞基质。在存在淋巴管、血管或胸膜浸润以及肿瘤坏死这几种情况时不应诊断为 MIA。如果一个肿瘤有多个微小病灶，最大浸润面积应以最大浸润直径来测量，且最大浸润直径应小于 5mm。此外，有研究者认为一个肿瘤如果有多个微小病灶，浸润大小不能用所有病灶的总和来计算，虽然美国病理学家测量乳腺癌多发病灶的浸润性成分时就采用了该方法[32]。另一种方法是通过乘以浸润区占总肿瘤大小的百分比来计算浸润程度。

此外，当浸润区域为低分化成分，如实性或微乳头状为主的腺癌，或由不满足多形肿瘤标准的巨大的梭形细胞组成时，MIA 患者是否能达到 5 年 100% 生存率还有待证实。

当存在多个肿瘤时，只有其他肿瘤均为原发性肿瘤而非肺内转移瘤时，才能使用 MIA 和 AIS 的标准。

在确诊 MIA 和 AIS 之前，所有肿瘤都需要进

行全面的组织学检查。因此，应鼓励研究机构购置组织冻存设备，有了这些设备，可能利用冰冻切片解决浸润性腺癌的诊断问题。

由于微浸润病灶很难观察到，因此进行 CT 复查将有助于评估鳞屑样肿瘤的大小以及浸润程度。

MIA 或 AIS 诊断过程中直径大于 3cm 的肿瘤建议进行鳞状上皮癌的补充诊断。这样做主要是因为建立 MIA 和 AIS 标准的文献中肿瘤直径都不超过 3cm。由于该分类是一个循证的过程，因此对于直径大于 3cm 的孤立性肿瘤，没有证据显示完全切除后 5 年生存率能达到 100%。因此对于 MIA 或 AIS 诊断过程中直径大于 3cm 的肿瘤，或不能排除浸润组分的组织样本，应使用鳞状上皮癌这一术语。

表 8.2 IASLC/ATS/ERS 推荐的小组织活检和细胞学分类方法

WHO 分类（2004）	小活检或细胞学：IASLC/ATS/ERS
腺癌 　混合型 　腺泡 　乳头状 　实性	腺癌形态模式清晰呈现：腺癌，描述可识别的模式（包括 2004 WHO 分类未提到的微乳头状模式） 如果是单纯性的鳞屑样生长方式，小样本中浸润组分不能排除
BAC（非黏液型）	鳞屑样生长方式腺癌（单纯性的，无特殊标注，浸润组分就被排除）
BAC（黏液型）	黏液腺癌（在模式图中展示）
胎儿型	带有胎儿型细胞特性的腺癌
黏液型（胶体样）	带有胶体样特性的腺癌
印戒细胞	带有印戒细胞特性的腺癌（在模式图中展示）
透明细胞	带有透明细胞特性的腺癌（在模式图中展示）
2004 WHO 对应的数据大多数都是实性腺癌	腺状细胞形态模式没有体现（特异性染色支持）：非小细胞癌，良性腺癌
鳞状细胞癌 　乳头状 　透明细胞 　小细胞 　基底细胞样	鳞状细胞形态病理展示：鳞状细胞癌
无 2004 WHO 对应数据	鳞状细胞形态模式没有体现（染色支持）：非小细胞癌，良性鳞状细胞癌
小细胞癌	小细胞癌
大细胞癌	非小细胞癌，不确定型
大细胞神经内分泌癌（LCNEC）	非小细胞癌伴神经内分泌形态（NE 阳性）可能是 LCNEC
带 NE 形态的大细胞癌	带 NE 形态的非小细胞癌（NE 阴性）– 见评论 评论：非小细胞癌，怀疑是 LCNEC，但却不能证明 NE 分化
腺鳞癌	鳞状细胞和腺癌形态模式存在：非小细胞癌，不确定型（腺状或鳞状组分存在） 评论：可能为腺鳞癌
2004 WHO 分类无对应数据	无鳞状细胞或腺癌形态模式存在，但免疫组化却显示独立的腺状或腺鳞状组分，NSCLC，不确定型 评论：可能为腺鳞癌
肉瘤样癌	低分化 NSCLC 伴梭形和（或）巨细胞癌（在腺癌或鳞状细胞癌中叙述）

*摘自参考文献 4。经 Lippincott Williams，Wilkins 许可

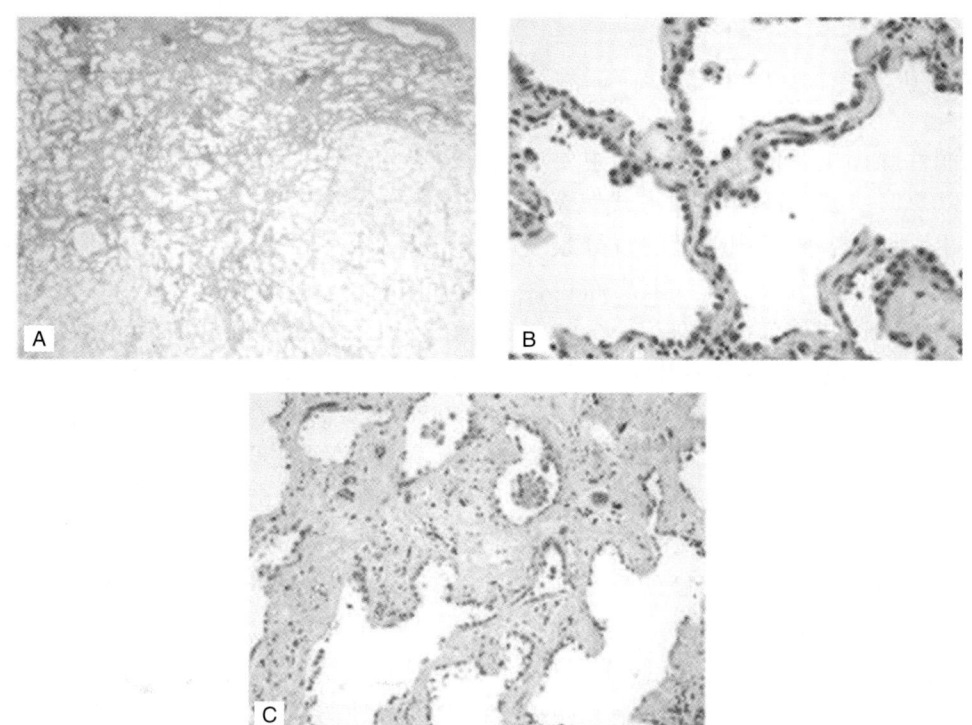

图 8.1（见彩插） 非黏液型 AIS。A. 限制性非黏液型肿瘤单纯鳞屑样生长且无浸润性。苏木精-伊红（H-E）染色×1.25。B. 鳞屑样生长或非典型细胞沿肺泡壁薄生长，H-E 染色×20。C. 肺泡壁薄纤维化增厚，但没有浸润，只存在鳞屑样生长，H-E 染色×20

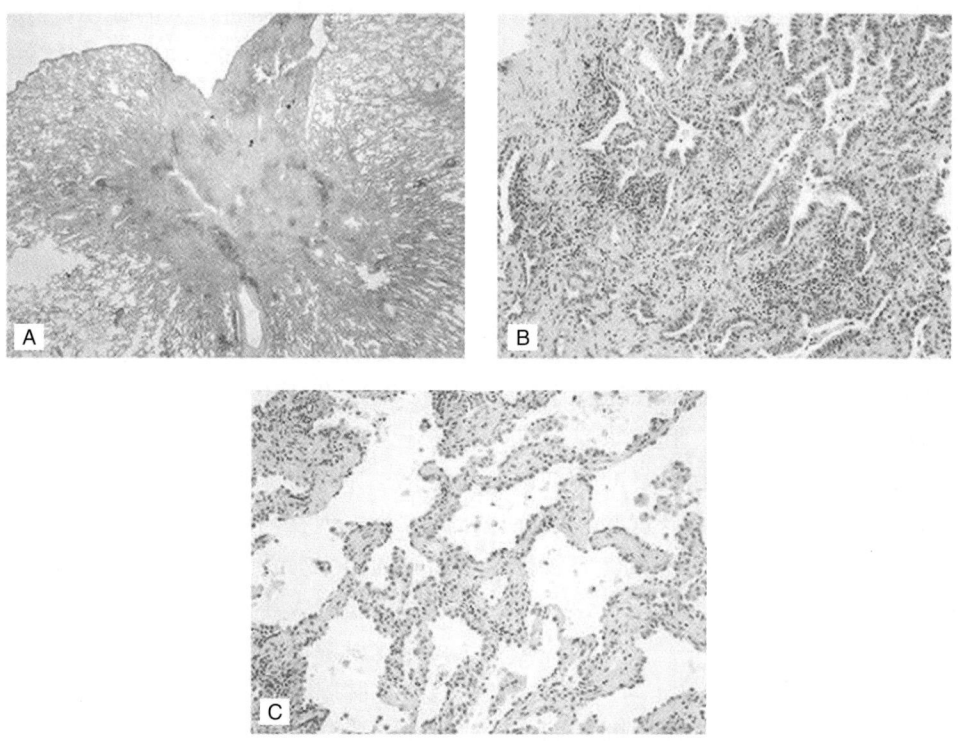

图 8.2（见彩插） 非黏液型 MIA。A. 腺癌鳞屑样生长方式为主且浸润灶小于 5mm，H-E 染色×1.25。B. 肿瘤细胞浸润肌纤维母细胞基质，H-E 染色×20。C. 其他区域表现为鳞屑样生长，肺泡壁薄生长，H-E 染色×20

浸润性腺癌

目前对浸润性腺癌主要依据肿瘤中的主要成分进行分类，以5%~10%增量半定量方式在综合组织分型估计出肿瘤中各种组织亚型的百分数之后，再依据主要成分进行分类。鳞状上皮癌包含之前的混合型肿瘤，这些混合型肿瘤有一个鳞屑样为主的生长方式（之前的非黏液型BAC），且浸润组织横径大于5mm或直径大于3cm（图8.3A~C）。其他主要类型包括腺泡样（图8.3D）、乳头状（图8.3E）、微乳头状（图8.3F）和实性生长方式为主的亚型（图8.3G）。微乳头状为主的亚型在多个研究中被报道且与早期腺癌预后不良有关（图8.3F）[4,29,33-34]。印戒细胞腺癌、透明细胞腺癌被记录为细胞学特性而不作为组织学亚型，只在百分比识别过程中被提到。透明细胞和印戒细胞的细胞特性改变主要见于实性生长方式为主的亚型，但有时也见于腺泡样和乳头状亚型[35-36]。

CT可见的毛玻璃样成分与固体成分之间存在较强的相关性，在活检中鳞屑样成分和浸润之间也有较强的相关性[29,37]。

浸润性腺癌的变异型

肺腺癌的变异型包括浸润性黏液型腺癌（之前的黏液型BAC）、胶样腺癌、胎儿型腺癌、肠型腺癌[4]。由于一些原因，浸润性黏液型腺癌（之前的黏液型BAC）与非浸润性黏液型腺癌被区分开。这些肿瘤常与KRAS基因突变、TTF-1表达缺失和多发性肺病变相关。这些肿瘤在组织学上显示了不同数量的鳞屑样、腺泡、乳头状或微乳头状生长，有不同水平的柱状细胞丰富的顶端黏蛋白和小基部面向核（图8.3H）[4]。这些肿瘤在CT下常表现为局部和多病灶合并的空气支气管征和大叶性实变。

切除样本腺癌亚型的预后

几项研究显示，本方法对切除样本的不同亚型腺癌的预后有影响，且亚型不同结果也不同[29,38-41]。Yoshizawa A等在一项514人参与的一期腺癌临床试验中，依据病理分型将受试者分为3组：①低级别AIS和MIA，其5年生存率为100%；②中间级别非黏液型鳞屑样为主、乳头状为主和腺泡为主的腺癌，其5年生存率分别为90%、83%和84%；③高级别浸润黏液型腺癌和胶体样为主、实性为主以及微乳头状为主的腺癌，其5年生存率分别为75%、71%、70%和67%[29]。其他两项研究也报道了类似结果[40-42]。在一项包含440例日本患者的队列研究中，Yoshizawa A等发现AIS和MIA的5年生存率为100%，鳞状上皮癌为94%，乳头状为主、腺泡样为主、实性为主以及微乳头状为主腺癌的5年生存率分别为88.67%、88.7%、43.3%和0，浸润性黏液型腺癌的5年生存率为88.8%[40]。Kadota等在一项包含540例一期肺腺癌患者的研究中报道AIS和MIA的5年生存率为100%，鳞状上皮癌为91%，腺泡样为主、乳头状为主、微乳头状为主及实性为主腺癌的3年生存率分别为87%、80%、59%以及69%，浸润黏液型腺癌和胶体样为主腺癌的3年生存率为62%[42]。

TNM分期：2011年腺癌分类的影响

2011年肺腺癌分类的提出，在两方面影响了肺腺癌的TNM分期。首先，形态学评估是决定腺癌两种代表性模式（转移性肿瘤和原发性肿瘤）的有力工具，即使用全面组织分型来比较组织生长形式的百分比，也可以用于细胞和基质特性的比较，这与分子和临床数据的区分有关[43-45]；其次，原发性肿瘤还是肺内转移肿瘤的鉴别对TNM分期和患者管理有很大影响，尤其是针对单叶和对侧肿瘤。

2012年UICC TNM的补充材料表明：当以尺寸作为T/pT分类标准时，需要测量浸润成分的大小[46]。传统的肺癌分期以肿瘤的总大小来决定T的大小，现在对于鳞屑样为主的浸润性肺癌，使用全面组织分型能帮助决定浸润成分的大小。浸润性肿瘤的大小可以用总大小减去鳞屑样成分的百分比计算，该方法在乳腺癌中已应用多年。所以早期肺腺癌的T因子大小最好通过浸润成分的大小而不是肿瘤总大小来决定，这样对生存时间的预测会更准确，且已有几个研究表明浸润成分的大小是一个非依赖性预后影响因子[29-30]。多项研究也表明依据浸润成分大小而不是肿瘤总大小

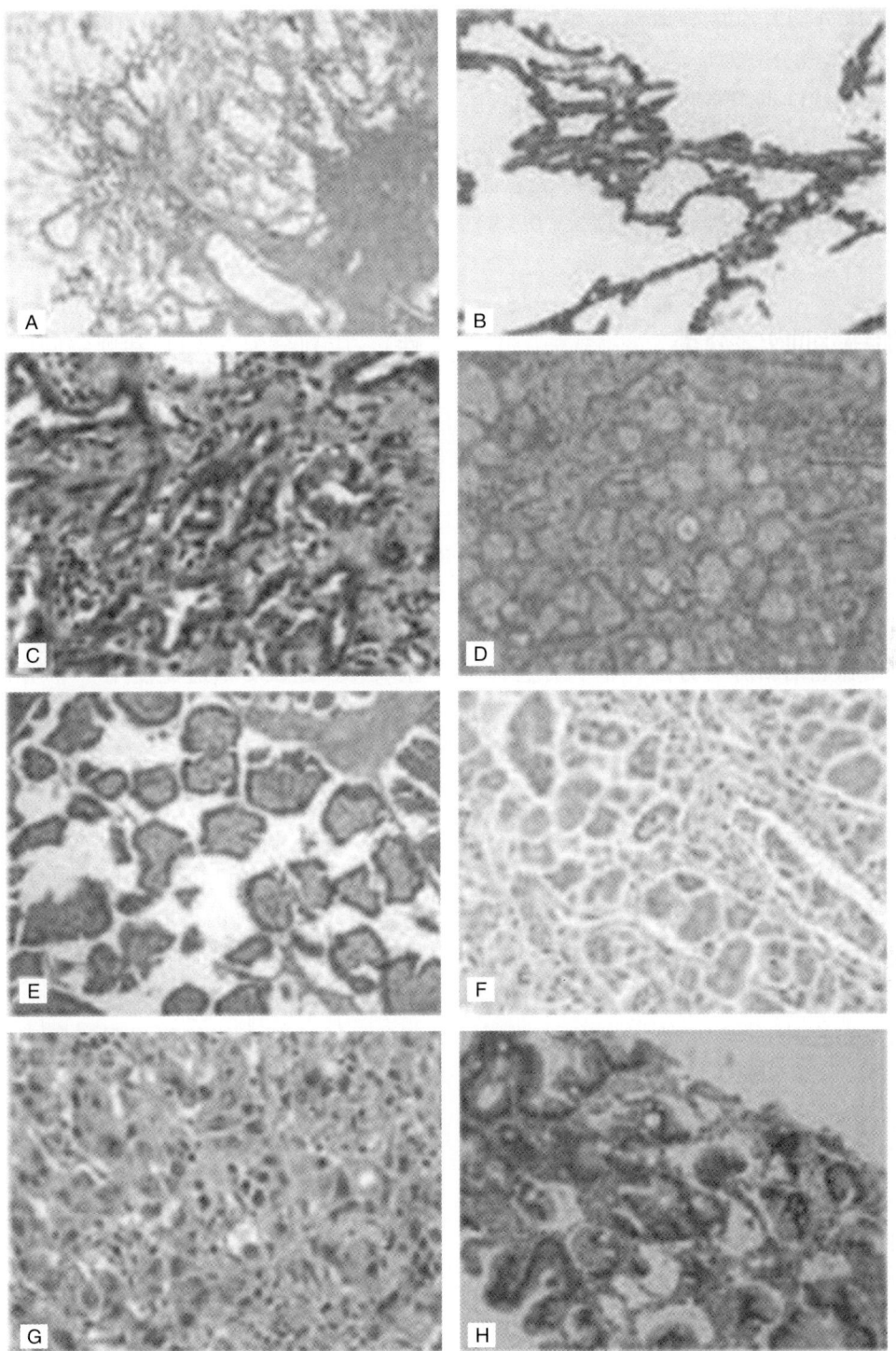

图 8.3（见彩插） 浸润性腺癌的主要组织模式。A. 鳞屑样为主的生长方式（左），以及浸润性腺泡样腺癌（右），H-E 染色 ×100。B. Ⅱ型肺泡上皮细胞和克拉拉细胞沿着肺泡壁表面的鳞屑样为主的生长方式，H-E 染色 ×200。C. 浸润性腺泡样腺癌区，H-E 染色 ×400。D. 包含圆至椭圆形恶性腺体的腺泡状腺癌浸润纤维间质，H-E 染色 ×200。E. 包含恶性立方体柱状肿瘤细胞的乳头状腺癌在纤维芯的表面生长，H-E 染色 ×100。F. 包含小乳头状腺细胞群的微乳头状腺癌在空间上的生长，其中大部分不显示纤维血管轴心，H-E 染色 ×200。G. 带有丰富胞质，以及明显核仁的泡状核的肿瘤细胞构成的实性腺癌被看到，而腺泡样、乳头状以及鳞屑样没有被看到，但多种细胞胞质内嗜碱性颗粒说明胞质内存在黏蛋白。H-E 染色 ×400。H. 浸润性黏液腺癌显示鳞屑样和腺泡样生长。肿瘤由柱状细胞构成，这些柱状细胞的顶端细胞质中被丰富的黏液填充，且能看见小基底核，H-E 染色 ×200

的 CT 测量的临床分期具有更好地预后预测价值，CT 中毛玻璃与实体成分就对应组织上的鳞屑样组成和浸润成分。当然这也需要利用 CT 来研究通过实体成分大小（而不是包括有毛玻璃成分的肿瘤总大小）是否能获得最佳的预测值[4,47-48]。总而言之，希望这些积累的数据能帮助解决以后的 TNM 分期问题。

活检和腺癌细胞学分类

肺癌分类的一个热点集中于活检和腺癌细胞学分类，这主要是因为该方法应用于 70% 的晚期非小细胞肺癌（NSCLC）患者[4]。NSCLC 的诊断方法已发生了重大转变，更多的注意力集中于活检和细胞的精准分类[3-6]。之所以对 NSCLC 进行细分如此重要，是因为现行的治疗方案依赖于组织学。例如依据腺癌的新分类方法，非小细胞癌、腺癌倾向和 NSCLC 不确定者应该进行 EGFR 突变检测。如发生突变，那么这些患者就适用 EGFR 酪氨酸激酶抑制剂[49-53]；如果没有发生突变，他们可能适用培美曲塞[54-57]和贝伐单抗联合化疗方案[58]。相反，对于肺鳞癌患者不需要进行 EGFR 突变检定，也不适用于上述治疗，但可能也会识别一些新的标志物，如 FRFR1 扩增和 DDR2 突变，他们有可能成为新的分子靶点[59-61]。这些新的治疗方法对肺癌分类的影响是深远的。

由于治疗方法的不断发展，2011 年 IASLC/ATS/ERS 的肺腺癌分类中对肺癌的活检和细胞学诊断发布了正式标准（表 8.2）[4]。腺癌从鳞癌中分离出来主要是由于如今的治疗多是组织依赖性的，也因此促使了新的术语和标准的产生。腺癌、NSCLC、腺癌倾向以及 NSCLC 不确定者相比于鳞癌都有 3 种治疗选择。晚期肺腺癌患者如有任何一种组织诊断就需要做 EGFR 突变检定，如果结果阳性，EGFR 酪氨酸激酶抑制剂治疗将有效提高治疗预测值及生存率[49-52]；如果没有 EGFR 突变，患者应测试是否有 ALK 重排，ALK 可预测克唑替尼的应答效果[62-63]。对于腺癌或 NSCLC 不确定者，组织检查是晚期肺癌患者应用培美曲塞的较好预测方法[54-57]。

新的分类建议，如果肿瘤在形态上没有明显的分化，就只使用腺癌（图 8.4A）和鳞癌这两个术语（图 8.4B）。然而，如果肿瘤只表现为癌症，而没有明显的鳞癌或腺癌特征，就建议通过腺癌和鳞癌细胞标志物使用免疫组化方法来区分，这种方法能区分大部分的肿瘤。目前腺癌和鳞癌最好的细胞标志物分别是 TTF-1 和 p40[4,64-66]。对于没有明确腺癌或鳞癌形态、但染色结果揭示腺癌的肿瘤（TTF-1 阳性，p63 阴性），应划分为 NSCLC 和腺癌倾向（图 8.4C 和 8.4D）。同样，如果细胞染色为鳞状细胞癌，则应该划分为 NSCLC 和鳞癌倾向（图 8.4E 和 8.4F）。如果肿瘤在光学显微镜下没有明显分化，也没有明显染色，或结果是矛盾的，则诊断为 NSCLC 不确定型。除了免疫组化，细胞学是对低分化 NSCLC 进行分类的另一种工具。相比于单纯活检，细胞学能更好地对一些肿瘤进行分型[3,67]。建议尽量避免使用"非鳞状细胞癌"这一术语及其他未提及的特异性诊断术语[4]。尽量避免使用 NSCLC，而多使用特异性诊断术语（腺癌或鳞癌）[4]。

由于并不是所有的肺肿瘤都是腺癌或鳞癌，因此病理学家在进行活检和细胞学诊断时就必须考虑 NSCLC 以外的诊断，如神经内分泌肿瘤（类癌、小细胞癌、大细胞神经内分泌癌）以及转移瘤（包括乳腺癌、恶性黑色素瘤和前列腺癌）[3]。因此初始诊断不能仅仅局限于腺癌或鳞癌，也应考虑其他诊断。

根据新的 IASLC/ATS/ERS 分类标准，结合免疫组化、细胞学诊断，NSCLC 诊断病例中 NSCLC 不确定性的比例应低于 5%[3,67]。过去晚期 NSCLC 诊断中 NSCLC 不确定型占 20%~40%，有研究报道这一数值会更高，但现在却发生了很大改变[56,58]。

对于每一个管理活检和细胞样本的机构，制订一个多学科策略计划是必需的。这些管理过程包括：①获得样本；②在病理实验室处理样本；③为分子诊断实验室提供样本；④得到结果获得病理报告及医学记录[3-4]。这个过程需要相关专家和肺癌患者充分交流，从而更好地保管样本，得到最可信的结果。临床科室的医生需获取足够的标本，以便用于诊断和分子研究（如放射科医

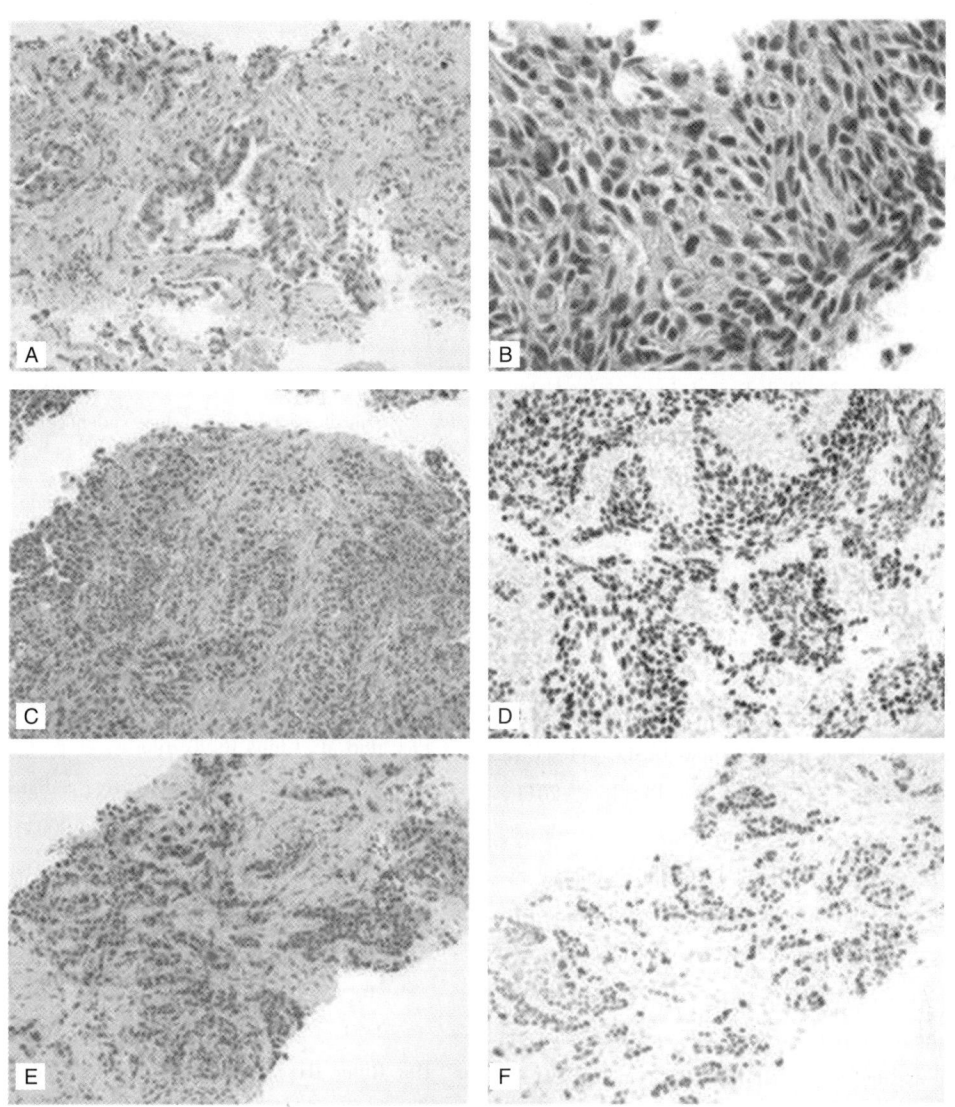

图 8.4（见彩插） A. 腺癌：肿瘤表现为腺泡样生长模式，H-E 染色 ×200。B. 鳞状细胞癌：肿瘤表现为角质化。C. NSCLC，良性腺癌：癌症细胞没有明显的鳞状或腺状分化，H-E 染色 ×200。D. TTF-1 染色阳性，从而可以诊断为 NSCLC，良性腺癌，H-E 染色 ×200。E. NSCLC，良性鳞状细胞癌：癌症细胞没有明显的鳞状或腺状分化，H-E 染色 ×200。F. p63 染色阳性，TTF-1 染色阴性（没显示），从而可以诊断为 NSCLC，良性鳞状细胞癌。p63 免疫组化 ×200

生、肺病或外科医生）。因此有计划的活检应能从样本组织的细胞学检查中获得核心组织或细胞成分[4,69]。对于肿瘤患者的大量胸水，为了能进行后续的免疫组化和分子研究，应该予以保存而不能丢弃。

为了能获得更多的样本进行分子研究，病理学家在临床实践中的另一个改变就是尽可能减少诊断和特异性固定过程中的组织样本的使用量[3-4]。为避免组织样本在多次处理过程中的损失，在研究可能需要进行分子测试的病例中，可一次切取多块样本[3]，包括腺癌以及那些需要进行特异性固定、经 H-E 染色为 NSCLC 不确定型。对于可疑腺癌，需进行 TTF-1 染色，如果结果是阳性，不仅能证实腺癌诊断，同时也能证明其为肺源性。对于形态上不确定的腺癌或鳞癌，最好依据新分类方法中的建议，选择一种腺癌（如 TTF-1）和鳞癌标志物（如 p40）进行鉴别[4,64]。少数病例中，有限的鉴定可能仍不能准确分类，这时需增加额外的鉴定指标来对肿瘤进行分类[3-4]。

（叶 欣 倪 阳 李庆玉 译）

参考文献

[1] Siegel R, Naishadham D, Jemal A. Cancer statistics. CA Cancer J Clin, 2013, 63 (1): 1-30.

[2] Howlader N, Noone AM, Krapcho M, et al. Lung cancer//SEER Cancer Statistics Review, 1975-2010. Bethesda, MD. National Cancer Institute. 2013. Internet Communication.

[3] Travis WD, Rekhtman N. Pathological diagnosis and classification of lung cancer in small biopsies and cytology: strategic management of tissue for molecular testing. Semin Respir Crit Care Med, 2011, 32: 22-31.

[4] Travis WD, Brambilla E, Noguchi M, et al. The New IASLC/ATS/ERS international multidisciplinary lung adenocarcinoma classification. J Thoracic Oncol, 2011, 6: 244-285.

[5] Travis WD, Brambilla E, Van SP, et al. Paradigm shifts in lung cancer as defined in the new IASLC/ATS/ERS lung adenocarcinoma classification. Eur Respir J, 2011, 38: 239-243.

[6] Travis WD, Rekhtman N, Riley GJ, et al. Pathologic diagnosis of advanced lung cancer based on small biopsies and cytology: a paradigm shift. J Thorac Oncol, 2010, 5: 411-414.

[7] Noguchi M. Stepwise progression of pulmonary adenocarcinoma-clinical and molecular implications. Cancer Metastasis Rev, 2010, 29: 15-21.

[8] Yoo SB, ChungJH, Lee HJ, et al. Epidermal growth factor receptor mutation and p53 overexpression during the multistage progression of small adenocarcinoma of the lung. J Thorac Oncol, 2010, 5: 964-969.

[9] Lantucjoul S, Salameire D, Salon C, et al. Pulmonary preneoplasia-sequential molecular carcinogenetic events. Histopathology, 2009, 54: 43-54.

[10] Travis WD, Brambilla E, Müller-Hermelink HK, et al. Pathology and Genetics: Tumours of the Lung, Pleura, Thymus and Heart. Lyon: IARC, 2004.

[11] Travis WD, Brambilla E. Pathology of lung preneoplasia//Hirsch FR, Bunn PA, Kato H, et al (eds). Textbook of Prevention and Detection of Early Lung Cancer. International Association for the Study of Lung Cancer. 1 ed. London and New York: Taylor&Francis, 2006: 75-89.

[12] Ruffini E, Bongiovanni M, Cavallo A, et al. The significance of associated pre-invasive lesions in patients resected for primary lung neoplasms. Eur J Cardiothorac Surg, 2004, 26: 165-172.

[13] Travis WD, Colby TV, Corrin B, et al. in collaboration with L. H. Sobin and pathologists from 14 countries Histological Typing of Lung and Pleural Tumors, 3rd edn. Berlin: Springer, 1999.

[14] Kitamura H, Kameda Y, Ito T, et al. Atypical adenomatous hyperplasia of the lung: Implications for the pathogenesis of peripheral lung adenocarcinoma. Am J Clin Pathol, 1999, 111: 610-622.

[15] Miller RR. Bronchioloalveolar cell adenomas. Am J Surg Pathol, 1990, 14: 904-912.

[16] Weng SY, Tsuchiya E, Kasuga T, et al. Incidence of atypical bronchioloalveolar cell hyperplasia of the lung: relation to histological subtypes of lung cancer. Virchows Arch A Pathol An at Histopathol, 1992, 420: 463-471.

[17] Mori M, Chiba R, Teztika F, et al. Papillary adenoma of type II pneumocytes might have malignant potential. Virchows Archr, 1996, 428: 195-200.

[18] Mori M, Chiba R, Takahashi T. Atypical adenomatous hyperplasia of the lung and its differentiation from adenocarcinoma: Characterization of atypical cells by morphometry and multivariate cluster analysis. Cancer, 1993, 72: 2331-2340.

[19] Ritter JH. Pulmonary atypical adenomatous hyperplasia. A histologic lesion in search of usable criteria and clinical significance. Am J Clin Pathol, 1999, 111: 587-589.

[20] Watanabe S, Watanabe T, Arai K, et al. Results of wedge resection for focal bronchioloalveolar carcinoma showing pure ground-glass attenuation on computed tomography. Ann Thorac Surg, 2002, 73: 1071-1075.

[21] Sakurai H, Dobashi Y, Mizutani E, et al. Bronchioloalveolar carcinoma of the lung 3 centimeters or less in diameter: A prognostic assessment. Ann Thorac Surg, 2004, 78: 1728-1733.

[22] Vazquez M, Carter D, Brambilla E, et al. Solitary and multiple resected adenocarcinomas after CT screening for lung cancer: histopathologic features and their prognostic implications. Lung Cancer, 2009, 64: 148-154.

[23] Yamato Y, Tsuchida M, Watanabe T, et al. Early results of a prospective study of limited resection for bronchioloalveolar adenocarcinoma of the lung. Ann Thorac Surg,

2001, 71: 971-974.

[24] Yoshida J, Nagai K, Yokose T, et al. Limited resection trial for pulmonary ground-glass opacity nodules: fifty-case experience. J Thorac Cardiovasc Surg, 2005, 129: 991-996.

[25] Koike T, Togashi K, Shirato T, et al. Limited resection for noninvasive bronchioloalveolar carcinoma diagnosed by intraoperative pathologic examination. Ann Thorac Surg, 2009, 88: 1106-1111.

[26] Noguchi M, Morikavva A, Kawasaki M, et al. Small adenocarcinoma of the lung. Histologic characteristics and prognosis. Cancer, 1995, 75: 2844-2852.

[27] Yim J, Zhu LC, Chiriboga L, et al. Histologic features are important prognostic indicators in early stages lung adenocarcinomas. Mod Pathol, 2007, 20: 233-241.

[28] Yamada S, Kohno T. Video-assisted thoracic surgery for pure ground-glass opacities 2 cm or less in diameter. Ann Thorac Surg, 2004, 77: 1911-1915.

[29] Yoshizawa A, Motoi N, Ricly GJ, et al. Impact of proposed IASLC/ATS/ERS classification of lung adenocarcinoma: prognostic subgroups and implications for further revision of staging based on analysis of 514 stage I cases. Mod Pathol, 2011, 24: 653-664.

[30] Borczuk AC, Qian F, Kazcros A, et al. Invasive size is an independent predictor of survival in pulmonary adenocarcinoma. Am J Surg Pathol, 2009, 33: 462-469.

[31] Suzuki K, Yokose T, Yoshida J, et al. Prognostic significance of the size of central fibrosis in peripheral adenocarcinoma of the lung. Arm ThoracSurg, 2000, 69: 893-897.

[32] Lester SC, Bose S, Chen YY, et al. Protocol for the examination of specimens from patients with invasive carcinoma of the breast. Arch Pathol Lab Med, 2009, 133: 1515-1538.

[33] Miyoshi T, Satoh Y, Okumura S, et al. Early-stage lung adenocarcinomas with a micropapillary pattern, a distinct pathologic marker for a significantly poor prognosis. Am J Surg Pathol, 2003, 27: 101-109.

[34] Tsutsumida H, Nomoto M, Goto M, et al. A micropapillary pattern is predictive of a poor prognosis in lung adenocarcinoma, and reduced surfactant apoprotein A expression in the micropapillary pattern is an excellent indicator of a poor prognosis. Mod Pathol, 2007, 20: 638-647.

[35] Cohen PR, Yoshizawa A, Motoi N, et al. Signet ring cell features (SRCF) in lung adenocarcinoma: a cytologic feature or a histologic subtype? Mod Pathol, 2010, 23: 400A.

[36] Deshpande CG, Yoshizawa A, Motoi N, et al. Clear cell change in lung adenocarcinoma: A cytologic change rather than a histologic variant. Mod Pathol, 2009, 22: 352A.

[37] Naidich DP, Bankier AA, MacMahon H, et al. Recommendations for the management of subsolid pulmonary nodules detected at CT: A statement from the Fleischner Society. Radiology, 2013, 266: 304-317.

[38] Russell PA, Wainer Z, Wright GM, et al. Docs lung adenocarcinoma subtype predict patient survival?: A clinicopathologic study based on the new International Association for the Study of Lung Cancer/American Thoracic Society/European Respiratory Society international multidisciplinary lung adenocarcinoma classification. J Thorac Oncol, 2011, 6: 1496-1504.

[39] Warth A, Mulcy T, Mcister M, et al. The novel histologic IASLC/ATS/ERS classification system of invasive pulmonary adenocarcinoma is a stage-independent predictor of survival. J Clin Oncol, 2012, 30: 1438-1446.

[40] Yoshizawa A, Sumiyoshi S, Sonobc M, et al. Validation of the IASLC/ATS/ERS lung adenocarcinoma classification for prognosis and association with *EGFR* and *KRAS* gene mutations: Analysis of 440 Japanese patients. J Thorac Oncol, 8: 52-61.

[41] Xu L, Tavora F, Battafarano R, et al. Adenocarcinomas with prominent lepidic spread: retrospective review applying new classification of the American Thoracic Society. Am J Sun Pathol, 2012, 36: 273-282.

[42] Kadota K, Suzuki K, D'Angelo SP, et al. Validation of the proposed IASLC/ American Thoracic Society (ATS) / European Respiratory Society (ERS) international multi-disciplinary classification of lung adenocarcinoma (ADC). Journal of Thoracic Oncology, 2011, 6: S286.

[43] Girard N, Deshpande C, Azzoli CG, et al. Use of epidermal growth factor receptor/Kirsten rat sarcoma 2 viral oncogene homolog mutation testing to define clonal relationships among multiple lung adenocarcinomas: comparison with clinical guidelines. Chest, 2010, 137: 46-52.

[44] Girard N, Deshpande C, Lau C, et al. Comprehensive

histologic assessment helps to differentiate multiple lung primary nonsmall cell carcinomas from metastases. Am J Surg Pathol, 2009, 33: 1752-1764.

[45] Girard N, Ostrovnaya I, Lau C, et al. Genomic and mutational profiling to assess clonal relationships between multiple non-small-cell lung cancers. Clin Cancer Res, 2009, 15: 5184-5190.

[46] Wittekind Ch, Compton CC, Brierley J, et al. UICCTNM Supplement, A Commentary on Uniform Use, 4th edn. Oxford, UK: Wiley-Blackwell, 2012.

[47] Tsutani Y, Miyata Y, Nakayama H, et al. Prognostic significance of using solid versus whole tumor size on high-resolution computed tomography for predicting pathologic malignant grade of tumors in clinical stage IA lung adenocarcinoma: a multicenter study. J Thorac Cardiovasc Surg, 2012, 143: 607-612.

[48] Yanagawa N, Shiono S, Abiko M, et al. New IASLC/ATS/ERS classification and invasive tumor size are predictive of disease recurrence in Stage I lung adenocarcinoma. J Thorac Oncol, 2013, 8: 612-618.

[49] Mok TS, Wu YL, Thongprasert S, et al. Gefitinib or carboplatin-paclitaxel in pulmonary adenocarcinoma. N Engl J Med, 2009, 361: 947-957.

[50] Mitsudomi T, Morita S, Yatabe Y, et al. Gefitinib versus cisplatin plus docetaxel in patients with non-small-cell lung cancer harbouring mutations of the epidermal growth factor receptor (WJTOG3405): an open label, randomised phase 3 trial. Lancet Oncol, 2010, 11: 121-128.

[51] Maemondo M, Inoue A, Kobayashi K, et al. Gefitinib or chemotherapy for non-small-cell lung cancer with mutated EGFR. A7 Engl J Med, 2010, 362: 2380-2388.

[52] Zhou C, Wu YL, Chen G, et al. Erlotinib versus chemotherapy as first-line treatment for patients with advanced EGFR mutation-positive non-small-cell lung cancer (OPTIMAL, CTONG-0802): a multicentre, open-label, randomised, phase 3 study. Lancet Oncol, 2011, 12: 735-742.

[53] Rosell R, Carcereny E, Gervais R, et al. Erlotinib versus standard chemotherapy as first-line treatment for European patients with advanced EGFR mutation-positive non-small-cell lung cancer (EURTAC): A multicentre, open-label, randomised phase 3 trial. Lancet Oncol, 2012, 13: 239-246.

[54] Ciuleanu T, Brodowicz T, Zielinski C, et al. Maintenance pemetrexed plus best supportive care versus placebo plus best supportive care for non-small-cell lung cancer A randomised, double-blind, phase 3 study. Lancet, 2009, 374: 1432-1440.

[55] Scagliotti G, Hanna N, Fossella F, et al. The differential efficacy of pemetrexed according to NSCLC histology: a review of two Phase III studies. Oncologist, 2009, 14: 253-263.

[56] Scagliotti GV, Parikh P, von PJ, et al. Phase III study comparing cisplatin plus gemcitabine with cisplatin plus pemetrexed in chemotherapy-naive patients with advanced-stage non-small-cell lung cancer. J Clin Oncol, 2008, 26: 3543-3551.

[57] Scagliotti G, Brodowicz T, Shepherd FA, et al. Treatment-by-histology interaction analyses in three phase III trials show superiority of pemetrexed in nonsquamous non-small-cell lung cancer. J Thorac Oncol, 2011, 6: 64-70.

[58] Johnson DH, Fehrenbacher L, Novotny WF, et al. Randomized phase II trial comparing bevacizumab plus carboplatin and paclitaxel with carboplatin and paclitaxel alone in previously untreated locally advanced or metastatic non-small-cell lung cancer. J Clin Oncol, 2004, 22: 2184-2191.

[59] Hammerman PS, Hayes DN, Wilkerson MD, et al. Comprehensive genomic characterization of squamous cell lung cancers. Nature, 2012, 489: 519-525.

[60] Dutt A, Ramos AH, Hammerman PS, et al. Inhibitor-sensitive EGFR1 amplification in human non-small cell lung cancer. PLoS One, 2011, 6: e20351.

[61] Hammerman PS, Sos ML, Ramos AH, et al. Mutations in the DDR2 Kinase gene identify a novel therapeutic target in squamous cell lung cancer. Cancer Discov, 2011, 1: 78-89.

[62] Sasaki T, Janne PA. New strategies for treatment of ALK rearranged non-small cell lung cancers. Clin Cancer Res, 2011, 17: 7213-7218.

[63] Shaw AT, Yeap BY, Solomon BJ, et al. Effect of crizotinib on overall survival in patients with advanced non-small-cell lung cancer harbouring ALK gene rearrangement: a retrospective analysis. Lancet Oncol, 2011, 12: 1004-1012.

[64] Bishop JA, Teruya-Feldstein J, Westra WH, et al. p40

[64] （DeltaNp63） is superior to p63 for the diagnosis of pulmonary squamous cell carcinoma. Mod Patholr, 2012, 25: 405-415.

[65] Rckhtman N, Ang DC, Sima CS, et al. Immunohistochemical algorithm for differentiation of lung adenocarcinoma and squamous cell carcinoma based on large senes of whole-tissue sections with validation in small specimens. Mod Pathol, 2011, 24: 1348-1359.

[66] Pelosi G, Fabbri A, Bianchi F, et al. DcltaNp63 (p40) and thyroid transcription factor-1 immunorcactivity on small biopsies or cellblocks for typing non-small cell lung cancer: A novel two-hit, sparing-material approach. J Thorac Oncol, 2012, 7: 281-290.

[67] ckhtman N, Brandt SM, Sigel CS, et al. Suitability of thoracic cytology for new therapeutic paradigms in non-small cell lung carcinoma: High accuracy of tumor sub typing and feasibility of EGFR and KRAS molecular testing. J Thoracic Oncol, 2011, 6: 451-458.

[68] Ou SH, Zell JA. Carcinoma NOS is a common histologic diagnosis and is increasing in proportion among non-small cell lung cancer histologics. J Thorac Oncol, 2009, 4: 1202-1211.

[69] Solomon SB, Zakowski MF, Pao W, et al. Core needle lung biopsy specimens: adequacy for EGFR and KRAS mutational analysis. AJR Am J Roentgenol, 2010, 194: 266-269.

第 9 章
多灶性细支气管肺泡癌的治疗

Howard West

Swedish Cancer Institute, Seattle, WA, USA

引 言

进展期细支气管肺泡癌（BAC）治疗前，我们首先要明确一个前提。在 IASLC/ATS/ERS 新修订的肺腺癌分期中，BAC 的定义已经改变，BAC 已不再被认定为一个独立的肺癌亚型[1]。过去，BAC 被定义为未侵犯基底膜或肺间质的腺癌。IASLC/ATS/ERS 在最新的肺腺癌分类中定义了非浸润性腺癌，分别包括单发病灶的 AIS，以及多中心生长的有相同组织学表型（非黏液型或黏液型）的贴壁生长为主的腺癌，后者既往被称为非黏液型和黏液型 BAC。

然而，过去权威病理学家的推荐和 BAC 等术语的临床应用一直存在差异[2]，新的分类能否被临床肿瘤学会广泛采纳仍有待观察。因为仍有病理学家继续使用 BAC 这一病理诊断，临床医生仍按以往的方法将 BAC 作为一种独立的疾病进行治疗和报道。在这一临床上坚持使用的定义范围内讨论 BAC 的临床管理仍有重大意义。

在这种情况下，推荐规范的管理时有必要注意一些事项。BAC 的定义被广泛用于人群，这类患者在组织学表现、自然病程、分子特征和对治疗的反应性上都存在异质性[2]，然而关于 BAC 的临床研究较少、研究样本量小，而且部分研究包含了多类人群以至于很难得出确定的结论，而且，尽管在公布的临床数据中没有明确特征，但是即便在同一患者，不同病灶的进展过程，侵袭性、影像学和分子学特征也可能表现出差异。当然，正如新的肺腺癌分类方法所示，没有基于 1 类证据的多灶性 BAC 的诊疗推荐，只有关于此类患者的重要临床经验和本领域专家的共识可供参考。

进展期 BAC 的异质性表现

在临床实践中，多灶性 BAC 是一种高度异质性疾病。其影像学表现多为缓慢进展的过程，包括一些散在的毛玻璃灶、广泛的粟粒样病灶，或很难与细菌性肺炎相鉴别的弥漫性肺实质浸润[3-4]。BAC 的临床进展速度可能数年基本无变化，也可能数周即出现致命性进展。在病理学上，BAC 不仅包含严格意义上的非浸润性成分（纯 BAC），也常包含微浸润成分。BAC 可能是黏液型、非黏液型或两种成分的混合型。正如其他的肺腺癌一样，黏液型 BAC 有时可出现 *EGFR* 基因突变、*KRAS* 基因突变、*ALK* 基因重排或其他少见的分子特征，这提示靶向治疗等全身治疗对其有效。

即使对于同一患者，不同部位病灶的进展速度、PET 扫描的代谢摄取率、影像表现中实性和非实性成分比例、病理学检查中的侵袭性，以及分子标志物特征也可能不尽相同。另外，一些惰性区域随着时间的变化可能转变为高侵袭性和快速进展区[5]。尽管多灶性 BAC 被简单划分为同一类型，对于不同的临床病理情况最好采取相对应的不同治疗策略。对于一个持续进展、广泛分布的多灶性粟粒表现、*EGFR* 基因突变阳性的 BAC，与一个在不同肺叶有 4~5 个病灶并且随访 3 年以上无明显增大的小毛玻璃表现的 BAC 病例相比，两者的最佳治疗方案并不一定相同。

我们现有的分期系统、公布的病例资料和临床试验数据不能够区分多灶性 BAC 的不同表现和自然病程（图 9.1）。然而，目前提倡的治疗思路是依据患者不同的临床表现给予个体化治疗，而非强制的一体化治疗。

由于这个疾病的异质性和潜在惰性，即使客观证据显示病情几乎无进展，患者也可能会因为自身或医生的焦虑而过度治疗、进行反复的射线扫描或分期诊断，这导致部分患者因为无进展、无症状的 BAC 或其他临床不相关的疾病而进行了反复的手术切除或者长期的全身治疗。相反，也有很多临床医生认为化疗对进展期 BAC 的作用甚微，或者反对局部治疗的概念，然而对于表现为多灶性生长，但实际只有一个快速进展的病灶，局部治疗是适宜的。

多灶性 BAC 的评估

尽管 BAC 最常以适宜手术切除的单发孤立结节被诊断（50%~85%），多灶性 BAC 也常以卫星灶的形式出现，位于单个肺叶内（60%~65% 多灶性疾病）、同侧肺的不同肺叶（20%~25%）、两侧肺（10%~15%）[6-8]。

鉴于表现形式的多样性、自然病程和患者疾病进展的异质性（可能存在疾病的一个或几个区域快速进展，而其他区域相对无明显变化），在制订和执行个体化治疗方案前对多灶性 BAC 的特点进行详细评估很重要。最初的肿瘤特征性描述应包含症状的仔细评估、肿瘤进程的评估、各病灶是否一致、尽最大可能进行病理评估，包括仔细评估肿瘤的侵袭性和明确有助于系统治疗的分子遗传学信息。

症 状

BAC 最常在无症状人群中进行术前检查或因其他非特异性症状进行胸部影像学检查时被发现。2/3 以上的 BAC 患者无论分期如何均无临床症状，伴有临床症状的患者最常表现为咳嗽（30%~50%）、呼吸困难（15%）、体重下降（10%~15%）、咯血（5%~10%）或者胸痛（5%~10%）[9-11]。

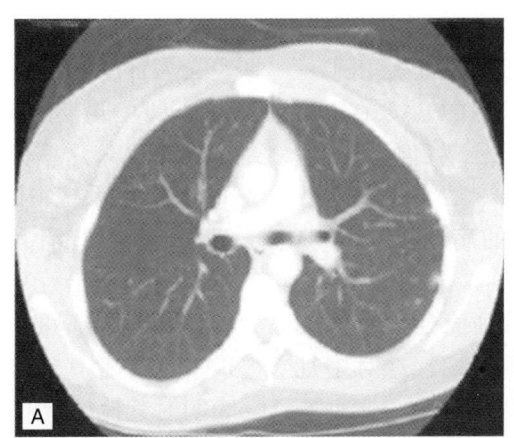

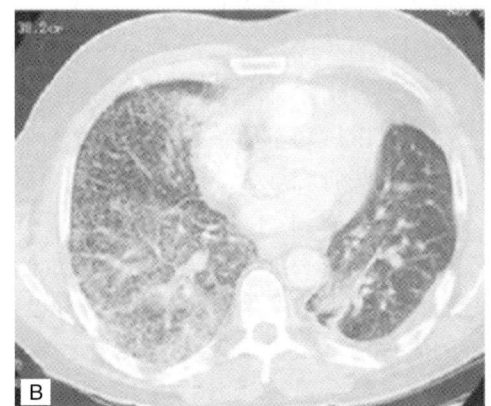
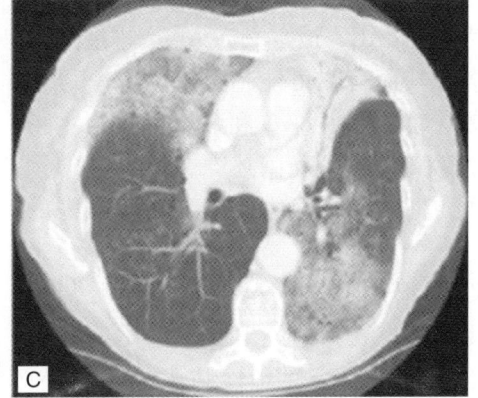

图 9.1 进展期 BAC 的病变范围实例。A. 一例无症状的女性，左肺下叶有散在的毛玻璃样结节。B. 粟粒型弥散的非黏液型 BAC 患者伴有严重的呼吸困难及干咳。C. 多叶融合型黏液型 BAC 患者伴有排痰性咳嗽及呼吸困难

支气管黏液溢见于5%~10%的多灶性BAC患者，其特征性表现为分泌大量黏稠、多泡的痰液。严重的病例每天可能产生超过1~2L的痰液，导致显著的电解质紊乱和因肺内分流所致的低氧血症[12-14]。对支气管黏液溢的特异性治疗将在下文中探讨。

自然病程和影像学表现

一般来说，进展期BAC的症状和影像学表现与炎性病灶相似，这导致了部分BAC患者在最初的数周甚至数月选用了抗生素、激素或联合方法的试验性治疗。直至经过一段时间的随访，临床症状和影像学表现仍无改善，才被诊断为BAC。BAC初始症状的严重程度和临床进程的多样性是选择初始治疗前需要考虑的。

PET扫描已广泛应用于肺结节和病因不明的肺浸润灶的检查，以及肺癌的常规分期。在PET扫描中，低代谢的肺部病灶通常被忽视或认为是非恶性肿瘤。BAC常表现为典型的惰性临床进程，肿瘤倍增时间长达1年或者数年[15-17]，因此在PET检查中BAC常因代谢率过低而漏诊[18]。亚厘米级的非实性病灶常因体积过小、细胞密度过低而无PET检查的意义。相应地，如果确诊或疑诊的BAC在PET检查中表现为高代谢状态，一般预示着肿瘤进入快速进展期，恶性程度更高，预后差[19-21]。

一般而言，PET检查低代谢的病灶在胸部CT中被认为是假阴性病灶[2,23]。然而，很多BAC在PET检查中表现低代谢常预示着肿瘤处于惰性临床进程，有更好的预后和多年生存期，这对多灶性BAC也是适用的[9-10,24]。在新分类中，这种有缓慢自然病程的孤立性肺病灶，也就是单发的非黏液型、非浸润性BAC，被定义为AIS。进展期肺癌的治疗策略对其而言很可能是过度治疗。尽管新分类的提议中对多灶性BAC和贴壁生长为主型肺腺癌的治疗意义没有明确阐述[1]，但更好的预后结果是新分类将其从肺腺癌中单独划分出来的重要原因[25]。

顾名思义，AIS的另外一层含义是指病灶局限在原位无外侵，常表现为单纯BAC，这是一种癌前病变，可能进展为侵袭性恶性肺腺癌。但是，即使这种情况属实[26]，非浸润性肺腺癌是否转变为浸润性肺腺癌仍未可知，因为一半以上的非浸润性腺癌病灶和同时存在的浸润性腺癌病灶有不同的K-ras基因突变[27]。

多灶性BAC的治疗干预

在确定多灶性BAC的最佳治疗方案前，有很多关键性问题亟待解决（图9.2）。

多灶性疾病是否位于一个肺叶或同侧肺内？

最新的非小细胞肺癌（NSCLC）的分期系统（第7版肺癌分期）显示，如无其他区域的病变，肺切除手术可能对同一肺叶内或同侧肺不同肺叶内的多发病灶有治疗意义[28-35]。

最新版的美国癌症联合委员会（American Joint Committee on Cancer，AJCC）NSCLC分期修订：如果没有淋巴结和远处转移，原发肿瘤同一肺叶内有转移结节划分为T3期，在第6版AJCC分期中被定义为ⅢB期，而在新分期中被定义为ⅡB期[36]。与之类似，若无淋巴结和远处转移，原发肿瘤同侧肺的不同肺叶中有转移结节在新分期中定义为T4期而非远处转移，新分期系统将其定义为ⅢA期，而在既往的分期系统中将其定义为NSCLC Ⅳ期[37]。

NSCLC这些分期的修订显示：相较于第6版AJCC分期系统中同期的其他情况，有转移结节的AIS或BAC患者预后更好。然而，分期的下降并不代表局部治疗就是此类疾病的最佳治疗方案。相比其他类型的NSCLC，组织学类型为AIS或BAC的患者有独特的临床进程和进展模式，这也表明对其他类型的NSCLC适用的治疗建议并不一定适用于AIS或BAC。但新分期方式并不是根据同侧肺的一或多个肺叶有AIS或BAC卫星结节的肺癌患者从手术中的获益情况制订的，新分期的确立仅以疾病术后整体生存期是否延长为基础。

一些研究显示，同一肺叶中有转移结节的患者适宜选择手术切除，而且术后多年无肿瘤复发[28,38-42]。然而对于一个几乎无进展的多灶性疾病，即使不进行手术治疗，患者也可能获得同样的生存期。因为缺乏手术治疗和保守治疗的对比数据，综合考虑治疗医生的判断、患者的意愿及身体条件、有无合并症以及疾病的模式来选择手术治疗、系统治疗或者随访观察是比较理性的。

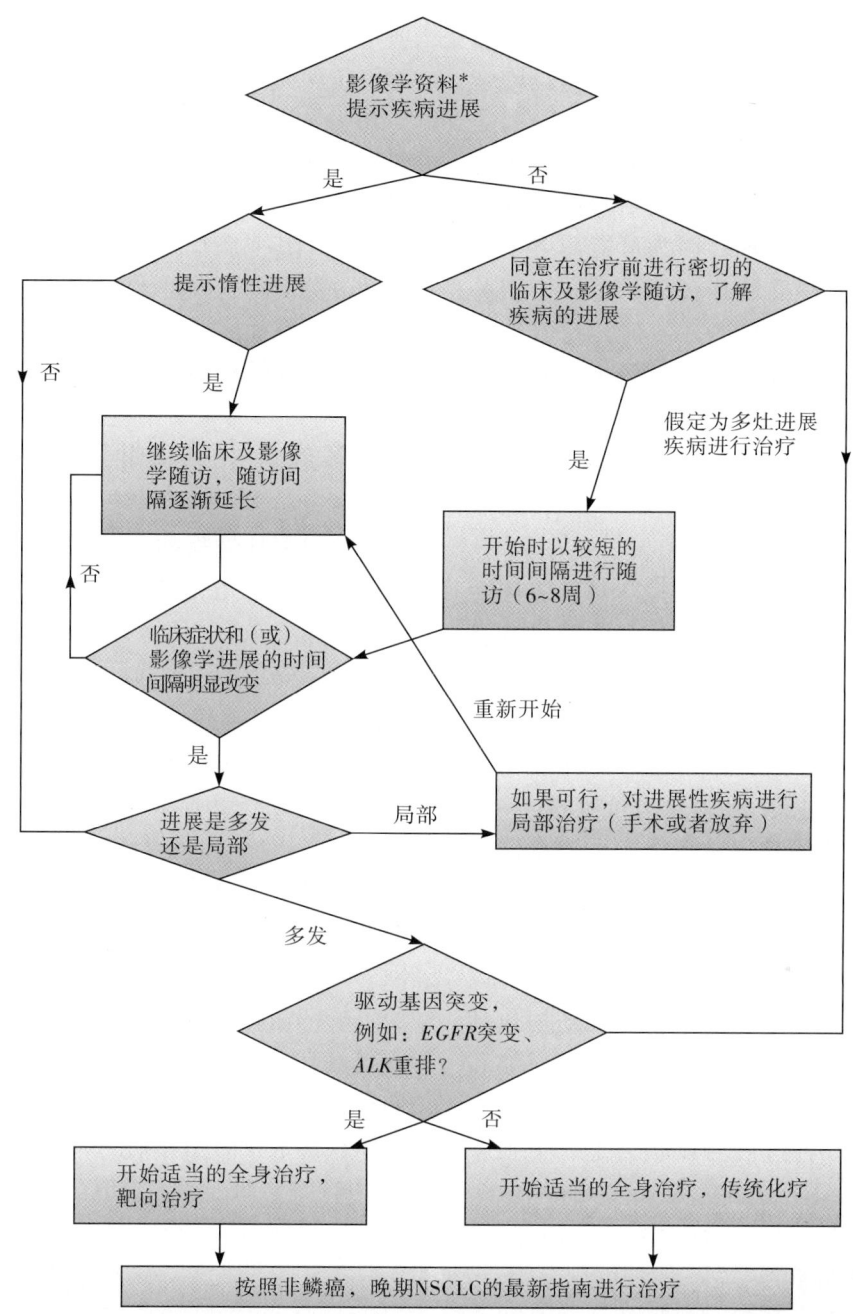

*影像学图片对比发现最短时间间隔改变，和（或）PET最大SUV很低

图 9.2　无症状的多灶性细支气管肺泡癌（BAC）治疗推荐

有无临床症状或明显的临床进程？

因为 AIS 或多灶性 BAC 的临床进展缓慢，首先明确是否需要治疗是很重要的。尽管进展期 BAC 可能出现临床症状，甚至部分呈现暴发性表现，多灶性 BAC 患者多数表现为无症状、散在、亚厘米级的毛玻璃样结节，这些毛玻璃样结节的倍增时间可能为数年，或者 1 到数年无变化。即使部分患者的影像学表现为较大和（或）广泛分布的肺结节，这些患者也可能无症状且多年随访观察病灶无明显变化。

对于有微小进展的多灶性 BAC 患者，很难衡量治疗作用和治疗副反应的利弊。多灶性 BAC 可能对多年以后的生存期有很小的影响，而治疗带给无症状患者的可能仅仅是生活质量的影响。一般来说，对于个体患者，评估选择个体治疗方案是适宜的。我们必须认识到多灶性 BAC 和 PET 高摄取、1 至数月即发生明显影像进展的侵袭性肺腺癌是完全不同的。

在很多病例中,患者是因为 PET 检查低 SUV 值或者多年一系列的影像学检查显示为慢性临床过程而得出临床组织学诊断。因为可能需要多年时间才可得出诊断,尽管临床证据显示肿瘤相关的症状很少,对生存期影响很小,但是初始治疗的选择经常基于患者和(或)医生的焦虑和下意识的决定,或者基于可能为癌的诊断。

如果出现明显的临床进展,这些进展是单灶性还是多灶性的?

鉴于多灶性 BAC 的异质性,尤其对于多灶性疾病,了解临床进展是单灶性还是多灶性很有意义。此外,如新修订的肺腺癌分期所着重强调的,鉴别数年或数十年可能无明显进展的慢性病程(如名词"原位"的解释)和快速出现肿瘤相关症状并威胁生命的快进展病程是很有价值的。

区分临床进程的关键意义在于,尽管总体病情是多灶性的,但存在单灶性进展时选择手术、放疗等局部治疗比较适宜(图 9.3)。在临床进程中出现与其他病灶不一致的更快的增长速度可以说明该病灶有独特的生物学特点,其他证据包括非实性病灶向实性病灶转变、PET 摄取率增加和(或)出现侵袭性生物学改变。

一般来说,单灶性进展可以认为是一个独立的病灶。当肿瘤组织学分类为Ⅳ期多灶性 BAC,而且仅适合全身治疗时,参考新修订的肺癌分期是有帮助的。对于广泛的癌前原位病变,尽管总体无明显变化,但出现有临床意义的单一进展灶时仍应局部治疗。关键问题是单一进展病灶是否对患者的预后起关键作用,或者说除进展的单发病灶外,其他病灶是否影响患者的生活质量和生存期。关键问题就是多灶性 BAC 中快速进展的主要区域和其他区域生长率的差异,如果差异显著,尽管是多灶性疾病,也适宜行局部治疗。

多病灶中单病灶进展的治疗方案

如果多灶性疾病仅单灶进展而其他病灶无明显临床进展,是否可以和其他单灶疾病患者一样选择手术、放疗、射频消融、冷冻治疗等局部治疗方法。一项最近发布的单中心系列研究[43]显示,在 39 个有"单独优势结节"的可疑多灶性 BAC 患者中,平均超过 30 个月的持续随访发现,只有 9 例(23%)患者显示出未切除结节的影像学进展。

相对于没有明显可见病变的患者,考虑到多灶性进展性 BAC 的主要风险,立体定向放射治疗因为并发症少和疗效显著成为很有吸引力的选择。假定局部治疗效果不佳,选择其他风险小的治疗方式也有特定的价值。类似于临床所描述的"早期转移",有时针对孤立性转移灶进行局部治疗后可以获得很长的生存期[44-45],这种情况与多灶性 BAC 的"早期进展"类似。

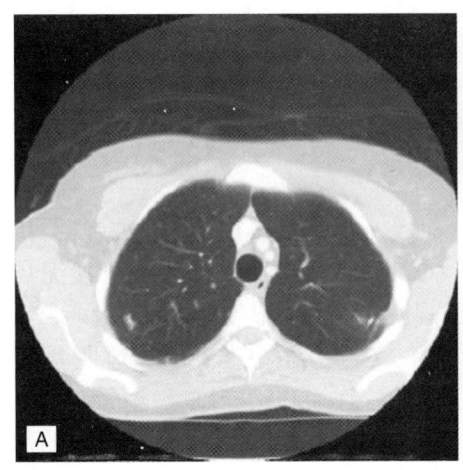
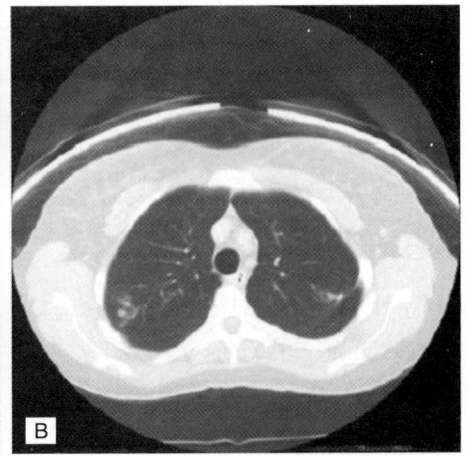

图 9.3 一例女性多灶性 BAC 患者,右肺上叶单病灶 17 个月内出现进展(A→B),其余病灶在这期间保持稳定。该患者单一进展的病灶接受了立体定向放疗

在微创胸腔镜手术和立体定向放疗广泛应用的时代，对随着时间发展表现出进展不一致的多灶性疾病选择一系列的局部治疗，可行性及吸引力均在逐渐增加。如果治疗间的时间间隔是以年来测量，并且治疗仅针对临床进展区域而非稳定的毛玻璃结节，局部治疗可能是非常合理的甚至是最优的方案。然而，对于在短短几个月内发生变化的弥散或多灶性病灶，临床实践中进行多次切除以及放疗则欠妥当。

必须承认，目前还没有基于临床数据的指南明确给出对于一系列局部治疗有利的倍增时间和治疗间隔。但是如果多灶性病变的进展在1年内出现，进行一系列局部治疗的价值是不确定的。进一步来说，一系列的局部治疗会导致更多有功能的肺组织损失，如果肺损伤较大肯定是有风险的。谨慎起见，对于高度怀疑为多灶性进展的病灶，切除两个肺叶或进行全肺切除术是不恰当的。

同样，一系列独立的小样本研究[46-51]显示对BAC及多灶性BAC进行肺移植手术是可能的。尽管这些研究的术后早期结果振奋人心，但长期随访结果发现肿瘤复发是这些患者的普遍结局[47,52]。然而，器官共享注册网站的数据显示，在多灶性BAC进行肺移植手术的总计29例患者中，5~7年的术后生存期为57%，而全人群肺移植患者术后生存期为50%。总体而言，肺移植术对于进展的BAC治疗效果并不明确，还不能作为可广泛应用的治疗策略。

如上文提到的，一些组织已经报道了多灶性肺结节进行同期或分期多次肺切除的可行性[28,38-42]，但是这些研究并没有区分病灶是明显增长的还是经长期随访没有或很少进展的。值得注意的是，手术文献所指的这些病例主要为独立的多原发性肿瘤，患者表现出良好预后的前提是这些肿瘤为独立的多原发癌，而不是无进展的多灶性疾病。遗憾的是，复发是多灶性疾病术后的普遍现象[34,53]。

必须认识到BAC是缓慢进展的疾病，无论是否进行干预或治疗，它在短期内预后都是很好的。此外，患者获得的干预措施很可能存在选择性偏差。并且由于患者年轻和身体状况较好，而且疾病进展缓慢，使其能够就诊于多家医院咨询治疗意见。而更多积极的治疗意见能否转化为临床获益，或者这些患者是否更倾向于选择通常疗效较好的治疗仍然是未知的，这些可能都会受到选择性偏差的显著影响。

在这种情况下，更应该重视治疗方式的选择。尽管很多患者和医生在选择有效治疗方案时会存在偏倚，即使局部治疗确实对多灶性进展的疾病无效，过度治疗也很可能是有害无益的。但是，如果我们对单个病例考虑具体的进展模式，通过谨慎选择病例，局部治疗可能成为多灶性BAC的最佳治疗方式。

姑息性手术

在一些罕见病例中，即使有多发的弥散性病灶，手术也可考虑作为一种姑息性的治疗措施。尤其在肺炎型BAC（一例患者的临床影像显示肺内广泛渗出性改变累及一个或多个肺叶，与肺炎表现一致；图9.1C）的特定情况下，手术可以考虑作为姑息性治疗方法来缓解患者的剧烈咳嗽、支气管黏液通气血流比失调导致的呼吸困难。尽管一些典型病例在术后早期即出现病情进展[54]，多个独立报道还是支持"在没有其他较好的治疗方案可选择的情况下，进行姑息手术来控制患者的严重症状"是可行的[55-56]。

多病灶BAC的系统治疗

由于AIS或BAC是一个慢性自然病程，首要问题在于明确是否应即刻采取全身治疗，即使患者合并多发病灶及弥漫性的进展模式。无论是无临床症状的亚厘米级的结节，或者是CT影像显示广泛的病变，对于无临床症状和有轻微临床症状的患者，若没有采取即刻治疗，应制订临床和影像学的随访间隔。AIS或BAC患者在6~8周内重复行CT检查通常不会有明显的影像学改变或者临床上的急剧恶化，缓慢的影像学改变有助于AIS或BAC的诊断。额外的观察对了解患者的自然病程很有价值，尽管焦虑的患者和医生会限制观察策略的实施，但许多患者仍可以避免因几个月或者几年的治疗带来的副作用。早期细心的随访，尤其是注意观察患者临床症状的变化，可以避免错过最佳的治疗时机。

同样，避免因可疑小结节的出现或者是现存结节的轻微进展而贸然放弃有效的治疗方案也是有益的。无论是由于有效的治疗，还是疾病的生理特性，或是二者兼具，如果多灶性 BAC 的自然病史长达数年，在患者病情恶化或者丧失进一步治疗的意愿之前制订出多种有效的治疗方案并不困难。尽管及时识别显著的临床进展，并停止明显无效的治疗是恰当的，但避免因临床不确定的可疑进展而中断耐受良好的治疗也是合理的。这些临床不确定的进展可以基于新出现的微小病变、最小生长间期或者 PET 显示肺部病变代谢增加来证实。

在晚期 NSCLC 的系统治疗试验中，多灶性 BAC 始终没有与 NSCLC 的其他亚型相区别。在多数病例中，多灶性 BAC 患者适用于广泛的 NSCLC 试验，与已转移的浸润性腺癌相比，多灶性 BAC 的预后更好[57]。

在 NSCLC 最新修订的 AJCC 分期系统中也体现了多灶性 BAC 患者的预后更好。该系统指出位于单侧肺外、但局限于胸内的 M1a 期肺癌预后好于远处转移的 M1b 期肺癌。这种变化反映了肿瘤局限于胸腔内（包括胸膜受累、胸膜种植）患者的生存优势，导致肺癌分期修订[37]的数据库中许多 M1a 期的 NSCLC 患者都被判定为多灶性 BAC，与 NSCLC 的其他亚型的Ⅳ期表现相比，BAC 的进展相对更慢且预后更好[57-59]。

重要的是，在回顾性和前瞻性全身治疗的临床试验中，BAC 的定义一般不严格遵循权威机构的组织学定义，而是依靠病理报告或者医生指定的组织学术语。向权威组织学机构提供肿瘤组织的研究清晰地表明，BAC 在临床实践中的定义有相当大的差异性，因此应考虑在更宽松的临床条件下，放宽 BAC 的病理学标准，而不仅仅是专家根据肺组织病理学来确定[2,60]。针对多病灶 BAC 的研究不断追求更宽松的 BAC 定义的应用，但权威组织学机构仍将其异质性划入晚期 NSCLC 试验内。此外，晚期 BAC 患者可能有非常多变的自然史和疾病负担，但可保留参与试验的资格。

普遍认为 BAC 对传统的化疗是耐药的，或者说与其他组织学类型的 NSCLC 相比，BAC 对化疗缺乏敏感性，在某种程度上，这可能和伴有快速细胞更新的化疗与疾病自然史有关[61]，但也可能在一定程度上与评估非实性、散发且可测量的肿瘤对化疗的反应比评估浸润性 NSCLC 对化疗的反应困难有关。

尽管肿瘤学普遍认为 BAC 对化疗不敏感，但有限的数据表明，常规化疗的反应率（RR）实际上与其他 NSCLC 组织学类型相同。一项在 Mayo 诊所进行的回顾性调查显示，BAC 患者化疗的反应率为 32%，而这一数据在其他 NSCLC 亚型为 33%[62]。

对于晚期 BAC 患者，有限的前瞻性试验数据也支持这一观点，BAC 患者对常规化疗的有效率与 NSCLC 患者一致。一项研究显示，58 例未接受过化疗的晚期 BAC 患者接受了 96h 的紫杉醇输注，总反应率为 14%，病情稳定率为 40%，中位生存时间为 12 个月[63]。另外一项相对小一些的研究中，对晚期 BAC 患者采用紫杉醇 3h 输注，结果总反应率为 11%，病情稳定率为 50%，中位生存时间为 8.6 个月[64]。最后，在法国 IFCT-0401 试验中 47 例采用吉非替尼作为一线治疗方案的患者，其中 43 例选择了化疗作为二线治疗方案[65]。具体的化疗药物包括 38 例采用含铂双药联合化疗（29 例同时采用紫杉烷，9 例同时采用吉西他滨），5 例患者接受单一化疗药物（3 例采用吉西他滨，2 例采用培美曲塞）。该治疗方案的反应率为 21%，中位无进展生存期（median progression-free survival, MPFS）为 3 个月。尽管样本量较小无法得出不同化疗方案优劣的结论，但有趣的是，铂 + 紫杉醇组合治疗的反应率为 28%，而铂 + 吉西他滨组合治疗的反应率为 0，两组都接受培美曲塞治疗的患者可以观测到长期反应（中位无进展生存期分别为 10 个月和 32 个月）。尽管只是单例报道，但其他人也注意到，一些晚期 BAC，包括符合肺炎临床影像学表现的黏液型 BAC 患者[66-67]，接受培美曲塞治疗获得了令人满意的结果。

早期口服表皮生长因子受体（EGFR）酪氨酸激酶抑制剂（TKI）如吉非替尼和厄洛替尼明确了 BAC 临床病理学的组织学特征与 EGFR TKIs 高概率的应答关系[68-69]。关于 BAC 患者对 EGFR TKIs 敏感并长期有效的频繁报道促使了晚期 BAC 多种试验的进展，并都取得了令人鼓舞的结果。在一项四中心的关于口服厄洛替尼的Ⅱ期临床试验中，

150 例患者中有 101 例晚期 BAC 患者，大部分未曾接受过其他治疗（N=74），反应率为 22%，中位生存期为 17 个月[60]。在多中心 SWOG Ⅱ 期临床试验中，136 例晚期 BAC 患者（101 例未接受化疗，35 例曾接受化疗）接受了每天 500mg 的单药吉非替尼治疗，未接受化疗和曾接受化疗的反应率分别为 17% 和 9%[70]。最后，一项法国研究中，99 例未接受过治疗的晚期 BAC 患者接受了每天 250mg 吉非替尼的治疗，反应率为 13%，病情稳定率为 16%[71]。

在过去的几年中，临床组织学已很大程度上被分子标志物替代，使得靶向治疗获得了巨大的临床收益，如 EGFR TKIs。例如，在 IPASS 试验中，无吸烟史和长期吸烟的亚洲肺癌患者进行吉非替尼和标准化疗的 EGFR 基因激活突变与 EGFR 野生型[72]相比差异显著，研究证实有无分子标记物在预测 EGFR TKI 的临床有效性方面要优于临床及病理指标。

根据抗血管增生剂贝伐单抗的应用前景，针对 S0126 单药吉非替尼治疗试验，SWOG 后续的 Ⅱ 期研究在 78 例 BAC 晚期患者中联合使用厄洛替尼与贝伐单抗[73]，反应率为 18%，中位无进展生存期为 5 个月，中位生存期为 17 个月。尽管并不优于 SWOG 先前进行单药吉非替尼的试验结果，但在该试验中无吸烟史的患者较少，哪种方案更有竞争力还有待进一步的研究证实。然而，在一项非前瞻性随机试验中，贝伐单抗对化疗或者 EGFR TKI 治疗的价值在 BAC 晚期患者中仍未确定。ECOG 4599 试验纳入了适合卡铂/紫杉醇联合或者不联合贝伐单抗治疗的患者，结果显示了这些活性药对改善生存质量的效果，它们也同样适用于其他合适的患者。

虽然数据有限，研究表明 EGFR TKI 对 BAC 最有效，因为晚期 BAC 患者 EGFR 突变丰富[74-75]，尤其是非黏液型 BAC[60,75-78]。86 例 BAC 患者中 EGFR 突变率为 26%，发生 EGFR 基因突变的均为非黏液型 BAC 患者（22/69 vs 0/17）[71]。在意大利人的较小型病例研究中也出现了类似的结果，30% 非黏液型 BAC 患者发生了 EGFR 基因突变，而黏液性 BAC 患者的 EGFR 基因的突变率为 0[54]。最后，日本 59 例 BAC 或肺腺癌患者中 44 例具有 BAC 特征，证实了 14% 的黏液型 BAC 患者和 58% 的非黏液型 BAC 发生了 EGFR 突变，KRAS 的突变率分别为 70% 和 29%[79]。然而，最近的报告还记录了同一例患者不同肺结节分子结构的变化[80-82]。

试验证实这些分子的差异与 EGFR TKI 治疗中不同的反应有关。在单药厄洛替尼的四中心试验中发现[60]，EGFR 基因突变患者的反应率为 87%，而 EGFR 野生型为 7%，中位无进展生存期分别为 13 个月和 2 个月。相反，这项研究中所有 EGFR 基因突变的患者 K-ras 基因没有突变，EGFR 未突变的患者中 K-ras 突变率为 32%，与普遍观察到的 EGFR TKI 低概率的客观反应或对 NSCLC 晚期患者的临床帮助是一致的[83-85]。

最近法国 IFCT-0504 的 Ⅱ 期试验中，未接受治疗的晚期 BAC 患者随机使用吉非替尼或者标准的卡铂或者紫杉醇进行化疗，所有患者在进展期使用培美曲塞作为三线治疗[86]。在 130 例合适的患者中，黏液型和非黏液型患者分别占 46% 和 41%，其余 13% 为不确定亚型。采用吉非替尼和化疗的反应率分别为 39% 和 53%，中位无进展生存期为 3.2 和 6.1 个月，中位生存期为 20.2 个月和 16.4 个月。亚组分析显示非黏液型 BAC 患者对吉非替尼和化疗的中位无进展生存期相近，而黏液性 BAC 患者对化疗更敏感（HR2.86）。然而，分子标记物研究并未报道，所以疗效的差异很有可能是由于非黏液型和黏液型 BAC 患者发生 EGFR 基因突变率不同造成的。

最近发现的肺癌发生的驱动基因是一个重排的退行性淋巴瘤激酶基因，口服 ALK 抑制剂克唑替尼最近被确认是 ALK 重排肺癌患者的最佳治疗方法[87]，现在克唑替尼已被 FDA 批准使用[88]。虽然最近才发现，对个体和相对少见的肺癌亚型的研究仍不足，一些报告强调 ALK 重排在 BAC 患者中发生的概率仍不清楚[89-90]。

总之，虽然受到多灶性 BAC 患者系统治疗数据的限制，对 EGFR TKI 长期有效的晚期 BAC 患者存在 EGFR 基因突变以及未发生 K-ras 基因突变表明这些患者的治疗应与其他 NSCLC 患者相同。具体而言，如果一例有症状的多灶性 BAC 患者无论有无进展都进行系统治疗，最佳的治疗方案可能应根据"驱动突变"存在与否决定，就像 Ⅳ 期非侵袭性腺癌患者的治疗标准一样。EG-

FR 基因突变或 ALK 基因重排的患者最可能表现出显著的客观疗效，并且口服 EGFR 和 ALK 抑制剂治疗的效果最好，而 EGFR 或者 ALK 野生型基因的 BAC 患者最适合直接采用传统的化疗作为初始治疗方法。重要的是，目前获得的临床数据不支持"化疗和 EGFR TKI 对治疗晚期 BAC 患者无效"这一观点。

支气管黏液溢

如前所述，支气管黏液溢是一种严重的症状，最常发生于 BAC 患者。虽然持续有效的治疗仍未被发现，一些治疗方法大部分以病例分析的形式取得了一定限度的成功，包括糖皮质激素[91-92]和非类固醇类抗炎药[93-94]。此外，最有效的干预和管理支气管黏液溢的方法是治疗潜在疾病，首先进行系统治疗，如 EGFR TKI 治疗[95-97]。对 ALK 阳性的黏液型 BAC 患者应用克唑替尼成功治疗支气管黏液溢在临床实践中也有个案报道。

在某些情况下，手术作为一种姑息性干预措施，有成功，也有失败[13,98]。

总之，支气管黏液溢仍然是一个很难控制的症状，除了有效治疗潜在的 BAC 进展外，目前仍没有其他公认有效的干预治疗措施。

总 结

尽管肺腺癌最新的分类[1]不提倡再使用"BAC"这一术语，但它只讨论了小的单发病灶，并且对临床诊断为晚期 BAC 的多灶性进展性疾病的资料很少。尽管 BAC 在自然病史及治疗效果上存在很大差异，但因其进展缓慢（即使多病灶也是如此）并且有相对较高的 EGFR 基因突变率，对 TKI 药物治疗有长期良好的疗效，因此临床上仍将其作为一类特征性疾病对待。

对于多病灶疾病在患者最初治疗前确定疾病进展速度是极具价值的，特别是在还未出现与癌症相关的重大疾病或者症状的患者。如果定期复查和随访诊断未发现明显的临床进展可以减轻患者和医生的焦虑，许多患者继续观察数月甚至数年都没有明显的临床进展，有些患者从不表现出疾病进展，也不会出现症状以及影响寿命。

一旦承认主观阈值的临床意义和进展的表现，通过质疑病程的进展是单发的（局限的）还是扩散的，对将晚期 BAC 与其他 NSCLC 区分开是有帮助的。许多多发灶的 BAC 患者可以表现为一个单发灶迅速进展，而其他病灶仍呈缓慢进展甚至没有变化。因为极惰性结节是没有临床价值的，如果基于患者病情的进展、身体状况和并发症不适合手术和放射治疗，则可以考虑局部治疗。

患者表现出弥散性和多灶性疾病的进展可以广义地定义为晚期 BAC，治疗建议和其他类型的晚期肺癌患者相同。目前能找到的最好的证据表明，晚期 BAC（尤其是非黏液型 BAC）对 EGFR TKI 的高反应率是由于这些患者的 EGFR 基因突变率高。因此，无论是临床或者是病理诊断为非黏液型还是黏液型 BAC，最好是通过检测分子驱动突变如 EGFR 突变和 ALK 重排来决定使用 EGFR TKI 或者是 ALK 抑制剂的全身治疗，如果当前临床驱动基因突变情况未明确，则可以选择以传统化疗为基础，联合应用贝伐单抗。

当前的证据表明晚期 BAC 患者对标准化疗的治疗效果与其他 NSCLC 晚期患者相比不敏感，但不建议患者放弃以化疗为基础的治疗受益机会。这在很大程度上是通过许多多发灶 BAC 患者化疗反应影像学评估的难易程度得出的结论。

总之，多发灶 BAC 是一种有显著医疗风险的临床疾病，无论局部还是全身性治疗直接产生的焦虑和反射性反应对患者是不利的。多灶性 BAC 的临床进程多变，可能不会威胁到患者的长期生活质量和生存，肺部病变可能无症状或者有轻微进展甚至无进展，这意味着我们应该把焦点聚集在有明确进展的疾病上，像其他类型的 NSCLC 一样。如果疾病进展十分有限，治疗策略应该考虑局部治疗，如果病情扩散进展，那么应根据临床相关分子标记物的检测结果决定全身治疗方案。

（任万刚　王功朝　彭忠民　译）

参考文献

[1] Travis WD, Brambilla E, Noguchi M, et al. International Association for the Study of Lung Cancer/Americal Thorac-

ic Society/Eruopean Respiratory Society international multidisciplinary classification of lung adenocarcinoma. J Thorac Oncol, 2011, 6（2）: 244 – 285.

[2] TravisWD, Garg K, Franklin WA, et al. Bronchiolalveolar carcinoma and lung adenocarcinoma: the clinical importance and research relevance of the 2004 World Health Organization Pathologic Criteria. J Thorac Oncol, 2006, 1（9）: S13 – S19.

[3] Akira M, Atagi S, Kawahara M, et al. Highresolution CT findings of diffuse brinchioloalveolar carcinoma in 38 patients. AJR Am J Roentgenol, 1999, 173: 1623 – 1629.

[4] Thompson W. Bronchioloalveolar carcinoma masquerading as pneumonia. Respir Care, 2004, 49: 1349 – 1353.

[5] Nakanishi K, Hiroi S, Kawai T, et al. Bronchogenic carcinoma and coexistent bronchioalveolar epithelial hyperplasia and adenocarcinoma of the lung. Hum Pathol, 1998, 29: 235 – 239.

[6] Grover FL, Piantidosi S. Lung Cancer Study Group. Recurrence and survival following resection of bronchioloalveolar carcinoma of the lung—the Lung Cancer Study Group experience. Ann Surg, 1989, 209: 779 – 790.

[7] Akata S, Fukushima A, Kakizaki D, et al. CT scanning of bronchioloalveolar carcinoma: specific appearances. Lung Cancer, 1995, 12: 221 – 230.

[8] Bonomo L, Storto ML, Ciccotosto C, et al. Bronchioloalveolar carcinoma of the lung. Eur Radiol, 1998, 8: 996 – 1001.

[9] Greco RJ, Steiner RM, Goldman S, et al. Bronchoalveolar cell carcinoma of the lung. Ann Thorac Surg, 1986, 41: 615 – 612.

[10] Dumont P, Gasser B, Rouge C, et al. Bronchioloalveolar carcinoma: histopathologic study of evolution in a series of 105 surgically treated patients. Chest, 1998, 113: 391 – 395.

[11] Daly RC, Trastek VF, Pairolero PC, et al. Bronchioloalveolar carcinoma: factors affecting survival. Ann Thorac Surg, 1991, 51: 368 – 377.

[12] Chetty K, Dick C, McGovern J, et al. Refractory hypoxemia due to intrapulmonary shunting associated with bronchiolalveolar carcinoma. Chest, 1997, 111（4）: 1120 – 1121.

[13] Falcoz PE, Hoan NT, Le Pimpec-Barthes F, et al. Severe hypoxemia due to intrapulmonary shunting requires surgery for bronchioloalveolar carcinoma. Ann Thorac Surg, 2009, 88（1）: 287 – 288.

[14] Venkata C, Mireles JA, Venkateshiah SB. Refractory hypoxemic respiratory failure due to adenocarcinoma of the lung with predominant bronchioloalveolar carcinoma component. Respir Care, 2009, 54（11）: 1496 – 1499.

[15] Wilson DO, Ryan A, Furhman C, et al. Doubling times and CT screen-detected lung cancers in the Pittsburgh Lung Screening Study. Am J Respir Crit Care Med, 2012, 185（1）: 85 – 89.

[16] Oda S, Awai K, Murao K, et al. Volumedoubling time of pulmonary nodules with groundglass opacity at multidetector CT: Assessment with computer-aided three-dimensional volumetry. Acad Radiol, 2011, 18（1）: 63 – 69.

[17] Lindell RM, Hartman TE, Swensen SJ, et al. Five-year lung cancer screening experience: CT appearance, growth rate, location, and histologic features of 61 lung cancers. Radiology, 2007, 242（2）: 555 – 562.

[18] Lee KS, Jeong YJ, Han J, et al. T1 non-small cell lung cancer: imaging and histopathologic findings and their prognostic implications. Radiographics, 2004, 24（6）: 1632 – 1636.

[19] Okada M, Tauchi S, Iwanaga K, et al. Associations among bronchioloalveolar carcinoma components, positiron emission tomographic and computed tomorgraphic findings, and malignant behavior in small lung adenocarcinomas. J Thorac CardiovascSurg, 2007, 133（6）: 1448 – 1454.

[20] Lee HY, Lee KS. Ground-glass opacity nodules: histopathology, imaging evaluation, and clinical implications. J Thorac Imaging, 2011, 26（2）: 106 – 118.

[21] Sun JS, Park KJ, Sheen SS, et al. Clinical usefulness of fluorodeoxyglucose（FDG）-PET maximal standardized uptake value（SUV）in combination with CT features for the differentiation of adenocarcinoma with a bronchioloalveolar carcinoma from other subtypes of non-small cell lung cancer. Lung Cancer, 2009, 66（2）: 205 – 210.

[22] Aquino SL, Halpern EF, Kuester LB, et al. FDGPET and CT features of non-small cell lung cancer based on tumor type. Int J Mol Med, 2007, 19（3）: 495 – 499.

[23] Huang TW, Lin LF, Hsieh CM, et al. Positron emission tomography in bronchioloalveolar carcinoma of the lung. Eur J Surg Oncol, 2012, 38（12）: 1156 – 1160.

[24] Storey CF, Knudtson KP, Lawrence BJ. Bronchiolar（"alveolar cell"）carcinoma of the lung. J Thorac Surg, 1953, 26: 331 – 406.

[25] Russell PA, Wainer Z, Wright G, et al. Does lung adenocarcinoma subtype predict survival? A clinicopathologic study based on the new International Association for the

Study of Lung Cancer/American Thoracic Society/European Respiratory Society international multidisciplinary lung adenocarcinoma classification. J Thorac Oncol, 2011, 6: 1496-1504.

[26] Wislez M, Beer DG, Wistuba I, et al. Molecular biology, genomics, and proteomics in bronchioloalveolar carcinoma. J Thorac Oncol, 2006, 1 (9): S8-S12.

[27] Westra WH, Baas IO, Hruban RH, et al. K-ras oncogene activation in atypical alveolar hyperplasias of the human lung. Cancer Res, 1996, 56 (9): 2224-2228.

[28] Nakata M, Sawada S, Yamashita M, et al. Surgical treatments for multiple primary adenocarcinoma of the lung. Ann Thorac Surg, 2004, 78 (4): 1194-1199.

[29] Osaki T, Sugio K, Hanagiri T, et al. Survival and prognostic factors of surgically resected T4 non-small cell lung cancer. Ann Thorac Surg, 2003, 75 (6): 1745-1751.

[30] Rao J, Sayeed RA, Tomaszek S, et al. Prognostic factors in resected satellite-nodule T4 nonsmall cell lung cancer. Ann Thorac Surg, 2007, 84 (3): 934-938.

[31] Pennathur A, Lindeman B, Ferson P, et al. Surgical resection is justified in non-small cell lung cancer patients with node negative T4 satellite lesions. Ann Thorac Surg, 2009, 87 (3): 893-899.

[32] Volpino P, Cavallaro A, Cangemi R, et al. Comparative analysis of clinical features and prognostic factors in resected bronchioloalveolar carcinoma and adenocarcinoma of the lung. Anticancer Res, 2003, 23 (6D): 4959-4965.

[33] Park JH, Lee KS, Kim JH, et al. Malignant pure pulmonary ground-glass opacity nodules: prognostic implications. Korean J Radiol, 2009, 10 (1): 12-20.

[34] Rusch VW, Tsuchiya R, Tsuboi M, et al. Surgery for bronchioloalveolar carcinoma and "very early" adenocarcinoma: an evolving standard of care? J Thorac Oncol, 2006, 1 (9 Suppl): S27-S31.

[35] Lin ZC, Long H, Rong TH, et al. Surgical treatment efficacy of bronchioloalveolar carcinoma: a retrospective analysis of 130 patients. Chinese J Cancer, 2006, 25 (9): 1123-1126.

[36] Goldstraw P, Crowley J, Chansky K, et al. The IASLC Lung Cancer Staging Project: proposals for the revision of the TNM stage groupings in the forthcoming (seventh) edition of the TNM classification of malignant tumours. J Thorac Oncol, 2007, 2 (8): 706-714.

[37] Rami-Porta R, Ball D, Crowley J, et al. The IASLC Lung Cancer Staging Project: proposals for the revision of the T descriptors in the forthcoming (seventh) edition of the TNM classification for lung cancer. J Thorac Oncol, 2007, 2 (7): 593-602.

[38] Roberts PF, Straznicka M, Lara PN, et al. Resection of multifocal non-small cell lung cancer when the bronchioloalveolar subtype is involved. J Thorac Cardiovasc Surg, 2003, 126 (5): 1597-1602.

[39] Mun M, Kohno T. Single-stage surgical treatment of synchronous bilateral multiple lung cancer. Ann Thorac Surg, 2007, 83 (3): 1146-1151.

[40] Mun M, Kohno T. Efficacy of thoracoscopic resection for multifocal bronchioloalveolar carcinoma showing pure ground glass opacities of 20 mm or less in diameter. J Thorac Cardiovasc Surg, 2007, 134 (4): 877-882.

[41] Battafarano RJ, Meyers BF, Guthrie TJ, et al. Surgical resection of multifocal non-small cell lung cancer is associated with prolonged survival. Ann Thorac Surg, 2002, 74: 988-993.

[42] Finley DJ, Yoshizawa A, Travis W, et al. Predictors of outcomes after surgical treatment of synchronous primary lung cancers. J Thorac Oncol, 2010, 5: 197-205.

[43] Gu B, Burt BM, Merritt MD, et al. A dominant adenocarcinoma with mutifocal ground glass lesions does not behave as advanced disease. Ann Thorac Surg, 2013, 96: 411-418.

[44] Tanvetyanon T, Robinson LA, Schell MJ, et al. Outcomes of adrenalectomy for isolated synchronous vs. metachronous adrenal metastases in non-small cell lung cancer: a systematic review and pooled analysis. J Clin Oncol, 2008, 26 (7): 1142-1147.

[45] Sofietti R, Ruda R, Mutani R. Management of brain metastases. J Neurol, 2002, 249 (10): 1357-1369.

[46] Zorn GL, McGifflin DC, Young KR, et al. Pulmonary transplantation for advanced bronchioloalveolar carcinoma. J Thorac Cardiovasc Surg, 2003, 125: 45-48.

[47] Garver RI Jr, Zorn GL, Wu X, et al. Recurrence of bronchioloalveolar carcinoma in transplanted lungs. N Engl J Med, 1999, 340: 1071-1074.

[48] de Perrot M, Chernenko S, Waddell TK, et al. Role of lung transplantation in the treatment of bronchogenic carcinomas for patients with end-stage pulmonary disease. J Clin Oncol, 2004, 22: 4351-4356.

[49] Etienne B, Bertocchi M, Gamondes J-P, et al. Successful double-lung transplantation for bronchioloalveolar cell carcinoma. Chest, 1997, 112: 1423-1424.

[50] Geltner C, Jamnig H, Bucher B, et al. Lung transplanta-

tion from bronchiolo-alveolar lung carcinoma. Lung Cancer, 2002, 37 (Suppl 1): S27.

[51] Paloyan EB, Swinnen LJ, Montoya A, et al. Lung transplantation for advanced bronchioloalveolar carcinoma confined to the lungs. Transplantation, 2000, 69: 2446-2448.

[52] Shin MS, Ho K-J. Recurrent bronchioloalveolar carcinoma after lung transplantation: Radiographic and histologic features of the primary and recurrence. J Thorac Imaging, 2004, 19: 79-81.

[53] Ebright MI, Zakowski MF, Martin J, et al. Clinical pattern and pathologic stage but not histologic features predict outcome for bronchioloalveolar carcinoma. Ann Thorac Surg, 2002, 74 (5): 1640-1646.

[54] Casali C, Rossi G, Marchioni A, et al. A single institution-based retrospective study of surgically treated bronchioloalveolar adenocarcinoma of the lung: clinicopathologic analysis, molecular features, and possible pitfalls in routine practice. J Thorac Oncol, 2010, 5 (6): 830-836.

[55] Barlesi F, Doddoli C, Thomas P, et al. Bilateral bronchioloalveolar lung carcinoma: Is there a place for palliative pneumonectomy? Eur J Cardiothorac Surg, 2001, 20: 1113-1116.

[56] Takao M, Takagi T, Suzuki H, et al. Resection of mucinous lung adenocarcinoma presenting with intractable bronchorrhea. J Thorac Oncol, 2010, 5 (4): 576-578.

[57] Breathnach OS, Ishibe N, Williams J, et al. Clinical features of patients with stage IIIB and IV bronchioloalveolar carcinoma of the lung. Cancer, 1999, 86 (7): 1165-1173.

[58] Zell JA, Ou SHI, Ziogas A, et al. Validation of the proposed International Association for the Study of Lung Cancer non-small cell lung cancer staging system revisions for advanced bronchioloalveolar carcinoma using data from the California Cancer Registry. J Thorac Oncol, 2007, 2 (12): 1078-1085.

[59] Chansky K, Sculier JP, Crowley JJ, et al. The International Association for the Study of Lung Cancer Staging Project: prognostic factors and pathologic TNM stage in surgically managed non-small cell lung cancer. J Thorac Oncol, 2009, 4 (7): 792-801.

[60] Miller VA, Riely GJ, Zakowski MF, et al. Molecular characteristics of bronchioloalveolar carcinoma and adenocarcinoma, bronchioloalveolar subtype, predict response to erlotinib. J Clin Oncol, 2008, 26 (9): 1472-1478.

[61] Chu E, DeVita VT. Principles of cancer management: Chemotherapy//VT DeVita, Jr, S Helman, SA Ronsenberg (eds). Cancer: Principals and Practice of Oncology, 6th edn. Philadelphia: LippincottWilliams &Wilkins, 2001: 289-306.

[62] Feldman ER, Eagan RT, Schaid DJ. Metastatic bronchioalveolar carcinoma and metastatic adenocarcinoma of the lung: clinical manifestations, chemotherapeutic responses, and prognosis. Mayo Clin Proc, 1992, 67 (1): 27-32.

[63] West HL, Crowley JJ, Vance RB, et al. Advanced brocnhioloalveolar carcinoma: A phase II trial of paclitaxel by 96-hour infusion (SWOG 9714). Annals of Oncology, 2005, 16: 1076-1080.

[64] Scagliotti GV, Smit E, Bosque L, et al. A phase II study of paclitaxel in advanced bronchioloalveolar carcinoma (EORTC trial 08956). Lung Cancer, 2005, 50: 91-96.

[65] Duruisseaux M, Baudrin L, Quoix E, et al. Chemotherapy effectiveness after first-line gefitinib treatment for advanced lepidic predominant adenocarcinoma (formerly advanced bronchioloalveolar carcinoma): exploratory analysis of the IFCT-0401 trial. J Thorac Oncol, 2012, 7 (9): 1423-1431.

[66] Garfield D Franklin W. Dramatic response to pemetrexed in a patient with pneumonic-type mucinous bronchioloalveolar carcinoma. J Thorac Oncol, 2011, 6 (2): 397-398.

[67] Okuda C, Kim YH, Takeuchi K, et al. Successful treatment with pemetrexed in a patient with mucinous bronchioloalveolar carcinoma: long-term response duration with mild toxicity. J Thorac Oncol, 2011, 6 (3): 641-642.

[68] Miller VA, Kris MG, Shah N, et al. Bronchioloalveolar pathologic subtype and smoking history predict sensitivity to gefitinib in advanced non-small-cell lung cancer. J Clin Oncol, 2004, 22 (6): 1103-1109.

[69] Hsieh RK, Lim HK, Kuo HT, et al. Female sex and bronchioloalveolar subtype predict EGFR mutations in non-small cell lung cancer. Chest, 2005, 128 (1): 317-321.

[70] West HL, Franklin W, McCoy J, et al. Gefitinib therapy in advanced bronchioloalveolar carcinoma: Southwest Oncology Group Study S0126. J Clin Oncol, 2006, 24 (12): 1807-1813.

[71] Cadranel J, Quoix E, Baudrin L, et al. IFCT-0401

Trial Group. IFCT – 0401 Trial: a phase II study of gefitinib administered as first-line treatment in advancedadenocarcinoma with bronchioloalveolar carcinoma subtype. J Thorac Oncol, 2009, 4 (4): 1126 – 1135.

[72] Mok TS, Wu Y-L, Thongprasert S, et al. Gefitinib or carboplatin-paclitaxel in pulmonary adenocarcinoma. New Engl J Med, 2009, 361: 947 – 957.

[73] West H, Moon J, Hirsch FR, et al. SWOG 0635 and S0636: Phase II trials in advanced-stage NSCLC or erlotinib (OSI – 774) and bevacizumab in bronchioloalveolar carcinoma (BAC) and adenocarcinoman with BAC features (adenoBAC), and in neversmokers with primary NSCLC adenocarcinoma. J Clin Oncol, 2012, 30 (suppl): A#7517.

[74] Marchetti A, Martella C, Felicioni L, et al. EGFR mutations in non-small-cell lung cancer: analysis of a large series of cases and development of a rapid and sensitive method for diagnostic screening with potential implications in pharmacologic treatment. J Clin Oncol, 2005, 23 (4): 857 – 865.

[75] Sun PL, Seol H, Lee HJ, et al. High incidence of *EGFR* mutations in Korean men smokers with no intratumoral heterogeneity of lung adenocarcinomas: correlation with histologic subtypes, EGFR/TTF – 1 expressions, and clinical features. J Thorac Oncol, 2012, 7 (2): 323 – 330.

[76] Garfield DH, Cadranel J, West HL. Bronchioloalveolar carcinoma: the case for two diseases. Clin Lung Cancer, 2008, 9 (1): 24 – 29.

[77] Matsumoto S, Iwakawa R, Kohno T, et al. Frequent *EGFR* mutations in noninvasive bronchioloalveolar carcinoma. Int J Cancer, 2006, 118 (10): 2498 – 2504.

[78] Sakuma Y, Matsukuma S, Yoshihara M, et al. Distinctive evaluation of nonmucinous and mucinous subtypes of bronchioloalveolar carcinomas in EGFR and K-ras gene-mutation analyses for Japanese lung adenocarcinomas: Confirmation of the correlations with histologic subtypes and gene mutations. Am J Clin Pathol, 2007, 128 (1): 100 – 108.

[79] Hata A, Katakami N, Fujita S, et al. Frequency of *EGFR* and *KRAS* mutations in Japanese patients with lung adenocarcinoma with features of the mucinous subtype of bronchioloalveolar carcinoma. J Thorac Oncol, 2010, 5 (8): 1197 – 1200.

[80] Chen Z-Y, Zhong W-Z, Chang X-C, et al. EGFR mutation heterogeneity and the mixed response to EGFR tyrosine kinase inhibitors of lung adenocarcinomas. Oncologist, 2012, 17: 978 – 985.

[81] Nakano H, Soda H, Takasu M, et al. Heterogeneity of epidermal growth factor receptor mutations within a mixed adenocarcinoma lung nodule. Lung Cancer, 2008, 60 (1): 136 – 140.

[82] Ikeda K, Nomuri H, Ohba Y, et al. Epidermal growth factor receptor mutations in multicentric lung denocarcinomas and atypical adenomatous hyperplasias. J Thorac Oncol, 2008, 3 (5): 467 – 471.

[83] Zhu CQ, da Cunha Santos G, et al. Role of KRAS and EGFR as biomarkers of response to erlotinib in National Cancer Institute of Cancer Clinical Trials Group Study BR. 21. J Clin Oncol, 2008, 26: 4268 – 4275.

[84] Linardou H, Dahbreh IJ, Kanaloupiti D, et al. Assessment of *K-RAS* mutations as a mechanism associated with resistance to EGFR-targeted agents: A systematic review and meta-analysis of studies in advanced non-small-cell lung cancer and metastatic colorectal cancer. Lancet Oncol, 2008, 9: 962 – 972.

[85] Brugger W, Triller N, Blasinka-Morawiec M, et al. Prospective molecular marker analysis of EGFR and KRAS from a randomized, placebo-controlled study of erlotinib maintenance therapy in advancednon-small cell lung cancer. J Clin Oncol, 2011, 29 (31): 4113 – 4120.

[86] Cadranel J, Gervais R, Wislez M, et al. IFCT – 0504 trial: Mucinous (M) and nonmucinous (NM) cytologic subtypes interaction effect in first line treatment of advanced bronchioloalveolar carcinoma (BAC) by erlotinib (E) or carboplatin/paclitaxel (C/P). J Clin Oncol, 2011, 29 (Suppl: abstr 7521): A#7521.

[87] Kwak EL, Bang YJ, Camidge DR, et al. Anaplastic lymphoma kinase inhibition in non-small-cell lung cancer. N Engl J Med, 2010, 363: 1693 – 1703.

[88] Pfizer I. Xalkori Prescribing Information, 2011. [2013 – 01 – 11] http://www.accessdata.fda.gov/drugsatfda_docs/label/ 2011/202570s000lbl.pdf.

[89] Inamura K, Takeuchi K, Togashi Y, et al. EML4 – ALK fusion is linked to histologic characteristics in a subset of lung cancers. J Thorac Oncol, 2008, 3 (1): 13 – 17.

[90] Sasaki T, Rodig SJ, Chirieac LR, et al. The biology and treatment of EML4 – ALK non-small cell lung cancer. Eur J Cancer, 2010, 46 (10): 1773 – 1780.

[91] Marom ZM, Goswami SK. Respiratory mucus hypersecretion (bronchorrhea): A case discussion-possible mechanisms (s) and treatment. J Allergy Clin Immunol,

1991, 87 (6): 1050-1055.

[92] Nakajima T, Terashima T, Nishida J, et al. Treatment of bronchorrhea by corticosteroids in a case of bronchioloalveolar carcinoma producing CA19-9. Intern Med, 2002, 41 (3): 225-228.

[93] Homma S, Kawabata M, Kishi K, et al. Successful treatment of refractory bronchorrhea by inhaled indomethacin in two patients with bronchioloalveolar carcinoma. Chest, 1999, 115 (5): 1465-1468.

[94] Tamaoki J, Kohri K, Isono K, et al. Inhaled indomethacin in bronchorrhea in bronchioloalveolar carcinoma (letter). Chest, 2000, 117: 1213-1214.

[95] Kitazaki T, Fukuda M, Soda H, et al. Novel effects of gefitinib on mucin production in bronchioloalveolar carcinoma: two case reports. Lung Cancer, 2005, 49 (1): 125-128.

[96] Milton DT, Kris MG, Gomez JE, et al. Prompt control of bronchorrhea in patients with bronchioloalveolar carcinoma treated with gefitinib. Support Care Cancer, 2005, 13 (1): 70-72.

[97] Yano S, Kanematsu T, Miki T, et al. A report of two bronchioloalveolar carcinoma cases which were rapidly improved by treatment with the epidermal growth factor receptor tyrosine kinase inhibitor ZD1839 ("Iressa"). Cancer Sci, 2003, 94 (5): 453-458.

[98] Yokouchi H, Murata K, Murakami M, et al. A case of diffuse pneumonic type of mucinous adenocarcinoma treated with reduction surgery. Gan To Kagaku Ryoho, 2012, 39 (12): 2396-2398.

第10章
放射学检查与肺癌筛查

Patricia de Groot[1], *Reginald F. Munden*[2]
[1]Department of Diagnostic Radiology, The University of Texas MD Anderson Cancer Center, Houston, TX, USA
[2]Department of Radiology, The Houston Methodist Hospital, Houston, TX, USA

引 言

肺癌是导致全球癌症死亡的主要原因之一，每年超过137万人死于肺癌[1]。在美国，每年肺癌的死亡人数占所有肿瘤死亡人数的1/4以上。尽管20世纪80年代以来美国男性肺癌的发病率有所下降，但死亡人数仍为前列腺癌的3倍，前列腺癌是导致男性肿瘤死亡的第二大病因。美国女性的肺癌死亡率几乎是乳腺癌的2倍[2]。在美国少数民族和教育程度低的人群中，肺癌的发病率高于普通人群[3]。在欧盟，男性肺癌患者每年的死亡人数约占肿瘤总死亡人数的25%，但男性的肺癌死亡率在过去的20年间一直呈下降趋势。相比之下，欧洲女性的肺癌死亡率自2009年以来增加了7%，预计将继续上升至2020年[4]。肺癌的5年生存率在欧盟的27个国家中差异很大，在发达国家中英国是最低的，约为8%[5-6]。在中国、韩国和一些非洲国家，随着近几十年来吸烟人数的增多，肺癌的发病率和死亡率也在上升[7]。

肺癌在形态、组织学以及生物学行为上都具有异质性[8]，其病理类型包括小细胞癌、鳞癌、腺癌及大细胞癌。目前医学研究的重点是肿瘤的基因组学和蛋白质组学，并有证据表明，肺癌的基因突变对于肿瘤的自然病程、对治疗的反应及预后有显著影响，即使在同一组织学类型的肺癌中也是如此[9]。

总体上肺癌的生存率较低，5年总体生存率为15%，且已保持了几十年，主要是由于大多数肺癌就诊时多为进展期（Ⅲ期或Ⅳ期）。而ⅠA期肺癌经有效治疗后5年生存率超过70%[10]，这也凸显了寻找一种能确诊早期肺癌的可靠方法的必要性。

筛查的概念

筛查的基本目的是通过筛选试验降低疾病特异性死亡率[11-12]。直到最近，所有肺癌筛查的尝试的统计学结果均显示未显著降低肺癌的死亡率[8]。合适的筛查试验必须满足一些沿用已久的标准，这样才是合理的，而目前还没有可用于肺癌的合适的筛查试验；对于成功的筛查，目标疾病必须有相当大的发病率和死亡率，而且必须在受筛查的人群中有较高的患病率；它必须有一个既定的临床前期，即在此期间患者没有相应的临床症状；另外，重要的是，处于临床前期的疾病能够在其病程中一个关键窗口期之前被该试验检测出来，而过了这个窗口期后其治疗和预后均较差；对于早期确诊的目标疾病必须有公认的有效治疗方法[11-12]。

此外，筛选试验必须对该种疾病有较好的灵敏度和特异度，以尽量减少假阳性和假阴性结果[11-12]，它必须准确、可重复性好。当然，有效的筛查也需要具有其他的社会心理和经济性特征。筛查过程应安全、无痛苦，更容易被患者和医生接受，还要操作简便，花费较低[12]。

偏 倚

确定筛查有效性的试验容易受几种偏倚的影响，导致人为的夸大或可能是相互矛盾的结果。

领先时间偏倚是指被筛检疾病检出时虽然处于临床前期，但结果与出现临床症状时被诊断出来是相同的。换言之，诊断和死亡之间的时间延长了，但对生存期并没有实际影响。病程长短偏倚是因为疾病进展率不同，一些惰性疾病有较长的临床前期，被筛检出的比例较高，这会导致在筛检人群中预后较好的低侵袭性肿瘤的检出率过高。定期重复筛查可检出两次筛查之间偶发的肿瘤，因而可以在一定程度上避免病程长短偏倚。

某些疾病的检出不会影响患者的预期寿命，而是某些目标疾病以外的因素实际导致患者死亡，即过度诊断偏倚[8,11]。然而，有人认为过度诊断的概念在肺癌上具有误导性[13-14]。有流行病学和病理学证据显示任何通过筛检发现的肺癌都有致命的可能[15,17]，即使死亡是由其他原因导致的。肺癌筛查人群有与烟草消费相关的共存病，包括肺气肿和心血管疾病。然而，最近对肺癌最常见的类型——腺癌的自然病程进展的研究显示，病程长短偏倚和过度诊断偏倚在肺癌中有重要意义。对于27%的患者，尤其是女性患者，表现为肺部纯毛玻璃影或部分实性病变影的腺癌的体积倍增时间可超过400d[18]。

为了处理在筛选试验中以上这些影响，公认的方法是随机对照临床试验。随机对照试验本身也会有缺点，包括参与者的不依从和交叉污染，或受试者从试验之外接受相关的临床治疗而造成的影响[8,11]。

另一种偏倚可能是志愿者筛选试验中固有的：一种选择偏倚，特别是选择参加和接受筛选的人的自我选择，它也被称为志愿者偏倚与参与偏倚。例如，最初接到邀请信的人中只有0.5%最后参加了美国国家肺筛查试验（the US National Lung Screening Trial, NLST）[19]。虽然这不会影响随机试验的研究组之间的比较，但也会对研究结果在全人群的推广造成影响。丹麦肺癌筛检试验（the Danish lung Cancer Screening Trial, DLCST）表明社会人口因素和社会心理因素影响志愿者参与筛检试验的意愿[19]。

历史的视角

1950年，Doll和Hill的试验无可争辩地确立了吸烟与肺癌之间的关系[20]，找出了肺癌的危险人群。根据目前WHO公布的数据估计，全球71%的肺癌死亡和22%的肿瘤死亡由吸烟引起[1]。试图证明在高危人群中实施筛选措施有效性的尝试始于20世纪50年代，目前仍在继续[21-22]。

放射学筛查

20世纪60年代，在一项55 000例受试者参与的大型试验中，依据接受胸部放射学检查的频次将受试者分为两组。结果显示，尽管更频繁的放射学检查能够发现更多的肺癌和更多可切除性病变，但对肺癌的整体死亡率无明显影响，两组非常相似[22]。

20世纪70年代开展的4项随机临床试验，其中3项由国家癌症研究所（the National Cancer Institute, NCI）资助，分别是Johns Hopkins肺项目、Sloan-Kettering肺项目和Mayo肺项目[23,25]。第四项试验是在捷克斯洛伐克进行的[26]。Johns Hopkins和Sloan-Kettering试验每年会对筛查试验组进行胸部X线检查和痰细胞学检查，对照组仅进行胸部X线检查。结果在检出肺癌的数量、病变的可切除性或者肺癌相关死亡率等方面未见差异。Mayo肺项目评估胸部X线摄影检查的频率并结合痰液分析进行筛检，但受限于患者不依从和组间交叉污染。其长期随访分析表明，肺癌死亡率在试验组（X线和痰）略高一些。然而，筛检组的5年和9年生存率提高了，这是因为肺癌在试验组的发病率较高，而不可测定的危险因素也影响了随机性[27]。捷克的研究基于筛检组和非筛检组在不同时间进行的胸部X线与痰细胞学检查结果，没有发现筛检能够降低肺癌的总体死亡率[26]。

20世纪90年代日本进行了4项政府资助的基于人群影像学筛查的病例对照研究，分别在宫城县、群马县、新泻市和冈山市开展[28]。在日本的老年人健康和医疗服务法制度下，自1987年起每年对所有40岁以上的人行微型氟摄影（1935开发的技术，类似于正面胸部平片）的癌症筛查，对于吸烟者每年行痰液细胞学检查[29]。甚至更早，依照20世纪50年代颁布的结核病控制法，日本居民每年都会接受大规模的微型胸部X线筛查[30]。然而，尽管有这些筛查项目，仍然没有足够的证据表明筛查能够降低肺癌死亡率，这促使了病例对照项目的启动[28]。4 项研究中有 3 项研究发现，每年的影像学筛查将显著减少肺癌的死亡人数。然而是否将这种模式应用于西方人口仍有待商榷[28]。

CT 筛查

技术的不断改进，特别是胸部计算机断层扫描（CT）的出现，建立了有效的筛查措施。众所周知，胸部 CT 在检出直径小于 1cm 的结节、实性结节及部分实性结节方面的敏感性优于 X 线平片[31-33]。低剂量 CT（low dose CT, LDCT）在研究过程中减少了患者的电离辐射剂量，使其更适用于有危险因素暴露但无已知疾病的患者。

在 20 世纪 90 年代早期到中期，日本进行了 3 项主要的 LDCT 肺癌筛查研究[33,35]，包括一项大型的为期 3 年的研究，这是利用移动式 CT 扫描仪在日本农村县区进行的基于人群的大规模筛查[29,33]。这些研究综合了在日本已有的项目下进行的胸部透视摄影与 LDCT 筛查。所有参与者使用相同的的筛查协议。对高危人群没有进行分类，吸烟者和非吸烟者都能够参与。在所有的研究中，诊断的病变中有很大一部分是ⅠA 期、可以手术切除的肺癌。他们同时还表明，LDCT 比胸片检出肺癌的敏感性更高。该项日本试验更重要的发现之一是在不吸烟的妇女中检出肺癌，主要是肺腺癌。这些观察性研究的结果表明，肺癌的 10 年生存率得到了改善[29]。

同时，早期肺癌行动计划（the Early Lung Cancer Action Project，ELCAP）是在美国发起的。这项研究还纳入传统的胸部 X 线和 LDCT，并论证 LDCT 与 X 线片相比有更高的灵敏度，这是在高危吸烟人群中得出的结论。它突出了 LDCT 在诊断早期肺癌中的价值，其中大部分（96%）可手术切除。研究预测，参与者的 5 年生存率至少为 80%；但是，这项研究样本量小，而且只有 1 组[15,36-37]。国际 ELCAP 颁布这种模式，并且到 2005 年为止，在对除美国之外的 8 个国家约 25 000 人进行 LDCT 筛查。在这个群体中，绝大多数检出的肺癌是Ⅰ期病变，有治愈的可能性[15]。

Mayo 的 CT 筛查研究开始于 20 世纪 90 年代末，在高危人群中连续 5 年采用 LDCT 筛查，每年进行一次痰细胞学、高危放血和呼吸量测定法筛查。虽然一些Ⅰ期肺癌在试验过程中被发现，但是研究得出的结论是，肺癌死亡率未得到改善[28]。此外，在研究的过程中还检出了非癌性的假阳性结节，可能是试验地区的地方性组织胞浆菌病导致的[38]。后续研究调查得出结论，依从方案，在有地方性真菌病的地区，CT 筛查有可能检出（肺癌），从而尽量减少良性活组织检查[39]。

使用 LDCT 早期试验未能改善疾病特异性死亡率或降低晚期肺癌的发病率[40]，因为他们是观察性研究而不是随机对照研究。

国家前列腺、肺、结直肠及卵巢（the National Prostate, Lung, Colorectal and Ovarian, PLCO）筛选试验开始于 1992 年，是一项评估 4 种恶性肿瘤筛查方法的大型试验。它纳入了 154 901 人参与肺癌筛查，其中对干预组中的不吸烟者进行 3 次胸片检查、吸烟者进行 4 次胸片检查，对照组只提供一般社区护理[41]。试验参与者中 50.5% 为女性，不吸烟者占约 45%，曾有吸烟史者占 42%，而现时吸烟者占 10%。这是唯一的随机对照肺癌筛查试验和唯一的在日本以外进行的包括了非吸烟者的试验。试验参与者的平均随访时间为 11.2 年[42]。在比较两个随机组间肺癌死亡率的初步分析中，还需评估参与者是否符合全国肺癌筛查试验入选标准。该试验得出的结论是，每年胸部 X 线检查不能降低肺癌死亡率[42]。

国家肺癌筛查试验

NLST 就是为了回答这个问题，即 LDCT 筛查能否降低肺癌的死亡率。2002 年开始了一项多中心随机对照试验，它是美国国家癌症研究所的肺癌筛查研究（the National Cancer Institute Lung Screening Study，LSS）中心与美国放射学会影像网络（the American College of Radiology Imaging Network，ACRIN）合作开展的[43-44]。53 454 名参与者被随机分为两组，结果显示，肺癌的特异性死亡率降幅为 20%[45]。

NLST 研究的主要终点是肺癌死亡率，几个次要终点也被纳入设计，包括肺癌的发病率与分期分布、肺癌的存活率和全因死亡率。此外，该 NLST-ACRIN 中心正在编制筛选效果和筛选结果对受试者吸烟习惯影响的数据调查表[44]。

试验设计

将 NLST 试验的参与者随机分到两个组中的 1 个，每年对患者行后前位胸片或胸部 LDCT 筛查。每个组有 1 次基线检查和两次额外筛查[44]。所有参与者中，26 732 人行胸片检查，26 722 人行 LDCT 筛查[46-47]。并对参与者进行随访，中位随访时间为 6.5 年，直到 2009 年 12 月 31 日[47]。

研究中使用的胸片根据不同试验中心的设备分为几种类型，包括增感屏胶片、计算机数字 X 线片。所有的 LDCT 检查使用多排螺旋 CT 完成，最初为 4 层 CT，但随着时间的推移也使用了 16 层和 64 层 CT。所有的 X 线片和 CT 系统都是经 NLST 认证的，符合试验方案要求和美国放射学会（American College of Radiology, ACR）指南[44]。试验方案中也包括一个严格的质量保障程序[43]。

每个试验中心对胸部 X 线片和 LDCT 检查结果进行评价的放射学医生都是经 NLST 资格认证的[44]。他们中的大多数是胸部放射学专家。他们接受了专门的培训以及对于筛查结果的阅片和报告质量控制培训[48]。

参与者队列

志愿者是通过发送针对性的邮件、公共电视、广播和报纸广告、网络广告和社区宣传招募的[46]。少部分志愿者是基于地域资料，通过指向明确的邮件、广告和社区大使等方式努力获得，目的是使试验人群能够代表全体有高风险患肺癌的美国人。

志愿者入选标准为：年龄在 55~74 岁，每年至少吸烟 30 包。既往每年吸烟达 30 包者，如果 15 年内已经戒烟也可以参加该试验[47]。排除标准为：过去 5 年内曾患肺癌，曾患除皮肤非黑色素瘤之外的癌，特定的原位癌以及曾经做过肺部手术者；参与了另一项癌症筛查试验、癌症预防试验或者过去 18 个月内做过胸部 CT 者；有家庭补氧和有金属植入物，如心脏起搏器者；有咯血症状，体重不明原因降低 15 磅，或之前 12 周内做过呼吸道感染治疗者[44]。

在 55 456 例参与者中，31 533 例（59%）为男性；39 234 例（73%）年龄 < 65 岁；总共有 27 677 例（52%）曾经吸烟，其余均为主动吸烟者；约 91% 的参与者为白人，4.4% 为黑人，1.7% 为西班牙裔或拉丁美洲人[46]。两组的随机分配产生相等的人口统计数据。与美国高危人群总体相比，试验参与者更年轻，更多的是曾经吸烟者，而不是现时吸烟者，并且受教育程度更高，有 32% 的志愿者具有至少 1 个大学学位。

结 果

3 轮筛选的每一轮，LDCT 组的阳性发现率均高于 X 线组。LDCT 检出的肺癌数为 1 060 处，X 线组检出 941 处，其中，LDCT 组的 367 处癌和胸部 X 线组的 525 处癌是在筛查结束后发生或者是筛查中未发现而在其后的几年内被诊断出来。之后胸部 X 线检出癌的数量更多，提示有些癌在 X 线片上漏诊了，而在 LDCT 上则不会漏诊。LDCT 组检出了更多的肺腺癌，尤其是贴壁为主的肺腺癌。LDCT 组第二和第三次筛查检出的 IV 期肺癌较少，所以关于治疗选择和预后有更好的分期分布[47]。

24% 的 CT 筛查结果提示肺癌，被归类为阳性筛查。这些病例中，96% 为假阳性筛查。此外，在 CT 组，在 39% 的参与者中至少有 1 个阳性 CT 结果。这些高阳性率引起了关于在总体人群中筛查有效性的担忧。NLST 肺癌筛查的成本效益目前正在审查，并可能回答这样的问题[47]。

CT 筛查诊断的癌症，52% 是 I A 期，11.2% 是 I B 期；而胸片筛查 33% 是 I A 期，15% 是 I B 期。CT 筛查的并发症非常低，只有 0.4%。总之，NLST 试验满足了有效试验的要求，这些项目正在全美国实施[47]。

LDCT 组的肺癌死亡人数较少，其肺癌特异性死亡率降低了 20%。在 LDCT 组，所有原因导致的死亡率均有所改善，与胸片组相比减少 6.7%。根据这些阳性结果，试验比原计划提前得出结论[47]。

正在进行的肺癌筛查试验和项目

世界范围内有一些 LDCT 的肺癌筛查试验。

试验人群、纳入和排除标准以及终点和随访量均不同。在欧洲，随机筛选研究包括荷兰和比利时的（Nederlands-Leuvens Longkanker Screening Onderzoek，NELSON）试验，丹麦肺癌筛查试验（the Danish Lung Cancer Screening Trial，DLCST），意大利的意大利肺癌 CT（Italian trials Italian Lung Cancer Computed Tomography，ITALUNG-Florence）、意大利多中心肺癌检测（Multicentric Italian Lung Detection，MILD）和 DANTE-Milan，以及德国的肺癌筛查干预（the German Lung Cancer Screening Interrention，LUSI）研究（评价多层 CT 检出肺癌有效性的欧洲试验的一部分）。在未来几年这些试验将公布最终结果[10,49]。法国的一项 X 线平片及 LDCT 筛查肺癌的预试验——Dépiscan，于 2007 年公布基线结果，为更大的 Grandepiscan 试验揭开序幕，有 20 000 人参与[49-50]。英国肺癌筛查（the United Kingdom Lung Cancer，UKLS）组正在进行包括 4 200 人参加的预试验，并将延续成为 10 年有 32 000 人参与的 UKLS 随机对照试验[51-52]。这些试验中的研究人员表示，所有的试验将继续，为了证实 NLST 的结果，并解决其他试验中许多关于理想目标人群、最佳方案和结果的处理，以及成本效益等方面的其他问题[52-53]。

在中国，研究者又出现了对胸部平片筛查肺癌新的兴趣[54-55]。胸部平片更容易操作，成本更低。最近的研究尝试通过将胸部平片与关于危险因素的详细自评调查问卷相结合来提高其准确性[54]，或与计算机辅助结节检测系统相结合[55]。在这两种情况下，都没有成熟的随访数据。

LDCT 肺癌筛查项目在日本已经存在了 10 年以上，经常由政府或雇主管理。雇主赞助的项目可能包括员工、退休人员和他们年龄在 50~69 岁的配偶，而其他项目是为社区居民提供的。吸烟史不是一个先决条件[56-57]。

美国的肺癌筛查建议

2012 年多个机构根据 NLST 阳性结果第一次发布了《肺癌筛查指南》。美国国家综合癌症网络（National Comprehensive Cancer Network，NCCN）建议对年龄在 55~74 岁、符合 NLST 纳入和排除标准的高危患者以及每年至少吸烟 20 包、伴有其他已知患肺癌危险因素中的一项、50 岁及以上的成年人每年进行 LDCT 筛查。NCCN 指南中筛查组不包括肺癌幸存者[58]。

NCCN 对中等危险或低度危险患者，即 2A 类患者不建议使用 LDCT 筛查肺癌。对年龄大于 50 岁，每年抽烟 20 包或者吸二手烟但没有其他危险因素者认为有中等危险；低度危险为年龄小于 50 岁和（或）每年吸烟小于 20 包[58]。

美国胸外科协会（American Association for Thoracic Surgery，AATS）在 2012 发表的指南有类似的建议，但将肺癌幸存者也作为高危人群纳入了筛查[59]。最高风险人群的一级指南是针对现时吸烟者或曾有每年 30 包吸烟史者，建议自 55 岁每年行 LDCT 筛查并持续到 79 岁。这被认为有 1 级证据支持[59]（图 10.1）。

AATS 肺癌幸存者 2 级指南建议肺癌治疗后没有复发或转移并且影像随访 4 年的患者每年行 LDCT 筛查。2 级指南也适用于年纪较轻、自 50 岁开始每年吸烟至少 20 包并且有使个体 5 年内患肺癌概率增加 5% 以上的其他因素的患者。风险因素包括环境或职业暴露、COPD、既往放射治疗或家族史。2 级指南得到了 2 级证据的支持，并得到 AATS 特别小组的一致同意[59]（图 10.2）。

其他机构也发布了建议，包括美国癌症协会（ACS）、美国肺脏协会（the American Lung Association，ALA）、美国胸科医师学会（the American College of Chest Physicians，ACCP）和美国临床肿瘤学会（the American Society of Clinical Oncology，ASCO）的联合建议。他们都采用了 NLST 的指导方针和建议，每年 LDCT 筛查只针对满足确切的 NLST 纳入和排除标准的高风险个人。此外，大多数这些机构建议，只能在能够为 NLST 参与者提供有经验的、多学科护理的中心筛选候选人[60]。

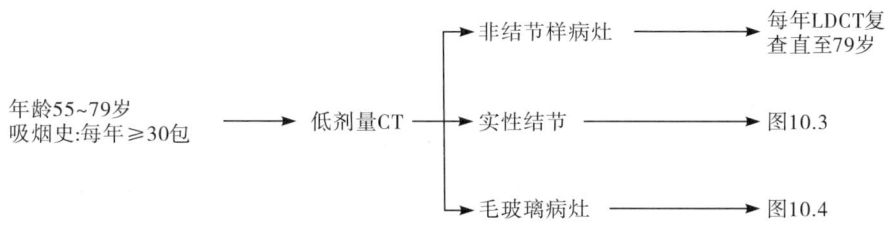

图 10.1 AATS 肺癌筛查指南 1 类最高风险

来源：经 Elsevier 许可，摘自 Jaklitsch MT, et al. The American for Thoracic Surgery guidelines for lung cancer screening using low-dose computed tomography scans for lung cancer survivors and other high-risk groups. J Thorac cardiovasc Surg, 2012, 144：35

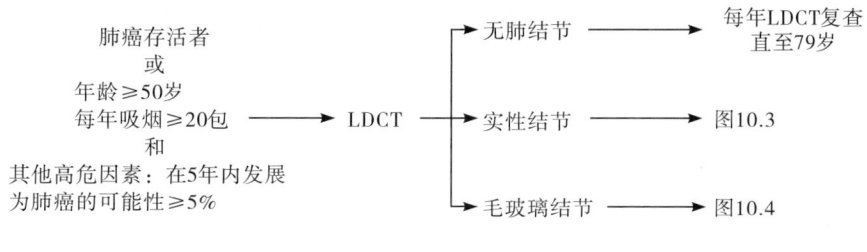

图 10.2 结合了风险与肺癌生存者的 AATS 肺癌筛查指南。CT：计算机体层摄影；LDCT：LDCT；COPD：慢性阻塞性肺疾病；FEV_1：第 1 秒用力呼气容积

来源：经 Elsevier 许可，摘自 Jaklitsch MT, et al. The American Association for Thoracic Surgery guidelines for lung cancer screening using low-dose computed tomography scans for lung cancer survivors and other high-risk groups. J Thorac Cardiovasc Surg, 2012, 144：35

结节的检出与处理

不管是在结节大小还是密度方面，LDCT 检出肺部异常的敏感性优于胸片[36]。对于直径小于 1cm 的结节 CT 显示更清晰，对于毛玻璃样结节、混合性毛玻璃样密度结节及实性结节也是如此。结节的恶变潜能与大小和密度相关。

小于 5mm 的非钙化实性结节的恶性概率小于 1%，直径 8～20mm 的结节的恶性概率为 18%，而直径大于 20mm 的实性结节的恶性概率为 50%[61]。随访间期结节增大是支持恶性病变的征象，尽管短时间内迅速增大也可能提示感染性病变。对于实性不确定性结节的随访方案已经得到确认[61-62]。Fleischner 学会推荐的有吸烟史的高危患者肺部结节≤4mm 者应当在基线检查之后 12 个月进行随访；如果结节无变化，就不必继续随访。对于结节直径＞(4～6)mm 者，如果无变化，分别在 6～12 个月和 18～24 个月随访。结节直径＞(6～8)mm 者应在 3～6 个月、9～12 个月及 24 个月时随访，明确两年内病变稳定。结节大于 8mm 患者的评估应在第 3、9 和 24 个月做 CT 和（或）动态灌注 CT，PET/CT 或活检[61]（见图 10.3 和图 10.4 的 AATS 结节处理指南）。

然而，整体而言，实性结节恶变可能性低，为 7%，毛玻璃结节为 18%。部分毛玻璃结节或部分实性结节恶变可能性最高，达 63%[16]。

越来越多的肺腺癌在 LDCT 上表现为毛玻璃样或部分实性结节，主要有 3 大类：①浸润前病变，与之相对应的是 Noguchi 分类 A 或 B 类肿瘤，包括 AAH 与 AIS；CT 表现从毛玻璃结节（ground glass nodules, GGO）到伴有内部肺泡塌陷的 GGO。许多这类病变倍增时间可长达两年（图 10.5）。②贴壁生长的 MIA 和浸润成分小于 5mm 的癌组织，常表现为伴有实性结节的 GGO。③所有亚型的浸润性腺癌（贴壁生长、腺泡状、乳头状、微乳头状），这些实性结节边缘可能有分叶、毛刺以及空气支气管征，与之对应的是 Noguchi C 类以及 D～F 类肿瘤[18,63]。

在影像随访期间直径持续大于10mm的纯GGO病变可能是AIS。对于这种病变，PET或CT检查结果往往为假阴性，针吸活检也容易出现取样误差。任何实性成分与GGO成分的混合性病变均是有潜在浸润性的恶性病变，建议及时处理[18,64]。基于病变的大小和密度，2013年Fleischner学会发布了以下建议：直径不超过5mm的纯GGO病变不需要随访；直径大于5mm的孤立性纯GGO病变需在3个月后复查CT，如果保持不变，应每年随访，至少3年；单发的实性成分直径大于5mm的部分实性结节应判定为恶性。如果怀疑有感染的可能，根据患者的危险因素，建议3个月后CT随访。当有多发GGO密度灶时，最初3个月的CT随访将确认是否为持续性GGO病变，然后根据占主导地位的病灶的特点进行处理[64]（见图10.3和10.4的AATS结节处理指南）。

过去30年间肺腺癌相对于肺鳞癌数量增多[65]，现在是北美最常见的组织学类型[66]。虽然与吸烟关系最密切的是肺鳞癌和小细胞肺癌（SCLC），但肺腺癌也与吸烟明显相关[67]。

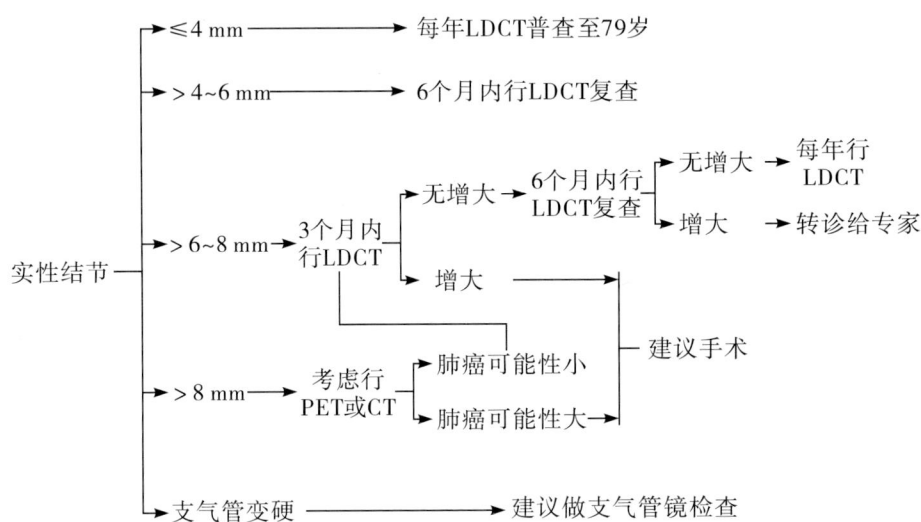

图10.3 AATS对LDCT上实性结节的肺癌筛查指南。PET或CT：正电子发射或计算机体层摄影
来源：经Elsevier许可，摘自Jaklitsch MT, et al. The American Association for Thoracic Surgery guidelines for lung cancer screening using low-dose computed tomography scans for lung cancer survivors and other high-risk groups. J Thorac Cardiovasc Surg, 2012, 144: 36

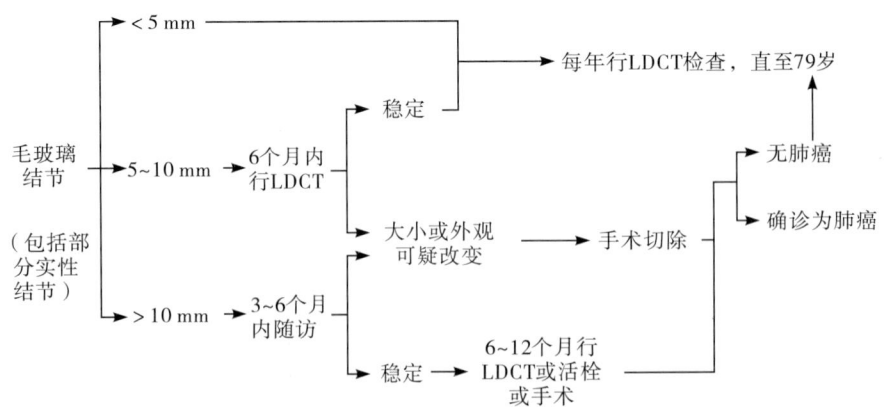

图10.4 AATS肺癌GGO筛查指南
来源：经Elsevier许可，摘自Jaklitsch MT, et al. The American Association for Thoracic Surgery guidelines for lung cancer screening using low-dose computed tomography scans for lung cancer survivors and other high-risk groups. J Thorac Cardiovasc Surg, 2012, 144: 36

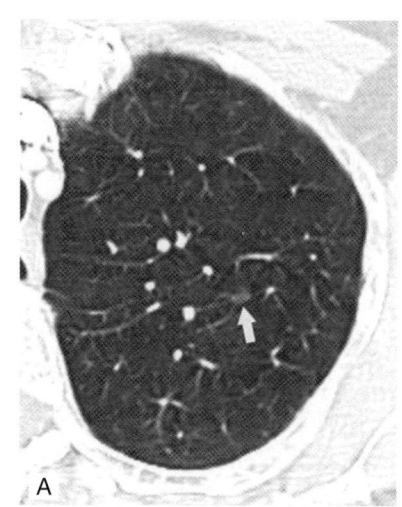
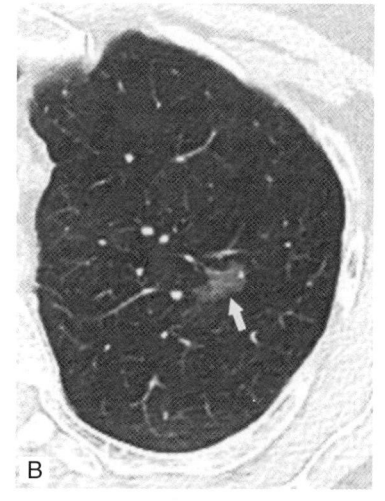

图 10.5 A. LDCT 肺窗显示左肺上叶 6mm 的 GGO（白箭头）。这个结节在普通胸部 X 线片上不能显示。B. 4 年后 LDCT 复查显示结节（白箭头）体积增大到 14×11mm。该患者做了左肺上叶切除，病理为中分化腺癌伴有明显的腺泡及鳞屑亚型

LDCT 筛查的风险

放射性风险

LDCT 筛查对患者每年检查的有效放射剂量约为 1.5mSv，低于美国每个人每年在日常活动中所累积的 3.5mSv 的平均背景辐射剂量。它可以和诊断性胸部 CT 比较，其有效辐射剂量是 8mSv，而 PET 或 CT 的有效辐射剂量为 14mSv[48]。

尽管单次 CT 检查对人所造成的致癌风险可以忽略，但是重复检查、患者的年龄和辐射的协同增效作用以及吸烟等因素却可能对相对危险度有影响[45,68]。使用 NLST 提供的数据得出的影响相关辐射增加癌症风险的模型预测显示，每 2500 例筛选者中有 1 例患癌症死亡[48]。高危人群每年筛查的辐射导致肺癌风险的预测表明，辐射导致的肺癌会使吸烟相关肺癌的人数增加：如果筛查从 50 岁开始，增加率为 1.8%；如果从 60 岁开始，该比为 0.8%[68]。由于辐射相关的癌变通常发生于受辐射后的 10~20 年，风险-效益比对于年轻人和低风险人群意义不大[48]。

心理学与检查程序风险

LDCT 发现的结节许多是良性的。据统计，超过 90% 的肺结节不是癌[48]。尽管如此，他们仍需要随访或明确诊断，并因此被归类为"阳性"发现。在一项研究中，一半的筛选参与者在等待 CT 结果时有恐惧和不适[69]。不确定的结果或者需要进一步检查可引起筛查参与者严重的焦虑情绪。

有创性诊断和治疗方法有致病和致死的风险。NLST 用 CT 筛查时的并发症发生率很低，只有 0.4%[47]。NLST 的调查结果包括 1.2% 的针吸活检或支气管镜检查、约 0.7% 行胸腔镜或开胸术或纵隔镜检查、未患肺癌的患者[48]。对于不是癌症的结节在诊断性干预之后，发生主要并发症或者死亡的风险为（4.1~4.5）/100 000 人。在筛查时肺癌患者手术的主要并发症发生率为 14%[48]。

LDCT 筛查的成本-效益

肺癌筛查计划的成本不仅包括 LDCT 的扫描成本，而且包括影像随访、诊断、治疗以及戒烟的服务成本。在美国大约有 700 万的高危吸烟者满足 NLST 标准，总计有 9 490 万的吸烟者和曾吸烟者。据估计在美国每年对 2 500 万名曾吸烟者进行 LDCT 筛查将花费 1 150 亿美元[70]。一些基于货币化估算寿命年和质量调整寿命年（quality-adjusted life year，QALY）的建模研究表明，LDCT 筛查才是提高成本-效益最好的方法，可使癌症死亡率下降超过 40%[45]。因此，建议只针对高危人群进行 CT 筛查[14]。筛查的参与率和依从性也将影响成本-效益比。

肺癌筛查与戒烟

医学界认为，戒烟计划和咨询在任何肺癌筛查计划中都应该被重视[58,60]。美国有5 490万主动吸烟者[71]。世界范围内，至少有13亿吸烟者[10]。就潜在及实际的筛查参与者的退出意愿，有研究发现了相互矛盾的证据[72-73]。尽管他们中的许多人在理论上都对戒烟服务感兴趣，但是一些研究发现高达1/5的吸烟者认为如果筛查结果阴性就无须担心，而继续吸烟[73-74]；还有3%的人表示，即使结果是阳性他们也将继续吸烟[73]。关于NELSON试验参与者的一项研究指出，虽然筛查结果不能确定需要随访的吸烟者会比阴性结果的吸烟者更努力地戒烟，但两年的随访结果显示戒烟率并没有统计学差异[75]。更多强化和综合性戒烟项目将是有益的[73]。

从试验到实践的转变

征 募

肺癌死亡率的改善和筛查成本-效益的提高依赖于对一个含有足够多的高危人群的成功筛查。对于乳腺癌和结直肠癌的大规模癌症筛查的经验揭示了一些患者方面或者是医疗保健机构方面的参与筛查的常见障碍[74]。肺癌筛查与普通的筛查不同，因为这种目标疾病与生活习惯关系更加密切，故肺癌筛查可能会增加吸烟者的抗拒态度。

虽然潜在的肺癌筛查在美国和其他国家的人群量是相当大的，但一些定性研究表明，主动吸烟者参与筛查的可能性小于预期[57,74,76]。一项报告显示只有23%的受访吸烟者认为他们有患肺癌的危险。吸烟者对肺癌表现出听天由命的态度，一般不理解早期检出和治疗会影响结果。一项调查显示，筛查试验的准确性对于吸烟者来说比不吸烟者更不重要，而试验成本对这两种人都很重要。对于LDCT筛查的误解包括预期会有疼痛和对于辐射引起癌症的恐惧，会对志愿者参与筛查的意愿产生不利影响。对于医疗服务提供者的不信任、焦虑和逃避行为也在抗拒筛查中起了一定作用[74,76]。

在一项在美国进行的研究中，大多数主动吸烟者为非白人、男性、受教育程度低并且是家中唯一的经济支柱。虽然他们有雇主提供的健康保险，但是比不吸烟者更可能没有指定的医疗保健机构。一部分人不太可能参加任何筛查，这正与这种人口结构相符合[57]。在英国，吸烟人群中有一个亚群很有趣，即中坚吸烟者。他们往往是白人、男性、年龄较大、受教育程度较低，为手工职业者和单身。他们不太相信吸烟会影响健康，更能抵抗社会戒烟的压力[77]。最近的一项研究评估了英国一个贫穷社区的社会营销宣传活动，专注于增强意识，即如果有持续性咳嗽症状应当去看医生并要求拍胸片。虽然干预的目的是促进肺癌的早期诊断并且这是针对50岁以上的男性吸烟者，但是在宣传材料中并没有特别提到癌症或者吸烟[6]。

既往吸烟者似乎更愿意参加筛查[57]，而且在NLST参与者中既往吸烟者比主动吸烟者略多一些[46]。在美国高风险人群是相当大的[71]。

从学术中心到社区医院

就像之前的许多肺癌筛查研究一样，NLST主要是在大型学术机构或以大学为基础的医疗中心开展的[44]，质量控制与结节处理算法也考虑在试验设计内[48]。研究由经过专科医师培训的放射科医生开展，手术均由经验丰富的外科和介入科医生完成，而且对患者的护理是在多学科团队合作下完成的。特别是，在试验范围内的手术并发症发生率显著低于其他报道[14,48]。若没有这些优势，很难开发出一种肺癌筛查方案，潜在的结果可能会受到影响。ACS在它的建议中提出了一条警告，即尽可能在一个有组织的肺癌筛查项目、有LDCT诊断经验以及有多学科临床专家的机构进行肺癌筛查[60]。

总 结

第一次有证据表明，LDCT筛查将减少肺癌死亡专率。虽然有些问题仍需要回答，目前的指导方针建议对某些高危人群进行筛查。努力协调和教育符合条件的主动吸烟者，可能有利于招募到足够的受试者。最后，应强调戒烟和预防的重要性。

（徐亮　黄勇译）

参考文献

[1] Cancer Fact Sheet N 297. World Health Organization, 2013. [2013-02-15]. http://www.who.int/ediacentre/factsheets/fs297/en/#.

[2] Siegel R, Naishadham D, Jemal A. Cancer statistics, 2013. CA: a Cancer Journal for Clinicians, 2013, 63: 11-30.

[3] Siegel R, Naishadham D, Jemal A. Cancer statistics, 2012. CA: a Cancer Journal for Clinicians, 2012, 62: 10-29.

[4] Malvezzi M, Bertuccio P, Levi F, et al. European cancer mortality predictions for the year 2013. Ann Oncol, 2013, 24 (3): 792-800, published online Feb. 12, 2013; doi: 10.1093/annonc/mdt010.

[5] Coleman MP, Forman D, Bryant H, et al. Cancer survival in Australia, Canada, Denmark, Norway, Sweden, and the UK, 1995-2007 (the International Cancer Benchmarking Partnership): An analysis of population-based cancer registry data. Lancet, 2011, 377: 127-138.

[6] Athey VL, Suckling RJ, Tod AM, et al. Early diagnosis of lung cancer: Evaluation of a community-based social marketing intervention. Thorax, 2012, 67: 412-417.

[7] Jemal A, Center MM, DeSantis C, et al. Global patterns of cancer incidence and mortality rates and trends. Cancer Epidemiol Biomarkers Prev, 2010, 19: 1893-1907.

[8] Patz EF, Jr., Black WC, Goodman PC. CT screening for lung cancer: not ready for routine practice. Radiology, 2001, 221: 587-591; discussion 98-99.

[9] Herbst RS, Heymach JV, Lippman SM. Lung cancer. New England Journal of Medicine, 2008, 359: 1367-1380.

[10] Jacobson FL, Jaklitsch MT. Lung cancer screening trials: The United States and beyond. Journal of Thoracic and Cardiovascular Surgery, 2012, 144: S3-S6.

[11] Lee JM. Screening issues for radiologists. Academic Radiology, 2004, 11: 162-168.

[12] Hulka BS. Cancer screening. Degrees of proof and practical application. Cancer, 1988, 62: 1776-1780.

[13] Stiles BM, Altorki NK, Yankelevitz DF. Screening for lung cancer: Challenges for thoracic surgery//Shields TW, Lo Cicero J, Reed CE, et al (eds). General Thoracic Surgery. 7th edn. Philadelphia: Wolters Kluwer Health/Lippincott Williams & Wilkins, 2009: 1299-1306.

[14] Ganti AK, Mulshine JL. Lung cancer screening. Oncologist, 2006, 11: 481-487.

[15] Henschke CI, Sone S, Markowitz S. International Early Lung Cancer Action Project (I-ELCAP): evaluation of low-dose CT screening//Proceedings of the Annual Meeting of the Radiologic Society of North America. Chicago, Illinois, 2004.

[16] Henschke CI, Wisnivesky JP, Yankelevitz DF, et al. Small stage I cancers of the lung: Genuineness and curability. Lung Cancer, 2003, 39: 327-330.

[17] Bianchi F, Hu J, Pelosi G, et al. Lung cancers detected by screening with spiral computed tomography have a malignant phenotype when analyzed by cDNA microarray. Clinical Cancer Research, 2004 (10): 6023-6028.

[18] Godoy MC, Naidich DP. Subsolid pulmonary nodules and the spectrum of peripheral adenocarcinomas of the lung: Recommended interim guidelines for assessment and management. Radiology, 2009, 253: 606-622.

[19] Hestbech MS, Siersma V, Dirksen A, et al. Participation bias in a randomized trial of screening for lung cancer. Lung Cancer, 2011, 73: 325-331.

[20] Doll R, Hill AB. Smoking and carcinoma of the lung; preliminary report. Br Med J, 1950, 2: 739-748.

[21] Boucot KR, Carnahan W, Cooper DA, et al. Philadelphia pulmonary neoplasm research project; preliminary report. J Am Med Assoc, 1955, 157: 440-444.

[22] Brett GZ. The value of lung cancer detection by six-monthly chest radiographs. Thorax, 1968, 23: 414-420.

[23] Frost JK, Ball WC, Jr., Levin ML, et al. Early lung cancer detection: Results of the initial (prevalence) radiologic and cytologic screening in the Johns Hopkins study. American Review of Respiratory Disease, 1984, 130: 549-554.

[24] Melamed MR, Flehinger BJ, Zaman MB, et al. Screening for early lung cancer. Results of the Memorial Sloan-Kettering study in New York. Chest, 1984, 86: 44-53.

[25] Marcus PM, Bergstralh EJ, Fagerstrom RM, et al. Lung cancer mortality in the Mayo Lung Project: Impact of extended follow-up. Journal of the National Cancer Institute, 2000, 92: 1308-1316.

[26] Kubik A, Polak J. Lung cancer detection: Results of a randomized prospective study in Czechoslovakia. Cancer, 1986, 57: 2427-2437.

[27] Strauss GM. The Mayo Lung Cohort: A regression analy-

sis focusing on lung cancer incidence and mortality. Journal of Clinical Oncology, 2002, 20: 1973 – 1983.

[28] Sagawa M, Nakayama T, Tsukada H, et al. The efficacy of lung cancer screening conducted in 1990s: Four case-control studies in Japan. Lung Cancer, 2003, 41: 29 – 36.

[29] Sone S, Nakayama T, Honda T, et al. Long-term follow-up study of a population-based 1996 – 1998 mass screening programme for lung cancer using mobile low-dose spiral computed tomography. Lung Cancer, 2007, 58: 329 – 341.

[30] Nakayama T, Baba T, Suzuki T, et al. An evaluation of chest X-ray screening for lung cancer in gunma prefecture, Japan: A population based case-control study. Eur J Cancer, 2002, 38: 1380 – 1387.

[31] Quekel LG, Kessels AG, Goei R, et al. Miss rate of lung cancer on the chest radiograph in clinical practice. Chest, 1999, 115: 720 – 724.

[32] Ko JP. Lung nodule detection and characterization with multi-slice CT. Journal of Thoracic Imaging, 2005, 20: 196 – 209.

[33] Sone S, Li F, Yang ZG, et al. Results of three year mass screening programme for lung cancer using mobile low-dose spiral computed tomography scanner. British Journal of Cancer, 2001, 84: 25 – 32.

[34] Kaneko M, Eguchi K, Ohmatsu H, et al. Peripheral lung cancer: Screening and detection with low-dose spiral CT versus radiography. Radiology, 1996, 201: 798 – 802.

[35] Nawa T, Nakagawa T, Kusano S, et al. Lung cancer screening using low-dose spiral CT: results of baseline and 1 – year follow-up studies. Chest, 2002, 122: 15 – 20.

[36] Henschke CI. Early lung cancer action project: Overall design and findings from baseline screening. Cancer, 2000, 89: 2474 – 2482.

[37] Henschke CI, Naidich DP, Yankelevitz DF, et al. Early lung cancer action project: initial findings on repeat screenings. Cancer, 2001, 92: 153 – 159.

[38] Swensen SJ, Jett JR, Hartman TE, et al. CT screening for lung cancer: five-year prospective experience. Radiology, 2005, 235: 259 – 265.

[39] Starnes SL, Reed MF, Meyer CA, et al. Can lung cancer screening by computed tomography be effective in areas with endemic histoplasmosis? Journal of Thoracic and Cardiovascular Surgery, 2011, 141: 688 – 693.

[40] Bach PB, Jett JR, Pastorino U, et al. Computed tomography screening and lung cancer outcomes. JAMA: The Journal of the American Medical Association, 2007, 297: 953 – 961.

[41] Prorok PC, Andriole GL, Bresalier RS, et al. Design of the Prostate, Lung, Colorectal and Ovarian (PLCO) cancer screening trial. Controlled Clinical Trials, 2000, 21: 273S – 309S.

[42] Oken MM, Hocking WG, Kvale PA, et al. Screening by chest radiograph and lung cancer mortality: The Prostate, Lung, Colorectal, and Ovarian (PLCO) randomized trial. JAMA, 2011, 306: 1865 – 1873.

[43] Gierada DS, Garg K, Nath H, et al. CT quality assurance in the lung screening study component of the National Lung Screening Trial: Implications for multicenter imaging trials. American Journal of Roentgenology, 2009, 193: 419 – 424.

[44] Aberle DR, Berg CD, Black WC, et al. The National Lung Screening Trial: overview and study design. Radiology, 2011, 258: 243 – 253.

[45] Chiles C. Lung cancer screening: achieving areduction in mortality. Seminars in Roentgenology, 2011, 46: 230 – 240.

[46] Aberle DR, Adams AM, Berg CD, et al. Baseline characteristics of participants in the randomized national lung screening trial. Journal of the National Cancer Institute, 2010, 102: 1771 – 1779.

[47] Aberle DR, Adams AM, Berg CD, et al. Reduced lung-cancer mortality with low-dose computed tomographic screening. New England Journal of Medicine, 2011, 365: 395 – 409.

[48] Bach PB, Mirkin JN, Oliver TK, et al. Benefits and harms of CT screening for lung cancer: A systematic review. JAMA, 2012, 307: 2418 – 2429.

[49] Nair A, Hansell DM. European and North American lung cancer screening experience and implications for pulmonary nodule management. European Radiology, 2011, 21: 2445 – 2454.

[50] Blanchon T, Brechot JM, Grenier PA, et al. Baseline results of the Depiscan study: A French randomized pilot trial of lung cancer screening comparing low dose CT scan (LDCT) and chest X-ray (CXR). Lung Cancer, 2007, 58: 50 – 58.

[51] Baldwin DR, Duffy SW, Wald NJ, et al. UK Lung Screen (UKLS) nodule management protocol: modelling of a single screen randomised controlled trial of low-dose CT screening for lung cancer. Thorax, 2011, 66: 308 – 313.

[52] Field JK, Baldwin D, Brain K, et al. CT screening for lung cancer in the UK: position statement by UKLS investigators

following the NLST report. Thorax, 2011, 66: 736-737.

[53] The European Lung Cancer Trials. The PISA Position Statement//State of the Art in Europe after Early Conclusion of the US National Lung Screening Trial: The European Lung Cancer Trials; March 4, 2011. Pisa, Italy.

[54] Chen B, Wang Y, Cao H, et al. Early lung cancer detection using the self-evaluation scoring questionnaire and chest digital radiography: A 3-year follow-up study in China. Journal of Digital Imaging, 2013, 26: 72-81.

[55] Xu Y, Ma D, He W. Assessing the use of digital radiography and a real-time interactive pulmonary nodule analysis system for large population lung cancer screening. European Journal of Radiology, 2012, 81: e451-e456.

[56] Nawa T, Nakagawa T, Mizoue T, et al. Longterm prognosis of patients with lung cancer detected on low-dose chest computed tomography screening. Lung Cancer, 2012, 75: 197-202.

[57] Silvestri GA, Nietert PJ, Zoller J, et al. Attitudes towards screening for lung cancer among smokers and their nonsmoking counterparts. Thorax, 2007, 62: 126-130.

[58] Wood DE, Eapen GA, Ettinger DS, et al. Lung cancer screening. Journal of the National Comprehensive Cancer Network, 2012, 10: 240-265.

[59] Jaklitsch MT, Jacobson FL, Austin JH, et al. The American Association for Thoracic Surgery guidelines for lung cancer screening using low-dose computed tomography scans for lung cancer survivors and other high-risk groups. The Journal of Thoracic and Cardiovascular Surgery, 2012, 144: 33-38.

[60] Wender R, Fontham ET, Barrera E, Jr., et al. American Cancer Society lung cancer screening guidelines. CA: a Cancer Journal for Clinicians, 2013, 63: 106-117.

[61] MacMahon H, Austin JH, Gamsu G, et al. Guidelines for management of small pulmonary nodules detected on CT scans: a statement from the Fleischner Society. Radiology, 2005, 237: 395-400.

[62] Stiles BM, Altorki NK. Screening for lung cancer: challenges for the thoracic surgeon. Surgical Oncology Clinics of North America, 2011, 20: 619-635.

[63] Travis WD, Brambilla E, Noguchi M, et al. International Association for the Study of Lung Cancer/American Thoracic Society/European Respiratory Society international multidisciplinary classification of lung adenocarcinoma. Journal of Thoracic Oncology, 2011, 6: 244-285.

[64] Naidich DP, Bankier AA, MacMahon H, et al. Recommendations for the management of subsolid pulmonary nodules detected at CT: A statement from the Fleischner Society. Radiology, 2013, 266: 304-317.

[65] Hoffmann D, Djordjevic MV, Hoffmann I. The changing cigarette. Preventive Medicine, 1997, 26: 427-434.

[66] Li YJ, Tsai YC, Chen YC, et al. Humanpapilloma virus and female lung adenocarcinoma. Seminars in Oncology, 2009, 36: 542-552.

[67] Yang P, Cerhan JR, Vierkant RA, et al. Adenocarcinoma of the lung is strongly associated with cigarette smoking: Further evidence from a prospective study of women. American Journal of Epidemiology, 2002, 156: 1114-1122.

[68] Brenner DJ. Radiation risks potentially associated with low-dose CT screening of adult smokers for lung cancer. Radiology, 2004, 231: 440-445.

[69] van den Bergh KA, Essink-Bot ML, Bunge EM, et al. Impact of computed tomography screening for lung cancer on participants in a randomized controlled trial (NELSON trial). Cancer, 2008, 113: 396-404.

[70] Mahadevia PJ, Fleisher LA, Frick KD, et al. Lung cancer screening with helical computed tomography in older adult smokers: A decision and cost-effectiveness analysis. JAMA, 2003, 289: 313-322.

[71] Patel JD. Lung cancer in women. Journal of Clinical Oncology, 2005, 23: 3212-3218.

[72] Schnoll RA, Bradley P, Miller SM, et al. Psychological issues related to the use of spiral CT for lung cancer early detection. Lung Cancer, 2003, 39: 315-325.

[73] Schnoll RA, Miller SM, Unger M, et al. Characteristics of female smokers attending a lung cancer screening program: A pilot study with implications for program development. Lung Cancer, 2002, 37: 257-265.

[74] Jonnalagadda S, Bergamo C, Lin JJ, et al. Beliefs and attitudes about lung cancer screening among smokers. Lung Cancer, 2012, 77: 526-531.

[75] van der Aalst CM, van den Bergh KA, Willemsen MC, et al. Lung cancer screening and smoking abstinence: 2 year follow-up data from the Dutch-Belgian randomised controlled lung cancer screening trial. Thorax, 2010, 65: 600-605.

[76] Patel D, Akporobaro A, Chinyanganya N, et al. Attitudes to participation in a lung cancer screening trial: a qualitative study. Thorax, 2012, 67: 418-425.

[77] Jarvis MJ, Wardle J, Waller J, et al. Prevalence of hardcore smoking in England, and associated attitudes and beliefs: cross sectional study. BMJ, 2003, 326: 1061.

第 11 章
肺癌影像学

Sonia L. Betancourt Cuellar, Edith M. Marom, Jeremy J. Erasmus
Department of Diagnostic Radiology, The University of Texas MD Anderson Cancer Center, Houston, TX, USA

引 言

影像学检查对非小细胞肺癌（NSCLC）的检测、诊断、分期、预后评估及监测肿瘤复发有重要作用。NSCLC 初诊时，我们常对其进行包括影像学在内的综合评估来明确肿瘤的进展程度。目前临床上采用第 7 版的美国癌症联合委员会（the American Joint Committee on Cancer, AJCC）TNM 分期系统[1-3]对 NSCLC 进行分期。本章节对 CT、MRI、FDG-PET 在 NSCLC 患者评估中的应用价值进行综述。

原发肿瘤的影像学评估（T）

原发肿瘤是依据其大小、部位和对局部的侵犯范围来描述的（表 11.1）。尽管胸部 X 线片对原发肿瘤的评估及检测胸腔内转移有一定作用，但 CT 检查对判断肿瘤对胸壁、纵隔、横膈的侵犯以及淋巴结转移、肺转移更可靠。需要强调的是，第 7 版 AJCC 的 T 分期系统中，对原发肿瘤的准确定义为：T1a（≤2cm）；T1b（>2cm，≤3cm）；T2a（>3cm，≤5cm）；T2b（>5cm，≤7cm）；T3 >7cm。并且指出，CT 为诊断原发肿瘤最理想的影像学检查方法。因此，相对较差的空间分辨率限制了 MR 和 PET 在评估原发灶方面的应用。另外，由于其广泛的实用性及经常用来指导 [如纵隔镜检查、支气管内镜超声（endobronchial ultrasound, EBUS）活检] 侵入性活检，并且能够指导外科手术采取合适的处理方法，因此 CT 普遍应用于 NSCLC 患者的病情评估。

尽管 CT 在确定肿瘤 T 分期方面具有较大价值，但在评估患者的病情时仍具有一定的缺陷。在这一点上，CT 和 MR 有利于确定较明显的胸壁（T3）及纵隔（T4）侵犯，但在显示其周围邻近解剖结构及微观浸润方面仍不够准确（图 11.1、11.2）。值得注意的是，尽管 T4 期的患者通常不能手术，但对于一些心脏、气管和椎体受侵、局部淋巴结无转移或仅同侧肺门淋巴结转移的患者，仍有手术治疗的可能。在这些认为可行外科手术治疗的患者中，MR 在显示椎体、大血管、心包及心脏的受侵程度方面，可作为 CT 重要的补充。另外，鉴于突出的软组织分辨力和多维的成像能力，MR 尤其适用于肺上沟癌的病情评估（图 11.3）[4-6]。MR 常应用于评测肺上沟癌对臂丛神经、锁骨下血管及椎体的侵犯程度[4-5]，重要的是对绝对手术禁忌证（对臂丛神经干或根的侵犯高于 T1 水平，侵犯 50% 以上的椎体，侵犯食管和气管）往往能够准确评估[7-8]。

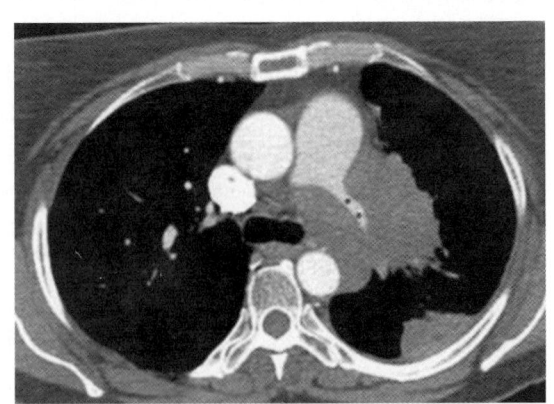

图 11.1 女性，54 岁，NSCLC 伴有纵隔侵犯，其增强 CT 显示有一较大、边界欠清的肿块包绕左肺动脉干并致其狭窄。纵隔侵犯定义为 T4，且不能手术切除。邻近胸膜的片状阴影为阻塞性炎症

除了评测原发肿瘤，T 分期的描述也能区分孤立性肺癌和伴有另外肺结节的肺癌。鉴于最近 AJCC 分期系统进行了修改，是否伴发肺结节及其位置可改变其 T 分期。特别指出的是，如果伴发的肺结节与原发灶位于同一肺叶，T 分期归为 T3；如果在同侧肺而不在同一肺叶，分期属于 T4；如果在对侧肺内，则属于 M1a。相对于 MR 与 PET，CT 的空间分辨力更高，更适用于肺组织及肺内转移的检查，尤其对肺内小病灶的检出效果更佳。尽管 CT 在检出肺结节方面起着重要作用，但是第 7 版 AJCC 将对侧的单一结节或多种结节均描述为 M1a。并且，肺内孤立性肿瘤及伴发的小结节可能是同时发生的多原发癌，或为原发肿瘤伴有肺转移（图 11.4）。就这一点而言，拥有 M1a 分期肺内单一的小结节（假设被看作双原发而不是转移）且无淋巴结转移的患者与肺内卫星灶与原发肿瘤（T3）在同一叶或不同叶（T4）行手术治疗后的患者，拥有相同的生存期[9]。

淋巴结的局部影像学（N）

淋巴结有无转移及转移位置在决定 NSCLC 患者的处理中起着重要作用（表 11.1）[2]。影像学评估淋巴结是否转移时，淋巴结的短径 >1cm 在胸片、CT 或 MR 中被认为异常。胸片对于淋巴结

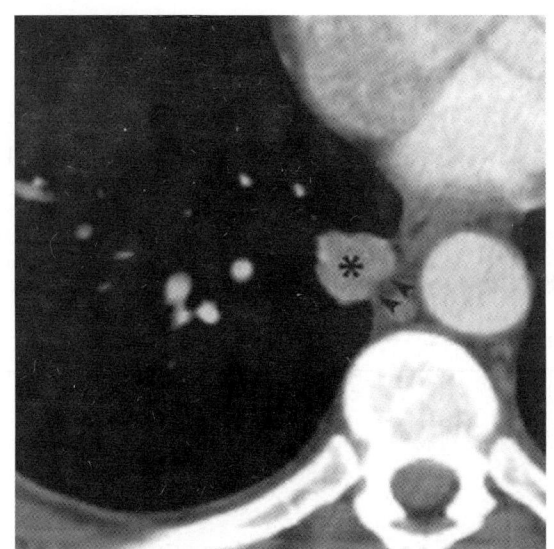

图 11.2　女性，54 岁，NSCLC 患者，慢性咳嗽病史，其增强 CT 示右肺下叶的结节与邻近胸膜紧贴。需注意该结节与邻近胸膜分界不清（箭头所示），会增加胸膜局部受侵的可能性，手术证实无胸膜侵犯

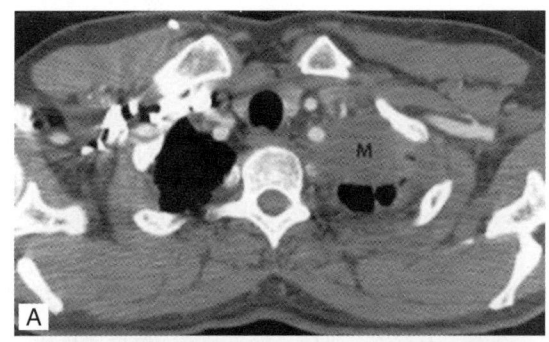

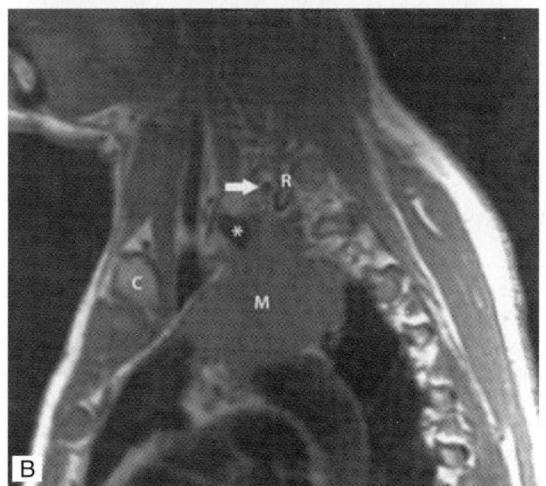

图 11.3　男性，47 岁，肺上沟癌（NSCLC）患者，有肩痛病史。A. 增强 CT 显示位于肺尖的肿块，无肋骨及椎体受侵。B. 矢状位的 MRI 显示肺上沟瘤（M），清晰显示邻近锁骨下动脉（*）及 C_8 神经根（箭头）。MR 可准确评估臂丛神经是否受侵，因此图显示 C_8 神经根没有受侵，所以该患者可行手术切除。C 为锁骨，R 为第一肋骨

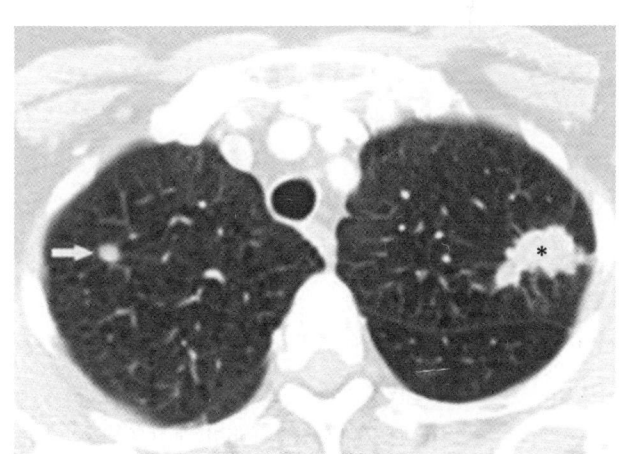

图 11.4　女性，66 岁，无任何症状，双肺均为鳞癌。增强 CT 显示左肺上叶结节（*）及右肺上叶结节（箭头），尽管分期为 M1a（不能行手术治疗），对其左肺上叶进行了切除手术，对右肺的恶性肿瘤进行了立体定向放疗。需注意的是分期定为 M1a 提示预后可能比预期更差

转移评测的特异度及灵敏度均不高。尽管 CT 和 MRI 对淋巴结是否转移的检测更优，但淋巴结的大小与转移之间没有明确的相关性，例如，增大的淋巴结可能是增生性反应，而一些小的淋巴结也可能转移。就此而言，Prenzel 报道了 256 例 NSCLC 患者的 2 891 个行手术切除的肺门及纵隔淋巴结：139 例无淋巴结转移的患者中，77% 的患者至少有 1 个淋巴结的直径 >1cm；而 127 例有淋巴结转移的患者中，12% 的患者淋巴结直径 ≤ 1cm[10]。Toloza 的一篇 meta 分析中指出了 CT 在评估 NSCLC 患者淋巴结转移方面的缺陷：对 3 438 例患者的评估中，总灵敏度为 57%，特异度为 82%，阳性预测值为 56%，阴性预测值为 83%[11]。

表 11.1 TNM 分期描述

原发肿瘤 T 分期	
Tx	原发肿瘤大小无法测量，或痰脱落细胞、支气管冲洗液中找到癌细胞，但影像学检查和支气管镜检查未发现原发肿瘤
T0	没有原发肿瘤的证据
Tis	原位癌
T1	肿瘤最大直径 ≤3cm，周围包绕肺组织及脏层胸膜，支气管镜见肿瘤侵犯叶支气管，未侵犯主支气管
T1a	原发肿瘤最大直径 ≤2cm
T1b	2cm < 原发肿瘤最大直径 ≤3cm
T2	3cm < 肿瘤最大直径 ≤5cm；侵犯主支气管（不常见的表浅扩散型肿瘤，不论体积大小，侵犯限于支气管壁时，虽可能侵犯主支气管，仍为 T1），但未侵及隆突；侵及脏层胸膜；有阻塞性肺炎或者部分肺不张。符合以上任何一个条件即归为 T2
T2a	3cm < 最大直径 ≤5cm
T2b	5cm < 最大直径 ≤7cm
T3	任何大小肿瘤有以下情况之一者：原发肿瘤最大直径 >7cm，累及胸壁或横膈或纵隔胸膜、支气管（距隆突 <2cm，但未及隆突）、心包；发生全肺不张或阻塞性肺炎；原发肿瘤同一肺叶出现卫星结节
T4	任何大小的肿瘤，侵犯以下器官之一者：心脏、气管、食管、大血管、纵隔、喉返神经、隆突或椎体；原发肿瘤同侧不同肺叶出现卫星结节
区域淋巴结 N 分期	
Nx	淋巴结转移情况无法评估
N0	无区域淋巴结转移
N1	同侧支气管或肺门或肺内淋巴结转移，包括直接浸润的淋巴结
N2	同侧纵隔和（或）隆突下淋巴结转移
N3	对侧纵隔和（或）对侧肺门，和（或）同侧或对侧前斜角肌或锁骨上区淋巴结转移
远处转移 M 分期	
M0	无远处转移
M1	远处转移
	M1a 原发肿瘤对侧肺叶出现卫星结节及胸膜播散（恶性胸腔积液、心包积液或胸膜结节）
	M1b 有远处转移（肺或胸膜除外）

说明：①任何大小的少见的表浅播散的肿瘤，只要其浸润范围局限于支气管壁，即使邻近主支气管，也定义为 T1a。②肿瘤大小 ≤5cm 或者大小无法确定的 T2 期肿瘤定义为 T2a，5cm < T2b 为肿瘤直径 <7cm。③大多数肺癌患者的胸腔积液（心包积液）由肿瘤引起，但有少数患者的胸腔积液（心包积液）多次细胞病理检查为阴性，非血性液，亦非渗出液。综合考虑以上因素，并确定与肿瘤无关时，积液将不作为分期依据，患者按照 T1、T2、T3、T4 进行分期

FDG-PET 在评估 NSCLC 中的应用越来越广泛，并且可提高淋巴结转移的检出率（图 11.5）。在一篇比较 PET 和 CT 对于 NSCLC 患者淋巴结分期的 meta 分析中，FDG-PET 对于淋巴结检查的特异度和灵敏度分别为 66%～100%（平均 83%）和 81%～100%（平均 92%），而 CT 检查的特异度和灵敏度分别为 20%～81%（平均 59%）和 44%～100%（平均 78%）。由于 NSCLC 患者的手术及新辅助治疗依赖于其 N 分期，因此对于 CT 检查无远处转移的患者均应行 PET 或 CT 检查[12-13]。

目前，FDG-PET 图像通常与 CT 图像融合扫描（而不是 PET 和 CT 分开扫描）。PET-CT 图像融合扫描可对局部 FDG 高摄取区域进行准确解剖定位，并且对肺门、纵隔及锁骨上淋巴结的 FDG 高摄取的定性有价值[14]。然而，在评估淋巴结是否转移时常会遇到这样的窘境：两幅图像显示不一致，例如 CT 所显示的增大淋巴结在 PET 图像上没有 FDG 高摄取，或者 CT 图像上的小淋巴结，PET 图像显示高摄取，在遇到这种 PET-CT 图像对淋巴结显示不一致的情况下，de Langen 关于淋巴结大小、FDG 高摄取区域以及病理的相关性报道可能有助于我们对这种情况的理解[15]：在一些 NSCLC 患者中，CT 显示淋巴结较小而 PET 显示高摄取时，分期为 N2 的概率为 62%；而当淋巴结直径 > 16mm，但 PET 无高摄取时，这一概率仅为 21%（图 11.6）；另外，当两者图像显示一致，即 PET 所示高代谢淋巴结，CT 亦显示增大时，概率为 90%。因此，由于 FDG-PET 在淋巴结评估方面的

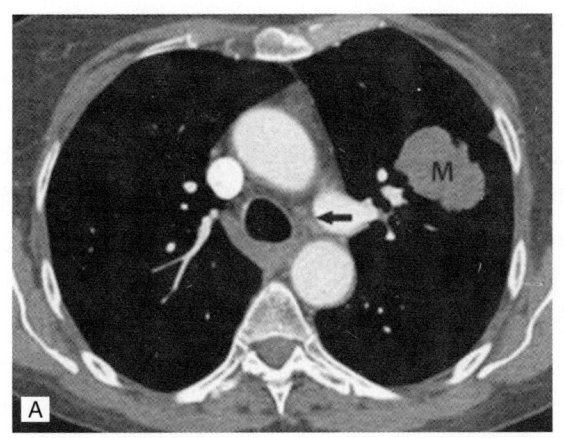
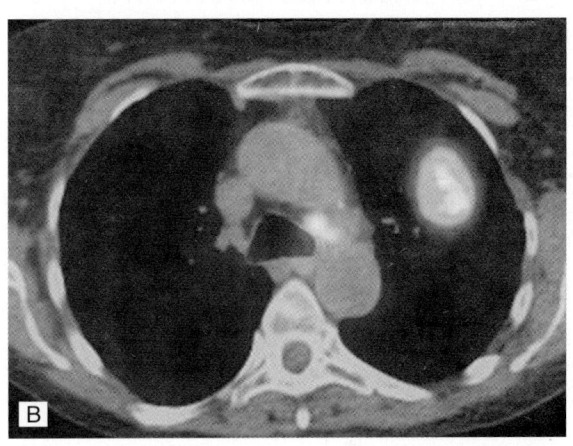

图 11.5 女性，58 岁，初步评估为可行手术切除的左肺上叶 NSCLC。A. CT 显示左肺上叶肿块（M）和同侧纵隔短径 < 1cm 的淋巴结（箭头）。B. 横轴位 PET 显示 FDG 高代谢的肿块及左下支气管旁的高摄取淋巴结。组织学检查显示该淋巴结转移，并且该患者的治疗方案修正为术前行辅助化疗

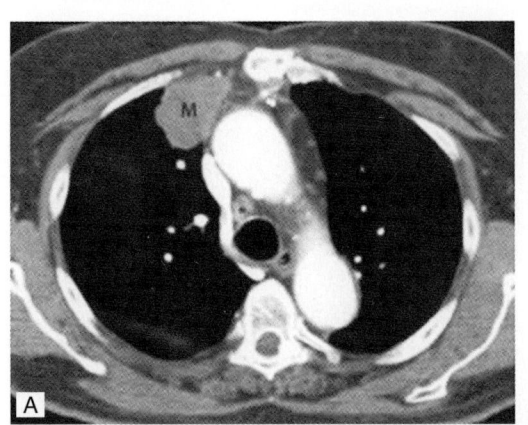
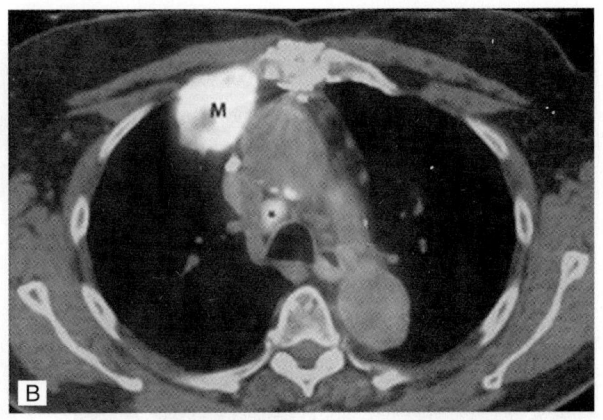

图 11.6 男性，78 岁，右肺上叶 NSCLC，初步评估可手术治疗。A. CT 显示右肺上叶的肿块和同侧纵隔短径 < 1cm 的淋巴结（*）。B. 横轴位的 PET 或 CT 显示位于右肺上叶 FDG 高摄取的肿块及右下气管旁同样高摄取的淋巴结（*）。组织学检查显示该淋巴结没有转移，患者可行手术切除。注意：对 NSCLC 患者，CT 显示的小淋巴结但 PET 高摄取，淋巴结转移概率为 62%

角色还未准确界定,FDG-PET 可用于指导淋巴结的侵入性采样,而不是作为侵入性手段的淋巴结分期替代检查。

远处转移的影像学特征(M)

NSCLC 常伴发对侧肺结节、胸膜结节、恶性胸腔或心包积液以及胸腔外的转移。然而,各种影像学检查手段在检测这些转移方面的作用并没有明确,通常一致的意见是:胸部 CT 为探测胸腔内或胸腔外转移的初级影像学检查,这一检查应常规包括肾上腺。在 CT 评估胸腔内的转移时(M1a),常见恶性胸腔积液,胸膜增厚或胸膜结节常提示转移,然而,即使没有胸膜增厚及胸膜结节,也不能除外胸膜转移。因此,仅依靠 CT 表现诊断胸膜转移比较困难。一些报道也指出,FDG-PET 对 NSCLC 患者胸腔积液的评估有一定价值[16-18]。然而,需要强调的是,FDG-PET 是 NSCLC 分期工具的一部分,而不是专门用于 NSCLC 患者胸腔积液的评估。

肾上腺病灶在 CT 或 MR 上表现典型。平扫 CT 所示低密度肾上腺结节或肿块(≤10HU)诊断为富含脂质的腺瘤,而高密度者则不易确定(图 11.7)[19]。不能明确诊断的肾上腺结节或肿块的进一步评估需要运用 MRI(化学位移分析或动态钆增强扫描)或增强 CT(肾上腺的强化及廓清)[20-21]。然而,近期的一项 meta 分析表明,FDG-PET 对于区分肾上腺结节的良恶性方面具有更高的敏感性和特异性,并且不需要再行其他影像学检查来进一步评估[22]。事实上,对于可能行手术切除的 NSCLC 患者,如果 PET 图像显示肾上腺 FDG 摄取正常,可以考虑对患者行根治性手术治疗,而不需要进一步的评估。如果肾上腺肿块在 PET 图像上显示 FDG 高摄取,则需要活检来明确是否转移。

与肾上腺的评估相比,影像学检查在检测其他器官,如肝脏、脑和骨的隐匿性转移方面存在更多变数。对于肺内局部晚期而无法手术或伴有其他脏器转移的 NSCLC,常会发生肝转移[23]。一项 meta 分析研究了影像学检查对一些没有出现相应症状的 NSCLC 患者的价值,仅有 3% 检测出了肝转移,对于肝脏的常规检查往往没有执行[24]。另外,尽管 FDG-PET 对于肝转移检测的特异度高,但灵敏度较低,因此不推荐 FDG-PET。

对于隐匿性脑转移的影像学检查目前尚存在争议。对于不具有神经症状的 NSCLC 患者,常规的神经学检查具有高的阴性预测值(79%~100%),并且仅有 0~10% 的患者的隐匿性脑转移可被 CT 或 MR 检测出[25]。然而,对于有神经症状的 NSCLC 患者,特别是对于腺癌患者,发生脑转移的可能性要比预期高[26]。另外,因为大脑常为转移的唯一部位,有将近 1/3 的患者病灶局限,具备手术机会,我们提议在 NSCLC 患者的初期分期评估中,将颅脑检查列为常规[27]。对于脑转移的影像学检查的重要性存在分歧可能归结于临床尚缺乏统一的实践指南。就这一点而言,美国胸部

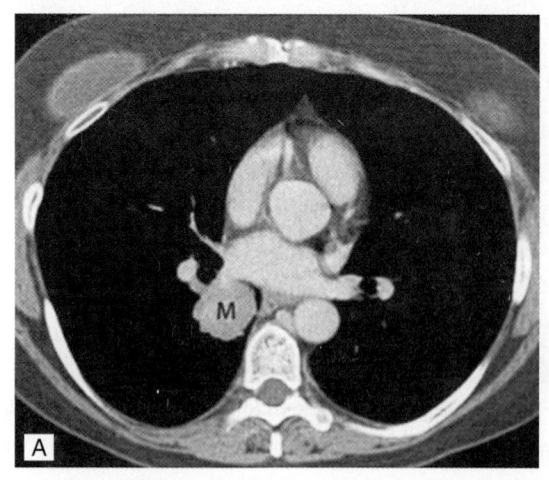
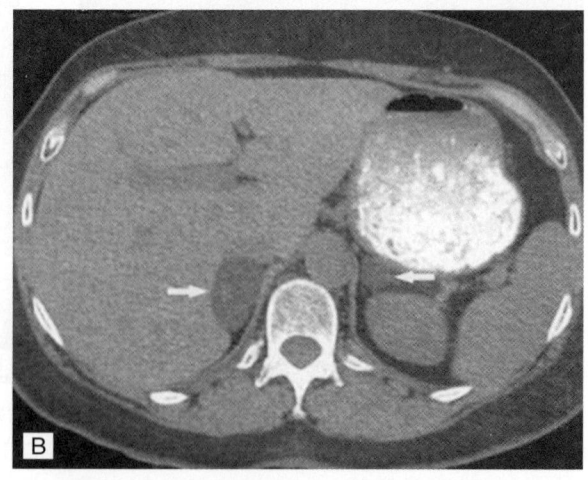

图 11.7 女性,60 岁,右肺下叶 NSCLC,伴右侧肾上腺腺瘤。A. 增强 CT 显示右肺下叶肿块(M)。B. 横轴位平扫 CT 显示边界清楚的富含脂质(平均 CT 值约为 2Hu)的肾上腺腺瘤(箭头)。平扫 CT 值 <10HU 可视为良性肿瘤的特征

协会（ATS）和欧洲呼吸协会（ERS）提倡对于无症状的患者，此项检查不列为常规，而美国临床肿瘤协会（the American Society of Clinical Oncology, ASCO）推荐对于无症状的Ⅲ期并将行局部治疗的 NSCLC 患者，应行颅脑 CT 或 MR 检查[28]。尽管 FDG-PET 偶尔也能发现脑转移，正常脑组织较高的 FDG 本底造成了其较低的灵敏度，因此不应常规应用。

胸片、TC-99m 骨扫描或 MR 很少检测到骨的隐匿性转移，所以对无相应症状的患者，这几项检查不列为常规。最近的一项研究将新确诊为 NSCLC 患者的全身 FDG-PET、CT 和 Tc-99m MDP（methylene diphosphonate）骨扫描进行了对比，这两项检查灵敏度相似（分别为 93.3% 和 93.5%），但是 PET、CT 拥有更高的特异度（分别为 94.1% 和 52.2%）[29]。作为检测骨转移的主要手段，如果 FDG-PET、CT 作为 NSCLC 分期检查的一部分，Tc-99m MDP 骨扫描并不能提供更多的信息。FDG-PET、CT 及 Tc-99m MDP 骨扫描检测骨转移的不一致性在 NSCLC 患者中的比例为 20%[30]。这种不一致性产生的很大一部分原因是 FDG-PET 可检测出早期骨转移，而 Tc-99m MDP 骨扫描不能检测出恶性肿瘤细胞对骨髓的早期浸润。然而，需要强调的是，对具有可能行手术治疗而 FDG-PET 检测出骨质存在病变的患者，进一步的组织学验证及其他影像学检查（如胸片、CT 或 MR）很有必要。

全身 FDG-PET 扫描在检测肾上腺、骨和胸腔外淋巴结转移方面比 CT 扫描具有更高的敏感性（图 11.8）。因此，FDG-PET 越来越广泛地用于检测远处转移，并且常应用于 CT 或其他影像学检查没有发现远处转移的患者。美国外科肿瘤学院（the American College of Surgeons Oncology Trial）报道了 PET 对于 M1 期肿瘤检测的灵敏度、特异度、阳性预测值（positive predictive value, PPV）和阴性预测值（negative predictive value, NPV）分别为 83%、90%、36% 和 99%[31]。重要的是，对于行标准的影像学检查及临床评估后，被认为能够行手术治疗的患者，全身 PET 图像在检测远处转移方面更有价值，据报道，FDG-PET、CT 可使 20% 的患者免于接受不恰当的手术治疗[31-32]。然而，由于 T 和 N 分期越高，PET 对发生转移的患者检出率也越高，所以 FDG-PET 对于早期肺癌的

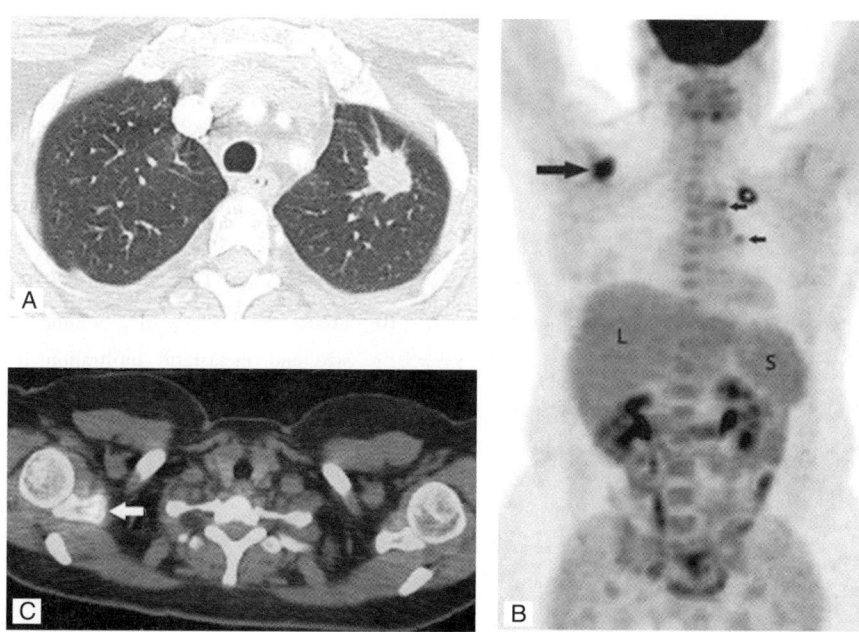

图11.8 女性，45岁，颈肩部疼痛，其左肺上叶为 NSCLC，并有孤立性骨转移。A. 增强 CT 显示有分叶的左肺上叶结节。全身 PET 最大密度投影图像显示左肺上叶结节 FDG 高摄取（*），左肺门及纵隔高摄取的淋巴结（短箭头所示）及右肩部 FDG 高摄取区（长箭头）。B. 代表 FDG 高代谢的膀胱；L = 肝脏，S = 脾。C. 横轴位的 PET、CT 显示肩胛骨喙突可疑转移（箭头）。组织学检查已确诊为转移，对该患者行姑息治疗

价值受到质疑[33-34]。一项随机临床试验显示，PET对于早期肺癌的检出率很低（<5%），因此，对于未检测出早期肺癌患者的处理实际上不会改变[34]。然而，参与这项研究的合作医院表明，PET检查会改变超过20%的患者后续的新辅助化疗（分期为ⅢA期N2的患者）方案。

尽管全身FDG-PET检查提高了肿瘤分期的准确性，但有时和NSCLC原发灶无关的胸腔外高摄取灶易被误认为是远处转移。因此，对所有可能改变患者治疗方式的胸腔外高摄取灶，应该行进一步的影像学检查或通过组织学活检来确定是否为转移灶。一项对新诊断为NSCLC并且肺外仅有1处FDG高摄取患者的前瞻性研究结果支持这一处理方案：这项研究入组的350例患者中，72例拥有孤立的FDG高摄取灶，其中，69例患者进行了活检组织学检查，有37例（54%）发生转移，另外32例患者（46%）的高摄取灶与NSCLC转移无关（为炎性或良性病灶；$n=26$），6例患者的高摄取灶被临床怀疑为第二原发肿瘤或肿瘤复发。

总 结

影像学检查是肿瘤TNM分期的重要组成部分，并且在决定NSCLC患者的治疗方案中起着重要作用。然而，在评估原发肿瘤、淋巴结及远处转移方面，影像学检查存在很大变数。胸部CT几乎广泛应用于NSCLC患者的分期，常用于评估原发肿瘤，指导侵入性采样，并且用来检测胸腔内或远处转移。MR主要对肺上沟瘤的评估具有独特价值。另外，当CT诊断存在疑问时，MR是重要的释疑手段。FDG-PET影像学检查在评估原发灶方面价值有限。全身FDG-PET影像学检查在诊断淋巴结和远处转移、改善肿瘤分期及决定最佳治疗方案方面均优于CT和MRI。

（郭延奕　黄勇 译）

参考文献

[1] Rami-Porta R, Ball D, Crowley J, et al. The IASLC Lung Cancer StagingProject: Proposals for the revision of the T descriptors in the forthcoming (seventh) edition of the TNM classification for lung cancer. J Thorac Oncol, 2007, 2 (7): 593-602.

[2] Rusch VW, Crowley J, Giroux DJ, et al. The IASLC Lung Cancer Staging Project: Proposals for the revision of the N descriptors in the forthcoming seventh edition of the TNM classification for lung cancer. J Thorac Oncol, 2007, 2 (7): 603-612.

[3] Postmus PE, Brambilla E, Chansky K, et al. The IASLC Lung Cancer Staging Project: proposals for revision of the M descriptors in the forthcoming (seventh) edition of the TNM classification of lung cancer. J Thorac Oncol, 2007, 2 (8): 686-693.

[4] Bruzzi JF, Komaki R, Walsh GL, et al. Imaging of nonsmall cell lung cancer of the superior sulcus: Part 2: initial staging and assessment of resectability and therapeutic response. RadioGraphics, 2008, 28 (2): 561-572.

[5] Bruzzi JF, Komaki R, Walsh GL, et al. Imaging of nonsmall cell lung cancer of the superior sulcus: Part 1: anatomy, clinical manifestations, and management. RadioGraphics, 2008, 28 (2): 551-560; quiz 620.

[6] Bolton WD, Rice DC, Goodyear A, et al. Superior sulcus tumors with vertebral body involvement: A multimodality approach. J Thorac Cardiovasc Surg, 2009, 137 (6): 1379-1387.

[7] Bilsky MH, Vitaz TW, Boland PJ, et al. Surgical treatment of superior sulcus tumors with spinal and brachial plexus involvement. J Neurosurg, 2002, 97 (3 Suppl): 301-309.

[8] Dartevelle P, Macchiarini P. Surgical management of superior sulcus tumors. Oncologist, 1999, 4 (5): 398-407.

[9] Finley DJ, Yoshizawa A, Travis W, et al. Predictors of outcomes after surgical treatment of synchronous primary lung cancers. J Thorac Oncol, 2010, 5 (2): 197-205.

[10] Prenzel KL, Monig SP, Sinning JM, et al. Lymph node size and metastatic infiltration in non-small cell lung cancer. Chest, 2003, 123 (2): 463-467.

[11] Toloza EM, Harpole L, Detterbeck F, et al. Invasive staging of non-small cell lung cancer: a review of the current evidence. Chest, 2003, 123 (1 Suppl): 157S-166S.

[12] Birim O, Kappetein AP, Stijnen T, et al. Meta-analysis of positron emission tomographic and computed tomographic imaging in detecting mediastinal lymph node metastases in nonsmall cell lung cancer. Ann Thorac Surg, 2005, 79 (1): 375-382.

[13] Gould MK, Kuschner WG, Rydzak CE, et al. Test performance of positron emission tomography and computed

tomography for mediastinal staging in patients with non-small-cell lung cancer: A meta-analysis. Ann Intern Med, 2003, 2; 139 (11): 879-892.

[14] Perigaud C, Bridji B, Roussel JC, et al. Prospective pre-operative mediastinal lymph node staging by integrated positron emission tomography-computerised tomography in patients with non-small-cell lung cancer. Eur J Cardiothorac Surg, 2009, 36 (4): 731-736.

[15] de Langen AJ, Raijmakers P, Riphagen I, et al. The size of mediastinal lymph nodes and its relation with metastatic involvement: A meta-analysis. Eur J Cardiothorac Surg, 2006, 29 (1): 26-29.

[16] Erasmus JJ, Goodman PC, Patz EF, et al. Management of malignant pleural effusions and pneumothorax. Radiol Clin North Am, 2000, 38 (2): 375-383.

[17] Gupta NC, Rogers JS, Graeber GM, et al. Clinical role of F-18 fluorodeoxyglucose positron emission tomography imaging in patients with lung cancer and suspected malignant pleural effusion. Chest, 2002, 122 (6): 1918-1924.

[18] Kim BS, Kim IJ, Kim SJ, et al. Predictive value of F-18 FDG PET/CT for malignant pleural effusion in non-small cell lung cancer patients. Onkologie, 2011, 34 (6): 298-303.

[19] Low G, Sahi K. Clinical and imaging overview of functional adrenal neoplasms. Int J Urol, 19 (8): 697-708.

[20] Remer EM, Obuchowski N, Ellis JD, et al. Adrenal mass evaluation in patients with lung carcinoma: a cost-effectiveness analysis. AJR Am J Roentgenol, Apr, 2000, 174 (4): 1033-1039.

[21] Low G, Dhliwayo H, Lomas DJ. Adrenal neoplasms. Clin Radiol, 67 (10): 988-1000.

[22] Boland GW, Dwamena BA, Jagtiani Sangwaiya M, et al. Characterization of adrenal masses by using FDG PET: A systematic review and meta-analysis of diagnostic test performance. Radiology, 2011, 259 (1): 117-126.

[23] Quint LE, Tummala S, Brisson LJ, et al. Distribution of distant metastases from newly diagnosed non-small cell lung cancer. Annals of Thoracic Surgery, 1996, 62: 246-250.

[24] Hillers TK, Sauve MD, Guyatt GH. Analysis of published studies on the detection of extrathoracic metastases in patients presumed to have operable nonsmall cell lung cancer. Thorax, 1994, 49 (1): 14-19.

[25] Silvestri GA, Gould MK, Margolis ML, et al. Noninvasive staging of non-small cell lung cancer: ACCP evidenced-based clinical practice guidelines (2nd edn). Chest, 2007, 132 (3 Suppl): 178S-201S.

[26] Sanchez de Cos J, Sojo Gonzalez MA, Montero MV, et al. Nonsmall cell lung cancer and silent brain metastasis: Survival and prognostic factors. Lung Cancer, 2009, 63 (1): 140-145.

[27] Yokoi K, Kamiya N, Matsuguma H, et al. Detection of brain metastasis in potentially operable non-small cell lung cancer. A comparison of CT and MRI. Chest, 1999, 115: 714-719.

[28] Pfister DG, Johnson DH, Azzoli CG, et al. American Society of Clinical Oncology treatment of unresectable non-small-cell lung cancer guideline: update 2003. J Clin Oncol, 2003, 22 (2): 330-353.

[29] Min JW, Um SW, Yim JJ, et al. The role of whole-body FDG PET/CT, Tc^{99m} MDP bone scintigraphy, and serum alkaline phosphatase in detecting bone metastasis in patients with newly diagnosed lung cancer. J Korean Med Sci, 2009, 24 (2): 275-280.

[30] Ak I, Sivrikoz MC, Entok E, et al. Discordant findings in patients with non-small-cell lung cancer: absolutely normal bone scans versus disseminated bone metastases on positron-emission tomography/computed tomography. Eur J Cardiothorac Surg, 2010, 37 (4): 792-796.

[31] Reed CE, Harpole DH, Posther KE, et al. Results of the American College of Surgeons Oncology Group Z0050 trial: The utility of positron emission tomography in staging potentially operable non-small cell lung cancer. J Thorac Cardiovasc Surg, 2003, 126 (6): 1943-1951.

[32] van Tinteren H, Hoekstra OS, Smit EF, et al. Effectiveness of positron emission tomography in the preoperative assessment of patients with suspected non-small cell lung cancer: The PLUS multicentre randomized trial. Lancet, 2002, 359 (9315): 1388-1393.

[33] MacManus MP, Hicks RJ, Matthews JP, et al. High rate of detection of unsuspected distant metastases by PET in apparent stage III non-small-cell lung cancer: Implications for radical radiation therapy. Int J Radiat Oncol Biol Phys, 2001, 50 (2): 287-293. Imaging Lung Cancer 201

[34] Viney RC, Boyer MJ, King MT, et al. Randomized controlled trial of the role of positron emission tomography in the management of stage I and II non-small-cell lung cancer. J Clin Oncol, 2004, 22 (12): 2357-2362.

[35] Lardinois D, Weder W, Roudas M, et al. Etiology of solitary extrapulmonary positron emission tomography and computed tomography findings in patients with lung cancer. J Clin Oncol, 2005, 23 (28): 6846-6853.

第 12 章
纵隔淋巴结分期

Mauricio Pipkin, *Shaf Keshavjee*
University of Toronto, CA

引 言

肺癌是导致人类因癌症死亡的首要原因。全世界每年死于肺癌的人数高于结肠癌、乳腺癌、前列腺癌死亡人数的总和[1]。肺癌的治疗是在 TNM 分期系统指导下进行的[2]。由于临床和病理分期的一致性较差，因此患者通常在临床上的分期普遍偏低[3]。无远处转移患者的纵隔淋巴结状态意味着有接受根治性治疗的可能。无纵隔受累的患者可能成为接受单纯根治性手术治疗的人选，而有纵隔淋巴结受累的患者通常预后较差，准确的淋巴结分期将有助于确定其治疗计划能否采用联合治疗模式，如新辅助放化疗。

影像学检查

作为一项基本检查，所有的可疑肺癌患者都应行胸部 CT 扫描。通常需行对比剂增强扫描以准确地评估淋巴结情况。临床普遍认为，如果 CT 横断面图像上的淋巴结短径 >1cm 则认为可疑淋巴结转移。然而，不是所有 >1cm 的淋巴结都是恶性的。大约有 40% 在 CT 上认为恶性的淋巴结实际为良性。此外，大约有 20% 在 CT 上认为"良性"的淋巴结实际为恶性[4]。对中央型肺癌或伴 N1 淋巴结增大、但纵隔阴性的肿瘤而言，其 N2～N3 淋巴结受侵犯的概率为 20%～25%[57]。最近有一篇汇总数据的综述报告了用 CT 评估纵隔转移的结果：灵敏度为 57%，特异度为 82%，阳性预测值为 56%，阴性预测值为 83%，这个结果与单个研究结果有显著差异[5]，其中周围型肺癌、肿瘤直径 <3cm 且淋巴结 <1cm 的亚组患者，其纵隔转移概率为 9%[6]。

PET 与 CT 相结合全面提高了单行 CT 的诊断准确率，这种结合模式在监测转移性淋巴结方面更加敏感和特异。一项 meta 分析显示 FDG-PET 较 CT 更加准确，PET 与 CT 的灵敏度分别为 79% 和 60%，特异度分别为 91% 和 77%[7]。但应当注意的是，单纯 PET 不如 PET-CT 相结合的优势明显。

一体化 PET-CT 提供了定性和解剖学上定位转移性淋巴结的能力。转移性淋巴结的解剖位置被标记在 FDG 摄取与 CT 相融合的图像中，以便有目的地进行活检以明确诊断[8-9]。一项前瞻性研究显示一体化的 PET-CT 较单纯 CT 特异度高，分别为 85% 与 61%[10]。而另一项研究显示一体化 PET-CT 较单纯 PET 灵敏度高，但特异度较低[11]。这凸显了组织学上（侵入性或创伤性分期方法）证实纵隔淋巴结转移的必要性。Cerfolio 等比较了 PET-CT 和单纯 PET 在 N2 组淋巴结中的诊断价值，结果显示，PET-CT 准确度较高，两者的诊断准确度分别为 96% 和 93%[12]。Darling 等报告了 PET-CT 在 cN0、cN1、cN2 患者中的假阳性率分别为 50%、20% 和 29%[13]。Ⅰ 期肿瘤患者的淋巴结大小正常时其纵隔转移风险较低，PET 扫描阴性的假阴性率仅为 5%[14]。其他报道也证实 cN0 患者的 PET 纵隔阴性结果通常可靠，其假阴性率为 3%[13]。因此，ACCP（美国胸科医生学会）建议对 Ⅰ 期肿瘤，CT 扫描结果为阴性及 PET 提示纵隔阴性患者，无须行纵隔镜。在目前（第 7 版）的 TNM 分期系统中，T2aN0 患者虽为 ⅠB 期，但不在上述建议之列[15]。

内镜检查

超声内镜引导下经支气管针吸活检（EBUS-TBNA 或 EBUS-FNA）是一种替代技术，它实现了在超声可视化下经支气管镜行纵隔及支气管周围淋巴结针吸活检的可能性[16]。此过程在镇静或者全身麻醉下进行，支气管镜经口、喉罩或气管内插管进入。通过超声成像检查进行定位和评估 N3、N2 和 N1 组淋巴结，使用一种特殊的超声下可见的针由支气管镜引入（图 12.1），一旦辨认出淋巴结既行针吸活检。理想情况下，活检取得的材料可由在场的细胞病理学专家进行评估，并确定所取组织是否足够（至少包含淋巴细胞）及肿瘤诊断是否成立。

EBUS-TBNA 在 2004 年首次被报道，作为评价纵隔和肺门淋巴结新型而微创的分期手段，其诊断准确度高[17]。创伤小、淋巴结实时定位和安全性是其主要优势。有趣的是，EBUS 还可以用微创的方式获取肺门、叶间和肺叶淋巴结——在该技术出现之前这是无法做到的[18]。一项 meta 分析显示 EBUS-TBNA 汇总的灵敏度为 93%，特异度为 100%。如果经选择患者均为 CT 或 PET 阳性者，则灵敏度上升至 94%。不经任何选择的患者亚组，灵敏度为 76%[19]。Adams 等发表了一篇系统性综述和 meta 分析比较了 EBUS-TBNA 和 CT 及 PET 的诊断能力。总共回顾了 10 项研究（$n=817$），显示 EBUS-TBNA 具有极佳的累积特异度 1.00 [95% CI（0.92，1.00）] 及良好的累积灵敏度 0.88 [95% CI（0.79，0.94）][20]。2011 年的一项研究表明，EBUS-TBNA 和纵隔镜在纵隔淋巴结分期上非常一致。EBUS-TBNA 和纵隔镜在纵隔淋巴结分期上的灵敏度、阴性预测值、诊断准确度分别为 81% 和 91%、93% 和 79%、90% 和 93%。当淋巴结转移被确定后，上述两种技术的特异度及阳性预测值均为 100%[21]。由此作者得出结论：两种技术结果相似，在肺癌的纵隔分期中 EBUS-TBNA 可替代颈部纵隔镜。然而，在高危患者中，EBUS-TBNA 针吸活检结果阴性的患者应再行纵隔镜检查确定。Andrade 等发表评论认为，EBUS-TBNA 应该由多学科肺癌团队中的内科医生实施[22]。

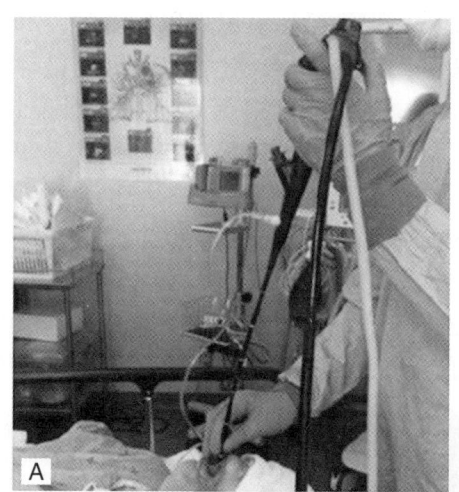
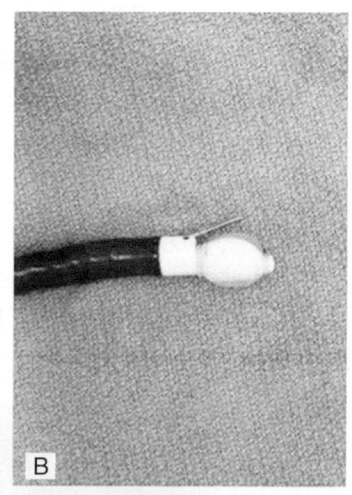
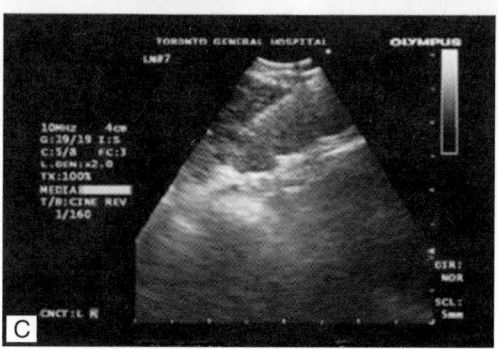

图 12.1 A. 正在进行的 EBUS-TBNA 检查。B. 内镜上针的一部分。C. 淋巴结活检的超声影像

超声内镜引导下经食管针吸活检（endoscopic esophageal ultrasound-guided fine meedle aspiration，EUS-FNA）是一种诊断方法，它提供了一种用于行2R、2L、3p、4R、4L组淋巴结活检的替代方法。然而除此之外，EUS-FNA可以到达更下方的部位，如5组、7组——尤其是7组后部和食管旁8组及9组淋巴结[23-24]。一项囊括了18项研究，1 201例患者的meta分析显示EUS-FNA的灵敏度为83%，特异度为97%[25]，对于未增大的淋巴结其灵敏度为58%[25]。将EBUS-TBNA和EUS-FNA结合使用可以对纵隔镜无法到达部位的淋巴结如3p组、8组和9组进行活检。Szlubowski发现二者结合使用其灵敏度为68%，特异度为98%，准确度为91%，阳性预测值（PPV）为91%，阴性预测值（NPV）为91%[26]。Herth等对139例被诊断为NSCLC的患者进行纵隔分期，结果显示EUS-FNA灵敏度为89%，而EBUS-TBNA的灵敏度为92%。二者结合使用时，灵敏度上升至96%，阴性预测值为95%[27]。因此可以认为，EBUS-TBNA与EUS-FNA结合使用是可行的[23,28-31]。然而，临床上并没有常规将二者结合使用的具体建议。当某个淋巴结区域在CT和PET上被识别出的情况下，需要注意和了解每种诊断方法的能力和局限性。从本质上讲，EBUS和EUS为外科医生提供了一种微创组织活检的途径，从而能对纵隔淋巴结站点进行定性和分期。

在Filho等进行的一项研究中，采用纵隔镜和电视辅助胸腔镜（video-assisted thoracoscopy，VATS）对后部淋巴结区域，尤其是后部隆突下区淋巴结进行检查，从而进行纵隔分期。共检查了62例患者，其中11例纵隔镜显示隆突下淋巴结未受侵犯，这些结果通过VATS途径得到了确认，得出的阳性预测值是89%，阴性预测值是94%，发生率为18%，灵敏度为73%，特异度为99%。这种方法可在未启用EBUS-TBNA和（或）EUS-FNA的机构中使用[32]。

纵隔镜

纵隔镜手术是一种在全身麻醉下进行的门诊手术。首先在胸骨上切迹做一长约3cm的皮肤切口，向下方分离至气管前筋膜，切开气管前筋膜以暴露气管，用手指钝性分离打开气管旁平面向下至隆突，通过手指触诊找到异常的淋巴结或肿块；之后将电视纵隔镜插入纵隔，在直视下行淋巴结活检。电视纵隔镜因其出色的可视性更受欢迎，尽管外科医生如有需要，也可通过传统方式直接通过纵隔镜下观察（图12.2）。使用纵隔镜解剖器（一种管状吸引装置，具有绝缘性，并有一个暴露的金属电极头，用于剖开组织和按需烧灼）进行系统的纵隔评价和纵隔解剖。每组淋巴结可以被系统地识别以便活检。2R组和4R组、7组、2L组和4L组可使用纵隔镜评估。1组和10组淋巴结也可根据需要使用纵隔镜进行评估和活检，而3组、5组、6组、8组和9组淋巴结不能使用纵隔镜评估。在理想的情况下，有5个淋巴结组别（2R组、4R组、7组、4L组和2L组）可以通过纵隔镜取到样本[15]（图12.3）。

影像技术的进步促进了颈部电视纵隔镜的发展。从概念上来说，这是一种传统的纵隔镜，具有

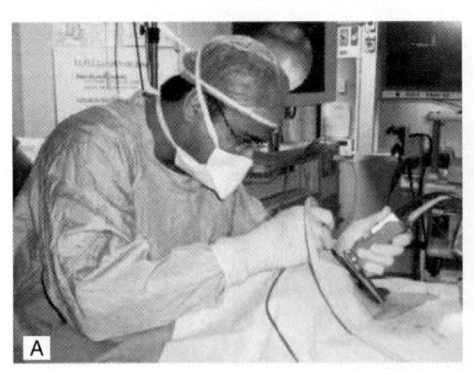
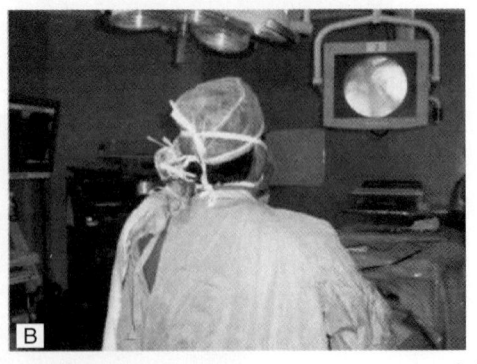

图12.2 电视纵隔镜：可在镜下直视（A）或通过HD（高清）监制器（B）[37]。来源：Yasufuku，2010[37]。经Lippincott Willams及Wilkins许可出版

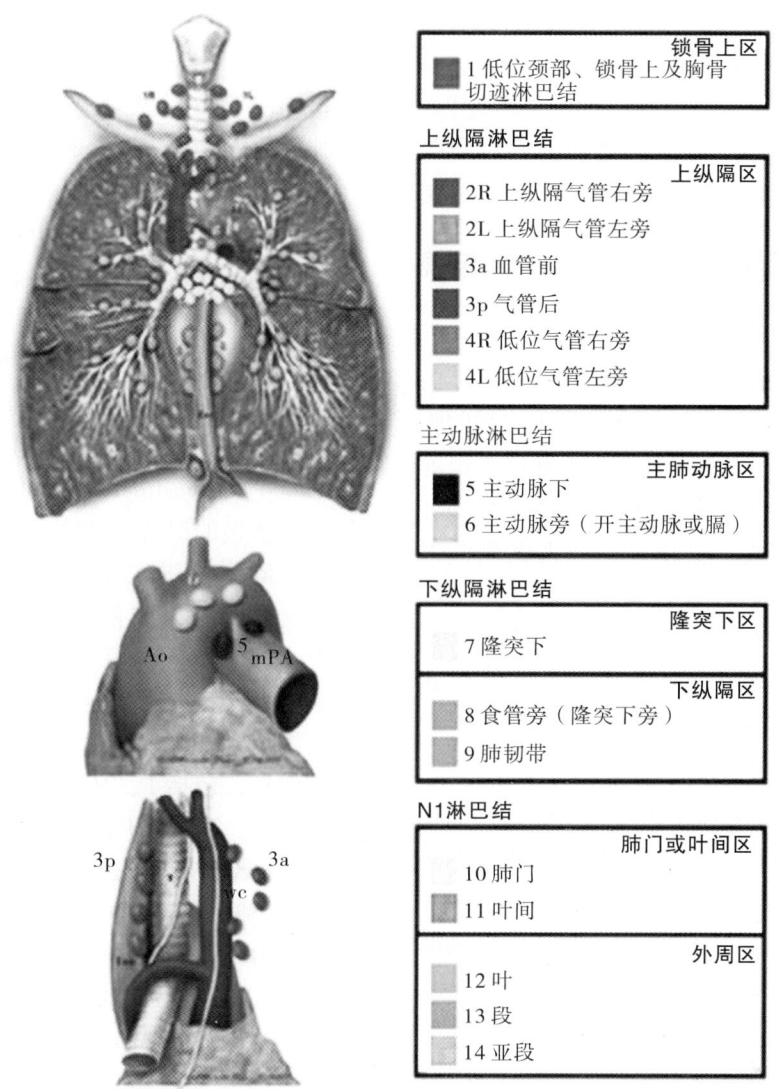

图12.3（见彩插） A~F：国际肺癌研究组织（IASLC）淋巴结示意图，用于CT扫描进行临床分期，横轴位（A~C）、冠状位（D）和矢状位（E、F）视野。右和左气管旁区之间的边缘可于A和B中显示。Ao：主动脉；AV：奇静脉；Br：细支气管；IA：无名动脉；IV：无名静脉；LA：动脉韧带；LIV：左无名静脉；LSA：左锁骨下动脉；PA：肺动脉；PV：肺静脉；RIV：右无名静脉；SVC：上腔静脉[55]。来源：Rusch, 2009[55]。经Lippincott Willams及Wilkins许可出版

高清摄像头并可将图像传输至屏幕。外科医生及其团队在手术室能通过视频监视器或直视下清楚地看到解剖过程[33]。清晰的可视化程度改善了手术的精确性和安全性。因为外科医生能清楚地看到和指导学习者进行手术操作，这也有利于教学。另外，因为可多人同时观看手术过程，电视纵隔镜允许快速学习和充分监督，同时不会降低安全性、延长手术时间或破坏手术过程的完整性[34]。一项研究比较了常规纵隔镜和电视纵隔镜，结果显示阴性预测值分别为0.81和0.83，准确度分别为83.8%和87.9%[35]。

若由有经验的外科医生操作，纵隔镜的并发症发生概率极低[36]，其发生率和死亡率分别为1.5%和0.4%[37]。并发症包括左侧喉返神经损伤、气胸和伤口感染，更严重的并发症包括气管支气管损伤、食管创伤和大血管或奇静脉损伤所致的出血。主要并发症是有潜在的生命威胁，且常需行正中胸骨切开术或右胸开胸手术来修复[38]。

颈部纵隔镜被认为是纵隔分期的金标准。一篇综述显示，颈部纵隔镜的灵敏度为72%~89%，差异较大，平均为81%，阴性预测值为91%[39]，并报道纵隔镜的特异度为100%。对于纵隔镜出现

假阴性的病例，一种解释为无法通过纵隔镜达到——通常为第5组或第6组，有时为第7组后部的位置；还有一种解释为由于操作者的技术原因，可能取得的淋巴结样本不完全。另一方面，高阴性预测值使其在排除纵隔转移上颇为可行[37]。

前路纵隔切开术，颈部纵隔镜扩大术，胸腔镜和再次纵隔镜检查

胸骨旁前路纵隔切开术的方法是1966年由McNeil和Chamberlain首次描述的[40]。在左侧前胸壁第2肋间隙做一个小切口可达第5组和第6组淋巴结（主-肺动脉窗和主动脉旁淋巴结），有些外科医生也会移除肋软骨，由切口处插入纵隔镜以进行解剖和活检。这个手术有效而安全，并发症发生率和死亡率均很低。有时使用电视纵隔镜（VATS）来评估第5组和第6组淋巴结。该模式的附加价值是同时可评估和活检第8、9、7组后部淋巴结及有可疑胸膜受侵时探查胸膜间隙。

颈部纵隔镜扩大术是由Robert Ginsberg首次描述的，这种术式可通过传统的颈部纵隔镜切口到达第5组和第6组淋巴结。采用钝性分离的方法在无名静脉后方、主动脉前方、左侧颈动脉和无名动脉之间创建一个间隙。实施这一过程具有挑战性，且当有其他技术可选择时很少采用这一方案。

再次纵隔镜检查可在某位患者新辅助治疗后，或有时为了对某患者的第二原发肺癌行分期时考虑实施。这两种情况均要求将之前已分期的纵隔进行重新分期。由于是在之前纵隔组织平面解剖分离的瘢痕上操作，因此这个过程颇具挑战性。累及无名动脉和静脉、奇静脉及肺动脉的粘连是格外值得关注的部分。在技术上，解剖分离一般自左侧向下进入纵隔并小心延伸至右侧。尽管再次纵隔镜检查在技术上更具挑战性，研究显示灵敏度可达73%，特异度100%，准确度达85%，阳性预测值和阴性预测值分别是100%和75%[41]。Mateu-Navarro等报告了24例新辅助治疗后行再次纵隔镜的N2期肺癌患者，50%的患者为阳性，灵敏度达70%，特异度达100%，准确度达80%[42]。DeWaele等的另一项报告显示，再次纵隔镜检查的患者有40例阳性和64例阴性，有17例为假阴性，灵敏度为71%，特异度为100%，准确度为84%[43]。在当今时代，我们更倾向于采用PET加EBUS-TBNA用于纵隔的首次分期，并计划在诱导治疗后行纵隔镜检查，以便能为这些有较高肿瘤风险的患者进行彻底而安全的分期。

电视辅助纵隔镜下淋巴结清扫术（VAMLA）——一种分期方法？

电视辅助纵隔镜下淋巴结清扫术（Video Assisted Mediastinoscopic Lymphadenectomy，VAMLA）和经颈部纵隔淋巴结扩大清扫术（Transcervical Extended Mediastinal Lymphadenectomy，TEMLA）是相对新兴的纵隔分期技术[44]。支持者主张不仅彻底清除纵隔淋巴结，也包括周围的脂肪组织，认为这样做可以改善其准确度[45]。在VAMLA技术中，淋巴结分离解剖与传统的纵隔镜相同，但是本质上是完成整块切除活检[46]。在TEMLA过程中需结合开胸和纵隔镜辅助技术进行广泛的淋巴结清扫：包括1、2R、4R、2L、4L、7、8、3A、3p、5、6、7、8组。Zielinski进行的一项入组了256例患者的研究报道了准确度为98%，在患者中N2~N3受侵犯的发生率为31.3%[47]。有报道称VAMLA的特异度为93.75%，灵敏度为100%[48]。两种方法均涉及"微创"或"混合型"的方法，尽管TEMLA与其他技术相比，采用的切口更大且胸骨内陷更严重。TEMLA和VAMLE的纵隔分离解剖均较广泛，且如文献中所指出，并发症发生率较其他纵隔分期方法高。喉返神经损伤是最常见的并发症，其发生率在TEMLA和VAMLA分别为3%和5%[49]。目前还不清楚这些技术带来的优势能否弥补其所引起的并发症。

讨论

纵隔分期是为肺癌患者制订治疗决策的先决条件。患者若有组织学诊断和在CT扫描上明显、广泛而无法手术切除的浸润时，即便没有远处转移，也不需要广泛的侵入或创伤性分期[14]。如果纵隔淋巴结肿大，则需要某种形式的侵入或创伤性分期手段。正如前面所讨论的，即便PET或CT显示淋巴结受侵，假阳性率仍高，且需在假定患者为进展期疾病之前获得组织学诊断来确认淋巴

结是否受侵。这可以通过几种方法来确认：纵隔镜仍是纵隔分期的金标准；但在前瞻性研究中分析得出 EBUS-TBNA 较纵隔镜在诊断准确度上有优势[21]。值得注意的是，这种内镜途径应该在有经验的中心开展，采用快速现场细胞学标本评估。EBUS-TBNA 和 EUS-FNA 相结合的方法显示灵敏度和特异度均提高，但二者都是依赖操作者技术的方法。因此，纵隔镜是否可被以上 1 种或相互结合的方法替代，仍未达成共识。

如果中央型肿瘤或疑似 N1 的情况下，纵隔淋巴结在 CT 上大小正常且 PET 阴性的患者，应行侵入性纵隔分期方法。此外，即便是 EBUS-TBNA 不能诊断或结果阴性，如果高度可疑，也应行纵隔镜以明确或排除 N2，尤其是 N3 病变。

外周型 T1 肿瘤、纵隔淋巴结大小正常而 PET 阳性的患者应行组织学检查确认 PET 阳性淋巴结以排除 PET 假阳性（EBUS-TBNA 或纵隔镜——EBUS-TBNA 在处理正常或小尺寸纵隔淋巴结上是有挑战性的）。然而，如果原发肿瘤是 PET 阳性（高代谢）且纵隔 PET 阴性时，可省去侵入性分期。

另外一个需要考虑到的问题是，使用 EBUS-TBNA 内镜的方法使我们相对容易地以微创的方式获得 N1 组淋巴结的标本，包括肺门和肺内淋巴结。当然，在 EBUS-TBNA 技术实现之前，是没有能力达到的。这提示了在术前确定 N1 病变的可能性，并有望在今后的试验中确定这项技术是否有助于肺癌患者判断预后或制订治疗计划。当然，当我们越来越多地考虑将 T1 肿瘤行亚段切除时，术前确认 N1 淋巴结阴性无疑将有助于制订手术计划，甚至有助于制订非手术治疗方法，如 SBRT 计划。此外，识别 N1 疾病的患者并对这部分患者行新辅助治疗可能被证明比辅助治疗更有益，尽管这还有待进一步研究。

N1 淋巴结取样也可用于获取组织衍生物标志物以用于预测靶向治疗的反应。我们对 N2 或 N3 肺癌患者行 EBUS-TBNA 的经验显示，可以通过 EBUS-TBNA 取得的组织标本进行以靶向治疗为目的的分子诊断、免疫组化以提供预后信息，以及化学灵敏度相关异常甲基化的评估等[37,50]。

一项系统性的综述对采用不同的方法进行 III 期 NSCLC 新辅助化疗后纵隔再分期进行了比较，结果表明，CT 和 PET 显示完全缓解的假阴性率分别为 50% 和 30%[53]。CT 和 PET 上纵隔淋巴结受累的假阴性率分别是 33% 和 25%，假阳性率均为 33%。侵入性分期的结果似乎更好一些。再次纵隔镜的假阴性率为 22%，EUS-FNA 为 14%，初次纵隔镜检查为 9%[53]。此外，降期的评估不应基于影像学检查能准确预测纵隔淋巴结的状态这一假设[53]。即使进行了系统的术前分期，仍有假阴性纵隔淋巴结受侵通过手术切除得到了证实[54]（图 12.4）。

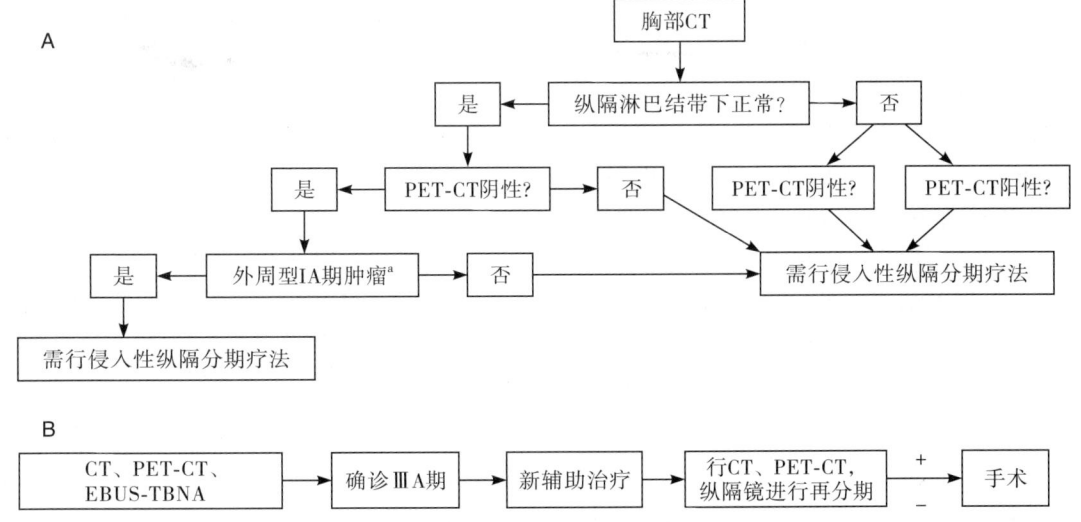

图 12.4 A. 临床分期为 T1～T4，N0～N3，无远处转移，潜在手术可切除的患者的纵隔分期流程图。ªT1：原发肿瘤直径≤3cm 且周围包绕肺或脏层胸膜，或叶支气管远端的支气管内肿瘤。Darling 等修改[14]。B. 针对 IIIA 期 N2 患者的纵隔分期途径

EBUS-TBNA 也是诱导治疗后分期的选择之一。Herth 等进行的一项回顾性研究中,将 124 例 N2 期 NSCLC 患者诱导化疗后进行重新分期。EBUS-TBNA 检测出 72% 的患者有肿大淋巴结。在这组患者中,35 例 EBUS-TBNA 纵隔分期阴性,其中 28 例在开胸手术中发现残留 N2 疾病。总体的 EBUS-TBNA 行诱导化疗后纵隔再分期的灵敏度、特异度、阳性预测值、阴性预测值和诊断准确度分别为 76%、100%、100%、20% 和 77%[51]。鉴于此,我们认为如果 EBUS-TBNA 呈阴性结果,由于其阴性预测值较低,在开胸手术前应行纵隔镜。Szlubowski 等进行了一项前瞻性研究,61 例患者经 EBUS-TBNA 进行了再分期;在 18 例(30%)患者中检测到纵隔受累;在 43 例阴性或不确定纵隔是否受累的患者中,行 TEMLA 并显示 9 例(15%)患者存在转移,其中 7 例(12%)患者在 EBUS-TBNA 可到达的淋巴结站点为阳性[52]。值得注意的是,活检假阴性结果仅出现于小淋巴结。同样,所有经 TEMLA 诊断的阳性 N2 淋巴结均只包含微转移灶。EBUS-TBNA 行再分期的诊断灵敏度、特异度、准确度、阳性预测值和阴性预测值分别为 67%、86%、80%、91% 和 78%。总之,EBUS-TBNA 似乎是纵隔再分期的一种有效技术。随着该技术临床经验的不断丰富,其性能可得到进一步的提高。

Ⅲa 期 N2 的患者应在完成新辅助治疗后进行再分期。众所周知,诱导放化疗后达到或接近完全病理缓解患者的远期预后极佳。由于 N3 手术切除的益处还未得到证实,因此纵隔再分期用于排除 N3 的存在尤其重要。再次强调,纵隔淋巴结阳性的存在可能导致一些高危患者放弃扩大切除的计划或其他患者考虑进一步的诱导治疗。我们更倾向于这些患者在诱导治疗前行 CT、PET 和 EBUS-FNA,诱导治疗后行 CT、PET 和纵隔镜进行纵隔分期,这可以避免再次行纵隔镜检查,正如前所述,纵隔镜在技术上更具挑战性,但灵敏度和诊断的准确度较低[24,28]。

(王银霞 黄伟 李宝生 译)

参考文献

[1] Siegel R, Naishadham D, Jemal A. Cancer statistics, 2012. CA Cancer J Clin, 2012, 62 (1): 10-29.

[2] Sobin LH, Gospodarowicz MK, Wittekind C. UICC TNM Classification of Malignant Tumours. 7th. New York: Wiley-Liss, 2009

[3] Santos PARD, Rocha RSD, Pipkin M, et al. Concordance between clinical and pathological staging in patients with stages I or II non-small cell lung cancer subjected to surgical treatment. J Bras Pneumol, 33 (6): 647-654.

[4] Silvestri GA, Gould MK, Margolis ML, et al. Noninvasive staging of non-small cell lung cancer: ACCP evidenced-based clinical practice guidelines. 2nd, 2007: 178S-201S.

[5] De Leyn P, Lardinois D, Van Schil PE, et al. ESTS guidelines for preoperative lymph node staging for non-small cell lung cancer. European Journal of Cardio-Thoracic Surgery, 2007J, 32 (1): 1-8.

[6] Tournoy KG, Keller SM, Annema JT. Mediastinal staging of lung cancer: novel concepts. Lancet Oncol, May; 2012, 13 (5): e221-229.

[7] Dwamena BAB, Sonnad SSS, Angobaldo JOJ, et al. Metastases from non-small cell lung cancer: mediastinal staging in the 1990s-meta-analytic comparison of PET and CT. Radiology, 1999, 213 (2): 530-536.

[8] Freudenberg LS, Rosenbaum SJ, Beyer T, et al. PET versus PET/CT dual-modality imaging in evaluation of lung cancer. Thorac Surg Clin, 2010, 20 (1): 25-30.

[9] Broderick SR, Meyers BF. PET Staging of mediastinal lymph nodes in thoracic oncology. Thorac Surg Clin, 2012, 22 (2): 161-166.

[10] Whitson BA, Groth SS, Maddaus MA. Recommendations for optimal use of imaging studies to clinically stage mediastinal lymph nodes in non-small-cell lung cancer patients. Lung Cancer, 2008, 61 (2): 9.

[11] Lee BE, Haag von D, Lown T, et al. Advances in positron emission tomography technology have increased the need for surgical staging in non-small cell lung cancer. J Thorac Cardiovasc Surg, 2007, 133 (3): 746-752.

[12] Cerfolio RJ, Ojha B, Bryant AS, et al. The accuracy of integrated PET-CT compared with dedicated pet alone for the staging of patients with nonsmall cell lung cancer. Annals of Thoracic Surgery, 2004, 78 (3): 1017-1023.

[13] Darling GEG, Maziak DED, Inculet RIR, et al. Positron emission tomography-computed tomography compared with invasive mediastinal staging in non-small cell lung cancer: Results of mediastinal staging in the early lung positron emission tomography trial. J Thorac Oncol, 2011, 6 (8): 1367-1372.

[14] Detterbeck FC, Jantz MA, Wallace M, et al. Invasive mediastinal staging of lung cancer: ACCP evidence-based clinical practice guidelines. 2nd. Chest, 2007, 132 (3suppl): 202S-220S.

[15] Darling GE, Dickie AJ, Malthaner RA, et al. Invasive mediastinal staging of nonsmall-cell lung cancer: A clinical practice guideline. Curr Oncol, 2011, 18 (6): e304-310.

[16] Nakajima T, Yasufuku K. The techniques of endobronchial ultrasound-guided transbronchial needle aspiration. Innovations (Phila), 2011, 6 (1): 57-64.

[17] Yasufuku K, Chiyo M, Sekine Y, et al. Real-time endobronchial ultrasound-guided transbronchial needle aspiration of mediastinal and hilar lymph nodes. Chest, 2004, 126 (1): 122-128.

[18] Ernst A, Eberhardt R, Krasnik M, et al. Efficacy of endobronchial ultrasound-guided transbronchial needle aspiration of hilar lymph nodes for diagnosing and staging cancer. J Thorac Oncol, 2009, 4 (8): 947-950.

[19] Gu P, Zhao Y-Z, Jiang L-Y, et al. Endobronchial ultrasound-guided transbronchial needle aspiration for staging of lung cancer: A systematic review and meta-analysis. Eur. J. Cancer, 2009, 45 (8): 1389-1396.

[20] Adams K, Shah PL, Edmonds L, et al. Test performance of endobronchial ultrasound and transbronchial needle aspiration biopsy for mediastinal staging in patients with lung cancer: Systematic review and meta-analysis. Thorax, 2009, 64 (9): 757-762.

[21] Yasufuku K, Pierre A, Darling G, et al. A prospective controlled trial of endobronchial ultrasound-guided transbronchial needle aspiration compared with mediastinoscopy for mediastinal lymph node staging of lung cancer. Journal of Thoracic and Cardiovascular Surgery, 2011, 142 (6): 1393-1400. e1.

[22] Andrade RS, Odell DD, D'Cunha J, et al. Endobronchial ultrasonography (EBUS) —its role in staging of non-small cell lung cancer and who should do it. Journal of Thoracic and Cardiovascular Surgery, 2012, 144 (3): S9-13.

[23] Kużdzał J, Szlubowski A. Ultrasound-guided transbronchial and transesophageal needle biopsy in the mediastinal staging of lung cancer. Thorac Surg Clin, 2012, 22 (2): 191-203.

[24] Groth SS, Andrade RS. Endobronchial and endoscopic ultrasound-guided fine-needle aspiration: A must for thoracic surgeons. Annals of Thoracic Surgery, 2010, 89 (6): S2079-2083.

[25] Micames CG. Endoscopic ultrasound-guided fine-needle aspiration for non-small cell lung cancer staging-a systematic review and metaanalysis. Chest, 2007, 131 (2): 539.

[26] Szlubowski AA, Zielinski MM, Soja JJ, et al. A combined approach of endobronchial and endoscopic ultrasound-guided needle aspiration in the radiologically normal mediastinum in non-small-cell lung cancer staging-a prospective trial. Eur J Cardiothorac Surg, 2010, 37 (5): 5.

[27] Herth FJF. Combined endoscopicendobronchial ultrasound-guided fine-needle aspiration of mediastinal lymph nodes through a single bronchoscope in 150 patients with suspected lung cancer. Chest, 2010, 38 (4): 90.

[28] Herth FJF. Nonsurgical staging of the mediastinum: EBUS and EUS. Semin Respir Crit Care Med, 2011, 32 (1): 62-68.

[29] Ohnishi R, Yasuda I, Kato T, et al. Combined endobronchial and endoscopic ultrasound-guided fine needle aspiration for mediastinal nodal staging of lung cancer. *Endoscopy*, ©Georg Thieme Verlag KG, 2011, 43 (12): 1082-1089.

[30] Hwangbo B. Transbronchial and transesophageal fine-needle aspiration using an ultrasound bronchoscope in mediastinal staging of potentially operable lung cancer. Chest, 2010, 138 (4): 795.

[31] Cerfolio RJ, Bryant AS, Eloubeidi MA, et al. The true false negative rates of esophageal and endobronchial ultrasound in the staging of mediastinal lymph nodes in patients with non-small cell lung cancer. Annals of Thoracic Surgery, 2010, 90 (2): 427-434.

[32] Filho DRDP, Avino AJGA, Brandao SLBS, et al. Joint use of cervical mediastinoscopy and video-assisted thoracoscopy for the evaluation of mediastinal lymph nodes in patients with non-small cell lung cancer. J Bras Pneumol, 2009, 35 (11): 1068-1074.

[33] Lerut T, De Leyn P, Coosemans W, et al. Cervical videomediastinoscopy. Thorac Surg Clin, 2010, 20 (2): 195-206.

[34] Martin-Ucar AE, Chetty GK, Vaughan R, et al. A prospective audit evaluating the role of video-assisted cervical mediastinoscopy (VAM) as a training tool. Eur J Cardiothorac Surg, 2004, 26 (2): 393-395.

[35] Leschber G, Sperling D, Klemm W, et al. Does videomediastinoscopy improve the results of conventional mediastinoscopy. Eur J Cardiothorac Surg, 2008, 33 (2): 289-293.

[36] Rami-Porta R, Call S. Invasive staging of mediastinal lymph nodes: Mediastinoscopy and remediastinoscopy. Thorac Surg Clin, 2012, 22 (2): 177 – 189.

[37] Yasufuku K, Keshavjee S. Staging non-small cell lung cancer. Clinical Pulmonary Medicine, 2010, 17 (5): 223 – 231.

[38] Lemaire A, Nikolic I, Petersen T, et al. Nine-year single center experience with cervical mediastinoscopy: complications and false negative rate. Annals of Thoracic Surgery, 2006, 82 (4): 1185 – 1189, discussion 1189 – 1190.

[39] Toloza EME, Harpole LL, Detterbeck FF, et al. Invasive staging of non-small cell lung cancer: A review of the current evidence. Chest, 2003, 123 (1 Suppl): 157S – 166S.

[40] McNeill TM, Chamberlain JM. Diagnostic anterior mediastinotomy. Annals of Thoracic Surgery. Soc Thorac Surgeons, 1966, 2 (4): 532.

[41] Van Schil P, van der Schoot J, Poniewierski J, et al. Remediastinoscopy after neoadjuvant therapy for non-small cell lung cancer. Lung Cancer, 2002, 37 (3): 281 – 285.

[42] Mateu-Navarro M, Rami-Porta R, Bastus-Piulats R, et al. Reme-diastinoscopy after induction chemotherapy in nonsmall cell lung cancer. ATS, 2000, 70 (2): 391 – 395.

[43] De Waele M, Serra-Mitjans M, Hendriks J, et al. Accuracy and survival of repeat mediastinoscopy after induction therapy for non-small cell lung cancer in a combined series of 104 patients. Eur J Cardiothorac Surg, 2008, 33 (5): 824 – 828.

[44] Rami-Porta R. Supermediastinoscopies: A step forward in lung cancer staging. J Thorac Oncol, 2007, 2 (4): 355 – 356.

[45] Zielinski M. Video-assisted mediastinoscopic lymphadenectomy and transcervical extended mediastinal lymphadenectomy. Thorac Surg Clin, 2012, 22 (2): 219 – 225.

[46] Yoo DG, Kim Y-H, Kim DK, et al. Clinical feasibility and surgical benefits ofvideo-assisted mediastinoscopic lymphadenectomy in the treatment of resectable lung cancer. Eur J Cardiothorac Surg, 2011, 40 (6): 4.

[47] Zielinski M. Transcervical extended mediastinal lymphadenectomy: Results of staging in two hundred fifty-six patients with non-small cell lung cancer. J Thorac Oncol, 2007, 2 (4): 370 – 372.

[48] Witte BB, Wolf MM, Huertgen MM, et al. Video-assisted mediastinoscopic surgery: Clinical feasibility and accuracy of mediastinal lymph node staging. ATS, 2006, 82 (5): 7.

[49] Yendamuri S, Demmy TL. Is VAMLA/TEMLA the new standard of preresection staging of non-small cell lung cancer. Journal of Thoracic and Cardiovascular Surgery, 2012, 144 (3): S14 – 17.

[50] Mohamed S, Yasufuku K, Nakajima T, et al. Analysis of cell cyclerelated proteins in mediastinal lymph nodes of patients with N2-NSCLC obtained by EBUS-TBNA: Relevance to chemotherapy response. Thorax, 2008, 63 (7): 642 – 647.

[51] Herth FJF, Annema JT, Eberhardt R, et al. Endobronchial ultrasound with transbronchial needle aspiration for restaging the mediastinum in lung cancer. J Clin Oncol, 2008, 26 (20): 3346 – 3350.

[52] Szlubowski A, Herth FJF, Soja J, et al. Endobronchial ultrasoundguided needle aspiration in non-small-cell lung cancer restaging verified by the transcervical bilateral extended mediastinal lymphadenectomy-a prospective study. European Journal of Cardio-thoracic Surgery, 2010, 37: 1180 – 1184.

[53] de Cabanyes Candela S, Detterbeck FC. A systematic review of restaging after induction therapy for stage IIIa lung cancer: prediction of pathologic stage. J Thorac Oncol, 2010, 5 (3): 389 – 398.

[54] Kirmani BH, Rintoul RC, Win T, et al. Stage migration: results of lymph node dissection in the era of modern imaging and invasive staging for lung cancer. European Journal of Cardio-Thoracic Surgery, 2013, 43 (1): 104 – 510.

[55] Rusch VW, Asamura H, Watanabe H, et al. The IASLC lung cancer staging project: A proposal for a new international lymph node map in the forthcoming 7th edition of the TNM classification for lung cancer. J Thorac Oncol, 2009, 4 (5): 568 – 577.

[56] Darling G, Dickie A, Malthaner R, et al. Invasive Mediastinal Staging of Exper Panel. Invasive Mediastinal staging of Non-small-cell Lung Cancer: A Clinical Practice Guideline, 2010. Toronto (ON): Cancer Care Ontario. Program in Evidence-based Care Evidence-based Series No. 17 – 6.

[57] Silvestri GA, Gonzalez AV, Jantz MA, et al. Methods for staging non-small cell lung cancer: diagnosis and management of lung cancer, 3nd: American College of Chest Physicians evidence-based clinical practice guidelines. Chest, 2013, 143 (5 Suppl): e211S – 250S.

第13章
孤立性肺结节的处理

Min P. Kim

Department of surgery, Division of Thoracic Surgery, Houston Methodist Hospital, Houston, TX, USA

引 言

孤立性肺结节是指在胸片上被肺组织包绕的直径≤3cm的单个高密度影。直径＞3cm的病灶称为肺肿块[1-3]。孤立性肺结节的成功诊断取决于对孤立性肺结节作为恶性病灶风险程度的准确评估,并根据风险评估提供适当的检查及干预措施。最终目的是为恶性肿瘤患者提供早期诊断及治疗,并降低有良性结节患者的发病率。应充分考虑患者的相关资料并提供能获得最佳治疗结果的方案。

孤立性肺结节可能是一种良性病变,如错构瘤、软骨瘤、肉芽肿病、肺炎、肺脓肿、类风湿关节炎、韦氏肉芽肿病、动静脉畸形、血管梗塞、血肿、先天性支气管闭锁或者为肺隔离症;也可能是恶性病变,如肺癌或者其他器官转移到肺的单个转移瘤[4]。临床表现及影像学特征可以提供信息以判断结节是否为恶性。

流行病学

美国肺癌筛查试验发现,可以通过低剂量计算机断层扫描(low-dose computed tomograply,LDCT)筛查肺癌高危人群[5]。研究表明,接受LDCT扫描进行肺癌筛查的人群,肺癌发病率相对减少20%。该试验入组超过50 000例年龄在55～74岁,在过去15年内每年至少吸烟30包的患者。排除既往被诊断为肺癌,18个月内接受过胸部CT扫描,近期咯血或者过去1年内体重减少15kg的患者。将入组患者随机分成两组:一组每年接受3次LDCT检查,另一组仅进行1次胸部影像学检查。在LDCT组,39%的患者中至少有1个阳性病灶,96%的阳性结果患者有良性病变。这项筛查最终在649例(2.4%)患者中发现肿瘤。但是,44例(0.2%)患者被漏诊;367例(1.4%)患者在筛查阶段后发展为肺癌。这项试验并没有发现能够判断肺结节良恶性的规律。放射科医生将结果告知试验的参与者或其监护人,但并没有明确的评估方法。最常见的方法是接受其他影像学检查,但是很少有患者接受有创检查[5]。

这项研究及其他大型研究表明[6-9],在筛查试验中确定的结节往往较小,并且恶性肿瘤的发病率较低。另外8项大型筛查试验的回顾性研究表明,被筛查人群中孤立性肺结节的发病率为8%～51%,其中恶性肿瘤占1.1%～12%[10]。然而,如果排除交界性或恶性可能性较大的结节,结节是恶性的概率可以高约55%[11]。

随着美国肺癌筛查试验证实LDCT筛查能够降低高危人群的发病率,更多的人将会被诊断为"孤立性肺结节"。目前还没有一套成熟的治疗原则来指导如何处理孤立性肺结节。然而,有一些指南可以平衡过度诊断程序和延迟癌症诊治。这些指南是根据临床表现和诊断成像特点,提供结节的恶性风险评估。

恶性风险

对于存在孤立性肺结节的患者,临床医生应根据临床及影像学特点来评估结节为恶性的可能性。孤立性肺结节的处理应依据此进行评估。

临床特点

以下几个临床特点可以增加单发结节的恶性

风险可能，其中包括患者的年龄、吸烟状况、职业暴露、COPD 史以及胸外恶性肿瘤病史。另一方面，近期有肺炎病史或者真菌感染病史的患者，结节为恶性的风险较小。

吸烟是肺癌最大的致病因素。因此，存在孤立性肺结节、有长期大量吸烟史的人，结节为恶性的可能性很大。与每天吸烟<1 包或者不吸烟的个体相比，当前吸烟频率高（>每天1包）的孤立性肺结节患者，结节恶性的风险最高[11]。戒烟<7年的患者较戒烟>7年的患者结节恶性的风险更高[11]。因此，戒烟患者的结节恶性危险程度低于现在仍吸烟的患者。

除了吸烟之外，患者的年龄也与孤立性肺结节的恶性概率有关。肺癌在 65~70 岁人群中的发病率很高，而 40 岁之前患者的发病率较低[12]。因此，65 岁相比 30 岁来说，孤立性肺结节为原发性肺癌的可能性更大。

个体病史亦与孤立性肺结节的恶性概率相关。有 COPD 病史的患者患恶性肿瘤的可能性更大[1]。石棉暴露是肺恶性肿瘤的高危因素[1]。最后，有胸外恶性肿瘤病史的患者在 CT 扫描中发现的孤立性肺结节，恶性可能性更大[13]。因此，结肠癌患者在 CT 扫描中发现的孤立性肺结节很可能诊断为转移性癌。但是，近期发生过真菌性肺炎的个体，恶性肿瘤的可能性小。应复查影像学检查，如果结节缩小或者消失，可能与肺炎有关。

放射学特征

CT 是评价孤立性肺结节放射学特征的最佳检查方法。通过胸部透视检查到孤立性肺结节时应再做胸部 CT 进一步评价结节的恶性可能。而且，应该根据之前所有的胸部影像学检查结果来计算结节的生长速度[14]。肿瘤大小、结节特征和生长速率会帮助医生明确恶性可能性的大小。

结节发展为肿瘤的可能性随其大小的增加而增大。在 8 项大型临床肺癌筛查研究中发现，直径 5mm 的结节发展为恶性的概率为 0~1%，5~10mm 的结节发展为恶性的概率为 6%~28%，11~20mm 的结节发展为恶性的概率为 33%~64%，>20mm 的结节发展为恶性的概率为 64%~82%[10,15]。因此，结节越大，其损害越大，恶性可能性也就越大。

结节的特征也能告诉我们其恶性可能性。6 项肺癌筛查研究发现，边缘光滑结节的恶性概率为 20%~30%，而边缘不规则、分叶状或针尖状结节的恶性概率为 33%~100%[10]。肺部边缘光滑的恶性肿瘤更容易转移到其他器官。孤立性肺结节的某种钙化模式表明它是良性的。弥散、中心分层、爆米花状的钙化结节可能是良性的，而斑点状、离心样的钙化结节则可能是恶性的[14]。

孤立性肺结节的生长速率也能预示其恶性可能性。大部分恶性孤立肺结节的大小在 40~400d 内翻倍。结节生长速度越快，其恶性可能性越大；生长速度越慢，其良性可能性越大[16-19]。肺部结节 2 年或 730d 以上稳定不变是预示良性的可靠指标[16,20]。然而，这并不是绝对的，这项指标的准确率只有 65%[17]。这可能是因为较小的孤立性肺结节的倍增时间很难估计。例如，5mm 的孤立性肺结节倍增后变成 6mm，而 CT 平扫不能发现这两种区别，显示它是稳定不变的。因此，如果单靠影像学标准，较小的结节可能要求长时间随访来确定其良恶性[17]。

治 疗

患者的意愿和决策制订共享

评价结节恶性可能性后，临床医生应该商讨每种治疗计划的利弊。一些患者担心结节恶变，不愿意定期随访；而另一些患者直到确定结节是恶性时，才同意手术切除。因此，制订每种治疗计划时都应将患者的意愿考虑在内[14]。

治疗计划

根据患者的临床病史和放射学研究，应该明确孤立性肺结节恶性可能性和提供个体化治疗计划。恶性可能性较低的结节应定期进行影像学检查；恶性可能性中等的结节应做无创性检查例如 FDG-PET，如果还不能明确，就应行结节样本活检；高度可疑恶性的结节应根据患者的手术指征和结节位置来制订治疗计划。

低度可疑恶性

评价恶性孤立性肺结节的风险后，如果其良

性可能较高，则应该定期做 CT 平扫，这种治疗的依据是恶性结节的倍增时间在 40～400d。因此，如果在 CT 平扫时发现结节倍增，则此结节恶性可能性增加，并且该患者应被划分为高危人群。定期随访的唯一缺点是有延误诊断恶性结节的风险[15]。因为存在这种可能，患者在最初发现肺结节时可以手术切除，而在随访时却发现了转移病灶。这使得可治愈的肺癌变得不可治愈，明显减少了总体生存率，考虑到这点，患者应定期行 CT 检查。

影像学检查没有标准的时间间隔，但有一般的指南和学会建议。Fleischner 学会（胸部影像与诊断学会）描述了较小结节（直径<8mm）的治疗策略[21]。有临床高危因素的患者，例如吸烟、结节直径<4mm 的患者 12 个月内应行一次 CT 随访，如果结节稳定不变，则不必再做后期随访。4～6mm 的结节患者应分别在 6～12 个月、18～24 个月做一次 CT 随访。6～8mm 的结节患者应在 3～6 个月、9～12 个月做定期随访，如果结节情况稳定，在第 24 个月再做一次 CT 随访。该建议发布 4 年后，大约 80% 的受访放射科医生知道这个建议并有 50% 的医生会将其应用于临床[22]。对于小结节（直径<8mm），Fleischner 学会的建议十分合理，但同时警告这仍有可能漏诊恶性结节。如果对于结节的状态有疑问，必要时可以间隔较长时间再次进行 CT 扫描以确定结节非恶性[17]。对于大的结节，应该缩短观察期来随访结节的生长。非恶性孤立性肺结节稳定的标准是 2 年。8～10mm 的孤立性肺结节合理的处理措施为至少 3、6、12、24 个月各随诊一次[14]。直径>1cm 的结节观察时间间隔更短，但是没有规定如何对结节进行检查。对于这种稍大的结节，通常需要 2～3 个月检查一次。在随后的检查中，如果结节体积增大，会增加恶性的风险。因此个体策略的制订应该基于下文所述的中度或高度可能性算法进行。

中度可疑恶性

临床及影像学检查显示结节为恶性的概率为中度概率，应该通过更长时间的观察来确定为恶性，包括 PDG-PET 加（或不加）组织活检，这种方式会增加或减少恶性孤立性肺结节的可能性。

FDG-PET

FDG-PET 扫描是将 ^{18}F 标记的脱氧葡萄糖（FDG）注射入患者体内，通过 FDG 的摄取量评估结节恶性的可能性。PET 对恶性结节的灵敏度高达 80% 和 100%，特异度为 40% 和 100%[10,23]。FDG-PET 特异度低是因为炎症及感染也会摄取葡萄糖，因此，肺炎的 PET 检查可能呈假阳性。最大摄取值（SUVmax）也可以提示结节恶性的可能性，SUVmax 为 0～2.5，恶性概率为 24%；最大摄取值为 2.6～4.0，恶性概率为 80%；SUVmax>4.1，恶性概率为 96%[24]。有研究显示，恶性肿瘤诊断最高精确值为孤立性结节的 SUVmax>4[25]。

若 PET 为阴性，则极大地降低了结节的恶性可能性，因此 PET 检查阴性患者仅行 CT 随访即可。在一项研究中，85% 的阴性患者进行了随诊，5% 的患者显示假阴性，但是此组患者的生存率与真阳性患者无显著差异[26]。PET 对小结节（<8mm）及特定转移肿瘤类型、特定肺癌不敏感，如类癌及支气管肺泡癌[24]。

如果为恶性结节，PET 对原发性肺癌的分期非常有益。在检测肺癌纵隔淋巴结转移中可以提高诊断准确度，为肺癌患者提供更好的术前分期[27]。虽然 PET 在孤立性肺结节的分期及处理方面花费较高，但整体看来物有所值[58]。

组织样本

PET 可以提高发现恶性结节的可能性，从中度可疑增加到高度可能性。然而，PET 检查后仍不能确定是否为恶性时，可行组织取样，依据部位，可以分开取样。

中心型病灶

中心型肺结节应依据支气管镜或超声内镜下（EBUS）活检确诊。支气管镜检通过支气管进行肺结节活检，而 EBUS 活检是针对近端气管及大支气管的病变。

支气管镜检及气管刷检活检的确诊率高达 74%[29]。然而，孤立性肺结节未行内镜气管组织活检的确诊率为 30%～40%[29-30]。活检的优势是可在患者清醒状态下给予镇静剂，且并发症少。

EBUS 活检是一种将直观查看气管和超声检测

气管周围组织相结合的技术，先在超声引导下确定孤立性肺结节的位置，然后再进行结节活检。EBUS 活检仅限于邻近主支气管的孤立性肺结节。总之，内镜活检是一种并发症少且诊断价值高的方法。另外，如果确定是恶性结节，患者在进行纵隔淋巴结分期的同时也完成了肺癌分期。EBUS 也能检测纵隔及一些肺门淋巴结。

中心至周围型病灶

CT 引导下经肺穿刺活检、经支气管活检两种方式可以进行中心型及周围型结节的诊断。前者诊断率较后者高，但是气胸发生率高。

肺组织活检

CT 引导下细针穿刺活检的诊断阳性率为 36%~86%，通常认为可达 80%[10,14]。患者在清醒状态和少量镇静剂及局部麻醉下进行操作。尽管诊断准确率高，但是会出现 30%~50% 的气胸[31-32]。CT 引导下细针穿刺活检的另一个缺点是如果肿瘤组织在一些特定部位，如中心病变或病变在缝隙中间则获取困难。气胸发生率与病变大小、肺气肿程度、结节与胸膜的距离及位置有关[33]。有研究报道，结节直径 > 1.5cm 与 < 1.5cm 诊断性样本中，气胸发生率分别为 73% 和 51%。总体诊断率为 68%，35% 的患者发生气胸，5% 的患者需要使用引流管[32]。

经支气管活检

目前有 3 种经支气管活检技术。通过这些技术，鞘管直接穿到肺结节位置，并借助穿刺针、活检钳和刷子进行活检。Meta 分析表明，与单纯应用支气管镜相比，电磁导航支气管镜（ENB；Super Dimension, Minneapolis, MN）、LungPoint 虚拟支气管镜导航（VBN；Broncus Technologies, Mountain View, CA）和径向支气管内超声（Olympus Medical, Tokyo, Japan）的诊断率可获得显著提高，可达 46%~80%，合并诊断率为 70%，气胸的总发生率为 1.5%[34]。

电磁导航支气管镜（ENB）可以引导鞘管放置到结节处，并且可以更换不同的工具进行活检取材。操作时首先要获得胸部 CT 薄层扫描并将其转换成肺的三维合成图像。然后，患者被放进一个电磁场，并将真正的支气管镜影像融合到计算机生成的虚拟图像中。通过一步步调整方向，引导鞘管到达单纯支气管镜不能看到的结节所在位置[35]。有几个因素可能会影响此项检查的诊断率，其中最重要的两点为结节的大小和 CT 图像上到达结节的气道显示情况[36]。这种技术也可以为那些确诊为肺癌但不能手术的患者放置（放疗）基准标记。这种技术可以只在镇静的情况下实施，当然，使用全身麻醉后更容易操作。总之，它诊断率非常好且气胸发生率非常低。

虚拟支气管镜导航（VBN）不使用由 ENB 提供的实时定位信息，而只利用 CT 扫描制作的支气管图像。Lungpoint 软件（Broncus Technologies）可以用薄层 CT 图像创建支气管图像[37]。虚拟图像叠加在实时支气管镜图像上，引导超细支气管镜到达结节位置[38]。根据病变的位置，可以使用标准支气管镜或超细支气管镜，并在 X 线透视下进行结节活检[37]。一项研究显示总诊断率为 63%，无气胸发生[37]。

径向支气管内超声引导（EBUS；Olympus Medical）鞘的放置和活检可以在患者清醒镇静后进行。首先进行标准的支气管镜检查，将一个小型径向 EBUS 经支气管镜插入并经鞘管引导至病灶位置；然后，退出 EBUS，使用一次性活检钳、细胞刷来获取活检组织；活检在透视下进行，以保证超声小探头未达到脏层胸膜以及活检钳正常工作。一项研究表明，此项技术的诊断灵敏度为 64%，气胸发生率为 1%[39]。径向支气管内超声可与 ENB 或 VBN 联合使用。在一项研究中，VBN 和径向 EBUS 联合应用的诊断准确率可达 80%，并且比单纯 EBUS 的定位速度更快[38]。

高度可疑恶性

对于具有高度可能的恶性孤立性肺结节患者，应根据其是否耐受手术确定处理原则。如果肺结节确实为原发性肺癌，应对患者进行标准心肺功能检查确定是否可以耐受手术治疗。即使不使用 FDG-PET 来确诊高概率恶性结节，对于可疑肺癌患者也应行 FDG-PET 检查来确定分期。如果 FDG-PET 显示其他位置的广泛转移，应在大多数可到达的位置进行活检并按照转移性肺癌治疗。如果 FDG-PET 显示只在肺结节区存在高摄取，应根据患者耐受手术的能力确定个体化治疗方案。

不能手术治疗的患者

如果患者被确定为不能手术，应尽力获得孤立性肺结节的明确诊断，上述几种方法均可以应用以获得诊断。根据病变的位置，可以使用支气管镜、径向 EBUS 或 CT 引导下经肺穿刺或经引导的经支气管结节活检术。对于不能手术的孤立性肺结节患者，引导支气管镜的优点是，早期肺癌患者可以放置放射治疗的基准标记。引导下支气管镜如电磁导航支气管镜，在放置基准标记方面具有非常高的成功率，并且很少发生位置移动[28]。高度可疑恶性的肺结节一旦确诊，应立即对肿瘤进行分期并采取适当的治疗措施。

适合手术治疗的患者

经心肺功能评估，如果患者适合手术，孤立性肺结节应根据病变位置进行处理。

周围型结节

对于周围型、经 FDG-PET 检查为高度可疑恶性的结节，如果患者可以耐受手术，应行 VATS 肺楔形切除术，如果病变为原发性肺癌，可行进一步肺叶切除和纵隔淋巴结清扫术。例如，一位 65 岁男性，有吸烟史，每年 40 包，肺周边位置发现一个 2cm、边缘毛刺的非钙化结节，经连续 CT 扫描 3 个月来体积不断增大，FDG-PET 上 SUVmax 为 8，没有转移征象并且可以耐受肺叶切除手术，手术可以使该患者在早期肺癌的诊断和治疗方面均有受益。

对于周围型结节，应对患者行对肺形态改变小的胸腔镜楔形切除术，术中进行结节的冷冻。VATS 肺楔形切除术的引入增加了良性病变的总体切除率[40]，但它比开胸肺切除术对肺形态改变小并且降低了死亡率[41]。如果结节是原发性肺癌，患者应接受全肺叶切除和纵隔淋巴结清扫术，因为这是 < 3cm 且无纵隔淋巴结转移证据肺癌的标准治疗方法，不仅可以明确诊断肿瘤[42]，还进行了治疗。如果胸腔镜楔形切除显示这是胸外恶性肿瘤的肺部转移，可以明确病变来源并且完成肺转移瘤的治疗；如果胸腔镜楔形切除术显示为良性结节，患者在明确诊断后就不再需要进行额外的 CT 扫描。

对于具有高风险恶性结节的患者，该方法避免了经胸或经支气管镜细针活检。这一策略的论点是，如果细针穿刺没有可诊断组织，患者会被安排进行胸腔镜楔形切除术。如果活检显示良性病变，仍有可能是穿刺没有取到恶性细胞，这是由技术错误或者细胞学检查的误读造成的，患者仍会被安排进行胸腔镜楔形切除术。如果穿刺证实为恶性，将对患者进行手术治疗。所以，不论穿刺结果如何，患者都将进行手术。因此，可疑恶性结节的穿刺结果并不会改变对患者的处理方法。最有可能的是，患者会承担所有的细针穿刺风险而获得最小的利益。然而，在没有证明存在恶性肿瘤的情况下，有些患者不愿意接受任何类型的手术干预，对这类患者应该行穿刺活检，先确认恶性肿瘤。

中部到中央的结节

高度可疑恶性结节如果位于肺中部到中央区域，需要行经支气管或经胸腔穿刺活检明确诊断后进行肺段或肺叶切除术。因为相比 VATS 肺楔形切除，VATS 肺段、肺叶切除术对肺组织的损伤更大，并有更高的死亡率，应对患者行穿刺活检以证实恶性肿瘤的存在。如果活检显示为早期肺癌，患者应接受胸腔镜或开胸肺叶切除术及纵隔淋巴结清扫术。

总　结

随着越来越多的医疗机构开展肺癌的筛查，孤立性肺结节的诊断必将有所增加。对这部分患者的处理应该基于临床危险因素的准确评估，如年龄、吸烟状况、职业暴露、胸外恶性肿瘤或慢性阻塞性肺疾病史。通过胸部 CT 扫描评估结节的大小、特点及生长速度。如果临床和影像学评估显示低度可疑恶性结节，患者应进行一系列 CT 扫描观察或制订随访策略；对于中度可疑恶性结节，患者应行 FDG-PET 检查，进行或不进行活检；对于高度可疑恶性结节，非手术患者应尽力取得组织样本；可进行手术的患者，对周围型结节应行胸腔镜肺楔形切除术，中部、中央区的结节应行经胸或经支气管镜取样。一旦确诊，患者将根据诊断结果得到适当的治疗。这种处理措施将为早期肺癌提供诊断和治疗策略，并减少良性结节诊治过程中带来的肺部损伤。

（陶恒敏　黄　伟　译）

参考文献

[1] Ost DE, Gould MK. Decision making in patients with pulmonary nodules. Am J Respir Crit Care Med, 2012, 185 (4): 363-372. PMCID: 3361350.

[2] Ost D. Fein AM, Feinsilver SH. Clinical practice. The solitary pulmonary nodule. New England Journal of Medicine, 2003, 348 (25b): 2535-2542.

[3] Gould MK, Fletcher J, Iannettoni MD, et al. Evaluation of patients with pulmonary nodules: when is it lung cancer: ACCP evidence based clinical practice guidelines. 2nd. Chest, 2007, 132 (3 Suppl): 108S-130S.

[4] Erasmus JJ, Connolly JE. McAdams HP, et al. Solitary pulmonary nodules: Part I. Morphologic evaluation for differentiation of benign and malignant lesions. Radiographia, 2000, 20 (1): 43-78.

[5] Aberle DR, Adams AM, Berg CD, et al. Reduced lung cancer mortality with low-dose computed tomographic screening. New England Journal of medicine, 2011, 365 (5): 395-409.

[6] Henschke CI, Yankelevitz DF, Naidich DP, et al. CT screening for lung cancer. Suspiciousness of nodules according to size on baseline scans. Radiology, 2004, 231 (1): 164-168.

[7] Gohagan J, Marcus P, Fagerstrom R, et al. Baseline findings of a randomized feasibility trial of lung cancer screening with spiral CT scan vs chest radiograph: The Lung Screenng Study of the National Cancer Institute. Chest, 2004, 126 (1): 114-121.

[8] Sone S, Li F, Yang ZG, et al. Results of three-year mass screeing programme for lung cancer using mobile low-dose spiral computed tomography scanner. Br J Cancer, 2001, 84 (1): 25-32. PMCID: 2363609.

[9] Swensen SJ. Jett JR, Hartman TE, et al. Lung cancer screening with CT: Mayo Clinic experience. Radiology, 2003, 226 (3): 756-761.

[10] Wahidi MM, Govert JA, Goudar RK, et al. Evidence for the treatment of patientswith pulmonary nodules when is it lung cancer: ACCP evidence-based clinical practice guidelines (2nd edn). Chest, 2007, 132 (3 Suppl): 94S-107S.

[11] Varoli F, Vergani C, Caminiti R, et al. Management of solitary pulmonary nodule. Eur J Cardiothorac Surg, 2008, 33 (3): 461-465.

[12] Parkin DM, Muir CS. Cancer Incidence in Five Continents Comparability and puality of data. IARC Sci Pub, 1992, 120: 45-173.

[13] Swensen SJ, Silverstein MD, Ilstrup DM, et al. The probability of malignancy in solitary pulmonary nodules, Application to small radiologically indeterminate nodules. Arch Intern Med, 1997, 157 (8): 849-855.

[14] Gould MK, Fletcher J, Iannettoni MD, et al. Evaluation of patients with pulmonary nodules: when is it lung cancer. ACCP evidence-based clinical practice guidelines. 2nd. Chest, 2007, 132 (3 Suppl): 108S-30S.

[15] Ost DE, Gould MK. Decision making in patients with pulmonary nodules. Am J Respir Crit Care Med, 2012, 185 (4): 363-372. PMCID: 3361350.

[16] Erasmus JJ, McAdams HP, Connolly JE. Solitary pulmonary nodules: Part II. Evaluation of the indeterminate nodule. Radiographics, 2000, 20 (1): 59-66.

[17] Yankelevitz DF, Henschke CI. Does 2-year stability imply that pulmonary nodules are benign. AJR Am J Roentgenol, 1997, 168 (2): 325-328.

[18] Howard TA, Woodring JH. Clinical and imaging evaluation of the solitary pulmonary nodule. Am Fam Physician, 1992, 46 (6): 1753-1759.

[19] Caskey CI, Templeton PA, Zerhouni EA. Current evaluation of the solitary pulmonary nodule. Radiol Clin North Am, 1990, 28 (3): 511-520.

[20] Good CA, Wilson TW. The solitary circumscribed pulmonary nodule; study of seven hundred five cases encountered roentgenologically in a period of three and one-half years. J Am Med Assoc, 1958, 166 (3): 210-215.

[21] MaMahon H, Austin JHM, Gamsu G, et al. Guidelines for management of small pulmonary nodules detected on CT scans: a statement from the Flecischner Society. Radiology, 2005, 237 (2): 395-400.

[22] Eisenberg RL, Bankier AA, Boiselle PM. Compliance with Flecischner Society guidelines for management of small lung nodules: a survey of 834 radiologists. Radiology, 2010, 255 (1): 218-224.

[23] Kubota K, Murakami K, Inoue T, et al. Additional effects of FDG-PET to thin-section CT for the differential diagnosis of lung nodules: a Japanese multicenter clinical study. Ann Nucl Med, 2011, 25 (10): 787-795.

[24] Bryant AS, Cerfolio RJ. The maximum standardized up-

为解剖标志以预警可能存在的变异动脉分支血管；最后需要处理的是右肺上叶支气管或后升支动脉，二者的处理顺序往往取决于解剖位置、动脉血管粗细以及切割吻合器放置角度。切除的肺叶应置于标本袋内移出以避免切口种植。所有切除的淋巴结应依据区域分组标记并单独送检。切除其他肺叶时术中肺门结构处理亦采取由前向后递进的相似流程，见图14.3～14.6。

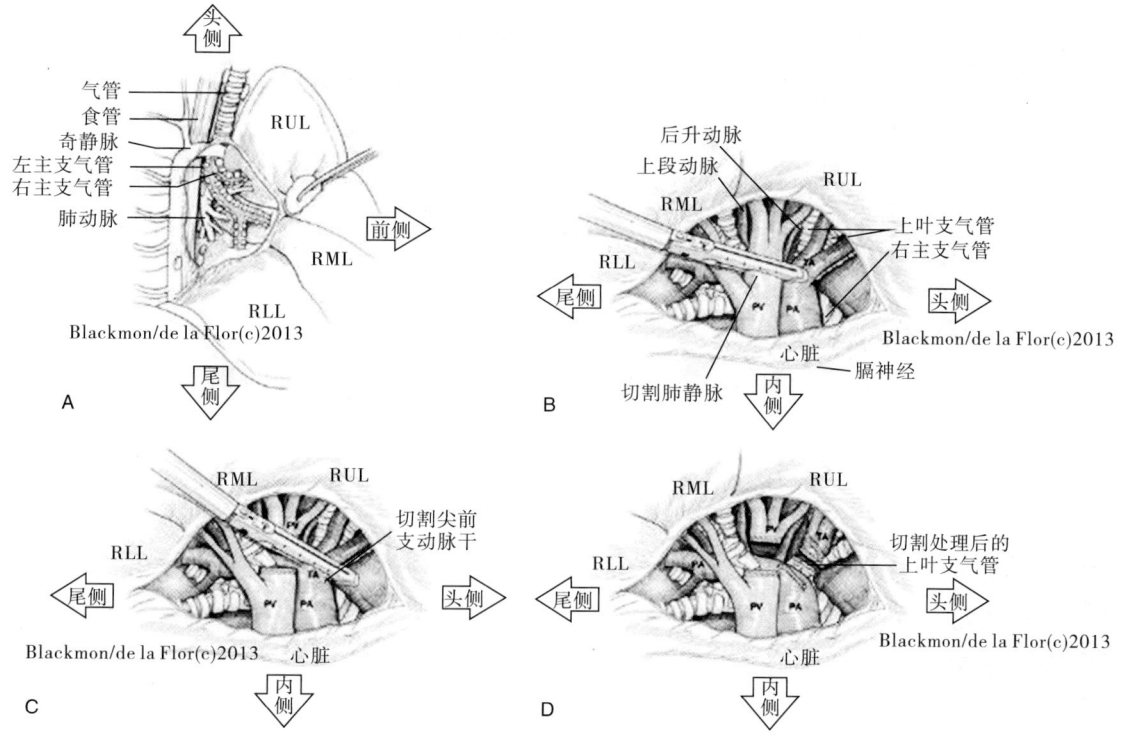

图14.2 A. 胸腔镜右肺上叶切除手术步骤：在肺门后方打开胸膜并解剖。B. 胸腔镜右肺上叶切除手术步骤：处理右肺上叶静脉。C. 胸腔镜右肺上叶切除手术步骤：处理右肺上叶尖前支动脉。D. 胸腔镜右肺上叶切除手术步骤：处理右肺上叶后升支动脉、上叶支气管。PA：肺动脉；PV：肺静脉；RLL：右肺下叶；RML：右肺中叶；RUL：右肺上叶；TA：尖前支动脉干

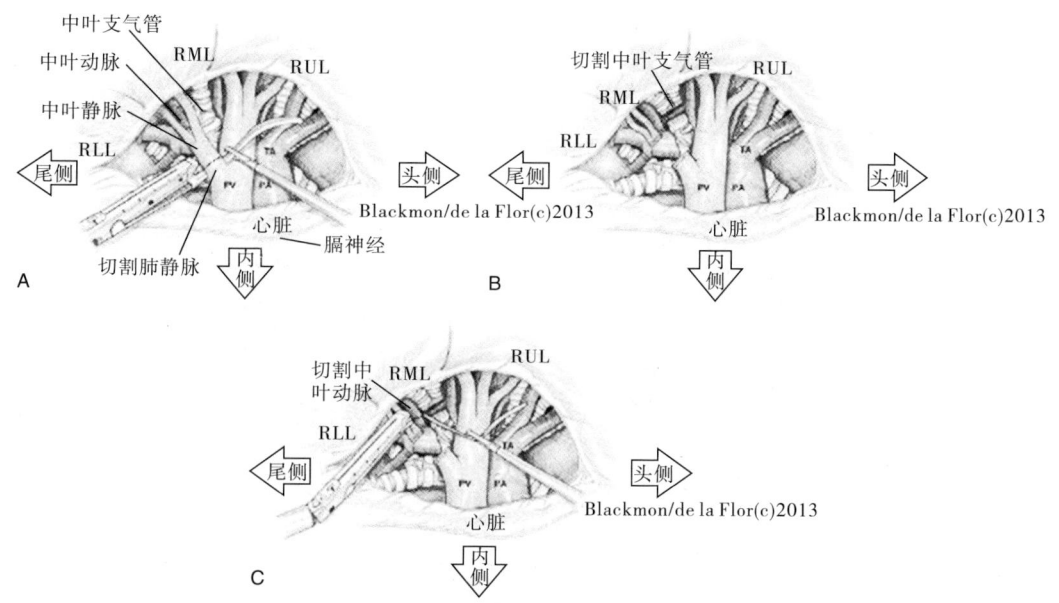

图14.3 胸腔镜右肺中叶切除术步骤。PA：肺动脉；PV：肺静脉；RLL：右肺下叶；RML：右肺中叶；RUL：右肺上叶；TA：尖前支动脉干

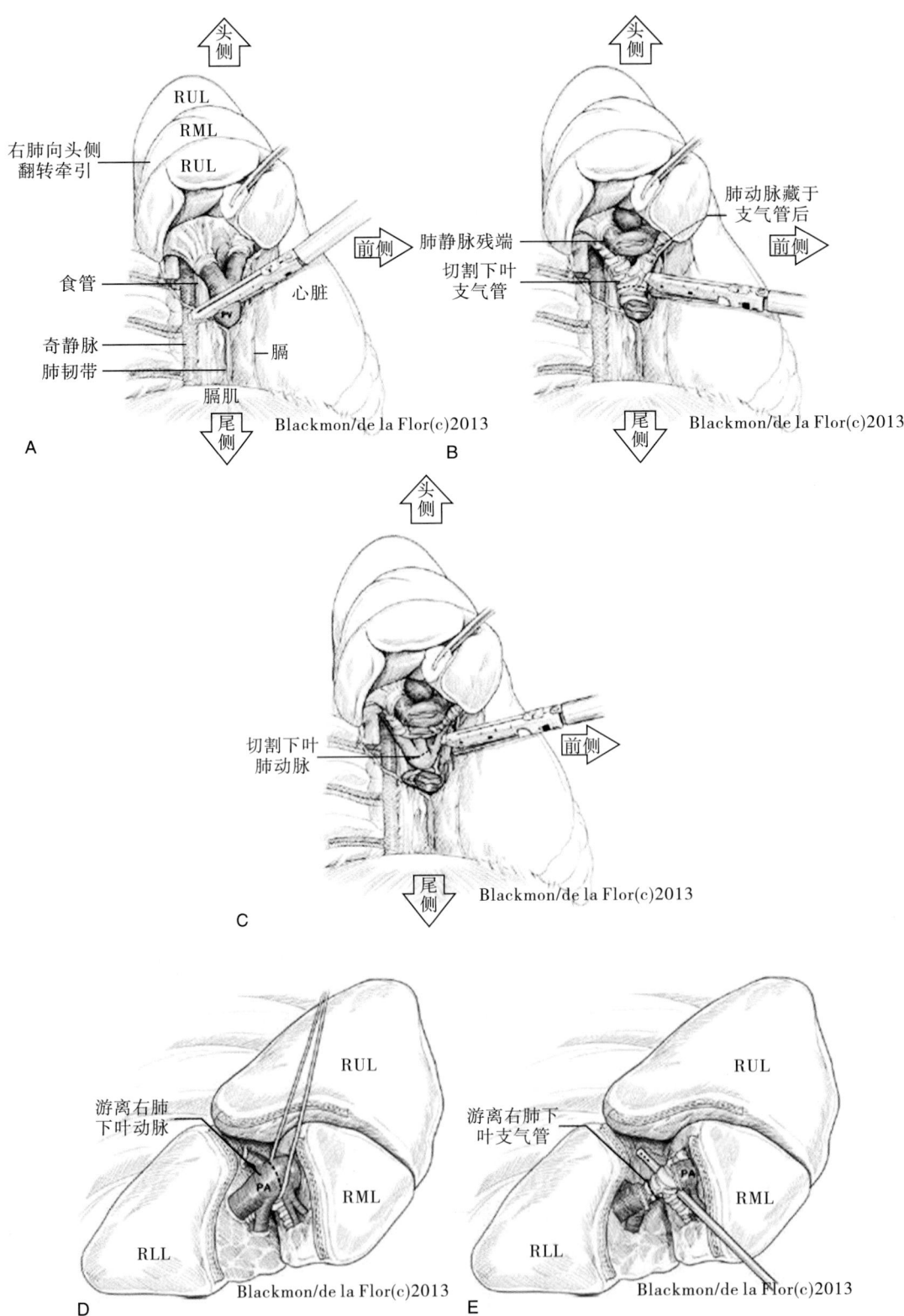

图14.4 胸腔镜右肺下叶切除术步骤。PA：肺动脉；PV：肺静脉；RLL：右肺下叶；RML：右肺中叶；RUL：右肺上叶

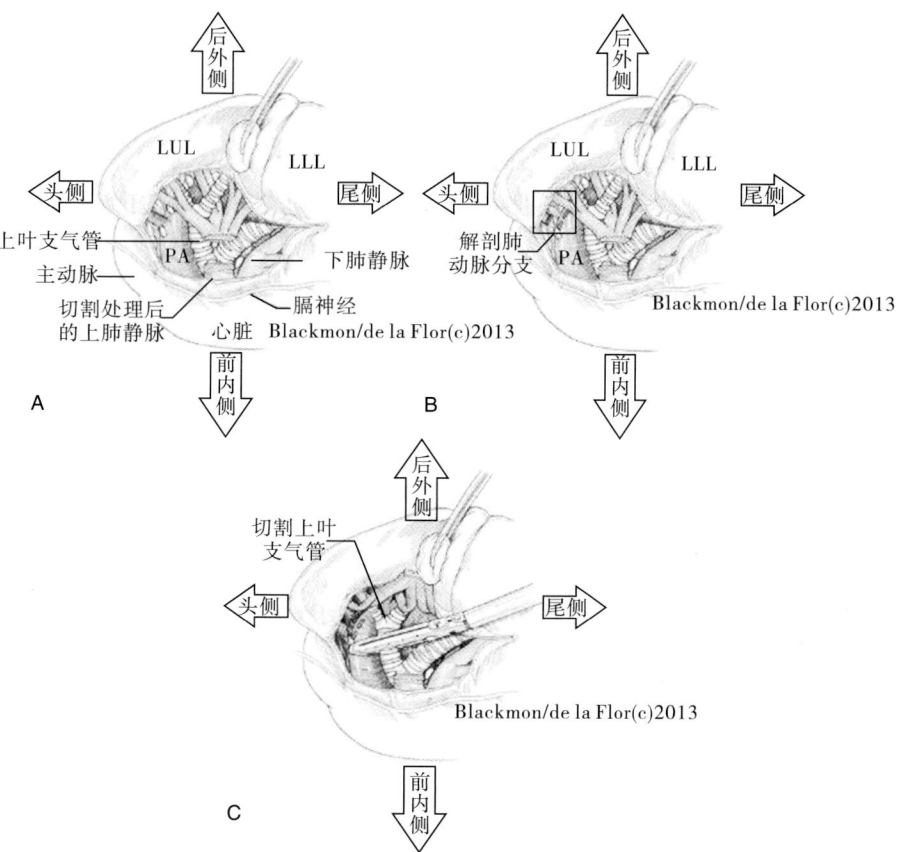

图 14.5 胸腔镜左肺上叶切除术步骤。LLL：左肺下叶；LUL：左肺上叶；PA：肺动脉；PV：肺静脉

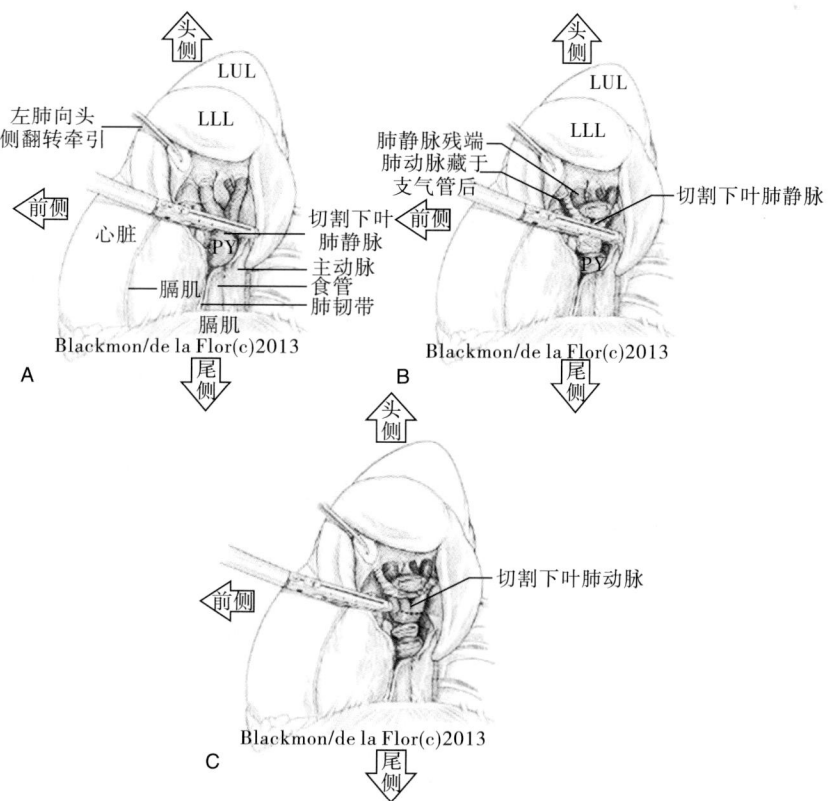

图 14.6 胸腔镜左肺下叶切除术步骤。LLL：左肺下叶；LUL：左肺上叶；PA：肺动脉；PV：肺静脉

胸腔镜肺叶切除术成功开展10余年来在整个胸外科领域广泛流行、传播，成为早期NSCLC治疗的标准术式[2-3]。已发表的4项随机对照临床试验研究中有3项显示胸腔镜肺叶切除术较开放肺叶切除术存在明显优势[5-8]，胸腔镜肺叶切除术也因此被明确纳入循证医学治疗指南中[4]。这些优势包括以下几点：减轻术后疼痛[9-11]，减少术中出血[5,8,10,12]，减轻炎症反应[13]，缩短胸管引流时间[9-10,13-15]，改善术后生活质量[14]，改善术后肺功能[16-19]，相当的手术持续时间[9,13-14,20]，缩短住院时间[2,3,5,13-15,21-24]，高性价比[16]以及提高术后辅助化疗的可行性[15,17]。近期一项关于胸腔镜肺叶切除术后并发症发生率、死亡率的评估研究显示其在很多其他方面也存在优势[18,20,25-30]。另外，胸外科医师协会普胸外科学组统计其认证胸外科医师的手术数据，结果显示从1999—2006年胸腔镜肺叶切除术占全部肺叶切除术的比例仅为20%[31]，因此胸腔镜肺叶切除术的优势和潜力更有待进一步研究。基于上述认识，胸腔镜肺叶切除术目前被认为是治疗早期NSCLC的金标准[32]。以下将对相关文献综述进行全面评价。

术后疼痛

Demmy等将胸腔镜肺叶切除术与常规开胸肺叶切除术患者分为两组，术后给予类似的镇痛治疗方案，结果腔镜组6%的患者诉剧烈疼痛，而开胸组为65%，同时腔镜组63%的患者诉轻微疼痛或者无疼痛，而开胸组该项数据仅为6%[32]。另有3项研究认为胸腔镜手术患者术后早期疼痛减轻或镇痛治疗需求减少[11,17-18]。并有研究证明其对术后疼痛的改善时效在1年以上[10]。

术中出血量和胸管引流

Tajiri等报道了胸腔镜组患者（n=168）较常规开胸组（n=61）患者的术中出血量更少[10]。另有研究报道了一致的结论或者二者无显著差异[5,8,10-11]。许多研究证明二者带管引流持续时间相当，部分研究显示腔镜手术在减少前3d引流总量方面较开胸组差异具有统计学意义[3,10,13-15]。

术后生活质量

肺叶切除患者术后如需依赖家庭保健或某项健康设备则说明其术后生活质量不佳，Demmy等发表了一项研究，通过分析这部分患者的比例发现胸腔镜手术患者术后生活质量相对有所改善[9]。进一步的研究显示胸腔镜手术患者更有机会恢复到术前的生活状态[14]。

肺功能

由于更多的患者可耐受创伤更小的胸腔镜肺叶切除术，传统观念认为的开胸手术肺功能低值或许不再适用。微创手术切口小、对胸壁破坏减小、术后疼痛减轻，理论上可保留更好的术后呼吸功能。具体评估需检测术后即刻以及术后3个月的肺功能指标。1996年，Tschernko等将47例胸腔镜肺叶切除术或腋下小切口开胸肺叶切除术患者纳入一项前瞻性临床对照试验，发现胸腔镜肺叶切除术组患者术后72h内血氧饱和度数值更高[17]。此外，FEV_1也被用来研究对比，Nagahiro等证实胸腔镜肺叶切除术患者术后2周时FEV_1恢复至术前水平的95%，而开胸肺叶切除组仅恢复了80%[11]。另一项日本学者的研究证实胸腔镜手术术后3个月时FEV_1恢复情况也存在优势，而Kaseda等报道了术后1年肺功能改善情况的阳性研究结果[18]。无论采取何种手术入路，肺功能差则意味着呼吸系统并发症的发生概率高，肺功能差的患者行开胸手术相比胸腔镜手术更容易出现呼吸系统并发症。因此，高危患者在评估手术可行性时更应慎重考虑应该采取何种术式或入路[33]。

手术及住院时间

假如主刀医生已完成学习曲线熟练掌握胸腔镜手术技巧并配备训练有素的团队，那么胸腔镜肺叶切除术与开胸肺叶切除术的总体手术时间不应有明显差异[5,9,13-14]。有研究总结了97项胸腔镜肺叶切除术的多中心临床数据[8]：死亡率为2%，平均手术时间为130min，平均术后住院时间为3d。3d的术后住院时间与其他已发表文献的结果一致[2,3,5,13-15,23-24]。Onaitis等报道了一项包含500例患者的连续开展的胸腔镜肺叶切除术研究[3]：术后30d内死亡率为1%，无术中死亡病例；中转开胸比例低于2%，且无紧急中转病例；中位带管引流时间为2d，术后平均住院时间为3d。总体来讲，大部分研究证实胸腔镜肺叶切除术缩短了术后住院时间[14-15]。

成本-效益

Burfeind等回顾性分析了2002—2004年行胸腔镜肺叶切除术或开胸肺叶切除术的113例患者的住院花费成本数据，通过使用生活质量评价量表并计算生活质量校正后的生存时间来评价分析每个纳入样本的成本或成本-效益[16]。开胸手术组的平均总花费为12 119美元，胸腔镜手术组的平均总花费为10 084美元，两者具有统计学差异（$P=0.0012$）。美国每年大约有50 000台肺叶切除手术，如果均采用微创手术方式则可节省1亿美元花费。

术后辅助化疗的依从性

胸腔镜肺叶切除术最具前景的优势之一在于可提高术后辅助化疗的依从性[15]。Petersen等对比研究了100例接受完全性肺叶切除手术的NSCLC患者，腔镜手术组（$n=57$）与开放手术组（$n=43$）相比在术后辅助化疗延期（18% vs 58%；$P=0.001$）及用药减量方面（26% vs 49%；$P=0.02$）更具优势，使得辅助化疗更具可行性，胸腔镜组患者接受拟定术后辅助化疗方案的比例更高（61% vs 40%；$P=0.03$）。另一项独立研究结果显示85%的胸腔镜手术组患者按计划接受了全周期化疗方案[17]。虽然这些研究的观察终点并非长期生存，但是其他类型肿瘤的相似研究发现接受术后化疗与生存质量改善呈正相关[34,36]。另外一些术后辅助化疗方面的研究显示，对照组传统开胸手术患者仅有55%~70%接受全部化疗方案，相比而言胸腔镜组在这方面优势更明显[37-38]。

并发症

最近，STS数据库大样本前瞻性病例匹配对照研究结果显示，胸腔镜肺叶切除术与传统开胸肺叶切除术相比术后并发症发生率更低[18,20,25-30]。近期一篇包含了21项探讨胸腔镜肺叶切除术后并发症、病死率对照研究（2项随机对照，19项非随机对照）的meta分析[35]结果显示，胸腔镜肺叶切除术在术后局部复发方面与开胸肺叶切除术无显著差异（$P=0.24$），全身复发率、5年存活率方面优势明显（P值分别为0.03、0.04）。

术中突发严重后果事件的概率低于1%[39]。尽管胸腔镜肺叶切除术中出现致死性并发症的情况并不多见，但是对于相关损伤、并发症发生可能性的认识是至关重要的，更主要的目的是预防并发症。术者扎实的解剖基础、仔细的游离操作、对潜在并发症清楚的认知、果断明智的中转开胸等有利于减少并发症出现并减轻并发症导致的损伤。

特殊情况

二次手术

胸腔镜肺叶切除手术的另一个优势体现在第二原发肺癌需要再次手术切除方面。腔镜手术创伤减轻，术后胸腔内及肺门处瘢痕组织增生减轻，故而可能使得再次手术更为可行。

腔镜手术推广发展的障碍

胸腔镜肺叶切除术的推广发展至今仍然存在障碍。对胸腔镜下肺动脉出血不可控制的认识是一种误解，这可能会阻碍胸外科医生考虑学习胸腔镜肺叶切除术。大多数美国执业胸外科医生在开展胸腔镜肺叶切除术之前都要接受培训，培训结业并进行资格认证是最普及的流程。美国大多数培训计划一般提供胸腔镜动物肺叶切除手术的机会，在患者身上开展实际手术的经验仍未知。美国胸外科委员会（the American Board of Thoracis Surgery）最近把胸腔镜肺叶切除术纳入必要的术式指标。当医院、协会等寻求培训老一辈的胸外科医生开展胸腔镜手术时，他们需要更高阶的培训路径及认证标准。

胸腔镜肺段切除术

Yang 等搜集并分析了肺段切除术后患者转归的相关研究，发现胸腔镜肺段切除术与开胸肺段切除术相比具有水平相当的肿瘤学结局，住院时间更短、围术期并发症发生率更低且花费更少[40]。而胸腔镜肺段切除术与胸腔镜肺叶切除术具有相近的并发症发生率、复发率及存活率。初步研究发现，胸腔镜肺段切除术相比胸腔镜肺叶切除术可以更好地保留肺功能及运动能力，但二者的总体肿瘤学结局是否存在差异仍未明确，需要比较其等效无复发存活期来证明。CALGB 140503 和 JCOG0802/WJOG4607L 是两项精心设计的旨在评价胸腔镜肺段切除术获益与否的前瞻性研究，其结果尚未公布。

胸腔镜全肺切除术

Nwogu 等回顾性分析了其单中心 6 年间接受肺切除手术的 70 例患者，发现与传统开胸全肺切除组相比，胸腔镜全肺切除组患者的住院时间缩短、术中出血量减少，二者的围术期并发症发生率及术后生存期方面水平相当[41]。

胸腔镜支气管成形重建术

尽管有个案研究及录像视频讨论如何实现在胸腔镜下完成支气管切除成形重建手术[42]，但其可行性尚无文献报道。这也是微创外科亟待突破的重要领域，未来机器人缝合技术以及精细关节头设备可能将大有作为。

胸腔镜胸壁切除术

尽管胸腔镜下开展肺叶或肺段切除等基本术式相比开放手术已经尽显优势，但是复杂胸壁切除或扩大切除手术方面的前景并不明确。胸壁切除手术需要更先进的胸腔镜器械，脊柱侧弯手术常用的微创骨科设备便极为适用，例如：内镜肋骨剪（现由 Medtronic 公司生产）、肋骨骨膜剥离器、线锯等。利用网格材料重建胸壁缺损时，全胸壁固定缝线、示踪设备、腹腔镜缝合器械都可便于安置和固定操作[43-44]。

胸腔镜淋巴结清扫术

Boffa 等利用美国胸外科医师协会数据库观察了 9 年间 11 531 例（传统开胸组 7 137 例，胸腔镜组 4 394 例）手术 N0 分期患者，研究他们的淋巴结转移情况以评价手术淋巴结清扫彻底与否[45]。临床分期 N0 患者行肺叶或肺段切除手术，胸腔镜组和开胸手术组纵隔淋巴结病理分期升期情况相当。另一方面，胸腔镜组 N0 升期为 N1 的比例相对更低，这似乎也预示着支气管旁、肺门淋巴结清扫完整性方面存在不稳定性。因此，随着越来越多的外科医生接受并开展胸腔镜手术，对于淋巴结切除完整性的关注也日益升温。部分医生在胸腔镜下做广泛淋巴结清扫时会觉得操作不舒适，进而可能会采取相对不彻底的淋巴结采样，机器人手术为此提供了一项可替代的微创技术，或许可以帮助避免上述操作。

机器人肺叶切除术

机器人胸外科手术是腔镜胸外科手术的一种替代术式，采用相似的视频导引下切除技术，其术野三维立体成像、多达 7 个自由度的机器人操作手臂、高精度成像、主-仆式远距离操作台等技术特点更为先进。机器人胸外科手术一般需要 3~4 个操作手臂，一项多中心研究统计了 325 例接受该术式的患者，中转开胸比例为 8%，围术期出现主要并发症的比例为 3.7%（$n=12$），其中出现 1 例院内死亡[46]。有些医疗中心报道这项新技术成本昂贵，尽管如此，其围术期并发症发病率、死亡率低，优势仍旧明显。正如之前研究胸腔镜微创手术与开胸手术对比的结果一样，机器人胸外科手术后分期特异性的长期生存期结果也是可以接受的。

总 结

早期 NSCLC 患者接受微创手术治疗是安全、有效、经济的。胸腔镜肺叶切除术可完整解剖肺门并对血管逐一处理，因此其总体肿瘤学结局与传统开胸肺叶切除手术相当。胸腔镜下解剖性切除手术的公认优势包括减少术后短期疼痛，缩短住院时间，快速恢复至完全活动能力，保留肺功能，减少术后并发症。此外，资料显示，胸腔镜肺叶切除术可改善患者术后辅助治疗的依从性，随机临床试验的验证是必要的，但具体实施的可能性不大。总之，胸腔镜肺叶切除术可作为早期肺癌患者的标准治疗选择。

（冯　振　刘　颖　彭忠民　译）

参考文献

[1] Siegel R, Naishadham D, Jemal A. Cancer statistics. CA Cancer J Clin, 2012, 62 (1): 10-29.

[2] McKenna RJ, Houck W, Fuller CB. Videoassisted thoracic surgery lobectomy: Experience with 1 100 cases. Ann Thorac Surg, 2006, 81: 421-426.

[3] Onaitis MW, Petersen PR, Balderson SS, et al. Thoracoscopic lobectomy is a safe and versatile procedure: Experience with 500 consecutive patients. Ann Surg, 2006, 244: 420-425.

[4] Ettinger DS, Akerly W, Bepler G, et al. National Comprehensive Cancer Network (NCCN). Non-small cell lung cancer clinical practice guidelines in oncology. J Natl Compr Canc Netw, 2008, 6: 228-269.

[5] Kirby TJ, Mack MJ, Landreneau RJ, et al. Lobectomy-video-assisted thoracic surgery versus muscle-sparing thoracotomy: A randomized trial. J Thorac Cardiovasc Surg, 1995, 109: 997-1001.

[6] Sugi K, Kaneda Y, Esato K. Video-assisted thoracoscopic lobectomy achieves a satisfactory long-term prognosis in patients with clinical stage IA lung cancer. World J Surg, 2000, 24: 27-31.

[7] Craig SR, Leaver HA, Yap PL, et al. Acute phase responses following minimal access and conventional thoracic surgery. Eur J Cardiothorac Surg, 2001, 20: 455-463.

[8] Shigemura N, Akashi A, Nakagiri T, et al. Complete vs. assisted thoracoscopic approach: a prospective randomized trial comparing a variety of video-assisted thoracoscopic lobectomy techniques. Surg Endosc, 2004, 18: 1492-1497.

[9] Demmy TL, Curtis JJ. Minimally invasive lobectomy directed toward frail and high-risk patients: A case control study. Ann Thorac Surg, 1999, 68: 194-200.

[10] Tajiri M, et al. Decreased invasiveness via two methods of thoracoscopic lobectomy for lung cancer, compared with open thoracotomy. Respirology, 2007, 12: 207-211.

[11] Nagahiro I, Andou A, Aoe M, et al. Pulmonary function, postoperative pain, and serum cytokine level after lobectomy: A comparison of VATS and conventional procedure. Ann Thorac Surg, 2001, 72: 362-365.

[12] Nomori H, Horio H, Naruke T, et al. What is the advantage of a thoracoscopic lobectomy over a limited thoracotomy procedure for lung cancersurgery. Ann Thorac Surg, 2001, 72 (3): 879-884.

[13] Yim APC, et al. VATS lobectomy reduces cytokine responses compared with conventional surgery. Ann Thorac Surg, 2000, 70: 243-247.

[14] Demmy TJ, et al. Discharge independence with minimally invasive lobectomy. Am J Surg, 2004, 188: 689-702.

[15] Petersen RP, Pham D, Burfeind WR, et al. Thoracoscopic lobectomy facilitates the delivery of chemotherapy after resection for lung cancer. Ann Thorac Surg, 2007, 83: 1245-1249.

[16] Burfeind W, Jaik N, Villamizar N, et al. A cost-minimization analysis of lobectomy: Thoracoscopic vs. posterolateral thoracotomy. Eur J Cardiothorac Surg, 2010.

[17] Tschernko E, Hofer S, Beiglmayer C, et al. Video-assisted wedge resection/lobectomy versus conventional axillary thoracotomy. Chest, 1996, 109: 1636-1642.

[18] Kaseda S, Aoki T, Hangai N, et al. Better pulmonary function and prognosis with video-assisted thoracic surgery than with thoracotomy. Ann Thorac Surg, 2000, 70: 1644-1646.

[19] Nakata M, et al. Pulmonary function after lobectomy: Video-assisted thoracic surgery versus thoracotomy. Ann Thorac Surg, 2000, 70: 938-941.

[20] Cattaneo SM, Park BJ, Wilton AS, et al. Use of video-assisted thoracic surgery for lobectomy in the elderly results in fewer complications. Ann Thorac Surg, 2008, 85: 231-236.

[21] Park BJ, Zhang H, Rusch VW, et al. Videoassisted thoracic surgery does not reduce the incidence of postoperative atrial fibrillation after pulmonary lobectomy. J Thorac Cardiovasc Surg, 2007, 133: 775-779.

[22] Nicastri DG, Wisnivesky JP, Litle VR, et al. Thoracoscopic lobectomy: report on safety, discharge independence, pain, and chemotherapy tolerance. J Thorac Cardiovasc Surg, 2008, 135: 642-647.

[23] Swanson SJ, Herndon JE, D'Amico TA, et al. Video-assisted thoracic surgery (VATS) lobectomy-report of CALGB 39802: a prospective, multiinstitutional feasibility

study. J Clin Oncol, 2007, 25: 4993 – 4997.

[24] Cajipe MD, Chu D, Bakaeen FG, et al. Videoassisted thoracoscopic lobectomy is associated with better perioperative outcomes than open lobectomy in a veteran population. Am J Surg, 2012, 204 (5): 607 – 612.

[25] Villamizar NR, Darrabie MD, Burfeind WR, et al. Thoracoscopic lobectomy is associated with lower morbidity compared to thoracotomy. J Thorac Cardiovasc Surg, 2009, 138: 419 – 424.

[26] Paul S, Altorki NK, Sheng S, et al. Thoracoscopic lobectomy is associated with lower morbidity than open lobectomy: A propensity-matched analysis from the STS Database. J Thorac Cardiovasc Surg, 2010, 139: 366 – 378.

[27] Berry MF, Hanna J, Tong BC, et al. Risk factors for morbidity after lobectomy for lung cancer in elderly patients. Ann Thorac Surg, 2009, 88: 1093 – 1099.

[28] Muraoka M, Oka T, Akamine S, et al. Videoassisted thoracic surgery lobectomy reduces the morbidity after surgery for stage I non-small cell lung cancer. Jpn J Thorac Cardiovasc Surg, 2006, 54: 49 – 55.

[29] Whitson BA, Andrade RS, Boettcher A, et al. Video-assisted thoracoscopic surgery is more favorable than thoracotomy for resection of clinical stage I nonsmall cell lung cancer. Ann Thorac Surg, 2007, 83: 1965 – 1970.

[30] D'Amico TA. Long-term outcomes after thoracoscopic lobectomy. Thorac Surg Clin, 2008, 18: 259 – 262.

[31] Boffa DJ, Allen MS, Grab JD, et al. Data from the Society of Thoracic Surgeons General Thoracic Surgery database: the surgical management of primary lung tumors. J Thorac Cardiovasc Surg, 2008, 135: 247 – 254.

[32] Hartwig MG, D'Amico TA. Thoracoscopic lobectomy: The gold standard for early-stage lung cancer. Ann Thorac Surg, 2010, 89 (6): S2098 – S2101.

[33] Ceppa DP, Kosinski AS, Berry MF, et al. Thoracoscopic lobectomy has increasing benefit in patients with poor pulmonary function: a Society of Thoracic Surgeons Database analysis. Ann Surg, 2012, 256 (3): 487 – 493.

[34] Bonadonna G, Valagussa P, Moliterni A, et al. Adjuvant cyclophosphamide, methotrexate, and fluorouracil in nodepositive breast cancer: the results of 20 years of follow-up. N Engl J Med, 332: 901 – 926.

[35] Yan TD, Black D, Bannon PG, et al. Systematic review and meta-analysis on safety and efficacy of VATS lobectomy for NSCLC. J Clin Oncol, 2009, 27: 2553 – 2562.

[36] Lohrisch, C, Paltiel, C, Gelmon, K, et al. Impact on survival of time from definitive surgery to initiation of adjuvant chemotherapy for early-stage breast cancer. J Clin Oncol, 2006, 24: 4888 – 4894.

[37] Strauss GM, Herndon J, Maddaus MA, et al. Randomized clinical trial of adjuvant chemotherapy with paclitaxel and carboplatin following resection in stage 1B non-small cell lung cancer (NSCLC): Report of Cancer and Leukemia Group B (CALGB) Protocol 9633. J Clin Oncol, 2004, 22 (suppl 14): 621s.

[38] Scagliotti GV, Fossati R, Torri V, et al. Randomized study of adjuvant chemotherapy for completely resected stage I, II, or IIIA non-small-cell lung cancer. J Natl Cancer Inst, 2003, 95: 1453 – 1461.

[39] Flores RM, Ihekweazu U, Dycoco J, et al. Video-assisted thoracoscopic surgery (VATS) lobectomy: catastrophic intraoperative complications. J Thorac Cardiovasc Surg, 2011, 142: 1412 – 1417.

[40] Yang CF, D'Amico TA. Thoracoscopic segmentectomy for lung cancer. Ann Thorac Surg, 2012, 94 (2): 668 – 681.

[41] Nwogu CE, Yendamuri S, Demmy TL. Does thoracoscopic pneumonectomy for lung cancer affect survival. Ann Thorac Surg, 2010, 89 (6): S2102 – 2106.

[42] Kamiyoshihara M, Ibe T, Takeyoshi I. Videoassisted thoracoscopic lobectomy with bronchoplasty for lung cancer: tip regarding bronchial anastomosis. Gen Thorac Cardiovasc Surg, 2008, 56 (9): 476 – 478.

[43] Demmy, TL, Nwogu CE, Yendamuri S. Thoracoscopic chest wall resection: What is its role. Annals of Thoracic Surgery, 2010, 89 (6): S2142 – 2145.

[44] Cerfolio RJ, Bryant AS, Minnich DJ. Minimally invasive chest wall resection: Sparing the overlying, uninvolved musculature of the chest. Ann Thorac Surg, 2012, 94 (5): 1744 – 1747.

[45] Boffa DJ, Kosinski AS, Paul S, et al. Lymph node evaluation by open or videoassisted approaches in 11 500 anatomic lung cancer resections. Ann Thorac Surg, 2012, 94 (2): 347 – 353; discussion 353.

[46] Park BJ, Melfi F, Mussi A, et al. Robotic lobectomy for non-small cell lung cancer (NSCLC): Longterm oncologic results. J Thorac Cardiovasc Surg, 2012, 143 (2): 383 – 389.

第 15 章
肺癌扩大切除术

Matthew A. Steliga[1], David C. Rice[2]
1. Division of Thoracic Surgery, University of Arkansas, Little Rock, AR, USA
2. Department of Thoracic and Cardiovascular Surgery, The University of Texas MD Anderson Cancer Center, Houston, TX, USA

引 言

肺癌是癌症所致死亡的主要原因，美国每年死于肺癌的人数达 16 万人，全球为 130 万人[1-2]。对高危人群进行筛查可发现更多早期局限的小肺癌，从而进行治疗。但目前筛查还没有普及，不符合筛查标准的人群仍有罹患肺癌的可能。尽管付出诸多努力，仍有许多肺癌患者发现时即表现为局部进展期。大多数进展期肺癌患者，尤其是伴有广泛纵隔淋巴结转移和远处转移者，不适合手术治疗。部分局部进展期肺癌患者仍可获得完全切除，而无法切除的局部进展期肺癌患者远期生存罕见。识别出可手术切除的局部进展期肺癌患者，使他们获得最大治愈可能，是所有肺癌专科医生关注的重点。

本章论述肺癌的扩大切除，即肿瘤和肺的解剖性切除，以及必要时对邻近结构的一并切除和重建。总的来说，临床指南[如非小细胞肺癌（NSCLC）指南[3]]有利于临床制订治疗方案，但即使指南有明确规定，仍需考虑患者的意愿、行为状态和医生的操作技能。病例选择极具挑战性，体现在临床决策过程中，对每一例生存期有可能延长的患者都应权衡手术治疗的风险与获益，同时避免不能带来生存获益的手术切除。本章重点讨论基于第 7 版 AJCC 分期标准的部分 T3 和 T4 局部进展期 NSCLC（表 15.1）的评估和治疗策略。

扩大切除的一般原则

一项基于胸外科医师协会数据库病例资料的回顾性研究表明，标准肺叶切除手术的死亡率约为 2%，并发症发生率约为 32%[5]。根据定义，局部进展期肺癌分期偏晚，易发生淋巴结转移和（或）血行转移，无论累及胸壁、大血管、大气道还是其他结构，虽可行扩大切除，但与标准肺叶切除相比，手术更复杂，围术期风险增大，术后更易发生远处转移和局部复发。因此，对局部进展期肺癌患者术前应进行全面、有效的评估。

一般来说，所有拟行扩大切除的患者都应行胸部 CT 增强扫描和 PET 评估肿瘤和周围结构的关系，以及淋巴结和远处转移情况。所有短轴 >1 cm 的纵隔淋巴结或 PET 显示标准化摄取值增加怀疑转移的患者，都必须经病理组织学证实。临床分期为 T4 的肿瘤，如术前发现 N2 或 N3 阳性，通常不适合行扩大切除手术，因这部分患者的手术治疗效果极差。即使影像学检查阴性，纵隔淋巴结活检仍至关重要，而且并发症发生率低，一旦证实转移，可避免开胸手术，尽快开始化疗和放疗。纵隔镜多年来一直是纵隔淋巴结分期的金标准，有时候还可用于肿瘤直接侵犯气管和纵隔情况的术前评估。支气管内镜超声（EBUS）和食管内镜超声（esophageal ultrasound，EUS）与纵隔镜相比，灵敏度、特异度类似，而侵袭性更小，正越来越多地代替纵隔镜检查。径向支气管内镜超声评估气管受侵的灵敏度优于 CT。更多纵隔分期方法的灵敏度和特异度的细节见第 12 章。

PET 发现颅内转移的灵敏度低，因此拟行扩大切除的患者术前应常规行脑部磁共振检查（MRI）。胸部 MRI 并非常规，但在了解肿瘤侵犯周围结构、肿瘤与脊柱和大血管关系时可选择性应用。

表 15.1　AJCC（第 7 版）局部进展期 NSCLC 分期[4]

T3	T4
累及：　胸壁	纵隔
膈肌	心脏
膈神经	大血管
纵隔胸膜	气管
心包壁层	喉返神经
主支气管，距隆突不足 2cm	食管
	椎体
阻塞性全肺不张	隆突
肿瘤所在肺叶结节	同侧不同肺叶结节

来源：AJCC 第 7 版局部进展期 NSCLC 分期[4]

无纵隔淋巴结转移的局部进展期肺癌，一旦出现远处转移，除极少数情况外，通常不考虑手术治疗。对侧肺孤立结节不一定是转移，有可能为同时性原发性肺癌，如果符合 Martini 和 Melamed [6] 所提出的标准，可分期手术切除或手术联合立体定向放射治疗。同样，无纵隔淋巴结转移的孤立性脑转移患者，如果脑转移可完全切除或伽马刀放疗控制，仍可考虑扩大切除，但这种情况比较罕见，需经胸部肿瘤多学科综合治疗组讨论，仔细权衡切除肺部病变的期望获益和潜在并发症的风险。

选择手术治疗的患者需经肿瘤学和生理学专家的仔细评估，传统标准是第 1 秒用力呼气容积（FEV_1）和肺一氧化碳弥散功能（diffusion capacity in the lungs for carbon monoxide，DLCO）大于预计值的 40%，但不达标并非所有患者手术切除的禁忌证，尤其在需切除局部进展期肿瘤所致的阻塞性肺病变的情况下。计算术后预测肺功能的方法对外科医生来说并不陌生，因此不在本章讨论的范畴，但术前定量肺通气或灌注扫描对于患者能否耐受手术的评估至关重要，因为局部进展期肺癌通常会影响拟切除肺组织的通气或血流情况。肺叶切除时 V/Q 扫描并非必要，但更晚期肿瘤尤其需全肺切除时 V/Q 扫描常常有助于外科医生评估手术的可行性。

明确患者适合根治性切除后，需要遵循若干手术原则。除肿瘤所致的阻塞性肺组织外，分别处理肺门动脉、静脉和支气管的解剖性切除以及显微镜下切缘阴性，是手术的目标和要求。此外，即使术前影像学和纵隔活检证实为阴性，纵隔淋巴结清扫仍然是标准肺癌手术的有机组成部分，尤其当肿瘤需行扩大切除时。Osarogiagbon 和同事最近发表的一项美国肺癌手术治疗病例的回顾性研究表明[7]，累及胸壁、隆突或其他结构的扩大性切除手术占比 5%，但令人失望的是竟有 54%（$n = 316/582$）的患者手术时未进行纵隔淋巴结清扫。纵隔淋巴结清扫可明确分期，有利于判断预后并依据循证医学证据给予合理的辅助治疗。即使术前充分的影像学和纵隔淋巴结活检明确为阴性，仍有部分患者手术时意外发现为镜下 N2，尤其是 T3N2 和 T4N2 的患者。当考虑到手术治疗预后差及扩大切除的风险时，通常会放弃手术。

胸壁侵犯

对胸外科医生而言，原发肿瘤直接侵犯胸壁的局部进展期肺癌最多见，适于手术切除。Coleman 于 1947 年最先报道了 7 例侵犯胸壁肺癌患者的手术治疗，其中 5 例行胸壁和肺联合切除[8]。如今，肺和胸壁的整块切除已成为直接侵犯胸壁的 T3N0 和 T3N1 肿瘤患者的标准治疗方法。胸壁受累的定义为 T3 期肿瘤[9]，指肿瘤侵犯壁层胸膜或更深层次胸壁，约占所有肺切除患者的 5%。

部分肿瘤侵犯胸壁患者的 CT 扫描可见明显的骨质破坏征象，但许多患者的影像学表现并不明显，尤其在肿瘤紧贴脏层胸膜表面时。明显的骨质破坏表明胸壁受累，胸壁受侵最敏感的 CT 征象是胸膜外脂肪间隙消失，灵敏度为 85%，而肋骨受侵的灵敏度仅为 16%[10]。侵犯胸壁的肿瘤为周围型，引起咳嗽、血痰和阻塞性肺炎罕见，最常见的症状为局限性胸痛。疼痛沿肋间神经支配区域或臂丛神经分布区域放射提示胸壁受侵犯。壁层胸膜和胸壁密布感觉神经纤维，不论 CT 征象如何，局限性胸痛对有无胸壁侵犯的判断更可靠[11]。胸壁受侵患者行 PET 检查有助于判断远处转移情况，但对发现局部侵犯不敏感。MRI 可明确局部侵犯情况，在评估肺上沟瘤侵犯臂丛神经和锁骨下血管时最有价值，低位胸壁受侵患者的术前评估并不常规应用。大部分侵犯胸壁患者应行经皮活检，而非支气管镜检查，有些怀疑胸壁受侵的患者活检时 CT 意外发现气胸致肿瘤和胸壁分离。超声检查时可通过动态观察胸膜和肺随呼吸运动情况判断有无胸壁受侵，经验丰富的医生检查的灵敏度和特异度分别为89%和95%，而CT检查的灵敏度和特异度分别为42%和100%[12]。低位胸壁受侵患者还可实时观察膈肌随呼吸运动情况，对判断胸壁受侵更有价值，而肺尖并不随呼吸运动。评估胸膜顶处胸壁受侵时超声的应用价值有限。术前超声检查评估胸壁受侵并非常规，原因在于胸壁受侵非根治性手术的禁忌证，具体切除策略在最终术中才能明确。

根据指南和拟行肺切除范围可前瞻性地计算出术后FEV_1或DLCO的预计值，如处于临界状态应引起重视，因为这种计算方法并没有考虑到胸壁切除对肺功能的影响[13]。单根肋骨切除对呼吸生理影响不大，如切除数根肋骨而没有进行重建，会出现胸壁反常呼吸运动，类似创伤所致连枷胸。肺功能处于临界状态的患者，胸壁切除后呼吸衰竭风险明显增加，更多患者需要机械通气。网状物和骨水泥重建恢复胸壁硬度可最大限度地减轻反常呼吸运动，临床医生应充分意识到，大块胸壁联合肺切除与单纯肺切除相比，患者术后呼吸功能紊乱更明显。Martin-Ucar等的研究表明，低体质指数、年龄>75岁、术前FEV_1<70%预计值会导致肺部并发症所致的手术死亡率增加[13]。少数肺功能真正处于临界状态的患者可能无法耐受同时胸壁切除，术前除了CT外，还应行MRI或超声检查以评估患者是否真正适合手术。

有时候良性粘连可使肺紧贴胸壁而没有肿瘤侵犯，而可疑胸壁受侵患者，外科医生需决定行全层胸壁切除还是胸膜外切除。如果患者无胸痛，肿瘤没有紧密固定于胸壁，结合影像学无明确侵犯胸壁征象或胸膜外脂肪间隙仍存在，首先开始胸膜外切除是合理的。一旦冰冻切片检查证实有更深层次的侵犯再转行胸壁全层切除，从而避免不必要的扩大切除。如果肿瘤确实侵犯胸壁，或镜下有更深层次的侵犯，胸膜腔解剖会导致肿瘤破溃，术后局部复发风险增加[11,14-15]。冰冻切片检查可确保完全切除。

肺癌胸壁侵犯手术治疗的目标是切缘阴性的整块切除，解剖性肺叶切除是标准，可通过传统开胸手术或胸腔镜完成肺门解剖和淋巴结清扫，后者切除胸壁时附加更加局限的开胸切口即可。胸膜种植罕见，一旦发生则无法完全切除，胸腔镜探查可及时发现，从而避免无益的开胸手术。远离肿瘤部位进入胸膜腔，镜下观察确定胸壁切缘，不再通过触摸决定，还可明确有无胸膜转移[16]。开胸手术时，术前仔细研究影像学检查资料，规划手术切口，远离肿瘤进入胸膜腔，避免肿瘤破溃；进入胸腔后，触摸探查肿瘤和胸壁受侵情况，决定切除范围。虽然有学者主张肉眼下1cm的切缘即足够[15]，但通常需切除胸壁侵犯部位上、下各一正常肋间隙，前后距离3~4cm[16-17]。肺癌侵犯胸壁切除的挑战之一是，固定于胸壁的团块状肿瘤影响肺门的暴露。有些患者可先行胸壁切除，再将肿瘤连同胸壁楔形切除，可极大地改善肺门的暴露，有利于剩余肺叶的解剖性切除和纵隔淋巴结清扫。

单根肋骨切除通常不需要重建，如切除多根肋骨会导致胸壁缺损范围超过5cm，某些部位的缺损重建可使患者获益；一些学者不常规重建胸壁缺损，报道显示并发症发生率并不高[17]。位于肺尖和后胸壁的缺损，因有肩胛骨和椎旁肌覆盖，即使切除不止一根肋骨通常也无须重建。前、侧和下胸壁缺损重建可避免畸形和大范围反常呼吸运动；肩胛下角或其稍上方的后胸壁缺损或需要重建，以避免肩胛下角嵌入，有时可切除肩胛下角来预防。一些医生习惯用聚四氟乙烯网（PTFE）重建胸壁缺损，硬度好，不渗透液体，但有组织不易长入与周围嵌合差的缺点。最常用的是聚丙烯网，比前者价廉，易于组织长入，抗感染能力强；愈合后网孔内长入的组织可增加重建的硬度；两层网片之间亦可灌注骨水泥塑形（"三明治"法），增加重建物的硬度（图15.1）。

Weyant等报道了262例胸壁切除患者的呼吸衰竭发生率仅为3.1%，归因于他们选择性应用网片重建胸壁，无论是否合并应用骨水泥；尽管患者的异质性明显，包含了不同类型的肿瘤，但重建可改善其呼吸生理并降低术后肺部并发症的发生率[19]。骨水泥尽管重塑了前侧胸壁缺损后的轮廓，增加了网片的硬度，减轻了反常呼吸运动的程度，但并不完美。呼吸和转动体位时，坚硬的重建物和肋骨直接接触会导致疼痛。通常应用骨水泥时，其周边不和肋骨边缘邻接或重叠。采用硅胶管内注入骨水泥并塑形成拟重建部位肋骨的形

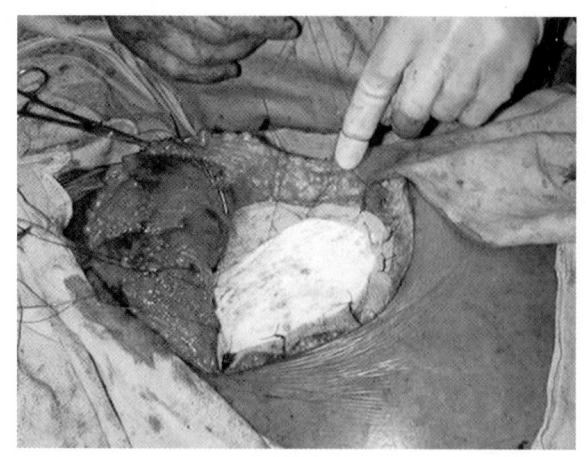

图 15.1（见彩插） 用聚丙烯网和骨水泥重建胸壁

状，变硬后与肋骨两断端缝合固定，再联合应用聚丙烯网重建胸壁的方法更符合解剖特点[20]。不含细胞的胶原蛋白补片是较新的重建材料，已用于胸壁肿瘤联合切除胸壁和椎骨后的重建[21]，与其他材料相比，可能更有利于抗感染，但费用更高，不易获得，张力亦随时间减弱，但用于重建胸壁与传统的聚丙烯网相比并不占优势。在网片和皮肤之间填充肌层可增进愈合并降低切口和网片感染的发生率。背阔肌、前锯肌和胸大肌血运丰富，均可旋转覆盖重建物，即使皮肤和皮下组织裂开，网片也不至外露。最好在开始手术前计划好要保留的胸壁肌层组织，随后开胸时进行游离和保护。网膜瓣和腹直肌瓣也可采用，需要合理规划手术切口。胸管的放置看起来简单，但置管部位应远离重建物以避免污染。最后，术中冰冻切缘检查仅限于软组织，骨组织需脱钙数天后才能进行病理检查。

侵犯胸壁的 T3 肿瘤手术治疗结果见表 15 - 2。有的研究包括了仅壁层胸膜受累行胸膜外切除的病例，而另外一些研究仅纳入了胸壁全层切除的病例，有的研究根据淋巴结转移情况进行了细分，有的研究将 N1 和 N2 混杂在一起[24-25,28]，因此无法直接比较。手术死亡率为 0 ~ 8%，5 年生存率为 22% ~ 61%；无淋巴结转移患者的预后最佳，5 年生存率为 78%；N2 患者的 5 年生存率仅为 0 ~ 20%[15,17-18,22-30]，提示术前纵隔分期的重要性。

表 15.2 肺癌侵犯胸壁的手术治疗效果

作者	年份	病例数	死亡率	总生存率	N0	N1	N2
Chapelier[18]	2000	100	2%	18%	22	9	0
Facciolo[17]	2001	104	0	61.4%	67	100	17
Magdeleniat[22]	2001	201	7%	21%	25	21	20
Elia[23]	2001	110	0	35%	47	0	
Burkhart[24]	2002	94	6.3%	38.7%	44	26*	26*
Riquet[15]	2002	125	7	22.5%	30.7	0	11.5
Rovario[25]	2003	146	0.7%	NS	78.5	7.2*	7.2*
Matsuoka[26]	2004	97	NS	34.2%	44.2	40.0	6.2
Doddoli[27]	2005	309	8%	30.7%	40	23.8	8.4
Volotini[28]	2006	68	4%	37%	42	17*	17*
Lin[29]	2006	42	NS	28.4%	39	17.1	
Lee[30]	2012	107	5%	26.3%	37.4	21.1	4.6

NS：未统计；*：淋巴结阳性患者的生存率，N1 和 N2 无区分

肺上沟瘤切除

影像医生 Henry Pancoast 首先注意到引起明显疼痛的胸顶部肿瘤，并以肺上沟瘤来描述，认为其可能起源于最后鳃裂残存的胚胎上皮，没有归类于侵袭性肺癌[31]。侵及邻近结构的肺尖部肿瘤历史上称为 Pancoast 肿瘤或肺上沟瘤，但一直到最近仍有争论，考虑到"肺上沟"这一概念并没有解剖学和影像学的相关性，因此，胸顶部肿瘤的命名更为准确[32]。尽管命名的观点不同，大部分文献仍采用肺上沟瘤的术语，本章仍继续沿用

这一命名。Shaw、Paulson 和 Kee1961 年首先采用放疗后手术切除治疗肺上沟瘤[33]，几十年来，这种扩大的后外侧开胸切口一直是治疗这种特殊类型肿瘤最常用的手术径路，如今在许多中心仍广泛采用。

尽管大多数学者认为这种局部进展期的侵袭性肿瘤应采用手术和放化疗，但存在不同治疗手段的组合和顺序。西南肿瘤协作组的Ⅱ期前瞻性临床研究（SWOG 9416），cT3-4N0-1 的肺上沟瘤术前采用同时性放化疗（依托泊苷+顺铂，45Gy 放疗），围术期死亡率为 1.8%，5 年生存率为 44%[34]。欧洲的一项研究包括了 31 例肺上沟瘤患者，部分为 N2 和 N3（cT3-4N0-3），3 周期化疗后同步放化疗达 45Gy，再分期后行手术切除，完全切除率为 94%，5 年生存率为 46%[35]。Toronto 多学科治疗组采用 SWOG9416 相同的诱导放化疗方案，手术死亡率为 5%，5 年生存率为 59%[36]。日本一项Ⅱ期临床研究同样采用基于铂类的同步诱导放化疗，放疗剂量为 45Gy，手术死亡率为 3.5%，5 年生存率为 56%，与 SWOG9416 相似。团块状的肺上沟瘤，如影像学怀疑肿瘤无法切除，术前放化疗具有理论上的优势：期望肿瘤治疗后缩小，增加完全切除率；为临床医生提供更多针对肿瘤个体化治疗方案疗效的信息；有些患者尽管给予了放化疗，病变仍进展并出现远处转移，提示这些患者可能存在未能发现的亚临床转移病灶，如果先手术，术后病变会快速进展，术前放化疗可避免无益的开胸手术以及相应的疼痛和并发症。尽管诱导治疗存在诸多优势，仍有一些中心对肺上沟瘤首先采用手术治疗，以避免放疗后所增加的挑战和并发症，因为放疗通常会导致组织间隙闭锁，组织放疗后的改变和肿瘤亦无法鉴别，从而增加手术难度。此外，放疗后手术，镜下或肉眼残存肿瘤难以再通过放疗有效控制。先手术再放疗的支持者认为，术后放疗可给予更大的放疗剂量；肺上沟瘤患者常有持续性疼痛，先手术可快速持久缓解症状[37]；最后，越来越多的证据支持 NSCLC 的辅助治疗，而非新辅助治疗。M. D. 安德森癌症中心最近的一项前瞻性Ⅱ期临床研究中，肺上沟瘤患者首先采用手术治疗，之后给予放疗，剂量为 60~64.8Gy，同时给予 2 个周期依托泊苷联合顺铂化疗，放疗结束后再给予 3 个周期的化疗，2 年、5 年和 10 年局部控制率为 84%、76% 和 76%，相应总生存率分别为 72%、50% 和 45%，与术前放疗的 45Gy 相比，这种综合治疗方案的放疗剂量明显增加[38]。

肿瘤累及锁骨下动脉或静脉在一些中心常规一并切除，这曾一度被认为是完全切除的禁忌证。Dartevelle 等描述的沿颈前胸锁乳突肌、越过锁骨后再向前胸壁延伸的手术径路可提供胸顶部的良好暴露，同时可控制大血管的近远端。Grunenwald 等将上述切口予以改良[39]，称为"活板门"切口，切断胸骨柄，保留胸锁关节和锁骨，旋转掀开整个锁骨及其附着肌肉。骨肌瓣的旋转可提供良好的暴露，切断的胸骨柄易于通过钢丝固定，这种颈胸切口的优势还在于可同时切除斜角肌淋巴结送检。在一些中心大多数肺上沟瘤均通过颈胸切口切除肿瘤和解剖肺门结构；有的中心除颈胸切口外，另外附加开胸切口或者联合胸腔镜进行肺门解剖，提供了更多的选择[40-41]。de Perrot 等提议将胸廓入口划分成不同的区域，肿瘤累及前方区域时，保留锁骨的前颈胸切口容易暴露，中心区域受累时切断锁骨暴露最好，而脊柱和神经根受累时从后方暴露更佳[42]。尽管观点不同，选择手术径路时还应考虑到手术医生的技能和对不同径路的熟悉程度。动脉和静脉切除重建在手术经验丰富的中心已成为常规，必要时可结扎处理锁骨下静脉，由于肩胛带有丰富的静脉侧支回流，患者应该可以耐受。考虑到有发生上肢水肿的风险，因此大多数医生会选择重建静脉。

椎体受累

单纯胸壁侵犯为 T3，而椎体受累为 T4（图 15.2），可表现为仅横突受累，或整个椎体几乎完全被肿瘤组织取代，有些病例可见肿瘤侵入椎管，即将压迫脊髓。椎体受累并非完全切除手术的禁忌证，但确实需仔细规划以达到安全切除。此类手术需在经验丰富的中心实施，并与脊柱外科医生合作。在有些中心，肿瘤侵犯椎体可通过部分

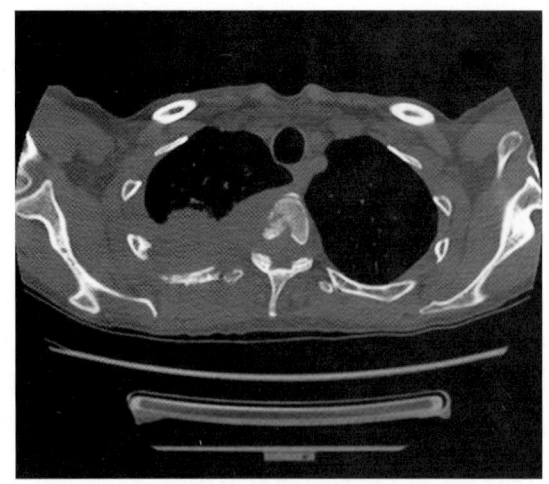

图 15.2　CT 扫描显示肋骨和椎体均受累

或全部椎体切除、重建修复稳定脊柱而治愈（图 15.3）[37, 43-45]。椎体切除通常以治愈为目的，一篇椎体切除的文献报道，为控制疼痛或仅限于解除脊髓压迫的姑息性手术占所有椎体切除手术的 10%（4/39）[37]。Bolton 等报道的 M.D. 安德森癌症中心纳入的 39 例累及椎体肺上沟瘤患者的回顾性研究中，手术切除后给予辅助放化疗，完全切除率为 56%（22/39），中位生存时间为 18 个月，5 年生存率为 27%，完全取决于淋巴结有无转移；淋巴结阴性患者的 5 年生存率为 41%，肺门或纵隔淋巴结转移者无长期存活者[37]。

胸壁、脊柱联合肺切除后除心律失常、肺炎、肺不张或漏气等常见并发症外，还有一些与胸壁和椎体切除重建有关的特异性并发症。一旦发生感染，PTFE 因组织不易长入往往需要移除。可能需要移除聚丙烯网，如部分和组织嵌合，可给予冲洗或采用负压感染伤口治疗装置，以促进肉芽组织长入网片并愈合。坚硬的骨水泥如与肋骨或胸骨直接接触会发出咔嚓声或爆裂音导致疼痛，有时需二次手术，最好的预防措施是避免坚硬的重建物和骨性结构直接接触。胸导管最终汇入左侧颈内静脉和锁骨下静脉交角，解剖左侧胸顶结构时应小心避免损伤；术野有淋巴液积聚时应警惕，术中发现任何淋巴液渗漏部位应予缝扎。术后少量淋巴液渗漏提示胸导管小分支损伤，可予保守治疗，如尽量避免经口进食，应用肠外营养和奥曲肽；如渗漏量大，保守治疗无效往往提示主干损伤，通常需再次手术结扎胸导管，胸腔镜下经右胸径路为佳。

切除后胸壁肿瘤有时需离断肋横突关节和肋椎关节，仔细识别神经根和肋间血管并予以结扎，但有时会发生脑脊液漏，原因在于解剖神经根近端时可能会损伤包裹神经根的硬脊膜外鞘。如果术后胸管引流液量大，患者出现严重的体位性头痛，直立位时加重，应高度怀疑脑脊液漏。一旦

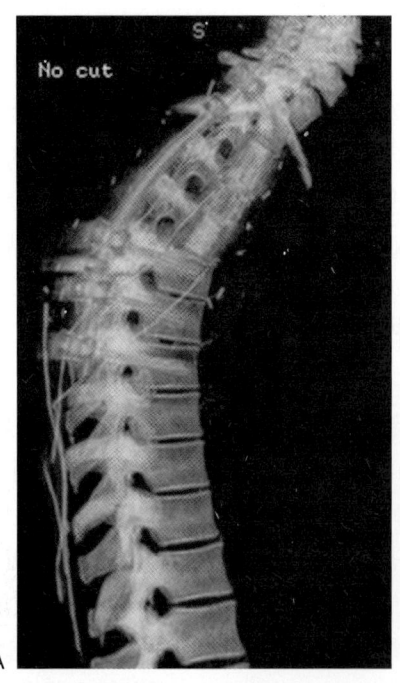
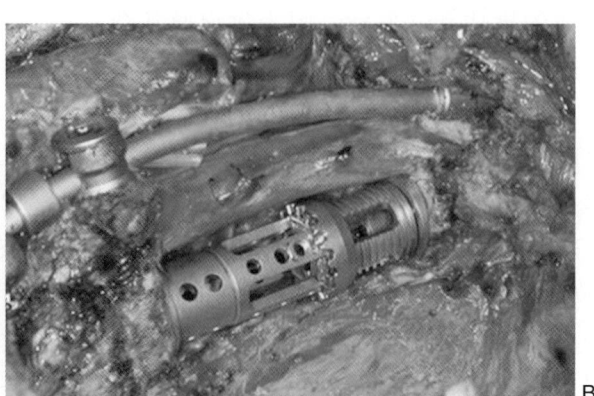

图 15.3（见彩插）　肿瘤侵犯脊柱行扩大切除后重建恢复稳定性。A. 术后影像学。B. 术中照片

发生，脑脊液的正压和胸膜腔负压使脑脊液漏的治疗极具挑战性，可放置腰椎脑脊液引流管或硬脊膜外腔注射自体静脉血，有时需再次手术。已有个案及另外 17 例相关病例文献报道肺上沟瘤开胸术后发生脑脊液漏会导致颅内积气，引发神经功能紊乱[46]。症状较轻者可自行吸收，严重神经功能障碍者需再次手术治疗。如椎体切除时发现硬脊膜撕裂，最好即刻修补并采用带蒂软组织瓣覆盖，如肋间肌瓣或前锯肌瓣。

膈肌受累

肺肿瘤直接侵犯膈肌并不常见，文献报道也少。恶性胸膜间皮瘤则常常侵犯膈肌，尽管 CT 或 MR 等影像学检查并不总能显示膈肌受侵的征象。肺癌侵犯膈肌多是术中发现，术前评估时并未引起怀疑。Weksler 等的单中心回顾性研究中，所有行肺癌手术的患者中，膈肌侵犯者仅占 0.2%（8/4668）[47]，说明这种情况比较罕见。膈肌部分切除后，小的缺损可选用不可吸收性材料如涤纶片，以不可吸收缝线行水平褥式缝合修补。缺损较大时，需采用网片修补，由于需要接触腹腔脏器，光滑且硬度佳的 PTFE 优于粗糙的聚丙烯网。文献报道膈肌受侵患者连同肺癌整块切除后的长期生存率为 20%～30%[48-49]，比其他 T3 期肿瘤患者差，原因很可能是膈肌的淋巴引流特性：不但直接引流至纵隔淋巴结，而且还可引流至内乳链和膈下腹主动脉旁淋巴结[50]。最后，呼吸生理紊乱的程度取决于膈肌切除部位和神经损伤程度，在临界肺功能患者应予考虑。

膈神经受累

肺肿瘤贴近纵隔且伴有同侧膈肌抬高提示膈神经受累。定量通气或灌注扫描显示受累侧肺功能较健侧减退。此外，吸气试验透视下可见受累侧膈肌出现矛盾运动。符合肿瘤学和生理学原则的肿瘤连同膈神经的整块切除可根治，没有必要保留无功能的膈神经。

术前膈肌位置正常，术中可意外发现膈神经受累。如果肿瘤没有直接侵犯膈肌，可仔细解剖保留膈神经，但血运受影响可导致短期甚至长期神经麻痹；如肿瘤直接侵犯膈肌，除外肺功能临界状态者，大部分患者可安全切除膈神经。Tokunaga 等报道了 13 例肺、纵隔肿瘤累及膈神经患者，6 例同时行膈神经切除和同侧膈肌折叠。13 例患者中，2 例（15%）术后机械通气时间超过 7d；6 例同时行肺肿瘤和膈神经切除患者中，2 例（33%）患者的机械通气时间超过 7d[51]。

喉返神经受累

右侧喉返神经起源于迷走神经后下行，勾绕右锁骨下动脉后位于气管食管沟，上行支配喉；左侧喉返神经于主动脉弓前方起源于左侧迷走神经后下行，勾绕主动脉弓下缘后同样上行于气管食管沟。患者出现声音嘶哑提示不仅喉返神经受累，而且锁骨下动脉、主动脉、食管或气管等往往受肿瘤直接侵犯。单纯神经受累不排除手术，但肿瘤如果直接侵犯邻近大血管、脏器或出现淋巴结或远处转移，则往往不能手术切除。术前检查喉返神经功能正常，有时术中发现肿瘤紧贴神经，如果二者间存在解剖层面，可保留神经。右侧喉返神经切断术后发生误吸风险高，患者需禁食，给予肠内或完全胃肠外营养。进食前需语音治疗师评估误吸风险，通常需要先行双重对比钡餐 X 线造影检查。如果患者存在误吸，可考虑患侧声带注射聚四氟乙烯或脂肪促进声带居中。术后早期声带注射可改善患者的发音质量、减少误吸、促进咳嗽清除呼吸道分泌物。术后 2~3 个月受累声带不再向侧方移位，耳鼻喉科医生再施行手术治疗，以达到确切和最理想化的患侧声带居中。

心包受累

肿瘤直接侵犯心包为 T3 期，适合手术；但影像学发现的心包积液往往为恶性，如确诊则分期为 M1a，不适合手术。不幸的是，肿瘤侵犯心包累及心外膜时影像学难以准确判断。肿瘤直接侵犯心包的手术治疗文献报道不多，需要遵循切缘阴性等原则，通常需要一并切除膈神经。心包部分切除后留有缺损，有可能发生心脏疝，尤其是右肺全切除术后。一旦发生，会导致心脏扭转，腔静脉回流受阻，发生快速循环衰竭造成患者死亡。大多数外科医生选择光滑的 PTFE 或软一些的可吸收材料，如聚乙醇酸或丙交酯双聚合物网修补心包缺损。采用 PTFE 修补时，心包多处开窗引流可避免心包内液体积聚导致心脏压塞。肺门处的团块状肿瘤打开心包后更容易切除，可在心包内解剖肺动静脉。关闭心包缺损操作简单，对于致命性心脏疝发生的预防至关重要。在左侧，即使全肺切除，心包缺损重建也并非必须，但需扩大缺损以避免部分心脏疝的发生。在右侧，如果术后保留足够多的肺组织，心包缺损通常不需要修补；中下叶切除后的心包缺损则需要修补，右全肺切除后心包缺损必须修补。

心脏大血管受累

肿瘤侵犯上腔静脉、主动脉或锁骨下动脉一度被认为无法治愈，但现在认为，肿瘤侵犯大血管的患者通常因为团块状淋巴结转移或远处转移而不适合手术治疗。在专科医学中心，经过严格挑选的部分 T4N0 或 T4N1 患者，在无远处转移和肺功能储备足够的情况下，仍可获得切缘阴性的完全性切除（图 15.4）而长期生存，并发症发生率亦可接受。

肿瘤直接长入上腔静脉者也可能完全切除，但制订合理的手术方案至关重要。在上腔静脉阻断过程中，需要在下肢建立大口径的静脉通路，

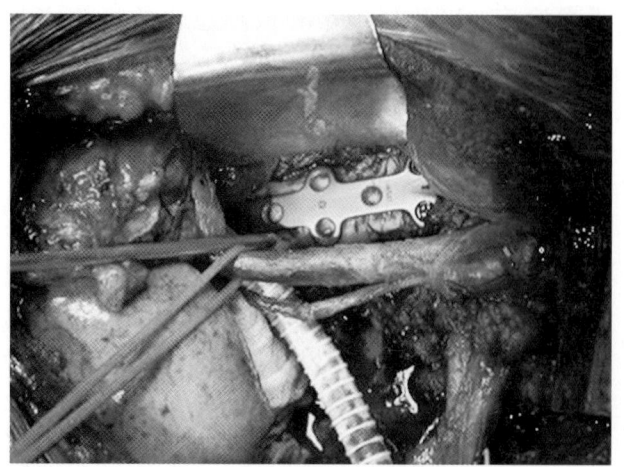

图 15.4（见彩插） 肺上沟瘤联合脊柱（可见固定装置）和锁骨下血管切除（聚四氟乙烯人工血管置换）

以保证输液和用药。根据肿瘤的部位和大小，可选择胸骨劈开，或部分胸骨劈开的前外侧开胸切口，即半蛤壳状切口，相比传统的开胸切口可更好地暴露上纵隔和肺门。切缘阴性的血管壁局部切除可直接修补，大的缺损需采用补片修补，如合成材料和心包、大隐静脉、奇静脉等自体组织。完全节段切除后采用涤纶、聚四氟乙烯或牛心包重建血管可行，效果好，但阻断上腔静脉会导致前负荷快速减少和低血压。通常膈神经需要一并切除。动脉低血压和快速静脉充血会导致脑水肿，静脉应用激素、肝素和血管收缩药物等保护性措施可降低这种风险[52]，需要切除上腔静脉的患者建立膈下静脉通路至关重要。切除上腔静脉的系列报道中，手术死亡率为 7.7%～14%，5 年生存率为 24%～31%[53-56]。对需要同时行隆突切除和上腔静脉重建的复杂病例务必将气道污染的可能性降至最小，以免发生移植血管感染这一灾难性的并发症。肿瘤侵犯上腔静脉可出现上腔静脉综合征，表现为面部和上肢充血肿胀，但无上腔静脉综合征并不意味着没有上腔静脉侵犯，如肿瘤进展缓慢，可形成侧支循环从而不出现面部肿胀。上腔静脉综合征患者没有纵隔淋巴结和远处转移、适合手术切除的情况比较少见。无法切除、症状明显的上腔静脉综合征患者，需行姑息性血管成形或放置支架以缓解静脉充血，或施行上腔静脉旁路手术。

过去认为 NSCLC 侵犯主动脉是手术禁忌证，但严格挑选的部分患者切除后可获得长期生存。患者如出现肩胛间区背痛，影像学上表现为肿瘤和主动脉间脂肪层次消失，增强扫描显示血管壁凹形变平坦或腔内不规则者提示主动脉侵犯。CT 和 MRI 显示主动脉侵犯不敏感，血管内超声检查灵敏度高，但不普及。最终有无主动脉侵犯需经验丰富的外科医生术中探查明确，大多数情况下，肿瘤只是邻近主动脉但没有侵犯。遇到肿瘤和降主动脉间的局限粘连，可沿血管壁仔细解剖分离，通常血管外膜下会有清晰的解剖层次。如肿瘤侵犯层次更深达血管中膜，则需全层切除和人工血管置换，单纯阻断主动脉会迅速增加左心室后负荷并导致下半身缺血，被动性动脉分流或搭建心房和降主动脉之间的旁路可避免阻断引起的血流动力学紊乱，并保证下本身的灌注。Misthos 等报

道了 13 例侵犯主动脉 T4 期肺癌患者的手术治疗，T4N0 亚组患者的 5 年生存率为 30.7%，无并发症发生[57]。Ohta 等报道了 16 例侵犯主动脉 T4 期患者的手术治疗，手术死亡率为 12.5%，并发症发生率为 31%。尽管围术期并发症发生率和死亡率高，但 pT4N0（$n=10$）患者的 5 年生存率高达 70%；另外 6 例患者的分期为 pT4N2~3，仅 1 例患者长期生存（5 年生存率为 17%）[58]。另有个案报道 1 例左下肺肿瘤侵犯降主动脉的 T4N1 患者，术前放置血管支架，随后开胸行左全肺切除，最终达到完全切除，患者存活，随访 23 个月仍无病生存，从而避免了阻断主动脉所引起的血流动力学紊乱和旁路手术相关的并发症[59]。

心肺转流术（cardiopulmonary bypass，CBP）可用于某些肿瘤的切除。最近的一篇综述纳入了 20 篇相关文献，讨论了心肺转流术在 NSCLC 切除中的应用，计划和非计划应用 CBP 患者的 5 年生存率存在统计学差异（54% vs 11%），总的 5 年生存率为 37%，90d 围术期死亡率为 1%，手术治疗的近期和远期生存情况完全可接受，对于严格挑选有潜在治愈可能的 NSCLC，CBP 的手术策略有较大的价值[60]。尽管 CBP 有利于复杂肿瘤的切除，但存在全身肝素化、体外循环所致炎症反应的相关风险和挑战，尤其是全肺切除后患者难以耐受的肺水肿。de Perrot 等报道了 7 例采用 CBP 切除的患者，2 例行隆突切除者均发生肺部并发症导致恢复缓慢，但确实得以生存[61]。另一篇文献报道了 19 例胸部进展期恶性肿瘤的 CBP 治疗，主要是肉瘤，1 例患者为原发性肺癌侵犯降主动脉，获得完全切除，随访 25 个月仍存活[62]。CBP 可应用于肺癌侵犯心脏、肺静脉或主肺动脉的手术治疗，或大气道切除重建时维持氧合，表面上看对患者有较大的侵袭性，但有些患者确实可获得长期生存。挑选合适的患者，CBP 治疗有可能使这些患者得以治愈。

肿瘤沿肺静脉浸润侵犯左心房局部的 T4 期肺癌适合手术治疗。Stella 等报道了 31 例侵犯心包内肺静脉或左心房肺癌患者的手术治疗，辅以术中超声心动图，完全切除率为 94%（29/31），无需 CBP；3 例死亡患者均为心包内右全肺切除；尽管切缘阴性、N2 患者仅占 26%（8/31），3 年生存率仅为 30%[63]。另一篇类似文献是 Wu 等报道的 46 例左心房切除的肺癌患者，无手术死亡患者，3 年生存率为 38%，5 年生存率为 22%[64]。

气管受累

气管和隆突切除在技术上具有挑战性，手术量大的医学中心具备处理此类患者的技能，挑选合适的患者可获得切缘阴性的完全切除和长期无病生存。气管和隆突切除的手术细节详见第 18 章。

同时性原发肺癌的外科观点

临床上不同肺叶或不同侧肺同时出现两个局限性肿瘤可通过手术治愈，但诊断和治疗决策具有挑战性，这类患者应由胸外科医生进行评估。虽然技术上的挑战远低于侵犯脏器的 T4 期肿瘤，治疗策略的挑战性却具有其独特性。术前分期至关重要，需要遵循前述 CT、PET 纵隔分期和 EBUS、EUS、纵隔镜活检的原则，以准确评估。不同组织学类型提示为双原发肿瘤，组织学类型相同有可能为孤立性转移或同时性原发肿瘤，分子检测有助于鉴别。但无论是双原发，还是孤立性转移，只要没有纵隔淋巴结和远处转移，这两种情况均可获得临床治愈。最近 AJCC 分期系统关于孤立性结节分期的定义调整如下：原发肿瘤所在肺叶内的卫星结节由 T4 降为 T3，适用于符合分期原则的肺叶切除；同侧不同肺叶内卫星结节为 T4，对侧肺内结节为 M1a，这两种情况均有可能通过手术治愈。

同侧不同肺叶内的病变，较大或更近肺门者行肺叶切除，较小或更外周者行亚肺叶切除。非同侧肺的双原发肿瘤，大多数外科医生选择分期切除，而不是一期切除双侧病变，主要考虑到双侧开胸手术所致的严重疼痛和呼吸功能减退。胸骨正中劈开切口可进入两侧胸膜腔，常规应用于双侧肺转移瘤的楔形切除，但解剖肺门行解剖性肺切除和系统纵隔淋巴结清扫受限，大多数胸外科医生基于这些考虑不选择胸骨正中切口治疗双侧肺癌。双侧 NSCLC 根据肿瘤部位和大小进行手术治疗时，如采用亚肺叶切除，肺段切除因更符合肿瘤学原则，优于非解剖性楔形切除。手术切除联合其他局部非切除消融技术也可以考虑，如立体定向放射治疗或经皮射频消融。考虑到双侧原发肿瘤并不多见，较大或靠近肺门的肿瘤行解剖性切除，较小或更外周者分期行消融可能是更好的选择。

单中心116例同时性原发肺癌患者的回顾性研究表明，同侧不同肺叶（T4）或对侧肺癌患者（M1a）的平均生存时间为65个月，优于AJCC分期中其他T4或M1a患者[65]。纳入6项独立研究的同时性双原发肺癌患者的手术治疗资料的系统评估分析了影响生存的预后因素，男性、高龄和淋巴结阳性者预后差；肿瘤位于双侧者死亡风险下降31%［HR=0.69；95% CI（0.50，0.94）］，中位生存时间52个月[66]。以上资料提示，尽管这些患者通常分期为ⅢB或ⅣA期，但完全切除后可获长期生存，优于其他ⅢB或ⅣA期患者，应常规评估手术治疗的可行性。

总 结

肺癌侵犯邻近器官为局部进展期，影响生存的关键因素并非肿瘤局部侵犯的程度，而是淋巴和血行转移情况，仅局部侵犯的肿瘤可获得有效的完全切除即是证明。全面的术前分期排除纵隔淋巴结或远处转移后，肿瘤连同邻近结构的整块切除是最有可能使患者长期生存的治疗措施。手术技术和围术期管理水平的提高，与其他专科医生的协作以及多学科综合治疗措施，扩大了局部进展期肺癌的手术适应证，使更多患者获得完全切除，生存期得以延长。

（杨 朋 王晓航 译）

参考文献

[1] Siegel R, Naishadham D, Jemal A. Cancer statistics, 2012. CA Cancer J Clin, 2012, 62: 10-29.

[2] Jemal A, Bray F, Center MM, et al. Global cancer statistics. CA Cancer J Clin, 2011, 61: 69-90.

[3] NCCN Clinical Practice Guidelines in Oncology. Non-Small Cell Lung Cancer Version 1. 2013. National Comprehensive Cancer Network, 2013. Available from: http://www.nccn.org/professionals/physician_gls/pdf/nscl.pdf (accessed Dec 15, 2012).

[4] Edge SB, Byrd DR, Compton CC, et al. AJCC Cancer Staging Manual. 7th. New York: Springer, 2010.

[5] Boffa DJ, Allen MS, Grab JD, et al. Data from the Society of Thoracic Surgeons General Thoracic Surgery Database: The surgical management of primary lung tumors. J Thorac Cardiovasc Surg, 2008, 135: 247-254.

[6] Martini N, Melamed MR. Multiple primary lung cancers. J Thorac Cardiovasc Surg, 1975, 70: 606-612.

[7] Osariogiagbon RU, Yu X. Mediastinal lymph node examination and survival in resected early stage non-small cell lung cancer in the Surveillance, Epidemiology, and End Results database. J Thorac Oncol, 2012, 7 (12): 1978-1806.

[8] Coleman FP. Primary carcinoma of the lung with invasion of the ribs: Pneumonecotmy and simultaneous block resection of the chest wall. Ann Surg, 1947, 126 (2): 156-168.

[9] Stoelben E, Ludwig C. Chest wall resection for lung cancer: Indications and techniques. Eur J Cardiothorac Surg, 2009, 35 (3): 450-456.

[10] Ratto GB, Piacenza G, Frola C, et al. Chest wall involvement by lung cancer: Computed tomography detection and results of operation. Ann Thorac Surg, 1991, 51: 182-188.

[11] Kawaguchi K, Mori S, Usami N, et al. Preoperative evaluation of the depth of chest wall invasion and the extent of combined resections in lung cancer patients, 2009, 64 (1): 41-44.

[12] Bandi V, Lunn W, Ernst A, et al. Ultrasound vs CT in detecting chest wall invasion by tumor. Chest, 2008, 133: 881-886.

[13] Martin-Ucar AE, Nicum R, Oey I, et al. En-bloc chest wall and lung resection for non-small cell lung cancer. Predictors of 60-day noncancer related mortality. Eur J Cardiothorac Surg, 2003, 23: 859-864.

[14] D'Andrilli A, Venuta F, Menna C, et al. Extensive resections: Pancoast tumors, chest wall resections, en bloc vascular resections. Surg Onc Clin N Am, 2011, 20: 733-756.

[15] Riquet M, Arame A, Barthes FLP. Non-small cell lung cancer invading the chest wall. Thorac Surg Clin, 2010, 20: 519-527.

[16] Berry MF, Onaitis MW, Tong BC, et al. Feasibility of hybrid thoracoscopic lobectomy and enbloc chest wall resection. Eur J Cardiothorac Surg, 2012, 41 (4):

888 – 892.

[17] Facciolo F, Cardillo G, Lopergolo M, et al. Chest wall invasion in non-small cell lung carcinoma: A rationale for en bloc resection. J Thorac Cardiovasc Surg, 2001, 121: 649 – 656.

[18] Chapelier A, Fadel E, Macchiarini P, et al. Factors affecting long-term survival after en bloc resection of lung cancer invading the chest wall. Eur J Cardiothorac Surg, 2000, 18: 513 – 518.

[19] Weyant MJ, Bains MS, Venkatraman E, et al. Results of chest wall resection and reconstruction with and without rigid prosthesis. Ann Thorac Surg, 2006, 81: 279 – 285.

[20] Dartevelle PG, Bedrettin Y, Mussot S. Extended resections for lung cancer//Roth JA, Cox J, Hong WK (eds). Lung Cancer. 3th. London: Blackwell Science, 2008: 195.

[21] Rocco G, Serra L, Fazioli F. The use of Veritas collagen matrix to reconstruct the posterior chest wall after costovertebrectomy. Ann Thorac Surg, 2011, 92: e17 – 18.

[22] Magdeleniat P, Ailfano M, Benbrahem C, et al. Surgical treatment of lung cancer invading the chest wall: Results and prognostic factors. Ann Thorac Surg, 2001, 71: 1094 – 1099.

[23] Elia S, Griffo S, Gentile M, et al. Surgical treatment of lung cancer invading the chest wall: A retrospective analysis of 110 patients. Eur J Cardiothorac Surg, 2001, 20: 356 – 360.

[24] Burkhart HM, Allen MS, Nichols FC, et al. Results of en bloc resection for bronchogenic carcinoma with chest wall invasion. J Thorac Cardiovasc Surg, 2002, 123: 670 – 675.

[25] Roviaro G, Varoli F, Grignani F, et al. Non-small cell lung cancer with chest wall invasion: evolution of surgical treatment and prognosis in the last 3 decades. Chest, 2003, 123: 1341 – 1347.

[26] Matsuoka H, Nishio W, Okada M, et al. Resection of chest wall invasion in patients with non-small cell lung cancer. Eur J Cardiothorac Surg, 2004, 26 (6): 1200 – 1204.

[27] Doddoli C, D'Journo B, Le Pimpec-Barthes F, et al. Lung cancer invading the chest wall: A plea for enbloc resection but the need for new treatment strategies. Ann Thorac Surg, 2005, 80: 2032 – 2040.

[28] Volotini L, Rapicetta C, Luzzi L, et al. Lung cancer with chest wall involvement: Predictive factors of long term survival after surgical resection. Lung Cancer, 2006, 52: 359 – 364.

[29] Lin YT, Hsu PK, Hsu HS, et al. En bloc resection for lung cancer with chest wall invasion. J Chin Med Assoc, 2006, 69 (4): 157 – 162.

[30] Lee CY, Byun CS, Lee JG, et al. The prognostic factors of resected non-small cell lung cancer with chest wall invasion. World J Surg Oncol, 2012, 10: 9.

[31] Pancoast HK. Superior pulmonary sulcus tumor. JAMA, 1932, 99: 1391.

[32] Van Schil PE, Sigal-Cinqualbre A, Dartevelle P, et al. Superior sulcus tumors: Do they really exist. J Thorac Oncol, 2012, 7 (5): 777.

[33] Shaw RR, Paulson DL, Kee JL. Treatment of the superior sulcus tumor by irradiation followed by resection. Ann Surg, 1961, 154 (1): 29 – 40.

[34] Rusch VW, Giroux DJ, Kraut MJ, et al. Induction chemoradiation and surgical resection for superior sulcus non-small cell lung carcinomas: Long term results of the Southwest Oncology Group Trial 9416 (Intergroup Trial 0160). J Clin Oncol, 2007, 25 (3): 313 – 318.

[35] Marra A, Eberhardt W, Pottgen C, et al. Induction chemotherapy, concurrent chemoradiation and surgery for Pancoast tumor. Eur Respir J, 2007, 29: 117 – 127.

[36] Fischer S, Darling G, Pierre AF, et al. Induction chemoradiation therapy followed by surgical resection for non-small cell lung cancer (NSCLC) invading the thoracic inlet. Eur J Cardiothorac Surg, 2008, 33: 1129 – 1134.

[37] Bolton WD, Rice DC, Goodyear A, et al. Superior sulcus tumors with vertebral body involvement: A multimodality approach. J Thorac and Cardiovasc Surg, 2009, 137 (6): 1379 – 1387.

[38] Gomez DR, Cox JD, Roth JA, et al. A prospective phase 2 study of surgery followed by chemotherapy and radiation for superior sulcus tumors. Cancer, 2012, 118: 444 – 451.

[39] Grunenwald MD, Spaggiari, MD. Transmanubrial osteomuscular sparing approach for apical chest tumors. Ann Thorac Surg, 1997, 63 (2): 563 – 566.

[40] Shikuma K, Miyahara R, Osako T. Transmanubrial approach combined with video-assisted approach for superior sulcus tumors. Ann Thorac Surg, 2012, 94 (1): e29 – 30.

[41] Truin W, Siebenga J, Belgers E, et al. The role of video-assisted thoracic surgery in the surgical treatment of superior sulcus tumors. Interact Cardiovasc Thorac Surg, 2010, 11 (4): 512 – 514.

[42] dePerrot M, Rampersaud R. Surgical approaches to apical thoracic malignancies. J Thorac Cardiovasc Surg,

2012, 144: 72-80.

[43] Fadel E, Missenard G, Chapelier A, et al. En-Bloc resection of non-small cell lung cancer invading the thoracic inlet and intervetrebal foramina. J Thorac Cardiovasc Surg, 2002, 123: 676-685.

[44] Grunenwald DH, Mazel C, Girard P, et al. Radical en bloc resection for lung cancer invading the spine. J Thorac Cardiovasc Surg, 2002, 123: 271-279.

[45] Bilsky MH, Vitaz TW, Boland PJ, et al. Surgical treatment of superior sulcus tumors with spinal and brachial plexus involvement. J Neurosurg, 2002, 97: 301-309.

[46] Navarro BO, Atance PL, Trueba AA. Pneumocephalus and cerebrospinal fluid fistula following removal of a superior sulcus tumor (Pancoast tumor). Arch Bronconeumol, 2004, 40 (9): 422-425.

[47] Weksler B, Bains M, Burt M, et al. Resection of lung cancer invading the diaphragm. J Thorac Cardiovasc Surg, 1997, 114: 500-501.

[48] Rocco G, Rendina EA, Meroni A. et al. Prognostic factors after surgical treatment of lung cancer invading the diaphragm. Ann Thorac Surg, 1999, 68: 2065-2068.

[49] Riquet M, Porte H, Chapelier A. Resection of lung cancer invading the diaphragm. J Thorac Cardiovasc Surg, 2000, 120 (2): 417-418.

[50] Brotons ML, Bolca C, Frechette E, , et al. Anatomy and physiology of the thoracic lymphatic system. Thorac Surg Clin, 2012, 22: 155-160.

[51] Tokunaga T, Sawabata N, Kadota Y, et al. Efficacy of intra-operative unilateral diaphragm plication for patients undergoing unilateral phrenicotomy during extended surgery. Eur J Cardiothorac Surg, 2010, 38: 600-603.

[52] D'Andrilli A, Venuta F, Menna C, et al. Extensive resections: Pancoast tumors, chest wall resections, en bloc vascular resections. Surg Onc Clin N Am, 2011, 20: 733-756.

[53] Shargall Y, de Perrot M, Keshavjee S, et al. 15 years single center experience with surgical resection of the superior vena cava for non-small-cell lung cancer. Lung Cancer, 2004, 45: 357-363.

[54] Suzuki K, Asamura H, Watanabe S, et al. Combined resection of superior vena cava for lung carcinoma: Prognostic significance of patterns of superior vena cava invasion. Ann Thorac Surg, 2004, 78: 1184-1189.

[55] Spaggiari L, Thomas P, Magdeleinat P, et al. Superior vena cava resection with prosthetic replacement for non-small cell lung cancer: long-term results of a multicentric study. Eur J Cardiothorac Surg, 2002, 21: 1080-1086.

[56] Yildizeli B, Dartevelle PG, Fadel E, et alResults of primary surgery with T4 non-small cell lung cancer during a 25-year period in a single center: The benefit is worth the risk. Ann Thorac Surg, 2008, 86: 1065-1075.

[57] Misthos P, Papagiannakis G, Kokotsakis J, et al. Surgical management of lung cancer invading the aorta or the superior vena cava. Lung Cancer, 2007, 56 (2): 223-227.

[58] Ohta M, Hirabayasi H, Shiono H, et al. Surgical resection for lung cancer with infiltration of the thoracic aorta. J Thorac Cardiovasc Surg, 2005, 129 (4): 804-808.

[59] Berna P, Bagan P, De Dominicis F, et al. Aortic endostent followed by extended pneumonectomy for T4 lung cancer. Ann Thorac Surg, 2011, 91 (2): 591-593.

[60] Muralidaran A, Detterbeck FC, Boffa DJ, et al. Long-term survival after lung resection for non-small cell lung cancer with circulatory bypass: A systematic review. J Thorac Cardiovasc Surg, 2011, 142: 1137-1142.

[61] de Perrot M, Fadel E, Mussot S, et al. Resection of locally advanced (T4) non-small cell lung cancer with cardiopulmonary bypass. Ann Thorac Surg, 2005, 79 (5): 1691-1696.

[62] Vaporciyan AA, Rice DC, Correa AM, et al. Resection of advancer thoracic malignancies requiring cardiopulmonary bypass. Eur J Cardio-Thorac Surg, 2002, 22: 47-52.

[63] Stella F, Dell'Amore A, Caroli G, et al. Surgical results and long-term follow-up of T4-non-small cell lung cancer invading the left atrium or the intrapericardial base of the pulmonary veins. Interactive Cardiovascular and Thoracic Surgery, 2012, 14: 415-419.

[64] Wu L, Xu Z, Zhao X, et al. Surgical treatment of lung cancer invading the left atrium or base of the pulmonary vein. World J Surg, 2009, 33: 492-496.

[65] Tanvetyanon T, Robinson L, Sommers KE, et al. Relationship between tumor size and survival among patients with resection of multiple synchronous lung cancers. J Thorac Oncol, 2010, 5: 1018-1024.

[66] Tanvetyanon T, Finley DJ, Fabian T, et al. Prognostic factors for survival after complete resections of synchronous lung cancers in multiple lobes: pooled analysis based on individual patient data. Ann Oncol, 2012, 7: 1-6.

第 16 章
肺癌的支气管镜干预

Donald R. Lazarus, George A. Eapen
Department of Pulmonary Medicine, The University of Texas MD Anderson Cancer Center, Houston, TX, USA

引 言

在美国，肺癌是癌症死亡的主要原因，每年有超过 15 万人死于肺癌[1]。60% 的非小细胞肺癌（NSCLC）患者在诊断时会出现与局部侵犯相关的症状[2]。在肺癌并发症中，大气道阻塞、咯血、支气管瘘可以通过支气管镜治疗得到缓解[3-5]。支气管镜技术也可以用来治疗早期中心型肺癌，但仅限于无法耐受标准疗法（包括手术和明确外部放疗）的患者[6-7]。能够使用支气管镜治疗的病变必须位于可曲式或硬性支气管镜所能触及的部位，主要包括气管、主支气管、中段支气管，有时也包括近段肺叶支气管[3,8-9]。在本章节，我们简要回顾能够通过支气管镜进行干预的中心气道病变（表 16.1），然后讨论支气管镜技术用于缓解和治疗肺癌中心气道疾病的更多细节。中心气道病变的原因不在本章讨论范围之内。

适用支气管镜技术的肺癌中心气道疾病

治疗性支气管镜技术应用于肺癌患者的最常见适应证是患者出现了中心气道受肿瘤侵犯的相关症状。应根据目前症状的类型，引起症状的病变性质及部位，以及当地可以获取的设备和医生的经验选择支气管镜治疗方法（图 16.1）。有 20%~30% 的肺癌患者会因为气管、主支气管的阻塞引起并发症，这些并发症包括呼吸困难、肺不张和阻塞性肺炎。在出现严重的狭窄之前，患者一般不会出现症状[8]。中心气道阻塞的类型决定了最有效、合理的治疗方式。Bolliger 等描述了 3 种气道狭窄：管腔内肿瘤生长所致的狭窄、管腔外压迫所致的狭窄以及上述两种因素都存在的狭窄[3]。腔内肿瘤生长引起的病变能够通过支气管镜得到最有效的治疗，使用机械和烧蚀方式破坏肿瘤可以恢复管腔通畅。气道腔外压迫如果导致了严重狭窄则需要支架扩张来恢复气道通畅。肿瘤腔内生长及腔外压迫同时存在的气道狭窄则需要联合方法治疗。咯血也是肺癌局部并发症之一。尽管，支气管食管瘘常见于食管癌，但也可以发生于肺癌[10]，它们常出现在放化疗期间。另外，持续的呼吸道污染会带来致命性伤害[5,10]。支气管内支架治疗可以减轻这些损害并且提高伴有气管食管瘘或支气管食管瘘肺癌患者的生活质量。

尽管大量咯血极其罕见，但 20% 的肺癌患者会发生次严重咯血[13]。大量咯血的定义存在争议，不同的作者主张 24h 内咯血量为 100~1 000mL，或

表 16.1 支气管镜干预在肺癌中的应用

机械干预
硬性支气管镜
球囊扩张术
气道支架
支气管镜显微切割
热干预
支气管镜激光
氩离子凝固
支气管内冷冻疗法
非机械，非热干预
光动力疗法
支气管内近距离放射治疗

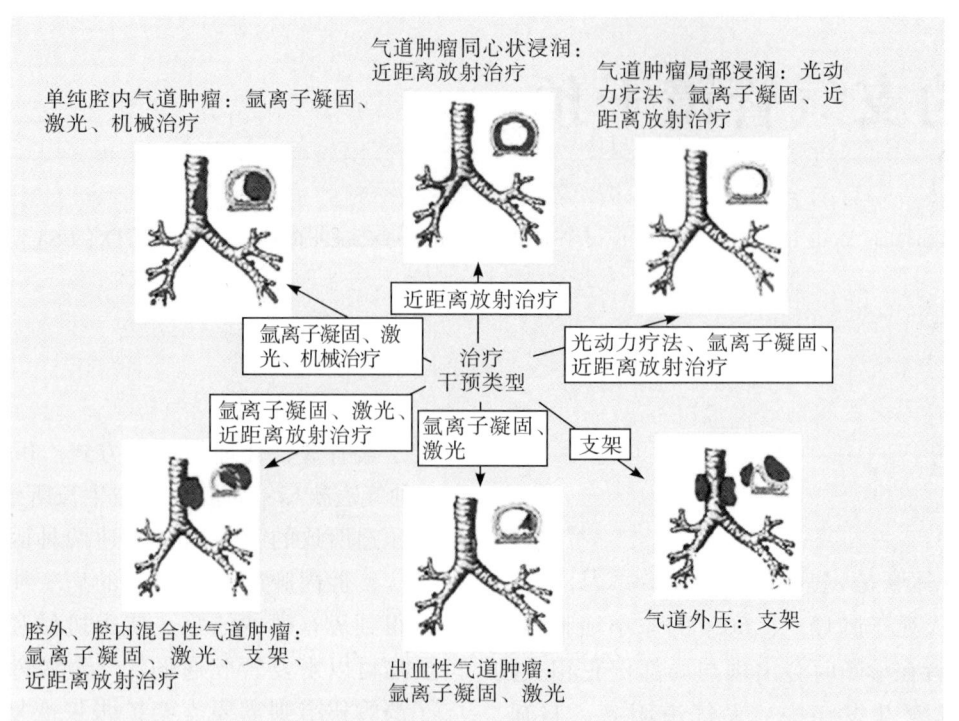

图 16.1（见彩插） 根据位置及病变类型选择适当的内镜治疗方法。经 Dr R. Morice 许可使用

者出血量 >100mL/h，从临床角度来看，大量咯血可以更好地定义为伴有呼吸功能不全或者血流动力学不足的咯血[14]。来源于可见中央气道独立病变的咯血可以接受支气管镜治疗。中央气道出血部位的定位需要使用影像学以及可曲式或者硬性支气管镜进行快速的临床评估。我们应当将影像和支气管镜技术互为补充，在同时使用的情况下，临床工作者可以有效定位出血来源[4,15]。如果出血量在 200mL/d 或者更大，支气管镜可以更有效地定位出血部位[16]。一旦出血部位明确，应该努力隔离出血部位以保护正常肺组织。有效技术包括放置出血面朝下，选择性地在不出血的主支气管插管，在出血部位安置支气管内封堵物来阻断出血。一旦患者情况稳定，中央气管的出血部位可以应用各种支气管镜得到控制，包括热疗技术、机械切除出血性肿瘤、光动力疗法和近距离放射治疗。通过支气管动脉栓塞和手术，大多数末梢出血可以得到更好的控制。

支气管内近距离放射治疗或光动力疗法可用于治疗目前只局限于中心气道的早期肺癌患者，或由于肿瘤的位置、肺功能低下或其他不良状况而不能使用标准手术和放化疗的患者。在这种条件下治疗的目的是治愈[9]。对以治愈为目的的支气管内治疗效果最佳的是直径 <1cm，未侵犯气管壁的软骨层，并且未出现区域淋巴结转移的病变[17]。近距离放射治疗和光动力学疗法也可以用于增强中心气道肿瘤传统放射治疗的疗效或用于治疗手术后支气管内肿瘤复发[9]。

支气管镜机械干预在肺癌中的应用

机械支气管镜可以用于切除支气管内肿瘤，扩张和加固气道梗阻肺癌患者受累狭窄的气管。这些技术包括硬性支气管镜、气管支架和纤维支气管镜微切割器。硬性支气管镜是其中可用于治疗所有 3 种有症状的中心气道病变最重要的工具。硬性支气管镜是有侧孔的中空金属管道，可用于通气和引导吸引以及将其他工具导入气道；也可以用它来建立安全气道，作为梗阻性气管肿瘤切除术前的通气策略；它不是容量循环通气而是喷射通气，可形成开放式回路，有利于手术器械便捷地通过工作通道。通常在支气管镜的尖端配备一个发光的望远镜，从而能够在长距离的气道中有良好的视野。硬性支气管镜备有不同的尺寸，外径 2~14mm。纤维支气管镜也能够通过硬镜，以便于观察更远端的支气管。相对大口径的硬性支气管镜的内部通道极其重要，可作为其他手术器械的导管。介入支气管镜操作者通常在同一时间内通过硬镜应用不止一种工具进行治疗，尤其是硅胶支架的放置必须通过硬性支气管镜。当进行介入操作时，硬性支气管镜操作者可保障气道安全，使氧合和通气便利。而且它有作为导管的功能，以便于其他治疗器械的进入，通过"打通"肿瘤，硬性支气管镜本身可用于治疗肺癌中央气道梗阻。应用最广泛的硬性支气管镜有一个斜面的尖端，术者可以应用硬性支气管镜尖端的斜刃来定位和切除腔内肿瘤。一个拧螺丝的动作就可以刮除肿瘤，再使用镊子和吸引器通过硬性支气管镜的通道移除肿瘤[18-19]。在气管内肿瘤切除术中，使硬性支气管镜保持恰当的方向很重要。如果支气管镜不能平行于气管壁，将有气道穿孔的风险。支气管镜管腔施加于气管壁上的压力有助于填塞压迫病灶和减少肿瘤切除后的出血[8]。在不切除腔内肿瘤的情况下硬性支气管镜也可用于扩张气管的狭窄部分。使用更大口径的硬性支气管镜，依次通过气管的狭窄部分，从而进行逐步的机械扩张，这种技术的缺点是当扩张气道时不能够直视黏膜并且与应用球囊导管连续扩张气道相比可能造成更多的黏膜损伤[8,18-19]。

支气管球囊成形术是治疗因外部肿瘤压迫导致支气管阻塞的另一项应用技术，在这项技术中，一个灵活、可膨胀的气囊导管通过可曲式或硬性支气管镜介入并膨胀，从而扩张气道狭窄部分。气囊导管的顶端应该超过狭窄部位，其扩张直径应该是狭窄气道直径的两倍，这样才能达到治疗效果。尽管球囊扩张术在改善因外部压迫导致的气管狭窄中的效果可信，但许多因恶性肿瘤导致气管狭窄的患者在球囊成形术后仍需要支架来维持气道通畅[20]（图16.2A~C）。

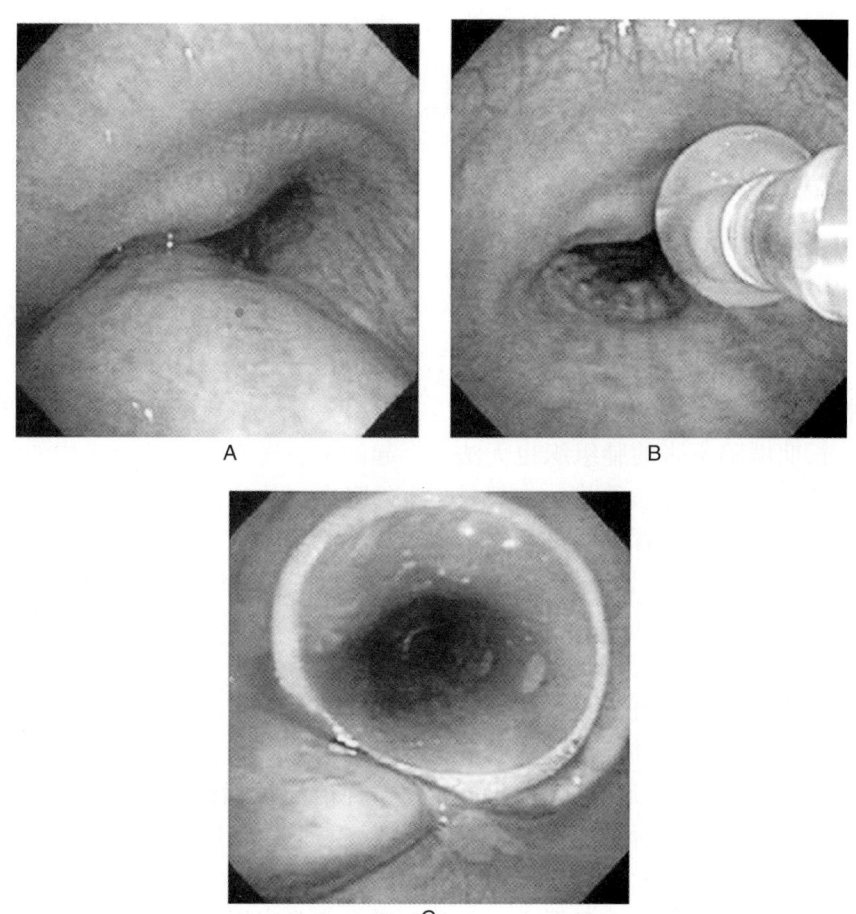

图16.2（见彩插） A. 69岁腺样囊性癌女性患者，表现为严重呼吸困难，肿瘤阻塞气管下段及双侧支气管主干。B. 球囊连续扩张气管下段狭窄。C. 球囊连续扩张，植入Y形气管支气管硅胶支架之后气道明显恢复

气管支架在减轻因恶性肿瘤导致气道狭窄方面受到越来越多的关注。目前最常用的支架是硅胶支架及可自动扩张金属支架。支气管镜下放置硅胶支架由Dumon发明并于1990年首次报道[21]。使用硬性支气管镜来放置可以使支架的移除或调整变的相对容易。相对于传统的直圆筒状，硅胶支架可塑形为"Y"字形以适应气管和双侧主支气管[22]。为减小移位的概率，大多数类型的硅胶支架外壁都具有螺栓排布[21]。硅胶支架可现场订制以最大限度地符合患者的气道并成功治疗更复杂的气道狭窄[23]。硅胶支架的缺点为放置困难，容易移位，与弯曲的气道吻合度差[22]。可自动扩张金属支架通常由合金制成，例如镍钛诺（镍和钛），比钢更具弹性，同时仍提供足够的径向力抵抗肿瘤的外源性压迫。一些可自动扩张的金属支架表面没有覆盖金属，一些表面部分或者全部覆盖聚亚安酯。与硅胶支架相比，可自动扩张金属支架更容易放置，并且能够在可曲式支气管镜下放置，另外，它们不易移位。虽然可自动扩张的金属支架不能当场塑形，但金属编织设计可以允许一些肿瘤通过支架壁生长并进入内腔，它们比硅胶支架更难以移除或者调整，更容易侵蚀穿透气管壁[22]。肺癌患者安装支架的适应证主要是减轻气道阻塞和封闭气道瘘管。支架不能有效减轻管腔内肿瘤引起的阻塞，但对管腔外（伴或不伴有管腔内肿瘤）压迫引起的气道阻塞效果最佳。还需要说明的是，对于支气管狭窄段远端气道不通畅或者没有正常肺组织的患者，支架是无效的。即使安放了支架，长期塌陷不张的肺组织也无法膨胀[22]。若肺癌患者伴有支气管食管瘘，支架是有效的姑息措施。食管支架比气管支架更普遍地应用于缓解气管食管瘘。但是它们可以侵蚀透支气管（重新形成瘘管）或者压迫气道（导致呼吸困难）[24]。气管和食管内同时置入双支架，或者首次治疗放一个气道支架，然后再置入一个食管支架，曾经被尝试用于避免这些并发症。硅胶支架和可自动扩张支架都成功地达到了这些目的。需要强调的是支气管瘘放置支架对不能耐受手术的患者来说顶多是姑息治疗，手术仍然是能够达到治愈效果的唯一方法[11-12,24-25]。一旦置入了气管支架，随访指导是非标准化的，主要基于当地的治疗经验。肺的清理至关重要，因为气道支架影响自然的黏膜纤毛清除率。目前还没有某种单一的方法被证明是最有效的。喷雾型支气管扩张剂、喷雾型高渗盐溶液和喷雾型乙酰半胱氨酸都曾被报道过[22]。一旦放置了支架，气道症状加重的患者则需要安排紧密的临床随访，即进行支气管镜检查。

纤维支气管镜微切割器是用于缓解支气管内肺癌症状的最新方法，这个设备由附着在有集成吸力中空金属管道上的旋转刀片组成。刀片切割的转速在1 000~5 000r/min，它由一个控制台和脚踏板控制。刀片可以通过一个单边的窗口直通向支气管壁，并且可以360°旋转。尽管最初的发明是为了治疗上呼吸道的疾病并且被耳鼻喉科医生运用，新型的纤维支气管镜微切割器通过加长管道已经可以穿过硬性支气管镜到达气管、主支气管并用于细支气管[26]。刀片可以到达气管、主支气管、中段支气管中的病灶，它可以非常精确地进行组织清除术。有集成吸力的管道可以迅速清除血液和组织碎片，以确保获得最佳的视野[27]。它的最佳适应证是切除近端气道管腔内的肿瘤组织并作为样本用于组织学诊断，而不是用热疗下烧焦的组织作为样本。它的缺点主要是不能到达末梢病灶并且有可能会损伤正常组织[26]。在接触气管支架时必须小心，因支架会被刀片损伤。

支气管镜热干预在肺癌中的应用

支气管镜热干预主要用于治疗由腔内肿瘤引起的中心气道梗阻及由于中心气道出血病灶引起的咯血。热疗法包括激光、电灼、氩离子凝固和冷冻治疗。

激光（Laser）是Light Amplified by Stimulated Emission of Radiation的各个单词的首字母缩写[8]。在这个过程中，原子被激发释放光子，释放的光子在同一轨道层和同一波长运动，这一过程可能会产生热能，这就是支气管内激光治疗的机制。这种治疗可做到靶组织的切除、凝固或气化[3]。激光长期以来用于治疗引起梗阻和咯血的支气管内病灶[28]。钕：钇铝石榴石（Nd：YAG激光器）激光普遍应用于支气管镜，这是因为它具有足够的功率来气化组织，同时可以保持极好的凝固作用。它的波长是1 064nm，而且具有精确、灵活的探头。肺癌患者的支气管激光治疗的适应证为明确的腔内肿物及邻近病变所产生的气道梗阻或咯血[3]。支气管激光治疗预后最好的是位于气管或主支气管且支气管末端腔内视野较好的外生型病变且血流动力学稳定的患者[19,29]。对于上叶支气管或段支气管内的外在压迫性病变或者气管腔内完全阻塞的患者来说，激光治疗效果较差[8,28]。光纤发射的激光延伸出支气管镜的前端，可见的引导激光可用于定位所期望的病灶。吸氧分数（FiO_2）必须保持在0.4左右，以降低气道烧伤风险的发生率。目标应该平行于气道，且机械清创后有明显的凝固发生[3]。许多小规模的研究已经表明，尽管尚未发现明确的存活优势，但是激光疗法对肺癌中心气道的梗阻有一定的缓和作用[8,29-30]。激光治疗的潜在并发症包括出血、缺氧、穿孔、气道烧伤、眼外伤（患者或医务人员在治疗过程中需要佩戴防护眼镜）和气体栓塞[3,18,19,28,31]。

支气管内电灼术需要高频率的电流来产生热量，这使得烧灼探头可以在接触点处切割或凝固组织[32]。组织效应受到电压、接触的持续时间、接触的面积及组织密度的影响[32-33]。高于40℃可以导致不可逆转的组织损伤，在70℃~100℃时可以导致组织凝固，高于200℃时就开始导致组织碳化和气化[32]。多个电灼工具可供选择，包括1个钝探头、1个平刀、烙钳和1个圈套[34]。气管内电灼术对减灭腔内肿瘤，圈套息肉状肿瘤和治疗咯血方面效果较好[3,32,35]。它需要器械和被烧灼的组织之间的直接接触，所以使用范围有限，只适用于可屈式支气管镜可以到达的那些气道。支气管内电灼术相当于Nd：YAG激光，可以有效治疗腔内肿瘤引起的气道阻塞，在某种程度上可以稍微降低治疗成本[34-35]。电灼的风险包括出血、穿孔、低氧血症、心脏起搏器故障和气道烧伤[3]。与支气管内激光疗法相比，FiO_2应保持在或低于0.4，以降低气道烧伤的风险。患者必须接地，并且不推荐带有起搏器或植入自动心脏除颤器的患者使用单极电灼术进行电灼[32]。

近几年来，氩离子凝固（argon plasma coagulation，APC）是一种非接触形式的电灼，已成为支气管内非常流行的一种治疗方法。氩气被电场电离，并导致均匀的单极电流从探头到达组织[32]。电流行进到最近的接触点，可以是探头的正前方，也可以不是，因为APC治疗可以进行侧面电灼[3,36]。与组织接触的电流被转换成热能后，导致组织表浅凝固并且可电灼至5mm或更小的深度[32,36]。一旦凝固达到一定深度，电流就会倾向于在组织表浅进行扩散，而不是继续更深的渗透，因为凝固的组织具有较大的阻力，这种特性降低了在APC治疗过程中穿孔的风险[36]。APC是通过将灵活的探头引入支气管镜的工作通道来使用的。患者必须接地，并且FiO_2应保持在0.4或更小，以减小气道烧伤的风险。探头从支气管镜的末端一直延伸到前端约1cm处，与靶组织保持3~4mm的距离。探头的头端应该比其他任何组织更接近靶组织，因为电流会流向接触的最近点，作用时间为3~4s。凝固过程中持续施加负压吸引可以帮助清理呼吸道的烟雾，降低气道发生烧伤的风险，并且保证气道内视野清晰[32,36]。目前发现APC的最大用途是治疗近端支气管内病变所致的咯血。它也可用于凝固和减灭腔内的肿瘤，作为机械减瘤的辅助治疗方法或单独应用[32,36]。APC的潜在并发症包括气道烧伤、穿孔、出血和气体栓塞[37-38]，但这些并发症非常罕见，所有APC过程中发生率不足3%[36-37]（图16.3A、B）。

冷冻疗法是另一种支气管镜热技术，通过冷冻技术重复进行冷冻和解冻循环来破坏组织[9]。缓慢解冻后快速冷冻，可以导致细胞内和细胞外冰晶的形成，导致细胞损伤和脱水。这个过程还导致局部血管损伤，包括血管收缩和毛细血管通透性增加。迟发的局部血栓形成导致组织发生梗死，在7~14d内引起非出血性坏死[39]。快速冷却，缓慢解冻，达到低于-40℃的低组织温度，并重复冷冻可以增加冷冻损伤的成功率[39-41]。冷冻疗法的效果还取决于组织类型，有更高含水量的组织，包括皮肤、黏膜、肿瘤和肉芽组织对冷冻治疗高度敏感。相反，一些组织，如脂肪、软骨和结缔组织，含水量较低，对冷冻治疗有一定的抵抗性[39-40]。支气管内冷冻治疗经由柔性触点探头通过输送管线连接到一个含有气瓶的控制台。当冷冻探头的尖端气体由高压降至低压时，气体迅速冷却。N_2O是支气管镜中最常用的冷却剂[9,41]。使用液氮在气道内进行喷雾冷冻疗法的安全性尚未确定，因此无法推荐使用，而且人们已经提出了对气体迅速膨胀造成气胸和心血管并

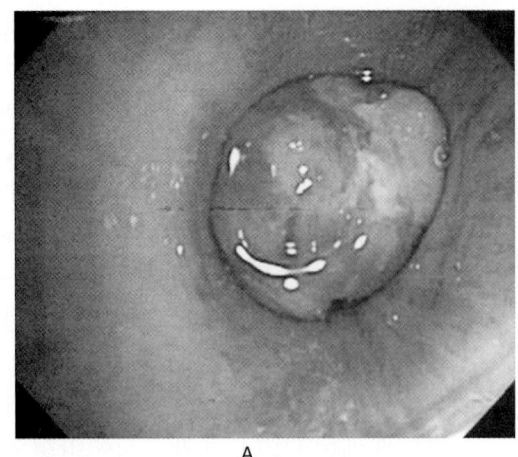 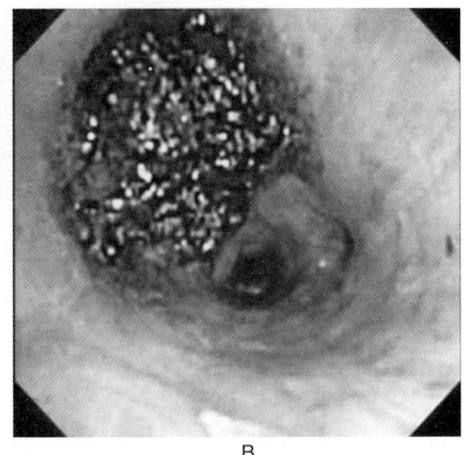

图 16.3（见彩插） A. 49 岁的右肺中叶腺癌女性患者，由于右中间支气管的完全性梗阻出现呼吸困难。B. 右中间支气管经过圈套电灼及氩离子血浆凝固治疗腔内肿瘤后完全再通

发症的担忧。一旦支气管镜定位到医生关注的病变部位，冷冻探头就会通过支气管镜的工作通道向前推进，直至探头尖端与视野的末端有一个安全的距离。然后将探头的尖端与靶病变接触，冷却剂被激活，大约冷冻 30s 之后，开始被动解冻。探头将被冻结到靶组织中直到解冻完成。第 1~3 次冻融循环是在直视下完成的，然后操作者移动探头到下一个位点，注意要与已治疗过的区域重叠，以确保肿瘤的整个表面都得到处理。如果需要，冷冻疗法可以重复进行[9]。支气管内冷冻疗法主要用于治疗管腔内肿瘤引起的气道阻塞。尽管其坏死效果延迟，但它可以通过冷冻阻塞气管的病变并在解冻发生之前移去探头，实现即时"低温再通"。处理过的肿瘤连同被冷冻的部分随探头一起除去，从而导致快速再通。这种技术可能导致出血，因此在必要的情况下操作员应准备干预措施[42]。无论是通过其延迟效应或通过"低温再通"，肺癌的冷冻疗法主要用于治疗气管支气管树的肿瘤阻塞[9,42-45]。它作为伴有支气管受侵犯肺癌常规疗法的辅助治疗措施也显示出一定的有效性，尤其是在与放射疗法结合应用时[45-46]。关于冷冻治疗的一个非常小规模的研究显示，早期表浅近端段肺癌的单一冷冻治疗表现出 1 年期的良好局部控制，但这种治疗方法目前仍然被视为一种试验[47]。冷冻疗法通常被认为是较为安全的，并且比其他大多数烧灼支气管内技术相对价格低廉，部分原因是没有气道火灾的风险（必要情况下患者需要在手术过程中保持 100% 氧气），也有部分原因是许多周围正常组织相对抗冷冻，不会被意外损伤。并发症主要限于出血、反应性水肿或坏死组织脱落，以及非常罕见的瘘[42,46]。

非热性及非机械性支气管镜干预治疗在肺癌中的应用

光动力疗法和近距离放射是使用非机械和非热机制来治疗和缓解气道受累肺癌的治疗方法。这两种方法都通过支气管镜进行，并且在精心筛选的案例中已经显示出缓解和治疗作用的有效性[9]。这两种方法都有延迟效应，因此不适用于需要立即缓解中央气道阻塞的患者。

光动力疗法（photodynamic therapy，PDT）是基于单独无害组分之间的相互作用而产生的组织损伤。这些组分包括光敏剂、光源和氧气[9,48]。特定波长的光可以激发出光敏化学物质，这种光敏化学物质是在从基态到激发态的肿瘤细胞中发现的。然后被激发的光敏剂与组织氧气相互作用以形成自由基和导致毒性的单线态氧。局部效应包括细胞膜和线粒体的直接细胞损伤、诱导细胞凋亡、局部血管损伤和肿瘤敏感的免疫和炎症反应[9,48-49]。理想的光敏剂应该对肿瘤有选择性，具有临床应用范围内的吸收光谱，并且具有单态氧的高产生率[49]。大多数市售光敏剂是从血卟啉衍生而来的。卟吩姆钠（光卟啉™；Axcan 制药；

Birmingham，AL）是美国最常用的光敏剂，是以 2mg/kg 进行缓慢注射。卟吩姆钠在注射后 72h 内从大多数正常组织中清除，但在肿瘤细胞、血管内皮细胞和皮肤中可以保留更长的时间。在 48h 的潜伏期后，波长为 630nm 的光作用于肿瘤，并激活该化合物。这可以使 5～10mm 深度的肿瘤被破坏[9,48-49]。光活化是通过一个非热光源，最常见的是激光来完成的。PDT 常用的激光器是氩泵浦染料激光器，钾氧钛磷酸盐（KTP）激光器和二极管激光器。光是光纤系统通过支气管镜的工作通道递送至肿瘤，光纤尖端的扩散器可以传播光[9]，经批准的光剂量为 200J/cm，光通常需要 8～12min 到达每个纤维的布置处[9,50]。PDT 的适应证为用于现有或即将出现症状的晚期中央型肺癌的缓解，由于其穿透深度最小，只适用于治疗主要为腔内成分的肿瘤。PDT 也适用于治疗以治愈为目的的早期中央型肺癌患者，这些患者不适用于手术或根治性放疗，但是对足够表浅的肿瘤进行 PDT 治疗也是有效的[9,50]。通过标准支气管镜或单独 CT 难以精确地评估肿瘤浸润的深度。径向探头支气管内超声（radial probe endobronchial ultrasound，RP-EBUS）已被证明可以精确地评估支气管肿瘤的浸润深度[51]。Miyazu 等采用 RP-EBUS 作为 18 例患者中的 PDT 良好候选人治疗前评估的一部分。队列中有一半患者尽管 CT 和标准支气管镜检查均发现只有表浅的侵袭，但通过 RP-EBUS 发现侵袭已超过软骨层，因此被确定为较差的 PDT 候选人[52]。因此，进行 PDT 之前需要通过支气管内超声谨慎地正式评估表浅支气管肿瘤的浸润深度，从而确定他们的治疗指征。因为 PDT 有延迟效应，所以不应当用于即将发生威胁生命的中央气道阻塞的患者。侵犯邻近的血管结构或对卟啉治疗过敏的肿瘤患者是 PDT 的其他禁忌证[50]。一旦适当的中心表浅病变被确定，就注入光敏剂。潜伏期之后，经过支气管镜检查，就可以看到待治疗的病灶。光纤维通过工作通道推进到气道，纤维头端的扩散器被嵌入肿瘤中。光线施加 8～12min 后，移除导管。在 24～48h 内建议重复做一次支气管镜检查以去除坏死的碎片。如果看到残存肿瘤，也可进行重复照射[9,50]。大多数评估 PDT 对缓解肺癌中心气道阻塞有效性的证据是通过病例报道的形式获得的。这些有限的研究表明，PDT 在减少腔内梗阻程度及减少呼吸困难症状上是有效的[9,50,53-55]。大多数小型研究显示，在以治愈为目的时，不适用于手术治疗的早期中央型肺癌患者使用 PDT 已经显示出 44%～100% 的局部控制率[52,56-60]。PDT 最常见的并发症是光敏性，其他包括咳嗽、治疗后肿瘤的延迟出血、胸部不适、气道反应性水肿和坏死性分泌物[50]。

支气管内近距离放射治疗使用一个放射源并将其置于非常接近靶肿瘤的位置，向周围组织提供低毒性的局部放射治疗。放射源放置在支气管内，伽马射线是主要的放射类型，可以用来破坏肿瘤细胞。平方反比定律表明放射的剂量率会随着距放射源中心距离的平方成反比减少；这允许邻近放射源的高放射剂量随着远离放射源，放射剂量快速减少。近距离放射治疗过程中发出的辐射不会直接杀死癌细胞，相反，它会损伤癌细胞的 DNA 导致细胞凋亡，降低细胞增殖。这种效果被延迟，并且在治疗后的 3～4 周达到最大值。与 PDT 不同，支气管腔内近距离放射治疗的一大优势是其更持续的效果和更深的穿透性——近距离放射治疗可以破坏软骨以外的组织[9]。近距离放射治疗的早期尝试受限于医务人员处理放射源时受到的放射暴露。自动远程后装机的引入增加了医务人员支气管内近距离放射治疗的安全性，并使其应用增加[61-62]。支气管内近距离放疗一般以高剂量率给予，即大于 12Gy/h，但通常是大于 100Gy/h。所使用的辐射源最常用的是铱-192。使用高剂量率近距离放疗需要的治疗时间短，可以在门诊治疗。治疗通常被分成 2～4 次，每次 5～15Gy[9,62-63]。近距离放射治疗的适应证为不适用体外放疗患者支气管内恶性病变相关症状的缓解（包括呼吸道梗阻、咯血和咳嗽），或者作为手术或体外放疗的辅助治疗方法。对于早期中心气道内肺癌患者来说，近距离放射治疗也可以作为治愈方法，上述患者的病灶应该可以通过支气管镜到达，但是不适用于进行手术或体外放射治疗[9]。近距离放射治疗之前，必须经支气管镜定位置入支气管后装导管。一旦操作者定位到肿瘤，应将后装导管放置到气管内并且其远侧的尖端至少超出肿瘤3cm，然后用胶带固定到鼻子上。虚拟导线引入后通过透视确认其位置，所需的照射长度也可以使用外用标签固定到皮肤进行标记。然后患者被输送到放射治疗的套房中，一个虚拟粒子被插入后装导管中，其正确位置通过X线确诊。虚拟粒子被移除后，敷料器与辐射源连接，在计算机控制下前进到适当的位置。它在每一个位置保持足够长的时间以应用规定的剂量，然后以5mm的间隔撤出。在治疗后导管被去除[9]。对于中心气道腔内梗阻为主的患者，近距离放射治疗用于缓解症状是有效的。一些研究表明，65%~85%的腔内病变为主的患者有症状上的改善。在一项大型的囊括了324例患者的队列研究中，67%的患者的病变可以成功缓解，不需要进一步的治疗[63-66]。对于主支气管有肿瘤阻塞的患者进行近距离放疗还可以增强体外放疗的作用[67]。当以治愈为目的时，结果则不太理想，且2年生存率为58%~78%[6,68-69]。近距离放射治疗的并发症较为常见，包括咯血、支气管狭窄、支气管软化和瘘管形成。咯血是近距离放射治疗最严重的并发症，其发病率在10%~50%。据报道，在进行近距离放疗的患者中，0~8%的患者发生致命性大咯血[9,66,70]。因为近距离放射治疗通常用于减轻咯血症状，所以我们难以确定有多少是由于治疗引起的，有多少是潜在的恶性肿瘤引起的。临床医生应该对进行近距离放射治疗的患者出现的咯血保持警惕。

总 结

支气管镜介入是肺癌患者中心气道受累时缓解症状的重要辅助治疗方法。对于近段中心气道阻塞和咯血来说这种方法最有效。选择最合适的干预方法应根据病灶的性质和位置、该症状的类型以及当地现有的设备和专业技术来确定。光动力疗法和支气管内近距离放射治疗也适用于以治愈为目的的早期中央气道的表浅肺癌的治疗，但只适用于患者不能耐受标准治疗的情况。应当强调的是，所有这些技术只能辅助而不是代替标准治疗如手术、化疗和放射治疗。

（于 洋 李 猛 王晓航 译）

参考文献

[1] Siegel R, Naishadham D, Jemal A. Cancer statistics. CA Cancer J Clin, 2013, 63 (1): 11-30.

[2] Numico G, Russi E, Merlano M. Best supportive care in non-small cell lung cancer: Is there a role for radiotherapy and chemotherapy. Lung Cancer, 2001, 32 (3): 213-226.

[3] Bolliger CT, Sutedja TG, Strausz J, et al. Therapeutic bronchoscopy with immediate effect: Laser, electrocautery, argon plasma coagulation and stents. Eur Respir J, 2006, 27 (6): 1258-1271.

[4] Hirshberg B, Biran I, Glazer M, et al. Hemoptysis: etiology, evaluation, and outcome in a tertiary referral hospital. Chest, 1997, 112 (2): 440-444.

[5] Schreiber J, Waldburg N. Bronchoesophageal fistula and fatal hemoptysis after bevacizumabcontaining chemotherapy without radiation in lung cancer. J Clin Oncol, 2012, 30 (32): e324.

[6] Perol M, Caliandro R, Pommier P, et al. Curative irradiation of limited endobronchial carcinomas with high-dose rate brachytherapy. Results of a pilot study. Chest, 1997, 111 (5): 1417-1423.

[7] Simone CB, 2nd, Friedberg JS, Glatstein E, et al. Photodynamic therapy for the treatment of non-small cell lung cancer. J Thorac Dis, 2012, 4 (1): 63-75.

[8] Ernst A, Feller-Kopman D, Becker HD, et al. Central airway obstruction. Am J Respir Crit Care Med, 2004, 169 (12): 1278-1297.

[9] Vergnon JM, Huber RM, Moghissi K. Place of cryotherapy, brachytherapy and photodynamic therapy in therapeutic bronchoscopy of lung cancers. Eur Respir J, 2006, 28 (1): 200-218.

[10] Burt M, Diehl W, Martini N, et al. Malignant esophagorespiratory fistula: management options and survival. Ann Thorac Surg, 1991, 52 (6): 1222-1228; discussion 8-9.

[11] Freitag L, Tekolf E, Steveling H, et al. Management of malignant esophagotracheal fistulas with airway stenting and double stenting. Chest, 1996, 110 (5): 1155-1160.

[12] Herth FJ, Peter S, Baty F, et al. Combined airway and oesophageal stenting in malignant airway-oesophageal fistulas: a prospective study. Eur Respir J, 2010, 36 (6): 1370-1374.

[13] Cahill BC, Ingbar DH. Massive hemoptysis. Assessment and management. Clin Chest Med, 1994, 15 (1): 147-167.

[14] Ibrahim WH. Massive haemoptysis: the definition should be revised. Eur Respir J, 2008, 32 (4): 1131-1132.

[15] Set PAK, Flower CDR, Smith IE, et al. Hemoptysis-comparativestudy of the role of Ct and fiberoptic bronchoscopy. Radiology, 1993, 189 (3): 677-680.

[16] Poe RH, Israel RH, Marin MG, et al. Utility of fiberoptic bronchoscopy in patients with hemoptysis and a nonlocalizing chest roentgenogram. Chest, 1988, 93 (1): 70-75.

[17] McWilliams A, Lam B, Sutedja T. Early proximal lung cancer diagnosis and treatment. Eur Respir J, 2009, 33 (3): 656-665.

[18] Bolliger CT, Mathur PN, Beamis JF, et al. ERS/ATS statement on interventional pulmonology. European Respiratory Society/American Thoracic Society. Eur Respir J, 2002, 19 (2): 356-373.

[19] Ernst A, Silvestri GA, Johnstone D. Interventional pulmonary procedures: Guidelines from the American College of Chest Physicians. Chest, 2003, 123 (5): 1693-1717.

[20] Hautmann H, Gamarra F, Pfeifer KJ, et al. Fiberoptic bronchoscopic balloon dilatation in malignant tracheobronchial disease: indications and results. Chest, 2001, 120 (1): 43-49.

[21] Dumon JF. A dedicated tracheobronchial stent. Chest, 1990, 97 (2): 328-332.

[22] Casal RF. Update in airway stents. Current Opinion in Pulmonary Medicine, 2010, 16: 321-328.

[23] Breen DP, Dutau H. On-site customization of silicone stents: Towards optimal palliation of complex airway conditions. Respiration, 2009, 77 (4): 447-453.

[24] Oida T, Mimatsu K, Kano H, et al. Double stents: airway stenting after esophageal-stent implantation for esophageal cancer. Hepatogastroenterology, 2011, 58 (112): 1985-1988.

[25] Kim KR, Shin JH, Song HY, et al. Palliative treatment of malignant esophagopulmonary fistulas with covered expandable metallic stents. AJR Am J Roentgenol, 2009, 193 (4): W278-282.

[26] Lunn W, Garland R, Ashiku S, et al. Microdebrider bronchoscopy: A new tool for the interventional bronchoscopist. Ann Thorac Surg, 2005, 80 (4): 1485-1488.

[27] Melendez J, Cornwell L, Green L, et al. Treatment of large subglottic tracheal schwannoma with microdebrider bronchoscopy. J Thorac Cardiovasc Surg, 2012, 144 (2): 510-512.

[28] Dumon JF, Shapshay S, Bourcereau J, et al. Principles for safety in application of neodymium-YAG laser in bronchology. Chest, 1984, 86 (2): 163-168.

[29] Desai SJ, Mehta AC, VanderBrug Medendorp S, et al. Survival experience following Nd: YAG laser photoresection for primary bronchogenic carcinoma. Chest, 1988, 94 (5): 939-944.

[30] Ross DJ, Mohsenifar Z, Koerner SK. Survival characteristics after neodymium: YAG laser photoresection in advanced stage lung cancer. Chest, 1990, 98 (3): 581-585.

[31] Tellides G, Ugurlu BS, Kim RW, et al. Pathogenesis of systemic air embolism during bronchoscopic Nd: YAG laser operations. Ann Thorac Surg, 1998, 65 (4): 930-934.

[32] Sheski FD, Mathur PN. Endobronchial electrosurgery: Argon plasma coagulation and electrocautery. Semin Respir Crit Care Med, 2004, 25 (4): 367-374.

[33] van Boxem TJ, Venmans BJ, Schramel FM, et al. Radiographically occult lung cancer treated with fibreoptic bronchoscopic electrocautery: A pilot study of a simple and inexpensive technique. Eur Respir J, 1998, 11 (1): 169-172.

[34] Coulter TD, Mehta AC. The heat is on: Impact of endobronchial electrosurgery on the need for Nd-YAG laser photoresection. Chest, 2000, 118 (2): 516-521.

[35] Boxem T, Muller M, Venmans B, et al. Nd-YAG laser vs bronchoscopic electrocautery for palliation of symptomatic airway obstruction: A costeffectiveness study. Chest, 116 (4): 1108-1112.

[36] Morice RC, Ece T, Ece F, et al. Endobronchial argon plasma coagulation for treatment of hemoptysis and neoplastic airway obstruction. Chest, 2001, 119 (3): 781-787.

[37] Reichle G, Freitag L, Kullmann HJ, et al. Argon plasma coagulation in bronchology: a new method-alternative or complementary. Pneumologie, 2000, 54 (11): 508-516.

[38] Reddy C, Majid A, Michaud G, et al. Gas embolism fol-

[39] Theodorescu D. Cancer cryotherapy: Evolution and biology. Rev Urol, 2004, 6 (Suppl 4): S9 – S19.

[40] Gage AA, Baust J. Mechanisms of tissue injury in cryosurgery. Cryobiology, 1998, 37 (3): 171 – 186.

[41] Gage AA, Guest K, Montes M, et al. Effect of varying freezing and thawing rates in experimental cryosurgery. Cryobiology, 1985, 22 (2): 175 – 182.

[42] Hetzel M, Hetzel J, Schumann C, et al. Cryorecanalization: A new approach for the immediate management of acute airway obstruction. J Thorac Cardiovasc Surg, 2004, 127 (5): 1427 – 1431.

[43] Walsh DA, Maiwand MO, Nath AR, et al. Bronchoscopic cryotherapy for advanced bronchial carcinoma. Thorax, 1990, 45 (7): 509 – 513.

[44] Mathur PN, Wolf KM, Busk MF, et al. Fiberoptic bronchoscopic cryotherapy in the management of tracheobronchial obstruction. Chest, 1996, 110 (3): 718 – 723.

[45] Asimakopoulos G, Beeson J, Evans J, et al. Cryosurgery for malignant endobronchial tumors: analysis of outcome. Chest, 2005, 127 (6): 2007 – 2014.

[46] Vergnon JM, Schmitt T, Alamartine E, et al. Initial combined cryotherapy and irradiation for unresectable nonsmall cell lung cancer. Preliminary results. Chest, 1992, 102 (5): 1436 – 1440.

[47] Deygas N, Froudarakis M, Ozenne G, et al. Cryotherapy in early superficial bronchogenic carcinoma. Chest, 2001, 120 (1): 26 – 31.

[48] Dolmans DE, Fukumura D, Jain RK. Photodynamic therapy for cancer. Nat Rev Cancer, 2003, 3 (5): 380 – 387.

[49] Pass HI. Photodynamic therapy in oncology: Mechanisms and clinical use. J Natl Cancer Inst, 1993, 85 (6): 443 – 456.

[50] Loewen GM, Pandey R, Bellnier D, et al. Endobronchial photodynamic therapy for lung cancer. Lasers Surg Med, 2006, 38 (5): 364 – 370.

[51] Kurimoto N, Murayama M, Yoshioka S, et al. Assessment of usefulness of endobronchial ultrasonography in determination of depth of tracheobronchial tumor invasion. Chest, 1999, 115 (6): 1500 – 1506.

[52] Miyazu Y, Miyazawa T, Kurimoto N, et al. Endobronchial ultrasonography in the assessment of centrally located early-stage lung cancer before photodynamic therapy. Am J Respir Crit Care Med, 2002, 165 (6): 832 – 837.

[53] Furukawa K, Okunaka T, Yamamoto H, et al. Effectiveness of photodynamic therapy and Nd-YAG laser treatment for obstructed tracheobronchial malignancies. Diagn Ther Endosc, 1999, 5 (3): 161 – 166.

[54] Moghissi K, Dixon K, Stringer M, et al. The place of bronchoscopic photodynamic therapy in advanced unresectable lung cancer: experience of 100 cases. Eur J Cardiothorac Surg, 1999, 15 (1): 1 – 6.

[55] Minnich DJ, Bryant AS, Dooley A, et al. Photodynamic laser therapy for lesions in the airway. Ann Thorac Surg, 2010, 89 (6): 1744 – 1748. discussion 8 – 9.

[56] Furuse K, Fukuoka M, Kato H, et al. A prospective phase II study on photodynamic therapy with photofrin II for centrally located early-stage lung cancer. The Japan Lung Cancer Photodynamic Therapy Study Group. J Clin Oncol, 1993, 11 (10): 1852 – 1857.

[57] Kato H. Photodynamic therapy for lung cancer review of 19 years' experience. J Photochem Photobiol B, 1998, 42 (2): 96 – 99.

[58] Cortese DA, Edell ES, Kinsey JH. Photodynamic therapy for early stage squamous cell carcinoma of the lung. Mayo Clin Proc, 1997, 72 (7): 595 – 602.

[59] Hayata Y, Kato H, Furuse K, et al. Photodynamic therapy of 168 early stage cancers of the lung and oesophagus: A Japanese multi-centre study. Lasers in Medical Science, 1996, 11: 255 – 259.

[60] McCaughan JS, Jr., Williams TE. Photodynamic therapy for endobronchial malignant disease: A prospective fourteen-year study. J Thorac Cardiovasc Surg, 1997, 114 (6): 940 – 946; discussion 6 – 7.

[61] Henschke UK, Hilaris BS, Mahan GD. Remote afterloading with intracavitary applicators. Radiology, 1964, 83: 344 – 345.

[62] Ung YC, Yu E, Falkson C, Haynes AE, et al. The role of high-dose-rate brachytherapy in the palliation of symptoms in patients with non-small-cell lung cancer: A systematic review. Brachytherapy, 2006, 5 (3): 189 – 202.

[63] Kelly JF, Delclos ME, Morice RC, et al. High-dose-rate endobronchial brachytherapy effectively palliates symptoms due to airway tumors: The 10-year M. D. Anderson cancer center experience. Int J Radiat Oncol Biol Phys, 2000, 48 (3): 697 – 702.

[64] Escobar-Sacristan JA, Granda-Orive JI, Gutierrez Jimenez T, et al. Endobronchial brachytherapy in the treatment of malignant lung tumours. Eur Respir J, 2004, 24 (3): 348 – 352.

[65] Paradelo JC, Waxman MJ, Throne BJ, et al. Endobronchial irradiation with 192Ir in the treatment of malignant endobronchial obstruction. Chest, 1992, 102 (4): 1072-1074.

[66] Gollins SW, Burt PA, Barber PV, et al. High dose rate intraluminal radiotherapy for carcinoma of the bronchus: Outcome of treatment of 406 patients. Radiother Oncol, 1994, 33 (1): 31-40.

[67] Langendijk H, de Jong J, Tjwa M, et al. External irradiation versus external irradiation plus endobronchial brachytherapy in inoperable non-small cell lung cancer: A prospective randomized study. Radiother Oncol, 2001, 58 (3): 257-268.

[68] Aumont-le Guilcher M, Prevost B, Sunyach MP, et al. High-doserate brachytherapy for non-small-cell lung carcinoma: A retrospective study of 226 patients. Int J Radiat Oncol Biol Phys, 2011, 79 (4): 1112-1116.

[69] Marsiglia H, Baldeyrou P, Lartigau E, et al. High-doserate brachytherapy as sole modality for early-stage endobronchial carcinoma. Int J Radiat Oncol Biol Phys, 2000, 47 (3): 665-672.

[70] Speiser BL. Brachytherapy in the treatment of thoracic tumors. Lung and esophageal. Hematol Oncol Clin North Am, 1999, 13 (3): 609-634.

第 17 章
原发性气管肿瘤

Francesco Sammartino[1], *Paolo Macchiarini*[2]
1. Department of General and Mininvasive Surgery, San Giovanni di Dio Hospital, Orbetello, Italy
2. Division Ear, Nose and Throat (CLINTEC), Karolinska University Hospital, Stockholm, Sweden

流行病学

由于发病率极低,很少有关于原发性气管肿瘤的流行病学报道。原发性气管肿瘤约占上呼吸道肿瘤的2%,占所有恶性疾病的0.1%~0.4%。气管肿瘤每年的发病率为2.7/1 000 000,占儿童新发肿瘤病例的8%[1-2]。成人90%的原发性气管肿瘤是恶性的,而在儿童恶性概率为30%[3-4]。

解剖和生理

为了减小气管手术的难度,必须明确上呼吸道的解剖和生理。从环状软骨到隆突的上缘,成人的气管长11~12cm。气管的远端2/3位于胸腔内,近端1/3在胸腔外的颈部区域,其全长由18~22个C型软骨环构成,每厘米大约2个软骨环[5]。气管的直径为1.5~2.5cm,以使气流在通过时不产生湍流或相关杂音。气管的后壁由嵌入气管肌的膜性部分组成,气管肌通过纵形肌和横形肌连接软骨环的两端及软骨间隙。气管的腔内部分覆以特有的气管黏膜,气管黏膜由假复层柱状上皮组成。在上皮的下面是纵行弹力纤维网、血管、淋巴组织、神经及黏液腺。

简单看来气管似乎就是一条单纯的传送气体的管道,但仔细研究起来它有许多功能。由于气管在颈部所处的位置,其侧向的韧性及纵向的弹性可以确保活动及吞咽时食管的扩张;气管具有足够的弹性确保其活动,但是也具有足够的韧性确保在呼吸时的正压及负压循环下避免塌陷;对含有尘粒及有害微生物的外界空气的暴露要求气管具有清洁功能及免疫功能。上述这些功能都由气管和支气管内的黏液腺完成,它们可以产生黏稠的黏液黏附细菌和外来颗粒,然后通过纤毛和咳嗽被运送到咽部清除。

气管的血管由毛细血管构成的网络组成[6]。气管侧面纵向血管的上半部分由甲状腺下动脉的分支供给,而来源于主动脉的支气管动脉为气管的下部及隆突供血。

手术操作时要特别注意气管周围的结构。支配喉内肌的双侧喉返神经沿气管两侧下行。食管沿着气管后壁与其紧密相连并提供毛细血管网。气管的前上部分覆以甲状腺并与双侧颈动脉关系密切。气管的下段首先与头臂干(又称无名动脉)交叉,然后与左侧头臂静脉交叉。在气管远端1/3处的前方有主动脉弓、上腔静脉及肺动脉绕行[3]。

在气管前、气管旁及隆突下多可见淋巴结。淋巴液的引流途径与肺癌相似,通常引流至离肿瘤最近的淋巴结[7]。

气管肿瘤的症状

因为诊断比较困难,大多数原发性恶性气管肿瘤患者在就诊时已到晚期或已不能手术。良性和恶性气管肿瘤最初的症状和体征通常是相同的,常见症状是干咳和喉部刺激感。随着病变在气管管腔内的生长,可能会出现气喘或喘鸣,经常被误诊为哮喘。症状和体征随肿瘤类型而不同,但与肿瘤部位无关[9-10]。鳞癌可以导致大量咯血,通常可以早期诊断[11];不足25%的腺样囊性癌患者会在其临床病程中出现咯血[2,8]。吞咽困难、声音嘶哑及声音的变化是疾病的进展期症状，但并不妨碍手术切除。这些症状的非特异度导致从出现症状到最后的诊断之间的间隔延长（最长达18个月），这时绝大多数患者已经处于疾病晚期。相比之下，鳞癌从出现症状到诊断的平均间隔时间仅为4个月。腺样囊性癌多通过气喘或喘鸣症状被发现，但是最突出的症状是呼吸困难。吞咽困难、声音嘶哑及声音改变的发生多是由直接浸润累及食管或喉返神经所导致。

诊断的延迟也归咎于气管管腔的功能储备，因为直到肿瘤堵塞管腔直径的50%~70%时才会出现症状。气喘常被错误地诊断为哮喘，它首先导致COPD或支气管炎。初始对抗生素治疗反应较好的患者经常伴有反复发作的单侧或双侧肺炎。原发性气管恶性肿瘤的症状总结见表17.1。

诊断和分期

气管镜是最重要和最常用的诊断工具。气管镜可以快速简便地获得一些关键信息，如为了手术设计需要获知气管和肿瘤的直径及位置，气管镜还可以为鉴别肿瘤获取活检组织（图17.1）。荧光支气管镜可以区分正常（绿色荧光）和非正常（棕色和红色）黏膜区域。自发荧光的缺失发生在异型增生、原位癌和浸润性癌，并且可以由此在早期发现支气管内肿瘤。

气管内超声检查（endotracheal ultrasonography，EU）涉及一个水囊遮盖的放射状探针或线型探针，前者可以提供超出气管和支气管壁结构的360°的视野，后者可以提供气管壁内或气管外远达4~5cm结构的纵向视野。EU可以显示气管壁的分层结构，并且可以精确地预测肿瘤的浸润情况。系统的纵隔评估对气管肿瘤患者也是必不可少的，EU可以提供关于纵隔和肺门淋巴结转移有价值的信息。如果细胞学为恶性，则对每个淋巴结采样1~3次，如果细胞学为良性或未获得诊断，则采样3次。采样超过3次通常不会确保获得可靠的病理诊断结果[12]。新的集成支气管镜具有线性排列的超声探头，可以对直径<5mm的纵隔淋巴结进行极为准确的评估，并可以在影像引导下进行细针穿刺活检。

螺旋CT扫描是影像学评估气管肿瘤时最常用的方法，因为憋一口气就可以快速获得整个胸腔的容积数据，使呼吸和心脏的运动伪影最小化。这些数据可以通过后续处理技术进行重建，使气管在轴位图像上变得直观。轴位图像可以评估气管的大小和形状，并且可以测量气管壁的厚度。气管邻近结构及外界压迫的存在可以被清晰地界定，尤其静脉造影增强以后格外明显。

冠状位和矢状位斜位多平面重建（coronal and sagittal oblique multiplanar reformats，MPRs）可以准确地判断气管病变的部位（离声带和隆突的距离）和长度、病变与解剖性标志物的关系、管腔狭窄的程度以及管腔外病变组织的生长。MPRs同样可以发现多灶性病变，在诊断的同时避免使1/3的患者接受不必要的手术治疗。二维和三维技术改进了气管肿瘤的手术设计以及治疗后的评估，创建了外部（CT支气管造影）和内部（虚拟支气管镜）CT扫描重建[13-14]。新的雾化造影剂或光谱技术的发展可以辨别良性和恶性黏膜组织，增强了虚拟支气管镜发现气道内侵袭前肿瘤的灵敏度和特异度。动脉CT成像可以在吸气和呼气时进行操作以便于发现气管软化患者气管直径的变化[15-16]。

MRI可用于评估经常因血管发育异常导致气管狭窄的小儿患者以及需要考虑放射剂量的患者[17]。氟代脱氧葡萄糖PET或CT成像既可以评估肿瘤的代谢活性，也可以评估其外侵范围及治疗后可能的复发，但在气管肿瘤中还没有得到广泛研究[18]。常规胸片会延迟疾病的确诊，因为气管肿瘤在胸片上看起来是正常的而经常被漏诊，使得胸片在追踪气管肿瘤时显得作用不大。

表17.1 原发性气管恶性肿瘤的症状及体征

气喘
喘鸣
呼吸困难
声音嘶哑
声音改变
咯血
吞咽困难
肺炎

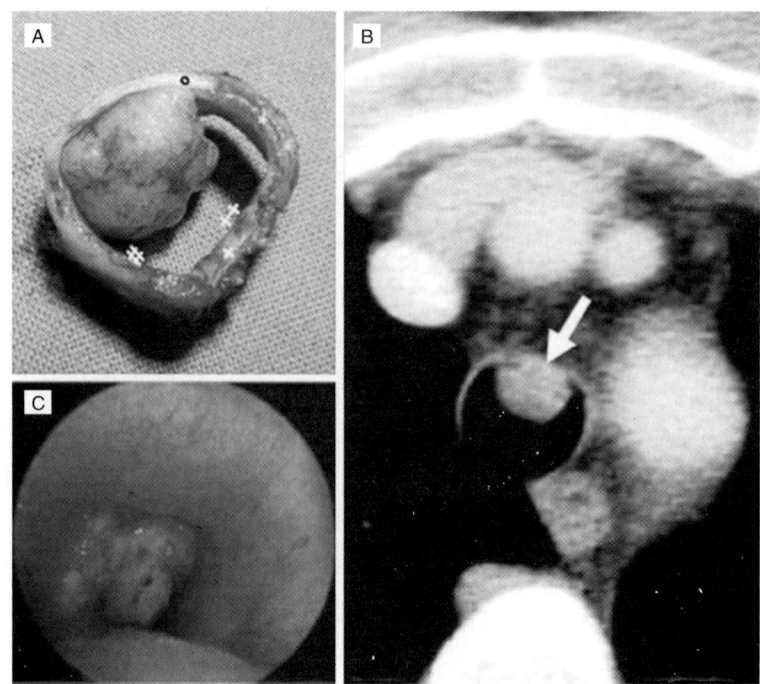

图 17.1 A. 气管肿瘤横截面。＊：黏膜下层，o：C 型软骨环，＋：气管膜部，＋＋：气管肌。B. CT 扫描显示气管前壁可见明显的肿瘤，白色箭头所示为肿瘤。C. 气管镜可见气管腔内肿瘤堵塞管腔

肿瘤的病理及分类

在原发性气管肿瘤中，恶性肿瘤在成人和儿童中的比例分别为 90% 和 30%[3-4,19]，起源于呼吸道上皮（上皮起源）、唾液腺（腺样起源）或间质结构（间质起源）。鳞癌和腺样囊性癌约占成人原发性气管肿瘤的 2/3，二者所占的比例相同。剩余的 1/3 由许多其他类型的肿瘤组成，大多是良性或低度恶性肿瘤如血管瘤、平滑肌瘤以及其他类型的肿瘤。所有原发性气管肿瘤的完整列表见表 17.2。

黑色素瘤、肾癌、乳腺癌及结肠癌通过血行转移到气管极为罕见。气管肿瘤血行转移到其他部位也少有发生，因为气管的血供比较单一，但是发生转移者多见于鳞癌。

气管鳞癌的生物学行为、病因、治疗效果与肺鳞癌相似。男性较女性多见（3:1），多发生于 60~80 岁的老年患者，且与吸烟明显相关。肿瘤可以是外生型或溃疡型，可以为多发且散布在较长的一段气管中。肿瘤生长较快，大约 1/3 的患者在诊断的同时已发生纵隔或肺转移，其在 CT 上的典型表现为多倍化、局灶固着病变、导致管腔偏心狭窄或环管壁周围增厚的肿物。

表 17.2 原发性气管肿瘤

上皮起源	
良性	乳头状瘤
	乳头瘤样增生
恶性	原位鳞癌
	鳞状细胞癌
	腺癌
	大细胞未分化癌
	神经内分泌癌
	典型或非典型类癌
	大细胞神经内分泌癌
	小细胞癌
腺体起源	
良性	多形性腺瘤
	黏液腺瘤
	肌上皮瘤
	大嗜酸粒细胞瘤
	其他
恶性	黏液表皮样癌
	腺样囊性癌
	多形性腺瘤癌变
间叶细胞起源	
良性	纤维瘤
	纤维瘤病
	良性纤维组织细胞瘤
	血管瘤

(续表 17.2)

	血管外皮细胞瘤
	副神经节瘤（化学感受组织瘤）
	管球瘤
	脂肪瘤
	平滑肌瘤
	颗粒细胞瘤
	施万细胞瘤
	软骨瘤
	成软骨细胞瘤
恶性	软组织肉瘤
	软骨肉瘤
	恶性淋巴瘤
	其他

来源：Macchiarini 2006[20]。经 Elsevier 许可使用

相反，腺样囊性癌在男性和女性中的发病率相同，多发生在 20~69 岁的患者，在 50~60 岁患者中的发病率稍高。它的进展相当缓慢，临床症状常为慢性过程，有时达数年。肿瘤常沿神经周围或黏膜下长距离扩散，仅有 10% 的患者发生区域淋巴结或远处转移。鉴于腺样囊性癌病程较长，其完整的临床定义无疑需要一个漫长的观察过程。肿瘤在 CT 上通常表现为一个腔内肿物或外形光滑的环周管壁增厚。在手术切除前，可以应用冠状 2D MPRs 及 3D CT 准确评估病变的长度。肿瘤的 F-FDG PET 摄取各不相同，与其分化程度有关。

在儿童，气管肿瘤发生在新生儿与 14 岁儿童之间，多位于颈段器官的后壁[4]。一些继发性肿瘤也可以累及气管，如喉、甲状腺、肺及食管，这时多建议姑息治疗。

由于气管肿瘤较为罕见，迄今为止仅有 2 项关于 TNM 分期分类的意见。Bhattacharyya N 在 2004 年提出了一项较为简便的 TNM 分类方法，紧接着 Macchiarini P 在 2006 年提出了一项更为广泛应用的 TNM 分期分类方法[20]。这些分类对预后和生存的影响有待临床进一步验证。表 17.3A 和 17.3B 列出了气管肿瘤的 TNM 分期分类。

表 17.3A TNM 分期

肿瘤分期	
Tx	无法评估
Tis	非浸润性肿瘤
T1a	<3cm 局限于黏膜
T1b	<3cm 局限于黏膜
T2*	任何肿瘤侵犯软骨或外膜
T3	任何肿瘤侵犯气管或喉
T4a	任何肿瘤侵犯隆突或主支气管
T4b	任何肿瘤侵犯邻近结构
淋巴结分期	
Nx	区域淋巴结无法评估
N0	无淋巴结转移证据
N1	局部淋巴结阳性（N1a<3cm；N1b<3cm）
上 1/3	纵隔最高淋巴结；上气管旁淋巴结；血管前及气管后淋巴结
中 1/3	上气管旁淋巴结；血管前及气管后淋巴结；下气管旁淋巴结；主动脉旁淋巴结（升主动脉或膈神经）
下 1/3	下气管旁淋巴结；血管前及气管后淋巴结；主动脉下淋巴结（主肺动脉窗）
N1A	上 1/3 1~3 个淋巴结阳性
N1B	上 1/3 <3 个淋巴结阳性
N2	区域淋巴结阳性
上 1/3	下气管旁淋巴结；主动脉下淋巴结（主肺动脉窗）
中 1/3	纵隔最高淋巴结；主动脉下淋巴结（主肺动脉窗）
下 1/3	上气管旁淋巴结；肺韧带淋巴结

(续表 17.3A)

转移		
	Mx	远处转移无法评估
	M0	无远处转移
	M1	N1、N2 之外的淋巴结转移
	M2	远处转移（例如：肺）

* 肿瘤侵犯部分膜部被认定至少为 T2，不考虑浸润深度
来源：Macchiarini[20]。经 Elsevier 许可使用

表 17.3B　分期系统（N：淋巴结分期；M：转移分期；T：肿瘤分期）

分期	T	N	M
0	Tis	N0	M0
Ⅰa	T1a	N0	M0
Ⅰb	T1b~2	N0	M0
Ⅱa	T1b~2	N1	M0
Ⅱb	T1b~2	N2	M0
Ⅲa	T3	N0	M0
Ⅲb	T3	N1~2	M0
Ⅳa	Any	N1~2	M1
Ⅳb	Any	N1~2	M0

来源：Macchiarini[20]。经 Elsevier 许可使用

治 疗

由于气管肿瘤较罕见，因此对患者进行治疗时没有明确的标准。气管切除并一期重建作为标准的手术治疗方法，应考虑用于良性肿瘤和局部恶性肿瘤的治疗。有的患者虽然肿瘤可以切除，但接受了姑息手术，如气管内支架植入、清创术或短距离放射疗法[21]，缩短了患者的预期寿命。治疗气管肿瘤最初的挑战来自气管切除，但其较低的发病率很难激励人们来系统性地面对这一问题。试验方面及临床方面的气管肿瘤治疗可以追溯到 19 世纪晚期，人们尝试了不同的治疗方法。原发性良性和恶性肿瘤可以通过开放手术或内镜切除以及放疗得到治疗。然而对于所有的良性及低级别恶性肿瘤来说，手术切除更安全有效，应该作为治疗的金标准。手术切除可以使患者永久解除气道狭窄以获得长期生存，并可以完整切除肿瘤以获得明确的病理诊断[22-23]和分期。

接受气管切除手术患者的生存可以得到改善，说明手术是最合适的治疗选择。并发症、年龄、一般状况、先前的治疗措施、组织学和肿瘤外侵等可能是限制患者手术切除适应证的因素，对这些患者在接受手术切除时应当慎重考虑。经过仔细挑选的手术患者的死亡率为 5%。为确保安全成功地完成一期重建，必须保留足够长的患者自身气管及充分的吻合口血供[3]。

关于上段气管肿瘤的治疗，喉、气管、隆突或肺切除的一些手术技巧都已经被报道过。气管切除的绝对禁忌证包括：出现阳性淋巴结；侵犯纵隔内不能切除的器官；纵隔接受过最大剂量超过 60Gy 的放疗或既往曾行手术治疗；鳞状细胞癌发生远处转移[3,8,23]。对于这些患者而言，激光手术外加支架植入可以延缓肿瘤的进程，但仅仅是一种姑息治疗方式。气管切除禁忌证的总结见表 17.4。

为了分期及评估气管肿瘤外侵的范围，必须行彻底的淋巴结清扫，注意避免损伤气管周围的血供。

对于不可切除的病变或者复发病变，短距离放射治疗可以作为肿瘤不完全切除术后的辅助治疗，可以减轻严重的症状。气管内清创术和支架植入可以被用于治疗不能行手术治疗的肿瘤或者保持气道开放缓解症状，直到可以进行进一步的治疗。

表 17.4　手术切除禁忌证

成人气管受累长度超过气管长度的 1/2
儿童气管受累长度超过气管长度的 1/3
纵隔淋巴结转移或全身转移
不可切除器官的纵隔侵犯
纵隔接受过 >60Gy 的放疗
鳞癌远处转移

当需要对气道狭窄的患者进行紧急治疗保持气道通畅时,建议行挽救性内镜下减瘤手术。任何妨碍进一步手术切除的治疗方法都应当尽量避免(如支架植入和气管造瘘术)。

如果怀疑病变侵犯食管,建议行食管镜检查和食管内镜超声检查。如果症状提示骨或脑转移,应当分别行骨扫描或头颅 MRI 检查。

关于继发性气管肿瘤,切除和重建的基本原理应遵循肿瘤学原则。对于技术比较熟练的外科医生而言,其手术风险并不高,手术也并不显得激进。

多年来,姑息手术一直是甲状腺癌侵犯气管患者最常见的手术方式。考虑到乳头状癌最后变得更具有侵袭性这一特性,削除术并不合适。完整切除,必要时切除范围包括气管和食管,似乎是侵袭性甲状腺癌唯一的根治性治疗方法。对表浅浸润患者,推荐气管重建经验并不丰富的外科医生使用削除术;对深部浸润患者,则推荐窗式切除术。然而,气管切除并行一期重建是这些患者目前的治疗方式,并显现出长期生存的改善。

手 术

所有的气管切除手术都需要对患者进行全身麻醉。气道控制至关重要,不能随意进行气管插管。维持气管插管超出狭窄部分可以避免呼吸骤停。

气道通气可以通过气管内插管伸入手术野并在气管横断后跨过狭窄部分来实现。另外可以通过周期性呼吸暂停进行 JET 通气或过度换气来实现气管内通气。在这方面,肺辅助装置(Lung assist devices iLA)可以作为一种替代选择在手术过程中清除 CO_2。在极端情况下,插管之前或插管过程中需要建立体外膜肺氧合(extracorporeal membrane oxygenation,ECMO),但是对于肺功能处于临界状态的患者,可以考虑应用最近出现的如静脉-静脉 ECMO 等技术。肿瘤的纵向延伸在成人达到一半,在婴儿或儿童达到 1/3 是手术的绝对禁忌证,因为此时残留气管的长度不足以进行一期重建。无论如何,必须在任何局部或全身治疗开始前考虑是否可以手术切除。最近,组织工程气管替代这项新技术为包括癌症在内的患有较长气管病变的患者提供了一种新的临床选择[24-25]。

技术:对于位于颈段或胸内气管最上段的肿瘤,通常采用颈领样切口联合胸骨小切口或全胸骨切口。牵拉开无名动脉、上腔静脉、无名静脉以及肺动脉,暴露远端气管。必须直接在气管上进行解剖游离,局限于狭窄部分,距离病变上下缘不超过 1~2cm 的正常气管,以便保留两侧的节段性血供。颈段气管可以通过低领状切口或领状切口联合胸骨上端部分切口得到暴露。如果存在气管造口,则并入领状切口或分别闭合。游离甲状腺峡部,在气管两侧暴露开。先在狭窄处下方正常气管处游离气管,紧贴气管后方游离出食管。在整个气管手术过程中,必须小心谨慎地游离两侧的喉返神经。此外,不能让血液灌入气管远端开口,一旦发生血液溢出,必须立即清理气道。接下来游离近端气管,当肿瘤的狭窄部分被去除后,经过手术野将交叉区域通气装置放入远端气管。在绝大多数患者,颈部向隆突屈曲及前伸可以保证颈段气管的无张力吻合。如果需要额外增加长度,可以采用 Montgomery 技术进行舌骨上肌喉松解并在术后大约 1 周保持颈部屈曲。为了使患者在术后保持连续的颈部屈曲,需要缝合或佩戴颈托以确保患者不会突然屈曲颈部。对位于气管下段的肿瘤,需行胸骨正中切口或较高位右后外侧开胸切口。一开始需游离奇静脉暴露隆突。游离出远端气管和左右主支气管。纤维支气管镜通过口腔气管插管可以引导切口进入远端气管。不管肿瘤位置如何,气道的重建技术是相同的。如果我们认为存在额外的吻合口张力,松解技术可用来帮助减小吻合口张力。通过解剖肺门环周的心包来游离肺韧带和松解肺门可以为远端气道提供 1~2cm 的额外活动度。舌骨上肌松解同样可以为隆突切除手术增加额外的长度。一旦做出了气道可以重建的决定,气管前非膜性部分需要行个体化环周吻合缝合,气管后膜性部分需要行连续缝合(成人用 4-0Vicryl 线,儿童用 5-0Vicryl 线;图 17.2)。所有的缝合都要求线结打在吻合口的外面。一旦后排连续缝合线结打紧,颈部即屈曲,术野内气管插管被移除,口内气管插管继续前插超过吻合口至左主支气管。然后打紧前排缝合线结,气管内插管向外退出至吻合口近端气管。当所有线结打紧后,必须检查吻合口是否密封良

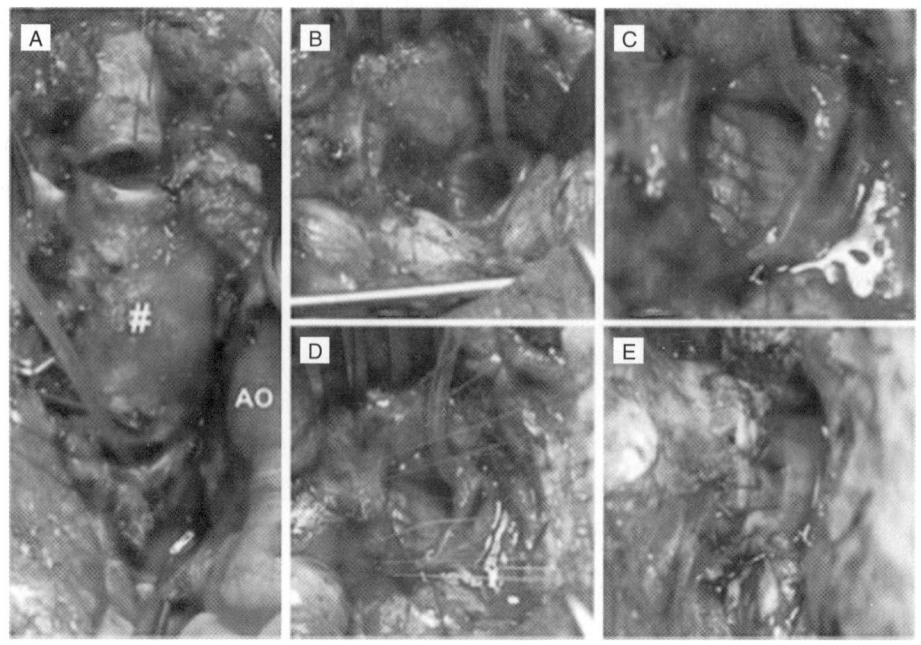

图 17.2（见彩插） A. 正面观：牵拉开主动脉（AO）后，胸腔内中段、远段气管。#：受肿瘤侵犯，需要切除的部分气管。B. 侧面观：切除肿瘤后，气管后壁行连续缝合。C. 收紧连续缝合线。D. 气管前壁间断缝合（7×缝线）。E. 收紧缝合线，吻合气管

好。麻醉医生给予患者 20cmH_2O、30cmH_2O 和 40cmH_2O（注：1cmH_2O = 0.098kPa）的通气压力。将手术野浸泡在生理盐水中以检查漏气情况。任何漏口都必须修补，如果漏口无法修补，甚至需要拆除整个吻合口重新吻合。一旦吻合口确认没有问题，需要用心包脂肪、胸膜或肋间肌的带蒂皮瓣遮盖吻合口。拔管前需要用气管镜检查吻合口。同样需要指出的是，在完成吻合之前需要送冰冻病理确保气管肿瘤已被完整切除。常建议行根治性淋巴结清扫术。气管切除术后会发生一些术后并发症，如吻合口裂开、吻合口肉芽组织形成、吞咽时误吸继而发生肺炎、喉返神经麻痹、气管-无名动脉漏、呼吸机辅助呼吸 >48h 以及可能需要气管切开。除肺功能障碍外，常见的并发症如切口感染或出血也可能发生。

预后情况

文献报道气管鳞癌患者的 5 年生存率约为 5%。手术联合放疗使腺样囊性癌的 5 年生存率有所提高，但因为局部复发和远处转移，10 年及以上的生存率持续降低。

总 结

气管原发性肿瘤较为罕见，由于其临床表现不具有特异性，通常在诊断时已处于晚期。但是对于经过高度选择的患者，可以行手术切除并重新吻合，联合辅助或新辅助治疗措施（取决于肿瘤类型），这些方法可能会使患者治愈。对于进展期气管肿瘤患者，治疗的选择尚有限，但是最新的进展带来了希望。气管肿瘤患者的治疗必须由多学科团队做出决定，包括诊断方法、分期、特殊的随访策略及详细的治疗方案。

（王 晖 王晓航 译）

参考文献

[1] Manninen MP, Antila PJ, Pukander JS, et al. Occurrence of tracheal carcinoma in Finland. Acta Otolaryngol, 1991, 111: 1162 – 1169.

[2] Bhattacharyya N. Contemporary staging and prognosis for primary tracheal malignancies: A population-based analysis. Otolaryngol Head Neck Surg, 2004, 131: 639 – 642.

[3] Grillo HC. Surgery of the trachea and bronchi//Grillo HC. Surgery of the Trachea and Bronchi. London: Hamilton, 2004: 208-247.

[4] Desai DP, Holinger LD, Gonzalez-Crussi F. Tracheal neoplasms in children. Ann Otol Rhinol Laryngol, 1998, 7: 790-796.

[5] Grillo HC, Dignan EF, Miura T. Extensive resection and reconstruction of mediastinal trachea without prosthesis or graft: an antomical study in man. J Thorac Cardiovasc Surg, 1964, 48: 741-749.

[6] Gelder CM, Hetzel MR. Primary tracheal tumours: A national survey. Thorax, 1993, 48: 688-692.

[7] Salassa JR, Pearson BW, Payne WS. Gross and microscopical blood supply of the trachea. Annals of Thoracic Surgery, 1977, 24: 100-107.

[8] Gaissert HA, Grillo HC, Shadmehr MB, et al. Long-term survival after resection of primary adenoid cystic and squamous cell carcinoma of the trachea and carina. Ann Thorac Surg, 2004, 78: 1889-1896.

[9] Hollingsworth HM. Wheezing and stridor. Clin Chest Med, 1987, 8: 231-240.

[10] Geffin B, Grillo HC, Cooper JD, et al. Stenosis following tracheostomy for respiratory care. JAMA, 1971, 216: 1984-1988.

[11] Gaissert HA. Primary tracheal tumors. Chest Surg Clin N Am, 2003, 13: 247-256.

[12] Andrade RS. Relevance of endobronchial ultrasonography to thoracic surgeons. Semin Thorac Cardiovasc Surg, 2010, 22: 150-154.

[13] LoCicero J, Costello P, Campos CT, et al. Spiral CT with multiplanar and three-dimensional reconstructions accurately predicts tracheobronchial pathology. Ann Thorac Surg, 1996, 62: 818-822.

[14] Remy-Jardin M, Remy J, Artaud D, et al. Volume rendering of the tracheobronchial tree: clinical evaluation of bronchographic images. Radiology, 1998, 208: 761-770.

[15] Gilkeson RC, Ciancibello LM, Hejal RB, et al. Tracheobronchomalacia: Dynamic airway evaluation with multidetector CT. AJR Am J Roentgenol, 2001, 176: 205-210.

[16] Zhang J, Hasegawa I, Hatabu H, et al. Frequency and severity of air trapping at dynamic expiratory CT in patients with tracheobronchomalacia. AJR Am J Roentgenol, 2004, 182: 81-85.

[17] Yedururi S, Guillerman RP, Chung T, et al. Multimodality imaging of tracheobronchial disorders in children. Radiographics, 2008, 28: e29.

[18] Lee EY, Litmanovich D, Boiselle PM. Multidetector CT evaluation of tracheobronchomalacia. Radiol Clin North Am, 2009, 47: 261-269.

[19] Gilbert JG, Kaufman B, Mazzarella LA. Tracheal tumors in infants and children. J Pediatr, 1949, 35: 63-69.

[20] Macchiarini P. Primary tracheal tumours. Lancet Oncol, 2006, 7: 83-91.

[21] Grillo HC. Primary tracheal tumours. Thorax, 1993, 48: 681-682.

[22] Grillo HC. Tracheal replacement: A critical review. Ann Thorac Surg, 2002, 73: 1995-2004.

[23] Mathisen DJ. Tracheal tumors. Chest Surg Clin N Am, 1996, 6: 875-898.

[24] Macchiarini P, Jungebluth P, Go T, et al. Clinical transplantation of a tissue-engineered airway. Lancet, 2008, 372: 2023-2030.

[25] Jungebluth P, Alici E, Baiguera S, et al. Tracheobronchial transplantation with a stem-cell-seeded bioartificial nanocomposite: A proof-of-concept study. Lancet, 2011, 378: 1997-2004.

第18章
肺癌手术后的辅助化疗

Kathryn A. Gold

Department of Thoracic/Head and Neck Medical Oncology, The University of Texas MD Anderson Cancer Center, Houston, TX, USA

引 言

手术切除是早期非小细胞肺癌（NSCLC）的标准治疗方式，但术后5年生存率仍不尽如人意：从ⅠA期的63%到ⅢA期的仅19%[1]。术后，10%~15%的患者出现局部复发，15%~60%发生远处转移，最终导致患者死亡。为了提高术后患者的局部及远处控制率和生存期，化疗和（或）放疗作为辅助治疗手段被应用并进行了大量研究。

尽管一些研究表明，术后辅助放疗能够提高局部控制率[2]，但大量的meta分析显示患者的生存期无明显改善[3]。因此对存在纵隔淋巴结受累或切缘阳性等局部复发高危风险因素的患者，术后放疗具有指征，但不常规应用于N0或N1期。

远处高转移率通常归因于手术时已存在无法识别的微转移灶，因此通过控制亚临床前的微转移病灶，理论上术后辅助化疗能够降低远处复发转移风险。对于包括乳腺癌和结肠癌在内的许多恶性肿瘤，辅助化疗已成为术后的标准治疗方法[4-5]，并在NSCLC中进行了广泛的探索研究。

辅助化疗的临床试验

在NSCLC辅助化疗的早期临床试验中，术后应用环磷酰胺或氮芥等烷化剂并未提高患者的生存期[6]。在后续的随机试验中，基于顺铂的术后辅助化疗亦未证实显著的临床获益[6]。对于上述试验研究，1995年的一篇meta分析进行了报道[6]，在8项研究中顺铂与多柔比星、环磷酰胺和长春地辛组合成多种方案，顺铂的剂量范围为$50 \sim 240 mg/m^2$，总的风险比（HR）为0.87（$P = 0.08$），化疗使死亡风险降低13%。该研究还显示化疗组2年及5年的绝对生存获益分别为3%（95%CI，0.5%的损害至7%的受益）和5%（95%CI，1%的损害至10%的受益）。这些结果尽管未达到统计学意义，但促使更多团队参与到基于顺铂的辅助化疗研究中。表18.1和18.2对这些研究进行了概括总结。

表18.1　近期以铂类为基础的辅助化疗随机试验汇总

试验	例数	分期	化疗方案	放射治疗	死亡风险比（95% CI）	P
ALPI[8]	1209	Ⅰ~ⅢA	MVP	可选择的	0.96（0.81，1.13）	0.589
IALT[9]	1867	Ⅰ~ⅢA	以顺铂为基础*	可选择的	0.89（0.76，0.98）	0.030
Big lung trial[11]	381	Ⅰ~ⅢA	以顺铂为基础*	可选择的	1.02（0.77，1.35）	0.900
JBR.10[12]	482	ⅠB~Ⅱ	顺铂+长春瑞滨	无	0.69（0.52，0.91）	0.040
ANITA[14]	840	ⅠB~ⅢA	顺铂+长春瑞滨	可选择的	0.80（0.66，0.96）	0.017
CALGB[15]	344	ⅠB	卡铂+紫杉醇	无	0.83（0.64，1.08）	0.120

＊研究者在几个方案之间进行选择：MVP、丝裂霉素、长春地辛、顺铂

表 18.2　在辅助化疗试验中常用的方案

试验	化疗方案 顺铂	化疗方案 其他	周期	依从性
ALPI[8]	100mg/m², d1	丝裂霉素 8mg/m² d1 和长春地辛 3mg/m² d1, d8	3d, 21d 为一个周期	69% 接受了 3 个周期
IALT[9]	80~120 mg/m², d1	长春地辛 3mg/m² wkly* 或长春花碱 4mg/m² wkly* 或长春瑞滨 30mg/m² wkly 或依托泊苷 100mg/m² d1, d2, d3	4d, 21d 为一个周期或 3d, 28d 为一个周期或 4d, 28d 为一个周期	74% 接受了 ≥ 240mg/m² 的顺铂
Big lung trial[11]	50~80mg/m², d1	丝裂霉素 6mg/m², 异环磷酰胺 3g/m², d1 或丝裂霉素 6mg/m², 长春花碱 6mg/m², d1 或长春地辛 3mg/m², d1, d8 或长春瑞滨 30mg/m², d1, d8	3d, 21d 为一个周期	64% 接受了 3 个周期化疗
JBR.10[12]	50mg/m², d1, d8	长春瑞滨 25mg/m², 每周 1 次	4d, 28d 为一个周期	58% 接受了至少 3 个周期化疗
ANITA[14]	100mg/m², d1	长春瑞滨 25mg/m², 每周一次	4d, 28d 为一个周期	50% 接受了所有 4 个周期化疗
CALGB[15]	无	卡铂 AUC6 和紫杉醇 200mg/m²	4d, 21d 为一个周期	86% 接受了所有 4 个周期化疗

*逐周调整的计划表：每周 1 次 ×4 周，之后每 2 周 1 次

日本临床肿瘤组织的 9304 试验

日本临床肿瘤组织（Japan Clinical Oncology Group, JCOG）9304 试验针对同侧纵隔淋巴结受累、手术完全切除的 NSCLC 患者，该研究的目标为 3 个周期的顺铂联合长春地辛的辅助化疗是否优于观察组[7]，受试人群于术后 6 周内开始化疗，具体用药方案为顺铂 80mg/m² 第 1 天 + 长春地辛 3mg/m² 第 1、8 天，每 4 周为 1 个周期，而术后放疗不予考虑。患者的入选标准为年龄 <75 岁、PS 评分 0~1 分、既往未经化疗或放疗者。治疗中心对患者进行了分层，以使两组之间达到良好的平衡，因为缓慢的入组率，该试验因未达到计划样本数而被终止。从 1994 年 1 月至 1998 年 7 月，共 119 例患者被随机分配到化疗组（59 例）和单纯手术组（60 例），58% 的患者完成了预期剂量的化疗，两组间的总生存期（overall survival, OS）和无病生存期（disease-free survival, DFS）无显著统计学差异，两组的中位生存时间为 36 个月，化疗组和对照组的 5 年生存率分别为 28% 和 36%（$P=0.89$），中位 DFS 则分别为 18 个月和 16 个月（$P=0.66$）。

意大利的辅助化疗项目（ALPI）

来自于意大利的辅助化疗项目（Adjuvant Lung Project Italy，ALPI）和欧洲癌症研究和治疗组织（the European Organization for Reasearch and Treatment of Cancer, EORTC）的研究者，将手术完全切除的Ⅰ、Ⅱ、ⅢA 期 NSCLC 患者，随机分配到 MVP 组（丝裂霉素 8mg/m² 第 1 天 + 长春地辛 3mg/m² 第 1、8 天 + 顺铂 80mg/m² 第 1 天，每 3 周为 1 个周期，连用 3 个周期）和观察组[8]。治疗于术后 42d 内启动，根据肿瘤近中心与否、大小、淋巴结受累数以及是否意图行放疗，对患者进行了分层。患者的放疗取决于每个参与中心的治疗策略并先于首个患者入组前决定。对于 MVP

组,患者的放疗于最后一次化疗结束后3~5周开始,而对照组的放疗于术后4~6周开始,主要研究重点为OS,次要研究终点为PFS和辅助化疗的相关毒副作用。该试验设计有80%的功效能够检测到死亡率20%的相对下降(使5年生存率从50%提高至57%),这与0.8的风险比相一致,双侧α值0.05。

从1994年1月至1999年1月该研究纳入1 209例患者,其中MVP组606例,对照组603例。两组间患者保持了良好的均衡:Ⅰ、Ⅱ、ⅢA期占比分别为39%、33%和28%,中位年龄61岁。尽管部分患者降低了药物剂量,MVP组中69%的患者完成了预期的3个周期的化疗。此外65%的MVP患者和82%的对照组患者接受了放射治疗。MVP组中与化疗相关的Ⅲ度或Ⅳ度中性粒细胞减少症发生率分别为16%和12%。研究中与治疗相关的死亡为10例,其中3例发生于化疗组,7例发生于对照组。64.5个月的中期随访显示两组间OS无显著统计学差异[HR = 0.96;95% CI(0.81,1.13);$P = 0.589$],两组间的PFS也未达统计学意义[HR = 0.89;95% CI(0.76,1.03);$P = 0.128$]。MVP组和对照组的中位OS分别为55个月和48个月,多因素分析表明生存期与病情分期、性别相关。K-ras、p53、Ki-67作为潜在的预测或预后标记物,但研究未发现这些生物标记物与患者的OS、DFS间存在明确相关。

国际肺癌辅助治疗试验(IALT)

国际肺癌辅助治疗试验(the International Adjuvant Lung Cancer Trial,IALT)协作组评估了基于顺铂的辅助化疗对完全切除的NSCLC患者生存期的影响[9]。1 867例完全切除的Ⅰ、Ⅱ或Ⅲ期NSCLC患者被随机分配到对照组或化疗组,后者需接受3~4个周期的含顺铂方案的化疗:顺铂($80 \sim 120 mg/m^2$,每3~4周1次)联合长春花生物碱类或依托泊苷(长春地辛$3mg/m^2$,每周1次,连续5周,后每2周1次;长春花碱$4mg/m^2$,每周1次,连续5周,后每2周1次;长春瑞滨$30mg/m^2$,每周1次;或依托泊苷$100mg/m^2$,每周1次)。因为无法确定术后最佳治疗方案和收益,每个参与中心自行确定病例分期、每周期所用顺铂剂量和顺铂联用的药物及术后放射治疗策略。年龄为18~75岁、完全切除的Ⅰ、Ⅱ、Ⅲ期NSCLC患者符合条件,依据治疗中心、手术类型及病例分期,于术后60d内被随机分配、分层入组。化疗于术后60d内开始,如有指征,可行纵隔淋巴结的放射治疗,剂量不超过60Gy。主要研究终点为OS,次要研究终点为DFS、第二原发癌及不良反应。该试验设计的目的是用于证实5%的绝对生存获益,使5年生存率从50%提高至55%。

试验从1995年2月开始注册入组,因进展缓慢筹备指导委员会于2000年12月31终止了试验入组。共有1 867例患者入组并被随机分配,这些患者来自于33个国家的148个中心。两组的试验患者得到了良好的均衡,IA、IB、Ⅱ和Ⅲ期占比分别为10%、27%、24%和39%,中位年龄59岁,女性占20%,40%为腺癌。3~4个周期的顺铂$100mg/m^2$联合依托泊苷是最常用的化疗方案,为49.3%的患者选择应用。化疗组中74%的患者承受了至少$240mg/m^2$剂量的顺铂。27%的患者接受了术后放疗。化疗组中23%的患者出现了3~4度的毒性作用,7例患者死于化疗相关毒副反应。化疗组中7.8%的患者未接受化疗。中位随访时间56个月,化疗组患者的总体生存率明显高于观察组[5年OS:44.5% vs 40.4%;HR = 0.86;95% CI(0.76,0.98);$P < 0.03$],化疗组患者的DFS也显著提高[HR = 0.83;95% CI(0.74,0.94);$P < 0.003$]。化疗组和对照组的中位OS分别为50.8个月和44.4个月,中位DFS分别为40.2个月和30.5个月,5年DFS比率分别为39.4%和34.3%。

在2009年发表的中位随访90个月的更新分析显示:化疗对总生存的获益仍持续存在,但未达统计学意义[HR = 0.91;95% CI(0.81,1.02);$P = 0.1$][10]。在化疗组中,非肺癌相关死亡风险有增加的趋势[HR = 1.34;95% CI(0.99,1.81);$P = 0.06$]。

英国肺癌试验(BLT)

英国肺癌试验(Big Lung Trial,BLT)小组将可手术切除的患者随机分配到基于顺铂的化疗组或对照组[11],术前予以化疗(新辅助化疗)或术后予以化疗可由主治医生自由掌握。临床医生可在下列 4 个化疗方案中选择：MIC（顺铂 50mg/m²、丝裂霉素 6mg/m² 及异环磷酰胺 3g/m²）、MVP（顺铂 50mg/m²、丝裂霉素 6mg/m² 及长春花碱 6mg/m²）、CV（顺铂 80mg/m² 及长春地辛 3mg/m²，第 1、8 天）和 NP（顺铂 80mg/m² 及长春瑞滨 30mg/m²，第 1、8 天），这些方案每 3 周应用 1 次，连用 3 个周期。

该试验的主要研究终点为 OS，这是一项检验力不足的研究——约有 20% 的效能检测到 5% 的生存差异——其目的是有助于一个更新的 meta 分析。共有 381 例患者随机入组，中位年龄 61 岁；其中男性占 69%；48% 为鳞状细胞癌，37% 为腺癌；Ⅰ期、Ⅱ期和Ⅲ期的患者比例分别为 27%、38% 和 34%。大约 95% 的患者达到肉眼完全切除，但 15% 的患者镜下切缘阳性。近 2/3 的化疗组患者按计划完成了 3 个周期的化疗，但这些患者中 40% 需要减量。分配到化疗组中的绝大多数（97%）患者接受了辅助化疗而不是新辅助化疗，只有少部分（14%）患者接受了术后放疗。中位随访 34.6 个月，化疗组的 OS 无显著获益（HR = 1.02；$P = 0.90$），手术联合化疗组和单纯手术组的中位 OS 分别为 33.9 个月和 32.6 个月，中位 PFS 分别为 27 个月和 24.7 个月。

JBR.10 试验

在这项北美组间的试验中，完全切除的 T2N0、T1N1 和 T2N1 期的 NSCLC 患者被随机分配到辅助化疗组和观察组[12]。这项试验由 NCIC CTG 在 1994 年启动，CALGB、SWOG、ECOG 于 1998 年加入。化疗组患者于术后 6 周内开始接受化疗，方案为：长春瑞滨 25mg/m² 每周 1 次，顺铂 50 mg/m² 第 1、8 天，每 4 周为 1 个周期，连用 4 个周期。根据淋巴结（N0 vs N1）和 *RAS* 突变（有、无和未知）状况对患者进行了分层，主要研究终点为 OS，次要研究终点包括无复发生存期、生活质量和毒性反应。

1994—2001 年，482 例患者被随机分配到化疗组（242 例）和观察组（240 例），两组患者均衡性良好，平均年龄为 61 岁。43% 的患者为腺癌，24% 存在 *RAS* 突变（*NRAS*、*KRAS* 或 *HRAS* 的 12、13 和 61 密码子位点）。仅有 45% 的患者能够按计划完成 4 个周期的化疗，7% 的化疗患者出现发热性中性粒细胞减少症，而治疗相关死亡率为 0.8%（2 例）。中位随访超过 5 年后，化疗组的中位 OS 较观察组显著提高（94 个月 vs 73 个月；HR = 0.69；$P = 0.011$），化疗组的无复发生存期也明显延长（未达到 vs 47 个月；HR = 0.6；$P = 0.0003$），两组的 5 年生存率分别为 69% 和 54%（$P = 0.03$）。亚组分析显示：化疗组ⅠB期患者的 OS 无显著改善，而Ⅱ期患者的中位 OS 明显提高（80 个月 vs 41 个月；$P = 0.004$）。在中位随访 9.3 年后，更新后的生存分析表明辅助化疗继续显示生存获益（HR = 0.78；$P = 0.04$），尽管这种收益似乎局限于淋巴结阳性的患者。

诺维本辅助化疗的国际相关研究（ANITA）

在诺维本辅助化疗的国际相关研究（the Adjuvant Navelbine International Trialist's Association，ANITA）试验中，研究者将手术完全切除的ⅠB、Ⅱ或ⅢA期 NSCLC 患者随机分配到化疗组或观察组[14]，入组患者来自于 14 个国家的 101 个研究中心，化疗组患者接受了 16 周的诺维本（30mg/m²，每周 1 次）联合顺铂（100mg/m²，每 4 周 1 次）的治疗方案，术后放疗根据每个中心的治疗策略实施，并推荐用于淋巴结阳性的患者。按照研究中心、分期和病史对患者进行了分层，主要研究终点为 OS，次要研究终点为 DFS 和安全性。该试验设计的目的是拥有 90% 的效力能够检测到 10% 的绝对生存改善，用于证实辅助化疗的得益，双侧 α 值为 0.05，试验计划的每组样本数为 400 例。从 1994 年 12 月至 2000 年 12 月，共有 840 例患者入组：化疗组 407 例，观察组 433 例。在这项研究中患者得到了很好的均衡，其中ⅠB、Ⅱ和ⅢA期占比分别为 36%、24% 和 39%，61% 的患者按计划完成了 3~4 个周期的化疗，化疗相关的Ⅲ~Ⅳ度中性粒细胞减少症发生率为 85%，发热性中性粒细胞减少症发生率为 9%，2% 的患者死于化疗的毒副作用。

两组的中位随访时间均超过 6 年，化疗组和观察组的中位 OS 分别为 65.7 个月和 43.7 个月 [HR = 0.80；95%CI（0.66，0.96）；$P = 0.017$]，化疗组的 5 年绝对生存获益为 8.6%，两组的 DFS 也有显著统计学差异（$P = 0.002$）。在亚组分析中，ⅠB期患者并未从辅助化疗中获益，而Ⅱ期和ⅢA期患者在统计学上有显著生存获益。

癌症和白血病组B-9633试验

在癌症和白血病组（the Cancer and Leukemia Group B，GALGB）9633试验中，完全切除的IB期（T2N0）肺癌患者被随机分配到单纯观察组和化疗组，后者接受4个周期的紫杉醇（200mg/m²）联合卡铂（AUC＝6）方案的辅助化疗[15]。经过34个月的随访后，该试验在2004 ASCO年会上初步显示出积极、肯定的趋势[16]，尽管最终的生存分析为阴性结果。患者于术后8周内开始接受化疗且无胸部放疗计划，试验于1996年9月启动并计划在3.5年内入组500例患者，因入组缓慢及其他试验结果的披露，在入组344例患者后该试验于2003年11月终止。

在年龄、性别、种族、体重下降、民族、组织学、肿瘤分化、手术类型方面，该试验对两组患者进行了良好的平衡。患者对辅助化疗的耐受性良好且无化疗相关死亡发生，35%的患者出现了Ⅲ或Ⅳ度的中性粒细胞减少症。随访74个月后，化疗组和观察组的OS和DFS无显著统计学差异，中位OS分别为95个月和78个月（HR＝0.83；P＝0.124），中位DFS分别为89个月和56个月（HR＝0.80；P＝0.065）。

在非计划的亚组分析中，CALGB的研究者发现肿瘤>4cm患者的OS和DFS获得显著改善，而<4cm患者的上述获益表现为下行趋势。与其他试验相比，该研究采用了卡铂-紫杉醇而非基于顺铂的化疗方案。

辅助化疗试验的汇总分析

在上述研究中，数个试验（ALPI、BLT和CALGB-9633）显示辅助化疗对患者无明显益处，但其他试验（IALT、JBR.10、ANITA）显示辅助化疗可显著改善患者的生存。部分试验如ALPI，采用较老且毒性较大的化疗方案；其他试验如BLT和CALGB-9633，在检验微小生存差异方面凸显势单力薄。因此一些meta分析汇集了单个随机试验数据以期得出更广泛明确的结论。

肺癌的顺铂辅助化疗评价（the Lung Adjuvant Cisplatin Evaluation，LACE）汇总分析了5个基于顺铂的个体随机试验数据（ALPI、IALT、ANITA、BLT和JBR.10）[17]，这些试验都是在1995年的meta分析后进行的[6]，共列入了4584例患者，病理分期囊括了ⅠA至Ⅲ期：ⅠA期8%，ⅠB期29%，Ⅱ期35%，Ⅲ期28%。辅助化疗使死亡风险降低了11%，5年绝对生存获益提高了5.4%，并具有显著的统计学差异（HR＝0.89，P＝0.005）。在前6个月接受化疗的患者死亡风险增加（化疗组74例患者死亡，对照组29例患者死亡），这主要归因于化疗的毒副作用和增多的心血管或肺意外。使用高剂量顺铂（计划剂量＞300mg/m²）有提高获益的趋势，但未达到统计学意义（P＝0.1）。化疗效果与分期有显著的交互作用，尽管人数很少，ⅠA期患者似乎未从化疗中获益[HR＝1.40；95% CI（0.95，2.06）]。ⅠB期患者的辅助化疗获益几乎微不足道[HR＝0.93；95% CI（0.78，1.10）]，但Ⅱ期和Ⅲ期患者的生存率显著提高并具有统计学意义[Ⅱ期HR＝0.83，95% CI（0.70，0.91）；Ⅲ期HR＝0.83，95% CI（0.72，0.94）]。一般状况良好的患者往往从化疗中获益，而处于边缘状况（PS＝2）患者的化疗效用尚不明确。

另一项由NSCLC meta分析协作组完成的大型meta分析包含了34项术后辅助化疗与单纯手术对比的随机试验、13项手术加放疗和化疗与手术加放疗对比的随机试验[18]。这项meta分析总共纳入了11 107例患者，该试验发现化疗使5年的绝对生存获益提高了4%。与LACE meta分析相比，化疗收益与肿瘤分期或一般状况之间无显著的交互作用。

患者对辅助化疗的选择

Ⅱ期和Ⅲ期肺癌

临床试验和meta分析表明，在OS和DFS方面，手术切除的Ⅱ期或Ⅲ期NSCLC患者均能从辅助化疗中获益。5年的绝对生存获益能够提高约5%[17-18]。对于一般状况良好和无禁忌证的患者，术后辅助化疗是标准的治疗方式。

ⅠA期肺癌

BLT、ALPI和IALT是仅有的几项包含ⅠA期患者的基于顺铂的辅助化疗试验[8-9,11]，总共347例该期患者被纳入了这些试验中，这些单个数据已被LACE汇集分析[17]。考虑到一些患者接受了毒性较大、较老的治疗方案，这项meta分析揭示辅助化疗不利于该亚组患者。尽管如此，仍没有明确的证据表明手术切除的NSCLC患者能够从辅助化疗中获益。

IB期肺癌

CALGB-9633是唯一重点针对IB期患者的基于铂类的大型辅助试验[15]。虽然初始结果良好，但最终分析显示患者未能从卡铂和紫杉醇的辅助化疗中获益。许多假说已经提出了针对本研究阴性结果的解释，这包括：与基于顺铂的两种药物方案相比，紫杉醇或卡铂方案活度较低。由于入组被提前终止，该试验缺乏足够的检验效力。在JBR.10和ANITA试验的亚组分析中，尽管统计检验显示化疗收益同疾病分期之间无明确的交互作用，但IB期患者仍未被观察到任何的化疗获益[12,14]。在LACE汇总分析中，辅助化疗曾报道有使患者获益的趋势，但未达到统计学意义[17]。

一项来自于CALGB-9633研究数据的非计划事后分析发现肿瘤直径>4cm能够预测化疗收益[15]，JBR.10研究也发现肿瘤大小和化疗获益间的类似关联。尽管这些亚组分析并未达到统计学意义，但肿瘤直径>4cm的患者往往能从化疗中受益，而肿瘤较小者则不能[13]。在我们机构，对于IB期患者的辅助化疗基于个人的基础情况决定，高风险特征的患者，如肿瘤直径>4cm、低分化、脏层胸膜受侵或血管浸润，建议接受化疗。

老年患者

肺癌患者呈现的中位年龄为70岁[19]，但在临床试验中老年患者的代表性较差。老年患者往往患有较多的并发症，可能难以耐受化疗。在JBR.10试验的亚组分析中，年龄超过65岁的患者在辅助化疗中有类似年轻患者的获益[HR=0.61；95% CI（0.38，098）；$P=0.04$]，尽管他们平均接受了较低剂量的化疗[20]。该试验只有23例可评价的大于75岁的患者，化疗使这些患者的存活率有降低的趋势[HR=2.35；95% CI（0.84，6.58）；$P=0.09$]。在LACE meta分析的4584例患者中，414例年龄在≥70岁[21]。年龄和化疗获益之间没有显著的统计学交互作用，但这些老年患者的OS有改善的趋势[HR=0.87；95% CI（0.68，1.11）]。尽管老年患者接受了较低剂量的顺铂，但总的不良事件同年轻患者相似。

在一相较大的观察性队列研究中，3324例年龄超过65岁且手术切除的Ⅱ期或Ⅲ期肺癌患者提取于SEER数据库[22]。只有21%的患者接受以铂类为基础的辅助治疗，类似于临床试验中的获益，化疗改善了患者的生存[HR=0.80；95% CI（0.72，0.89）]，尽管因严重不良事件提高了住院治疗率。

基于这些结果，尽管需要考虑并发症，但不应仅凭患者的年龄来决定是否使用辅助化疗和选择方案。

功能状态不佳的患者

对于WHO功能状态（performance statws, PS）评分为2分或以上的患者，辅助化疗的获益尚不清楚。JBR.10和CALGB 9633只允许PS 0或1的患者入组[12,15]，而其他试验只纳入了少量PS不佳的患者。在LACE meta分析的4584例患者中，只有183例的PS为2，辅助化疗有使这些患者有向恶化发展的趋势[17]。

辅助化疗方案的选择

顺铂 vs 卡铂

对于转移性肺癌患者，大多数研究表明顺铂或卡铂为基础的两药联合方案具有相似的PFS和OS[23-24]，虽然一项荟萃分析表明基于顺铂的治疗具有更高的反应率[25]。在辅助治疗研究中，以顺铂为基础的方案已被用于最大的临床试验，这包括纳入LACE meta分析的所有试验[17]。唯一应用基于卡铂方案的大型试验是CALBG-9633，但试验结果未能证实辅助化疗会带来显著的生存获益[15]。因此顺铂被认为是辅助治疗首选的药物，但以卡铂为基础的化疗方案也可用于无法耐受顺铂的患者。

第二种药剂的选择

研究最多的辅助化疗方案是顺铂和长春瑞滨，它被用于 ANITA 和 JBR.10 试验的所有患者及 IALT 和 BLT 试验的部分患者[9,11-12,14]。对于疾病转移者，顺铂联合新的药物如多西紫杉醇、吉西他滨或培美曲塞，同联合长春瑞滨相比，具有类似或更高的反应率和生存率[23,26-27]。这些更新的治疗方案通常具有较好的耐受性，虽然它们还没有在辅助治疗中进行随机试验研究，但已常用于临床实践。可选择用于辅助治疗的方案包括顺铂联合吉西他滨、顺铂联合多西紫杉醇、顺铂联合培美曲塞（仅限于非鳞状细胞癌）。如果患者无法耐受顺铂，在 CALGB-9633 中应用过的卡铂联合紫杉醇是一种合适的方案[15]。

未答复的问题

预测及预后的生物标志物

目前还没有验证的生物标志物来确定哪些特殊的亚组人群能够从辅助治疗中获益。通过分析细胞毒性药物应答和耐药的生物标记物来制订治疗决策十分有价值，这可以确保从辅助化疗中可能获益的患者接受恰当的治疗，不太可能获益的患者免遭药物毒性。许多研究已试图确认具有预测性或预后性的生物标志物，在已发表的辅助治疗试验中，常见的分子改变如 p53 基因突变、p53 蛋白表达或 KRAS 突变，还没有被证明有一致的预后或预测价值[8,28-30]。

切除修复交叉互补 1（the excision repair cross-complementation group 1, ERCC1）酶在核苷酸切除修复途径中起着关键的作用，作为一种化疗耐药标志物已被广泛研究。IALT 分析了 761 例肿瘤的 ERCC1 蛋白表达情况，以顺铂为基础的化疗能明显延长 ERCC1 阴性患者的生存期［占病例数的 56%，HR = 0.65；95% CI（0.50，0.86）；P = 0.002］，而辅助化疗对 ERCC1 阳性者无效［HR = 1.14；95% CI（0.84，1.55）；P = 0.40］[31]。ERCC1 的测定在技术上存在困难，而且其他研究显示了不一致的结果[32]。

一些团队已经使用基因表达数据来创建风险预测模型，但这些研究的结果并不一致，且没有得到前瞻性的验证[33-36]。目前，应用生物标志物来选择辅助化疗仍为试验性的，应在临床试验中进行更好的验证。

辅助化疗和靶向治疗的应用

靶向治疗在 NSCLC 中的应用日益广泛，表皮生长因子受体（EGFR）抑制剂厄洛替尼和吉非替尼被积极用于 NSCLC 的治疗，尤其是 EGFR 突变的患者[37-39]。一些使用这些药物作为辅助治疗的试验启动了，在加拿大 BR.19 研究中，503 例手术切除的 IB 至 ⅢA 期肺癌患者被随机分配到吉非替尼组（250mg，口服，每天 1 次）或安慰剂组，在临床主治医生的酌情处理下患者可以接受辅助放疗或化疗。这项研究仅以抽象形式呈现，但初步结果并不乐观——吉非替尼治疗组的 DFS 和 OS 有缩短的趋势[40]，这一总生存期缩短的趋势也在 EGFR 突变的亚组人群中出现。RADIANT 是一项 Ⅲ期随机临床试验，针对 IB 至 ⅢA 期切除的 NSCLC 患者——或每天口服厄洛替尼 150mg 或安慰剂。符合条件的患者必须为肿瘤 EGFR 的免疫组化或 FISH 检测阳性者，这项研究的入组工作已完成，但尚未公布结果。SELECT 试验是一项单臂的 Ⅱ期研究，目前正在招募 EGFR 突变的 NSCLC 患者，所有患者要接受每天口服厄洛替尼 150mg，预期入组 100 例。

贝伐单抗是一种抗血管内皮生长因子（antivascular endothelial grouth factor, VEGF）抗体，它已被批准应用于非鳞状 NSCLC 患者的一线治疗，可联合卡铂和紫杉醇[41]。E1505 为一个进行中的组间试验，正招募手术切除的 IB 至 ⅢA 期的 NSCLC 患者而不考虑组织学亚型，该试验将患者随机分配或接受 4 个周期的化疗或接受 4 个周期的化疗联合贝伐单抗，随后贝伐单抗维持 1 年，计划入组 1 500 例。

目前，靶向治疗在肺癌辅助治疗中的作用尚不完全明确，这些方法只能应用于临床试验中。

总 结

- 4 个周期以顺铂为基础的辅助化疗是一般状况良好的 Ⅱ期或 ⅢA 期 NSCLC 患者术后的标准治

疗方案。
- 辅助化疗不常规推荐用于 IA 期肺癌患者。
- 伴有不良特征的 IB 期肺癌患者可能从辅助化疗中获益。
- 研究最多的辅助化疗方案为顺铂联合长春瑞滨，但顺铂联合多西他赛、培美曲塞或吉西他滨也是可行的治疗方案。
- 若无禁忌证，首选以顺铂为基础的化疗方案而非基于卡铂的方案。
- 目前尚没有成熟的生物标志物来预测能否从辅助化疗中获益。
- 靶向治疗在辅助治疗中的作用正处于积极的研究中，但这些药物并非标准治疗，而主要在临床试验中使用。

（黄广慧 译）

参考文献

[1] van Rens MT, de la Riviere AB, Elbers HR, et al. Prognostic assessment of 2 361 patients who underwent pulmonary resection for nonsmall cell lung cancer, stage I, II, and IIIA. Chest, 2000, 117（2）：374-379.

[2] The Lung Cancer Study Group. Effects of postoperative mediastinal radiation on completely resected stage II and stage III epidermoid cancer of the lung. The Lung Cancer Study Group. N Engl J Med, 1986, 315（22）：1377-1381.

[3] PORT Meta-analysis Trialists Group. Postoperative radiotherapy in non-small-cell lung cancer：systematic review and meta-analysis of individual patient data from nine randomised controlled trials. PORT Meta-analysis Trialists Group. Lancet, 1998, 352（9124）：257-263.

[4] International Multicentre Pooled Analysis of Colon Cancer Trial（IMPACT）Investigators. Efficacy of adjuvant fluorouracil and folinic acid in colon cancer. International Multicentre Pooled Analysis of Colon Cancer Trials（IMPACT）investigators. Lancet, 1995, 345（8955）：939-944.

[5] Early Breast Cancer Trialist's Collaborative Group. Systemic treatment of early breast cancer by hormonal, cytotoxic, or immune therapy. 133 randomised trials involving 31 000 recurrences and 24 000 deaths among 75 000 women. Early Breast Cancer Trialists' Collaborative Group. Lancet, 1992, 339（8785）：71-85.

[6] Non-small Cell Lung Cancer Collaborative Group. Chemotherapy in non-small cell lung cancer：a meta-analysis using updated data on individual patients from 52 randomised clinical trials. BMJ, 1995, 311（7010）：899-909.

[7] Tada H, Tsuchiya R, Ichinose Y, et al. A randomized trial comparing adjuvant chemotherapy versus surgery alone for completely resected pN2 non-small cell lung cancer（JCOG9304）. Lung Cancer, 2004, 43（2）：167-173.

[8] Scagliotti GV, Fossati R, Torri V, et al. Randomized study of adjuvant chemotherapy for completely resected stage I, II, or IIIA non-small-cell Lung cancer. J Natl Cancer Inst, 2003, 95（19）：1453-1461.

[9] The International Adjuvant Lung Cancer Trial Collaborative Group. Cisplatin-based adjuvant chemotherapy in patients with completely resected non-small-cell lung cancer. NEngl J Med, 2004, 350（4）：351-360.

[10] Arriagada R, Dunant A, Pignon JP, et al. Long-term results of the international adjuvant lung cancer trial evaluating adjuvant Cisplatin-based chemotherapy in resected lung cancer. J Clin Oncol, 2010, 28（1）：35-42.

[11] Waller D, Peake MD, Stephens RJ, et al. Chemotherapy for patients with non-small-cell lung cancer：the surgical setting of the Big Lung Trial. Eur J Cardiothorac Surg, 2004, 26（1）：173-182.

[12] Winton T, Livingston R, Johnson D, et al. Vinorelbine plus cisplatin vs. observation in resected non-small-cell lung cancer. N Engl J Med, 2005, 352（25）：2589-2597.

[13] Butts CA, Ding K, Seymour L, et al. Randomized phase III trial of vinorelbine plus cisplatin compared with observation in completely resected stage IB and II nonsmall-cell lung cancer：updated survival analysis of JBR-10. J Clin Oncol, 2010, 28（1）：29-34.

[14] Douillard JY, Rosell R, De Lena M, et al. Adjuvant vinorelbine plus cisplatin versus observation in patients with completely resected stage IB-IIIA nonsmall-cell lung cancer（[Adjuvant Navelbine International Trialist Association（ANITA）]：a randomised controlled trial. Lancet Oncol, 2006, 7（9）：719-727.

[15] Strauss GM, Herndon JE, 2nd, Maddaus MA, et al. Adjuvant paclitaxel plus carboplatin compared with observation in stage IB non-small-cell lung cancer：CALGB 9633 with the Cancer and Leukemia Group B, Radiation Therapy Oncology Group, and North Central Cancer Treatment Group Study Groups. J Clin Oncol, 2008, 26（31）：5043-5051.

[16] Strauss GM, Herndon JE, Maddaus MA, et al. Randomized clinical trial of adjuvant chemotherapy with paclitaxel

and carboplatin following resection in stage IB non-small cell lung cancer: report of Cancer and Leukemia Group B (CALGB) protocol 9633. J Clin Oncol. Annual Meeting Proceedings, 2004; 22 (14S): 7019.

[17] Pignon JP, Tribodet H, Scagliotti GV, et al. Lung adjuvant cisplatin evaluation: A pooled analysis by the LACE Collaborative Group. J Clin Oncol, 2008, 26 (21): 3552-3559.

[18] Arriagada R, Auperin A, Burdett S, et al. Adjuvant chemotherapy, with or without postoperative radiotherapy, in operable non-small-cell lung cancer: two meta-analyses of individual patient data. Lancet, 2010, 375 (9722): 1267-1277.

[19] Siegel R, DeSantis C, Virgo K, et al. Cancer treatment and survivorship statistics, 2012. CA Cancer J Clin, 2012, 62 (4): 220-241.

[20] Pepe C, Hasan B, Winton TL, et al. Adjuvant vinorelbine and cisplatin in elderly patients: National Cancer Institute of Canada and Intergroup Study JBR.10. J Clin Oncol, Apr 20, 25 (12): 1553-1561.

[21] Fruh M, Rolland E, Pignon JP, et al. Pooled analysis of the effect of age on adjuvant cisplatin-based chemotherapy for completely resected non-small-cell lung cancer. J Clin Oncol, 2008, 26 (21): 3573-3581.

[22] Wisnivesky JP, Smith CB, Packer S, et al. Survival and risk of adverse events in older patients receiving postoperative adjuvant chemotherapy for resected stages II-IIIA lung cancer: observational cohort study. BMJ, 2011, 343: d4013.

[23] Schiller JH, HarringtonD, Belani CP, et al. Comparison of four chemotherapy regimens for advanced non-small-cell lung cancer. N Engl J Med, 2002, 346 (2): 92-98.

[24] Ohe Y, Ohashi Y, Kubota K, et al. Randomized phase III study of cisplatin plus irinotecan versus carboplatin plus paclitaxel, cisplatin plus gemcitabine, and cisplatin plus vinorelbine for advanced non-small-cell lung cancer: Four-Arm Cooperative Study in Japan. Ann Oncol, 2007, 18 (2): 317-323.

[25] Ardizzoni A, Boni L, Tiseo M, et al. Cisplatin-versus carboplatin-based chemotherapy in first-line treatment of advanced non-small-cell lung cancer: an individual patient data meta-analysis. J Natl Cancer Inst, 2007, 99 (11): 847-857.

[26] Fossella F, Pereira JR, von Pawel J, et al. Randomized, multinational, phase III study of docetaxel plus platinum combinations versus vinorelbine plus cisplatin for advanced non-small-cell lung cancer: The TAX 326 study group. J Clin Oncol, 2003, 21 (16): 3016-3024.

[27] Scagliotti GV, Parikh P, Von Pawel J, et al. Phase III study comparing cisplatin plus gemcitabine with cisplatin plus pemetrexed in chemotherapy-naive patients with advanced-stage non-small-cell lung cancer. J Clin Oncol, 2008, 26 (21): 3543-3551.

[28] Schiller JH, Adak S, Feins RH, et al. Lack of prognostic significance of p53 and K-ras mutations in primary resected non-small-cell lung cancer on E4592: A laboratory ancillary study on an eastern cooperative oncology group prospective randomized trial of postoperative adjuvant therapy. J Clin Oncol, 2001, 19 (2): 448-457.

[29] Tsao MS, Aviel-Ronen S, Ding K, et al. Prognostic and predictive importance of p53 and RAS for adjuvant chemotherapy in non small-cell lung cancer. J Clin Oncol, 2007, 25 (33): 5240-5247.

[30] Cuffe S, Bourredjem A, Graziano S, et al. A pooled exploratory analysis of the effect of tumor size and KRAS mutations on survival benefit from adjuvant platinumbased chemotherapy in node-negative non-small cell lung cancer. J Thorac Oncol, 2012, 7 (6): 963-972.

[31] Olaussen KA, Dunant A, Fouret P, et al. DNA repair by ERCC1 in non-small-cell lung cancer and cisplatin-based adjuvant chemotherapy. NEngl J Med, 2006, 355 (10): 983-991.

[32] Hubner RA, Riley RD, Billingham LJ, et al. Excision repair cross-complementation group 1 (ERCC1) status and lung cancer outcomes: a metaanalysis of published studies and recommendations. PLoS ONE, 2011, 6 (10): e25164.

[33] Shedden K, Taylor JMG, Enkemann SA, et al. Gene expressionbased survival prediction in lung adenocarcinoma: a multi-site, blinded validation study. Nature Medicine, 2008, 14 (8): 822-827.

[34] Gold KA, Lee JJ, Ping Y, et al. Biologic risk model for recurrence in resected early-stage non-small cell lung cancer. J Clin Oncol: ASCO Annual Meeting Proceedings, 2011, 29 (15s): 7053.

[35] Zhu CQ, Ding K, Strumpf D, et al. Prognostic and predictive gene signature for adjuvant chemotherapy in resected nonsmall-cell lung cancer. J Clin Oncol, 2010, 28 (29): 4417-4424.

[36] Kratz JR, He J, Van Den Eeden SK, et al. A practical molecular assay to predict survival in resected non-squa-

mous, non-smallcell lung cancer: Development and international validation studies. Lancet, 2012, 379 (9818): 823-832.

[37] Shepherd FA, Pereira JR, Ciuleanu T, et al. Erlotinib in previously treated non-small-cell lung cancer. NEngl J Med, 2005, 353 (2): 123-132.

[38] Lynch TJ, Bell DW, Sordella R, et al. Activating mutations in the epidermal growth factor receptor underlying responsiveness of non-small-cell lung cancer to gefitinib. N Engl J Med, 2004, 350 (21): 2129-2139.

[39] Mok TS, Wu Y-L, Thongprasert S, et al. Gefitinib or carboplatin-paclitaxel in pulmonary adenocarcinoma. NEngl J Med, 2009, 361 (10): 947-957.

[40] Goss GD, Lorimer I, Tsao MS, et al. A phase III, randomized, double-blind, placebo-controlled trial of the epidermal growth factor receptor inhibitor gefitinib in completely resected stage IB-IIIA non-small cell lung cancer. J Clin Oncol: ASCO Annual Meeting Proceedings, 2010, 28 (18s): LBA7005.

[41] Sandler A, Gray R, Perry MC, et al. Paclitaxel-carboplatin alone or with bevacizumab for non-small-cell lung cancer. N Engl J Med, 2006, 355 (24): 2542-2550.

第19章
可手术非小细胞肺癌的新辅助化疗

Christopher G. Azzoli[1], Katherine M. W. Pisters[2]
1. Department of Medicine, Harvard Medical School, Massachusetts General Hospital, Boston, MA, USA
2. Department of Thoracic/Head and Neck Medical Oncology, The University of Texas MD Anderson Cancer Center, Houston, TX, USA

引 言

2012年美国新发大约226 160例肺癌患者；死亡160 340例[1]。肺癌是男性和女性癌症相关死亡的首要因素，其中非小细胞肺癌（NSCLC）约占90%[2]。近期采用低剂量螺旋CT筛查重度吸烟者可早期发现肺癌从而降低肺癌相关死亡率[3]。然而，肺癌筛查尚未普及，大部分肺癌患者确诊时仍为进展期，丧失了治愈机会[4]。

对于早期NSCLC，手术可能治愈。然而即使手术成功，癌症5年复发和死亡的概率对于术后病理分期pⅠA、pⅠB、pⅡA、pⅡB、pⅢA、pⅢB者高达27%、42%、54%、64%、76%、91%[5]。临床或术前分期通常低估疾病的严重程度，尤其是未采用FDG-PET及纵隔镜进行分期时。据估计对于特定临床分期的生存率较相应手术或病理分期更差（表19.1）[5]。考虑到单纯手术的生存率较低，研究者已经引入辅助治疗如化疗或胸部放疗，以期提高患者的生存期。

表19.1 可切除NSCLC临床及病理分期相关5年生存率

分期	TNM	5年生存率	
		病理分期	临床分期
ⅠA	T1N0M0	73%	50%
ⅠB	T2N0M0	58%	43%
ⅡA	T1N1M0	46%	36%
ⅡB	T2N1M0, T3N0M0	36%	25%
ⅢA	T3N1M0, T1-3N2M0	24%	19%

来源：Goldstraw 2007[5]，已获得批准使用

多年来绝大多数辅助化疗相关临床试验并未证实辅助化疗具有生存获益。1995年进行的一项meta分析探讨了辅助化疗的作用[6]。该meta分析部分分析了术后辅助化疗的作用并与单纯手术进行比较。研究发现含顺铂方案的化疗有生存获益，这一结果与多数研究一致。Meta分析发现顺铂为基础的化疗具有5年5%的净生存获益（$P=0.08$）。这一结果促使后续进行的多项大型、随机临床试验采用顺铂为基础的联合化疗作为辅助化疗方案。直到2003年，第一项也是最大样本量的临床试验发布，该试验证实可手术切除的NSCLC患者术后辅助化疗具有生存获益[7-10]。之后术后辅助化疗成为Ⅱ~Ⅲ期NSCLC的标准治疗方法。术后辅助化疗在本书第18章中已有详细阐述。

本章的重点在于新辅助化疗，也称术前化疗或诱导化疗在可切除NSCLC中的应用。30多年来，因为手术切除后患者生存不佳并且2003年前缺乏辅助化疗的证据，对术前化疗进行了诸多探索。20世纪90年代早期，基于局部进展期、未切除的NSCLC在胸部放疗前进行化疗较单纯放疗具有生存获益的研究[11-12]，新辅助治疗成为研究焦点，此外多种理论均支持术前化疗具有优势的观点。与辅助化疗相比，手术前进行化疗可以评估肿瘤对于化疗的影像学和病理学反应，早期治疗临床未检出微转移病灶，并提高药物利用率[13-14]。

尽管较早引起密切关注，除ⅢA/N2患者外新辅助化疗仍处于研究阶段，这主要是由新辅助化疗相关Ⅲ期临床试验开始时间决定。术后或辅助化疗先于大型、随机比较新辅助化疗后手术对比单纯手术的临床试验进行，结果是多数大型新辅

助化疗相关临床试验在辅助化疗证实具有生存获益后提前终止[15-17]。此外，目前尚无一项样本量足够大的临床试验对比辅助化疗与新辅助化疗的生存获益[14]。

多项随机化临床试验经历了 8 年时间（1995—2003），最终验证了顺铂辅助化疗对于可切除 NSCLC 具有生存获益这一假说。随着新化疗药物年复一年的出现，临床试验必须更侧重于合适患者对应合适药物，而非关注术前治疗的时间。新辅助化疗相关Ⅲ期临床试验同样经历了 8 年时间才证实新辅助化疗的安全性并且具有生存获益。

本章将对这些数据进行分析并通过案例证实新辅助化疗能更快速地治疗微转移病灶，提高药物渗透性，最重要的是提供有效终点，例如影像学表现、病理反应及降低肿瘤分期，从而为更进一步将新型化疗药物更快应用于可切除 NSCLC 提供数据支持。

可切除Ⅲ期疾病的Ⅱ期临床试验

评估Ⅲ期 NSCLC 新辅助化疗的Ⅱ期临床试验最早开始于 20 世纪 80 年，之前斯隆-凯瑟琳纪念肿瘤医院（Memorial Sloan-Kettering Cancer Center，MSKCC）研究证实上述患者单纯手术后预后不良[18]。Martini 等证实存在同侧纵隔淋巴结转移的患者术后 5 年生存率高达 24%，但对于同侧巨大纵隔淋巴结转移的亚组（X 线检查可见重大淋巴结或支气管镜下隆突偏斜）3 年生存率仅为 8%[18]。基于上述观察，一项由丝裂霉素、长春碱类（长春地辛、长春新碱）、大剂量顺铂组成的方案（MVP）用于预后不良、巨块型的 N2 患者。一项纳入 136 例患者的大型Ⅱ期临床试验，MSKCC 的研究者证实影像学有效率高达 77%，其中 65% 的患者接受完全手术切除[19]。病理学上，14% 的患者达到完全缓解，手术切除标本完全没有肿瘤存活证据。136 例患者的中位生存时间为 19 个月。完全切除患者的 3 年生存率为 41%，较既往单纯手术患者 8% 的 3 年生存率显著提高。

加拿大的研究者进行了另一项确认临床试验[20]。多伦多研究组纳入了 65 例纵隔镜证实的ⅢA 期NSCLC 患者，术前行丝裂霉素、长春地辛及顺铂方案化疗 2 个周期，之后进行开胸手术，术后行两个周期的同方案辅助化疗。诱导化疗的有效率为 68%，54% 的患者接受手术切除。全组患者的中位生存时间为 18.6 个月，5 年生存率为 29%，10 年生存率为 22%。

一系列其他Ⅱ期临床试验完整地评估了ⅢA 期患者术前新辅助化疗包括或不包括放疗的作用[21-24]。这些研究证实，辅助化疗的影像学有效率明显高于Ⅳ期 NSCLC 患者，新辅助化疗后进行手术切除是可行的，并且部分患者获得病理学完全缓解，部分出现临床降期。单纯采用新辅助化疗的临床试验中，病理学完全缓解率（pathologic complete response，path CR）高达 18%，而采用化疗及放疗的临床试验病理学完全缓解率高达 26%[20,24]。病理学获得完全缓解的患者具有显著生存时间延长。这些研究的另一项重大发现在于影像学缓解与病理学缓解无关，术中疾病状况可能比影像学更多，也可能更少。最后，与单独采用新辅助化疗的患者相比，采用放化疗联合的患者生存无显著差异。该书中其他章节对术前及术后放疗进行了更详细的阐述。

美国协作组试图开展一项临床试验对比可切除ⅢA 期/N2 NSCLC 新辅助放化疗与单纯新辅助化疗（RTOG0412/西南肿瘤协作组 S0332）的临床试验。该试验开始于 2005—2006 年，但因为试验设计缺陷提前终止。研究者发现内科医生及患者对于这一分期的治疗选择倾向特别明显，因此内科医生和患者均对随机分组不满意。Ⅲ期 NSCLC 多学科治疗方法中新辅助放疗的应用在该书中其他部分进行了详细阐述。

近期部分Ⅱ期临床试验中研究者在新辅助治疗中检验新型化疗药物的疗效。部分研究采用两药方案，而其他则采用三药联合方案。部分研究仅关注ⅢA 期/N2 患者，而其他研究选择性纳入部分ⅢB 期患者。这些Ⅱ期临床试验在患者选择及后续手术或胸部放疗的应用方面存在差异，因此和单一随机化临床试验相比结果可能受影响，但研究仍然证实两药及三药联合方案、老药与新药无显著差异。

对Ⅲ期 NSCLC 患者相关Ⅱ期临床试验的总结见表 19.2。瑞士的 Betticher 及其同事研究多西他赛和顺铂在ⅢA/N2 NSCLC 患者中的应用[23]。该研究中，90 例具有潜在可手术切除的ⅢA 期/N2

表19.2 可切除Ⅲ期NSCLC新辅助治疗相关前瞻性Ⅱ期临床试验

研究	分期	方案	N	客观有效率	R0	中位生存时间（月）	1年生存率	病理CR
Betticher[23]	ⅢA～N2	DP	90	66%	48%	33%	65%	19%/75切除
Van Zandwijk[25]	ⅢA～N2	GP	47	70%	NR	19%	69%	NR
Migliorino[26]	ⅢA～N2/ⅢB	GP	70	57%	41%	15%	67%	3%
Garrido[27]	ⅢA/B	DGP	136	72%	50%	16%	NR	NR
Esteban[28]	ⅢA～B	GPVn	62	65%	NR	NR	NR	25%
		GP	66	61%	NR	NR	NR	18%
Lorent[29]	ⅢA～N2	VdIP	131	54%	47%	24%	(21% 5年)	5%
Cappuzzo[30]	ⅢA～N2/ⅢB	GPacP	42	71%	38%	22%	92%	7%
De Marinis[31]	ⅢA～N2	GPacP	49	74%	55%	23%	85%	16%

DP：多西他赛，顺铂；GP：吉西他滨，顺铂；DGP：多西他赛，吉西他滨，顺铂；GPVn：吉西他滨，顺铂，长春新碱；GPacP：吉西他滨，紫杉醇，顺铂；NR：未报道；VdIP：长春地辛，异环磷酰胺，顺铂

NSCLC患者接受3个周期的顺铂联合多西他赛化疗，化疗耐受性良好，96%的患者完成了3个周期的化疗。影像学有效率为66%，并且48%的患者接受了完整切除。截止随访期满，完整切除患者的中位生存时间为5.2年（0.3～6.3年）。

Van Zandwijk及其同事评估了顺铂联合吉西他滨新辅助化疗在ⅢA期/N2 NSCLC患者中的应用效果（EORTC 08955）[25]。患者在评估前接受新辅助化疗（3个周期）并作为EORTC 08941临床试验的一部分随机分至手术组或化疗组。EORTC 08941临床试验的结果详见文中其他重点探讨Ⅲ期NSCLC手术及放疗的章节。EORTC 08955中，47例入组患者中影像学有效率为70%。37例[70%；95% CI（55，83%）]获得客观缓解。53%的患者纵隔淋巴结肿瘤完全消失。诱导化疗后接受开胸手术治疗的患者中有71%完整切除。

意大利的研究者同样探讨了吉西他滨联合顺铂在ⅢA期/N2型及部分ⅢB期NSCLC患者中的应用效果[26]。一项纳入70例患者的Ⅱ期临床试验，影像学有效率为57%。28例（41%）患者可接受完全切除，2例患者病理学完全缓解。中位随访时间16个月，中位生存时间为15个月。

西班牙研究者对由多西他赛、顺铂和吉西他滨组成的三联方案进行了探讨[27]。试验纳入纵隔镜证实的N2（ⅢA）或T4N0-1（ⅢB）期患者。129例可评价疗效的患者中，影像学有效率为56%；可手术患者的总体完全切除率为69%（其中ⅢA期为72%，ⅢB期为66%）；可评估患者的总体完全切除率为48%。62例完全切除患者中8例（12.9%）病理完全缓解；中位生存时间为16个月；3年生存率为37%，5年生存率为21%，并且ⅢA期与ⅢB期生存率无显著差异。62例完全切除患者的中位生存时间为48个月，13例未完全切除患者为13个月，15例未手术患者为17个月（$P = 0.005$）。完全切除、不完全切除和未手术患者的5年生存率分别为41%、11%和0。多因素分析显示完全切除（$HR = 0.35$；$P < 0.0001$），临床有效（$HR = 0.32$；$P < 0.0001$）及年龄<60岁（$HR = 0.64$；$P = 0.027$）是最主要的预测因子。

意大利的另一组研究者探讨了顺铂联合吉西他滨加或不加长春瑞滨作为诱导化疗在Ⅲ期NSCLC中的作用[28]。该研究共纳入154例患者，两药和三药联合方案在影像学有效率方面无差异（65% vs 61%）。三药联合组的血液学毒性和疲乏略常见，但差异无统计学意义。两组多数患者接受放疗作为局部治疗。这些行手术切除的患者中，病理学完全缓解率在两药方案组为18%，三药方案组为25%。中位无进展生存时间在两药方案组为368d，三药方案组为322d，提示两组的疗效相似。

比利时的研究者对ⅢA期/N2型NSCLC患者给予3个周期的长春地辛、异环磷酰胺和顺铂联合方案新辅助化疗[29]。影像学完全缓解见于54%的患者，所有患者的中位生存时间为24个月，5年生存率为21%。75例患者接受手术，完全切

除率为47%。尽管全组患者的总生存似乎与化疗疗效相关，对于接受完全切除的患者上述影响不存在。部分患者的切除率更低；但是，作者强调完全切除后的长期生存见于部分未达到影像学评估有效的患者。

吉西他滨、紫杉醇及顺铂同样作为诱导化疗方案进行了研究。一项研究中，42例ⅢA期/N2和ⅢB期NSCLC患者接受三药方案化疗[30]，影像学有效率为71%；21例患者接受开胸手术，16例完全切除（38%）。病理学完全缓解率为7%；较短中位随访时间内（14个月），总生存时间为22个月。该方案作为诱导化疗方案同样应用于49例ⅢA期/N2 NSCLC患者[31]。该研究纳入的49例患者中，74%获得影像学缓解，55%完全切除。在这一小样本研究中，8例（16%）达到病理学完全缓解。中位随访时间15.6个月，总生存时间为23个月。

早期患者Ⅱ期临床试验

在证实诱导化疗对Ⅲ期NSCLC患者具有应用潜力后，研究者设计了部分临床试验验证诱导化疗对早期NSCLC患者的作用，研究汇总详见表19.3。第一项上述研究为BLOT（Bimodality Lung Oncology Team）试验[13]，该试验序贯纳入两组临床分期为ⅠB、Ⅱ及ⅢA期的患者。采用CT检查进行临床分期，所有患者均要求进行纵隔镜检查。该研究中不常规进行PET检查。纵隔镜检查证实为N2或肺上沟癌者不纳入研究。患者术前及术后接受卡铂联合紫杉醇方案化疗（第一组：术前2个周期及术后3个周期；第二组：术前3个周期和术后4个周期）。两组综合分析，影像学有效率为51%，完全切除率为86%，病理学完全缓解率为5%。3年及5年生存率分别为61%和42%。两组间的患者特征或结果无统计学差异。基于上述理想数据的支持，随后研究者开始了一项随机化Ⅲ期临床试验（S9900），该试验结果将在后文中进行阐述。

日本临床肿瘤协作组（Japan Clinical Oncology Group，JCDG）进行了一项随机化Ⅱ期临床试验对比多西他赛顺铂联合方案与单纯多西他赛方案诱导化疗的作用[32]。该研究中80例临床分期ⅠB和Ⅱ期的NSCLC患者接受两药治疗后生存改善。2例接受多西他赛-顺铂化疗的患者出现病理学完全缓解，联合治疗组的影像学有效率高于单纯多西他赛组（45% vs 15%）。联合治疗组的1年、2年、4年无病生存率分别为78%、65%和57%，而单药治疗组分别为62%、44%和36%。

一项研究对由吉西他滨、卡铂、紫杉醇组成的三药方案在可手术的ⅠB、Ⅱ或ⅢA期患者中的应用进行了探讨[33]。21d为1个周期，用药包括吉西他滨1 000mg/m²第1天和第8天，卡铂第1天应用，AUC为5，紫杉醇第1天为175mg/m²。纳入44例患者的影像学有效率为76%；36例患者接受了完全肿瘤切除，其中5例患者达到病理学完全缓解并且病理学证实切除肿瘤无活性；1年生存率为86%。作者因此得出结论：三药联合细胞毒药物作为新辅助化疗方案对于可手术的NSCLC患者安全有效。

一项由吉西他滨和长春瑞滨组成的不含铂方案用于ⅠB~Ⅲ期的NSCLC患者，术前共进行两个周期的化疗[34]。该研究纳入了62例患者，影像学有效率较低，仅为34%；77%的患者接受了完整切除，并且3%的患者病理学完全缓解；1年、2年生存率分别为80%、65%；中位生存时间为38个月。该研究证实与含铂两药联合方案相比，不含铂方案的总生存率相似，但是影像学有效率及病理学有效率均低。

表19.3 早期可手术NSCLC前瞻性Ⅱ期新辅助化疗临床试验

研究	分期	方案	病例数	ORR	RO	OS	Path CR
Pisters等[13]	ⅠB~ⅢA	PacCbp	134	51%	86%	（42%）5年	5%
Kuniton等[32]	ⅠB~Ⅱ	DP	40	45%	95%	NR	5%
		D	39	15%	85%	NR	0%
Abratt等[33]	ⅠB~ⅢA	PacGCb	44	75%	82	NR	11%
Ramnath等[34]	ⅠB~Ⅲ	GVn	62	34%	77%	（65%）2年	3%

DP：多西他赛，顺铂；D：多西他赛；GVn：吉西他滨，长春瑞滨；NR：未报道；PacCb：紫杉醇，卡铂；PacGCb：紫杉醇、吉西他滨、卡铂；ORR：影像学有效率；RO：完全切除率；OS：总生存；Path CR：病理学完全缓解率

随机化Ⅱ期和Ⅲ期临床试验

基于早期Ⅱ期临床试验关于新辅助化疗的数据支持，随后开展了多项评估新辅助化疗联合手术对比单纯手术的随机化临床试验。这些试验详细归纳于表19.4。这些新辅助化疗相关临床试验并开始于2003年以前，同年辅助化疗个体化研究的第一项阳性结果问世。2003年Ⅱ~Ⅲ期NSCLC患者进行单纯手术治疗已不符合伦理，多数包括Ⅰ~Ⅲ期患者的大型临床试验提前终止，导致样本量太小不足以进行统计学分析。

然而，最早期设计的单纯针对Ⅲ期NSCLC患者的临床试验虽样本量小但足以证明新辅助化疗的显著获益。Roth及其同事开展了一项随机化Ⅲ期临床试验，该试验中可手术切除的ⅢA期NSCLC患者接受环磷酰胺、依托泊苷和顺铂三药新辅助化疗后行手术治疗或单纯手术治疗[35]。化疗组患者接受3个周期的新辅助化疗，有效患者再行3个周期的辅助化疗。中期分析结束，因研究已证实新辅助化疗组具有显著生存获益，在纳入60例患者后研究提前终止。之后在中位时间长达82个月的随访后仍可见新辅助化疗的显著生存获益。化疗组的中位生存时间为21个月，5年生存率为36%；而单纯手术组的中位生存时间为14个月，5年生存率为15%。

表19.4 可手术的NSCLC新辅助化疗随机临床试验

研究	分期	方案	病例数	客观有效率	R0	中位生存时间（月）	1年生存率	病理CR
Roth[35]	ⅢA	CEP	28	35%	39%	21	36%	0
		对照	32		31%	14	15%	
Rosell[36]	ⅢA	MIP	30	60%	77%	22	17%	3%
		对照	30		90%	10	0	
Pass[37]	ⅢA/N2	EP	13	62%	85%	29	46%（2年）	8%
		对照	14		86%	16	21%（2年）	
Zhou[38]	Ⅲ	Varied	414	73%	94%	NR	34%	15%
		对照	310		92%	NR	24%	
Nagai[39]	ⅢA/N2	VdP	31	28%	65%	17	10%	NR
		手术	31		77%	16	22%	
DePierre[41]	ⅠB、Ⅱ、ⅢA	MIP	179	64%	92%	37	41%	11%
		手术	176		86%	26	3%	
Sorensen[43]	ⅠB、Ⅱ、ⅢA	PacCb	44	46%	79%	34	36	NR
		手术	46		70%	23	24%	
Pisters[15]	ⅠB、Ⅱ、ⅢA	PacCb	168	41%	94%	47	69%（2年）	NR
		手术	167		89%	40	63%（2年）	
Gilligan[16]	ⅠA~ⅢB	P/Cb-based	258	49%	82%	54	75%	4%
		手术	261		80%	55	75%	1*
Scagliotti[17]	ⅠB、Ⅱ、ⅢA	GP	129	35%	88%	94	68%（3年）	5
		手术	141		84%	58	60%（3年）	1*
Felip[14]	ⅠA（>2cm）、	PacCb pre	201	53%	87%	NR	47%（5年）	10.5%
	ⅠB、Ⅱ、	PacCb post	211		90%	NR	46%（5年）	
	ⅢA（T3N1）	手术	212		90%	NR	44%（5年）	

CEP：环磷酰胺，依托泊苷，顺铂；DP：多西他赛，顺铂；EP：依托泊苷，顺铂；GP：吉西他滨，顺铂；MIP：丝裂霉素，异环磷酰胺，顺铂；NR：未报道；PacCb：紫杉醇，卡铂；P/Cb-based：顺铂/卡铂为基础；VdP：长春地辛，顺铂。*：两项临床试验中各有1例单纯手术组患者病理分期为T0N0

巴塞罗那的 Rosell 及其同事开展了一项类似的Ⅲ期临床试验[36]。该试验中，临床分期为ⅢA期的 NSCLC 患者随机接受手术或术前 3 个周期的丝裂霉素、异环磷酰胺、顺铂联合新辅助化疗后再手术。两组分别进行纵隔放疗 50Gy。纳入 60 例患者后随访 24 个月进行的中期分析证实新辅助化疗具有显著生存获益，入组提前终止。随访 7 年再次分析证实化疗组的中位生存时间为 22 个月，5 年生存率为 17%，而单纯手术组的中位生存时间为 10 个月，5 年生存率为 0。

NCI 进行了另一项诱导治疗相关的Ⅲ期临床试验。该研究将ⅢA 期/N2 患者随机化分为两组，一组接受顺铂联合依托泊苷方案新辅助化疗后再手术（如化疗有效再行 4 个周期的辅助化疗），另一组接受单纯手术，两组均行 54～60Gy 的纵隔放射治疗。4 年合计 27 例患者纳入该研究。1992 年公布的中期分析证实，化疗组具有提高生存期的趋势，中位生存时间围 29 个月 vs 16 个月，$P = 0.095$。

一项来自中国的Ⅲ期 NSCLC 新辅助化疗的大型随机化临床试验以摘要形式进行了报道[38]。12 年共纳入 724 例患者，所有患者随机化接受新辅助化疗后采用手术或单纯手术。414 例患者接受了 2 个周期的化疗，21 例接受了支气管动脉介入化疗（数据未公布），另外 393 例患者接受了静脉化疗（130 例患者给予顺铂联合吉西他滨；68 例给予丝裂霉素、长春碱、顺铂；67 例给予顺铂联合依托泊苷；36 例给予环磷酰胺、多柔比星、顺铂；32 例给予长春地辛、顺铂；30 例给予紫杉醇、长春新碱；30 例给予紫杉醇、顺铂）。73% 的患者诱导化疗有效，15% 的患者病理学完全缓解；化疗组的完全切除率为 94%，单纯手术组为 92%；手术并发症及手术相关死亡两组间无统计学差异；5 年、10 年生存率为 34%、29% 与 24%、22%（$P < 0.01$）。该临床试验的有效率、切除率、生存率、病理学完全缓解率均高于其他临床试验，并且不同诱导化疗方案的上述指标存在显著差异。

日本临床肿瘤协作组的肺癌手术研究小组的 Nagai 及其同事近期公布了关于ⅢA 期/N2 NSCLC 患者的随机化Ⅲ期临床试验结果[39]。该试验计划 3 年内入组 200 例患者，然而因为进展缓慢（5 年入组 62 例患者）提前终止。研究者指出对患者有益的补偿不足，诱导化疗组的住院时间延长和国内媒体广泛报道 NSCLC 化疗无效是入组缓慢的主要原因。中位随访时间 6.2 年，两组间的总生存无显著差异，中位生存时间或 5 年生存率（化疗组 17 个月和 10% vs 单纯手术组的 16 个月和 20%）

至于早期 NSCLC（例如不含纵隔淋巴结受累者），第一项对新辅助化疗的报道来自英国伦敦的皇家 Brompton 医院[40]。该研究在 22 例早期（IB、Ⅱ、ⅢA）可切除 NSCLC 患者中进行。将患者随机化分为行丝裂霉素、长春碱和顺铂化疗后行手术治疗组（$n = 11$）或单纯手术治疗组（$n = 11$）。40 例潜在入组患者中，22 例最终同意入组。化疗组患者的耐受性良好，并且手术并发症和死亡率无增加。基于这一有限的经验，作者建议在所有可手术的 NSCLC 和支持权责发生制的医学研究委员会的肺组试验——the UK BLT 的患者进行大样本多中心Ⅲ期临床试验。

2002 年报道了一项关于可切除 IB、Ⅱ 和 ⅢA 期 NSCLC 丝裂霉素、异环磷酰胺和顺铂诱导化疗的随机化Ⅲ期临床试验[41]；355 例可入组患者随机化分配接受单纯手术或 2 个周期的新辅助化疗后再行手术治疗。有效患者（影像学或病理学有效）再接受 2 个周期的辅助化疗。除临床 N2 期患者较少分配至单纯手术组外（28% vs 40%；$P = 0.65$），两组患者的特征均衡性良好。化疗组的术后并发症更多，但无统计学差异（24/167 vs 22/171）。化疗组的术后死亡率为 6.7%，而手术组为 4.5%（$P = 0.38$）。术后第 4 年中位生存时间 11 个月（37 个月 vs 26 个月）。化疗组生存率提高 8.6%，但比较无统计学差异。亚组分析显示，化疗获益主要局限于 N0～N1 患者，死亡的相对风险为 0.68，$P = 0.027$。治疗阶段联合治疗组死亡患者更多，但无统计学差异。诱导化疗的影响更多在于生存获益。两组间的局部复发风险无差异。化疗组远处转移的相对风险为 0.54，$P = 0.01$。2003 年该研究的随访数据公布，最小随访间隔为 60 个月[42]。3 年和 5 年生存的差异稳定在 10%（第 3 年，$P = 0.04$；第 5 年，$P = 0.06$）。N0 - 1 亚组统计学的显著获益仍然存在，5 年生存率为 49% 与 34%（$P = 0.02$）。

斯堪的纳维亚人公布了关于临床分期 IB、Ⅱ 和 ⅢA（除外 N2 患者）期患者采用新辅助紫杉醇联合卡铂化疗的临床试验[43]，该研究因入组缓慢提前终止（6年入组90例患者）。44例随机接受化疗的患者影像学有效率为46%，完全切除率为79%。46例接受单纯手术的患者完全切除率为70%，化疗组的中位生存时间为34个月，5年生存率为36%；而对照组的总生存时间为23个月，5年生存率为24%，两组间无统计学差异。

西南肿瘤协作组临床试验S9900是一项比较紫杉醇联合卡铂3个周期诱导化疗后手术与单纯手术治疗临床分期IB、Ⅱ和ⅢA NSCLC（除外肺上沟癌和N2患者）患者的Ⅲ期临床试验[15]。该研究旨在纳入600例患者从而证实生存时间增加33%或5年生存率提高10%。在完全切除NSCLC辅助化疗随机化临床试验证实具有生存获益后，该试验终止，共入组354例患者。两组间患者的特征均衡性良好。随机化分配至化疗组的患者，影像学有效率为41%，94%完全切除，并且无预期外毒副反应。单纯手术组的中位生存时间为41个月，而新辅助化疗组为62个月[HR=0.79；95% CI（0.60, 1.06）；$P=0.11$]；单纯手术组的中位PFS为20个月，而新辅助化疗组为33个月[HR=0.80；95% CI（0.61, 1.04）；$P=0.10$]。

一项由英国医学研究院和欧洲癌症研究与治疗组织发起的一项欧洲多中心临床试验（LU22/NVALT2/EORTC 08012）随机化纳入519例手术切除分期Ⅰ~Ⅲ期的NSCLC患者，分别给予单纯手术治疗或3个周期铂类为基础的化疗后行手术治疗[16]。随机化前，研究者确定了6种标准治疗方案，其中4种含顺铂，2种含卡铂（联合紫杉醇或多西他赛）。多数患者（61%）为Ⅰ期，包括17% IA期，Ⅲ期仅占7%。多数化疗组患者（75%）完成所有3个周期的化疗，49%有效，31%临床降期。与卡铂方案相比，研究者更多采用顺铂方案（78%顺铂，12%卡铂）。两组间手术成功率相近（单纯手术与化疗后手术相比，肺叶切除成功率：56% vs 60%；完全切除成功率：80% vs 82%）。化疗组术后并发症并未增加，生活质量同样未受影响。最终分析显示，并无PFS[HR=0.96；95% CI（0.77, 1.21）；$P=0.74$]或OS[HR=1.02；95% CI（0.80, 1.31）；$P=0.86$]获益的证据。

与LU22/NVALT 2/EORTC 08012缺乏有效性相比，一项欧洲独立进行的临床试验更具潜力。Ch. E. S. T.（早期NSCLC化疗临床试验）是一项随机化Ⅲ期临床试验，该研究对比3个周期的新辅助顺铂联合吉西他滨化疗后手术与单纯手术[17]。该研究的终点为无进展生存时间（progress free survial, PFS），并且该研究最初计划随机纳入700例患者。与S9900相似，Ch. E. S. T. 研究在纳入270例患者后因辅助化疗临床试验阳性结果的出现而提前终止。与LU22相比，Ch. E. S. T. 仅纳入ⅠB~ⅢA期患者，IB期患者仅占47%。单纯手术组IB/ⅡA期患者稍多（55% vs 49%）。化疗有效率为35%，PFS和总生存期（overall survial, OS）的HR分别为0.70[95% CI（0.50, 0.97）；$P=0.003$]和0.63[95% CI（0.43, 0.92）；$P=0.02$]，且化疗联合治疗组具有生存获益。ⅡB/ⅢA期亚组具有最大获益（3年PFS率：36.1% vs 55.4%；$P=0.002$），无额外副反应。

NATCH试验是一项Ⅲ期临床试验，该研究直接比较早期可切除NSCLC新辅助化疗联合手术、手术联合辅助化疗以及单纯化疗的作用[14]。624例IA（肿瘤直径>2cm）、IB、Ⅱ或T3N1期患者随机化接受单纯手术、3个周期新辅助紫杉醇+卡铂化疗后手术或手术后行紫杉醇联合卡铂化疗，主要研究终点是无病生存期（DFS）。新辅助组，97%的患者开始预定方案化疗，影像学有效率为53%；辅助化疗组，66%的患者开始预定方案化疗，94%的患者接受手术；三组间的手术过程和术后死亡率相似。与单纯化疗患者相比，新辅助化疗组患者的DFS更长，但无统计学差异（5年DFS 38% vs 34%；HR=0.92；$P=0.176$）；辅助化疗组的5年DFS率为37%，而单纯手术组为34%（HR=0.96；$P=0.74$）。尽管NATCH研究证实多种治疗方案在DFS方面无显著统计学差异，但更趋向于新辅助治疗，与辅助化疗相比，更多患者能接受新辅助化疗。

新辅助化疗的meta分析

考虑到验证新辅助化疗联合手术对比单纯手术的临床试验存在阳性与阴性结果，有时研究早期终止或不足以检测新辅助化疗的获益，因此meta分析就显得异常重要。截至目前，共4项meta分析探讨诱导化疗在可切除NSCLC中的作用，所有来自数据分析而非个体患者数据[6, 44-46]。这些meta分析的结果总结于表19.5。

表 19.5 可手术 NSCLC 新辅助化疗随机临床试验荟萃分析

	Berghmans[44]	Burdett[45]	Gilligan[16]	Song[46]
临床试验数	6	7	8	13
病例数	590	988	1507	3224
风险比	0.66（0.48，0.93）	0.82（0.69，0.97）	0.88（0.76，1.01）	0.84（0.77，0.92）
纳入试验	Dautzenberg[73]	Dautzenberg[73]	Dautzenberg[73]	Dautzenberg[73]
	Rosell[36]	Rosell[36]	Rosell[36]	Rosell[36]
	Roth[35]	Roth[35]	Roth[35]	Roth[35]
	Depierre[41]	Depierre[41]	Depierre[41]	Depierre[41]
	Nagai[39]	Nagai[39]	Nagai[39]	Nagai[39]
	Pass[37]	Sorensen[43]	Sorensen[43]	Sorensen[43]
		Pisters[13]	Pisters[13]	Pisters[13]
			Gilligan[16]	Gilligan[16]
				Zhou[38]
				Liao[74]
				Li[75]
				Yao[76]
				Scagliotti[17]

Berghmans 等进行的第一项 meta 分析纳入 1965 年至 2004 年 6 月所有新辅助与辅助化疗的随机化临床研究[44]。研究发现进行新辅助化疗的 HR 为 0.66［95% CI（0.48，0.93）］，进行辅助化疗的 HR 为 0.84［95% CI（0.78，0.89）］。该 meta 分析中纳入的随机化新辅助方案在上文中已阐述，共纳入 6 项临床试验共 590 例患者。当对临床Ⅲ期 NSCLC 新辅助化疗的有效性进行分析时，HR 变为 0.65［95% CI（0.41，1.04）］，尽管Ⅲ期患者具有采用化疗的较强倾向，但无统计学差异。

Burdett 等进行的第二项 meta 分析数据同样来自于随机化临床试验的摘要或原文[45]，共检索 12 项合格随机对照临床试验，其中 5 项因不能从发表结果中提取足够数据而排除在外。该 meta 分析中剩余 7 项合格临床试验共包括 988 例患者。研究者发现新辅助化疗能提高患者的生存率，［HR = 0.82；95% CI（0.69，0.97）；$P = 0.02$］，等同于 5 年 6% 的净生存获益。同样根据采用的化疗方案进行了一组分析。所有患者接受铂类为基础的化疗——顺铂或卡铂——联合其他药物，其他药物包括：长春碱类或依托泊苷，紫杉类或其他。不同化疗组间疗效无明显差异。作者得出的结论为与未接受新辅助化疗的患者相比，接受新辅助化疗的 NSCLC 患者具有显著生存获益。

考虑到 LU22/NVALT2/EORTC 08012 研究的阴性结果，该研究的作者 Burdett 等更新了 meta 分析的结果。并且添加他们的临床试验并采用摘要统计的方法重新评估 HR。当试验的结果加入 Burdett meta 分析后，新辅助化疗仍有显著总体获益［$P = 0.07$；HR = 0.88；95% CI（0.76，1.01）］，$n = 1507$。

最新 meta 分析与最初 3 个 meta 分析类似，但并非个体患者数据 meta 分析[46]。该研究纳入 Burdett 等采纳的临床试验，并额外加入 6 项。新辅助化疗组 NSCLC 患者的总生存显著优于单纯手术组［混合 HR = 0.84；95% CI（0.77，0.92）；$P = 0.0001$］，$n = 3224$。当仅考虑Ⅲ期 NSCLC 时，结果类似［混合 HR = 0.84；95% CI（0.75，0.95）；$P = 0.005$］。

对手术相关并发症及死亡的影响

所有新辅助化疗对比单纯手术的研究均有一项

高度一致并反复证实的结论，即新辅助化疗不影响手术安排，不增加手术风险。如前详述，多个临床试验均报道患者接受新辅助化疗与接受相同的手术方式（肺叶切除或全肺切除）相比，其完全切除率、手术相关并发症发生率和死亡率相同[14-17]。

独立的回顾性研究同样探讨了这一问题，来自 M. D. 安德森肿瘤中心的 Siegenthaler 等报道了关于 380 例 NSCLC 患者接受肺叶切除或更大范围切除的系列研究。随访除 45 例患者（既往肺癌病史、胸部放疗或放化疗、恶性肿瘤等）外，来自 MDACC 胸外科数据库的 335 例合格病例（259 例行单纯手术，76 例新辅助化疗后手术）纳入该研究。基于临床分期、术后分期或切除程度，新辅助化疗并不影响患者的发病率或死亡率。总体或亚组死亡率或发病率包括肺炎、急性呼吸窘迫综合征、再插管、气管切开、伤口并发症或住院时间均无统计学差异。

MSKCC 对 1993—1999 年所有新辅助化疗后进行开胸手术的患者进行了总结，共纳入 470 例患者，采用单因素及多因素 logistic 回归模型识别副反应相关预测因子。总体而言，MSKCC 手术相关死亡率为 3.8%，显著优于其他初始手术的研究。总体并发症及严重并发症发生率分别为 38% 和 27%，这与既往初始手术的研究相似。作者因此得出结论，采用新辅助化疗并不影响总体并发症发生率。值得注意的是，该研究发现，新辅助化疗后进行右肺全切术患者的手术相关死亡率高达 24%，显著高于既往未采用新辅助化疗相关临床试验的死亡率。因此作者指出，新辅助化疗后必须慎重选择右肺全切术，仅在没有其他可切除办法时才进行。

第 3 项来自法国的系列研究纳入 114 例新辅助化疗后开胸的患者[49]。该研究中，55 例行全肺切除术的患者仅有 1 例死亡。总体并发症发生率为 29%，这与其他手术研究相似。作者因此得出结论：新辅助化疗并不增加术后并发症的发生率和死亡率。

新辅助试验中的替代疗效终点

新辅助化疗的一大优势在于它不仅为Ⅳ期患者，同时还能为较早期的肺癌患者提供新药的测试平台。对于在术前接受化疗的患者，其疗效可通过多种替代疗效终点来进行评价，这些终点主要包括影像学反应、病理学反应及降期。这些评价指标临床易于获得，并可能预测如 PFS 及总生存期在内的远期疗效，而通常这些远期指标需要数年时间来进行评测。另外，在新辅助化疗期间的疗效观察在理论上也能用于筛选需进一步行术后辅助治疗的患者。

问题并不在于在新辅助临床试验中是否应用替代疗效终点，而是在于如何将其作用最优化。而由于在新辅助及Ⅳ期患者中缺乏对影像学疗效、FDG-PET 疗效或病理学疗效的通用定义，因此该问题还有一定的复杂性[50-52]。在Ⅳ期 NSCLC 患者中，影像学反应是评价药物有效最可靠、直观及久经试验的指标，因此在新辅助药物研究中，如实体瘤疗效评价标准（response evaluation criteria in solid tumors，RECIST）标准在内的标准影像学评价标准仍广泛使用[53-54]。然而，评价病理疗效的方法和指标尚未在各个临床试验中标准化[55]。Path CR 表示在手术时未见肿瘤。Path CR 是已获得较好验证的研究终点。法国的两项接受铂类新辅助化疗的连续临床试验中，492 例患者的回顾性分析显示，Path CR 率达到了 8%，可降低 60% 以上的死亡风险［RR = 0.34；95% CI（0.18，0.64）][56]。然而，新辅助临床试验中 Path CR 率仍较低（3%~17%），依赖该疗效终点会错过部分病理有效带来的临床获益[55]。

在 NATCH 试验中，研究人员比较了单独手术、术前卡铂及紫杉醇化疗与术后卡铂及紫杉醇化疗，其 5 年无病生存率在单独手术组为 34%，术前化疗组为 38%，术后化疗组为 37%[14]。术前化疗组中，达到影像学有效的 106 例患者的 5 年无病生存率达到 51%，而达到 Path CR 的 19 例患者的 5 年无病生存率则达到了 59%。该研究并未提供两组间差异的统计学比较。其他多项新辅助化疗的Ⅲ期临床试验也未报道螺旋 CT 显示的新辅助化疗影像学有效率能否预测患者的远期生存获益[15-17]。

在食管 - 胃肿瘤中，FDG-PET 检查被常规用于评价新辅助化疗的疗效[57]。FDG-PET 扫描能否用于评价可切除 NSCLC 新辅助化疗的疗效是一个研究热点。FDG-PET 的主要问题在于缺乏扫描的持续性，标准摄取值（standardized uptake value，SUV）的测量，以及对 PET 反应最佳截断值的争议。最近一篇对 9 项前瞻性研究的综述显示，应用 PET 记录临床有效性或生存期，拥有较为宽泛的有效性、特异度、阳性预测值及阴性预测值[58]。新辅助化疗后对 N2 重新分区的合并数据显示，总灵敏度为 64%［95% CI（53%，74%）］，总特异度为 85%［95% CI（80%，89%）］。作者总结 FDG-PET 在新辅助化疗后重新分区中的作用优于普通 CT，但不可接受的假阳性率及假阴性率使其难以成为评估新辅助化疗疗效的唯一常规工具[58]。CT 扫描、超声内镜引导下活检及纵隔镜检查应被用于明确疗效及降期，特别是当结果会影响下一步手术计划时。除了 FDG-PET，包括 MRI、外周循环肿瘤细胞及其他血清肿瘤标志物检测等新技术，可提高新辅助化疗中新疗法的评估效能[59-60]。

无论何种生物标志物，其作为替代疗效终点指标在预测 NSCLC 手术患者的无病生存期及总生存期上的检测效能不如临床或病理分期稳定，但考虑到新辅助化疗临床试验的结果时，不同分期患者的混合是目前为止影响人群生存期预测的最重要因素。鉴于不同临床及病理分期患者间治疗结局的差异（表 19.1），新辅助化疗临床试验的一个主要问题在于入组时患者模糊或错误的分期。术前应用 FDG-PET、支气管超声内镜活检（明确淋巴结转移）以及纵隔镜（除外淋巴结转移）等技术进行谨慎分期，将会有效避免临床试验及日常临床实践中分期的混乱不清。

除了这些潜在的难以解决的问题，替代疗效终点指标已被证实可有效预测多项新辅助治疗前瞻性研究中患者的总生存期。这些观察指标在分期配对的临床试验中尤其有意义。例如，Betticher 等人报道的 II 期临床试验中，研究人员通过纵隔镜确诊可手术切除的 III A/N2 期 NSCLC 患者，并进行多西他赛/顺铂方案的新辅助化疗[61]。在 75 例化疗后成功进行手术的患者中，一些因素与总生存期及无病生存期密切相关，这些因素包括完全（R0）切除、影像学疗效、病理学疗效以及纵隔降期。这些替代疗效终点指标在后续的新辅助研究中仍有重要作用。

机会试验窗

迄今为止，肺癌药物治疗最重要的发现是 *EGFR* 突变阳性的 IV 期 NSCLC 患者口服表皮生长因子受体（EGFR）酪氨酸激酶抑制剂的疗效显著优于传统化疗[62]，该内容已在本书其他章节中详细阐述。不吸烟或既往少量吸烟者、女性、亚裔、腺癌 IV 期患者的 *EGFR* 阳性突变率更高。

继这项发现之后不久，一项在 MSKCC 进行的 II 期临床试验检测了早期 NSCLC 中 EGFR-TKI 药物，吉非替尼的疗效[63]。吸烟指数小于 15 的 I 期及 II 期手术切除 NSCLC 患者在术前接受 21d 的吉非替尼。吉非替尼治疗期间评价影像学疗效，并分析相关分子标志物。共有 50 例 I、II 期患者接受治疗。在术前 21d 的吉非替尼治疗结束后，50 例患者中有 21 例（42%）可观测到 25% 及以上的有效性。21 例有效患者中有 17 例表达 *EGFR* 突变，而其余 4 例则没有突变（$P = 0.0001$）。对吉非替尼治疗有影像学疗效或表达 *EGFR* 阳性突变的半数患者术后继续服用吉非替尼。中位随访时间为 44.1 个月，并未达到中位无病生存及总生存，各临床亚组间的 2 年无病生存期未见显著差异（如 *EGFR* 突变/未突变，辅助吉非替尼组）。因此作者总结新辅助治疗为早期 NSCLC 新药应用提供了新的平台。

由荷兰 4 家医院进行的另一项 II 期临床试验纳入 60 例可手术的早期 NSCLC 患者，并在术前给予 3 周的厄洛替尼[64]，同时应用 PET 扫描、CT 扫描及切除标本的组织学检查来评价治疗效果。PET 扫描显示 16 例患者代谢改变（下降幅度 >25% 标准摄取值）；CT 扫描显示 3 例（5%）患者有 CT 图像改变；而组织病理学检查显示 14 例（23%）患者中有超过 50% 的部位坏死，而其中 3 例（5%）有 95% 以上的组织坏死。在 *EGFR* 突变阳性或突变阴性的患者中均可观察到影像学或组织学获益的证据。作者总结新辅助治疗平台应对早期患者研制新药，特别是明显有效且低毒性的治疗方式至关重要。

另一项 IV 期 NSCLC 患者的治疗进展是贝伐单抗的应用。贝伐单抗作为一类单克隆抗体可直接阻断血管生成蛋白-血管内皮生长因子（VEGF）。

在Ⅳ期非鳞状细胞癌的 NSCLC 患者中，贝伐单抗联合化疗能显著提高患者的总生存期[65]。在 MSKCC 中研究新辅助吉非替尼的同一研究团队也在早期 NSCLC 患者中评估了贝伐单抗联合顺铂或多西他赛方案新辅助化疗的有效性及安全性，并对特定患者给予术后辅助治疗[66]。该研究的另一项新意是其在第 1 个周期给予贝伐单抗单药治疗，并评估了贝伐单抗单药治疗的影像学评效。由于顾及抗血管药物可能影响伤口愈合，患者在其新辅助化疗最后一个周期中停用贝伐单抗以便术前清除体内残留药物。该研究的主要观察终点是病理降期（术前临床至术后病理分期的下降），共纳入 50 例患者，34 例（68%）为临床ⅢA 期。主要研究终点——分期下降率为 38%［95% CI（23%，53%）］，这并未达到预先设定的 50% 的标准[66]（N. A. Rizvi，个人交流）。次级观察终点包括对化疗的影像学反应率（45%），术前并发症发生率（12%）与历史数据相当。单药贝伐单抗未能达到部分缓解，但 18% 的患者出现瘤内空洞并有病理有效的趋势（57% vs 21%；$P = 0.07$）。病理有效率与 3 年生存率相关（100% vs 49%；$P = 0.01$）。KRAS 突变 NSCLC 均未见病理缓解（1/10），而突变型 KRAS 缓解率则为 11/31。作者因此总结贝伐单抗联合化疗的新辅助治疗并不推荐在未经选择的患者中应用。

Jones 等完成了一项有关可手术的 NSCLC 患者术前新辅助 vorinostat（组蛋白去甲基化抑制剂）联合硼替佐米（蛋白酶抑制剂）的Ⅰ期临床试验[67]。21 例患者纳入研究，其中 20 例接受手术治疗。硼替佐米的最大可耐受剂量为 $1.3 mg/m^2$，伏立诺他 300mg，每天 2 次。治疗后 30% 的患者（6/20）瘤体内出现 60% 以上区域的组织学坏死，其中 2 例存在≥90% 区域的组织学坏死。实验室检查包括肿瘤转移测定、20S 蛋白酶活性、特定蛋白表达以及治疗前后基因表达序列分析。作者得出结论：术前采用这些靶向药物治疗可行，并可作为一个用于检测上述药物对细胞信号通路影响的平台。

Altoriki 等对 29 例术前接受两个周期紫杉醇联合卡铂方案化疗的 IB～ⅢA 期 NSCLC 患者，术后每天给予塞来昔布治疗[68]。总体临床有效率为 65%（48% 部分缓解，17% 完全缓解）；18 例（62%）患者出现Ⅲ度或Ⅳ度中性粒细胞减低；28 例患者肿瘤完全切除。与单纯紫杉醇联合卡铂方案相比，在紫杉醇及卡铂方案治疗后使用塞来昔布，原发灶 PGE2 水平显著提高。作者得出结论：化疗联合 COX2 抑制剂是未来治疗的保证，但是一项 Ⅳ期 NSCLC 患者相关的Ⅲ期临床试验中塞来昔布活性消失使得对该通路研究的热情下降[69-70]。

Altorki 等的另一项研究中，早期可切除 NSCLC 接受口服抗血管生存抑制剂——帕唑帕尼[71]。患者随机至口服治疗组，术前接受帕唑帕尼 800mg，每天 1 次，治疗 2～6 周。共纳入 35 例患者，33 例（94%）为临床Ⅰ期 NSCLC，2 例（6%）为临床Ⅱ期 NSCLC。中位治疗持续时间为 16d（3～29d）。30 例（86%）患者给予帕唑帕尼治疗后出现影像学肿瘤体积减小。2 例患者的肿瘤体积缩小≥50%，3 例患者依据 RECIST 评效为 PR（partial response）。帕唑帕尼耐受性良好，高血压、腹泻和疲乏的发生率与预期一致。1 例患者术后 11d 发生肺栓塞。治疗后数个帕唑帕尼基因及其他血管生存因子出现异常调整。连续血浆细胞因子分析证实术后血浆中 SVEGFR2 及白介素 - 4（IL - 4）变化与肿瘤退缩显著相关。基线白介素 - 12（IL - 12）及数个其他细胞因子与肿瘤退缩相关。采用多因素分析方法，由肝细胞生长因子及 IL - 12 构成的基线特征与肿瘤对帕唑帕尼的反应相关，并且其预测准确性高达 81%。作者认为未来需采用更简单的平台评估帕唑帕尼的临床疗效。

总 结

自 19 世纪 80 年代以来大量针对可切除 NSCLC 术前新辅助化疗的Ⅱ期及Ⅲ期临床试验公布，尚无研究证实对于Ⅰ～Ⅱ期 NSCLC 具有显著统计学差异生存获益。多项Ⅲ期、随机化新辅助化疗相关临床试验在 2003 年辅助化疗确认具有生存获益后提前终止。即便如此，部分基本情况已达成一致。

所有前瞻性Ⅲ期临床试验均证实新辅助化疗与手术间无相互干扰，两组间的 R0 切除率、手术并发症发生率及死亡率无显著差异[14-17]。新辅助化疗后手术是纵隔镜证实可切除ⅢA/N2期NSCLC的标准治疗方法[35-36]。N2期患者是否行新辅助化疗尚存在争议，其他章节将会对该内容进行阐述。至于meta分析，新辅助化疗与辅助化疗的获益相似[46]。与辅助化疗类似，新辅助化疗的主要获益者为临床Ⅱ~Ⅲ期NSCLC。仅有一项小样本研究直接对比新辅助化疗与辅助化疗，新辅助化疗的有效率似乎更高，药物弥散性更好。

对比新辅助化疗与辅助化疗的随机化临床试验是明确这一问题的关键。然而，这一方案难以施行。已有证据表明内科医生及患者选择性较强，因此很难接受随机化治疗方案。部分外科医生及患者希望尽快进行肺癌切除，以避免延误手术时机。另外一部分临床医生关注于术后较高的肺癌术后复发风险——尤其是巨大肿瘤或术前EBUS证实的N1期患者，对于这部分患者，更推荐进行术后辅助化疗。

最后，也许是最重要的，新辅助机会窗试验可作为可切除NSCLC患者的新药检测平台，采用足够有效的终点如影像学有效率、病理反应率及降期等。可切除Ⅱ~Ⅲ期NSCLC患者顺铂辅助化疗方案可延长生存时间的结论历经8年，共纳入4 500例患者才得以最终证实。随着药物的快速更新，Ⅳ期NSCLC患者的化疗新药不断涌现，可切除NSCLC患者不可接受的较高的复发和死亡风险下降，筛查所伴随的可手术NSCLC患者增加。临床医生必须尽快开发新型新辅助平台，发现新型标志物及治疗策略以促进可切除NSCLC患者新药的发现。在头对头辅助化疗临床试验中检测所有新型、更有效的药物是很难实现的，值得高兴的是，有证据表明新辅助化疗用于检测上述药物也是允许的。

（危志刚　译）

参考文献

[1] Siegel R, Naishadham D, Jemal A. Cancer statistics, 2012. CA Cancer J Clin, 2012, 62: 10-29.

[2] Govindan R, Page N, Morgenszstern D, et al. Changing epidemiology of small-cell lung cancer in the United States over the last 30 years: analysis of the surveillance, epidemiologic, and end results database. J Clin Oncol, 2006, 24: 4539-4544.

[3] Aberle DR, Adams AM, Berg CD, et al. Reduced lung-cancer mortality with low-dose computed tomographic screening. N Engl J Med, 2011, 365: 395-409.

[4] Bach PB, Mirkin JN, Oliver TK, et al. Benefits and harms of CT screening for lung cancer: a systematic review. Jama, 2012, 307: 2418-2429.

[5] Goldstraw P, Crowley J, Chansky K, et al. The IASLC Lung Cancer Staging Project: Proposals for the revision of the TNM stage groupings in the forthcoming (seventh) edition of the TNM Classification of malignant tumours. J Thorac Oncol, 2007, 2: 706-714.

[6] Chemotherapy in non-small-cell lung cancer: A meta analysis using updated data on individual patients from 52 randomised clinical trials. Non-small Cell Lung Cancer Collaborative Group. BMJ, 311: 899-909.

[7] Arriagada R, Dunant A, Pignon JP, et al. Longterm results of the international adjuvant lung cancer trial evaluating adjuvant Cisplatin-based chemotherapy in resected lung cancer. J Clin Oncol, 2010, 28: 35-42.

[8] Winton T, Livingston R, Johnson D, et al. Vinorelbine plus cisplatin vs. observation in resected non-small-cell lung cancer. N Engl J Med, 2005, 352: 2589-2597.

[9] Douillard JY, Rosell R, De Lena M, et al. Adjuvant vinorelbine plus cisplatin versus observation in patients with completely resected stage IB-ⅢA nons-mall-cell lung cancer [Adjuvant Navelbine International Trialist Association (ANITA)]: A randomised controlled trial. Lancet Oncol, 2006, 7: 719-727.

[10] Pignon JP, Tribodet H, Scagliotti GV, et al. Lung adjuvant cisplatin evaluation: A pooled analysis by the LACE Collaborative Group. J Clin Oncol, 2008, 26: 3552-3559.

[11] Dillman RO, Herndon J, Seagren SL, et al. Improved survival in stage Ⅲ non-small-cell lung cancer: seven-year follow-up of cancer and leukemia group B (CALGB) 8433 trial. J Natl Cancer Inst, 1996, 88: 1210-1215.

[12] Sause WT, Scott C, Taylor S, et al. Radiation Therapy Oncology Group (RTOG) 88-08 and Eastern Cooperative Oncology Group (ECOG) 4588: Preliminary results of a phase Ⅲ trial in regionally advanced, unresectable non-small-cell lung cancer. J Natl Cancer Inst, 1995, 87: 198-205.

[13] Pisters KM, Ginsberg RJ, Giroux DJ, et al. Induction chemotherapy before surgery for earlystage lung cancer: A

novel approach. Bimodality Lung Oncology Team. J Thorac Cardiovasc Surg, 2000, 119: 429 - 439.

[14] Felip E, Rosell R, Maestre JA, et al. Preoperative chemotherapy plus surgery versus surgery plus adjuvant chemotherapy versus surgery alone in early-stage non-small-cell lung cancer. J Clin Oncol, 2010, 28: 3138 - 3145.

[15] Pisters KM, Vallieres E, Crowley JJ, et al. Surgery with or without preoperative paclitaxel and carboplatin in early-stage non-small-cell lung cancer: Southwest Oncology Group Trial S9900, an intergroup, randomized, phase III trial. J Clin Oncol, 2010, 28: 1843 - 1849.

[16] Gilligan D, Nicolson M, Smith I, et al. Preoperative chemotherapy in patients with resectable non-small cell lung cancer: Results of the MRC LU22/NVALT 2/EORTC 08012 multicentre randomised trial and update of systematic review. Lancet, 2007, 369: 1929 - 1937.

[17] Scagliotti GV, Pastorino U, Vansteenkiste JF, et al. Randomized phase III study of surgery alone or surgery plus preoperative cisplatin and gemcitabine in stages IB to IIIA non-small-cell lung cancer. J Clin Oncol, 2012, 30: 172 - 178.

[18] Martini N, Flehinger BJ, Zaman MB, et al. Prospective study of 445 lung carcinomas with mediastinal lymph node metastases. JThoracCardiovasc Surg, 1980, 80: 390 - 399.

[19] Martini N, Kris MG, Flehinger BJ, et al. Preoperative chemotherapy for stage IIIa (N2) lung cancer: The Sloan-Kettering experience with 136 patients. Ann Thorac Surg, 1993, 55: 1365 - 1373; discussion 1373 - 1374.

[20] Burkes RL, Shepherd FA, Blackstein ME, et al. Induction chemotherapy with mitomycin, vindesine, and cisplatin for stage IIIA (T1 - 3, N2) unresectable non-small-cell lung cancer: final results of the Toronto phase II trial. Lung Cancer, 2005, 47: 103 - 109.

[21] Albain KS, Rusch VW, Crowley JJ, et al. Concurrent cisplatin/etoposide plus chest radiotherapy followed by surgery for stages IIIA (N2) and IIIB non-small-cell lung cancer: mature results of Southwest Oncology Group phase II study 8805. J Clin Oncol, 1995, 13: 1880 - 1892.

[22] Elias AD, Skarin AT, Leong T, et al. Neoadjuvant therapy for surgically staged IIIA N2 non-small cell lung cancer (NSCLC). Lung Cancer, 1997, 17: 147 - 161.

[23] Betticher DC, Hsu Schmitz SF, Totsch M, et al. Mediastinal lymph node clearance after docetaxelcisplatin neoadjuvant chemotherapy is prognostic of survival in patients with stage IIIA pN2 non-small-cell lung cancer: A multicenter phase II trial. J Clin Oncol, 2003, 21: 1752 - 1759.

[24] Eberhardt W, Wilke H, Stamatis G, et al. Preoperative chemotherapy followed by concurrent chemoradiation therapy based on hyperfractionated accelerated radiotherapy and definitive surgery in locally advanced non-small-cell lung cancer: mature results of a phase II trial. J Clin Oncol, 1998, 16: 622 - 634.

[25] Van Zandwijk N, Smit EF, Kramer GW, et al. Gemcitabine and cisplatin as induction regimen for patients with biopsy-proven stage IIIA N2 non-small-cell lung cancer: a phase II study of the European Organization for Research and Treatment of Cancer Lung Cancer Cooperative Group (EORTC 08955). J Clin Oncol, 2000, 18: 2658 - 2664.

[26] Migliorino MR, De Marinis F, Nelli F, et al. A 3-week schedule of gemcitabine plus cisplatin as induction chemotherapy for Stage III non-small cell lung cancer. Lung Cancer, 2002, 35: 319 - 327.

[27] Garrido P, Gonzalez-Larriba JL, Insa A, et al. Long-term survival associated with complete resection after induction chemotherapy in stage IIIA (N2) and IIIB (T4N0-1) non small-cell lung cancer patients: the Spanish Lung Cancer Group Trial 9901. J Clin Oncol, 2007, 25: 4736 - 4742.

[28] Esteban E, de Sande JL, Villanueva N, et al. Cisplatin plus gemcitabine with or without vinorelbine as induction chemotherapy prior to radical locoregional treatment for patients with stage III non-small-cell lung cancer (NSCLC): Results of a prospective randomized study. Lung Cancer, 2007, 55: 173 - 180.

[29] Lorent N, De Leyn P, Lievens Y, et al. Longterm survival of surgically staged IIIA-N2 non-small-cell lung cancer treated with surgical combined modality approach: analysis of a 7-year prospective experience. Ann Oncol, 2004, 15: 1645 - 1653.

[30] Cappuzzo F, De Marinis F, Nelli F, et al. Phase II study of gemcitabine-cisplatin-paclitaxel triplet as induction chemotherapy in inoperable, locallyadvanced non-small cell lung cancer. Lung Cancer, 2003, 42: 355 - 361.

[31] De Marinis F, Nelli F, Migliorino MR, et al. Gemcitabine, paclitaxel, and cisplatin as induction chemotherapy for patients with biopsy-proven Stage IIIA (N2) nonsmall cell lung carcinoma: A Phase II multicenter study. Cancer, 2003, 98: 1707 - 1715.

[32] Kunitoh H, Kato H, Tsuboi M, et al. A randomised phase II trial of preoperative chemotherapy of cisplatin-docetaxel or docetaxel alone for clinical stage IB/II non-small-cell lung cancer results of a Japan Clinical Oncology Group trial (JCOG 0204). Br J Cancer, 2008, 99: 852–857.

[33] Abratt RP, Lee JS, Han JY, et al. Phase II trial of gemcitabine-carboplatin-paclitaxel as neoadjuvant chemotherapy for operable non-small-cell lung cancer. J Thorac Oncol, 2006, 1: 135–140.

[34] Ramnath N, Sommers E, Robinson L, et al. Phase II study of neoadjuvant chemotherapy with gemcitabine and vinorelbine in resectable non-small-cell lung cancer. Chest, 2005, 128: 3467–3474.

[35] Roth JA, Atkinson EN, Fossella F, et al. Longterm follow-up of patients enrolled in a randomized trial comparing perioperative chemotherapy and surgery with surgery alone in resectable stage IIIA non-small-cell lung cancer. Lung Cancer, 1998, 21: 1–6.

[36] Rosell R, Gomez-Codina J, Camps C, et al. Preresectional chemotherapy in stage IIIA non-small-cell lung cancer: A 7-year assessment of a randomized controlled trial. Lung Cancer, 1999, 26: 7–14.

[37] Pass HI, Pogrebniak HW, Steinberg SM, et al. Randomized trial of neoadjuvant therapy for lung cancer: interim analysis. Ann Thorac Surg, 1992, 53: 992–998.

[38] Zhou Q, Liu L, Li L, et al. A randomized clinical trial of preoperative neoadjuvant chemotherapy followed by surgery in the treatment of stage III non-small-cell lung cancer. Lung Cancer, 2003, 41: S45–S46.

[39] Nagai K, Tsuchiya R, Mori T, et al. A randomized trial comparing induction chemotherapy followed by surgery with surgery alone for patients with stage IIIA N2 non-small cell lung cancer (JCOG 9209). J Thorac Cardiovasc Surg, 2003, 125: 254–260.

[40] de Boer RH, Smith IE, Pastorino U, et al. Preoperative chemotherapy in early stage resectable nonsmall-cell lung cancer: a randomized feasibility study justifying a multicentre phase III trial. Br J Cancer, 1999, 79: 1514–1518.

[41] Depierre A, Milleron B, Moro-Sibilot D, et al. Preoperative chemotherapy followed by surgery compared with primary surgery in resectable stage I (except T1N0), II, and IIIa non-small-cell lung cancer. J Clin Oncol, 2002, 20: 247–253.

[42] Depierre A, Westeel V, Milleron B, et al. 5-year results of the French randomized study comparing preoperative chemotherapy followed by surgery and primary surgery in resectable stage I (except T1N0), II and IIIA non-small cell lung cancer. Lung Cancer, 2003, 41: S62.

[43] Sorensen J, Riska H, Ravn J, et al. Scandinavian phase III trial of neoadjuvant chemotherapy in NSCLC stages IB-IIIA/T3. J Clin Oncol, 2005, 23.

[44] Berghmans T, Paesmans M, Meert AP, et al. Survival improvement in resectable non-small cell lung cancer with (neo) adjuvant chemotherapy: results of a meta-analysis of the literature. Lung Cancer, 2005, 49: 13–23.

[45] Burdett S, Stewart LA, Rydzewska L. A systematic review and meta-analysis of the literature: Chemotherapy and surgery versus surgery alone in non-small cell lung cancer. J Thorac Oncol, 2006, 1: 611–621.

[46] Song WA, Zhou NK, Wang W, et al. Survival benefit of neoadjuvant chemotherapy in non-small cell lung cancer: an updated meta-analysis of 13 randomized control trials. J Thorac Oncol, 2010, 5: 510–516.

[47] Siegenthaler MP, Pisters KM, Merriman KW, et al. Preoperative chemotherapy for lung cancer does not increase surgical morbidity. Ann Thorac Surg, 2001, 71: 1105–1111; discussion 1111–1112.

[48] Martin J, Ginsberg RJ, Abolhoda A, et al. Morbidity and mortality after neoadjuvant therapy for lung cancer: the risks of right pneumonectomy. Ann Thorac Surg, 2001, 72: 1149–1154.

[49] Perrot E, Guibert B, Mulsant P, et al. Preoperative chemotherapy does not increase complications after nonsmall cell lung cancer resection. Ann Thorac Surg, 2005, 80: 423–427.

[50] Mandrekar SJ, Qi Y, Hillman SL, et al. Endpoints in phase II trials for advanced non-small cell lung cancer. J Thorac Oncol, 2010, 5: 3–9.

[51] Soria JC, Massard C, Le Chevalier T. Should progression-free survival be the primary measure of efficacy for advanced NSCLC therapy? Ann Oncol, 2010, 21: 2324–2332.

[52] Lara PN, Jr., Redman MW, Kelly K, et al. Disease control rate at 8 weeks predicts clinical benefit in advanced non-small-cell lung cancer: Results from Southwest Oncology Group randomized trials. J Clin Oncol, 2008, 26: 463–467.

[53] Oxnard GR, Morris MJ, Hodi FS, et al. When progressive disease does not mean treatment failure: reconsidering the criteria for progression. J Natl Cancer Inst,

[54] Eisenhauer EA, Therasse P, Bogaerts J, et al. New response evaluation criteria in solid tumours: revised RECIST guideline (version 1.1). Eur J Cancer, 2009, 45: 228–247.

[55] Pataer A, Kalhor N, Correa AM, et al. Histopathologic response criteria predict survival of patients with resected lung cancer after neoadjuvant chemotherapy. J Thorac Oncol, 2012, 7: 825–832.

[56] Mouillet G, Monnet E, Milleron B, et al. Pathologic complete response to preoperative chemotherapy predicts cure in early-stage non-small-cell lung cancer: combined analysis of two IFCT randomized trials. J Thorac Oncol, 2012, 7: 841–849.

[57] Lordick F, Ott K, Krause BJ, et al. PET to assess early metabolic response and to guide treatment of adenocarcinoma of the oesophagogastric junction: The MUNICON phase II trial. Lancet Oncol, 2007, 8: 797–805.

[58] Rebollo-Aguirre AC, Ramos-Font C, Villegas Portero R, et al. Is FDG-PET suitable for evaluating neoadjuvant therapy in non-small cell lung cancer? Evidence with systematic review of the literature. J Surg Oncol, 2010, 101: 486–494.

[59] Ohno Y, Koyama H, Yoshikawa T, et al. Diffusion-weighted MRI versus 18F-FDG PET/CT: performance as predictors of tumor treatment response and patient survival in patients with non-small celllung cancer receiving chemoradiotherapy. AJR Am J Roentgenol, 2012, 198: 75–82.

[60] Punnoose EA, Atwal S, Liu W, et al. Evaluation of circulating tumor cells and circulating tumor DNA in non-small cell lung cancer: association with clinical endpoints in a phase II clinical trial of pertuzumab and erlotinib. Clin Cancer Res, 2012, 18: 2391–2401.

[61] Betticher DC, Hsu Schmitz SF, Totsch M, et al. Prognostic factors affecting long-term outcomes in patients with resected stage IIIA pN2 non-small-cell lung cancer: 5-year follow-up of a phase II study. Br J Cancer, 2006, 94: 1099–1106.

[62] Mok TS, Wu YL, Thongprasert S, et al. Gefitinib or carboplatin-paclitaxel in pulmonary adenocarcinoma. N Engl J Med, 2009, 361: 947–957.

[63] Rizvi NA, Rusch V, Pao W, et al. Molecular characteristics predict clinical outcomes: prospective trial correlating response to the EGFR tyrosine kinase inhibitor gefitinib with the presence of sensitizing mutations in the tyrosine binding domain of the EGFR gene. Clin Cancer Res, 2011, 17: 3500–3506.

[64] Schaake EE, Kappers I, Codrington HE, et al. Tumor response and toxicity of neoadjuvant erlotinib in patients with early-stage non-small-cell lung cancer. J Clin Oncol, 2012, 30: 2731–2738.

[65] Sandler A, Gray R, Perry MC, et al. Paclitaxelcarboplatin alone or with bevacizumab for non-small-cell lung cancer. N Engl J Med, 2006, 355: 2542–2550.

[66] Price K, Kris MG, Rusch V, et al. Phase II study of induction and adjuvant bevacizumab in patients with stage IB-IIIA non-small cell lung cancer (NSCLC) receiving induction docetaxel and cisplatin. J Clin Oncol, (abstract 7531), 2009, 27.

[67] Jones DR, Moskaluk CA, Gillenwater HH, et al. Phase I trial of induction histone deacetylase and proteasome inhibition followed by surgery in non-small-cell lung cancer. J Thorac Oncol, 2012, 7: 1683–1690.

[68] Altorki NK, Keresztes RS, Port JL, et al. Celecoxib, a selective cyclo-oxygenase-2 inhibitor, enhances the response to preoperative paclitaxel and carboplatin in early-stage non-small-cell lung cancer. J Clin Oncol, 2003, 21: 2645–2650.

[69] Groen HJ, Sietsma H, Vincent A, et al. Randomized, placebo-controlled phase III study of docetaxel plus carboplatin with celecoxib and cyclooxygenase-2 expression as a biomarker for patients with advanced non-small-cell lung cancer: The NVALT-4 study. J Clin Oncol, 2011, 29: 4320–4326.

[70] Koch A, Bergman B, Holmberg E, et al. Effect of celecoxib on survival in patients with advanced nonsmall cell lung cancer: A double blind randomised clinical phase III trial (CYCLUS study) by the Swedish Lung Cancer Study Group. Eur J Cancer, 2011, 47: 1546–1555.

[71] Altorki N, Lane ME, Bauer T, et al. Phase II proof-of-concept study of pazopanib monotherapy in treatment-naive patients with stage I/II resectable non-small-cell lung cancer. J Clin Oncol, 2010, 28: 3131–3137.

[72] Nikolinakos PG, Altorki N, Yankelevitz D, et al. Plasma cytokine and angiogenic factor profiling identifies markers associated with tumor shrinkage in earlystage non-small cell lung cancer patients treated with pazopanib. Cancer Res, 2010, 70: 2171–2179.

[73] Dautzenberg B, Benichou J, Allard P, et al. Failure of the perioperative PCV neoadjuvant polychemotherapy in resectable bronchogenic non-small cell carcinoma. Re-

sults from a randomized phase II trial. Cancer, 1990, 65: 2435-2441.

[74] Liao ML, Zhou YZ, Ding JA, et al. The study of peri-operative chemotherapy in stage I-IIIa NSCLC. Zhonghua Yi Xue Za Zhi, 2003, 83: 962-966.

[75] Li Q, Song YH, Zheng ZY. Clinical evaluation of preoperative short course chemotherapy in treatment of stage III non-small cell lung cancer. Chin J Cancer Prev Treat, 2005, 10: 505-507.

[76] Yao K, Xiang MZ, Min JX. A randomized clinical trial of preoperative neoadjuvant chemotherapy in the treatment of stage III non-small cell lung cancer. J Clin Oncol China, 2004, 31: 611-613

第 20 章
图像引导的放射治疗

Kenneth E. Rosenzweig, Sonal Sura
Department of Radiation Oncology, Icahn School of Medicine at Mount Sinai, New York, NY, USA

引　言

非小细胞肺癌（NSCLC）有两种主要的治疗方法：早期肺癌立体定向放射治疗（stereotactic body radiation therapy，SBRT）和局部晚期肺癌放化疗。

美国肿瘤放射治疗协作组织（the Radiation Therapy Oncology Group，RTOG）0236 试验彻底证实了 SBRT 的临床疗效，RTOG 0236 试验是一项多中心 II 期临床研究，该研究证实 I 期 NSCLC 不可手术患者的 3 年肿瘤局部控制率达到 97.6%[1]。SBRT 的特点是在每分次放疗中给予很高的剂量。RTOG 0236 试验采用每分次 18Gy（校正密度异质性）至少隔天 1 次的治疗方案。由于该方案剂量大且治疗次数较少（共 3~5 次），许多中心采用图像引导放疗（intensity modulated radiation therapy，IGRT）来保证治疗的精确性。

局部晚期 NSCLC 患者的放疗往往分次多、治疗时间长，其局部控制率和生存率仍然是主要的挑战。虽然有三维适形放疗（three-dimensional conformal radiation therapy，3D-CRT）和调强放疗（intensity modulated radiation therapy，IMRT）这样的新技术出现[2-8]，但是据报道其 2 年局部失败率仍然在 22%~50%[4,7]。最近，RTOG 0617 试验报道了其初步研究结果，该试验比较了 60Gy 和 74Gy 同步化疗联合或不联合西妥昔单抗治疗局部晚期 NSCLC 的疗效。74Gy 试验组的总生存率和局部控制率均不如 60Gy 标准剂量组。74Gy 组和 60Gy 组的局部失败率分别是 34% 和 25%[9]。

传统上肿瘤的大小、位置、几何结构、患者的解剖结构都是通过治疗前的 X 线透视或静态 CT 扫描来确定。然而，传统的成像形式如 CT 并不能使疾病充分可视化。一项改善肿瘤界线的措施是将 FDG-PET 扫描引入治疗计划。这样，既提供了肿瘤的解剖图像也提供了代谢图像。

胸部肿瘤放疗的另一个挑战是呼吸过程中肿瘤和周期正常器官的运动。不论是从定位扫描到实际治疗时还是每分次放疗过程中，运动都会改变肿瘤的确切位置。

IGRT 指治疗开始前在放射治疗室中获取图像。这些图像是 CT 扫描的三维图像或 X 线产生的二维图像，以骨骼、解剖结构、肿瘤内或周围的标记物为辅助标志[10]。现在有许多技术可以提供这样的图像。

传统模拟定位方式与基于 CT 的模拟定位方式对比

在现代放疗中，随着 CT 模拟定位机的引入，放射肿瘤学领域已经从二维治疗计划时代跨越到三维时代。Chen 等人回顾性分析了 SEER 数据库中行根治性放疗的 III 期 NSCLC 患者。他们报道了 3D-CRT 应用的快速趋势：在 1994 年，该根治性放疗的患者中有 2.4% 采用 3D-CRT，到 2000 年达到了 34%，而到 2005 年研究结束时，3D-CRT 的使用率已经增长到了 77.4%。从统计学和临床角度，CT 模拟定位比传统模拟定位拥有更低的死亡率（$P<0.01$）[11]。

PET 和 PET-CT 在放疗计划中的应用

肺癌放疗计划制订过程中的一个重要步骤是

肿瘤的精确勾画。局部晚期肺癌患者的病灶常常不能被 CT 检测到,而在 PET 图像上会因为发生形变不能准确地反映肿瘤区域。有研究对比了 PET 图像、手术和纵隔镜检测纵隔淋巴结病变及分期情况。在两项 meta 分析中,PET 检测 NSCLC 淋巴结分期的灵敏度和特异度分别为 84%~88% 和 89%~92%[12-13]。多项研究表明 PET 有很好的淋巴结阴性预测值,其范围在 87%~100%[14-16],而淋巴结阳性预测值则低于 80%[14,16-17]。Li 等的多中心研究入组了 200 例术前行 FDG PET-CT 扫描的肺癌患者,用组织病理学来检测 PET-CT 淋巴结预测的准确性。结果表明,PET-CT 预测纵隔淋巴结转移的特异度达到 83%,阴性预测值达到 91%。结论:PET-CT 上纵隔淋巴结转移的阴性结果是作为单独用 SBRT 初始治疗肿瘤的充分证据[18]。

FDG-PET 图像应用于放疗计划的效应/价值已经得到研究(图 20.1)。为评估基于 CT 或 X 线图像制订放疗计划的放射野覆盖度,Kiffer 等人将以隆突为基准点将 PET 图像和前后方位模拟定位图像进行配准。在基于 AP 图像制订放疗计划的 15 例患者中,有 4 例患者的放射野覆盖不充分,原因是 PET 检测到的异常纵隔淋巴结没有在 CT 上呈现[19]。Munley 等的一系列研究表明,当把 PET 和 CT 结合起来定义靶区时,PET 使 34% 患者的靶区(在射束孔径方向)增加 15mm[20]。Nestle 等回顾性评估了 PET 改变 AP/PA 方向靶区的大小。35% 的患者初始 CT 方案的靶区体积或形状发生改变,多数是体积的缩小,并且多数发生在肺不张患者中[21]。Schmuecking 等报道,由于 PET 数据引入计划系统后,能够明显区分肿瘤组织和肺不张,能使计划靶体积(plan target volum, PTV)降低 21%,这能明显降低正常肺组织的受照体积(V_{20})[22]。Hellwig 等报道,由于 FDG 能明显区分转移淋巴结,故 PET-CT 能明显改变照射野的大小。CT 检测纵隔淋巴结转移的灵敏度是 56%,而 PET-CT 对所有分期检测的灵敏度是 83%,当 CT 显示淋巴结增大时,PET 检测的灵敏度是 91%,对正常大小淋巴结,检测的灵敏度是 70%[23]。在一篇关于 PET-CT 在 NSCLC 放疗计划中应用的综述中,进一步强调了 PET-CT 在制订更精确放疗计划中的地位[24]。

在放疗计划的制订中使用软件配准的 PET-CT 图像也得到了广泛的研究。Caldwell 等评估了 30 例接受根治性放疗的 NSCLC 患者,这些患者的 CT 扫描都显示有肺不张。大多数患者在 PET 和 CT 融合图像上勾画的 PTV 都比单独用 CT 勾画的 PTV 小,这能明显降低正常肺组织和脊髓的受量[25]。在一项包含 11 例 NSCLC 患者的研究中,Erdi 等发现,在所有患者中,配准后的 PET-CT 都能明显改变原来在 CT 上勾画的 PTV。体积的增加是因为检测到了 CT 上没有检测到的阳性淋巴结,体积的降低是因为肺不张组织的排除[26]。Bradley 等研究了在 CT 和 PET-CT 融合图像上勾画的 GTV 的差异。在 24 例接受 3D-CRT 放疗的患者中,有 14 例因为 PET 信息的引入,改变了其肿瘤和淋巴结区域的勾画,其中有 2 例患者的临床靶区(clinical target volume, CTV)降低,原因是 PET 从肿瘤区域中区分出了肺不张组织。在这些患者中,预测正常组织毒性的参数,如肺平均受量(mean Lung dose, MLD)、食管平均受量(mean esophageal dose, MED)和接受剂量 >20Gy 的体积(V20)也相应降低,理论上降低了放射性肺炎和放射性食管炎的发生风险[27]。Giraud 等将双探头符合线路显像得到的 PET 图像与定位 CT 图像以体外标记点为基

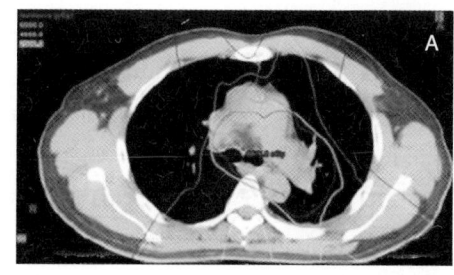 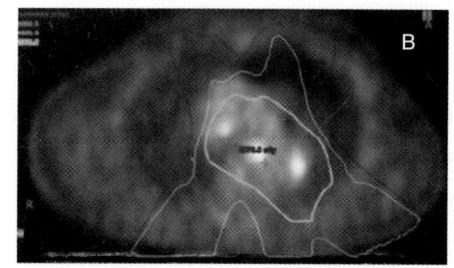

图 20.1(见彩插) 一例患有ⅢB 期不可手术 NSCLC 的 62 岁女性患者。该部位安全地接受了 60Gy/30f 剂量。治疗计划基于 PET-CT 融合图像制定。A. 计划 CT 的一个层面,PTV 以红色勾画。B. 相同层面的 FDG-PET 图像。6 000cGy、4 000cGy、2 000cGy 等剂量线分别以绿色、蓝绿色和蓝色标注

准进行融合，也得到与这些研究相一致的结果[28]。以上各项研究表明，PET 的应用能够潜在改善患者的结局，既能确定 CT 上看不到的病灶边界，也能降低靶区内正常肺组织的体积并因此降低发生肺损伤的风险。

同样，Shirvani 等研究了 PET 在局限期小细胞肺癌（SCLC）患者中的应用。在该研究中，其照射剂量分布在 PET-CT 的高代谢区域，而没有对选择性淋巴结区域进行预防照射。62 例患者都根据 PET-CT 阳性结果制订调强放疗计划，忽略了 PET-CT 显示阴性的区域；基于 PET-CT 勾画靶区，接受每天 2 次，每次 30min，共 45Gy 的治疗方案。结果显示，62 例患者中只有 1 例在未照射的选择性淋巴结区域出现复发。多数患者复发发生在远处区域或高剂量照射区域，而没有发生在初始 PET 显示阴性的选择性淋巴结区域。这表明即使在 SCLC 中，基于 PET-CT 的放疗计划可以不行选择性淋巴结预防照射。然而作者认为，虽然 PET 定义的纵隔淋巴结放疗区域看起来是安全的，但是 PET 检测的假阳性率高达 30%，更理想的方法是获得 PET 阳性纵隔淋巴结的病理学证据[29]。

由于将 PET 图像纳入肺癌治疗计划的研究展现了良好的前景，RTOG 发起了进一步研究其应用的试验。RTOG 0515 试验是一项研究 PET 对放疗计划制订产生影响的 II 期前瞻性临床试验。纳入的 47 例患者均勾画了 2 个 GTV，一个仅用 CT 图像勾画，另一个用 PET-CT 勾画。两者间的差异量化为 GTV 的大小，包含淋巴结的个数和位置、肺平均受量，超过 20Gy 的体积（V_{20}）和食管平均受量。结果显示，基于 PET-CT 勾画的 GTV 明显较小，肺平均受量也稍微低一些，而其他指标无显著差异。51% 的患者淋巴结勾画发生改变。这项试验表明 PET 的应用改变了绝大多数患者的 GTV，并倾向于降低 GTV 值[30]。

在治疗中使用 PET-CT 扫描的自适应放疗方案源于头颈部的相关研究，但现在已经开始在肺癌治疗的相关研究中得到广泛应用。有两项试验研究了放疗 5~6 周后行治疗中 PET 扫描的患者，评估了靶区体积的变化，目标是降低后续接受高剂量照射的体积。研究结果显示，虽然正常组织并发症平均获益只有约 2%，但接受全部处方剂量照射的靶体积降低了 20%~40%[31-32]。

肿瘤的运动

治疗胸部恶性肿瘤的一个重要方面是控制放疗中呼吸运动的影响。对于不能耐受手术或根据分期或肿瘤位置不能手术切除的患者，放疗是首选，且通常与化疗联合[33]。呼吸引起的器官运动会限制肿瘤放疗时的精确性。一些研究者的研究结果表明，使用传统的放疗技术，肿瘤的剂量欠缺高达 30%[34]。Stevens 等和其他学者的研究显示，自由呼吸状态下肺部肿瘤的运动范围在 5~10mm，而个别患者这一数值高达 4.5cm[35]。解决这些问题的方法是在 GTV 的基础上增加大的外扩边界来得到 PTV。由于考虑到正常组织毒性，靶体积的增大会使基于 V_{20} 等参数设定的剂量很难达到肿瘤杀伤剂量[36]。

淋巴结也容易受呼吸运动的影响。Donnelly 等的研究显示，纵隔和肺门淋巴结的呼吸动度平均在 2.5~5.2mm，最大值是 14.4mm[37]。在类似的研究中，Pantarotto 等评估了 100 个淋巴结的运动，其平均动度为 6.8mm（范围：1.7~16.4mm）[38]。两项研究都表明，下纵隔淋巴结的呼吸动度显著高于上纵隔。因此，在制订治疗计划和治疗过程中，减少器官和肿瘤运动造成的影响会有助于提高放疗的精确性，并且能在可接受的毒性范围内推送更高的剂量，获得更有利的生存结果。

目前有两种能显著降低呼吸运动效应的技术得到了应用。一种是在患者自由呼吸的条件下用控制射线投射的设备来检测呼吸运动，通过控制直线加速器，使其在特定的呼吸时相投射射线[39]。另一种技术是呼吸控制，要么是患者主观控制，要么是使用阀门装置，如 Wong 等发明的主动呼吸控制技术（active breathing control，ABC）[40-41] 或深吸气末屏气技术（the deep inspiration breath hold，DIBH）[42]。

STIC 2003 是一项在法国开展的可比较、非随机、多中心的前瞻性试验[43]。该试验对 401 例 NSCLC 患者未进行呼吸门控时的适形放疗计划与进行呼吸门控的适形放疗计划进行了比较，其结果显示了呼吸门控计划的心、肺和食管受量均有降低。

展生存期和总生存期[76-77]。过去几十年间，SABR用于治疗来自不同原发肿瘤的不能手术的肺部寡转移瘤。部分医疗机构也用SABR治疗身体各部位（肺、纵隔、肝、骨、肾上腺等）局限或转移性肿瘤，以期提高Ⅳ期NSCLC患者的无进展生存期[78]。作为一种减瘤手段使肿瘤更适于全身治疗，根据诺顿-西蒙假说，Kavanagh、Timmerman及同事们开展了一项针对一线全身化疗失败的Ⅳ期NSCLC患者的Ⅱ期临床试验。这部分患者最多有6个颅外转移灶，将所有已知转移灶给予SABR同步厄洛替尼治疗，24例计划入组的患者均同意入组治疗。最终结果虽尚在评估，但似乎令人鼓舞。从目前研究的早期结果来看，相比传统二线全身治疗方案，这部分患者获得了更长的PFS和OS[79]。

在未来的治疗中，SABR可能也适用于另外两类人群——多发早期原位肿瘤和放疗后出现复发的患者。对多个肺部小肿瘤患者，SABR可能会成为肺多次或扩大切除的替代方式[80-81]。SABR也是治疗NSCLC常规分割放疗后复发的安全、有效的方式[82]。

总　结

SABR主要是工程学和物理学研究发展的产物。更重要的是，他们促进了放射生物学的进步，如关于局部控制率生物因素的探索[83]。通过给予远高于常规分割的总剂量或分次剂量杀灭肿瘤，最终改善疗效。物理技术学的发展和生物学的创新两方面的有机结合给肺癌患者带来了新的希望。

由于全身治疗疗效的改进，放疗将会有选择性地应用于晚期肿瘤全身治疗后残留病灶的治疗[2]。目前，放疗主要局限于Ⅰ~Ⅲ期肺癌的根治性治疗。将来，放疗可能更多地用于Ⅳ期肺癌的巩固治疗或全身治疗后残留病灶的治疗。随着物理技术和生物学的进一步发展，通过放疗改善晚期肿瘤的局部控制率将是一种有效、经济的理想治疗方式。

放射肿瘤学包括放疗技术、生物学、临床等方面的研究，以及该学科与外科学、内科学的合作，目的是促进实现"自适应"治疗[84-86]。在这种治疗模式下，治疗方式的选择基于综合治疗前的各种诊断信息，包括影像资料的分析、分期、组织样本（蛋白质、基因等）以及其他预测指标等。选择正确的治疗方式后，开始对患者治疗的同时监测治疗过程。及早评估治疗实施的正确性、肿瘤反应、代谢的变化、耐受性等，有利于在治疗过程中及时更改治疗方案[87-89]。治疗结束后，影像学和代谢指标的评价可用于指导是否需要辅助化疗或者避免治疗毒性。与"一刀切"的治疗模式不同，自适应治疗采用个体化治疗模式，在治疗过程中不断进行评估，根据治疗反应不断调整治疗方案，以期达到更好的疗效。而在实现这个目标之前，需要继续募集患者进行前瞻性临床试验，从而使SABR发挥其最大潜力。

（赵　倩　朱　健　黄　伟　译）

参考文献

[1] Potters L, Steinberg M, Rose C, et al. American Society for Therapeutic Radiology and Oncology and American College of Radiology practice guideline for the performance of stereotactic body radiation therapy. Int J Radiat Oncol Biol Phys, 2004, 60 (4): 1026-1032.

[2] Timmerman R, Papiez L. Stereotactic body radiation therapy: rationale, techniques, applications, and optimization of an emerging technology. Oncology, 2004, 18 (4): 474-477.

[3] Leksell L. The stereotaxic method and radiosurgery of the brain. Acta Chir Scand, 1951, 102 (4): 316-319.

[4] Hamilton AJ, Lulu BA, Fosmire H, et al. Preliminary Clinical Experience with Linear Accelerator-based Spinal Stereotactic Radiosurgery. Neurosurgery, 1995. 36 (2): 311-319.

[5] Lax I, Blomgren H, Naslund I, et al. Stereotactic radiotherapy of extracranial targets Z Med Phys, 1994, 4 (2): 112-113.

[6] Blomgren H, Lax I, Naslund I, S et al. Stereotactic high dose fraction radiation therapy of extracranial tumors using an accelerator: clinical experience of the first thirty-one patients. Acta Oncol, 1995, 34 (6): 861-870.

[7] Shirato H, Shimizu S, Shimizu T, et al. Real-time tumour-tracking radiotherapy. Lancet, 1999, 353 (9161): 1331-1332.

[8] Uematsu M, Shiod, A Tahara K, et al. Focal, high dose, and fractionated modified stereotactic radiation thera-

py for lung carcinoma patients. Cancer, 1998, 82 (6): 1062-1070.

[9] Herfarth KK, Debus J, Lohr F, et al. Stereotactic single-dose radiation therapy of liver tumors: results of a phase I/II trial. J Clin oncl, 2001, 19 (1): 164-170.

[10] Wulf J, Hadinger U, Oppitz U, et al. Stereotactic radiotherapy of targets in the lung and liver. Strahlenther Onkol Dec, 2001, 177 (12): 645-655.

[11] NagataY, Negoro Y, Aoki T, et al. Clinical outcomes of 3D conformal hypofractionated single high-dose radiotherapy for one or two lung tumors using a stereotactic body frame. Int J Radiat Oncol Biol Phys, 2002, 52 (4): 1041-1046.

[12] Timmerman R, Papiez L, McGarry R, et al. Extracranial stereotactic radioablation: results of a phase I study in medically inoperable stage I non-small cell lung cancer. Chest, 2003, 124 (5): 1946-1955.

[13] Guerrero M, Li X. Extending the linear-quadratic model for large fraction doses pertinent to stereotactic radiotherapy. Phys Med Biol, 2004, 49 (20): 4825.

[14] Curtis SB. Lethal and potentially lethal lesions induced by radiation—a unified repair model. Radiat Res, 1986, 106 (2): 252-270.

[15] Benedict SH, Lin PS, Zwicker RD, et al. The biological effectiveness of intermittent irradiation as a function of overall treatment time: development of correction factors for linac-based stereotactic radiotherapy. Int J Radiat Oncol Biol Phys, 1997, 37: 765-769.

[16] Fowler IF, Welsh JS, Howard SE. Loss of biological effect in prolonged fraction delivery. Int J Radiat Oncol Biol Phys, 2004, 59 (1): 242-249.

[17] Wolbarst AB, Chin LM, Svensson GK. Optimization of radiation therapy: integral-response of a model biological system Int J Radiat Oncol Biol Phys, 1982, 8 (10): 1761-1769.

[18] Yaes RJ, Kalend A. Local stem cell depletion model for radiation myelitis. Int J Radiat Oncol Biol Phys, 1988, 14 (6): 1247-1259.

[19] Nevinny-Stickel M, Sweeney RA, Bale RJ, et al. Reproducibility of patient positioning for fractionated extracranial stereotactic radiotherapy using a double-vacuum technique. Strahlenther onkol, 2004, 180 (2): 117-122.

[20] Fuss M, Salter J, Rassiah P, et al. Repositioning accuracy of a commercially available double-vacuum whole body immobilization system for stereotactic body radiation therapy. Technol Cancer Res Treat, 2004, 3 (1): 59-67.

[21] Hof H, Herfarth KK, Munter M, et al. The use of the multislice CT for the determination of respiratory lung tumor movement in stereotactic single-dose irradiation. Strahlenther onkol, 2003, 179 (8): 542-547.

[22] Nagata Y, Negoro Y, Aoki T, et al. Three-dimensional conformal radiotherapy for extracranial tumors using a stereotactic body frame, Igaku butsuri, 2000, 2 (1): 28-34.

[23] Fairclough-Tompa L, Larsen T, Jaywant SM. Immobilization in stereotactic radiotherapy: the head and neck localizer frame. Med Dosm, Fall, 2001, 26 (3): 267-273.

[24] Alheit H, Dornfeld S, Dawel M, et al. Patient position reproducibility in fractionated stereotactically guided conformal radiotherapy using the BrainLAB Mask system. Strahlenther onkol, 2001, 177 (5): 264-268.

[25] Negoro Y, Nagata Y, Aoki T, et al. The effectiveness of an immobilization device in conformal radiotherapy for lung tumor: reduction of respiratory tumor movement and evaluation of the daily setup accuracy. Int J Radiat Oncol Biol Phys, 2001, 50 (4): 889-898.

[26] Wulf J, Hadinger U, Oppitz U, et al. Stereotactic radiotherapy of extracranial targets: CT-simulation and accuracy of treatment in the stereotactic body frame. Radiother Oncol, 2000, 57 (2): 225-236.

[27] Takacs H, Kishan A, Deogaonkar M, et al. Respiration induced target drift in spinal ste-reotactic radiosurgery: evaluation of skeletal fixation in a porcine model. Stereotactic and functional neurosurgery, 1999, 73 (1-4): 70.

[28] Herfarth KK, Debus J, Lohr F, et al. Extracranial stereotactic radiation therapy: set-up accuracy of patients treated for liver metastases. Int J Radiat Oncol Biol Phys, 2000, 46 (2), 329-335.

[29] Lohr F, Debus J, Frank C, et al. Noninvasive patient fixation for extracranial stereotactic radiotherapy. Int J Radiat Oncol Biol Phys, 1999, 45 (2): 521-527.

[30] Bale RI, Sweeney R, Vogele M, et al. Nichtinvasive Kopffixation für externe Bestrahlung von Tumoren im Kopf-Hals-Bereich. Strahlenther onkol, 1998, 174 (7): 350-354.

[31] Lax I, Blomgren H, Larson D, et al. Extracranial stereotactic radiosurgery of localized targets. Journal of Radiosurgery, 1998, 1 (2): 135-148.

[32] Lax I, Blomgren H, Naslund I, et al. Stereotactic radiotherapy of malignancies in the abdomen: methodological aspects. Acta Oncol, 1994, 33 (6): 677-683.

[33] Takai Y, Mituya M, Nemoto K, et al. Simple method of stereotactic radiotherapy without stereotactic body frame for extracranial tumors. Nihon Igaku Hoshasen Gakkai zasshi, 2001, 61 (8): 403-407.

[34] Wang LT, Solberg TD, Medin PM, et al. Infrared patient positioning for stereotactic radiosurgery of extracranial tumors. Comput Biol Med, 2001, 31 (2): 101-111.

[35] Uematsu M, Shioda A, Suda A, et al. Intrafractional tumor position stability during computed tomography (CT) -guided frameless stereotactic radiation therapy for lung or liver cancers with a fusion of CT and linear accelerator (FOCAL) unit. Int J Radiat Oncol Biol Phys, 2000, 48 (2): 443-448.

[36] Uematsu M, Sonderegger M, Shioda A, et al. Daily positioning accuracy of frameless stereotactic radiation therapy with a fusion of computed tomography and linear accelerator (focal) unit: evaluation of z-axis with a z-marker. Radiother Oncol, 1999, 50 (3): 337-339.

[37] Kimura T, Hirokawa Y, Murakami Y, et al. Reproducibility of organ position using voluntary breath-hold method with spirometer for extracranial stereotactic radiotherapy. Int J Radiat Oncol Biol Phys, 2004, 60 (4): 1307-1313.

[38] O'Dell WG, Schell MC, Reynolds III, et al. Dose broadening due to target position variability during fractionated breath-held radiation therapy. Med Phys, 2002, 29 (7): 1430-1437.

[39] Murphy MJ, Martin D, Whyte R, et al. The effectiveness of breath-holding to stabilize lung and pancreas tumors during radiosurgery. Int J Radiat Oncol Biol Phys, 2002, 53 (2): 475-482.

[40] Yin F, Kim JG, Haughton C, et al. Extracranial radiosurgery: Immobilizing liver motion in dogs using high-frequency jet ventilation and total intravenous anesthesia. Int J Radiat Oncol Biol Phys, 2001, 49 (1): 211-216.

[41] Kini VR, Vedam SS, Keall PJ, et al. Patient training in respiratory-gated radiotherapy. Medl Dosim, 2003, 28 (1): 7-11.

[42] Vedam SS, Keall PJ, Kini VR, et al. Determining parameters for respiration-gated radiotherapy. Med Phys, 2001, 28 (10): 2139-2146.

[43] Hara R, Itami J, Aruga T, et al. Development of stereotactic irradiation system of body tumors under respiratory gating. Nihon Igaku Hoshasen Gakkai Zasshi, 2002, 62 (4): 156-160.

[44] Kuriyama K, Onishi H, Sano N, et al. A new irradiation unit constructed of self-moving gantry-CT and linac. Int J Radiat Oncol Biol Phys, 2003, 55 (2): 428-435.

[45] Kitamura K, Shirato H, Seppenwoolde Y, et al. Tumor location, cirrhosis, and surgical history contribute to tumor movement in the liver, as measured during stereotactic irradiation using a real-time tumor-tracking radiotherapy system. Int J Radiat Oncol Biol Phys, 2003, 56 (1): 221-228.

[46] Sharp GC, Jiang SB, Shimizu S, et al. Prediction of respiratory tumour motion for real-time image-guided radiotherapy. Phys Med Biol, 2004, 49 (3): 425.

[47] Schweikard A, Shiomi H, Adler J. Respiration tracking in radiosurgery. Med Phys, 2004, 31 (10): 2738-2741.

[48] Papiez L, Timmerman R, Desrosiers C, et al. Extracranial stereotactic radioablation physical principles. Acta Oncol, 2003, 42 (8): 882-894.

[49] Liu R, Wagner TH, Buatti JM, et al. Geometrically based optimization for extracranial radiosurgery. Phys Med Biol, 2004, 49 (6): 987.

[50] Cardinal R, Wu Q, Benedic H, et al. Determining the optimal block margin on the planning target volume for extracranial stereotactic radiotherapy. Int J Radiat Oncol Biol Phys, 1999, 45 (2): 515-520.

[51] Papie, L. On the equivalence of rotational and concentric therapy. Phys Med Biol, 2000, 45 (2): 399.

[52] Hadinger U, Thiele W, Wulf J. Extracranial stereotactic radiotherapy: evaluation of PTV coverage and dose conformity. Z Med Phys, 2002, 12 (4): 221-229.

[53] Papiez L, Moskvin V, Timmerman R. Radiation Therapy. Stereotactic body radiation therapy, 2005, 29 (3): 57.

[54] Mayer R, Williams A, Frankel T, et al. Two-dimensional film dosimetry application in heterogeneous materials exposed to megavoltage photon beams. Med Phys, 1997, 24 (3): 455-460.

[55] McGarry RC, Papiez L, Williams M, et al. Stereotactic body radiation therapy of early-stage non-small-cell lung carcinoma: Phase I study. Int J Radiat Oncol Biol Phys, 2005, 63 (4): 1010-1015.

[56] Timmerman R, McGarry R, Yiannoutsos C, et al. Excessive toxicity when treating central tumors in a phase II study of stereotactic body radiation therapy for medically ino-perable early-stage lung can-cer. J Clin Oncol, 2006, 24 (30): 4833-4839.

[57] Baumann P, Nyman J, Lax I, et al. Factors important for

efficacy of stereotactic body radiotherapy of medically inoperable stage I lung cancer A retrospective analysis of patients treated in the Nordic countries. Acta Oncol, 2006, 45 (7): 787-795.

[58] Fritz P, Kraus HJ, Mühlnickel W, et al. Stereotactic, single-dose irradiation of stage I non-small cell lung cancer and lung metastases. Radiat Onco, 2006, 1 (1): 30.

[59] Nyman J, Johansson KA, Hulten U. Stereotactic hypofractionated radiotherapy for stage I non-small cell lung cancer—mature results for medically inoperable patients. Lung Cancer, 2006, 51 (1): 97-103.

[60] Zimmermann F, Geinitz H, Schil S, et al. Stereotactic hypofractionated radiation therapy for stage I non-small cell lung cancer. Lung Cancer, 2005, 48 (1): 107-114.

[61] Wulf J, Baier K, Mueller G, et al. Dose-response in stereotactic irradiation of lung tumors. Radiother Oncol, 2005, 77 (1): 83-87.

[62] Timmerman RD, Park C, Kavanagh BD. The North American experience with stereotactic body radiation therapy in non-small cell lung cancer. Journal of Thoracic Oncology, 2007, 2 (7): S101-S112.

[63] Nagata Y, Takayama K, Matsuo Y, et al. Clinical outcomes of a phase I/II study of 48 Gy of stereotactic body radiotherapy in 4 fractions for primary lung cancer using a stereotactic body frame. Int J Radiat Oncol Biol Phys, 2005, 63 (5): 1427-1431.

[64] Xia T, Li H, Sun Q, et al. Promising clinical outcome of stereotactic body radiation therapy for patients with inoperable Stage I/II non-small-cell lung cancer. Int J Radiat Oncol Biol Phys, 2006, 66 (1): 117-125.

[65] Hara R, Itami J, Kondo T, et al. Clinical outcomes of single-fraction stereotactic radiation therapy of lung tumors. Cancer, 2006, 106 (6): 1347-1352.

[66] Nagata Y, Hiraoka M, Shibata T, et al. A phase II trial of stereotactic body radiation therapy for operable T1N0M0 non-small cell lung cancer: Japan Clinical Oncology Group (JCOG0403). Int J Radiat Oncol Biol Phys, 2010, 78 (3): S27-S28.

[67] Timmerman R, Paulus R, Galvin J, et al. Stereotactic body radiation therapy for inoperable early stage lung cancer. JAMA, 2010, 303 (11): 1070-1076.

[68] Palma D, Visser O, Lagerwaard FJ, et al. Impact of introducing stereotactic lung radiotherapy for elderly patients with stage I non-small-cell lung cancer: A population-based time-trend analysis. J Clin Oncol, 2010, 28 (35): 5153-5159.

[69] Chang JY, Balter PA, Dong L, et al. Stereotactic body radiation therapy in centrally and superiorly located stage I or isolated recurrent non-small-cell lung cancer. Int J Radiat Oncol Biol Phys, 2008, 72 (4): 967-971.

[70] Lagerwaard F, Haasbeek C, Smit E, et al. Outcomes of risk-adapted fractionated stereotactic radiotherapy for stage I non-small-cell lung cancer. Int J Radiat Oncol Biol Phys, 2008, 70 (3): 685-692.

[71] Register SP, Zhang X, Mohan R, et al. Proton stereotactic body radiation therapy for clinically challenging cases of centrally and superiorly located stage I non-small-cell lung cancer. Int J Radiat Oncol Biol Phys, 2011, 80 (4): 1015-1022.

[72] Onishi H, Araki T, Shirato H, et al. Stereotactic hypofractionated high-dose irradiation for stage I nonsmall cell lung carcinoma. Cancer, 2004, 101 (7), 1623-1631.

[73] Fowler JF. The linear-quadratic formula and progress in fractionated radiotherapy. The British journal of radiology, 1989, 62 (740): 679-694.

[74] Ginsberg RJ, Rubinstein LV. Lung Cancer Study Group, Randomized trial of lobectomy versus limited resection for T1 N0 non-small cell lung cancer. The Annals of Thoracic Surgery, 1995, 60 (3): 615-623.

[75] Timmerman RD, Paulus R, Pass HI, et al. RTOG 0618: Stereotactic body radiation therapy (SBRT) to treat operable early-stage lung cancer patients In ASCO. Annual Meeting Proceedings, 2013, 31 (15): p7523.

[76] Milano MT, Katz AW, Schell MC, et al. Descriptive analysis of oligometastatic lesions treated with curative-intent stereotactic body radiotherapy. Int J Radiat Oncol Biol Phys, 2008, 72 (5): 1516-1522.

[77] Milano MT, Philip A, Okunieff P. Analysis of patients with oligometastases undergoing two or more curative-intent stereotactic radiotherapy courses. Int J Radiat Oncol Biol Phys, 2009, 73 (3): 832-837.

[78] Salama JK, Hasselle MD, Chmura SJ, et al. Stereotactic body radiotherapy for multisite extracranial oligometastases. Cancer, 2012, 118 (11): 2962-2970.

[79] Iyengar P, Kavanag BD, Smith I, et al. A phase II trial of stereotactic body radiation therapy combined with erlotinib for patients with limited but progressive metastatic non-small-cell lung cancer. J Clin Oncol, 2014, 32 (34): 3824-3830.

[80] Chang JY, Liu YH, Zhu Z, et al. Stereotactic ablative

radiotherapy: a potentially curable approach to early stage multiple primary lung cancer. Cancer, 2013, 119 (18): 3402-3410.

[81] Kelly P, Balter PA, Rebueno N, et al. Stereotactic body radiation therapy for patients with lung cancer previously treated with thoracic radiation. Int J Radiat Oncol Biol Phys, 2010, 78 (5): 1387-1393.

[82] Liu H, Zhang X, Vinogradskiy YY, et al. Predicting radiation pneumonitis after stereotactic ablative radiation therapy in patients previously treated with conventional thoracic radiation therapy. Int J Radiat Oncol Biol Phys, 2012, 84 (4): 1017-1023.

[83] Timmerman RD, Story M. Stereotactic body radiation therapy: a treatment in need of basic biological research. The Cancer Journal, 2006, 12 (1): 19-20.

[84] Martinez AA, Yan D, Lockman D, et al. Improvement in dose escalation using the process of adaptive radiotherapy combined with three-dimensional conformal or intensity-modulated beams for prostate cancer. Int J Radiat Oncol Biol Phys, 2001, 50 (5): 1226-1234.

[85] Bortfeld T, Paganetti H. The biologic relevance of daily dose variations in adaptive treatment planning. Int J Radiat Oncol Biol Phys, 2006, 65 (3): 899-906.

[86] Song W, Schaly B, Bauman G, et al. Image-guided adaptive radiation therapy (IGART): Radiobiological and dose escalation considerations for localized carcinoma of the prostate. Med Phys, 2005, 32 (7): 2193-2203.

[87] Yan D, Lockman D, Brabbins D, et al. An off-line strategy for constructing a patient-specific planning target volume in adaptive treatment process for prostate cancer. Int J Radiat Oncol Biol Phys, 2000, 48 (1): 289-302.

[88] Wu C, Jeraj R, Olivera GH, et al. Reoptimization in adaptive radiotherapy. Phys. Med Biol, 2002, 47 (17): 3181.

[89] Brahme A. Biologically optimized 3-dimensional in vivo predictive assay-based radiation therapy using positron emission tomography-computerized tomography imaging. Acta Oncol, 2003, 42 (2): 123-136.

第 22 章
质子治疗

Joe Y. Chang, James D. Cox
Department of Radiation Oncology, The University of Texas MD Anderson Cancer Center, Houston, TX, USA

引 言

非小细胞肺癌（NSCLC）患者占所有肺癌患者的80%，其中只有20%~25%早期NSCLC患者能够接受手术治疗，有相当一部分患者因合并症无法耐受手术。对于这部分患者来说，基于光子（X线）的放射治疗被认为是标准治疗手段，近50%处于局部进展期的患者需要接受包括放疗在内的综合治疗。对于Ⅰ期NSCLC患者，接受传统剂量的放疗能够使局部小病灶得到长达两年的有效控制[1-3]。然而，对Ⅲ期患者，放化疗仅能达到50%~60%局部控制率，中位生存期为15~17个月，5年生存率为10%~15%[4]。

局部控制不佳是远处转移的一个重要原因，也是治疗失败的一个重要因素，因此，彻底根治肿瘤是十分必要的。大量临床证据表明，NSCLC患者的生存率与局部控制率之间存在剂量-效应关系[5-8]。然而，射线剂量越高，毒副作用越大，特别对于同步放化疗，高剂量放疗的毒副作用尤其明显[4]。

RTOG 7301试验显示生存获益剂量为>60Gy，因此，目前肺癌的光子放疗标准剂量定为60~66 Gy[9]。然而，60~66Gy的剂量仍然不能保证对肿瘤的局部控制率超过50%。Cox等人[10]开展的RTOG 8311试验表明，单纯行总剂量为69.6Gy、单次剂量为1.2Gy的放疗可以提高生存率。然而，RTOG 9410试验表明，放化疗同步时，69.6Gy的放疗剂量比60Gy导致更严重的放疗副反应，而生存并没有明显改善。RTOG 0617试验结果也指出，同步放化疗时，相比60Gy，74Gy的（光子）放疗剂量将引起更严重的副反应并带来更低的生存率[11]。

20世纪80年代诊断影像的发展推动了个体化放疗的进步。从此，放疗不再以解剖图谱为依据，而是基于患者本身的解剖结构。X射线计算机断层扫描（computed tomography, CT）等成像扫描技术可以在三维空间展示肿瘤与周围正常组织的解剖关系。三维放疗的剂量的计算越来越精确，例如多叶准直器已广泛应用于医用直线加速器中。这些工具实现了从射束路径上对肿瘤的观察以及对肿瘤高度适形的辐射剂量分布。

20世纪90年代，商业化的放射治疗计划系统将三维适形放疗（3D conformal radiation theraphy, 3D-CRT）引入肿瘤治疗。与二维治疗计划相比，计算机模拟剂量分布清楚地显示了3D-CRT使瘤区得到更高剂量的照射，并使正常组织避免或减少受照。3D-CRT之所以能够被迅速接受并推广开来，主要由于计划系统的使用有效减少了正常组织的受照体积。实际上，Ⅲ期NSCLC患者行同期放化疗时，3D-CRT能够使照射剂量由63Gy增加到74Gy[12,13]。

不同强度的X线小野使高剂量区形状具有更高的可塑性。物理师对不同的剂量强度进行优化，并通过使用动态多叶光栅实现调强放疗（intensity-modulated radiation therapy, IMRT）。与3D-CRT相比，IMRT的认可程度及推广速度相对较慢。虽然此项技术能够有效减小放疗副反应，但使用IMRT时，医生、物理师与剂量师需要在治疗计划的制订上耗费大量时间及人力。这种精确程度需要更精细的靶区勾画、计划设计以及质量保障。而且，由于分次治疗间及治疗过程中（如呼吸时）都存在位置误差，导致肿瘤脱离照射范围。因此，有必要于每次治疗前对患者进行体位影像学验证。因此，"影像引导放射治疗"同时涵盖了每天的影像学验证、3D CRT 以及 IMRT 三个概念。

尽管 3D CRT 或 IMRT 能减少正常组织放疗并发症，但 X 射线的高投射特点限制了治疗剂量的进一步提升。而质子束是由有能量的粒子组成，这些粒子由已规定好的角度射入组织。当质子束射入体内，粒子运动开始变慢，并且在接近轨迹尽头处沉积自身大部分的能量。这种射束中心轴深度剂量分布称为"布拉格峰（Bragg peak）"。通过调制布拉格峰的能量及时间，即"拉长的布拉格峰"（spread-out Bragg peak，SOBP），靶区能够得到一个充分、局部非扩散、均匀的剂量照射，并且使周围正常组织免受照射。当保留器官功能作为优先考虑条件时，质子束治疗应被作为首选，尤其对于肺癌患者[14-15]。在本章节，我们将对以下内容进行综述：质子束治疗计划的基本原理、肺癌患者的质子治疗及其预后。

质子的相对生物效应及生物学研究

高能粒子放疗（如质子或碳原子核高能粒子）是直接离子化的，因为他们自身的能量使加速运动的粒子通过库仑力与原子中的电子相互作用。与光子不同，这些粒子属于高线性能量传递（linear energy transfer，LET）射线质，因此，他们与组织相互作用时，不仅直接损伤细胞中 DNA，而且调动其运动轨迹上的次级电子，导致自由基增多，而这些自由基也导致 DNA 损伤。在临床中使用 SOBP 时，通常认为在百分深度剂量（percentage depth dose，PDD）曲线的平台区，射线对细胞的损伤是几乎恒定的。但实际上，粒子运动轨迹中的细胞损伤程度是不断变化的。

尽管带电粒子放疗中所用到的不同的原子核有大致相同形状的百分深度剂量曲线，但他们的放射生物学效应最终依赖于所使用粒子的 LET 特征。因此，改变 SOBP 对于剂量分布是有效的，但是肿瘤的放射损伤程度依赖于射线的另一特性——相对生物效应（relative biological effectiveness，RBE）。这一特性被定义为达到同样生物学效应时，标准射线（一般为 X 线）所需的剂量与所测定射线达到同样生物学效应所需剂量的比值。如果某粒子束的 RBE 高，则该粒子束被吸收的单位能量能造成极大的损伤，也就是说该粒子的品质高。值得注意的是，RBE 在不同组织中也不同，其随细胞的增殖速度与剂量的变化而变化（剂量越低 RBE 越高）。

质子的 RBE 接近光子。Paganetti 等总结了一系列质子试验数据并得出质子的 RBE 约为 1.1 的结论[16]。这意味着质子在放射生物效应上接近光子，并使射线效能提高 10%。然而重离子拥有相当大的相对生物效应，如碳离子的 RBE 接近 3，与中子相似。尽管碳离子的高 RBE 似乎在控制乏氧肿瘤中有优势，但这对于正常组织来说却是劣势。

另一个值得一提的放射生物学现象，是关于带电粒子在放疗中的相对优势。在光子治疗中，乏氧或是细胞处于射线不敏感周期（如 S 期）都能降低或抵消癌细胞的放射灵敏度。在这二者中，放射灵敏度的改变使细胞能够修复射线对 DNA 的破坏，并且在乏氧环境、姐妹染色单体以及特定细胞周期时相的 DNA 修复酶存在时，这种修复能力增强。然而，即使存在以上 3 种放射生物学修复方式，DNA 损伤中单链、双链断裂也难以被修复。因为高线性能量传递的粒子（例如碳离子）更容易引起这类损伤，所以肿瘤组织的氧合作用、细胞周期效应就变得不那么重要。重离子的这种能力能使他们克服自身的射线抵抗性质，在理论上比光子更有优势。实际上，在放射生物学中的这种差异就是区别重离子与质子的一个重要性质，即二者中谁在放射生物学中更类似于光子。然而肿瘤组织学和剂量分割方式不同可以使质子的 RBE 产生变化[17-18]。由于一些实际使用中的原因，治疗模型没有考虑 RBE 的变化。然而，随着带电粒子使用的增加，考虑特殊条件下的 RBE 变化越来越有必要性。

质子治疗的另一个优势在于，他们能优先作用于可导致局部复发以及远处转移的肿瘤干细胞。近期，一项临床前期研究指出，在射线照射有抵抗作用的 NSCLC 细胞株时，质子比相同剂量的光子靶向杀灭肿瘤干细胞更加有效，而这种细胞杀伤作用不会发生在正常支气管上皮细胞株[19]。以上研究表明，在预防治疗对射线抵抗的肿瘤干细胞导致的局部复发及远处转移方面，质子比光子更有优势，但此结论有待经过临床试验验证。进一步研究 DNA 损伤修复的分子生物学机制以及质子引起的信号传导机制将有助于阐明质子治疗的最佳方式[20]。另外，质子治疗、化疗、分子靶向治疗的联合将开辟提高肿瘤治疗增益比的新天地[21]。

质子治疗的原理

如前所述，质子在肿瘤治疗中的优势在于其高度聚集的剂量分布，而不是其增强的生物学效应。肿瘤靶区能够受到高治疗剂量质子束照射，同时周围易受射线损伤的正常组织能够免于照射，尤其可保护射线方向远端的正常组织。当复杂因素相同或者所用治疗技术相同时，质子照射所致的正常组织受照剂量为 X 线的一半或更少[22]。更高的剂量应该能提高肿瘤局控率。

质子束的基本特性在于其经过靶肿瘤远端表面后，可以在几微米的距离内停止运动，而 X 射线则将其能量沉积在正常组织和器官中，然后从进入患者体内的对面射出，这些正常组织与器官位于靶区外的射线路径上。这使质子较 X 线显示出巨大优势。此外，在人体内靶区外射线束路径上的正常组织与器官中，质子比 X 线沉积更少的剂量。由于质子束的物理学特点（如布拉格峰），更高剂量的质子在放疗中引起的正常组织副作用与较低剂量的光子在放疗中引起的副作用相同。因此，质子放疗比包括 IMRT 的常规光子放疗在控制肿瘤及提高生存率方面均有优势[14-15]。

质子治疗计划与实施

质子束的物理学特点

如所有重粒子（氦离子、碳离子、负 π 介子等）一样，质子有独特的剂量深度分布，即通常所说的布拉格峰。这种剂量深度的特点是，入射剂量较低（约为最大剂量的 30%~40%），随之而来的是一个剂量峰值，此时剂量迅速升高形成一个狭窄的峰（布拉格峰），然后迅速下降到 0。布拉格峰的深度取决于射线所穿透的材料组成以及质子的能量。图 22.1A 展示了一个典型的布拉格峰。

布拉格峰很窄，以至于无法针对除临床最小靶区以外的任何病灶进行治疗，这些靶区的深度基本为 20cm。通常，向布拉格峰后追加较小的能量和较低的权重，调整照射范围，就可产生一个宽大的剂量均一区，称为 SOBP（图 22.1B）。通过在射线束中放置一个射程调制轮（动态调强）或一个脊形过滤器（被动调强），或改变加速器的能量，或在调整每个布拉格峰的权重时调整能量选择系统，都可以获得 SOBP。通过选择合适的射程平衡锤和每个原始布拉格峰的权重，都可以得到深度均一的射线。为了在肿瘤靶区内得到横向均匀的剂量，射线束必须横向分布，要么通过一个被动的双散射系统、要么通过磁性驱动射束点进行扫描，来得到均匀的剂量投射。通常来说，需要生产不同深度的 SOBP，以适应不同的靶区体积。值得注意的是，SOBP 深度增加的时候，表面剂量也随之增加。质子治疗需要能量在 70Mev 至（230~250）MeV 的质子束，这样能使穿透人体的深度在 7cm 至（30~37）cm。剂量率应接近 2Gy/min。

被动散射系统

目前，被动散射体系是质子放疗技术中获得横向射束分布的标准方法。在这一体系内，质子束首先穿过一级散射装置射程调制轮，再穿过使射线束侧向展开的二级散射装置射程分配器，并且在射入人体之前穿过定制射程补偿器。经过这样一个双散射系统（使用射程调制轮一级散射器和二级散射器），可以在最后出射口中产生一束宽而平坦的射线束。射程分配器决定了质子的最大穿透深度，射程调制轮可扩展布拉格峰，形成既包括肿瘤靶区同时又可避开周围正常组织的均匀剂量分布。定制射程补偿器可修整靶区远端表面的剂量分布，使其与靶区远端边缘及随后的拖尾相匹配，从而校正患者解剖结构与补偿器之间的细微误差。在设计射程补偿器时，治疗计划系统要计算患者体表至计划靶区（planning target volume，PTV）远端的等效水射程深度，因此需要计算射程补偿器每一点的厚度以校正患者体表的形状以及体表至 PTV 之间的所有不均匀性，以及 PTV

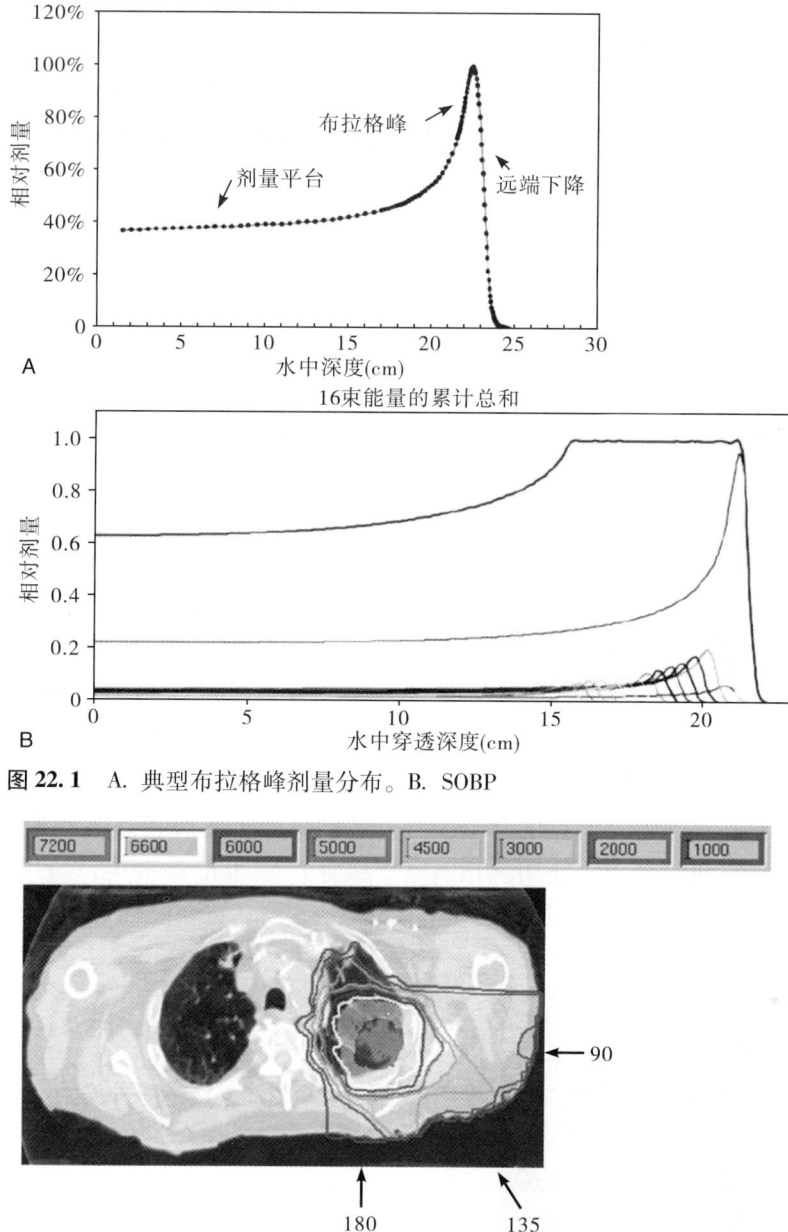

图 22.1 A. 典型布拉格峰剂量分布。B. SOBP

图 22.2（见彩插） 典型被动散射质子放疗计划射束排布。内在肿瘤靶区（internal gross tumor volume，iGTV）标为红褐色；附近临床靶区（CTV）为卡其色（绿）；计划靶区（PTV）为蓝色。箭头指示射束角度。顶部不同颜色数字指示等剂量曲线（cGy）

后表面的形状。使用被动散射系统的质子治疗技术，需要在照射靶区的同时减少危及器官的受照剂量，因此，射线数量及入射角度对于使用被动散射系统的质子放疗也很重要。图22.2列出了肺癌质子放疗中传统射线束数量及入射角度。

被动散射系统安全、简单，对加速器的时间构造灵敏度相对较低。尽管该系统能够满足既定目标，但也存在一些问题，最明显的就是射线利用率低。在散射系统和射线束限制装置中浪费了20%~40%质子。与回旋加速器相比，以同步加速器为基础的质子治疗的剂量率被限制得更多，质子的大量浪费是其中的一大问题。同时，被动散射系统对射线束位置的变化也很敏感。不仅如此，当质子被散射系统或装置拦截时，他们产生二级中子，这将增加患者的整体受照剂量。中子拥有高 RBE，并且被认为会导致继发肿瘤[23]。该系统的另一个缺点是，它针对整个靶区产生一个扩展布拉格峰，这样在治疗不规则、厚薄不均匀的大靶区时，高剂量区就会落在正常组织上。基于这个因素，被动散射技术的剂量适形特性被称为"2.5维"。动点扫描系统是解决这些问题的有效手段，将会在后文详述。

动点束点扫描系统

在动态束点扫描系统中，进入治疗喷管的窄射线束受磁力作用以穿过靶区的横断面并在纵深上实现既定剂量分布。射线束可以是连续的，也可以停在某个特定时间或特定位置，直到达到预定剂量。然后，在离散点扫描中，需关闭射线束及磁场，移动下一射线束照射点至预定位置[24]。通过选择合适的能量扫描最深一层，当该层扫描完毕、能量衰减，再扫描下一层。这样，整个靶区都能被照射，以类似于被动扫描的方法使每个野的剂量分布一致，或每个野的剂量分布不一致但把各野汇总时总剂量分布一致，这被称为调强质子治疗（intensity modulated proton therapy，IMPT）。图22.3为一个典型的动态扫描系统。使用连续扫描时，射线束的强度可随入射点的移动而不同，从而产生不一致的剂量分布。使用离散式扫描时，束点在每个三维像素停留的时间不同，将导致剂量分布不同。

动态点扫描有如下优点：它为整个靶区调整剂量分布模式；无须其他设备如剂量限制孔径或射程补偿器；几乎不浪费质子，射线利用率高；产生中子量少。该方法的缺点是难以在肿瘤运动时进行照射。然而射线束门控技术，如呼吸门控质子放疗（于"肿瘤移动因素"部分详述）可以降低治疗中的不确定性。尽管实际上每层的重复扫描次数是有限制的，但是每层扫描多次或增加治疗分次，便会减少由器官运动所带来的剂量误差。IMPT所需时间应该与X射线的IMRT所需时间相差无几，具有可比性。

质子治疗与光子治疗计划

与X线和电子线放疗相同，质子放疗亦使用多个治疗野行开放的非共面照射，以合理限制皮肤受量及射束路径中正常组织免于受照。然而，因为质子有其特性，治疗方案中所用的质子与X线、电子有很大不同。例如，在质子治疗中，质子剂量分布在射程远端迅速下降，质子束可以直接穿过临床正常结构，与X线和电子治疗不同，此二者均在重要结构中产生毒副反应。然而，这存

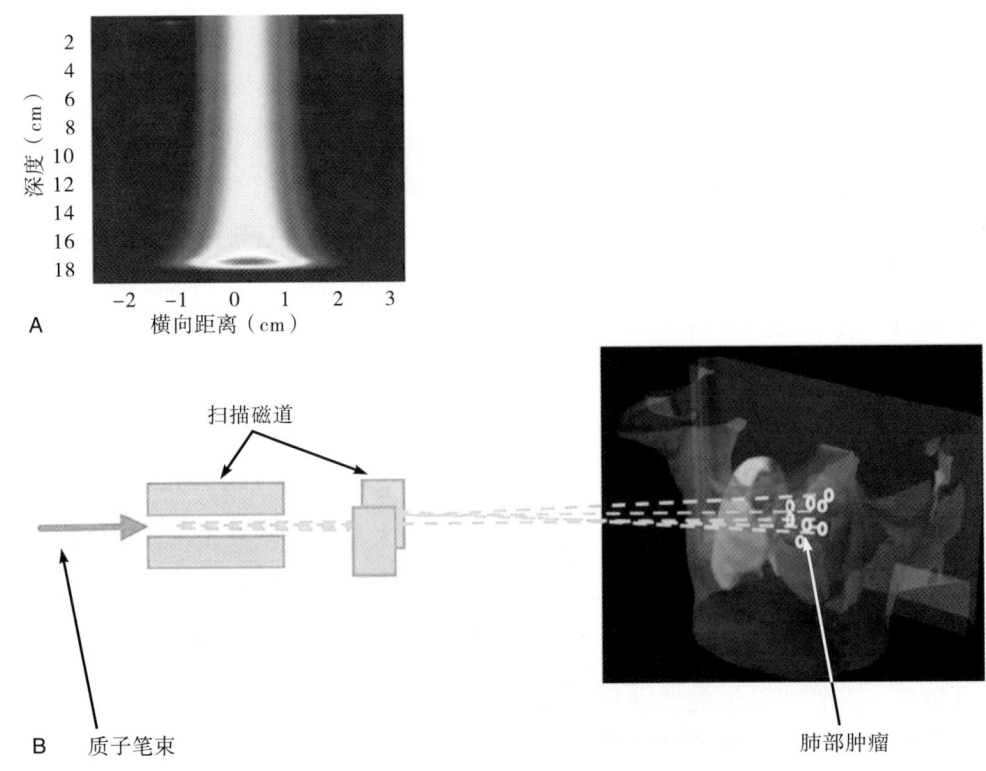

图22.3（见彩插） A. 典型动态点扫描。B. 散射束剂量喷涂示意图

在着一种不确定性,即靶区远端边缘的质子剂量和扩展布拉格峰末端边缘 RBE 可能增加。导致这些不确定性的原因必须被考虑进去。

因此,质子治疗中需要对质子束的不确定性有更深刻的了解,尤其是与质子束停止点相关的不确定性。CT 数据的错误或治疗计划及实施中的错误都将导致质子束的停止,造成质子束过早消失(靶区欠量)或射线束传递太远(肿瘤后方重要组织过度照射)。基于 CT 所反映出的已知组织拦截能力测量,可用于建立 CT 值与质子质量阻止能力的关系,由此计算质子在组织中的传递范围[25]。如前所述,RBE 的不确定性是另一个需要考虑的问题。前期计算结果证实,质子束的 RBE 随组织特点、剂量、剂量率、能量、照射深度[16]不同而不同,而不随其固有值的改变而改变。

X 线与质子治疗的另一个重要区别在于,X 线放疗定义靶区的外扩时,将临床靶区(clinical target volume,CTV)扩展为计划靶区(PTV)。质子束有 3 个边界,2 个横向半影由 Coulomb 多重散射导致,远端剂量下降由射程离散导致。因为多重散射及射程离散均依赖质子束的射程(能量),所以质子剂量分布有 3 个面,每个面都具有随深度变化的剂量梯度。同样,侧面半影对深度的依赖比 X 线对 17cm 以下等效水的依赖更强烈;而在更浅的深度上,质子横向半影比 X 线小。总之,每一次治疗射线束必须有其自身的边界,这一边界依赖于射线束穿越组织的深度。因此,在质子治疗中,将 CTV 扩展为 PTV 不是一个直接的途径,并且这种扩展也强烈依赖于射线的方向。事实上,PTV 的概念在质子治疗计划中是无用的。

对于质子治疗计划中的被动散射系统最严格的限制,源自于穿过靶区的布拉格峰(SOBP)宽度的不一致,这将导致一些周边正常组织受到高剂量照射。然而,这一问题可以通过使用多射线束、点扫描技术和调强治疗计划来解决。随着动态束点扫描技术的出现,质子治疗向前迈出了关键的一步。如本章节前文所述,点扫描带来了可调强度的治疗计划及照射实施技术,极大地改善了质子剂量分布,这正如 IMRI 在 X 线治疗中的应用。

通过"逆"治疗计划系统,IMPT 计划得到了优化,与逆 IMRT 相似[26-27]。然而,IMPT 也有其他的复杂之处,因为除了射线能量之外,每一束射线强度和剂量都可变,这增加了优化的自由度,也增加了 IMPT 剂量适形的潜能,不过这需要以更复杂的计算及治疗为代价。

对于有相同复杂程度的治疗计划来说,IMPT 计划依然优于 IMRT 计划,尤其是在解决了运动不确定性情况下的正常组织保护方面[28]。IMPT 与 IMRT 的靶区覆盖情况基本相同(图 22.4)。平均来看,IMRT 计划在对辐射敏感的器官上有两倍于 IMPT 计划的整体剂量,因此后者在根本上更好地保护了重要的脏器[23,28]。

影像引导的质子照射

质子剂量分布是高度准确的,因为扩展布拉格峰(SOBP)高剂量区之后剂量急剧降为 0。然而,当计划设计、患者摆位或剂量投射未得到优化、不准确时,这一优点(与 X 线相比)将消失殆尽。质子束的照射范围内的一个错误会导致靶区远端体积无法接受照射(如果射野太短)或正常重要结构被超量照射(如果射野太长)。加速器机载影像引导、实时监控以及施照过程的质量控制可以保障患者摆位及治疗的准确性。

多数质子治疗系统包括 3 个互相垂直的影像系统(X 线球管和平板成像装置)、影像分析系统

IMPT 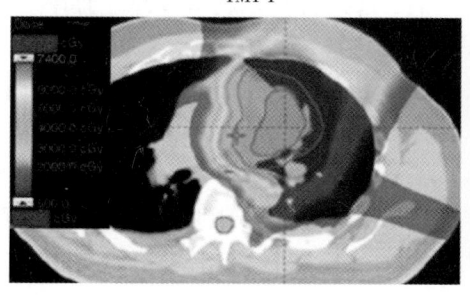 IMRT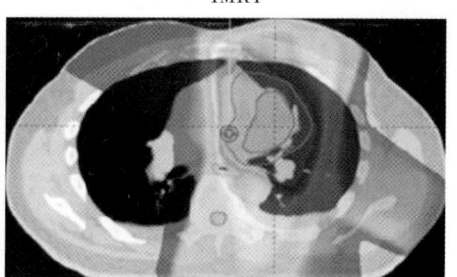

图 22.4 Ⅲ期 NSCLC 调强光子放疗和调强质子治疗剂量分布对比

和数字化的6维床。更加现代化的质子治疗系统装备机载的容积成像影像引导系统,包括锥形束CT或滑轨CT。这些立体定位技术的使用保证了患者治疗体位的正确性,纠正了摆位误差,并能够确认每分次治疗中每个照射野执行的准确性。

肿瘤运动因素

多种因素导致了肺癌质子放疗的复杂性,其中最棘手的便是治疗过程中肿瘤随呼吸运动。心跳也能引起肿瘤运动,但与呼吸相比,其幅度较小。多级探测器及快速成像技术的发展使我们可以获得患者呼吸时的实时图像,并通过使用4维CT测量肿瘤及器官的运动度。

将4维CT影像应用于4维治疗计划更有趣、更有挑战性。4维治疗计划可以计算自由呼吸时的实际剂量分布[29-30]。这一过程中,每一呼吸时相中的剂量分布都可以计算出来,然后与图像进行形变配准。这样合成的剂量分布与剂量-体积直方图可以反映出患者以4维CT影像中的呼吸方式呼吸时的实际受量。

为确保所有肿瘤细胞均可被质子束照射,M.D.安德森癌症中心[29]和麻省总医院的研究者们[30]使用4维CT引导的治疗计划评估靶区内及周围正常组织中的质子剂量-体积分布。这些计划包括通过融合不同呼吸时相的靶体积以产生内靶体积(internal target volume,ITV)。M.D.安德森癌症中心的研究者们使用ITV产生最大密度投影(maximal intensity projection,MIP),并在此基础上设计了一个质子治疗中所需的补偿器[30]。这项技术使计划的剂量分布更接近实际投射的剂量分布。相比于Mo-yers建议在高活动度的肺癌治疗中使用大外扩边界[31],ITV技术的外扩边界更小,从而可以在更好地保护正常组织的同时,使几乎整个肿瘤都能受到最大剂量的照射。这样,便可以用个体化的基于肿瘤实际运动的ITV来设计补偿器[30]。当肿瘤移动出照射野时,这一技术可以减轻肿瘤后方正常组织的过度照射,而且无论肿瘤在不同的呼吸时相中移动到何处,它都可以保证整个肿瘤受到合理的治疗。

对比于IMRT或被动散射质子治疗,IMPT对运动更敏感。在目前的临床实践中,我们建议肿瘤移动幅度<1cm者可以用IMRT治疗或被动散射质子治疗。为了尽量减小运动引起的不确定性,肿瘤运动≤5mm者应该使用IMPT治疗。呼吸时,大概有50%的肺部肿瘤运动距离接近5mm,30%~40%的运动距离接近5~10mm,10%的运动距离>1cm[32]。对于随呼吸运动幅度较大的肿瘤,在接受质子治疗时辅助以呼吸门控技术就显得十分必要。

自适应质子治疗

质子治疗不仅对分次内的肿瘤运动敏感,而且对分次间的肿瘤运动和解剖学的改变也很敏感。研究者近期开始研究分次治疗间肿瘤的运动及解剖学改变对质子放疗剂量分布的影响。在一项研究中,8例局部进展的NSCLC患者接受了质子治疗,Hui和Chang等人[33]获取了他们每周的4D CT扫描图像。他们为每例患者设计了适形被动散射质子治疗计划,并且将其与7周为一个周期的IMRT计划相比较。对其中一例患者来说,如果使用质子治疗,整个疗程中随着治疗次数的增加,其正常组织受照射的剂量增加,而CTV的剂量则被迫妥协(降低了近8%)。但是,这一改变在IMRT治疗中则不那么显著。因此,对于一些正在接受质子治疗的患者来说,应该实施分次的自适应计划。随后,这一团队又在同一组患者基础上开展了另一项临床研究,结果表明,20%的Ⅲ期NSCLC患者接受质子放疗[74Gy(RBE)/37f]与紫杉醇、卡铂同步治疗后,需要实施自适应质子治疗,因为随着时间的推移,解剖结构的变化将会影响到放疗剂量对肿瘤靶区的覆盖,并且超出剂量阈值[34]。自适应计划可以减少正常组织的受量、避免靶区遗漏,尤其适用于肿块大且在治疗过程中缩小的患者。即使对肿瘤体积大的患者,自适应计划仍可以使毒副作用减少到可接受的范围内,并且达到与非自适应计划相似的局部控制率、远处转移控制率和总生存率。

正常组织受量:质子治疗 vs 其他放疗技术

与3D-CRT、IMRT或体部立体定向放射治疗(SBRT)相比,质子治疗可降低正常组织受量

如前所述,剂量增加对于肺癌病变的局部控

制十分重要。人们始终致力于减少正常组织的无意暴露，与二维放疗相比，3D-CRT技术在该领域前进了一大步。IMRT有加速放疗的优点，同时不引起一些肺癌患者周围正常组织更大的毒副作用[35-37]。然而，在治疗肺癌中IMRT的运用一直被推迟，因为IMRT的焦点少，但是与其他放疗手段相比，更多的正常肺组织会受到破坏性剂量的照射。肿瘤随呼吸运动也是剂量学与IMRT照射技术上的复杂因素[38-39]。实际上，一项研究表明，IMRT比3D-CRT使患者肺组织受量≥5Gy的体积（V_5）增加[35-36]。然而，至少对于局部进展期患者来说，相比于3D-CRT，IMRT在不明显增加副反应发生的情况下，可以增加更大的剂量[35-37,40-41]。

我们推测质子治疗相比3D-CRT或IMRT能更好地使重要器官免受照射，我们比较了Ⅰ期或ⅢA/B期的NSCLC患者的剂量体积直方图（dose volume histogram，DVH），他们均接受了标准剂量的3D-CRT、IMRT或简单、无调强的三维被动散射质子治疗，这些方式均不采用调强技术，且采用标准或提升后的剂量[14]。比较结果表明，质子治疗使整个肺15%~17%或更多的体积免受照射，使对侧肺19%~23%或更多的体积免于照射。这部分免于暴露的体积有望大大减少肺部放疗副反应。与标准剂量的光子治疗相比，质子治疗也降低了食管、脊髓、心脏的受量，在大剂量分割的质子治疗中也是如此。而且，质子治疗使非靶体积的累积剂量改善了33%~60%，这在疾病早期以及对侧肺的射线暴露方面最明显。质子治疗可以明显降低心脏和脊髓的受量，提高患者的生活质量、延长其生命、使再次质子治疗成为可能。再重申一次，质子治疗使重要正常组织免于照射，这样便可以在肺癌治疗中施行大剂量照射、加速照射或二者并行，以提高局部控制率及生存率，并不增加治疗相关的副反应。近5年来，IMRT最优化和自动计划系统的发展大大提高了IMRT的适形度。然而，被动散射质子治疗更明显地减少心脏、脊髓、同侧及对侧肺的受量。但是，被动散射质子治疗中肺部V_{20}、全肺平均受量、食管剂量值的改善（毒副反应的减少可能也与以上进步有关）可能不是在所有的病例中都很明显，尤其是解剖结构复杂的个案，例如对侧肺门或锁骨上淋巴结受累、肿瘤紧邻食管或脊髓的患者。因为被动散射质子治疗中，射野个数有限，治疗野需要足够的边界以应对治疗中的不确定性，所以传递治疗剂量到复杂形状或位置的肿瘤靶区非常困难，例如肿瘤环形围绕敏感的重要结构生长。这样的案例需要在剂量上做出妥协以避免使正常组织结构受到破坏性的照射。另一个更有效的替代技术是IMPT，该技术使用扫描束治疗，通过构建包含靶区和正常组织约束项的目标函数，可以同时优化笔形射束的强度和能量。Zhang，Chang以及其他人比较了接受IMPT、被动散射质子治疗和IMRT的Ⅲ期NSCLC患者的剂量-体积直方图（DVH），以探索根治性个体化放疗的可能性[28]。这一对比结果显示，IMPT比IMRT使更多的肺、心脏、脊髓和食管免于照射，并同时将剂量由63Gy增加至83.5Gy，而IMRT的平均最大耐受剂量仅74Gy。与被动散射质子治疗相比，在相同或减少正常组织暴露的情况下，IMPT可以使处方剂量从74Gy增加至平均最大耐受剂量84.4Gy（范围是79.4~88.4Gy）。不仅如此，IMPT避免了复杂肿瘤治疗中可能出现的靶区欠量情况。临床上肺癌的IMPT治疗正在M.D.安德森癌症中心开展，但同时该技术仍有待进一步研究，因为还存在很多与肿瘤运动相关的不确定性和计划制定、质量保障方面复杂的问题。

对于中心型或超局限Ⅰ期的肺癌来说，质子治疗仍然能比立体定向放疗产生更少的毒副作用（后者是另一种以光子为基础的技术），因为质子的大部分能量沉积在质子束运动轨迹的末端。M.D.安德森癌症中心的研究员们也通过治疗计划比较被动散射质子治疗与立体定向放疗的相对优点[42]，并得出以下结论：与光子立体定向放疗相比，质子治疗（尤其是IMPT）可定向传递剂量到靶体积上，并且使周边正常组织的受量明显减少。

临床试验

几项NSCLC的质子治疗临床试验已经开展。早期试验关注的是早期疾病的大剂量或加速质子治疗，结果喜人，其治疗效果可与手术切除的ⅠA期患者的治疗结果相媲美。Bush等[43]纳入68例临床Ⅰ期患者，以51钴Gray当量（cobalt gray equivalents，CGE）2周分10次或60CGE 2周分10

次进行治疗。无 1 例出现放射性肺炎或晚期食管反应或心脏毒性症状。3 年局部控制率与疾病相关生存率分别为 74% 和 72%。T1（87%）期和 T2（49%）期患者的局部控制率显著升高，同时表现出提高生存率方面的趋势。局部控制方面，质子治疗后的 3 年 DFS 预期优于普通放疗。Shioyama 等[44]研究了 55 例 NSCLC 患者，他们接受平均剂量为 76Gy 的质子治疗，平均单次剂量为 3Gy。9 例 IA 期患者的 5 年生存率为 70%，19 例 IB 期的患者为 16%（$P<0.05$）。5 年野内局部控制率：IA 期（89%）优于 IB 期（39%）。47 例患者（92%）的急性肺损伤不大于 1 级，3 例为 2 级，1 例为 3 级，无患者表现为 4 级或更严重的损伤。这项研究中几乎没有出现晚期损伤患者。随后，Nihei 等[45]报道称，他们的初步试验结果显示 37 例 I 期 NSCLC 患者接受了 70~94CGE 治疗，分 20 次照射，2 年无进展生存率和总生存率分别为 80% 和 84%。IA 期患者的 2 年无局部复发生存率为 79%，IB 期为 60%。无严重急性放疗损伤发生，只有 3 例患者发生了 2 级或 3 级慢性肺损伤。近期，Chang 与其同事[46]报道了一项 I/II 期前瞻性研究，该研究纳入了中心型或超局限 IA~II 期 NSCLC 患者。早期结果表明（平均随访时间为 16.3 个月），总剂量 87.5CGE、分次剂量为 2.5CGE 的质子放疗在 67% 患者中产生了 2 级皮炎，44% 患者发生 2 级疲乏，11% 发生 I 期肺炎，6% 发生 2 级食管炎，6% 发生 2 级胸壁痛。无 4 级或 5 级副反应发生，局部控制率为 88.9%。以上发现与前述 Shioyama 与其同事的发现相似[44]，后者的 IA 期患者的 5 年局部控制率为 89%，仅 1 例出现 3 级急性放射损伤。

以上临床试验表明，对于早期 NSCLC 患者而言，质子治疗是安全且有效的。然而，目前还没有明确的最优方案。另外，以上研究均采用了简单的三维质子治疗，而 IMPT 和 IGRT 均未严格采用。目前，III 期 NSCLC 质子治疗的临床数据仍然很少，而该期肺癌最需要放射治疗。在一项回顾性研究中，35 例 II 或 III 期 NSCLC 患者接受质子治疗（平均剂量为 78.3CGE，范围为 67.1~91.3CGE），同期行化疗，Nakayama 与其同事[47]研究发现 1 年总生存率与无局部进展生存率分别为 81.8% 和 93.3%，2 年总生存率与无向部进展生存率为 58.9% 和 65.9%。令人惊讶的是，无 3 级或更严重的毒副反应发生。Sejpal 与其同事[48]也分析了 62 例局部进展的 NSCLC 患者，他们接受同步质子放化疗，化疗以铂类或多西他赛为基础方案，研究者将其预后与接受光子治疗患者的预后做了比较。质子治疗的平均总剂量为 74CGE，2 个光子治疗组的剂量为 63Gy。尽管质子治疗的剂量更高，质子治疗组的肺炎、食管炎、骨髓副反应发生率却比光子治疗组还低。最后，Chang 与其同事完成了一项 I 期试验，该试验纳入 44 例 III 期 NSCLC 患者，他们接受 74CGE 治疗，常规分割（单次剂量为 2CGE），同期每周行卡铂与紫杉醇治疗[49]。尽管治疗强度大，但几乎没有患者表现出 3 级放射损伤反应：5 例患者发生 3 级食管炎，5 例患者发生了 3 级皮炎，只有 1 例患者发生 3 级肺炎。没有出现 4 级、5 级放射损伤反应。局部控制率为 80%，总生存时间为 29.4 个月。总体来说，以上试验表明，对局部进展的肺癌患者来说，质子治疗可以减少副反应的发生，不仅可提高生活质量，而且可延长寿命。

我们迫切期待其他正在开展的研究结果。包括一项 I 期随机试验，该试验将 III 期 NSCLC 患者的 IMRT 与质子治疗［74Gy（RBE）］同期行化疗进行对比；另一项随机试验将中心型或复发的 NSCLC 的立体定向光子放疗与立体定向质子放疗进行对比。其他正在进行中的研究包括一项由 M.D. 安德森癌症中心与麻省总医院联合开展的，由美国国家卫生局支持的研究，以探究优化质子治疗，包括对不确定性的合理管控、结合门控技术的质子治疗和 IMPT。

（董原利　朱　健　李宝生　译）

参考文献

[1] Kaskowitz L, Graham M, Emami B, et al. Radiation therapy alone for stage I non-small cell lung cancer. Int Radiat Oncol Biol Phys, 1993, 27: 517-523.

[2] Dosoretz D, Kann M, Blitzer P, et al. Medically inoperable lung carcinoma: the role of radiation therapy. Semin Radiat Oncol, 1996, 6: 98-104

[3] Dosoretz D, Galmarini D, Rubenstein J, et al. Local control in medically inoperable lung cancer: an analysis of its

importance in outcome and factors determining the probability of tumor eradication. Int J Radiat Oncol Biol Phys, 1993, 27: 507-516.

[4] Curran WJ, Paulus R, Langer CJ, et al. Sequential vs. concurrent chemoradiation for stage III non-small cell lung cancer: Randomized phased III trial RTOG 9410. J Natl Cancer Inst, 2011, 103 (19): 1452-1460.

[5] Rosenman J, Halle J, Socinski M. High-dose conformal radiotherapy for treatment of stage IIIA/IIIB non-small-cell lung cancer: technical issues and results of a phase I/II trial. Int J Radial Oncol Biol Phys, 2002, 54 (2): 348-356.

[6] Kong E, Ten Haken R, Schipper M. et al. High-dose radiation improved local tumor control and overall survival in patients with inoperable/unresectable non-small-cell lung cancer: long-term results of a radiation dose escalation study. Int J Radial Oncel Biol Phys, 2005, 63 (2): 324-333.

[7] Choi N, Doucette J. Improved survival of patients with unresectable non-small-cell bronchogenic carcinoma by an innovated high-dose en-bloc radiotherapeutic approach. Cancer, 1981, 48: 10l-109.

[8] Machtay M, Bae K, Movsas B, et al. Higher biologically effective dose of radiotherapy is associated with improved outcomes for locally advanced Non-Small Cell Lung Carcinoma treated with chemoradiation: An analysis of the Radiation Therapy Oncology Group. Int J Radiat Oncol Biol Phys, 2012, 82 (1): 425-434.

[9] Perez C, Bauer M, Edelstein S, et al. Impact of tumor control on survival in carcinoma of the lung treated with irradiation. Int J Radiat Oncol Biol Phys, 1986, 12: 539-547.

[10] Cox J, Azarnia N, Byhardt R, et al. A randomized phase I/II trial of hyperfrctionated radiation therapy with total doses of 60.0 Gy to 79.2 Gy: Possible survival benefit with greater than or equal to 69.6 Gy in favorable patients with Radiation Therapy Oncology Group stage III non-small-cell lung carcinoma: report of Radiation Therapr Oncology Group 83-11. J Clin Oncol, 1990, 8 (9): 1543-1555.

[11] Bradley JD, Paulus R, Komaki R, et al. Randomized phase III comparison of standard-dose (60 Gy) versus high-dose (74 Gy) conformal chemoradiotherapy ± cetuximab for stage IIIA/IIIB non-small cell lung cancer: Preliminary findings on radiation dose in RTOG 0617, Presented at the 53rd Annual Meeting of the American Society for Radiation Oncology (ASTRO). Miami, FL, 2011, 3: 2011.

[12] Schild S, McGinnis W, Graham D, et al. Results of a phase I trial of concurrent chemotherapy and escalating doses of radiation for unresectable non-small cell lung cancer. Int J Radiat Oncol Biol Phys, 2006, 65 (4): 1106-1111.

[13] Belderbos J, Heemsbergen W, De Jaeger K, et al. Final results of a phase I/II dose escalation trial in non-small-cell lung cancer using three-dimensional conformal radiotherapy, Int Radial Oncol Biol Phys, 2006, 66 (1): 126-134.

[14] Chang JY, Zhang X, Wang X, et al. Significant reduction of normal tissue dose by proton radiotherapy compared with three-dimensional conformal or intensity-modulated radiation therapy in stage I or stage III non-small-cell lung cancer. Int J Radiat Oncol Biol Phys, 2006, 65: 1087-1096.

[15] Ruvsscher DK, Chang JY. Proton therapy for thoracic tumors. Semin Radiat Oncol, 2013, 23 (3): 115-119.

[16] Paganetti H, Niemierko A, Ancukiewiez M, et al. Relative biological effectiveness (RBE) values for proton beam therapy. Int J RadiatOncolBiol Phys, 2002, 53 (2): 407-421.

[17] Carabe A, Moteabbed M, Depauw N, et al. Range-uncertainty in proton therapy due to variable biological effectiveness. Phys Med Biol, 2012, 57 (5): 1159-1172.

[18] Paganetti H. Nuclear interactions in proton therapy: Dose and relative biological effect distributions originating from primary and secondary particles. Phys Med Biol, 2002, 47 (5): 747-764.

[19] Zhang X, Lin SH, Fang B, et al. Therapy-resistant cancer stem cells have differing sensitivity to photon versus proton beam radiation. J Thordac Oncol, 2013, 8 (12): 1484-1491.

[20] Halperin E. Particle therapy and treatment of cancer. Lancet Oncol, 2006, 7 (8): 676-685.

[21] Baumann M. Keynote comment: radiotherapy in the age of molecular oncology. Lancet Oncol, 2006, 7: 786-787.

[22] Lomax A, Bortfeld T, Goitein G, et al. A treatment planning inter-comparison of proton and intensity modulated photon radiotherapy. Radiother Oncol. 1999, 51 (3): 237-271.

[23] Hall E. Intensity-modulated radiation therapy, protons, and the risk of second cancers, Int I Radiat Oncol Biel Phys. 2006, 65 (1): 1-7.

[24] Kanai T, Kawachi K, Kumamoto Y, et al. Spot scanning system for proton radiotherapy. Med PhyS, 1980, 7 (4): 365-369.

[25] Schneider U, Pedroni E, Lomax A, et al. The calibration of CT Hounsfield units for radiotherapy treatment planning. Phys Med Biol, 1996, 41: 111-124.

[26] Oelfkc U, Bortfeld T. Inverse planning for photon and proton beams, Med Dosim, 2001, 26 (2): 113-124.

[27] Bortfeld T. An analytical approximation of the Bragg curve for therapeutic proton beams. Med Phys, 1997, 24: 2024-2033.

[28] Zhang X, Li Y, Pan X, et al. Intensity-modulated proton therapy reduces the dose to normal tissue compared with intensity-modulated radiation therapy or passive scattering proton therapy and enables individualized radical radiotherapy for extensive stage ⅢB non-small-cell lung cancer: a virtual clinical study. Int J Radiat Oncol Biol Phys, 2009, 77 (2): 357-366.

[29] Kang Y, Zhang X, Chang JY, et al. 4D Proton treatment planning strategy for mobile lung tumors. Int J Radiat Oncol Biol Phys, 2007, 67 (3): 906-914.

[30] Engelsman M, Rietzel E, Kooy HM. Four-dimensional proton treatment planning for lung tumors. Int J Radiat Oncol Biol Phys, 2006, 64 (5): 1589-1595.

[31] Movers M, Miller D, Bush D, et al. Methodologies and tools for proton beam design for lung tumors. Int J Radiat Oncol Biol Phys, 2001, 49 (5): 1429-1438.

[32] Chang JY, Dong L, Liu H, et al. Image-guided radiation therapy for non-small cell lung cancer. J Thorac Oncol, 2008, 3: 177-186.

[33] Hui Z, Zhang X, Starkschall G, et al. Effects of interfractional motion and anatomic changes on proton therapy dose distribution in lung cancer. Int J Radiat Oncol Biol Phys, 2008, 72 (5): 1385-1395.

[34] Koay EJ, Lege D, Mohan R, et al. Adaptive/nonadaptive proton radiation planning and outcomes in a phase II trial for locally advanced non-small cell lung cancer. Int J Radiat Oncol Biol Phys, 2012, 84 (5): 1093-1100.

[35] Murshed H, Liu H, Liao Z, et al. Dose and volume reduction for normal lung using intensity-modulated radiotherapy for advanced-stage non-small-cell lung cancer. Int J Radial Oncol Biol PhyS, 2004, 58 (4): 1258-1267.

[36] Liu H, Wang X, Dong L, et al. Feasibility of sparing lung and other thoracic structures with intensity-modulated radiotherapy for non-small-cell lung cancer. Int. J Radiat Oncol Biol Phys, 2004, 58 (4): 1268-1279.

[37] Grills I, Yan D, Martinez A, et al. Potential for reduced toxicity and dose escalation in the treatment of inoperable non-small-cell lung cancer: A comparison of intensity-modulated radiation therapy (IMRT), 3D conformal radiation, and elective nodal irradiation. Int Radial-Oncol Biol Phy, 2003, 57 (3): 875-890.

[38] Chul C, Yorke B, Hong L. The effects of intrafraction organ motion on the delivery of intensity-modulated field with a multileaf collimator. Med Phys, 2003, 30 (7): 4736-4746.

[39] Bortfeld T, Jokivarsi K, Goitein M, et al. Effects of intra-fraction motion on IMRT dose delivery Statistical analysis and simulation. Phys Med Biol, 2002, 47 (13): 2203-2220.

[40] Yom SS, Liao Z, Liu HH, et al. Initial evaluation of treatment-related pneumonitis in advanced-stage non-small-cell lung cancer patients treated with concurrent chemotherapy and intensity-modulated radiotherapy. Int Radiat Oncol Biol Phys, 2007, 68 (1): 94-102.

[41] Jiang ZQ, Yang K, Komaki R, et al. Long-term clinical outcome of intensity-modulated radiotherapy for inoperable non-small cell lung cancer: The MD Anderson experience. Int J Radiat Oncol Biol Phys, 2012, 83 (1): 332-339.

[42] Register SP, Zhang X, Mohan R, et al. Proton stereotactic body radiation therapy for clinically challenging cases of centrally and superiorly located stage I non-small-cell lung cancer. Int J Radiat Oncol Biol Phys, 2011, 80 (4): 1015-1022.

[43] Bush D, Slater J, Shin B, et al. Hypofractionated proton beam radiotherapy for stage I lung cancer. Chest, 2004, 126 (4): 1198-1203.

[44] Shioyama Y, Tokuuye K, Okumura T, et al. Clinical evaluation of proton radiotherapy for non-small-cell lung cancer. Int J Radiat Oncol Biol Phys, 2003, 56 (1): 7-13.

[45] Nihei K, Ogino T, Ishikura S, et al. High-dose proton beam therapy for stage I non-small-cell lung cancer. Int J Radiat Oncol Biol Phys, 2006, 65 (1): 107-111.

[46] Chang JY, Komaki R, Wen HY, et al. Toxicity and patterns of failure of adaptive/ablative proton therapy for early-stage, medically inoperable non-small cell lung cancer. Int J Radiat Oncol Biol Phys, 2011, 80 (5): 1350-1357.

[47] Nakayama H, Satoh H, Sugahara S, et al. Proton beam therapy of stage Ⅱ and Ⅲ non-small-cell lung cancer. Int J Radiat Oncol Biol Phys, 2011, 81 (4): 979-984.

[48] Sejpal S, Komaki R, Tsao A, et al. Early findings on toxicity of proton beam therapy with concurrent chemotherapy for nonsmall cell lung cancer. Cancer, 2011, 117 (13): 3004-3013.

[49] Chang JY, Komaki R, Lu C, et al. Phase 2 study of high-dose proton therapy with concurrent chemotherapy for unresectable stage Ⅲ nonsmall cell lung cancer. Cancer, 2011, 117 (20): 4707-4713.

第23章
非小细胞肺癌的放化联合治疗

Daniel Gomez[1], Zhongxing Liao[1], Pierre Saintigny[2], Ritsuko U. Komaki[1]
1. Department of Radiation Oncology, The University of Texas MD Anderson Cancer Center, Houston, TX, USA
2. Department of Thoracic/Head and Neck Medical Oncology, The University of Texas MD Anderson Cancer Center, Houston, TX, USA

引 言

许多局部进展期的非小细胞肺癌（NSCLC）患者失去了根治性手术切除的机会。对于这部分患者，序贯或同步放化综合治疗成为一个可行的选择。过去20年间，许多研究通过评价和对比这些治疗方法，证实了基于患者一般情况、照射剂量、系统性治疗模式及化疗和放疗的时间安排等因素造成的毒副反应发生率及疗效的不同。总之，这些试验结果确定了同步放化疗作为目前不可手术的NSCLC的标准疗法。本章节阐述了放化联合治疗的依据并综述了形成当今肺癌治疗模式的相关研究，并且总结了与放化联合治疗相关的各种毒副反应及远期预后。

放化联合治疗的依据

通常来说，放化联合治疗提高疗效的依据有以下4点：不同的抗肿瘤机制，正常组织保护，空间协同作用及肿瘤治疗反应增强作用，其中，只有空间协作及肿瘤治疗反应增强作用适用于NSCLC的治疗[1]。空间协同的本质很明确（如放疗针对局限的肿瘤病灶，化疗则针对远处转移），但肿瘤治疗反应增强作用则不然。因为专业术语（如放射增敏）对不同的研究者意义也有所不同，我们更倾向于使用Steel和Peckham推荐的术语[1]。

Eberhardt及其同事对放、化疗联合治疗的依据进行了详尽准确的综述[2]。该综述的重点总结如下：电离辐射通过产生自由基破坏肿瘤细胞并导致其坏死和凋亡[3]，同样，全身治疗通过打乱信号通路导致肿瘤细胞死亡并降低增殖能力[4]。当序贯治疗时，化疗与放疗的作用理论上能互补，射线控制局部区域病灶，化疗控制全身微小转移的恶性细胞。当选择序贯治疗时，两种治疗方法都能给予较高的剂量，所以更有效。

相反，当同步治疗时，不止通过放化疗各自及相关的细胞杀伤能力作用于同一细胞来增加疗效，而且还能作用于不同的细胞导致DNA损伤、杀死特异性细胞并能降低增殖速度[1,5]。如Eberhardt所说："理论上，超相加效应能通过适当处理对两种治疗的修复过程的抑制来达到，以实现不同治疗方式的抗肿瘤潜能互补"[1-2,5]。举例来说，细胞周期同步能增加电离辐射引起的细胞死亡。

然而，尽管治疗理论各有不同，导致大多数不可手术的NSCLC患者死亡的原因却归结于局部肿瘤的治疗不当。许多临床证据支持这个观点。首先，单纯放疗与局部肿瘤控制后再加放疗的患者相比预后差，这与放射野内肿块残留或进展相关[6-7]。其次，仅接受姑息放疗或单药化疗的患者死于胸内病变者多于胸外转移，尤其是鳞状细胞癌[8]。再次，更多接受几次大分割放疗的局限期不可手术患者死于胸内肿瘤并发症的远多于远处转移（72% vs 15%）[9]。但是Perez等却发现改善局部肿瘤控制率增加了远处转移的发生率[10]。最终另外一个研究团队发现同步放化疗提高了肿瘤局部控制率，而这反过来改善了预后[11]。

序贯放化疗

如前所述,放疗前的诱导化疗有两个优点:①诱导化疗能直接攻击所有肿瘤细胞,包括临床证实的和亚临床病灶;②如果诱导化疗有效,就为放疗期间或之后继续应用化疗提供了依据。尽管许多前瞻性随机临床试验得到的数据有混杂,但有3项基于铂类化疗和≥60Gy放疗的研究报道的总生存率有获益(表23.1)[12-16]。

这3个试验中最有名的一个由癌症和白血病B组报道,其结果显示诱导化疗有明确的生存获益。这项编号CALGB8433的试验对两种治疗方式进行了比较,第1种治疗方式为铂类(100mg/m²)联合长春花碱(每周5mg/m²,连用5周)诱导化疗,然后自第50天起序贯放疗(每次2Gy,每周5次,总剂量60Gy)。第2种治疗方式为自治疗第1天起单纯放疗。这项研究在达到计划收益之前就提前关闭了,关闭当时诱导化疗就已显示出优越的中位生存期和5年生存率,长期随访显示患者仍有生存获益[13]。Le Chevalier及其同事报道的包括353例患者的第2项临床试验证实了CALGB试验振奋人心的结果[14,18-19]。在CALGB试验开始阶段,患者被随机分为诱导化疗后联合放疗组或单纯放疗组,诱导化疗组先接受了3次/月,一个周期的长春地辛(第1~2天1.5mg/m²),环磷酰胺(第2~4天200mg/m²),顺铂(第2天100mg/m²)和洛莫司汀(75mg/m²)化疗,然后自第75~80天开始放疗(2.5Gy/次,每周4次,总剂量65Gy);另一组仅接受单纯放疗。结果再次证实诱导化疗的生存获益更大,而且远处转移率下降,但未发现局部控制率有所改善。实际上,由于法国协作组的研究者在治疗开始后3个月常规用纤维支气管镜活检原发肿瘤灶,所以他们能证明两组治疗方式的肿瘤局部失败(高达80%以上),并且诱导化疗对局部控制率没有改善。这些结果

表23.1 局部进展期NSCLC序贯放化疗的临床试验

研究	病例数	照射剂量(Gy)	化疗方案	中位生存时间(月)	局部区域控制率(%) 3年	局部区域控制率(%) 5年	总生存率(%) 3年	总生存率(%) 5年
Dillman等, 1996[13]	77	60	—	9.7	6	5	11	7
	79	60	顺铂联合长春花碱	13.8	18	6 (P=0.026)	23	19 (P=0.012)
Brodin等, 1996[12]	164	56(分程照射)	—	未报道	未报道	3(4年)	6	1.4
	163	56(分程照射)	CE	未报道	未报道	7(4年; P=0.07)	13	3 (P=0.16)
Morton等, 1991[15]	58	60	—	9.6	未报道		未报道	7
	56	60	氨甲蝶呤、阿霉素、环磷酰胺、洛莫司汀	10.4	未报道	未报道	未报道	5
Le Chevalier等, 1992[14]	177	65	—	10.0	17(1年)	未报道	4	3
	176	65	长春地辛、环磷酰胺、顺铂、洛莫司汀	12.0	15(1年)	未报道	12	6 (P<0.02)
Sause等, 2000[16]	149	60	顺铂联合长春花碱	11.4	未报道	未报道	11	5
	151	60		13.2	未报道	未报道	17	8
	152	69.5(每天2次)	0	12	未报道	未报道	14	6 (P=0.04)

导致RTOG（肿瘤放射治疗组）和ECOG（美国东部肿瘤协作组）合作发起了一项三臂临床试验（即RTOG88-08，又称为ECOG4588）。这项试验比较了NSCLC常规分割放疗、序贯放化疗（如CALGB模式）和超分割放疗（总剂量69.6Gy）生存率的不同[16,20]。结果显示序贯放化疗组明显优于常规分割放疗和超分割放疗组，后两者的生存率相似。随后Komaki等分析了这项试验的失败模式[21]，发现只有鳞状细胞癌患者的远端转移控制得到改善，并且化疗对局部肿瘤影响不显著[22]，这个结果与法国试验一致。

CALGB试验结束后，Dillman和合作者对试验数据进行了回顾性质控综述[13,17]，发现大量病例（23%）的放射野并不能完全覆盖原发肿瘤，并且上述所有试验中诱导化疗后的放疗技术均为二维放射治疗计划，如今看来是不规范的。

从上述试验可以得出以下推论：第一，如果可行，序贯化疗后联合放疗比单纯放疗好；第二，至少在某些情况下，化疗确实能控制鳞癌的远处转移播散，这与临床前研究的结论一致；最后，放射野内原发灶的控制比预想的差，诱导化疗对此也无增益。

同步放化疗

为提高局部控制率并降低远处转移率，研究者努力探索其他治疗策略，包括放疗同步铂类为基础的化疗、化疗联合超分割放疗及化疗新药、靶向药联合放疗。单药化疗联合放疗的目的是改善局部控制率。

Byhardt报道了首个RTOG同步放化疗的临床试验[23]，即RTOG 90-15，这项试验联合了来自CALGB8433试验的顺铂-长春碱方案化疗和Cox等报道的剂量寻觅试验中具有优越性的超分割放疗方案（1.2Gy/f，每天2次，每周5d，共69.6Gy）[24]。尽管只有个别患者预后因素好，中位生存期仍达到12.2个月，该数据令人鼓舞[23]。值得注意的是，RTOG 90-15试验进行的同时，超分割放疗方案也与RTOG 8808/ECOG 4588试验中的常规分割方案进行了比较。

RTOG90-15后续试验，又被称为RTOG90-16，与前者设计相同，不同的是比较了放疗期间每天口服依托泊苷联合顺铂是否比长春碱类联合顺铂更有效[25]。具体方案为：超分割放疗期间，自第1天联合顺铂（第1天和第9天75mg/m^2，静脉滴注）及依托泊苷（第1~14天，第29~43天50mg，口服，每天2次）化疗。这种联合治疗的毒性值得关注，尤其是食管毒性。然而，它带来的生存获益也非常显著：对有良好预后因素的患者，中位生存期为21个月，两年生存率为42%。来自阿维尼翁的Rebort等在随后的一项研究中报道了确切的结果，这个研究与之前的化疗方案相似，但用的是常规分割放疗[26]。

为了降低RTOG91-06方案的急性毒性，随后的Ⅰ、Ⅱ期临床试验RTOG92-04微调了化疗方案[27]，具体为每周末不放疗的时间取消了依托泊苷（50mg，口服），这样就将服用依托泊苷由28d降至20d。这个方案的结果非常复杂，尽管调整后的化疗方案降低了非血液系统毒性，代价却是提高了局部肿瘤进展率。而且中位生存期和1年生存率也没有明显提高（分别为15.5个月 vs 14.1个月，65% vs 58%）。

许多研究比较了NSCLC同步放化疗和单纯放疗的疗效。一项包括19项随机试验、2 728例患者的meta分析对比了NSCLC同步放化疗和单纯放疗疗效，结果显示同步放化疗显著提高了总生存率、无进展生存率和局部区域无进展生存率。而且，与单纯放疗相比，同步放化疗与3级以上放射性肺炎及晚期肺、食管毒性的发生率不相关。然而，同步化疗组急性食管反应及血液系统毒性更严重，如白细胞减少和贫血。最后，亚组分析显示同步放化疗每天1次的分割模式较每天2次的获益更大[28]。

序贯与同步放化疗的比较

许多研究通过对比序贯和同步放化疗的疗效来确定局部进展期NSCLC的最佳治疗模式。正如前述，序贯治疗的潜在优势包括毒性低和单纯化疗药物浓度更高。另一方面，同步治疗能通过互补机制发挥化疗的放疗增敏作用，因此理论上能提高局部疾病控制率（disease control rate，DCR）。至少有7个临床试验就序贯和同步放化疗的PFS

和 OS 进行了比较[29-35]。这些试验的放化疗方案多种多样，但化疗都以铂类为基础。总的来说，这些试验的结果显示同步放化疗的生存获益更大，但毒性也更大。如 RTOG94-10 比较了 3 种化放综合治疗方案：①顺铂联合长春花碱化疗序贯放疗 1.8Gy/f，每天 1 次，共 63Gy；②顺铂联合长春花碱化疗同步放疗 1.8Gy/f，每天 1 次，共 63Gy；③顺铂联合依托泊苷化疗同步放疗 1.2Gy/f，每天 2 次，共 69.6Gy。第二组的中位生存期（17 个月）优于另外两组（第一组和第三组分别为 14.6 个月和 15.2 个月），但每天 2 次放疗的毒性更大[29]。同样，法国一项研究发现顺铂联合依托泊苷化疗同步放疗，后续顺铂联合长春花碱巩固化疗的中位生存期（16.3 个月 vs 14.5 个月）、两年总生存期（overall survival，OS）、4 年 OS 均优于顺铂联合长春花碱化疗序贯放疗。同步放化疗的食管毒性更明显。

另外两个关于序贯和同步放化疗的试验观察了新型化疗药组合卡铂联合紫杉醇的疗效[34-35]。两项试验均未发现同步治疗有生存获益。但是 Huber 等的报道提示可能有中位生存获益。另外，Belani 等的报道也提示之前的同步化疗组较其他组的中位生存期延长了 3 个月。

Auperin 等和 O'Rourke 等进行了两个不同的 meta 分析，评价了 6 项关于同步与序贯放化疗的Ⅲ期随机试验生存和毒性的不同[28,37]。结果显示同步放化疗有显著的 OS 获益 [HR = 0.74；95% CI（0.62，0.89）]，3 年、5 年绝对获益分别为 5.7% [95% CI（18.1%，23.8%）] 和 4.5%。同步放化疗还降低了局部区域进展，但对远处转移无改善，说明这种生存获益得益于良好的局部区域控制（图 23.1）。同步两联或三联化疗看上去比单药治疗的 PFS 获益更大 [HR = 0.83；95% CI（0.72，0.95）] vs [HR = 1.15；95% CI（0.90，1.48）]，P = 0.02。同步与序贯治疗相比，治疗相关死亡人数更多（4% vs 2%），但没有统计学差异。同步治疗组严重食管炎的发生率明显增加 [RR = 4.96；95% CI（2.17，11.37）][28]。

总之，来自这些多中心临床试验的结果为局部晚期 NSCLC 应用基于铂类的同步放疗提供了依据和保证。这项治疗手段显示出目前最好的 5 年生存率，可作为不能手术的ⅢA、ⅢB 期 NSCLC 的根治性治疗手段之一。

同步放化疗后手术切除

另一种同步治疗方案是诱导放化疗后再行手术切除。这种方案适用于以下两种患者：①胸外科医生对手术切除有争议；②患者愿意接受手术风险。不幸的是，大多数临床试验都未明确ⅢA 期 N2 的 NSCLC 人群中适合这种治疗的亚组及入组标准。这些研究中受侵淋巴结的大小和数目异质性明显，并且一些研究建议有微小纵隔结节受侵的最好行术前化疗[38]。这些异质性限制了该方法的广泛临床应用。

西南肿瘤协作组（SWOG）的一项Ⅱ期临床试验 SWOG 8805 评价了同步放化疗后手术的疗效。这些研究纳入了 126 例精心挑选的ⅢA 或ⅢB 期患者，并且转移淋巴结都经过活检或经皮细针抽吸证实[39]。治疗方案为前 5 周为顺铂（第 1、8、29、36 天的剂量为 50 mg/m^2）联合静脉依托泊苷（第 1~5 天，第 29~33 天的剂量为 50 mg/m^2）。化疗同步放疗（1.8Gy/f，每周 5 次，共 45Gy），2~4 周后行胸廓切开肿瘤切除术。中位生存期为 15 个月，2 年 OS 为 40%。在放疗前 N2 期患者有超过 50% 降期为 N0；然而几乎 40% 的患者出现局部复发，并且大部分患者有远处转移。3 年总 OS 为 27%，在放化疗后纵隔病变消失患者的生存率明显高于病变残留患者（44% vs 18%）。

这些振奋人心的结果促使了另一项随机试验的开展，这项试验对比了手术与放化疗联合对 N2 期 NSCLC 的治疗效果，其最终结果发表于 2005 年（INT 0139 试验也被称为 RTOG 9309 和 ECOG/SWOG 9336 试验）[40]。类似于 SWOG 8805，所有患者先进行了为期 5 周的诱导化疗联合放疗，然后随机分配，其中一般患者在 2~4 周后手术探查，另一半继续原方案放化疗（总剂量达 61.0Gy/33 次）。手术组的无进展生存期（progression-free survival，PFS）略长（12.8 个月 vs 10.5 个月；P = 0.017），但中位生存期无显著差异（23.6 个月 vs 22.6 个月；P = 0.24）。治疗相关死亡率在手术组和非手术组分别为 8% 和 2%。最后，

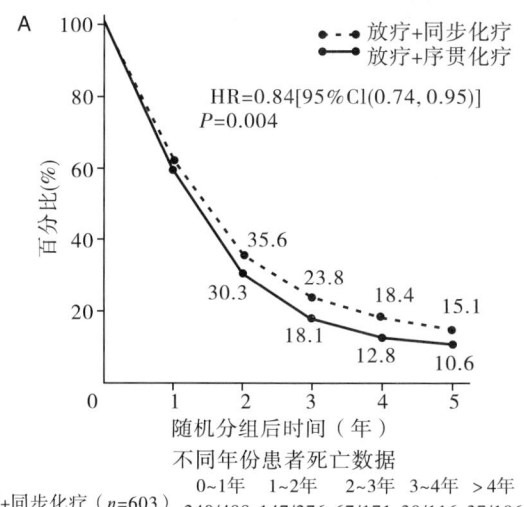 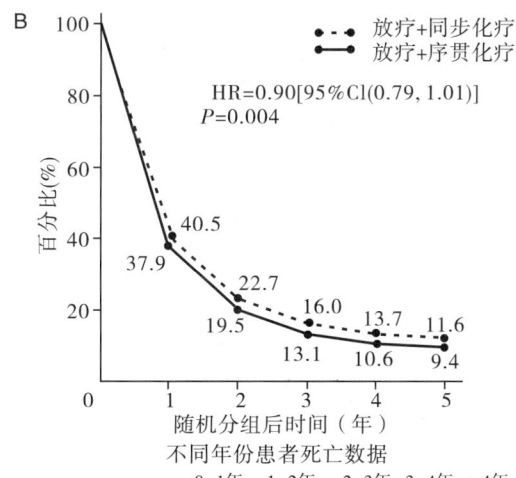

图 23.1 局部进展期 NSCLC 同步与序贯放化疗的 meta 分析中的总生存和无进展生存曲线

探索性分析显示接受肺叶切除的患者生存率优于单纯行放化疗者,但全肺切除的则不然[41]。这项研究的结果提示,对于局部进展期患者,根治性同步放化疗(理论上同步进行)或诱导化疗联合或不联合放疗后续手术都是可行的。M. D. 安德森肿瘤中心的一个多学科小组对这类病例进行了回顾性分析,一般来说,一般情况和肺功能较好,无巨大淋巴结和单个淋巴结受侵的患者,不需要行全肺切除,推荐根治性肺叶切除。这些标准与 2012 年 NCCN 的指南一致[42]。

放疗

放疗剂量在肿瘤局部控制率中的重要性

如前所述,局部进展期 NSCLC 根治性放化疗失败的一个主要原因是局部复发[13,16]。最终有超过 90% 的患者局部复发;影像学检查仅能发现 45%~52% 的病例,但活检却证实 85% 的患者局部治疗失败[13,43-44]。

局部区域疾病的有效控制非常重要,因为不受控制的局部病灶能引起严重的症状,如阻塞性肺炎、出血、疼痛,甚至能导致死亡。对接受同步放化疗的患者来说,局部区域疾病的良好控制能转换为生存获益[36]。提高肿瘤局部控制率的一种方法就是强化局部区域治疗;对于不能手术切除的肿瘤患者来说,增加放疗剂量是一种合理的办法。尽管还没有研究证实放疗剂量增加有确切的生存获益,2012 年发表的一篇包括 7 项同步放化疗的前瞻性临床试验的综述证实局部区域控制情况与总生存期有强关联(图 23.2A)[44]。该综述中将局部区域控制明确定义为两种情况:①无局部区域进展,即随机化时所有患者的局部区域病灶都受到了控制;②反应(疗效)控制,即影像学必须证实原发肿瘤至少达到 PR,如果未达到 PR,随机化时这些患者即被视为局部区域失败。只有 46% 的患者在治疗结束时就达到 PR。随着时间的延长,局部区域控制率下降,分别为 1 年 28%,2 年 17%,5 年 8%(图 23.2B)。而且,接受更高生物等效剂量(biological equralent dose,BED)的放疗与局部区域控制和生存强关联,$P<0.0001$(图 23.2C)。在一项纳入近 1 400 例患者的研究中,患者接受同步放化疗,放疗剂量达 60~69.6Gy,其中 BED 随时间调整每增加 1Gy,就有约 4% 的生存获益和约 3% 的局部区域控制获益[44]。这个结论证实了分割放疗后高剂量放疗能提高局部区域控制和总生存的假说。

然而,RTOG 0617 试验的结果却让大家对高剂量射线是否有生存获益产生了质疑,这项Ⅲ期临床试验的最初设计目的是观察Ⅲ期 NSCLC 患者同步放化疗加或不加西妥昔单抗对疗效的影响,其中放疗剂量为 60Gy 或 74Gy。2011 年 6 月的一项临时中期分析显示两组(高剂量比低剂量放疗)结果无差异,意味着高剂量放疗与低剂量相比,基本不可能改善预后。在撰写本章节时,两组的毒性还没有被证实有明显差异,并且对于高剂量放疗没有生存获益的原因还未找到。对于高剂量和

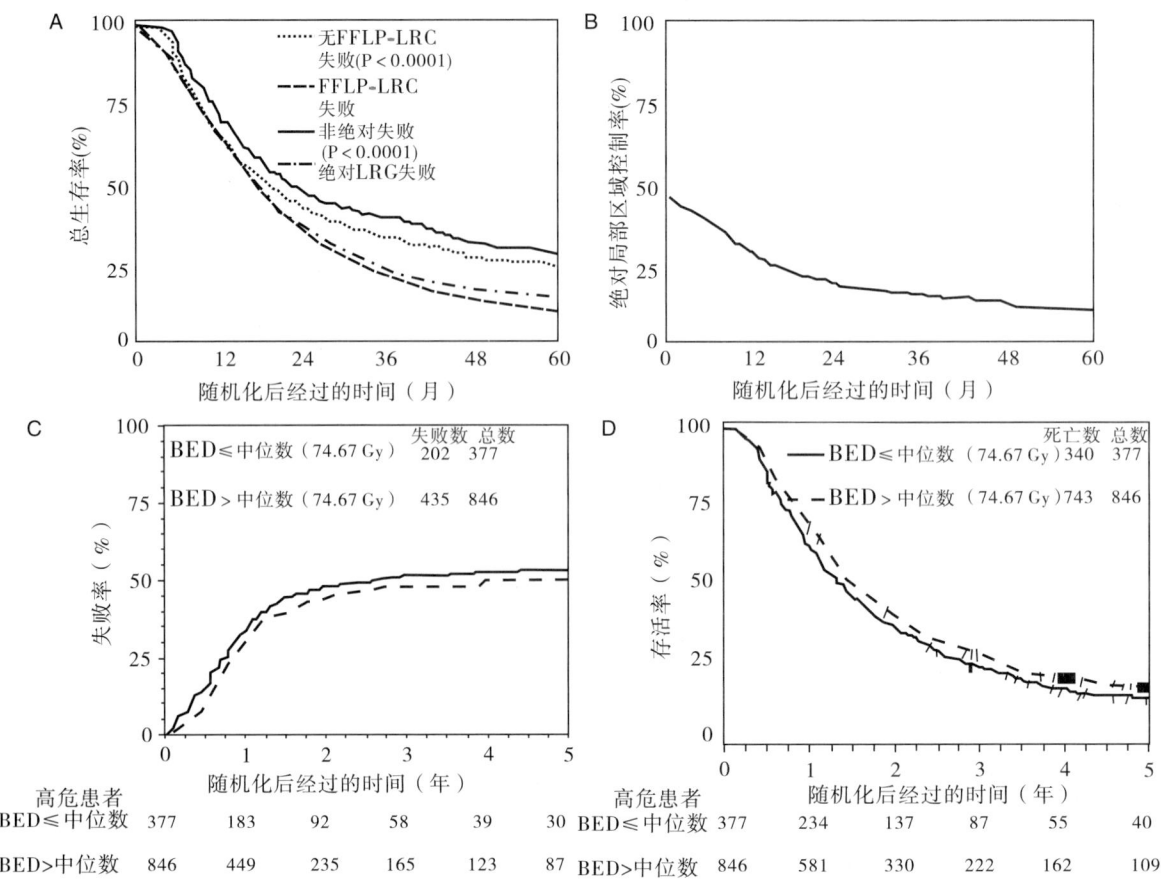

图 23.2 A. 接受根治性放疗的患者局部区域控制的改善转化为总生存获益。B. 1 390 例患者局部区域控制率的下降，由治疗后的 46% 将为 5 年时的 8%。FFLP：局部区域进展；LRC：局部区域控制；BED：等效生物剂量。C. IMRT 失败率的下降和总生存获益（经 Elsevier 同意，摘自 Machtay M, Paulus R, Moughan J, et al. Defining local-regional control and it's importance in locally advanced non-small-cell lung carcinoma. J Thorac Oncol, 2012, 7: 716-722[44]）

正常剂量放疗组对比的研究正在进行，可能可以部分解释上述结果。

放疗靶区的设计与勾画

许多因素影响 NSCLC 治疗靶区确认及照射野的设置。这些因素包括原发肿瘤的大小和部位、肺门和纵隔淋巴引流区域、组织学类型、可用设备及射束能量。以往传统放疗的照射野需要外扩边界很大才能覆盖照射范围。随着高度适形技术的出现，我们推荐应用适形放疗，抛弃传统放疗。

选择性淋巴结照射

许多医生认为手术和外照射的疗效相似。这两种治疗方式都是为了局部控制。因此，多年来，除少数个例，美国的标准放疗模式一直是特定区域淋巴结预防性照射 40~50Gy（如同侧肺门、同侧及对侧纵隔和锁骨上淋巴结区），复位缩野后原发肿瘤再补充照射 20Gy[45-50]。这种选择性淋巴结照射（elective nadal irradiatian, ENI）的主要争议在于射野内局部复发率高。如果射线连肿块本身都控制不好，那为何还要扩大照射体积？只为覆盖可能发生微转移的地方？然而，自 RTOG 7301 试验最初建立放疗剂量体积标准以来，肺癌治疗的几项重大变革，特别是化放联合治疗、3D CRT 的出现和 PET 用于 NSCLC 的分期，很大程度上解决了这个疑问。

最近的一些临床试验发现选择性治疗的淋巴结失败率很低，因此，当先进技术用于诊断、分期和放疗时，可见病变外的照射野对疾病的控制没有益处。如一项早期 NSCLC 根治性放疗失败模式的综述显示，孤立的区域失败发生率不超过 15%[51]，说明即便不用 ENI，也能有效控制局部射野内病变。

Zhang 及其同事观察了支气管肺癌只照射原发肿瘤不照射淋巴结的预后，发现 3 年和 5 年生存率分别为 55% 和 32%[45]。Dosoretz 等的另一项试验发现射野大小与疾病转归不相关,根据肿块大小分层分析的结果仍然如此。第三项试验,Krol 及其同事报道了 108 例接受根治性放疗但未行 ENI 的 I 期肺癌患者的预后,放疗靶区为原发肿瘤。3 年及 5 年 OS 分别为 31% 和 15%,值得注意的是,这项研究的 3 年、5 年疾病特异性生存率分别为 42% 和 31%[48]。这些数据与靶区包括传统射野及区域淋巴引流区的疗效相当。这些结果也被 Senan 及其同事的研究证实[46],他们报道未行选择性淋巴结照射的 III 期患者有类似的低失败率。

其他研究进一步验证了 ENI 的失败率低。Rosenzweig 等对接受 3D CRT 患者 ENI 的失败率进行了系列报道,发现失败率在 5% ~ 10%[47-52]。Yuan 等报道了一项纳入 200 例不可手术的 NSCLC 患者的随机临床试验,治疗方式为 4~6 个周期以顺铂为基础的化疗及 3D CRT。患者被随机分为累及野放疗组和 ENI 组,剂量为每次 1.8~2.0Gy,前者总剂量为 68~74Gy,后者总剂量为 60~64Gy。ENI 组的靶区包括原发肿瘤、同侧肺门、双侧纵隔,如果有上纵隔转移还包括锁骨上区。结果显示,累及野放疗的总生存率更高,放射性肺炎的发生率更低[53]。提醒一下,解读这项研究结果需要注意两组间放疗剂量的差异及是否诱导化疗产生的不确定性。尽管如此,最近的一个关于 ENI 的专家共识建议:根据患者的具体情况来制订治疗方案,如分期及安全的放射剂量等。这样,在某些情况下是可以考虑 ENI 的[54]。至少有两个可能的原因来解释 ENI 试验中低于预期的区域淋巴结失败率。首先,即使不刻意照射,同侧肺门、气管旁和隆突下淋巴结区域也会接受 40~50Gy 的附带照射[55];第二,肺癌患者经常面对竞争死因(如局部失败、原位失败或者其他并发疾病),即便没有发现选择性淋巴结失败,这些病变也能导致死亡。

三维适形放疗

3D CRT 较传统放疗有几个明显的优势:改善了肿瘤与正常组织的勾画质量;图像分割与展示;精确的剂量计算;能操纵射束几何形状及通过正向计划加权。对靶区勾画改善的重要性不能过高估计。一旦患者摆好治疗体位进行 CT 扫描,放射肿瘤医生就可以三维勾画肿瘤部位及相邻的组织;选择能最大限度覆盖肿瘤的射束角度,同时使暴露于射线的正常组织面积最小化;改变射束权重;通过改变床角达到非共面照射。这种适形技术还能融合其他互补的成像模式,如 PET-CT 来帮助勾画肿瘤部位和单光子发射计算机断层来选择射束角度。

NSCLC 3D CRT 的计划制定很大程度上得益于国际辐射单位委员会(International Commission on Radiation Units,ICRU)出版的靶区定义指南应用[56]。根据这个指南,大体肿瘤体积(grass tumer volume,GTV)定义为原发肿瘤和淋巴结转移。临床肿瘤体积(clinical tumor volume,CTV)定义为隐藏微转移灶的解剖学定义区域(肺门/纵隔淋巴结或大体可见肿瘤的周围区域)。计划靶体积(planning target volume,PTV)覆盖治疗过程中器官的生理运动及分次治疗过程中的每日摆位误差。为了保证 GTV 的适形高剂量照射并使周围正常组织(特别是肺)的受照剂量最小化,通过射野形状设置、射束设定及权重分配,三维治疗计划也就完成了。

实施 3D CRT 非常重要的一点就是不能超过敏感组织的最大耐受剂量,对肺癌来说,包括正常肺组织、食管、脊髓和心脏。不幸的是,正常组织的部分容积耐受不是很明确。在可能的情况下,要特别注意限制正常肺组织的照射剂量(例如,不超过 20Gy,未修正的不均匀性)。需要生成所有正常胸部器官的剂量 - 体积直方图(dose-volume histogram,DVH)并分析受照剂量及体积。尽管 DVH 的分析仍在不断发展,它对预测肺炎等并发症和优化治疗计划的确有用[55,57-59]。图 23.3 显示了右肺上叶 T2N2 期鳞状细胞癌 IMRT 应用的典型图像。

将射线引起的正常组织毒性最小化

过去几十年,美国国立癌症研究所指定的工作组综合文献,并征求了经验丰富的放射肿瘤医生的意见后,制订了器官对射线的部分容积耐受性[60]。1991 年工作组的研究发表时,许多医生仍沿用 5 年并发症发生率来估计器官的耐受剂量(如被照射组织的毒性评价终点定义为 5 年内并发症发生率为 5% 或 5 年内并发症发生率为 50%)。然而,工作组承认这些指标,特别是关于正常胸部组织的,是在生物调节剂、同步放化疗或 3D CRT 出现之前,缺乏足够信息的情况下汇集的。

之后,对正常组织毒性的认识有了长足的进

步。这些研究被总结为一系列共识文件并在 2010 年出版于《临床正常组织效应的定量分析（Quantitative analyses of Normal Tissue Effects in the Clinic, QUANTEC)》。这些研究总结性地概括了可用的文献，并对各种正常组织结构的剂量限制提供了建议。这些文献对肺癌的临床治疗提供了完善、基于循证医学的剂量限制模式（表 23.2）[61-65]。肺和食管的剂量限制情况见下文。

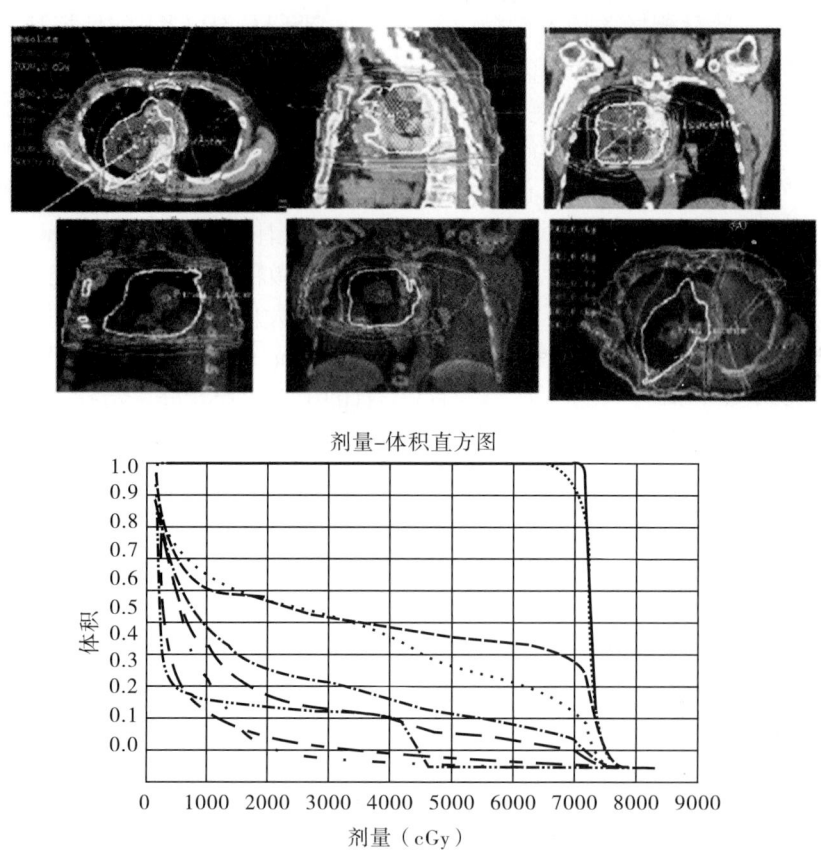

图 23.3（见彩插）　Ⅲ期 NSCLC 放疗计划典型的剂量分布图和剂量体积直方图。上图：基于 CT 图像的 IMRT；中图：基于肺单侧 PET/CT 图像的 IMRT 计划；下图：一个典型的剂量体积直方图。直方图中不同的颜色代表不同的器官结构

表 23.2　常规分割放疗（如单次照射剂量 <3Gy）时胸部恶性肿瘤的推荐限制剂量（来源于 QUANTEC 推荐剂量）[61-64]

	单纯放疗	化疗联合放疗	术前放化疗
脊髓[1]	最大剂量 <45Gy	最大剂量 <45Gy	最大剂量 <45Gy
肺[2]	平均肺剂量 ≤20Gy	平均肺剂量 ≤20Gy	平均肺剂量 ≤20Gy
	$V_{20} \leq 40\%$	$V_{20} \leq 35\%$	$V_{20} \leq 30\%$
		$V_{10} \leq 45\%$	$V_{10} \leq 40\%$
		$V_5 \leq 65\%$	$V_5 \leq 55\%$
心脏	$V_{30} \leq 45\%$	$V_{30} \leq 45\%$	$V_{30} \leq 45\%$
	平均剂量 <26Gy	平均剂量 <26Gy	平均剂量 <26Gy
食管	最大剂量 ≤80Gy	最大剂量 ≤80Gy	最大剂量 ≤80Gy
	$V_{70} < 20\%$	$V_{70} < 20\%$	$V_{70} < 20\%$
	$V_{50} < 50\%$	$V_{50} < 40\%$	$V_{50} < 40\%$
	平均剂量 <34Gy	平均剂量 <34Gy	平均剂量 <34Gy
肾脏[3]	剂量为 20Gy 时双侧肾暴露体积 <32%	剂量为 20Gy 时双侧肾暴露体积 <32%	剂量为 20Gy 时双侧肾暴露体积 <32%
肝脏	$V_{30} \leq 40\%$	$V_{30} \leq 40\%$	$V_{30} \leq 40\%$
	平均剂量 <30Gy	平均剂量 <30Gy	平均剂量 <30Gy

Vx：暴露于 X 照射剂量时的器官体积百分比

肺

射线引起的肺损伤与剂量和体积效应均相关。急性或亚急性射线引起的肺损伤表现为放射性肺炎，慢性期则为肺纤维化。两种并发症均能造成严重的器官衰竭甚至致命。

肺损伤的发生率为 13%～44%，这个幅度反映了所用的标准不一致、患者个体异质性、治疗方案和放疗技术的不同[59,66-70]。可以作为预测肺炎的临床因素有：体力差[71]、放疗前肺功能差[72-73]、COPD[74]、下叶肿瘤[75]、同步化疗[75]、放疗剂量高和分次照射剂量高等。能预测肺炎的剂量参数包括平均肺受量（mean lung dose, MLD）[74,76-78]和接受超过预计量时的肺体积（百分比；$V_{剂量}$）[57,70,72,76,78-80]。可预测的剂量参数从简单到复杂。MLD 既简单又实用，同样有效的参数还有照射剂量为 20Gy 或以上时全肺的受照体积（V_{20}）[81]。事实上，QUANTEC 小组推荐 V_{20} 不超过 30%～35%，MLD 不超过 30Gy（常规分割放疗时），因为很多研究证实这两个参数与肺损伤的发生有关。使用这些指标应该能使接受根治性放疗的 NSCLC 患者发生肺损伤的风险减少到不超过 20%。其他涉及更复杂算法的变量有 DVH 逆向还原（器官的 DVH 逆向还原为单一有效的均衡剂量）、肺的有效体积（effective volume, Veff）、正常组织并发症发生率（normal tissue complication probability, NTCP）模型[82-84]和 Niemierko 的功能亚单位模型[85]。

治疗 NSCLC 和评价剂量限制的一个关键问题是哪一个对肺毒性更强，是小区域的高剂量照射还是大区域的低剂量照射[86]？似乎需要分析 DVH 的一系列重要参数。例如，Graham 等分析了 99 例接受根治性治疗的不可手术的 NSCLC 患者的 DVH 图，所有患者都接受了三维适形治疗，发现 V_{20} 和 MLD 都与≥2 级的放射性肺炎发生相关[57]。然而，另一项关于 DVH 图的分析研究中，49 例患者接受了胸部 3D CRT（其中 48 例还接受了化疗），18 例发生了肺炎。射线剂量被分为低剂量（≤10Gy）、中等剂量（10～40Gy）和高剂量（>40Gy），肺作为一个单元和单独的器官（同侧和对侧）进行剂量分析。通过分析，作者发现高剂量的影响最重要，因为剂量超过 10Gy 就能增加 10%～50% 的肺炎风险。这些研究为 NSCLC 治疗的标准剂量限制，如 V_{10}、V_{20} 时和 MLD 的组合应用提供了进一步的支持。

食 管

胸部恶性肿瘤的放射治疗通常会将食管暴露于高剂量射线中，在 2～3 周的常规分割放疗后，患者经常会有不舒服的急性反应，如吞咽困难、吞咽疼痛或两者都有。这些反应引起脱水和体重下降的发生率很高，甚至被迫中断治疗。食管对射线的晚期反应一般表现为纤维化，能导致食管狭窄。患者可能发生不同程度的消化不良并可能需要做内镜下扩张术来扩张食管。极少数情况下，急性和晚期反应还可引起食管穿孔和梗阻。

过去几十年，急性和慢性食管炎的临床和剂量学预测因素是一个研究热点。许多因素增加了食管炎的发病风险，包括食管受照体积、是否整个食管都在照射野内、放疗分割模式（每天 1 或 2 次，每次剂量）、既往有食管并发症（如食管狭窄、最大食管受量、平均受量及纵隔淋巴结受侵[87-93]）。

我们最近发表了一项评价≥3 级食管炎预测因子的临床研究，纳入了 652 例接受放疗的 NSCLC 患者。在这项研究中，我们运用 Lyman-Kutcher-Berman 模型，根据单次分割食管的 DVH 参数和作为剂量调整因子的各种临床因素来分析放射性食管炎的发生。我们发现小体积高剂量照射较整个食管的平均剂量更具预测性，如将同步化疗作为一项剂量调整因子，则能显著提高该模型的预测性。我们还发现同步紫杉醇化疗有增加食管炎发生的可能[94]。

QUANTEC 小组还发表了一些关于放射性食管炎发生的共识建议。首先，他们承认食管感染（如念珠菌病和单纯疱疹病毒）类似于食管炎，并且推荐临床医生在治疗时考虑到这种相似性；第二，他们强调胃食管反流病等能加重放射性食管炎的症状；第三，肺下叶肿瘤放疗时应考虑放射性胃炎和食管炎的可能，因为射野内可能包括部分胃；第四，也可能是最重要的，即对食管炎症状的评分为有差异，因为某些判断标准取决于主治医生。例如，通用不良事件术语标准认为 2 级食管炎需要静脉输液治疗，3 级食管炎需要入院治疗。两例患者的食管炎尽管症状相似，也有可能被分为不同级别。因此该小组得出结论：需要建立基于生活质量或分子终点的更为可靠的评分系统。最后，QUANTEC 小组的作者承认，目前不能确定食管放疗最佳的体积参数阈值，尤其因为接受超过预剂量照射时广泛的肺体积百分比与严重急性食管炎的发生密切相关。M. D. 安德森癌症中心所用的剂量限制（平均食管受量 <34Gy，食管 V_{70} <20%，最大受量 <80Gy）是部分基于其他研究报道的结果[95]。并且，与评价肺毒性一样，许多模型被用来预测食管毒性，包括正常组织并发症概率模型、Lyman-Kutcher-Berman 模型（即相对连续性模型）。在预测算法的选择上，QUANTEC 的作者推荐医生和研究者采用最有经验的研究所采用的模型。他们进一步强调这些分析报告的任何新内容都需要经过回顾性或前瞻性研究的证实。

在某些情况下，NSCLC 的放疗不可避免地会波及食管，特别是中心型或有明显纵隔淋巴结受侵的患者。对于这类患者，Dana-Farber 癌症研究所/布莱根妇女医院提出了一个新参数，即"野内食管（$Esoph_{in}$）"来预测食管炎发生风险。在 2000—2006 年的一项纳入了 109 例接受同步放化疗的局部进展期 NSCLC 的研究中，发现这个参数与食管狭窄的发生发展密切相关。具体来说，$Esoph_{in}$ 的 V_{55} <50% 是预测食管炎发生的最佳临界值[96]。类似这样的进一步研究将有益于获得适宜和个体化的剂量限制数据。

新型放疗技术

调强放疗

过去几十年，IMRT 普遍用于 NSCLC 的治疗。IMRT 较 3D CRT 的优势包括逆向计划和动态多叶准直器，能使临床医生在设计射束前就对肿瘤区域和正常组织的剂量限制设定标准，还能通过变换射束的通量来形成高剂量陡降的高度适形计划。M. D. 安德森癌症中心的研究者通过几项涉及治疗计划的对比研究，证实了 IMRT 较 3D 适形放疗的优越性。有这样的一项研究，对所有 I～III 期 NSCLC 病例的研究均发现，IMRT 与 3D CRT 相比，肺的 V_{20} 和 MLD 都更低。但是，因为应用了多条射束来实现高适形度，V_5 和 V_{10} 在 IMRT 更高[97]。来自 William Beaumont 医院的另一项研究显示，IMRT 特别有益于 NSCLC 淋巴结受侵的患者，研究者强调只有 IMRT 技术才可能将放疗剂量提高至 70Gy 以上[98]。

迄今为止，IMRT 对 3D-CRT 的优势分析可能来自于 M. D. 安德森癌症中心，这里的学者回顾性分析了约 500 例患者，其中 318 例接受了不考虑呼吸运动的 3D CRT，其余的患者接受了考虑呼吸运动引起的肿块运动 IMRT，图像引导的 IMRT 计划降低了严重放射性肺炎的发生率（从 25% 降至 10%），并且还有总生存获益[99]。目前，图像引导的 IMRT 计划（考虑呼吸运动）已成为 M. D. 安德森癌症中心根治性放疗的标准手段。

质子束治疗

过去 5～10 年，质子束疗法（proton beam therapy, PBT）越来越多地用于各种类型癌症的治疗，包括 NSCLC。PBT 的剂量学优势来源于质子优越的剂量分布，即"布拉格峰"。许多有关治疗计划对比的剂量学研究已证实 PBT 较 3D-CRT 和 IMRT 的优越性。特别的是，来自 M. D. 安德森癌症中心的学者评价了早期和局部进展期 NSCLC 的正常组织参数，发现 PBT 对肺的 V_5、V_{10} 和 V_{20}、食管、脊髓和心脏的受量都有很大程度的剂量学改善[100]。其他研究单位的剂量学分析进一步验证了 PBT 的潜在优势[101-102]。

最近一些研究也显示这种潜在的剂量学优势转化成了临床获益。Sejpal 及同事在一项研究中证实 PBT 与 3D-CRT 或 IMRT 相比，即使靶区的照射剂量更高，放射性肺炎和食管炎的发生率反而更低[103]。Chang 及同事报道了一项纳入 44 例 III 期 NSCLC 患者的 II 期临床试验，所有患者都接受了 74Gy 的高剂量 PBT 同步每周方案的紫杉醇联合卡铂化疗，结果显示中位随访时间为 19.7 个月时中位生存期为 29.4 个月[104]，这比之前报道的一项光子治疗的类似治疗方案的 III 期试验的时间长得多。毒性反应的发生率和严重程度都在合理范围，只有 5 例患者出现了 3 级食管炎，1 例出现了 2 级肺炎。当写作本章时，一项局部进展期 NSCLC 的对比 PBT 与 IMRT 同步化疗的 III 期多中心试验正在进行。这项试验的研究终点为放射性肺炎和局部区域控制，预计在 2013 年 6 月完成。

小细胞肺癌（SCLC）的放化疗

系统治疗是局限期和广泛期小细胞肺癌（small-cell lung cancer, SCLC）的重要组成部分。20多年前，一项具有里程碑意义的meta分析显示，局限期SCLC增加化疗与单纯放疗相比，3年总生存率有5%的获益（20% vs 15%，$P<0.15$），25%的局部控制率改善[105]。因此，除了少数T1-T2N0的病例推荐术后系统治疗外，放化疗已经成为局限期SCLC的标准疗法。接下来大部分的论述集中在局限期疾病的化疗放上，如局限于一侧肺伴随或不伴随纵隔或同侧肺门淋巴结受侵的病变。

局限期疾病的序贯放化疗

4~6个周期的系统治疗常用于局限期SCLC。化疗与放疗的顺序有两种：早放疗，系统治疗一开始就开始放疗；晚放疗，化疗几个周期后再开始放疗，并且是序贯治疗。两种治疗方式各有理论优势。早放疗的总治疗时间缩短，理论上提高了患者的依从性并减少了肿瘤的加速再群体化。与NSCLC一样，这种方式能提高治疗强度，甚至能发挥两种方式的协同作用。晚放疗的毒性小，如果序贯放疗，在肿瘤对化疗有效的情况下，可能会减少放疗的体积。最后，推迟放疗能评价化疗疗效，这有可能影响后续局部治疗的选择，进一步引起放化疗毒性。

许多早和晚放疗的对比研究产生了有争议的结果。在一项国家癌症中心加拿大临床试验小组进行的研究中，308例患者被随机分为早放疗组，即放疗同步第一周期化疗，或晚放疗组，即最后一个周期化疗时开始放疗。化疗方案由环磷酰胺+表柔比星+长春新碱与依托泊苷+顺铂交替组成。照射剂量为40Gy、15次，所有患者都接受了预防性脑照射（prophylactic cranial irradiation, PCI）。早放疗组的无进展生存期（$P=0.036$）和总生存期都有获益（$P=0.008$）[106]。然而，伦敦肺癌小组开展的类似临床试验中，化疗方案和放疗剂量都相同，早、晚放疗分别定义为自第2和第6周期化疗开始同步放疗，结果显示，早放疗与晚放疗相比，并没有明显获益[107]。

尽管单个临床试验的结果有争议，meta分析的建议将有助于确定SCLC的治疗方案。这些meta分析报道显示，与晚放疗相比，早放疗虽然毒性增加，但确有微小的生存获益。2004年Fried[108]与2006年de Ruysscher[109]发表的2篇著名文章报道了每天2次放疗联合基于铂类的化疗可以提高生存获益。2012年美国临床肿瘤协会报道的一项Ⅲ期临床试验的早期结果发现，无论放疗（52.5Gy，每天1次，每次2.1Gy）开始于化疗的第1周期或第3周期（顺铂70mg/m² 联合依托泊苷100mg/m²），总生存率无显著差异。尽管从第3周期开始放疗，发热性中性粒细胞减少的发生率低[110]。M.D. 安德森癌症中心的现行办法是大多数患者在第3个周期化疗前就开始放疗。

化疗方案

目前SCLC的标准化疗方案是基于铂类的方案，局限期病变联合依托泊苷，广泛期病变联合依托泊苷或伊立替康。选择这个方案是因为更强效的化疗药物，如烷化剂或蒽环霉素，与该方案疗效相似，但毒性更大[111-112]。日本的一项随机临床试验证实，伊立替康联合卡铂可作为广泛期SCLC的治疗方案，因为该方案与依托泊苷联合顺铂相比，有更好的总生存期和无进展生存期[113]。但是随后的随机试验却没有显示出明显的获益[114-115]。实际上，比日本的研究纳入更多患者的SWOG试验显示出更高的胃肠道副反应发生率，但血液学毒性较低[115]（图23.4）。值得注意的是，SWOG试验还包括人群相关的药物遗传学研究，显示伊立替康-顺铂相关腹泻和中性粒细胞减少的分子预测将对以后的研究有帮助。

目前，卡铂和顺铂都是化疗中常用的铂类。通常，顺铂发生胃肠道反应（恶心）、周围神经病变和肾毒性的风险更高，卡铂发生骨髓抑制的风险更高。许多小型临床试验对卡铂和顺铂的疗效进行了对比，但最近一项纳入近700例患者，4项随机试验的meta分析证实了两种药物的总生存期和无进展生存期相似（图23.5），毒性与上述小型试验中的结果吻合[116]。

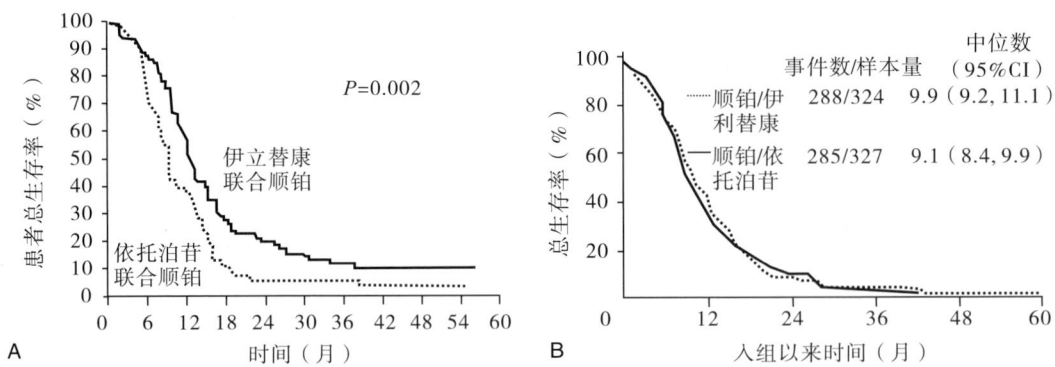

图 23.4 广泛期 SCLC 对比 IP 方案（伊立替康联合顺铂）和 EP 方案（依托泊苷联合顺铂）的两项Ⅲ期试验。来自日本的研究显示，与 EP 方案相比，IP 方案的总生存和无疾病生存率更高（A 图），西南肿瘤小组的一项更大的试验并未显示出任何优势（B 图），美国国家综合癌症网络认为两种方案都可以用于广泛期疾病

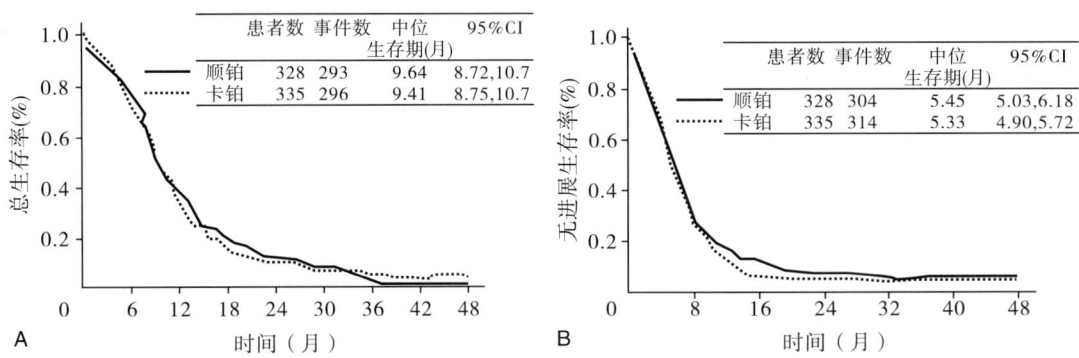

图 23.5 SCLC 卡铂与顺铂的疗效比较。纳入 663 例患者，4 个随机试验的 meta 分析显示两者的总生存期（A 图）或无进展生存期（B 图）无显著差异，但两者的毒性反应不同（见正文）

放疗剂量和分割模式

目前局限期 SCLC 的治疗有 3 种与化疗联合的常用放疗方案，每种方案都有研究报道和高级别证据支持。最常用的方案是每次 1.5Gy，每天 2 次，共 45Gy。支持这个方案的证据来自于 INT-0096，它是由 Turrisi 等进行的一项临床试验。患者接受了 EP 方案化疗联合放疗，放疗模式为上述方式或每次 1.8Gy，每天 1 次，共 45Gy。结果显示，每天 2 次放疗和每天 1 次放疗的生存率分别为 26% 和 16%（P<0.05）。当然，每天 2 次放疗的严重食管炎（≥3 级）发生率更高（27% vs 11%；P<0.001）[117]。

第二种放疗方案来源于 Berger 发表的 CALGB 研究，纳入了 63 例患者，都接受了同步化疗和胸部放疗。化疗方案为 2 个周期紫杉醇联合拓扑替康诱导化疗，后续 3 个周期卡铂联合依托泊苷化疗联合胸部放疗，其中完全缓解或部分缓解的患者接受了 PCI。结果显示两年总生存率为 48%，两年无进展生存率为 31%，与 INT-0096 试验相比，血液学毒性相似，食管炎发生率低（21% vs 32%）[118]。

第 3 种放疗方案来源于 RTOG 97-12，该试验纳入了 64 例患者，治疗方案为 4 个周期顺铂（60mg/m²）联合依托泊苷（120mg/m²，随后改为 240mg/m²），自治疗第 1 天加入放疗。放疗采用剂量提升模式，CTV 每次 1.8Gy，每天 1 次，自第 3 天起，GTV 按照每天 2 次照射，分别在第 5、7、9 及 11 天增加剂量（相对应的总剂量为 50.4Gy、54.0Gy、57.6Gy、61.2Gy 和 64.8Gy）。最大耐受剂量为 61.2Gy，18 个月生存率为 82%[119]。

这 3 个治疗方案的疗效和毒性促使了自 2008 年开始的一项Ⅲ期随机试验的开展，以比较 3 种治疗方案的效果（CALGB 30610/RTOG 0538）。所有患者都接受了早期放疗（化疗一开始或 1 个周期后），化疗方案为顺铂 80mg/m² 联合依托泊苷 100mg/m²，21d 为 1 个周期，共 4 个周期。完全缓解或接近完全缓解的患者都接受了 PCI，主要研究终点为总生存期。截至 2012 年 12 月，试验数据在全国范围内持续累积，其结果将为优放化疗方案或治疗方案提供 I 类证据。

放疗靶区和剂量限制

像 NSCLC 的治疗一样，现代的 3D 或 4D 成像技术出现之前，SCLC 的照射靶区也很大。如 INT-0096 试验的照射靶区包括原发肿瘤、双侧纵隔、同侧肺门淋巴结，如果隆突淋巴结受侵，还包括隆突下 5cm[117]。然而过去几年间，PET、CT 等更敏感的成像技术的使用改善了肿瘤分期并使放疗靶区缩小为累及野照射。上述关于 3D CRT 计划的 CALGB30610/RTOG0538 试验，以及 4D 放疗计划中 CTV 定义为 GTV 外扩不超过 1.0cm 的要求反映了这种转变。然而，唯一需要进行选择性照射的区域是同侧肺门。这种常用、重点考虑同侧肺门累及淋巴结的照射方法，目前在 M.D. 安德森癌症中心常用。

SCLC 胸部放疗的剂量限制与 NSCLC 相似，但每天 2 次放疗有 2 个明显的例外：首先，脊髓的受照剂量不超过 36Gy；其次，食管的剂量阈值还未确定，但鉴于严重食管炎的高发生率，应受到特别重视。虽然放疗不会对靶区造成损害，但患者应被告知有发生严重治疗相关并发症的风险，甚至需要根据食管受量和患者的一般情况行插鼻饲管。

广泛期病变的巩固性胸部放疗

来自 II 期临床试验的证据支持对化疗效果好的广泛期疾病患者可以行胸部放疗。Jeremic 报道了一项类似的研究，该研究纳入了 210 例患者，接受了 3 个周期顺铂（80mg/m²）联合依托泊苷（80mg/m²）化疗。原发灶局部和远处转移灶均完全缓解，或局部部分缓解而转移灶完全缓解的患者随后被随机分为两组，一组接受超分割放疗（54Gy/36f，每天 2 次）同步卡铂联合依托泊苷化疗。另一组则继续给予 4 个周期顺铂联合依托泊苷化疗。接受巩固性胸部放疗的患者的中位生存期明显延长（17 个月 vs 11 个月；$P=0.041$），但无转移生存率无显著差异[121]。

在 M.D. 安德森癌症中心，对达到上述疗效的患者，我们通常推荐巩固性胸部放疗。2009 年 RTOG 开放了一个随机 II 期试验，广泛期 SCLC 患者先接受了 4~6 个周期铂类为基础的化疗，后续治疗为 PCI 加原发病变灶包括胸部的巩固性放疗，或单纯 PCI（REOG 0937）。这个研究结果将有助于阐明广泛期 SCLC 综合放疗的重要性。

预防性脑照射

过去几十年，许多研究评价了 PCI 在局限期和广泛期 SCLC 中的重要性。这些研究中，一部分关键性的研究证实 PCI 能降低特定患者亚组的颅内转移并能提高总生存期，其中影响局限期 SCLC 的关键研究是 Auperin 等发表的一篇 meta 分析，该文纳入了来自 7 项随机试验的 1 000 例患者，对于 CR 的患者是否进行 PCI 进行了对比。结果显示，接受 PCI 的患者总生存率提高了 5.4%；另外，复发风险及脑转移的累计发生率均下降[122]。Slotman 等报道的一项广泛期 SCLC 的重要研究，该研究中在 4~6 个周期化疗后至少达到部分缓解的患者被随机分为不同剂量的 PCI 组和未行 PCI 组。结果显示 PCI 组的中位总生存期延长（从 5.4 个月至 6.7 个月）并且 1 年总生存率增加（从 13.3% 增加至 27.1%；$P<0.05$）。PCI 还能降低颅内转移发生率并能延长无病生存期（PFS）[123]。

对于 PCI 的最佳剂量选择，研究者争论了一段时间，特别是对于无明显病变、正在进行全脑放疗的患者，PCI 发生严重副反应的风险较高。来自一个多中心协作组的研究成果可能有助于解决这个问题。这项研究纳入了 720 例局限期 SCLC 患者，所有患者在完全缓解后随机分为 2 组接受 PCI，一组剂量为每次 2.5Gy，共 10 次；另一组剂量为每次 2.0Gy，共 18 次。两组的预后无显著差异，但高剂量组出现了 5 例严重并发症（1 例死于神经功能恶化，1 例癫痫大发作，1 例脑血管事件，1 例双眼白内障，还有 1 例死于癫痫大发作），标准剂量组未出现严重并发症。毒性反应如头痛、疲劳和恶心也在高剂量组多见[124]。随后的跟踪分析对患者的神经功能和生活质量进行了评价,结果显示随着时间的推移,患者的交流能力、智力障碍和记忆力都有轻微恶化。虽然严重并发症的发生率低,但笔者强调应该事先向准备做 PCI 的患者说明有发生这些副作用的风险,特别是年迈和已有认知功能障碍的患者[125]。

总 结

迄今为止,NSCLC 放化联合治疗取得的进展虽然不太大,但却保证了这种治疗策略的延续。仍有几个主要问题需要解决,包括手术在可切除肿瘤治疗中的作用、新化疗方案的选择和新放疗技术的应用。Ⅰ期毒性试验后紧接着迅速进行Ⅱ期试验而不是进行对比性的Ⅲ期试验,这种试验方法将会持续阻碍 NSCLC 治疗的进步。使用更新更有效的药物,更快地从Ⅰ期研究过渡到Ⅲ期试验应该能加快 NSCLC 的治疗进展,同时也为制订对比和临床试验通用的标准提供了基础。

对于 SCLC 的主要治疗进展包括确立了不同化疗方案的疗效和毒性,确立了放疗和化疗的最佳时机,并且阐明了 PCI 在局限期和广泛期疾病中的地位。需要进一步研究确定最有效的放疗分割模式及巩固性放疗在广泛期 SCLC 局部控制率中的作用。与 NSCLC 一样,分子治疗的进展将成为改善 SCLC 患者生存及预测特殊毒性发生的关键,这样才能真正实现对患者的个体化治疗。

(王 娟 黄 伟 李宝生 译)

参考文献

[1] Steel GG, Peckham MJ. Exploitable mechanisms in combined radiotherapy-chemotherapy: the concept of additivity. Int J Radiat Oncol Biol Phys, 1979, 5 (1): 85-91.

[2] Eberhardt W, Pottgen C, Stuschke M. Chemoradiation paradigm for the treatment of lung cancer, Nat Clin Pract Oncol, 2006, 3 (4): 188-199.

[3] Weichselbaum RR, Beckett MA, Vokes EE, et al. Cellular and molecular mechanisms of radioresistance. Cancer Treat Res, 1995, 74: 131-140.

[4] Chabner BA. Biological basis for Cancer treatment. Ann Intern Med, 1993, 118 (8): 633-637.

[5] Tannock IF. Treatment of cancer with radiation and drugs, J Clin Oncol, 1996, 14 (12): 3156-3174.

[6] Perez CA, Bauer M, Edelstein S, et al. Impact of tumor control on survival In carcinoma of the lung treated with irradiation. Int J Radiat Oncol Biot Phys, 1986, 12 (4): 539-547.

[7] Eiscrt DR, Cox JD, Komaki R. Irradiation for bronchial carcinoma: reasons for failure. I Analysis of local control as a function of dose, time, and fractionation. Cancer, 1976, 37 (6): 2665-2670.

[8] Cox JD, Byhardt R, Komaki R, et al. Interaction of thoracic irradiation and chemotherapy on local control and survival in small cell carcinoma of the lung. Cancer Treat Rep, 1979, 63 (8): 1251-1255.

[9] Saunders MI, Barltrop MA, Rassa PM, et al. The relationship between tumor response and survival following radiotherapy for carcinoma of the bronchus. Int J Radiat Oncol Biol Phys, 1984, 10 (4): 503-508.

[10] Perez CA, Pajak TF, Rubin P, et al. Long-term observations of the patterns of failure in patients with unresectable non-oat cell carcinoma of the lung treated with definitive radiotherapy. Report by the Radiation Therapy Oncology Group. Cancer, 1987, 59 (11): 1874-1881.

[11] Schaake-Konning C, Van Den Bogaert W, Dalesio O, et al. Effects of concomitant cisplatin and radiotherapy on inoperable non-small-cell lung cancer. New England Journal of Medicine, 1992, 326 (8): 524-530.

[12] Brodin O, Nou E, Metrcle C, et al. Comparison of induction chemotherapy before radiotherapy with radiotherapy only in patients with lacally advanced squamous cell carcinoma of the lung. The Swedish Lung Cancer Study Group. Eur J Cancer, 1996, 32A (11): 1893-1900.

[13] Dillman RO, Herndon J, Seagren SL, et al. Improved survival in stage Ⅲ non-small-cell lung cancer Seven-year follow-up of cancer and leukemia group B (CALGB) 8433 trial. Journal of the National Cancer Institute, 1996, 88 (17): 1210-1215.

[14] Le Chevalier T, Arriagada R, Tarayre M, et al. Significant effect of adjuvant chemotherapy on survival in locally advanced non-small-cell lung carcinoma. J Natl Cancer Inst, 1992, 84 (1): 58.

[15] Morton RF, Jett JR, Mc Ginnis WL, et al. Thoracic radiation therapy alone compared with combined chemoradiatherapy for locally unresectable non-small cell lung canc-

er. A randomized, phase Ⅲ trial. Ann intern Med, 1991, 115 (9): 681-686.

[16] Sause W, Kolesar P, Taylor SI, et al. Final results of phase Ⅲ trial in regionally advanced unresectable non-small cell lung cancer Radiation Therapy Oncology Group. Esstern Cooperative Oncology Group, and southwest Oncology Group. Chest, 2000, 117 (2): 358-364.

[17] Dillman RO, Scagren SL, Propert KJ, et al. Easton of induction chemotherapy plus high-dose radiation versus radiation alone in stage Ⅲ non-small-cell lung cancer, see comments. New England Journal of Medicine, 1990, 323 (14): 940-945.

[18] Arriagada R, Le Chevalier T, Quoix E, et al. ASTRO (American Society for Therapeutic Radiology and Oncology) plenary: Effect of chemotherapy on locally advanced non-small cell lung carcinoma: a randomized study of 353 patients. GETCB (Groupe d'Etude et Traitement des Cancers Bronchiques), FNCLCC (Fed-eration Nationale des Centres de Lutte contre le Cancer) and the CEBI trialists. Int J Radiat Oncol Biol Phys, 1991, 20 (6): 1183-1190.

[19] Le Chevalier T, Arriagada R, Quoix E, et al. Radiotherapy alone versus combined chemotherapy and radiotherapy in nonresectable non-small-cell lung cancer First analysis of a randomized trial in 353 patients. Journal of National Cancer Institute, 1991, 83: 417-423.

[20] Sause WT, Scott C, Taylor S, et al. Radiation Therapy Oncology Group (RTOG) 88-08 and Eastern Cooperative Oncology Group (ECOG) 4588: Preliminary results of a phase Ⅲ trial in regionally advanced, unresectable non-small-cell lung cancer. Journal of the National Cancer Institute, 1995, 87 (3): 198-205.

[21] Komaki R, Scott CB, Sause WT, et al. Induction cisplatin/vinblastine and irradiation vs. irradiation in unresectable squamous cell lung cancer. Failure patterns by cell type in RTOG 88-08/ECOG 4588. Radiation Therapy Oncology Group. Eastern Coopcrative Oncology Group, see comments. International Journal of Radiation Oncology. Biology, Physics, 1997, 39 (3): 537-544.

[22] Komaki R, Scott CB, Sause WT, et al. Induction cisplatin/vinblastine and irradiation vs. induction in unresectable squamous cell lung cancer failure patterns by cell type in ETOG 88-08/ECOG 4588. Radiation Therapy Oncology Group. Eastern Cooperative Oncology Group. Int J Radiat Oncol Biol Phys, 1997, 36 (3): 537-544.

[23] Byhardt RW, Scott CB, Ettinger DS, et al. Concurrent hyperfractionated irradiation and chemotherapy for unresectable nonsmall cell lung cancer. Results of Radiation Therapy Oncology Group 90-15. Cancer, 1995, 75 (9): 2337-2344.

[24] Cox JD, Azarnia N, Byhardt RW, et al. A randomized phase Ⅰ/Ⅱ trial of hyperfractionated radiation therapy with total doses of 60.0 Gy to 79.2 Gy: possible survival benefit with greater than or equal to 69.6 Gy in favorable patients with Radiation Therapy Oncology Group saige Ⅲ non-small-cell lung carcinoma: report of Radiation Therapy Oncology Group 83-11. Journal of Clinical oncology, 1990, 8 (9): 1543-1555.

[25] Lee JS, Scott C, Komaki R, et al. Concurrent chemoradiation therapy with oral etoposide and cisplatin for locally advanced inoperable non-small-cell lung cancer: Radiation therapy oncology group protocol 91-06. Journal of Clinical Oncology, 1996, 14 (4): 1055-1064.

[26] Reboul F, Brewer Y, Vincent P, et al. Concurrent cisplatin, etoposide, and radiothcrapy for unresectable stage Ⅲ nonsmall cell lung cancer: A phase Ⅱ study. Int J Radiat Oncol Biol Phys, 1996, 35 (2): 343-350.

[27] Komaki R, Scott C, Ettinger D, et al. Randomized study of chemotherapy/radiation therapy combinations for favorable patients with locally advanced inoperable nonsmall cell lung cancer: Radiation Therapy Oncology Group (RTOG) 92-04. Int J Radiat Oncol Biol Phys, 1997, 38 (1): 149-155.

[28] O'Rourke N, Roque IFM, Farre Bernado N, et al. Concurrent chemoradiothcrapy in non-small cell lung cancer. Codhrane Database Syst Rev, 2010, 6: CD00214.

[29] Curran WJ. Sequential versus concurrent chemoradiation in unresected stage Ⅲ NSCLC: RTOG 94-10 initial report. Journal of Clinical Oncology, 2000, 19: 484a.

[30] Fournel P, Robinet G, Thomas P, et al. Randomized phase Ⅲ trial of sequential chemoradiotherapy compared with concurrent chemoradiotherapy in locally advanced non-small-cell lung cancer: Groupe Lyon-Saint-Etienne d'Oncologie Thoracique-Groupe Fransais de Pneumo-Cancerologie NPC 95-01 Study. J Clin Oncol, 2005, 23 (25): 5910-5917.

[31] Rao CZ. study of concurrent versus sequential chemoradiotherapy with vinorelbine and cisplatin in stage Ⅲ non-small cell lung cancer. Chinese Journal of Cancer Preven-

tion and Treatment, 2007, 14 (12): 942-943.
[32] Reinfuss MS, Kowalska T, Glinski B, et al. Evaluation of efficacy of combined chemoradiotherapy in locoregional advanced, inoperable non-small cell lung cancer. Nowotwory, 2005, 55 (3): 200-206.
[33] Zatloukal P, Petruzelka L, Zemanova M, et al. Concurrent versus sequential chemoradiotherapy with cisplatin and vinorelbine in locally advanced non-small cell lung cancer: A randomized study. Lung Cancer, 2004, 46 (1): 87-98.
[34] Belani CP, Choy H, Bonomin P, et al. Combined chemoradiotherapy regimens of paclitaxel and carboplatin for locally advanced non-small-cell lung cancer: A randomized phase II locally advanced muiti-modality protocol. J Clin Oncol, 2005, 23 (25): 5883-5891.
[35] Huber RM, Flentje M, Schmindt M, et al. Simultaneous chemoradiotherapy compared with radiotherapy alone after induction chemotherapy in inoperable stage IIIA or IIIB non-small-cell lung cancer. Study CTRT99/97 by the Bronchial Carcinoma Therapy Group. J Clin Oncol, 2006, 24 (27): 4397-4404.
[36] Auperin A, Le Pechoux C, Rolland E, et al. Meta-analysis of concomitant versus sequential radiochemotherapy in locally advanced non-small-cell lung cancer. J Clin oncol, 2010, 28 (13): 2181-2190.
[37] O'Rourke N, Macbeth F. Is concurrent chemoradiation the standard of care for locally advanced non-small cell lung cancer? A review of guidelines and evidence. Clin Oncol (R Coll Radiol), 2010, 22 (5): 347-355.
[38] Andre F, Grunenwald D, Pignon JP, et al. Survival of patients with resected N2 non-small-cell lung cancer evidence for a subclassification and implications. J Clin Oncol, 2000, 18 (16): 2981-2989.
[39] Albain KS, Rusch VW, Crowley JJ, et al. Concurrent cisplatin/etoposide plus chest radiotherapy followed by surgery for stages IIIA (N2) and IIIB non-small-cell lung cancer: mature results of Southwest Oncology Group phase II study 8805. J Clin Oncol, 1995, 13 (8): 1880-1892.
[40] Albain K, Swann R, Rusch V, et al. Phase III study of concurrent chemotherapy and radiotherapy (CT-RT) vs. CT/RT followed by surgical resection for stage IIIA (pN2) non-small-cell lung cancer (NSCLC): Outcomes update of North American Intergroup 0139 (RTOG 9309). Proceedings of American Society of Clinical Oncology, 2005, 23 (16s): 624s.
[41] Albain KS, Swann RS, Rusch VW, et al. Radiotherapy plus chemotherapy with or without surgical resection for stage III non-small-cell lung cancer: A phase III randomized controlled trial. Lancet, 2009, 374 (9687): 379-386.
[42] National Comprehensive Cancer Network guidelines, www.nccn.org, 2012.
[43] Kong FM, Ten Haken RK, Schipper MJ, et al. High-dose radiation improved local tumor control and overall survival in patients with inoperable/unresectable non-small-cell lung cancer: long-term results of a radiation dose escalation study. Int J Radiat Oncol Biol Phys, 2005, 63 (2): 324-333.
[44] Machtay M, paulus R, moughan J, et al. Defining local-regional control and its importance in locally advanced non-small-cell lung carcinoma. J Thorac oncol, 2012, 7 (4): 716-722.
[45] Zhang HX, Yin WB, Zhang LJ, et al. Curative radiotherapy of early operable non-small-cell lung cancer. Radiother Oncol, 1989, 14 (2): 89-94.
[46] Senan S, Burgers S, Samson MJ, et al. Can elective nodal irradiation be omitted in stage III non-small-cell lung cancer? Analysis of recurrences in a phase II study of induction chemotherapy and involved-field radiotherapy. Int J Radiat Oncol Biol phys, 2002, 54 (4): 999-1006.
[47] Rosenzweig KE, Sim SE, Mychalczak B, et al. Elective modalirradiation in the treatment of non-small-cell lung cancer with three-dimensional conformal radiation therapy. Int J Radiat Oncol Biol Phys, 2001, 50 (3): 681-685.
[48] Krol AD, Aussems P, Noordijk EM, et al. Local irradiation alone for peripheral stage I lung cancer: Could we omit the elective regional nodal irradiation? Int J Radiat Oncol Biol Phys, 1996, 34 (2): 297-302.
[49] Dosoretz DE, Katin MJ, Blitzer PH, et al. Medically inoperable lung carcinoma: The role of radiation therapy. Seminars in Radiation Oncology, 1996, 6 (2): 98-104.
[50] Dosoretz DE, Galmarini D, Rubenstein JH, et al. Local control in medically inoperable lung cancer: an analysis of its importance in outcome and factors determining the probability of tumor eradication. Int J Radiat Oncol Biol Phys, 1993, 27 (3): 507-516.
[51] Jeremic B, Casas F, Wang L, et al. Radiation therapy for early stage (I/II) non-small-cell lung cancer.

Front Radiat Ther Oncol, 2010, 42: 87-93.

[52] Rosenzweig KE, Sura S, Jackson A, et al. Involved-field radiation therapy for inoperable non-small-cell lung cancer. J Clin Oncol, 2007, 25 (35): 5557-5561.

[53] Yuan S, Sun X, Li M, et al. A randomized study of involved-field irradiation versus elective nodal irradiation in combination with concurrent chemotherapy for inoperable stage III non-small-cell lung cancer. Am J Clin Oncol, 2007, 30 (3): 239-244.

[54] Belderbos JS, Kepka L, Kong FM, et al. Elective nodal irradiation (ENI) in locally advanced non-small-cell lung cancer (NSCLC): Evidence versus opinion? Int J Radiat Oncol Biol Phys, 2009, 74 (1): 322.

[55] Martel MK, Strawderman M, Hazuka MB, et al. Volume and dose parameters for survival of non-small-cell lung cancer patients. Radiother Onco, 1997, 44 (1): 23-29.

[56] International Commission on Radiation Units and Measurements (ICRU), www.icru.Org, 2012.

[57] Graham M, Purdy J, Emami B, et al. Clinical dose-volume histogram analysis for pneumonitis after 3D treatment for non-small-cell lung cancer (NSCLC). Int J Radiat Oncol, 1999, 45: 323-329.

[58] Graham MV, Matthews JW, Harms WB, et al. Three-dimensional radiation treatment planning study for patients with carcinoma of the lung. Int J Radiat Oncol iol Phys, 1994, 29 (5): 1105-1117.

[59] Martel M, Ten Haken R, hazuka M. Dose-volume histogram and 3-D treatment planning evaluation of patients with pneumonitis. Int J Radiat Oncol, 1994, 28: 575-581.

[60] Emami B, Lyman J, Brown A, et al. Tolerance of normal tissue to therapeutic irradiation. Int J Radiat Oncol Biol Phys, 1991, 21 (1): 109-122.

[61] Kirkpatrick JP, van der Kogel AJ, Schultheiss TE. Radiation dose-volume effects in the spinal cord. Int J Radiat Oncol Biol Phys, 2010, 76 (3): S42-49.

[62] Werner-Wasik M, Youke E, Deasy J, et al. Radiation dose-volume effects in the esophagus. Int J Radiat Oncol Biol Phys, 2010, 76 (3): S86-S93.

[63] Marks LB, Bentzen SM, Deasy JO, et al. Radiation dose-volume effects in the lung. Int J Radiat Oncol Biol phys, 2010, 76 (3): 70-76.

[64] Gagliardi G, Consitne LS, Moiseenko V, et al. Radiation dosevolume effects in the heart. Int J Radiat Oncol Biol Phys, 2010, 76 (3): S77-S85.

[65] Bentzen SM, Constine LS, Deasy JO, et al. Quantitative Analyses of Normal Tissue Effects in the Clinic (QUANTEG): An introduction to the scientific issues. Int J Radiat Oncol Biol Phys, 2010, 76 (3): S3-S9.

[66] Oetzel D, Schraube P, Hensley F, et al. Estimation of pneumonitis risk in three-dimensional treatment planning using dose-volume histogram analysis. Int J Radiat Oncol, 1995, 33 (2): 455-460.

[67] Marks LB, Munley MT, Bentel GC, et al. Physical and biological predictors of changes in whole-lung function following thoracic irradiation. Int J Radiat Oncol, 1997, 39 (3): 563-570.

[68] Armstrong J, Raben A, Zelefsky M, et al. Promising survival with three-dimensional conformal radiation therapy for non-small-cell lung cancer. Radiotherapy and Oncology, 1997, 44: 17-22.

[69] Kwa S, Lebesque J, Theuws J, et al. Radiation Pneumonitis as a function of mean lung dose. An analysis of pooled data of 540 patients. Int J Radiat Oncol, 1998, 42: 1-9.

[70] Fu X, Huang H, Bentel G, et al. Predicting the risk of symptomatic radiation-induced lung injury using both the physical and biologic parameters V (30) and transforming growth factor beta. Int J Radiat Oncol, 2001, 50: 899-908.

[71] Robnett TJ, Machtay M, Vines EF, et al. Factors Predicting severe radiation pneumonitis in patients receiving definitive chemoradiation for lung cancer. Int J Radiat Oncol, 2000, 48 (1): 89-94.

[72] Hernando ML, Marks LB, Bentel GC, et al. Radiation-induced pulmonary toxicity: S dose-volume histogram analysis in 201 patients with lung cancer. Int J Radiat Oncol, 2000, 51 (3): 650-659.

[73] Johansson S, Bjermer L, Franzen L, et al. Effects of ongoing smoking on the development of radiation-induced pneumonitis in breast cancer and oesophagus cancer patients. Radiotherapy and Oncology, 1998, 49 (1): 41-47.

[74] Rancati T, Ceresoli GL, Gagliardi G, et al. Factors Predicting radiation pneumonitis in lung cancer patients: a retrospective study. Radiotherapy and Oncology, 2003, 67 (3): 275-283.

[75] Yamada M, Kudoh S, Hirata K, et al. Risk factors of pneumonitis following chemoradiotherapy for lung cancer. European Journal of Cancer, 1998, 34 (1): 71-75.

[76] Claude L, PerolPérol D, Ginestet C, et al. A prospective

[76] study on radiation pneumonitis following conformal radiation therapy in non-small-cell lung cancer: clinical and dosimetric factors analysis. Radiotherapy and Oncology, 2004, 71 (2): 175-181.

[77] Kim TH, Cho KH, Pyo HR, et al. Dose-volumetric parameters for predicting severe radiation pneumonitis after three-dimensional conformal radiation therapy for lung cancer. Radiology, 2005, 235 (1): 208-215.

[78] Willner J, Jost A, Baier K, et al. A Little to a lot or a lot to a little? An analysis of pneumonitis risk from dose-volume histogram parameters of the lung in patients with lung cancer treated with 3-D conformal radiotherapy. Strahlentherapie Onkologie, 2003, 179: 548-556.

[79] Armstrong J, Zelefsky M, Leibel S, et al. Strategy for dose escalation using 3-dimensional conformal radiation therapy for lung cancer. Annals of Oncology, 1995, 6: 693-697.

[80] Tsujino K, Hirota S, Endo M, et al. Predictive value of dosevolume histogram parameters for predicting radiation pneumonitis after concurrent chemoradiation for lung cancer. Int J Radiat Oncol, 2003, 55: 110-115.

[81] Munley MT, Lo JY, Sibley GS, et al. A Neural network to prediet symptomatic lung injury. Physics in Medicine and Biology, 1999, 44 (9): 2241-2249.

[82] Seppenwoolde Y, Lebesque J, De Jaeger K, et al. Comparing different NTCP models that predict the incidence of radiation pneumonitis. Int J Radiat Oncol, 2003, 55 (3): 724-735.

[83] Lyman JT. Complication probability as assessed from dose-volume histograms. Radiat Res Suppl, 1985, 8: S13-S19.

[84] Kutcher GJ, Burman C. Calculation of complication probability factors for non-uniform normal tissue irradiation: The effective volume method. Int J Radiat Oncol Biol Phys, 1989, 16 (6): 1623-1630.

[85] Niemierko A. Reporting and analyzing dose distributions: A concept of equivalent uniform dose. Med Phys, 1997, 24 (1): 103-110.

[86] Willner J, Jost A, Baier K, et al. A little to a lot or a lot to a little? An analysis of pneumonitis risk from dose-volume histogram parameters of the lung in patients with lung cancer treated with 3-D conformal radiotherapy. Strahlenther Onkol, 2003, 179 (8): 548-556.

[87] Ahn SJ, Kahn D, Zhou S, et al. Dosimetric and clinical predictors for radiation-induced esophageal injury. Int J Radiat Oncol Biol Phys, 2005, 61 (2): 335-347.

[88] Bradley J, Deasy JO, Bentzen S, et al. Dosimetric correlates for acute esophagitis in patients treated with radiotherapy for lung carcinoma. Int J Radiat Oncol Biol Phys, 2004, 58 (4): 1106-1113.

[89] Kim TH, Cho KH, Pyo HR, et al. Dose-volumetric parameters of acute esophageal toxicity in patients with lung cancer treated with three-dimensional conformal radiotherapy. Int J Radiat Oncol Biol Phys, 2005, 62 (4): 995-1002.

[90] Maguire PD, Sibley GS, Zhou SM, et al. Clinical and dosimetric predictors of radiation-induced esophageal toxicity. Int J Radiat Oncol Biol Phys, 1999, 45 (1): 97-103.

[91] Takeda K, Nemoto K, Saito H, et al. Dosimetric correlations of acute esophagitis in lung cancer patients treated with radiotherapy. Int J Radiat Oncol Biol Phys, 2005, 62 (3): 626-629.

[92] Wei X, Liu HH, Tucker SL, et al. Risk factors for acute esophagitis in non-small-cell lung cancer patients treated with concurrent chemotherapy and three-dimensional conformal radiotherapy. Int J Radiat Oncol Biol Phys, SDepl; 2006, 66 (1): 100-107.

[93] Werner-Wasik M, Pequignot E, Leeper D, et al. Predictors of Severe esophagitis include use of concurrent chemotherapy, but not the length of irradiated esophagus: A multivariate analysis of patients with lung cancer treated with nonoperative therapy. Int J Radiat Oncol Biol Phys, 2000, 48 (3): 689-696.

[94] Gomcz DR, Tucker SL, Martel MK, et al. Predictors of high-grade esophagitis after definitive threedimensional conformal therapy, intensity-modulated radiation therapy, or proton beam therapy for non-small-cell lung cancer. In J Radiat Oncol Biol Phys, 2012, 84 (4): 1010-1016.

[95] Singh AK, Lockett MA, Bradley JD. Predictors of radiation-induced esophageal toxicity in patients with non-small-cell lung cancer treated with three-dimensional conformal radiotherapy. Int J radiat Oncol Biol Phys, 2003, 55 (2): 337-341.

[96] Caglar HB, Othus M, Allen AM. Esophagus infield: a new predictor for esophagitis. Radiother Oncol, 2010, 97 (1): 48-53.

[97] Liu HH, Wang X, Dong L, et al. Feasibility of sparing lung and other thoracic structures with intensity-modulated radiotherapy for non-small-cell lung cancer. Int J Radiat Oncol Biol Phys, 2004, 58 (4): 1268-1279.

[98] Grills IS, Yan D, Martinez AA, et al. Potential for re-

duced toxicity and dose escalation in the treatment of inoperable non-small-cell lung cancer a comparison of intensity-modulated radiation therapy (IMRT), 3D conformal radiation and elective nodal irradiation. Int J Radiat Oncol Biol Phys, 2003, 57 (3): 875-890.

[99] Liao ZX, Komaki RR, Thames HD, et al. Influence of technologic advances on outcomes in patients with unresectable, locally advanced non-small-cell lung cancer receiving concomitant chemoradiotherapy. Int J Radiat Oncol Biol Phys, 2010, 76 (3): 775-781.

[100] Chang JY, Zhang X, Wang X, et al. Significant reduction of normal tissue dose by proton radiotherapy compared with threedimensional conformal or intensity-modulated radiation therapy in Stage I or Stage III non-small-cell lung cancer. In J Radiat Oncol Biol Phys, 2006, 65 (1): 1087-1096.

[101] Nichols RC, Huh SN, Henderson RH, et al. Proton radiation therapy offers reduced normal lung and bone marrow exposure for patients receiving dose escalated radiation therapy for unresectable stage iii non-small-cell lung cancer: a dosimetric study. Int J Radiat Oncol Biol Phys, 2012, 83 (1): 158-163.

[102] Vogelius IR, Westerly DC, Aznar MC, et al. Estimated radiation pneumonitis risk after photon versus proton therapy alone or combined with chemotherapy for lung cancer. Acta Oncol. 2011, 50 (6): 772-776.

[103] Sejpal S, Komaki R, Tsao A, et al. Early findings on toxicity of proton beam therapy with concurrent chemotherapy for nonsmall cell lung cancer. Cancer, 2011, 117 (13): 3004-3013.

[104] Chang JY, Komaki R, Lu C, et al. Phase 2 study of high-dose proton therapy with concurrent chemotherapy for unresectable stage III nonsmall cell lung cancer. Cancer, 2011, 117 (20): 4707-4713.

[105] Pignon JP, Arriagada R, Ihde DC, et al. A meta-analysis of thoracic radiotherapy for small-cell lung cancer. N Engl J Med, 1992, 327 (23): 1618-1624.

[106] Murray N, Coy P, Pater JL, et al. Importance of timing for thoracic irradiation in the combined modality treatment of limited-stage small-cell lung cancer. The National Cancer Institute of Canada Clinical Trials Group. J Clin Oncol, 1993, 11 (2): 336-344.

[107] Spiro SG, James LE, Rudd RM, et al. Early compared with late radiotherapy in combined modality treatment for limited disease small-cell lung cancer. A London Lung Cancer Group multicenter randomized clinical trial and meta-analysis. J Clin Oncol, 2006, 24 (24): 3823-3830.

[108] Fried DB, Morris DE, Poole C, et al. Systematic review evaluating the timing of thoracic radiation therapy in combined modality therapy for limited-stage small-cell lung cancer. J Clin Oncol, 2004, 22 (23): 4837-4845.

[109] De Ruysscher D, Pijls-Johannesma M, Bentzen SM, et al. Time between the first day of chemotherapy and the last day of chest radiation is the most important predictor of survival in limited-disease small-cell lung cancer. J Clin Oncol, 2006, 24 (7): 1057-1063.

[110] Park KS, Kim S-W, Ahn M-j, et al. Phase III trial of concurrent thoracic radiotherapy (TRT) with either the first cycle or the third cycle of cisplatin and etoposide chemotherapy to determine the optimal timing of TRT for limited disease small-cell lung cancer. J Clin Oncol, suppl, 2012: 7005.

[111] Laurice SA, Logan D, Markman BR, et al. Practice guideline for the role of combination chemotherapy in the initial management of limited-stage small-cell lung cancer. Lung Cancer, 2004, 43 (2): 223-240.

[112] Sundstrom S, Bremnes RM, Kaasa S, et al. Cisplatin and etoposide regimen is superior to cyclophosphamide, epirubicin, and vincristine regimen in small-cell lung cancer: Results from a randomized phase III trial with 5 years' follow-up. J Clin Oncol, 2002, 20 (24): 465-472.

[113] Noda K, Nishiwaki Y, Kawahara M, et al. Irinotecan plus cisplatin compared with etoposide plus cisplatin for extensive small-cell lung cancer. N Engl J Med, 2002, 346 (2): 85-91.

[114] Hanna N, Bunn PA, Jr., Langer C, et al. Randomized phase III trial comparing irinotecan/cisplatin with etoposide/cisplatin in patients with previously untreated extensive-stage disease small-cell lung cancer. J Clin Oncol, 2006, 24 (13): 2038-2043.

[115] Lara PN, Jr., Natale R, Crowley J, et al. Phase III trial of irinotecan/cisplatin compared with etoposide/cisplatin in extensive-stage small-cell lung cancer: Clinical and pharmacogenomic results from SWOG S0124. J Clin Oncol, 2009, 27 (15): 2530-2535.

[116] Rossi A, Di Maio M, Chiodini P, et al. Carboplatin-or cisplatinbased chemotherapy in first-line treatment of small-cell lung cancer. The COCIS meta-analysis of individual patient data. J Clin Oncol, 2012, 30 (14):

1692-1698.

[117] Turrisi AT, 3rd, Kim K, Blum R, et al. Twice-daily compared with once-daily thoracic radiotherapy in limited small-cell lung cancer treated concurrently with cisplatin and etoposide. N Engl J Med, 1999, 340 (4): 265-271.

[118] Bogart JA, Herndon JE, 2nd, Lyss AP, et al. 70 Gy thoracic radiotherapy is feasible concurrent with chemotherapy for limited-stage small-cell lung cancer. Analysis of Cancer and Lenkemia Group B study 39808. Int J Radiat Oncol Biol Phys, 2004, 59 (2): 460-468.

[119] Komaki R, Swann RS, Ettinger DS, et al. Phase I study of thoracic radiation dose escalation with concurrent chemotherapy for patients with limited small-cell lung cancer: Report of Radiation Therapy Oncology Group (RTOG) protocol 97-12. Int J Radiat Oncol Biol Phys, 2005, 62 (2): 342-350.

[120] Bradley JD, Dehdashti F, Mintun MA, et al. Positron emission tomography in limited-stage small-cell lung cancer. A prospective study. J Clin Oncol, 2004, 22 (16): 3248-3254.

[121] Jeremic B, Shibamoto Y, Nikolic N, et al. Role of radiation therapy in the combined-modality treatment of patients with extensive disease small-cell lung cancer: A randomized study. J Clin Oncol, 1999, 17 (7): 2092-2099.

[122] Auperin A, Arriagada R, Pignon JP, et al. Prophylactic cranial irradiation for patients with small-cell lung cancer in complete remission. Prophylactic Cranial Irradiation Overview Collaborative Group. N Engl J Med, 1999, 341 (7): 476-484.

[123] Slotman B, Faivre-Finn C, Kramer G, et al. Prophylactic cranial irradiation in extensive small-cell lung cancer. N Engl J Med, 2007, 357 (7): 664-672.

[124] Le Pechoux C, Dunant A, Senan S, et al. Standard-dose versus higher-dose prophylactic cranial irradiation (PCI) in patients with limited-stage small-cell lung cancer in complete remission after chemotherapy and thoracic radiotherapy (PCI 99-01, EORTC 22003-08004, RTOG 0212, and IFCT 99-01): A randomized clinical trial. Lancet Oncol, 2009, 10 (5): 467-474.

[125] Le Pechoux C, Laplanche A, Faivre-Finn C, et al. Clinical neurological outcome and quality of life among patients with limited small-cell lung cancer treated with two different doses of prophylactie cranial irradiation in the intergroup phase III trial (PC199-01, EORTC 22003-08004, RTOG 0212 and IFCT 99-01). Ann Oncol, 2011, 22 (5): 1154-1163.

第24章
基于剂量提升与非常规分割的个体化放疗在非小细胞肺癌中的应用

Heath D. Skinner, Ritsuko U. Komaki, Joe Y. Chang, James D. Cox
Department of Radiation Oncology, The University of Texas MD Anderson Cancer Center, Houston, TX, USA

引 言

在过去的十几年中，放疗是肺癌的主要治疗方式，其中包括根治性放疗与辅助性放疗。在这期间，放疗技术的进步使得临床医生在提高肿瘤控制率的同时，还可以降低周围正常组织的毒性。最近的两篇 meta 分析[1-2]均证明针对非小细胞肺癌（NSCLC），肿瘤的局部控制率与患者的生存期明显相关。在许多临床病例中，肿瘤的局部控制是通过放疗加速分割方式或剂量提升方式实现的。然而，最近的研究开始关注剂量提升能否让 NSCLC 患者获益。本章节将针对由于身体条件无法手术或手术无法切除的 NSCLC 患者，回顾近年来在剂量提升和加速分割方面的一些研究，包括能够实现剂量提升的放疗新技术与其应用的临床试验。同时还会简单讨论关于剂量提升与多种复杂的影像、照射剂量、生物靶区等因素相关性研究。

剂量提升与非常规分割放疗的发展历史

20 世纪 60 年代，对于无法手术或手术无法切除的 NSCLC 患者来说，二维放疗技术（单次照射 2Gy，照射 20 次，放疗剂量共 40Gy）是主要的治疗手段。而这种放疗方式的效果往往不能让人满意[3]。一些学者开始探索放射剂量提高到 50～60Gy 的可能性，另外一些学者开始使用大分割分段治疗方式。这些有争议性的观点促成了 RTOG 73-01 随机研究的开展。RTOG 73-01 包括 4 组不同的放疗方式：常规分割 40Gy（2Gy×20次）、50Gy（2Gy×25次）、60Gy（2Gy×30次）及非常规分割 40Gy（4Gy×10次，治疗中间休息 2 周）；常规组 3 年的局部复发率为 52%、42% 及 33%，非常规组为 44%。3 年的局部控制率或复发率是两个相对概念分别为 52%、42%、33% 及 44%，同时患者的生存期也随着剂量的提升而获益。尽管之后几年的研究未观察到随着剂量提升患者的生存期延长，但这些研究均认为患者接受单独放疗时，给予常规分割的剂量提升能够延长患者的生存期。对于能够长期存活的患者进行观察，发现正常组织损伤毒性在可以接受的范围，特别是 3 级放射性肺炎、食管炎发生率均低于 15%[6]。

20 世纪 70 年代，研究者的目光主要集中在大分割放疗技术在治疗局部进展期 NSCLC 患者方向上[7-9]。但随着 RTOG III 期临床试验（6Gy，每周 2 次，共 36Gy）[7]的结果公布，这种与放射增敏剂醚醇硝唑（misonidazole）联合应用的大分割放疗方式研究最终结束。RTOG III 期临床试验观察到，不仅醚醇硝唑对局部控制率及生存期无任何益处，而且其 3 级放射损伤发生率明显高于 RTOG 73-01 试验，同时未显示出更好的局部控制率和生存获益。

基于上述研究，RTOG 及美国均认为 60Gy（2Gy×30次）为局部进展期 NSCLC 患者的标准放射治疗方案。该协助组与其他的进一步研究主要集中在基于上述的剂量提升与辅助化疗方案的研究上。对于化疗协同放疗的 NSCLC 患者的研究将在其他章节进行讨论。本章节主要讨论剂量提升和非常规分割的进一步研究。

继 RTOG 73-01 研究之后，更加安全的剂量提升方案引起了人们的注意，一种可能实现的方式是超分割放疗。由于毒性反应被过去和现在均认为是给予更高放疗剂量的主要限制性因素，因此超分割放疗方式在放射生物学方面更具优势。理论上讲，超分割放疗在肿瘤继续发生损伤的同时，正常组织可以进行修复。针对局部进展期 NSCLC 患者的 RTOG 81-08 临床 I 期试验显示了使用超分割放疗的可行性和安全性，其具体放疗总剂量最大可达 74.4Gy，每天 2 次[10]。随后进行的 RTOG 83-11，是随机的 I、II 期临床试验，利用超分割方式给予剂量爬升试验[11]，具体方案为总剂量从 60Gy 开始，逐步增加 4.8Gy，最终达到 79.2Gy，所有的放疗计划均是每天 2 次，每次 1.2Gy，放疗间隔 6h。69.6Gy 剂量组患者的中位生存期为 13.7 个月，明显高于低剂量组，但总剂量超过 69.6Gy 组无明显生存获益。同时，69.6Gy 剂量组的 3 级或 3 级以上放射损伤发生率为 8.5%，与其他剂量组无显著差异。这一结果明显优于同时期其他队列研究，包括单独放疗 60Gy（2Gy×30 次）剂量组研究与 60Gy（2Gy×30 次）+序贯化疗 CALGB（Cancer and Leukemia Group B）84-33 研究[12-13]。

连续超分割加速放射治疗（Continuous, Hyperfractionated, Accelerated Radiation Treatment, CHART）这一概念随即被提出。在一项关于 CHART 的初步研究中，给予 23 例局部进展期 NSCLC 患者单纯放疗，每天 3 次，每次 1.4Gy，总剂量 50.4Gy[14]。当发现患者可以耐受毒性时，剂量提升至每天 3 次，每次 1.5Gy，总剂量 54Gy。当 54Gy CHART 剂量组与 60Gy 常规分割剂量组对比时，CHART 组 1 年存活率达到 64%[15-16]，2 年存活率 CHART 组明显高于常规分割剂量组（30% vs 21%），但是治疗 3 个月后放射性急性食管炎（19% vs 3%）及症状性放射性肺炎（19% vs 10%）发生率明显高于常规分割剂量组[15]。

上述发现提示，通过剂量提升及超分割放疗方式可以提高患者的生存期，其他一些同时含有化疗方案的研究取得了同样的结果，这些研究直接导致了 RTOG 88-08 研究的开展[17]。RTOG 88-08 是一项 III 期临床研究，包含了 3 种治疗方案：单纯放疗总剂量 60Gy 组（每天 1 次，每次 2Gy，共 30d）；上述标准 60Gy 方案加序贯化疗组（顺铂+长春花碱）；放疗总剂量 69.6Gy 组（每天 2 次，共 58 次，每次 1.2Gy）。结果显示放疗序贯化疗组的生存期明显延长，但 69.6Gy 剂量组的中位生存期亦能达到 12 个月。

继 RTOG 88-08 研究后，随后的两项独立研究都显示加入化疗与超分割放疗均能使患者获益[18-19]。I 期临床研究 RTOG 90-15 及 II 期临床研究 RTOG 91-06 探讨超分割放疗 69.6Gy 加入化疗方案，其结果显示加入化疗较单纯超分割明显提高了生存期（中位生存期 18.9 个月 vs 10.6 个月），但明显增加了毒性反应，近 60% 的患者出现了 4 级血液毒性，3.9% 的患者出现了治疗相关性死亡[19]。这种超分割放疗方式明显增加了放射性食管毒性，53% 的患者出现了 3 级或以上放射性食管炎。然而，由于这种超分割的方式明显提高了生存期，故接下来的一些试验继续对其进行研究[20-21]。为了探讨化疗与放疗的先后顺序，RTOG 94-10 对比了常规分割 63Gy 剂量组与超分割 69.6Gy 剂量组，两组均使用同步化疗方案，发现两组之间的生存期无显著差异，但超分割放疗组较严重的放射性食管炎发生率明显增加（45% vs 22%）。另外的一些试验研究运用常规分割给予上述两组同样的总剂量，亦显示两组间的生存期无显著差异[22-23]。令人感兴趣的是，另外一项 RTOG 的研究中，尽管患者入组人数较少，其结果显示超分割加入化疗组较常规分割组的生存期明显改善（中位生存期 22 个月 vs 14 个月），而毒性无明显增加[24]。但最近的一项研究对比了常规分割 60Gy 组（6 周完成）与超分割 60Gy（3 周完成）组，显示两组之间的生存期无显著差异[25]。食管放射毒性在超分割组明显增加。

对于局限进展期 NSCLC 患者的治疗，关于剂量提升及非常规分割方式研究的复杂性增加了（表 24.1），主要体现在其毒性反应。然而，观察这些研究结果发现，一些放疗技术的进步可以减轻剂量提升带来的毒性反应，接下来我们将就这一话题继续展开讨论。

表 24.1 NSCLC 剂量提升和超分割 III 期临床试验

临床试验	入组人数	入组标准	入组放疗方案	入组化疗方案	结论	毒性反应
RTOG 73-01(4)	447	III 期	①40Gy,分段照射 ②40Gy,单次2Gy,每天1次 ③50Gy,单次2Gy,每天1次 ④60Gy,单次2Gy,每天1次	无	治疗方案 4 与其他对比,局部控制率提高 33%;各治疗方案远期生存无明显差异	15%患者发生 3 级和 3 级以上放射性肺炎和食管炎
RTOG 83-11(11)	884	II~IV 期(无远处转移,KPS>50%)	下列所有放疗方案均为单次1.2Gy,每天2次 ①60Gy ②64.8Gy ③69.6Gy ④74.4Gy ⑤79.2Gy	无	治疗方案 3 与 1、2 对比,远期生存明显改善	每个治疗方案约10%的患者出现 3 级及以上毒性反应
CHART(14-16)	563	非手术患者,PS 0~1	①60Gy,单次2Gy,每天1次 ②54Gy,单次1.5Gy,每日3次	无	治疗方案 2 与 1 对比,远期生存改善	治疗方案 2 中 19%患者出现验证的放射性肺炎及食管炎
RTOG 88-08(17)	458	II、IIIA~B 期,KPS>70,体重减轻<50%	①60Gy,单次2Gy,每天1次 ②60Gy,单次2Gy,每天1次 ③69.6Gy,单次1.2Gy,每天2次	诱导(顺铂+长春花碱)仅方案 2	治疗方案 2 远期生存改善	各治疗方案无明显差别
Jeremic 研究(24)	131	III 期,KPS>50	①69.6Gy,单次1.2Gy,每天2次	放化疗同步(卡铂+依托泊苷)(方案 2)	治疗方案 2(24 个月)远期生存改善	各治疗方案无明显差别
RTOG 94-10(21)	610	II~III 期,KPS>70,体重减轻<50%	①63Gy,单次1.8 或 2Gy,每天1次 ②63Gy,单次1.8 或 2Gy,每天1次 ③69.6Gy,单次1.2Gy,每天2次	顺铂+长春花碱序贯放疗(治疗方案 1)或顺铂+长春花碱同步放化疗治疗方案 2、3	治疗方案 2(17 个月)和 3(15.2 个月)远期生存明显改善	同步化疗组患者出现明显急性毒性反应
澳大利亚(25)	204	非手术患者,PS 0~1	临床配对:60Gy,每次2Gy,每天1次 vs 60Gy,每次2Gy,每天2次,联合化疗或单纯放疗	卡铂	远期生存各治疗方案组无统计学差异,但治疗方案 1 组远期生存较好(20.3 个月)	治疗方案 2 组出现严重的毒性反应
RTOG-0617(51)	423	IIIA~B 期,PS 0~1,1 秒用力呼气容积≥1.2L/s	临床配对:60Gy,单次2Gy,每天1次 vs 74Gy,单次2Gy,每天1次	卡铂+紫杉醇,联合西妥昔单抗或单次化疗	治疗方案 2 组由于临床交叉分析,提前终止	各治疗方案无明显差别

KPS:卡式评分;LRF:局部失败率;PS:体力状态

放疗技术与放疗适形度进展

在过去的二三十年间，放疗技术的进步在肺癌放疗计划制定及实施方面提供了更好的适形度。尽管一些技术在其他章节已经深入讨论，但在剂量提升方面，图像引导放疗发挥了非常重要的作用。CT 的出现，使放疗在真正的三维放射计划中得以实施，使放疗具备更好的适形度，特别是在 NSCLC 的治疗中，在保护正常肺组织及食管的同时，提高局部控制率[26]。随着 4D-CT 的出现，图像引导放疗已经取得了长足的进步。4D-CT 在监控正常呼吸时相的同时，能够利用植入基准点标记使肿瘤运动可视化，能够在治疗中通过屏气或呼吸门控实现控制肿瘤的运动[27-29]。在呼吸运动过程中，肿瘤靶区的位置在某一特定时相是固定的，制订放疗计划时就可以减少靶区外扩边界，正常组织亦可以减少受照剂量[30]。

从以往的标准靶区验证图像到现在的基于千伏级高质量图像或 CT 验证图像引导的放疗技术，使患者在多次治疗过程中，都能保证体位的准确性。对于上述技术的研究能减少肿瘤外扩边界和保护周围正常组织。

最后，放疗在照射剂量传输方面亦取得了巨大的进步。调强放疗（IMRT）的出现能够更好地保护正常组织。在一些回顾性研究中，IMRT 被证实具有剂量学与减轻毒性方面的优势[31-34]。尽管关于 IMRT 与其他放疗技术的前瞻性对比研究相对较少，但基于这些研究，IMRT 已经成为 NSCLC 及其他肿瘤放疗的主要治疗方式。另外，一些学者已经开始利用质子放疗技术治疗肿瘤。在一项临床 II 期研究中，对于局部进展期接受同步放化疗的 NSCLC 患者，质子治疗组（RBE 74Gy）发生 3 级及以上毒性的概率低于常规 X 线治疗组（63Gy）[35]。

所有放疗新技术尽量都减少正常组织受量。另外，一些剂量参数被证实与正常组织急性和远期毒性相关[36-37]。由于能够辅助选择治疗方式和筛选出符合剂量提升放疗方式的患者并减少毒性反应，剂量参数 V_{20}（接受至少 20Gy 剂量的正常肺组织体积）和肺组织平均受量（mean lung dose，MLD）作为参数评价指标已运用在放疗计划评价和剂量提升中。

总之，对于局部进展期 NSCLC 放疗，多种新技术的开展能够减少放射毒性反应，又一次引出剂量提升这一放疗方式是否具有可行性和安全性的问题。这一话题将在下一部分进一步阐释。

局部进展期患者剂量提升放疗的新研究

由于上述关于 CHART 及能够提高放疗适形度的新技术研究获得了成功，一些研究开始着眼于在 CHART 的基础上加入化疗。到目前为止，这些研究进展缓慢，甚至部分研究提前关闭。ECOG 2597 试验研究诱导化疗后序贯放疗，对比 CHART 组及常规分割组的放疗效果。尽管研究发现 CHART 组的中位生存期为 20.3 个月，但严重毒性反应为 10%，与常规分割组对比，未显示较好的结果[23]。另外一项独立研究诱导化疗后 CHART 放疗，中位生存期为 25 个月，毒性反应可以接受，但这些研究在 43 例患者入组后关闭[38]。CHARTWEL 试验研究了相同放疗剂量与分割方式随机分组，发现总体局部控制率无明显改善，而亚组分析发现，对于肿瘤分期较晚的患者或接受化疗的患者，运用 CHART 可以提高局部控制率，但急性毒性反应较重。

因为缺乏患者受益及加入化疗后明显增加相关的毒性反应的研究结果，目前看来 CHART 方案的实施应当慎重。

相反，在标准分割的基础上进行剂量提升越来越受到人们的重视，许多研究机构在治疗局部进展期 NSCLC 患者，剂量接近或超过 70Gy。如果治疗计划中未超出相关危及器官的剂量限定且未产生明显放疗毒性，上述治疗方案则被认为是可以接受的[36-37]。回顾性分析提示当放疗剂量超过 67~74Gy 时，患者的生存状况较好[40-43]。这些回顾性研究结果被北卡罗莱纳大学主导的 I、II 期临床试验进一步验证，其研究对象为局限进展期 NSCLC 接受诱导或同步化疗的患者。在这一研究中，患者接受的放疗剂量经过 4 次剂量提升，从常规分割 60Gy 到 74Gy。3 级及以上放射食管炎发生率为 8%，中位生存期为 24 个月。同课题组的另外一项Ⅰ期临床试验，放疗剂量提高至90Gy[46]，其严重的食管炎放射率为16%，2例患者死于咳血；同时，中位生存期同样为24个月，与上一项研究相比无延长。这一系列研究值得我们注意的是，尽管接受超过66Gy放射剂量的患者中位生存期接近25个月，但严重晚期并发症的发生率为24%[47]。

上述结果提示，剂量提升可以改善生存期及可控的急性毒性反应，促成了RTOG临床Ⅰ、Ⅱ期试验的开展，其给予常规分割74Gy，并接受同步化疗[48-49]。Ⅰ期试验得到的结果与北卡罗来纳大学的研究相似[44-45,48]，55例患者全部接受74Gy剂量放疗，其中位生存期为25.9个月，3级及以上放射性肺炎的发生率为22%，严重的非血液放射毒性发生率为61%。相同的结果出现在CALGB 30105研究中，该试验为Ⅱ期随机临床试验，患者接受两组不同方案的化疗，两组接受放疗剂量均为74Gy[50]。在这项研究中，使用吉西他滨被发现明显增加了毒性，故导致了研究提前关闭。虽然中位生存期接近25个月，但严重的放射性肺炎与食管炎的发生率均为16%。尽管发生了较高的毒性反应，从生存结果来看值得进一步研究，故RTOG进行了临床Ⅲ期试验，给予常规分割60Gy与74Gy，并加入了传统的全身治疗；同时还研究了联合西妥昔单抗的有效性[51]。在RTOG 0617试验中，临床分期为Ⅲ期的500例NSCLC患者分为4组，常规分割60Gy、74Gy、60Gy+西妥昔单抗、74Gy+西妥昔单抗，所有患者接受卡铂+紫杉醇周方案同步化疗。423例患者完成治疗后，此研究由于其无效性提前终止（90例发生在高剂量组）。另外，研究发现1年存活率在低剂量组较高（81% vs 74%）。撰写本章节的同时，低剂量组入组研究仍在开放，已无患者进入到高剂量组。

RTOG 0617试验给肿瘤放疗界留下了很多的疑问，可能直到此研究完成后才会有确定的答案，但是对目前得到的数据进行分析也是非常重要的。例如，高剂量组与低剂量组在放疗相关毒性发生率方面统计学差异不显著，高剂量组中7例患者死于放疗相关毒性，低剂量组中3例患者死于放疗相关毒性。这一发现引发了剂量越高毒性越大与上述结果冲突的猜想。

最近发表的2篇关于NSCLC放疗的meta分析结论增加了对于上述疑问解释的复杂性，这两篇meta分析均得到剂量提升有益于患者的结论[52-53]。需要特别指出的是，Partridge和其团队分析了16项临床试验发现，在照射剂量转化为生物等效剂量（biologically equivalent dose，BED）后，剂量与治疗反应成明显相关性[52]。另外一项meta分析中，Machtay及其团队分析了RTOG试验的1 356例局限进展期NSCLC患者，所有患者接受放疗及化疗（包括序贯或同步），证实了BED与生存及局部-区域控制率相关[53]。值得注意的是，BED每增加1，生存率增加约4%，局部-区域控制率增加约3%。这些大的临床数据与RTOG 0617的结果相反。然而，在结果公布的时，RTOG试验的标准剂量为常规分割60Gy、分30次，与RTOG 88-08试验相同。

个体化放疗计划

综上所述，关于剂量提升、非常规分割联合同步化疗的未来研究必须考虑治疗所带来的毒性反应。如我们所观察到的，这一章节所回顾的一系列阳性结果表明放疗剂量的提高带来正常组织放疗损伤的增加，而最终止于阴性结果研究RTOG 0617。那么我们应该如何选择将来的放疗方式呢？

如我们上文所提到的，基于NSCLC的放疗技术的进步使开展更好的适形度及个体化放疗成为可能。随着基于图像放疗计划的制订及图像引导放疗的广泛应用，使最大限度的保护周围正常组织并减少放疗相关毒性越来越成为可能。而且，当先进的放疗照射技术（IMRT、质子放疗）成为标准治疗方法时，个体化放疗将成为趋势。我们期望的是随着放疗技术的进步，可以减少放疗相关毒性的同时安全提高放疗剂量。

另外一种技术，即自适应放疗技术的应用，能够真正实现个体化的剂量提升。自适应放疗计划包括放疗中肿瘤的重复影像，当肿瘤在治疗过程中缩小的同时放疗野也相应缩小，并能对肿瘤组织进行准确覆盖。目前，基于FDG PET/CT的自适应放疗计划，能够提高肿瘤放疗剂量分布，尤其对于邻近重要组织的肿瘤[54]。例如，在给予常规分割45Gy时，重复的FDG PET/CT能够反映实体肿瘤的治疗效果。结合这一信息，制定自适应放疗计划应考虑 PET 所反映的治疗效果。事实上，上述放疗方式就是 RTOG 1106 试验的研究目的。RTOG 1106 试验是正在进行的随机Ⅱ期临床试验，针对试验组患者在治疗过程中，调整基于 PET、CT 的放疗计划。根据 PET、CT 反映的治疗效果，在各项参数处于正常范围的情况下，肿瘤放射剂量可提升至 85.5Gy。

最后，基于生物信息的剂量提升引起了我们的关注。这一放疗方式的理论基础为，并非肿瘤的各个部位均对放疗敏感，还有部分区域为放疗抵抗的区域，特别是乏氧区域。因此，假如知道肿瘤的哪一部分为放疗抵抗区域，并且这部分区域能被观察到，我们就可以给予这部分区域更高的放疗剂量，这样就最大限度地减少了肿瘤的高剂量区，减轻了放疗相关毒性。例如，高 SUV 区被认为是放疗抵抗和肿瘤复发的区域[57]，如果这一区域给予较高的剂量，那么我们在提升剂量获益的同时，并没有增加毒性反应。其他的一些成像方式基本上是标记缺氧区域，利用与上述相似的方式已经被提出应用于放疗，并值得我们进一步研究[58]。

总　结

在过去的二三十年间，关于 NSCLC 放疗的放疗剂量提升与非常规分割放疗研究取得了一些进展，但是最近遇到了较大的困难。将来的研究方向，是在了解放疗可以带来明显的正常组织毒性的同时，研究基于影像及生物靶区的剂量提升技术，以找到有效性与毒性的平衡点。

（刘　佳　黄　伟　李宝生　译）

参考文献

[1] Aupérin A, Le Péchoux C, Rolland E, et al. Meta-analysis of concomitant versus sequential radiochemotherapy in locally advanced non-small-cell lung cancer. Journal of Clinical Oncology, 2010, 28（13）：2181 – 2190.

[2] O'Rourke N, Roqué I, Figuls M, et al. Concurrent chemoradiotherapy in non-small cell lung cancer. The Cochrane Library, 2010.

[3] Roswit B, Patno ME, Rapp R, et al. The Survival of Patients with Inoperable Lung Cancer：A Large-Scale Randomized Study of Radiation Therapy Versus Placebo 1. Radiology, 1968, 90（4）：688 – 697.

[4] Lee RE, Carr DT, Childs DS Jr. Comparison of split-course radiation therapy and continuous radiation therapy for unresectable bronchogenic carcinoma：5 year results. American Journal of Roentgenology, 1976, 126（1）：116 – 122.

[5] Perez CA, Pajak TF, Rubin P, et al. Long-term observations of the patterns of failure in patients with unresectable non-oat cell carcinoma of the lung treated with definitive radiotherapy report by the radiation therapy oncology group. Cancer, 1987, 59（11）：1874 – 1881.

[6] Kong F-M, Hayman JA, Griffith KA, et al. Final toxicity results of a radiation-dose escalation study in patients with non-small-cell lung cancer（NSCLC）：Predictors for radiation pneumonitis and fibrosis. International Journal of Radiation Oncology, Biology, Physics, 2006, 65（4）：1075 – 1086.

[7] Simpson JR, Bauer M, Wasserman TH, et al. Large fraction irradiation with or without misonidazole in advanced non-oat cell carcinoma of the lung：a phase Ⅲ randomized trial of the RTOG. Radiation Therapy Oncology Group. Int. J Radiat Oncol Biol Phys, 1987, 13（6）：861 – 867.

[8] Jakobsson M, Taskinen PJ, Kylmämaa T. Misonidazole combined with radiotherapy in the treatment of non-small cell lung cancer. A randomized double-blind trial. Strahlentherapie and Onkol, 1987, 163（2）：90 – 93.

[9] Panduro J, Kjaer M, Wolff-Jensen J, et al. Misonidazole combined with radiotherapy in the treatment of inoperable squamous cell carcinoma of the lung a double-blind randomized trial. Cancer, 1983, 52（1）：20 – 24.

[10] Cox JD, Pajak TF, Herskovic A, et al. Five-year survival after hyperfractionated radiation therapy for non-small-cell carcinoma of the lung（NSCCL）：results of RTOG protocol 81 – 08. American journal of clinical oncology, 1991, 14（4）：280 – 284.

[11] Cox JD, Azarnia N, Byhardt RW, et al. A randomized phase Ⅰ/Ⅱ trial of hyperfractionated radiation therapy with total doses of 60.0 Gy to 79.2 Gy：possible survival benefit with greater than or equal to 69.6 Gy in favorable patients with Radiation Therapy Oncology Group stage Ⅲ non-small-cell lung carcinoma：report of Radiation Therapy Oncology Group 83 – 11. Journal of Clinical Oncology, 1990, 8（9）：1543 – 1555.

[12] Dillman RO, Herndon J, Seagren SL, et al. Improved survival in stage III non-small-cell lung cancer: seven-year follow-up of cancer and leukemia group B (CALGB) 8433 trial. Journal of the National Cancer Institute, 1996, 88 (17): 1210-1215.

[13] Scott C, Sause WT, Byhardt R, et al. Recursive partitioning analysis of 1592 patients on four Radiation Therapy Oncology Group studies in inoperable non-small cell lung cancer. Lung Cancer, 1997, 17: S59-S74.

[14] Saunders M I, Dische S. Continuous, hyperfractionated, accelerated radiotherapy (CHART) in non-small cell carcinoma of the bronchus. International Journal of Radiation Oncology, Biology, Physics, 1990, 19 (5): 1211-1215.

[15] Saunders M, Dische S, Barrett A, et al. Continuous hyperfractionated accelerated radiotherapy (CHART) versus conventional radiotherapy in non-small-cell lung cancer: a randomized multicentre trial. The Lancet, 1997, 350 (9072): 161-165.

[16] Saunders M, Dische S, Barrett A, et al. Continuous, hyperfractionated, accelerated radiotherapy (CHART) versus conventional radiotherapy in non-small cell lung cancer: mature data from the randomized multicentre trial. Radiotherapy and oncology, 1999, 52 (2): 137-148.

[17] Sause W, Kolesar P, Taylor S IV, et al. Final results of phase III trial in regionally advanced unresectable non-small cell lung cancer: Radiation Therapy OncoloGy Group, Eastern Cooperative Oncology Group, and Southwest OncoloGy Group. Chest Journal, 2000, 117 (2): 358-364.

[18] Byhardt RW, Scott CB, Ettinger DS, et al. Concurrent hyperfractionated irradiation and chemotherapy for unresectable nonsmall cell lung cancer. Results of radiation therapy oncology group 90-15. Cancer, 1995, 75 (9): 2337-2344.

[19] Komaki R, Scott C, Lee JS, et al. Impact of Adding Concurrent Chemotherapy to Hyperfractionated Radiotherapy for Locally Advanced Non-Small Cell Lung Cancer (NSCLC): Comparison of RTOG 83-11 and RTOG 91-06. American journal of clinical oncology, 1997, 20 (5): 435-440.

[20] Komaki R, Scott C, Ettinger D, et al. Randomized study of chemotherapy/radiation therapy combinations for favorable patients with locally advanced inoperable nonsmall cell lung cancer: Radiation Therapy Oncology Group (RTOG) 92-04. International Journal of Radiation Oncology. Biology. Physics, 1997, 38 (1): 149-155.

[21] Curran WJ, Scott CB, Langer CJ, et al. Long-term benefit is observed in a phase III comparison of sequential vs. concurrent chemo-radiation for patients with unresected stage III NSCLC: RTOG 9410. Proc Am Soc Clin Oncol, 2003, 22 (S1): 2499.

[22] Furuse K, Fukuoka M, Kawahara M, et al. Phase III study of concurrent versus sequential thoracic radiotherapy in combination with mitomycin, vindesine, and cisplatin in unresectable stage III non-small-cell lung cancer. Journal of Clinical Oncology, 1999, 17 (9): 2692-2692.

[23] Belani CP, Choy H, Bonomi P, et al. Combined chemoradiotherapy regimens of paclitaxel and carboplatin for locally advanced non-small-cell lung cancer: A rando mized phase II locally advanced multi-modality protocol. Journal of clinical oncology, 2005, 23 (25): 5883-5891.

[24] Jeremic B, Shibamoto Y, Acimovic L, et al. Hyperfractionated radiation therapy with or without concurrent low-dose daily carboplatin/etoposide for stage III non-small-cell lung cancer: a randomized study. Journal of clinical oncology, 1996, 14 (4): 1065-1070.

[25] Ball D, Bishop J, Smith J, et al. A randomised phase III study of accelerated or standard fraction radiotherapy with or without concurrent carboplatin in inoperable non-small cell lung cancer: Final report of an Australian multi-centre trial. Radiotherapy and oncology, 1999, 52 (2): 129-136.

[26] Fang LC, Komaki R, Allen P, et al. Comparison of outcomes for patients with medically inoperable Stage I non-small-cell lung cancer treated with two-dimensional vs. three-dimensional radiotherapy. International Journal of Radiation Oncology, Biology, Physics, 2006, 66 (1): 108-116.

[27] Nehmeh SA, Erdi YE, Pan T, et al. Four-dimensional (4D) PET/CT imaging of the thorax. Medical physics, 2004, 31 (12): 3179-3186.

[28] Rosenzweig KE, Hanley J, Mah D, et al. The deep inspiration breath-hold technique in the treatment of inoperable non-small-cell lung cancer. International Journal of Radiation Oncology, Biology, Physics, 2000, 48 (1): 81-87.

[29] Ramsey CR, Scaperoth D, Arwood D, et al. Clinical efficacy of respiratory gated conformal radiation therapy. Medical Dosimetry, 1999, 24 (2): 115-119.

[30] Chang JY, Dong L, Liu H, et al. Image-Guided Radiation Therapy for Non-small Cell Lung Cancer. Journal of

[31] Yom SS, Liao Z, Liu HH, et al. Initial evaluation of treatment-related pneumonitis in advanced-stage non-small-cell lung cancer patients treated with concurrent chemotherapy and intensity-modulated radiotherapy. International Journal of Radiation Oncology, Biology, Physics, 2007, 68 (1): 94-102.

[32] Liao ZX, Komaki RR, Thames HD Jr, et al. Influence of technologic advances on outcomes in patients with unresectable, locally advanced non-small-cell lung cancer receiving concomitant chemoradiotherapy. International Journal of Radiation Oncology, Biology, Physics, 2010, 76 (3): 775-781.

[33] Bezjak A, Rumble RB, Rodrigues G, et al. Intensity-modulated radiotherapy in the treatment of lung cancer. Clinical oncology, 2012, 24 (7): 508-520.

[34] Govaert SLA, Troost EGC, Schuurbiers OCJ, et al. Treatment outcome and toxicity of intensity-modulated (chemo) radiotherapy in stage III non-small cell lung cancer patients. Radiat Oncol, 2012, 7: 150.

[35] Chang J Y, Komaki R, Lu C, et al. Phase 2 study of high-dose proton therapy with concurrent chemotherapy for unresectable stage III nonsmall cell lung cancer. Cancer, 2011, 117 (20): 4707-4713.

[36] Marks LB, Yorke ED, Jackson A, et al. Use of normal tissue complication probability models in the clinic. International Journal of Radiation Oncology, Biology, Physics, 2010, 76 (3): S10-S19.

[37] Marks LB, Bentzen SM, Deasy JO, et al. Radiation dose-volume effects in the lung. International Journal of Radiation Oncology, Biology, Physics, 2010, 76 (3): S70-S76.

[38] Hatton M, Nankivell M, Lyn E, et al. Induction chemotherapy and Continuous Hyperfractionated Accelerated Radiotherapy (CHART) for patients with locally advanced inoperable non-small-cell lung cancer: The MRC INCH randomized trial. International Journal of Radiation Oncology, Biology, Physics, 2011, 81 (3): 712-718.

[39] Baumann M, Herrmann T, Koch R, et al. Final results of the randomized phase III CHARTWEL-trial (ARO 97-1) comparing hyperfractionated-accelerated versus conventionally fractionated radiotherapy in non-small cell lung cancer (NSCLC). Radiotherapy and Oncology, 2011, 100 (1): 76-85.

[40] Rengan R, Rosenzweig KE, Venkatraman E, et al. Improved local control with higher doses of radiation in large-volume stage III non-small-cell lung cancer. International Journal of Radiation Oncology, Biology, Physics, 2004, 60 (3): 741-747.

[41] Bradley JD, Ieumwananonthachai N, Purdy JA, et al. Gross tumor volume, critical prognostic factor in patients treated with three-dimensional conformal radiation therapy for non-small-cell lung carcinoma. International Journal of Radiation Oncology, Biology, Physics, 2002, 52 (1): 49-57.

[42] Kong FM, Ten Haken RK, Schipper MJ, et al. High-dose radiation improved local tumor control and overall survival in patients with inoperable/unresectable non-small-cell lung cancer: Long-term results of a radiation dose escalation study. International Journal of Radiation Oncology, Biology, Physics, 2005, 63 (2): 324-333.

[43] Wang L, Correa CR, Zhao L, et al. The Effect of Radiation Dose and Chemotherapy on Overall Survival in 237 Patients With Stage III Non-Small-Cell Lung Cancer. International Journal of Radiation Oncology, Biology, Physics, 2009, 73 (5): 1383-1390.

[44] Socinski MA, Rosenman JG, Halle J, et al. Dose-escalating conformal thoracic radiation therapy with induction and concurrent carboplatin/paclitaxel in unresectable stage III A/B nonsmall cell lung carcinoma. Cancer, 2001, 92 (5): 1213-1223.

[45] Rosenman JG, Halle JS, Socinski MA, et al. High-dose conformal radiotherapy for treatment of stage III A/III B non-small-cell lung cancer: technical issues and results of a phase I/II trial. International Journal of Radiation Oncology, Biology, Physics, 2002, 54 (2): 348-356.

[46] Socinski MA, Morris DE, Halle JS, et al. Induction and concurrent chemotherapy with high-dose thoracic conformal radiation therapy in unresectable stage III A and III B non-small-cell lung cancer: A dose-escalation phase I trial. Journal of clinical oncology, 2004, 22 (21): 4341-4350.

[47] Lee CB, Stinchcombe TE, Moore DT, et al. Late complications of high-dose (≥66 Gy) thoracic conformal radiation therapy in combined modality trials in unresectable stage III non-small cell lung cancer. Journal of Thoracic Oncology, 2009, 4 (1): 74-79.

[48] Bradley JD, Moughan J, Graham MV, et al. A phase I/II radiation dose escalation study with concurrent chemotherapy for patients with inoperable stages I to III non-small-cell lung cancer: phase I results of RTOG 0117. International Journal of Radiation Oncology, Biolo-

gy, Physics, 2010, 77 (2): 367-372.

[49] Bradley JD, Bae K, Graham MV, et al. Primary analysis of the phase Ⅱ component of a phase Ⅰ/Ⅱ dose intensification study using three-dimensional conformal radiation therapy and concurrent chemotherapy for patients with inoperable non-small-cell lung cancer: RTOG 0117. Journal of Clinical Oncology, 2010, 28 (14): 2475-2480.

[50] Socinski MA, Blackstock AW, Bogart JA, et al. Randomized phase Ⅱ trial of induction chemotherapy followed by concurrent chemotherapy and dose-escalated thoracic conformal radiotherapy (74, Gy) in stage Ⅲ non-small-cell lung cancer: CALGB 30105. Journal of Clinical Oncology, 2008, 26 (15): 2457-2463.

[51] Bradley JD, Paulus R, Komaki R, et al. A randomized phase Ⅲ comparison of standard-dose (60 Gy) versus high-dose (74 Gy) conformal chemoradiotherapy +/- cetuximab for stage ⅢA/ⅢB non-small cell lung cancer: preliminary findings on radiation dose in RTOG 0617. 53rd annual meeting of the American Society of Radiation Oncology, 2011: 2-6.

[52] Partridge M, Ramos M, Sardaro A, et al. Dose escalation for non-small cell lung cancer: analysis and modelling of published literature. Radiotherapy and Oncology, 2011, 99 (1): 6-11.

[53] Machtay M, Bae K, Movsas B, et al. Higher biologically effective dose of radiotherapy is associated with improved outcomes for locally advanced non-small cell lung carcinoma treated with chemoradiation: An analysis of the radiation therapy oncology group. International Journal of Radiation Oncology, Biology, Physics, 2012, 82 (1): 425-434.

[54] Sonke J-J, Belderbos J. Adaptive radiotherapy for lung cancer. Seminars in radiation oncology. WB Saunders, 2010, 20 (2): 94-106.

[55] Kong F-MS, Frey KA, Quint LE, et al. A pilot study of [18F] fluorodeoxyglucose positron emission tomography scans during and after radiation-based therapy in patients with non-small-cell lung cancer. Journal of clinical oncology, 2007, 25 (21): 3116-3123.

[56] Feng M, Kong F-M, Gross M, et al. Using fluorodeoxyglucose positron emission tomography to assess tumor volume during radiotherapy for non-small-cell lung cancer and its potential impact on adaptive dose escalation and normal tissue sparing. International Journal of Radiation Oncology, Biology, Physics, 2009, 73 (4): 1228-1234.

[57] Klopp AH, Chang JY, Tucker SL, et al. Intrathoracic patterns of failure for non-small-cell lung cancer with positron-emission tomography/computed tomography-defined target delineation. International Journal of Radiation Oncology, Biology, Physics, 2007, 69 (5): 1409-1416.

[58] Bollineni VR, Wiegman EM, Pruim J, et al. Hypoxia imaging using positron emission tomography in non-small cell lung cancer: implications for radiotherapy. Cancer treatment reviews, 2012, 38 (8): 1027-1032.

第25章
分子靶向治疗与肺癌个体化放疗

Steven H. Lin, Ritsuko U. Komaki
Department of Radiation Oncology, The University of Texas MD Anderson Cancer Center, Houston, TX, USA

放疗技术的进步提高了治疗有效率

放疗技术的进步已经显著提高了治疗效果，传统放疗使用旧式技术，在正常组织剂量限制下，肿瘤得不到足够的根治剂量，因而不能获得满意的效果[1]。适形治疗如3D适形放疗、剂量调强放疗（IMRT）和质子放疗等，放射技术及实施方法的进步，实现了在给予更高剂量放射线的同时减少邻近组织的放射性照射损伤[2]。立体定向放射治疗（stereotactic body radiation therapy，SBRT）相对于传统分次放疗治疗早期肺癌更有效，这些技术的进步可以提高放疗治愈率。大量临床经验及前瞻性临床试验得到的数据显示，SBRT的局部控制率非常好（>95%），远处转移率与手术患者相似，为25%~30%[3-4]。一项纳入了行SBRT或肺叶切除术肺癌患者的Ⅲ期临床试验正在全世界范围内开展，以对比SBRT与手术治疗的临床有效率。在可手术的Ⅲ期N2非小细胞肺癌（NSCLC）患者中，术后辅助分次放疗相对其他旧技术可改善治疗后的复发率或死亡率，从而提高生存率[1]。然而，小细胞肺癌（SCLC）和局部进展期（Ⅱ~Ⅲ期临床或技术不可切除）NSCLC，放疗和化疗是主要治疗手段。这些疾病的病变程度往往不适用于SBRT，而是需要经过6~7周的传统分割放疗。复发以转移性为主时通常是肿瘤的主要死因，所以加强非转移性Ⅲ期N2肺癌的局部控制率可以提高总生存率。一项创新性研究RTOG 7301显示，相对于较低剂量放疗，较高剂量的放疗（60Gy）可改善局部控制率和总生存期。为了对抗肿瘤细胞的加速再分布以进一步改善上述结果，CHART（连续超分割加速放射治疗，每周连续7d，每天3次）在不联合化疗的情况下对比了传统分割放疗的效果[5]。虽然CHART可改善局部控制率和总生存期，但难以改变临床实践，因为在美国很难将CHART加入标准临床实践中。在肺癌治疗中将化疗与放疗联合可达到最大获益。20世纪80年代开展的多项随机临床试验表明，在传统分割放疗后行序贯化疗可以改善生存率[6]。另外，一些关键研究比较了序贯化疗与同步化疗，显示同步化疗的获益更大，但毒性也较高[7]。

突破放疗效果的瓶颈

虽然细胞毒性化疗同步联合放疗相对单纯放疗可提高放疗效果并改善总治疗效果，但至今没有进一步的突破。到目前为止，不同模式的同步放化疗之间差异并不大，无论是诱导化疗还是巩固化疗，彼此之间很少或者没有优势（有时甚至有害）[8-9]。改良的分割放疗联合化疗（CHART-WEL）与标准的放化疗方案的疗效相当，但代价是急性毒性增加[10]。剂量提升的Ⅰ、Ⅱ期临床试验使用先进的放疗实施方法，在改善局部控制率和生存期方面显示出很好的可行性和稳定性[11-13]。但是一项Ⅱ期随机临床试验对比了标准剂量（60Gy）和高剂量（74Gy）的同步放化疗，结果显示高剂量组的局部控制率和总生存期更差[14]。所以尽管放疗经历了多年的研究和进步，局部进展期肺癌的结果仍然较差，中位生存期为17~24个月，5年总生存率为15%~20%。据此表明，目前我们所采取的治疗手段治疗肺癌得到的结果止步不前，并且在改善疗效方面处于一个瓶颈期（图 25.1A）。为了提高治愈率，生物技术的创新必不可少，最终使得治愈率曲线左移（图 25.1B），其效应必须特异性地针对肿瘤，同时正常组织的反应非常小。这是因为肿瘤细胞存在基因缺陷，使他们对放射线共同作用的药物敏感。尽管可靠的数据来自单臂Ⅱ期试验，但将靶向药物同步联合当前的标准治疗，如放疗或放化疗，有希望提高放疗的效果。

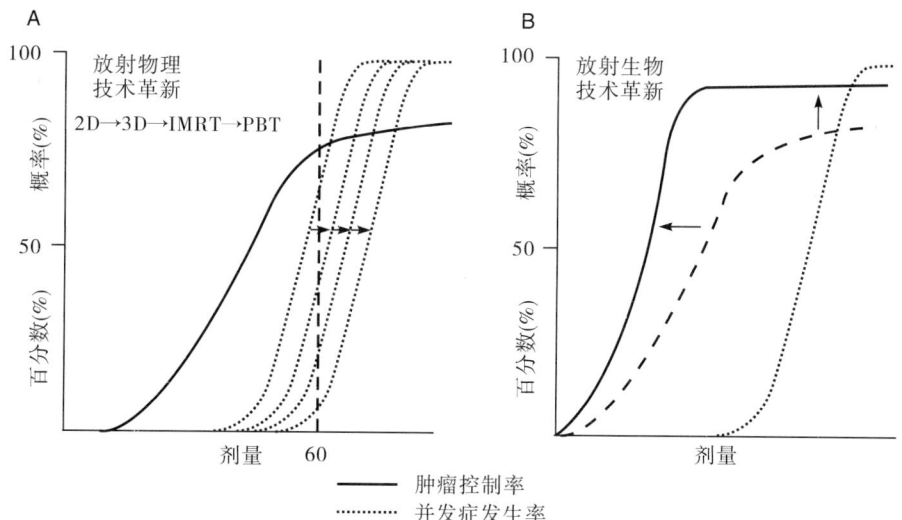

图 25.1 肺癌治疗结果的改善需要物理和生物技术的改进。该图代表治愈指数曲线，体现每一种成功的技术革新及其对应的理论上结果改善的提高程度。然而，虽然这些技术的毒性下降，但生物效应达到一个瓶颈期。为了改善疾病治疗结果，需要分子靶向药物联合放疗使得生物效应曲线左移

靶向治疗联合放疗：过去的成功与失败

细胞毒性化疗与放疗协同作用杀死肿瘤细胞，但这两种治疗选择性不强，正常组织的毒性反应也较严重，因此，多种治疗策略使用分子靶向治疗联合放疗来增强肿瘤细胞的放射效应。这些方法利用肿瘤或微环境的特性以达到放射线特异性靶向作用于肿瘤。过去已经开发了很多种方案，如靶向作用于乏氧肿瘤、肿瘤血管以及 EGFR 通路。

乏氧靶向治疗

多年来乏氧靶向治疗一直是肿瘤放射治疗中的经典方案。众所周知，乏氧会引起肿瘤细胞对放射线明显的抗拒[15]。因为肿瘤内血供增加，血管生成和抗血管生成平衡异常，所以在大多数肿瘤中都会观察到坏死及乏氧区域。临床前模型和临床实践中也发现乏氧会造成治愈率下降[16-17]。主要有两个方面的因素：第一，放疗发挥细胞毒性作用关键在于分子氧对 DNA 的化学固定作用；第二，细胞保护机制会诱导肿瘤对化疗和放疗产生抵抗，主要由该过程中关键转录因子 HIFI-α 介导，诱导许多乏氧诱导基因表达，从而提高了细胞在乏氧压力下的抵抗力[18]。临床制订了一些治疗策略用来对抗乏氧效应，例如使用生物活性药物[19]、乏氧细胞毒素如替拉扎明（Tirapazamine）[20]、或者 HIFI-α 拮抗剂[21]，但绝大多数尝试集中在头颈肿瘤放疗中，也没有可靠的结论[19]或在临床中得到成熟的应用[21]。在肺癌中仅有一项乏氧靶向治疗方案取得了一定的临床经验，即使用卡波金（carbogen）提高肿瘤的氧摄取率。卡波金由 95% 的 O_2 和 5% 的 CO_2 组成，在每次放疗前后各吸入 1 次，通过增加血氧浓度来加强肿瘤放射效应。临床前研究显示该方案可比较有效地提高肿瘤对放射线的反应，特别是在加入烟酰胺（维生素 B_3）后，后者可以通过微血管交换增强肿瘤灌注和再氧合[22]。但这项肺癌Ⅲ期 ARCON 临床试验（加速放疗联合高氧和烟酰胺）因为获益甚微被很快终止，没有证据显示 ARCON 优于传统放疗[23]。对比加速放疗，只有 cT2-4 喉鳞状细胞癌中的一项Ⅲ期 ARCON 试验的结果为阳性[24]。该试验共纳入 345 例患者，虽然局部控制率无差

异,在区域控制率上 ARCON 组明显更好(93% vs 86%,P=0.04);更重要的是,获益很大程度上受限于乏氧肿瘤而不是富氧肿瘤(100% vs 55%,P=0.01);两组的毒性相当。该试验使用加速放疗作为标准对照,所以卡波金/烟酰胺联合放化疗治疗头颈部肿瘤能否获益仍不清楚。由于当前标准治疗为同步放疗,卡波金的加入是否影响护理标准,尤其在肺癌治疗中是否会影响正常护理并不确定。

血管靶向治疗

氧化作用在放疗抗肿瘤效应中十分关键,肿瘤血流灌注会明显影响疗效。肿瘤内血管促生成因子和血管抑制因子的不正常表达导致了不正常且紊乱的血管结构[25]。目前,抗血管生成药物如贝伐珠单抗可以使肿瘤血管结构正常化,从而增加化疗药物的输送,提高肿瘤氧浓度。这种"血管结构正常化"同样增强了肿瘤对放射线的反应。影响这个效应的机制可能很多,但抗血管药物联合放疗对于肿瘤治疗是一项有前途的举措[26-27]。多种血管靶向药物已用于活体的临床前研究中,并证实了血管正常化效应,但当这些药物定时并按顺序同步联合放疗时,放疗增强效应并不是持续存在[26,28]。而后,在多种肿瘤中进行了大量的临床试验,包括胃肠道肿瘤、头颈肿瘤、直肠肿瘤、胰腺肿瘤等,在Ⅰ、Ⅱ期临床试验获得了肯定的结果,显示了一定的临床效果[29]。然而在多种药物的联合试验中观察到了胃肠道出血和穿孔事件发生率为6%~7%,这提示在使用任何抗血管生成药物联合试验中都必须小心监测这些事件。在 NSCLC 的一项Ⅲ期随机临床试验中,贝伐珠单抗联合卡铂/紫杉醇作为ⅢB~Ⅳ期 NSCLC 的一线治疗方案,同样发现部分患者出现致死性咯血,尤其是在中心型或鳞状细胞癌中,导致在此类患者中禁用上述方案[30]。此类药物联合放化疗现已得到更多的关注。一项局限期 SCLC 的Ⅱ期临床研究中将贝伐珠单抗联合放化疗,在纳入29例患者后因为2例患者出现气管食管瘘(tracheoesophageal fistula, TEF)和1例患者出现致死性消化道出血而终止。在一项独立的Ⅱ期临床试验中,贝伐珠单抗同步联合放化疗治疗局部进展期 NSCLC,在纳入5例患者后因2例患者出现进展的 TEF 而停止。最近,Socinski 及其同事报道了一项 NSCLC Ⅲ期临床试验,该试验将贝伐珠单抗和厄洛替尼联合同步化疗和高剂量放疗(74Gy),其中放疗选择2D放疗技术并行选择性淋巴结照射[31]。但其结果令人失望,不仅毒性较大(29%患者出现3级或4级食管炎,1例患者出现3级 TEF),而且生存率无改善。这项试验再次表明贝伐珠单抗联合放疗并不安全。鉴于上述报道提及的毒性反应,若要继续在 NSCLC 中开展此类药物联合同步放化疗的方案需要特别警惕,并需要更多的研究[32]。其他种类的血管靶向药物(如恩度,目前在中国用于联合放疗治疗局部晚期 NSCLC)是否有不同的毒性反应尚无定论。要想继续研究必须了解怎样去联合此类药物与放疗或放化疗才是最合理的。

EGFR 靶向治疗

EGFR 受体家族(ERBB 1~4)是一类重要的酪氨酸激酶生长因子受体(receptor tyrosine kinase, RTK),参与肿瘤的生长及存活,其在几乎全部头颈部肿瘤和大部分其他肿瘤包括 NSCLC 中过度表达。这些 RTKs 种类繁多,但在某一特定肿瘤中,某一类 RTK 往往要比其余种类更重要,例如头颈部肿瘤和 NSCLC 中的 ERBB1,乳腺癌和上消化道肿瘤中的 ERBB2/Her-2,这些受体可激活多个细胞内的信号通路,包括 RAS 和 PI3K 通路,从而刺激生长,提高 DNA 损伤修复和组织凋亡[33-34]。可与细胞外结构域结合,抑制受体活性的抗体(例如西妥昔单抗→ERBB1/EGFR,赫赛汀→ERBB2/Her2),以及可抑制激酶活性的 ATP 竞争性拮抗剂(例如厄洛替尼、拉帕替尼),当两者分别都有效时,RTKs 就是良好的药物靶点。而且,无论是 NSCLC 中 EGFR 突变后肿瘤基因依赖,还是基因扩增,靶向药物的特异性和有效性最终依赖于肿瘤对 RTKs 的依赖程度。EGFR 靶向治疗作为放疗增敏剂已被证实有效。其中最著名的例子是 Harari 等[36]和 Ang 等[37]在19世纪90年代在头颈部肿瘤细胞系中实施的一项联合西妥昔单抗与放射治疗的重要研究,这些临床前研究最终引出了一项关键临床试验。试验结果显示,相对于单纯放疗,在治疗头颈部肿瘤时西妥昔单抗联合到放疗能得到 10% 的 OS 获益[38]。不幸的是，在 RTOG 0522 试验中，放化疗与西妥昔单抗联合方案中，后者带来的获益可以忽略不计[39]。RTOG 0324 作为一项Ⅱ期临床试验，首次探索西妥昔单抗在与放化疗联合的地位。该研究的患者的中位生存期为 22.7 个月，2 年总生存率为 49.3%[40]。另一项Ⅱ期随机临床试验 RTOG 0617 评价了西妥昔单抗的获益，它采用 2×2 因子设计，随机将标准剂量（60Gy）或高剂量（74Gy）与加入（或不加入）西妥昔单抗配对，结果发现加入西妥昔单抗并不能获益（HR = 0.99；P = 0.4838）[41]。另外在西妥昔单抗组，2~5 级的毒性反应更多见。当肿瘤行 EGFR 表达染色时（H-评分），高 H-评分肿瘤相对于评分低者更能从西妥昔单抗治疗中获益（P = 0.02）[41]。另一种 EGFR 靶向治疗方案是小分子 EGFR 靶向 TKI。M. D. 安德森癌症中心开展了一项Ⅱ期临床试验，在Ⅲ期 NSCLC 中厄洛替尼联合放化疗，显示中位生存期为 34.1 个月，2 年生存率为 68%，未出现 4~5 级急性毒性反应[42]。但其局限性与 RTOG 0617 类似，上述试验是在非选择性患者中进行的，所以，EGFR 的标志物或许能帮助患者选择从哪种治疗方案中获益。虽然有一项Ⅲ期试验 RTOG 1306 仅仅是根据 NSCLC 患者中 *EGFR* 突变或 *EML4-ALK* 易位检测在 CRT 后决定行厄洛替尼或克里唑替尼治疗，目前尚无基于标志物的试验在 EGFR 靶向联合同步放化疗中开展。

肺癌新型靶向药物联合放疗指南

大多数传统治疗是将 NSCLC 作为一种疾病来治疗，最近几年依据肿瘤的病理机制逐渐采取不同的化疗方案，包括腺癌（培美曲塞）和鳞癌（吉西他滨）[43]。然而，通过对肺癌进行高通量基因测序发现，NSCLC 中存在基因异质性[44-45]。而且腺癌的基因改变与鳞癌差异显著[46]。事实上，NSCLC 不是单一的疾病而是有着不同基因谱的一系列疾病[46-47]。60% 的 NSCLC 有着致病性基因突变，并可用于靶向药物治疗，但仍然存在相当一部分肿瘤并没有确切或可用于靶向治疗的基因改变。*EGFR*、*ALK* 及 *ROS1* 基因变化提供了一个直接治疗的机会，但在其他更普遍的基因突变如 *TP53*、*LKB1*、*KRAS* 可否使用靶向治疗尚无结果。同样，在 SCLC 治疗中发现的靶点非常少。为了促进该领域的发展，特别是提高不可切除 NSCLC 和 SCLC 的治愈率，我们需要继续努力将分子靶向药物与放疗联合。如果一种药物可以同时选择性增强肿瘤化疗及放疗效果，将会极大地提高这些肿瘤的治愈率。但是临床试验要求系统进行，缺乏设计则无法提供证据。

最近许多综述总结了多种方案以筛选出靶向药物联合放疗的最佳方案。这些方案在引用中列出[48-50]。我们对这些方案进行了总结，思考如何最优化地联合分子靶向治疗与放疗。

能够联合放疗的潜在药物

在接受放疗时，许多信号通路参与放射保护机制，如修复过程或肿瘤激活通路中。理论上联合抑制这些通路的药物可以更好地杀伤肿瘤细胞。这在许多临床前研究中已经得到证实，总结如图（图 25.2A）。

DNA 损伤修复靶向药物

自从证实单链及双链 DNA（dsDNA）断裂是放射杀伤细胞的主要机制后，提高 DNA 损伤修复（DNA damage repair, DDR）是对抗放疗修复效应最直接的方法。DsDNA 断裂事件会影响细胞周期进程及 DNA 修复活动，并诱导进入复杂信号通路，DDR 通路蛋白便在其中[51]。利用敲除的方法从细胞中剔除这些蛋白可有效增强细胞对放射的灵敏度。由于这些蛋白许多都属于 PI3K 激酶家族，大量药物被开发用于抑制该通路，其中包括 PARP、ATM/ATR 和 DNA-PK 抑制剂。许多此类药物，尤其是 PARP 抑制剂，无论在体内及体外模型中与放疗联合，均显现出潜在细胞杀伤能力[52-53]。同时，许多此类药物正处于早期临床试验阶段。ABT-888 属于 Abbott 的 PARP 抑制剂，是此类药物中最早开发、最有效的药物，在临床试验中显示出可用于多个肿瘤包括 NSCLC 中行联合放化疗。最近的 SWOG Ⅰ、Ⅱ期临床试验（S1206）在不可切除的Ⅲ期 NSCLC 中应用了 ABT-888 联合放化疗，以检验其安全性及前期效

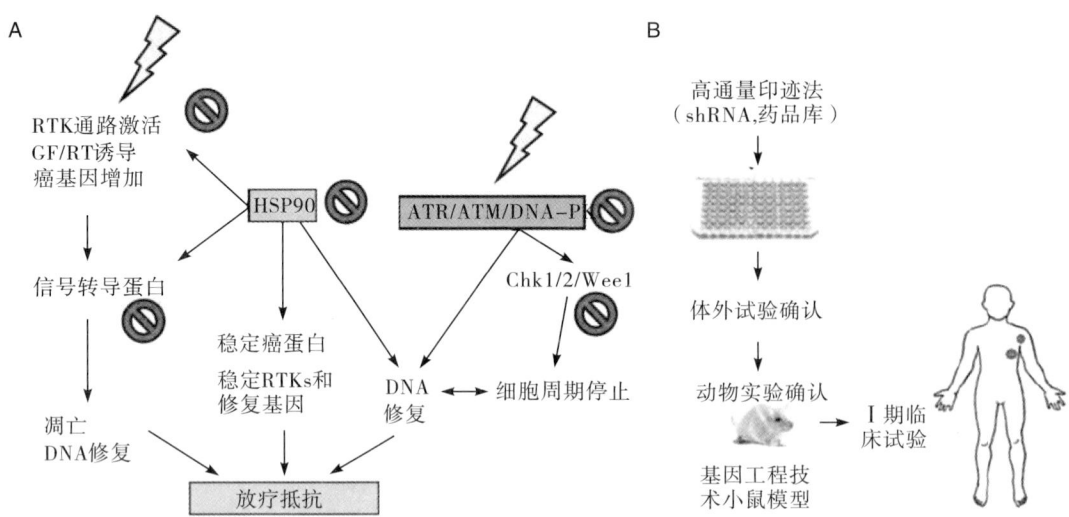

图 25.2 如何识别靶向药物并应用于临床试验。A. 基于信号通路的方案需要正确理解放疗 DDR 与细胞通路的相互作用，才能在临床试验中得到最优候选药物。这些通路展示了其中一个经临床证实的例子，他们与放疗的相互作用至关重要，其中带有红色斜线的圆圈代表了已知的抑制剂，可以提高放射线的灵敏度。B. 鉴别基因或药物对放疗的综合致死量的方法。体外试验探索和后续研究证实是临床试验的必要步骤。GEMM（Genetically Engineering Mouse Model）：基因驱动的小鼠模型

果。ATM 和 DNA-PK 抑制剂类药物均已开发，目前在小型早期临床试验中进行了评估。此类药物的临床应用潜力在特定的肿瘤亚型患者中效果最佳，其基因突变会增加药物联合放疗杀伤的敏感性。上述为一个联合杀伤的例子，而且许多临床试验揭示 PARP 抑制剂在 BRCA1 或 BRCA2 肿瘤中尤为有效，因为这类肿瘤同源重组修复功能有缺陷。

细胞周期检查点抑制剂

放射线引起的 DNA 损伤如果一直得不到修复，就会损害细胞。当一系列的信号转导事件影响到细胞周期及有丝分裂纺锤体蛋白时，细胞周期进程被阻止，而后修复开始。由 ATM/ATR 传向 Chk1/2 和磷酸酶或细胞周期依赖性激酶的信号可诱导细胞周期停止在 G1/S 和 G2/M 期。P53 是调节细胞周期的关键蛋白，通过诱导 WAF/D21 表达，直接抑制 Cyclin-CDK2，导致停留在 G1/S 期。其他蛋白由蛋白激酶如 Chk1/2 和 Wee1 介导激活，在 G2/M 转折点上形成阻碍，调节进入有丝分裂。有丝分裂的转折点一般由一系列的 polo 样激酶和 Aurora 激酶诱发。在细胞周期中，还存在另外一个关键点调节有丝分裂而影响细胞周期，在遭受应激如 DNA 损伤时，这些节点受到任何干扰均会导致细胞没有时间进行充分的 DDR 而进入细胞分裂，最终因分裂障碍导致细胞死亡。所以这些通路为肿瘤联合同步放疗提供了机会[56]。临床前研究已经揭示了这些药物联合放疗的效果，尤其是 TP53 缺陷的肿瘤。TP53 缺陷的细胞经历应激时无法进入 G1/S 间歇，因此 DNA 损伤修复依赖于 G2/M 期或有丝分裂阻滞。许多药物如 Chk1（AZD7762）、Wee1（MK1775）和 Aurora 激酶 A 抑制剂（MLN8237，VX-680），在 TP53 突变肿瘤中已被证实可选择性增强化疗和放疗的细胞毒性[56-57,59-61]。早期试验在进展期肿瘤中进行此类药物联合化疗的研究。然而，此类药物联合放疗才是临床发展中最令人期待的领域。

信号转导抑制剂

GF 受体或肿瘤基因通路激发引起信号转导级联反应，对于帮助癌细胞存活非常关键，包括增强修复和抵抗凋亡。这些抑制剂或许潜在作用于 RTKs 或 GCPRs 信号下游，发挥更广泛的抗肿瘤作用。在 I～Ⅲ期药物试验中，这些药物往往作为单一药物或联合化疗进行测试。前面提到一项厄洛替尼联合放化疗治疗不可切除Ⅲ期 NSCLC 的Ⅱ期试验已经完全结束，结果 2 年生存率为 66%。

其他如 PI3K、AKT、mTOR、MEK 的抑制剂正在临床前研究中，显示出一定的放疗增敏作用，为此类药物应用于临床提供了必要的证据。

表观遗传药物

甲基化或染色体集合引起异常表观遗传改变，进而造成异常基因表达，是肿瘤的一大特点。在血液恶性肿瘤中使用去甲基化药物具有一定的临床效果，但在实体肿瘤中获益有限。美国 FDA 批准了 HDAC 抑制剂如 Vorinostat 治疗复发皮肤 T-细胞淋巴瘤，并且在实体肿瘤中联合化疗进行了大量试验，获益良多。但遗憾的是，上述任何一个试验都没有成为治疗实体瘤的标准。临床前研究显示联合表观基因药物有一定的放疗增敏作用[62-64]，但其机制是通过 DNA 损伤和基因表达效应实现，缺乏特异性[65]。目前，虽然有多个姑息性盆腔肿瘤放疗联合伏利诺他治疗转移性胃肠道肿瘤的 I 期试验[66]和一项使用丙戊酸联合放疗治疗胶质母细胞瘤的 II 期试验（NCT00302159），但 HDAC 抑制剂联合放疗治疗肺癌的试验尚未进行。

HSP90 抑制剂

热休克蛋白（heat shock protein，HSP）是一大族类蛋白质，在蛋白质折叠和打开过程中扮演伴侣蛋白的功能。在细胞应激如热休克时，它们表达上调，帮助细胞在蛋白错误折叠所造成的细胞毒效应下存活下来。HSP90 是一类高保守的分子伴侣蛋白，帮助超过 200 种被称为"客户蛋白"的蛋白质成熟，其中许多是肿瘤蛋白，他们在肿瘤细胞中突变并维持癌变状态。因此靶向 HSP90 治疗是在肿瘤全身治疗中一个有潜力的位点[67]。许多报道显示此类药物有潜在的放疗增敏效应，能够增强凋亡及诱导有丝分裂障碍[68]。尽管这些药物有潜在的抗肿瘤效应，17-AAG 和 NVP-AUY922 两项临床试验分别因肝毒性和眼毒性而被终止。被寄予厚望的药物 SAT-9090 是二代 HSP90 抑制剂，在所有已进行的 I、II 期试验中显示出比 17-AAG 更小的眼毒性[69]。这些药物联合放疗的前景非常广阔。

免疫治疗

肿瘤能够存活的一个关键因素是肿瘤细胞可以逃避免疫系统，肿瘤微环境的免疫抑制性会抑制细胞杀伤 T 细胞正确杀伤肿瘤细胞[70]。有学者使用抗体结合关键免疫分子如 CTLA[71]或将激活的自体免疫细胞回输[72]，在进展期黑色素瘤和前列腺癌中分别显示出生存改善，并得到美国 FDA 批准使用。当前，其他检查点阻断抑制剂使用针对 PD-1、PDL1 和其他分子的单克隆抗体，正于多种进展期肿瘤包括 NSCLC 中进行早期试验。许多早期临床试验在大剂量治疗后，进展的 NSCLC 得到显著持续的反应，总反应率为 14%~28%[73-74]。这些治疗手段被期望能逐步应用于其他肿瘤，且因为治疗作用机制不同，免疫治疗联合其他治疗有望获得更长久的疗效[75]。随着越来越多已知和未知的基因正在被研究是否参与免疫调节，如何获得最佳联合治疗方式、提高肿瘤杀伤力并最小化治疗相关的致死性过敏反应和自身免疫反应，这些都需要更多的研究来解答。

众所周知，放射线诱导的细胞死亡同样依赖于 $CD8^+$ 细胞，如果去除动物体内 $CD8^+$ 细胞或将肿瘤细胞接种于免疫抑制的动物体内，放疗的作用会减弱[76]。放疗诱导的细胞毒性作用与免疫系统相互作用引起远隔效应，这是因为放疗损伤导致肿瘤裂解诱发全身免疫反应，从而表现出肿瘤细胞的系统性效应。放疗患者中已观察到远隔效应，但过去因该反应较弱且不可复制而存在争议[77]。现在，远隔效应在临床前研究中被证实是一个 CD8-T 细胞介导的过程，而且免疫治疗联合放疗可揭示这个效应[78]。最近，部分研究报道，该效应在患者接受免疫检查点阻滞或细胞因子治疗时可被重复实现[79-80]。因此，它有希望联合消融放疗增强 IV 期肿瘤治疗的效果，提高早期肿瘤接受 SBRT 或局部进展期肿瘤放疗后的治愈率。将来需要更多研究筛选出免疫治疗联合放疗的最佳方案。

将药物引入临床试验的思考

药物联合放疗的综合致死效应

越来越多的药物被开发用于治疗肿瘤，将它们联合放疗进行临床试验是一项巨大的挑战。如何决定某一类药物的适应证需要两个步骤。第一是设计合理的方案，这需要详细评估可能影响放疗效果的途径，包括对抗放射损伤效应的细胞保护机制，综合致死的基因易感性（如选择 BRCA1 或 BRCA2 突变 PARP 抑制剂），然后选择作用于这些途径的药物，其中部分步骤已在图 25.2A 中列出。不可否认，虽然部分药物存在放疗增敏现象，但其机制仍未明确。因此第二步是靶点识别，使用高通量筛选技术识别放疗敏感的关键基因，同时完成药物库的功能性筛选，以得到与放疗协同作用的新靶点和未知通路（图 25.2B），这两种方案均可选择药物用于临床试验。

临床优先开发的药物

在大量具有潜在放疗增敏作用的药物中，只有一小部分得以开发最终应用于临床，其中因素很多，如安全性、系统有效性、经济因素均会影响药物开发，因为后者难以预测，所以安全性将是一种药物应用于临床的重要因素。幸运的是，许多药物在多种肿瘤中已经进行了单药或联合其他多种细胞毒性药物的 I、II 期临床试验，来确定剂量、安全应用方法及系统活性。

关于肿瘤治疗易感靶点的临床前研究

由于目前对药物主要评价系统有效性，所以需要一些临床试验验证药物的放疗协同作用。首先，至少要在易感疾病（如肺癌、乳腺癌、胰腺癌）的细胞系水平得到证实，而克隆存活试验是获得此类证据的金标准[81]。体外培养试验得到的数据并不能充分反映肿瘤在一个完整器官内的生长，所以要有选择性的在恰当的肿瘤模型中进行试验，即便某一个模型优于其他所有模型，但仍不足以完全反映人类体内环境。因此，大多数指南要求药物联合放疗的试验至少在两种体外细胞系和至少一种动物模型中进行。

患者标志物的选择

只有患者体内存在特定的突变可以激活肿瘤基因通路，应用靶向治疗药物才会得到最佳效果。患者的选择最好基于标志物预测，使得患者从药物治疗中获益最大。同样的标准适用于选择联合放疗的药物。许多药物靶向作用于 RAS 的下游如 PI3K 和 MEK 抑制剂，或部分选择作用于 RAS 突变[82-83]。最近一项关于 KRAS 突变型肺癌应用 MEK 抑制剂的 II 期临床试验显示，多西他赛联合 AZD6244 组的患者无进展生存期优于单药多西他赛[84]。TP53 有助于预测细胞周期药物的有效性，如 Chk1、Wee1、Aurora 激酶 A 和 PLK1 抑制剂[85]。在同步联合放疗或序贯治疗中，若肿瘤存在 EGFR 突变或 EML4-ALK 易位，可用于决定患者接受厄洛替尼还是克里唑替尼。但是部分药物并没有可用于预测的生物标志物，因此在进行上述试验的同时，也要将寻找活检标本的标志物作为研究目的之一。开发可靠（或相关的）标志物预测临床反应，帮助患者从治疗中利益最大化，并可将后期的大型 III 期临床试验用于患者的选择和分组。

临床试验的设计

I 期试验必须确保这些药物联合放疗过程中的安全性。由于部分药物存在交叉毒性，例如黏膜炎、食管炎或肺炎，因此要着重检测每个位点的灵敏度，而在何种疾病中并不重要（如盆腔肿瘤、喉癌）。典型的剂量提升试验可用来研究常规治疗（放疗或放化疗）同步联合靶药物，以得到药物标准化的最大耐受量（maximum tolerated dose，MTD）。剂量限制毒性（DLT）的评估可以帮助限定 MTD。这需要一个合适的窗口评估急性或亚急性毒性，如放射治疗中的食管炎和治疗后的肺炎。大多数放疗试验规定在完成放疗 DLT 的评估后，自治疗起始后至少第 10 周作为第 1 个随访点，但这仅仅是一个预期因素，特别的毒性反应如气管食管瘘、肺炎和食管狭窄，可能只有在治疗的最后才发生。所以传统的 3+3 试验设计应用于此类试验时，必须采取评估措施如 TiT6 CRM，以确保试验进行过程中的有效性和安全性。

在可能治愈的患者中进行 I 期试验是一个伦理问题。由于此类药物联合放疗的试验未曾实施过，可能存在潜在的剂量限制毒性，不能给予可治愈患者同等剂量，所以此类研究的患者队列应慎重选择，必须充分权衡这些治疗可能带来的获益及风险。例如，药物联合放疗应针对那些最可能获益的患者，如患者携带某个突变并有相对应的抑制剂（如厄洛替尼→EGFR 突变，MEK 抑制剂→*KRAS* 突变），对这些患者使用研究中的药物是不可取的，所以要充分确认这些治疗可能带来的风险。但是，在靶向药物单独联合放疗的保守设定中，标准需纳入早期研究，但这并不像一个长期药物开发理想的设定，更像是在人体中临床验证药物联合放疗的综合效应，和评估联合后的毒性。这将为在治疗组开发药物提供早期数据。

经典的 3+3 Ⅰ期试验设计中，3~6 例患者常接受 1 个特定的剂量水平来观察放疗毒性。由于评价放疗毒性需要长期评估，直到毒性在一个特定药物剂量水平得到充分评估，试验剂量才会停止递增。

这种设计在病例数积累缓慢的单个机构研究中可能足够应付，但在积累快速的多中心研究中效果不明显，那么使用 Master template 法同步评估多种药物或许是更有效的设计方案。不同分组的患者应签署相应的知情同意书，这可总结为"ping-pang"或"flip-flop"试验类型[86]，即患者的分组要随着试验的进行而变化（图 25.3A）。如果超过 1 种药物分组需要完成，根据药物的种类，采用"rolling"法随机分配方式将患者纳入不同药物分组。这种设计可以同步持续积累患者，同时维持等同于"3+3"试验的安全性。

为了使药物联合放疗或放化疗的叠加毒性最小，Ⅱ期试验推荐剂量应依据指南执行，如单独药物试验，应遵循药物效应的最大剂量，例如肿瘤细胞激酶抑制剂试验中的蛋白磷酸化过程。这些过程，对于某些可以通过针吸活检获取组织的肿瘤来说易于达到，但由于完成放疗前、中、后期活检难度较大，所以在胸部肿瘤中执行困难。

一旦在感兴趣药物联合放疗试验中确定了其 MTD，在继续行安全性评估时，Ⅱ期试验可提供一些关于治疗有效性的证据（图 25.3B）。Ⅱ期试验常用无进展生存期作为首要评估点，总生存率作为次要评估点。由于单纯放疗或放化疗的临床反应率较高，肿瘤生长动力学不同，评估反应的最佳时间也不确定，而且原发疾病的炎症性改变难以区别，所以放疗试验中反应率不是一个有效的研究终点。除了无进展生存期，其他评估点包括 1 年局部控制率、图像反应特征（如 FDG-PET 反应）或病理反应（新辅助放疗后行手术切除）。由于组织学证据不容易获得，所以未来有关新放疗方式的Ⅱ期临床试验应作为随机对照试验进行。由于病理对照不能准确反映治疗反应，即便有好的

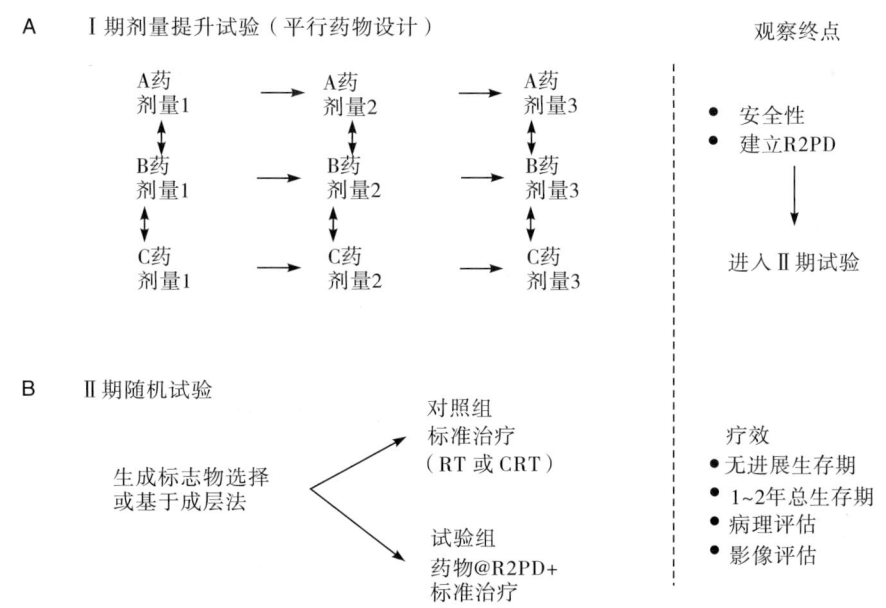

图 25.3 Ⅰ/Ⅱ期试验用来设计将靶向药物引入联合放疗的临床试验
A. Ⅰ期试验决定最大耐受剂量。某一特定药物联合放疗，经典的"3+3"剂量提升试验设计中，3 例患者在任意时间进入到某一种药物 X 组，同时与其他药物进行对比。这种平行药物试验设计采用的是"Master template"法。B. 在确定药物 X 的 MTD 之后，患者进入Ⅱ期试验。给予某一特定明确的标志物或基于相关标志物进行分层，然后随机分配对照组和试验组（药物 X+放疗）。评价标准主要包括无进展生存期、1~2 年生存率、病理或影像表现

染色方法和技术进步，病理对照也不能作为充分对照（传统的单臂Ⅱ期试验）。这种情况长久阻碍了一些Ⅱ期试验，这些试验在组织学上得到了很好的结果，但Ⅲ期试验中相对随机对照组结果却是阴性[87]。

靶向药物联合放疗临床发展的挑战与机遇

靶向药物联合放疗快速发展的主要挑战是要克服传统药物试验的实施方法，传统方案首先测试单一药物的安全性和治疗反应，然后在Ⅱ、Ⅲ期试验中联合成熟的细胞毒性化疗方案。此类做法也适用于Ⅳ期患者接受多线治疗失败后姑息治疗。虽然某些药物能够改善治疗效果，并最终通过 FDA 审核，但是肿瘤无病生存期或总生存期的微小改善会受到过长且复杂的试验干扰。药企及官方管理部门应意识到并调查治疗组中药物的潜力，如果这些药物作为单药或联合化疗显示出系统活性，并有放疗增敏证据，那么这些靶向药物联合放疗很有希望改善所有的疾病研究终点。由于靶向药物主要负责控制不可见的微小转移灶而不是影像可见病灶，所以患者的局部控制率得到改善并减少了远处转移复发。这样，对比同步标准治疗方案可得到更大的生存获益，并且用来区分生存差异所需的患者数也会减少。这还会产生经济效益，因为转移组中使用的许多药物往往不能获得同等的经济效益。假如有人提出将某药物由保守组提到治疗组，将会加速药物的开发和批准。使用替代终点评估如影像或病理反应或许也有助于药物尽快获得批准。

总 结

随着放疗技术的进步，药物联合放疗得到了越来越广泛的临床应用。高剂量放疗联合药物的叠加效应与毒性成正相关，但低剂量放疗不存在这种现象。由于药企在药物开发过程中投入了大量资金，大量不同作用和安全谱特性的药物有机会覆盖肿瘤细胞的每一条通路。抑制这些通路可与放疗损伤效应协同作用，并阻止交叉抵抗的发生。如果在局部进展期肺癌中给予某药物治疗，应努力寻找这些药物放疗增敏的临床前证据，并尽早投入到Ⅰ、Ⅱ期临床试验中，是改善疾病结局的关键。药企及管理部门应当关注这些药物带来的获益。通过这些努力，有希望改善局部进展期肺癌患者的生存期。

（安典政　黄　伟译，李宝生　审）

参考文献

[1] Liao ZX, Komaki RR, Thames Jr HD, et al. Influence of technologic advances on outcomes in patients with unresectable, locally advanced non-small-cell lung cancer receiving concomitant chemoradiotherapy. International Journal of Radiation Oncology Biology Physics, 2010, 76 (3): 775-781.

[2] Berman AT, Rengan R. New approaches to radiotherapy as definitive treatment for inoperable lung cancer. Seminars in Thoracic and Cardiovascular Surgery, 2008, 20 (3): 188-197.

[3] Onishi H, Shirato H, Nagata Y, et al. Hypofractionated stereotactic radiotherapy (HypoFXSRT) for stage I non-small cell lung can-cer: Updated results of 257 patients in a Japanese multi-institutional study. Journal of Thoracic Oncology, 2007, 2 (7 suppl, 3): S94-Sl00.

[4] Timmerman R, Paulus R, Galvin J, et al. Stereotactic body radiation therapy for inoperable early stage lung cancer. JAMA, 2010, 303 (11): 1070-1076.

[5] Saunders M, Dische S, Barrett A, et al. Continuous, hyperfractionated, accelerated radiotherapy (CHART) versus conventional radiotherapy in non-small cell lung cancer: Mature data from the randomized multicenter trial. Radiotherapy and Oncology, 1999, 52 (2): 137-148.

[6] DillmanRO, Seagren SL, Propert KJ, et al. A randomized trial of induction chemotherapy plus high-dose radiation versus radiation alone in Stage Ⅲ non-small-cell lung cancer. New England Journal of Medicine, 1900, 323 (14): 940-945.

[7] Curran Jr WJ, Paulus R, Langer CJ, et al. Sequential vs concurrent chemoradiation for stage Ⅲ non-small-cell lung cancer: Randomised phase Ⅲ trial RTOG 9410. Journal of the National Cancer Institute, 2011, 103 (19): 1452-1460.

[8] Vokes EE, Herndon Ii JE, Kelley MJ, et al. Induction chemotherapy followed by chemoradiotherapy compared with chemoradiotherapy alone for regionally advanced unre-

sectable stage Ⅲ non-small-cell lung cancer: Cancer and leukemia group B. Journal of Clinical Oncology, 2007, 25 (13): 1698-1704.

[9] Yamamoto S, Tsujino K, Ando M, et al. Is consolidation chemotherapy after concurrent chemoradiotherapy beneficial for locally advanced non-small cell lung cancer? A pooled analysis of the literature. J Clin Oncol, 2012, 30 (suppl: adstr7000).

[10] Baumann M, Herrmann T, Koch R, et al. Final results of the randomized phase Ⅲ CHARTWEL-trial (ARO 97-1) comparing hyperfractionated-accelerated versus conventionally fractionated radiotherapy in non-small cell lung cancer (NSCLC). Radiotherapy and Oncology, 2011, 100 (1): 76-85

[11] Belderbos JSA, De Jaeger K, Heemsbergen WD, et al. First results of a phase Ⅰ/Ⅱ dose escalation trial in non-small cell lung cancer using three-dimensional conformal radiotherapy. Radiotherapy and Oncology, 2003, 66 (2): 119-126.

[12] Kong FM, Ten Haken RK, Schipper MJ, et al. High-dose radiation improved local tumor control and overall survival in patients with inoperable/unresectable non-small-cell lung cancer: Long-term results of a radiation dose escalation study. International Journal of Radiation Oncology Biology Physics, 2005, 63 (2): 324-333.

[13] Bradley JD, Moughan J, Graham MV, et al. A phase Ⅰ/Ⅱ radiation dose escalation study with concurrent chemotherapy for patients with inoperable stages Ⅰ to Ⅲ non-small-cell lung cancer: Phase Ⅰ results of RTOG 0117. International Journal of Radiation Oncology Biology Physics, 2010, 77 (2): 367-372.

[14] Bradley J, Paulus R, Komaki R, et al. A randomized phase Ⅲ comparison of standard-dose (60 Gy) versus high-dose (74 Gy) conformal chemoradiotherapy +/- Cetuximab for Stage ⅢA/ⅢB non-small cell lung cancer: Preliminary findings on radiation dose in RTOG 0617. Proceedings of the American Society for Radiation Oncology Annual Meeting. 2011, PL 01.

[15] Vaupel P, Mayer A. Hypoxia in cancer: Significance and impact on clinical outcome. Cancer anf Metastasis Reviews, 2007, 26 (2): 225-239.

[16] Brizel DM, Sibley GS, Prosnitz LR, et al. Tumor hypoxia adversely affects the prognosis of carcinoma of the head and neck. International Journal of Radiation, Oncology, Biology Physics, 1997, 38 (2): 285-289.

[17] Nordsmark M, Overgaard M, Overgaard J. Pretreatment oxygenation predicts radiation response in advanced squamous cell carcinoma of the head and neck. Radiotherapy and Oncology, 1996, 41 (1): 31-39.

[18] Carmeliet P, Dor Y, Herber JM, et al. Role of HIF-1α in hypoxiamediated apoptosis, cell proliferation and tumor angiogenesis. Nature, 1998, 394 (6692): 485-490.

[19] Overgaard J, Hansen HS, Overgaard M, et al. A randomized double-blind phase Ⅲ study of nimorazole as a hypoxia radiosensitizer of primary radiotherapy in supraglottic larynx and pharynx carcinoma. Results of the Danish Head and Neck Cancer Study (DAHANCA) Protocol 5-85. Radiotherapy and Oncology, 1998, 46 (2): 135-146.

[20] Rischin D, Peters LJ, O'Sullivan B, et al. Tirapazamine, cisplatin, and radiation versus cisplatin and radiation for advanced squamous cell carcinoma of the head and neck (TROG 02.02, headstart): A phase Ⅲ trial of the trans-tasman radiation oncology group. Journal of Clinical Oncology, 2010, 28 (18): 2989-2995.

[21] Schwartz DL, Powis G, Thitai-Kumar A, et al. The selective hypoxia inducible factor-1 inhibitor PX-478 provides in vivo radiosensitization through tumor stromal effects. Molecular Cancer Therapeutics, 8 (4): 947-958.

[22] Chaplin DJ, Horsman MR, Trotter MJ. Effect of nicotinamide on the microregional heterogeneity of oxygen delivery within a murine tumor. Journal of the National Cancer Institute, 1990, 82 (8): 672-626.

[23] Bernier J, Denekamp J, Rojas A, et al. ARCON: Accelerated radiotherapy with carbogen and nicotinamide in non small cell lung cancer: A phase Ⅰ/Ⅱ study by the EORTC. Radiotherapy and Oncology, 1999, 52 (2): 149-156.

[24] Janssens GO, Rademakers SE, Terhaard CH, et al. Accelerated radiotherapy with carbogen and nicotinamide for laryngeal cancer: results of a phase Ⅲ randomized trial. Journal of Clinical Oncology, 2012, 30 (15): 1777-1783.

[25] Jain RK. Normalization of tumor vasculature: an emerging concept in antiangiogenic therapy. Science, 2005, 307 (5706): 58-62.

[26] Mauceri HJ, Hanna NN, Beckett MA, et al. Combined effects of angiostatin and ionizing radiation in antitumour therapy. Nature, 1998, 394 (6690): 287-291.

[27] Lee CG, Heijn M, Di T E, et al. Anti-Vascular endothelial growth factor treatment augments tumor radiation

response under normoxic or hypoxic conditions. Cancer Research, 2000, 60 (19): 5565-5570.

[28] Williams KJ, Telfer BA, Brave S, et al. ZD6474, a potent inhibitor of vascular endothelial growth factor signaling, combined with radiotherapy: schedule-dependent enhancement of antitumor activity. Clinical Cancer Research, 2004, 10 (24): 8587-8593.

[29] Ranpura V, Hapani S, Wu S. Treatment-related mortality with bevacizumab in cancer patients: a meta-analysis. JAMA, 2011, 305 (5): 487-494.

[30] Sandler A, Gray R, Perry MC, et al. Paclitaxel-carboplatin alone or with bevacizumab for non-small-cell lung cancer. New England Journal of Medicine, 2007, 355 (24): 2542-2550.

[31] Socinski MA, Stinchcombe TE, Moore DT, et al. Incorporating bevacizumab and erlotinib in the combined-modality treatment of stage III non-small-cell lung cancer: results of a phase I/II trial. Journal of Clinical Oncology, 2012, 30 (32): 3953-3959.

[32] Spigel DR, Hainsworth JD, Yardley DA, et al. Tracheoesophageal fistula formation in patients with lung cancer treated with chemoradiation and bevacizumab. Journal of Clinical Oncology, 2010, 28 (1): 43-48.

[33] Normanno N, De Luca A, Bianco C, et al. Epidermal growth factor receptor (EGFR) signaling in cancer. Gene, 2006, 366 (1): 2-16.

[34] Mendelsohn J, Baselga J. Epidermal growth factor receptor targeting in cancer. Seminars in oncology, 2006, 33 (4): 369-385.

[35] Ciardiello F, Tortora G. Drug therapy: EGFR antagonists in cancer treatment. New England Journal of Medicine, 2008, 358 (11): 1160-1174, 1096.

[36] Harari PM, Huang SM. Head and neck cancer as a clinical model for molecular targeting of therapy: combining EGFR blockade Physics, 2001, 49 (2): 427-433.

[37] Milas L, Mason K, Hunter N, et al. In vivo enhancement of tumor radioresponse by C225 antiepidermal growth factor receptor antibody. Clinical Cancer Research, 2000, 6 (2): 701-708.

[38] Bonner JA, Harari PM, Giralt J, et al. Radiotherapy plus cetuximab for locoregionally advanced head and neck cancer: 5-year survival data from a phase 3 randomised trial, and relation between cetuximab-induced rash and survival. The Lancet Oncology, 2010, 11 (1): 21-28.

[39] Numico G, Franco P, Cristofano A, et al. Is the combination of Cetuximab with chemo-radiotherapy regimens worthwhile in the treatment of locally advanced head and neck cancer? A review of current evidence. Critical Reviews in Oncology/Hematology, 2013, 85 (2): 112-120.

[40] Blumenschein Jr GR, Paulus R, Curran WJ, et al. Phase II study of cetuximab in combination with chemoradiation in patients with stage IIIA/B non-small-cell lung cancer: RTOG 0324. Journal of Clinical Oncology, 2011, 29 (17): 2312-2318.

[41] Bradley J, Masters G, Hu C, et al. An intergroup randomized phase III comparison of standard-dose (60 Gy) versus high-dose (74 Gy) chemoradiotherapy (CRT) +/- cetuximab (cetux) for stage III non-small cell lung cancer (NSCLC): Results on cetux from RTOG 0617. Journal of Thoracic Oncology, 2013, 8 (2).

[42] Komaki R, Allen PK, Wei X, et al. Value of adding erlotinib to thoracic radiation therapy with chemotherapy for stage III non-small cell lung cancer: a prospective Phase II study. Journal of Thoracic Oncology, 2013, 8 (2).

[43] Scagliotti GV, Parikh P, Von Pawel J, et al. Phase III study comparing cisplatin plus gemcitabine with cisplatin plus pemetrexed in chemotherapy-naive patients with advanced-stage non-small-cell lung cancer. Journal of Clinical Oncology, 2008, 26 (21): 3543-3551.

[44] Lee W, Jiang Z, Liu J, et al. The mutation spectrum revealed by paired genome sequences from a lung cancer patient. Nature, 2010, 465 (7297): 473-477.

[45] Gerlinger M, Rowan AJ, Horswell S, et al. Intra-tumor heterogeneity and branched evolution revealed by multiregion sequencing. New England Journal of Medicine, 2012, 366 (10): 883-892.

[46] Weir BA, Woo MS, Getz G, et al. Characterizing the cancer genome in lung adenocarcinoma. Nature, 2007, 450 (7171): 883-892.

[47] Govindan R, Ding L, Griffith M, et al. Genomic landscape of non-small cell lung cancer in smokers and never-smokers. Cell, 2012, 150 (6): 1121-1134.

[48] Harrington KJ, Billingham LJ, Brunner TB, et al. Guidelines for preclinical and early phase clinical assessment of novel radiosensitisers. British Journal of Cancer, 2011, 105 (5): 628-639.

[49] Lawrence YR, Vikram B, Dignam JJ, et al. NCI-RTOG Translational Program Strategic Guidelines for the Early-Stage Development of Radiosensitizers. Journal of the National Cancer Institute, 2013, 105 (1): 11-24.

[50] Lin SH, George T, Ben-Josef E, et al. Opportunities

and challenges in the era of molecularly targeted agents and radiation therapy. Journal of the National Cancer Institute. In press, 2013.

[51] Hall EJ (ed). Radiobiology for the Radiologist, 7th edn. Lippincott/Williams & Wilkins, 2012.

[52] Veuger SJ, Curtin NJ, Richardson CJ, et al. Radiosensitization and DNA repair inhibition by the combined use of novel inhibitors of DNA-dependent protein kinase and poly (ADP-ribose) polymerase-1. Cancer Research, 2003, 63 (18): 6008-6015.

[53] Donawho CK, Luo Y, Penning TD, et al. ABT-888, an orally active poly (ADP-ribose) polymerase inhibitor that potentiates DNA-damaging agents in preclinical tumor models. Clinical Cancer Research, 2007, 13 (9): 2728-2737.

[54] Farmer H, McCabe N, Lord CJ, et al. Targeting the DNA repair defect in BRCA mutant cells as a therapeutic strategy. Nature, 2005, 434 (7035): 917-921.

[55] Fong PC, Boss DS, Yap TA, et al. Inhibition of poly (ADP-ribose) polymerase in tumors from BRCA mutation carriers. New England Journal of Medicine, 2009, 361 (2): 123-134.

[56] Luo Y, Leverson JD. New opportunities in chemosensitization and radiosensitization: modulating the DNA-damage response. Expert Review of Anticancer Therapy, 2005, 5 (2): 333-342.

[57] Bridges KA, Hirai H, Buser CA, et al. MK-1775, a novel Wee1 kinase inhibitor, radiosensitizes p53-defective human tumor cells. Clinical Cancer Research, 2011, 17 (17): 5638-5648.

[58] Li J, Wang Y, Sun Y, et al. Wild-type TP53 inhibits G2-phase checkpoint abrogation and radiosensitization induced by PD0166285, a WEE1 kinase inhibitor. Radiation Research, 2002, 157 (3): 322-330.

[59] Chen Z, Xiao Z, Gu WZ, et al. Selective Chk1 inhibitors differentially sensitize p53-deficient cancer cells to cancer therapeutics. International Journal of Cancer, 2006, 119 (12): 2784-2794.

[60] Moretti L, Niermann K, Schleicher S, et al. MLN8054, a small molecule inhibitor of aurora kinase A, sensitizes androgen-resistant prostate cancer to radiation. International Journal of Radiation Oncology Biology Physics, 2011, 80 (4): 1189-1197.

[61] Wan XB, Fan XJ, Chen MY, et al. Inhibition of Aurora—A results in increased cell death in 3-dimensional culture microenvironment, reduced migration and is associated with enhanced radiosensitivity in human nasopharyngeal carcinoma. Cancer Biology and Therapy, 2009, 8 (15).

[62] Zhang F, Zhang T, Teng ZH, et al. Sensitization to γ-irradiation-induced cell cycle arrest and apoptosis by the histone deacetylase inhibitor trichostatin A in non-small cell lung cancer (NSCLC) cells. Cancer Biology and Therapy, 2009, 8 (9): 823-831.

[63] Zhang Y, Jung M, Dritschilo A, et al. Enhancement of radiation sensitivity of human squamous carcinoma cells by histone deacetylase inhibitors. Radiation Research, 2004, 161 (6): 667-674.

[64] Brieger J, Mann SA, Pongsapich W, et al. Pharmacological genome demethylation increases radiosensitivity of head and neck squamous carcinoma cells. International Journal of Molecular Medicine, 2012, 29 (3): 505-509.

[65] Zhu WG, Hileman T, Ke Y, et al. 5-Aza-2'-deoxycytidine activates the p53/p21Waf1/Cip1 pathway to inhibit cell proliferation. Journal of Biological Chemistry, 2004, 279 (15): 15161-15166.

[66] Ree AH, Dueland S, Folkvord S, et al. Vorinostat, a histone deacetylase inhibitor, combined with pelvic palliative radiotherapy for gastrointestinal carcinoma: the Pelvic Radiation and Vorinostat (PRAVO) phase 1 study. The Lancet Oncology, 2010, 11 (5): 459-464.

[67] Isaacs JS, Xu W, Neckers L. Heat shock protein 90 as a molecular target for cancer therapeutics. Cancer Cell, 2003, 3 (3): 213-217.

[68] Camphausen K, Tofilon PJ. Inhibition of Hsp90: a multitarget approach to radiosensitization. Clinical Cancer Research, 2007, 13 (15): 4326-4330.

[69] Ying W, Du Z, Sun L, et al. Ganetespib, a unique triazolone-containing Hsp90 inhibitor, exhibits potent antitumor activity and a superior safety profile for cancer therapy. Molecular Cancer Therapeutics, 2012, 11 (2): 475-484.

[70] PardollDM. Immunology beats cancer: a blueprint for successful translation. Nature Immunology, 2012, 13 (12): 1129-1132.

[71] Hodi FS, O'Day SJ, McDermott DF, et al. Improved survival with ipilimumab in patients with metastatic melanoma. New England Journal of Medicine, 2010, 363 (8): 711-723.

[72] Kantoff PW, Higano CS, Shore ND, et al. Sipuleucel-T immunotherapy for castration-resistant prostate cancer.

[73] Topalian SL, Hodi FS, Brahmer JR, et al. Safety, activity, and immune correlates of anti-PD-1 antibody in cancer. New England Journal of Medicine, 2012, 366 (26): 2443-2454.

[74] Brahmer JR, Tykodi SS, Chow LQM, et al. Safety and activity of anti-PD-L1 antibody in patients with advanced cancer. New England Journal of Medicine, 2012, 366 (26): 2455-2465.

[75] Wolchok JD, Kluger H, Callahan MK, et al. Nivolumab plus ipilimumab in advanced melanoma. New England Journal of Medicine, 2013, 369 (2): 122-133.

[76] Lee Y, Auh SL, Wang Y, et al. Therapeutic effects of ablative radiation on local tumor require CD8 + T cells: changing strategies for cancer treatment. Blood, 2009, 114: 589-595.

[77] Kaminski J M, Shinohara E, Summers J B, et al. The controversial abscopal effect. Cancer treatment reviews, 2005, 31 (3): 159-172.

[78] Demaria S, Ng B, Devitt M L, et al. Ionizing radiation inhibition of distant untreated tumors (abscopal effect) is immune mediated. International Journal of Radiation Oncology Biology Physics, 2004, 58 (3): 862-870.

[79] Postow MA, Callahan MK, Barker CA, et al. Immunologic correlates of the abscopal effect in a patient with melanoma. New England Journal of Medicine, 2012, 366 (10): 925-931.

[80] Seung SK, Curti BD, Crittenden M, et al. Phase 1 study of stereotactic body radiotherapy and interleukin-2—tumor and immunological responses. Science translational medicine, 2012, 4 (137).

[81] Franken NAP, Rodermond HM, Stap J, et al. Clonogenic assay of cells in vitro. Nature Protocols, 2006, 1 (5): 2315-2319.

[82] Wee S, Jagani Z, Xiang KX, et al. PI3K pathway activation mediates resistance to MEK inhibitors in KRAS mutant cancers. Cancer Research, 2009, 69 (10): 4286-4293.

[83] Williams TM, Flecha AR, Keller P, et al. Cotargeting MAPK and PI3K signaling with concurrent radiotherapy as a strategy for the treatment of pancreatic cancer. Molecular Cancer Therapeutics, 2012, 11 (5): 1193-1202.

[84] Jänne PA, Shaw AT, Pereira JR, et al. Selumetinib plus docetaxel for KRAS-mutant advanced non-small-cell lung cancer: a randomised, multicentre, placebo-controlled, phase 2 study. Lancet Oncology, 2013, 14 (1): 38-47.

[85] Sur S, Pagliarini R, Bunz F, et al. A panel of isogenic human cancer cells suggests a therapeutic approach for cancers with inactivated p53. Proceedings of the National Academy of Sciences, 2009, 106 (10): 3964-3969.

[86] Choy H, Jain AK, Moughan J, et al. RTOG 0017: a phase I trial of concurrent gemcitabine/carboplatin or gemcitabine/paclitaxel and radiation therapy ("ping-pong trial") followed by adjuvant chemotherapy for patients with favorable prognosis inoperable stage ⅢA/B non-small cell lung cancer. Journal of Thoracic Oncology, 2009, 4 (1): 80-86.

[87] Hanna N, Neubauer M, Yiannoutsos C, et al. Phase Ⅲ study of cisplatin, etoposide, and concurrent chest radiation with or without consolidation docetaxel in patients with inoperable stage Ⅲ non-small-cell lung cancer: The Hoosier Oncology Group and US Oncology. Journal of Clinical Oncology, 2008, 26 (35): 5755-5760.

[88] Pazdur R. Endpoints for assessing drug activity in clinical trials. Oncologist, 2008, 13 (2): 19-21.

第26章
EGFR 酪氨酸激酶抑制剂与单克隆抗体：相关临床试验回顾

Kathryn F. Mileham[1], Edward S. Kim[1], William N. William Jr[2]

1. Solid Tumor Oncology, Levine Cancer Institute, Carolinas HealthCare System, Charlotte, NC, USA
2. Department of Thoracic/Head and Neck Medical Oncology, The University of Texas MD Anderson Cancer Center, Houston, TX, USA

背 景

1962 年，Stanley Cohen 在切牙和眼睑迅速生长的新生小鼠中分离出了一种新型蛋白[1]。由于发现了此类我们现在称之为表皮生长因子（EGF）的蛋白，Cohen 于 1986 年被授予诺贝尔奖。此后，EGF 及其家族相关受体在癌症发生发展中的作用日益显著，以 EGF 信号通路为靶点的药物目前正广泛应用于临床。

目前广泛应用于非小细胞肺癌（NSCLC）患者的表皮生长因子受体（EGFR）拮抗药物主要有两种：酪氨酸激酶抑制剂（tyrosine kinase inhibitors，TKIs）及单克隆抗体（monoclonal antibodies，mAbs）。并且，以吉非替尼、厄洛替尼为代表的酪氨酸激酶抑制剂已被批准用于晚期 NSCLC。

在该章节中，我们将回顾多项 EGFR 靶向药物治疗复发或转移性 NSCLC 的临床试验，这些临床试验分别评价了 EGFR 靶向药物作为一线治疗（联合化疗、化疗后序贯治疗或单药治疗）、维持治疗、挽救治疗以及 EGFR 轴的一些新药物在 NSCLC 中的作用。

一线治疗：抗 EGFR 治疗联合化疗在分子非选择性 NSCLC 患者中的作用

两项大型多中心、随机对照试验评价了厄洛替尼联合铂类一线治疗晚期 NSCLC 的有效性。

在 TRIBUTE Ⅲ 期临床试验中，受试的晚期 NSCLC 患者被随机分为两组，试验组给予150mg/d 剂量的厄洛替尼，对照组服用安慰剂，两组均联用最多 6 个周期的卡铂 - 紫杉醇化疗，随后继续服用厄洛替尼或安慰剂[2]。所有 1 059 例患者中，两组的中位总生存期（主要终点）、客观缓解率及进展时间（次级终点）均无统计学差异［中位总生存期：厄洛替尼组 10.6 个月 *vs* 对照组 10.5 个月；HR = 0.99；95% CI（0.86，1.16）；P = 0.95］。然而，由于 EGFR-TKIs 在非吸烟肺癌患者中相关数据的发布，TRIBUTE 试验在破盲前调整了统计计划，并依据吸烟史观察患者总生存期的差异。结果显示，厄洛替尼治疗的不吸烟患者的中位生存期显著延长（22.5 个月 *vs* 10.1 个月），且该差异与肿瘤组织学无关。

TALENT 是另一项多中心随机对照双盲Ⅲ期临床试验，评价了厄洛替尼（150mg/d）联合 6 个周期顺铂 - 吉西他滨方案化疗序贯厄洛替尼维持治疗作为晚期 NSCLC 一线治疗的有效性和安全性[3]。值得注意的是，出现疾病进展的患者仍能继续接受研究治疗（厄洛替尼或安慰剂）联合或不联合二线治疗，或只接受二线治疗。两组间总生存期（主要终点）、疾病进展时间、有效率、反应持续时间、生活质量（次级终点）均无显著差异。厄洛替尼组与安慰剂组的中位总生存期分别为 43 周和 44.1 周（HR = 1.06）。一项 TALENT 研究中非吸烟患者的回顾性研究（N = 18）显示其总生存期及无进展生存期显著延长，与 TRIBUTE 试验结果吻合。

多项Ⅲ期临床试验亦未能证实吉非替尼联合铂类化疗能带来临床获益，这也与厄洛替尼联合铂类化疗在 TRIBUTE 和 TALENT 试验中的结果一致[4-5]。在 INTACT-1 与 INTACT-2 这两项国际间、双盲、随机对照试验中，超过 2 100 例既往未接受过化疗的患者被随机分组，分别接受顺铂-吉西他滨（INTACT-1）或卡铂-紫杉醇（INTACT-2）联合 250mg/d 或 500mg/d 剂量的吉非替尼或安慰剂。在 INTACT-1 中的无进展生存期分别为 5.8 个月 vs 5.5 个月 vs 6.0 个月（$P=0.76$）；而 INTACT-2 中无进展生存期则分别为 5.3 个月 vs 4.6 个月 vs 5.0 个月（$P=0.06$）。两项研究均未显示总有效率和中位生存期有所提高。

总之，TRIBUTE、TALENT、INTACT-1 及 INTACT-2 试验显示，在未经选择的患者中，厄洛替尼或吉非替尼联合化疗不能带来临床获益，该治疗模式不推荐作为晚期 NSCLC 的一线治疗。

西妥昔单抗是一种阻断 EGFR 信号通路的嵌合型单克隆 IgG1 抗体。有两项Ⅲ期临床试验研究了西妥昔单抗联合铂类化疗在晚期 NSCLC 中的治疗作用。

FLEX 是在表达 EGFR 的晚期 NSCLC 患者中进行的一项跨国、多中心、开放性的Ⅲ期临床试验，该研究评估了顺铂-长春瑞滨联合西妥昔单抗或单用顺铂-长春瑞滨化疗作为一线治疗的疗效[6]。患者首先接受最多 6 个周期的化疗，随后给予西妥昔单抗（每周 1 次）序贯治疗直至疾病进展或发生不可耐受的毒副反应。对 112 例随机患者的意向-治疗分析显示，顺铂-长春瑞滨联合西妥昔单抗治疗组的中位总生存期（主要终点）优于单纯化疗组[11.3 个月 vs 10.1 个月；HR = 0.871；95% CI（0.762，0.996）；$P=0.044$]。

BMS099 是另一项纳入 676 例晚期 NSCLC 患者的多中心、开放性随机对照Ⅲ期临床试验，该试验不限制患者的病理类型及 EGFR 表达或突变状态，评估了紫杉烷类-卡铂联合西妥昔单抗或单用紫杉烷类-卡铂化疗一线治疗的疗效[7]。化疗方案中使用紫杉醇或多西他赛由研究者依据情况自行决定。与 FLEX 类似，化疗最多应用 6 个周期，序贯每周 1 次的西妥昔单抗，直至出现疾病进展或发生不可耐受的毒副反应。紫杉烷类-卡铂联合西妥昔单抗组的客观缓解率有显著提高（25.7% vs 17.2%；$P=0.007$）；但该指标只是次级终点。由独立放射学审查委员会（independent radiologic review committee，IRRC）观测的结果显示：主要终点-无进展生存期并未因联用西妥昔单抗而不同。IRRC 观测化疗联用西妥昔单抗的中位无进展生存期为 4.40 个月，而单独化疗组为 4.24 个月[HR = 0.902；95% CI（0.761，1.069）；$P=0.236$]。西妥昔单抗组的中位总生存期有所提高，但未达到统计学显著差异[9.69 个月 vs 8.39 个月；HR = 0.890；95% CI（0.754，1.051）；$P=0.169$]。值得注意的是，该结果与 FLEX 临床试验中总生存期的提高相类似。

尽管 BMS099 试验未达到无进展生存期的观察终点，但 BMS099 与 FLEX 有相类似的结果。它们均显示化疗联合西妥昔单抗能显著提高客观缓解率，且能带来 1.3 个月的中位总生存期的延长（尽管 BMS099 试验的结果统计学差异不显著）。这些结果与 EGFR-TKIs 联合化疗的结果有显著差异，可能是由单克隆抗体的作用机制不同导致。尽管在 FLEX 临床试验中获得阳性结果，但西妥昔单抗尚未获批应用于 NSCLC 的治疗。

两种单克隆抗体（拮抗 VEGF 的贝伐单抗与拮抗 EGFR 的西妥昔单抗）的联用，在临床试验 SWOG0536 中显示出了良好疗效[8]。在这项评估有效性及安全性的单臂Ⅱ期临床试验中，大约 100 例晚期 NSCLC 患者接受了卡铂、紫杉醇、贝伐单抗及西妥昔单抗作为一线治疗。患者首先接受至多 6 个周期的化疗，续以贝伐单抗及西妥昔单抗直至疾病进展。该研究顺利达到了可行性观察终点，次级观察终点包括客观缓解率、无进展生存期、总生存期及毒副作用。客观缓解率为 53%，无进展生存期为 7 个月，总生存期为 14 个月。在这些结果基础上，一项大型Ⅲ期临床试验 SWOG 0819 正在进行，该试验将在晚期 NSCLC 患者中评估卡铂-紫杉醇+贝伐单抗联合西妥昔单抗的疗效。

一线治疗：化疗间插抗 EGFR 治疗

由于临床前数据显示酪氨酸激酶抑制剂诱导的细胞周期阻滞可能与化疗的周期特异性抗肿瘤

作用产生拮抗作用[9-11]，因此化疗与 EGFR-TKI 的序贯给药被作为另一种一线治疗模式在多项临床试验中进行了测试。

FAST-ACT 是一项评估该治疗模式的 II 期随机临床试验[12]。该研究中的 154 例患者在第 1 天和第 8 天接受吉西他滨 - 铂类化疗后，在第 15~28 天接受 150mg/d 的厄洛替尼或安慰剂（每 4 周 1 次）。治疗有效的患者继续接受厄洛替尼或安慰剂直至出现疾病进展或不可耐受的毒副作用。主要终点是在治疗第 8 周的无进展率（包括完全缓解 + 部分缓解 + 稳定患者，RECIST 标准）。厄洛替尼组第 8 周的无进展率为 80.3%，安慰剂组为 76.9%。因为联用厄洛替尼显著延长了无进展生存期(29.4 周 vs 23.4 周；校正 HR = 0.47；$P = 0.000\ 2$)，所以开展了一项评估化疗后序贯应用厄洛替尼的名为 FAST-ACT II 的 III 期随机对照临床试验。这项纳入 451 例患者的双盲、随机对照临床试验显示，厄洛替尼能显著延长无进展生存期（主要终点），厄洛替尼组和安慰剂组的中位无进展生存期分别为 7.6 个月与 6.0 个月 [HR = 0.57；95% CI (0.46, 0.70)；$P < 0.000\ 1$][13]。厄洛替尼组的客观缓解率也较安慰剂组显著提高 (42.9% vs 17.8%；$P < 0.000\ 1$)。总生存期是该研究的另一个次级终点，但安慰剂与二线厄洛替尼间的交叉作用为较大混杂因素。对 283 例患者的生物标记物分析显示，EGFR 突变阳性患者表现出对一线化疗间插厄洛替尼最优的无进展生存期获益[14]。

另一项临床试验并未获得关于化疗间插厄洛替尼治疗的有利结果[15]。在该项纳入 143 例患者的随机对照 II 期临床试验中，其中一组接受 150mg/d 的厄洛替尼，另一组接受 4 个周期（21d 为一个周期）卡铂 - 紫杉醇方案化疗间插 150mg/d 的厄洛替尼（第 2~15 天），并在 4 个周期的化疗 - 厄洛替尼治疗结束后继续应用厄洛替尼直至疾病进展。化疗联合厄洛替尼组的 6 个月无进展生存率（主要终点）为 26%，而单用厄洛替尼组为 31%。中位无进展生存期分别为 4.57 个月与 2.69 个月。所以，这项规模较小的 II 期临床试验结果并不支持化疗间插 EGFR-TKIs 治疗方案。

一线治疗：抗 EGFR 单药治疗

由于 TKIs 单药治疗在二线及三线治疗中获得了令人鼓舞的结果，因此一些 II 期临床试验开始评价 TKIs 一线治疗晚期 NSCLC 的有效性。在未行分子选择的患者中的相关研究结果均不令人满意[16-17]。但是，当基于 EGFR 突变状态来评估疗效时，EGFR 突变患者则能达到更好的临床效果[17-20]。另一些 II 期临床试验观察了一般情况差的患者单药 TKIs 一线治疗的疗效，但这些肺癌患者也未进行 EGFR 突变状态选择。在这些研究中，治疗有效率均较低，且无进展生存期和中位总生存期未获得显著延长[21-22]。

III 期临床试验 TOPICAL[23]纳入了 670 例未行且不适合化疗的患者（一般情况差或有严重并发症），并随机分别接受厄洛替尼或安慰剂。两组的中位总生存期（主要终点）无显著差异 [厄洛替尼组与安慰剂组分别为 3.7 个月与 3.6 个月；HR = 0.94；95% CI (0.81, 1.10)；$P = 0.46$]。

这些 II 期及 III 期临床试验表明，并无证据支持在未经选择的不适用化疗的肺癌患者中首选 EGFR-TKIs 治疗。

也有一些研究评估了在未经选择的老年肺癌患者中一线应用单药表皮生长因子受体酪氨酸激酶抑制剂（EGFR-TKIs）的有效性。一项开放、多中心 II 期临床试验评估了 70 岁以上未经化疗的晚期 NSCLC 患者中厄洛替尼（150mg/d）的疗效[24]。该研究中有 80 例患者得到治疗，中位总生存期（主要终点）为 10.9 个月，1 年、2 年生存率（主要终点）分别为 46% 和 19%。EGFR 突变阳性与疾病控制率、肿瘤进展时间的延长以及生存率相关。作者总结该单药治疗有效且耐受性好。该研究结果与另一项同为评估 TKI 治疗 70 岁以上未化疗的晚期 NSCLC 老年患者的开放、多中心 II 期临床试验——INVITE 的结果形成对比[25]，该研究的不同之处在于患者随机接受化疗（长春瑞滨）或 250mg/d 的吉非替尼而不是厄洛替尼。作为主要终点的无进展生存期在吉非替尼组是 2.7 个月，在长春瑞滨组是 2.9 个月 [HR = 1.19；95% CI (0.85, 1.65)；$P = 0.310$]。治疗有效率及总生存期虽未得到提高，但吉非替尼组的生活质量及不良反应发生率要优于化疗组。

TORCH 是另一项在加拿大和意大利进行的国际间、多中心、开放、随机对照 III 期临床试验，该研究计划在晚期 NSCLC 患者中评估厄洛替尼一线治疗并于进展后行顺铂-吉西他滨化疗的治疗模式，并比较该治疗模式与相反给药顺序的经典治疗模式对总生存期的作用[26]。但该试验在计划时，根据厄洛替尼在 BR.21 试验所有患者中的有效性，其已在未经选择的患者中注册，因此 TORCH 试验未应用某些临床或生物标记物来筛选患者。在首个计划的临时分析中，厄洛替尼序贯化疗的疗效要亚于化疗序贯厄洛替尼疗法，因此该研究被终止了。标准组的中位总生存期为 11.6 个月，而试验组为 8.7 个月。试验组未校正的死亡风险比为 1.22 [95% CI (1.03, 1.44)]。

因此，目前的数据显示在未经选择的人群，即使对那些一般情况差、高龄的患者，一线应用 EGFR-TKIs 不能带来有效率、无进展生存期或总生存期延长等临床获益。

随着多项临床试验的结束以及 EGFR 突变和酪氨酸激酶抑制相关知识的发展，明确提示后续试验需要相应调整以达到 EGFR-TKIs 治疗的有效率、无进展生存期或总生存期的提高。作为晚期 NSCLC 的二线或三线治疗，单药 TKIs 相较于最佳支持治疗[27-28]及化疗[29]的试验结果充满希望，包括女性、不吸烟者、亚洲人群及腺癌病理类型这些特征的治疗有效亚组得到确定[30]。最终，进一步的研究显示，这些患者 EGFR 突变的发生率较高，并且研究表明，EGFR-TKIs 一线治疗突变的肺癌患者能显著提高客观缓解率和无进展生存期[31-32]。

截至 2010 年 12 月，已报道了 4 项比较吉非替尼联合铂类一线治疗晚期 NSCLC 的随机对照Ⅲ期临床试验，包括 IPASS, First-SIGNAL, WJ-TOG3405 及 NEJ002[33-36]。

IPASS 旨在比较晚期 NSCLC 中的特定人群（不吸烟或既往少量吸烟的肺腺癌患者）按 1:1 的比例随机分组接受卡铂/紫杉醇化疗或吉非替尼一线治疗的疗效差异。在这项纳入 1 217 例东亚患者的开放、随机对照Ⅲ期临床试验中，吉非替尼组不仅在主要研究终点无进展生存期上不亚于卡铂/紫杉醇化疗组 [5.7 个月 vs 5.8 个月；HR = 0.741；95% CI (0.651, 0.845)；$P < 0.000\ 1$]，并且在 12 个月无进展生存率上显著优于化疗组（24.9% vs 6.7%；HR = 0.74；$P < 0.000\ 1$）。在 437 例（35.9%）中 EGFR 突变阳性者 261 例（59.7%），其中，140 例为外显子 19 缺失，111 例为外显子 21（L858R）突变，11 例为外显子 20（T790M）突变，10 例为其他类型突变并且有 11 例同时存在多种类型突变。EGFR 突变与吉非替尼疗效相关。阳性突变患者接受吉非替尼治疗后无进展生存期显著延长 [HR = 0.48；95% CI (0.36, 0.64)；$P < 0.000\ 1$]；而阴性突变患者接受吉非替尼治疗后的无进展生存期则显著缩短 [HR = 2.85；95% CI (2.05, 3.98)；$P < 0.000\ 1$]。同样，EGFR 突变患者亚组中吉非替尼治疗的有效率为 71.2%，显著优于卡铂/紫杉醇组的 47.3%（$P = 0.000\ 1$）。吉非替尼组患者的生活质量显著提高，毒副反应可耐受。总体来说，IPASS 试验突出了 EGFR 突变肺癌患者的特质及其对 TKI 治疗的有效应答。

继 IPASS 之后，First-SIGNAL, WJTOG3405 及 NEJ002 是 3 项后续在 EGFR 突变晚期 NSCLC 患者中进行的比较吉非替尼与化疗作为一线治疗疗效的Ⅲ期临床试验（表 26.1）。First-SIGNAL 试验纳入了 313 例韩国不吸烟肺腺癌患者，随机接受 250mg/d 的吉非替尼或吉西他滨-顺铂化疗[34]。两组的总生存期（重要终点）相似，并未达到预想的吉非替尼对总生存期的治疗优势 [吉非替尼组 22.3 个月 vs 吉西他滨-顺铂组 22.9 个月；HR = 0.932；95% CI (0.716, 1.213)；$P = 0.604$]。但吉非替尼组的治疗有效率（55% vs 46%）及 1 年无进展生存率（16.7% vs 2.8%）均显著优于化疗组[37]。在 First-SIGNAL 中，仅 96 例患者检测了 EGFR 突变状态，其中 42 例突变阳性。在该亚组中，接受吉非替尼治疗的患者无进展生存期显著延长 [8.4 个月 vs 6.7 个月；HR = 0.613；95% CI (0.308, 1.221)；$P = 0.084$][34]。

两项由日本研究机构开展的在晚期 NSCLC 患者中比较了吉非替尼与化疗一线治疗疗效的Ⅲ期临床试验均显示吉非替尼能延长 EGFR 突变肺癌患者的无进展生存期。NEJ002 研究在 EGFR 突变阳性的日本患者中比较了吉非替尼与卡铂/紫杉醇作为一线治疗疗效的差异[36]。中期分析中，吉非替尼可带来无进展生存期的显著获益，因此该研究在纳入 230 例患者后便不再纳入新受试者。对 228 例患者进行最终分析后，吉非替尼组的中位无进展生存期为 10.8 个月，卡铂/紫杉醇组为 5.4 个月 [HR = 0.30；95% CI (0.22, 0.41)；$P < 0.001$]。

总有效率上也是吉非替尼组显著占优势（73.7% vs 30.7%；P<0.001）。后续研究更新了生存数据，显示两组总生存期无显著差异[38]。该结果很可能是由于两组间存在极高的交叉率，96% 化疗患者后续接受吉非替尼治疗且 90% 接受吉非替尼患者后续进行了卡铂/紫杉醇的二线治疗。吉非替尼组的中位总生存期为 27.7 个月，化疗组为 26.6 个月 [HR = 0.887；95% CI（0.634，1.241）；P=0.483]，亚组分析显示总生存期无显著差异。

WJTOG3405 是一项开放性Ⅲ期临床试验，在日本纳入了 177 例既往未接受化疗且表达 EGFR 突变（19 外显子缺失或 L858R 点突变）的晚期 NSCLC 患者[35]。由于进行了分子选择，所以被研究人群中有超过 2/3 的患者是女性和从未吸烟者，并且有相当大比例的肺腺癌。患者被随机分为两组，分别接受 250mg/d 剂量的吉非替尼或顺铂-多西他赛化疗。该研究达到了包括无进展生存期在内的主要研究终点。在纳入生存分析的 172 例患者中，吉非替尼组相较于顺铂-多西他赛组的无进展生存期显著延长 [9.2 个月 vs 6.3 个月；HR=0.489；95% CI（0.336，0.710）；P<0.000 1]。

两项Ⅲ期临床试验评估了厄洛替尼一线治疗 EGFR 突变阳性 NSCLC 患者的疗效。由西班牙肺癌组开展的 EURTAC 是一项前瞻性、随机对照Ⅲ期临床试验，比较了厄洛替尼与铂类化疗一线治疗 EGFR 突变阳性的晚期 NSCLC 的疗效差异[39]。173 例患者中有 99% 为欧美白人。化疗方案包括顺铂-多西他赛，顺铂-吉西他滨，卡铂-多西他赛及卡铂-吉西他滨，每 3 周 1 次，连用 4 周。厄洛替尼组的无进展生存期（主要研究终点）显著优于化疗组 [9.7 个月 vs 5.2 个月；HR=0.37；95% CI（0.25，0.54）；P<0.000 1]。同时，厄洛替尼也有效提高了治疗有效率（58% vs 15%），但两组的中位总生存期无显著差异 [22.9 个月 vs 18.8 个月；HR=0.80；P=0.42]。

OPTIMAL 为另一项在中国开展的开放性、随机对照Ⅲ期临床试验，比较了厄洛替尼与吉西他滨-卡铂化疗一线治疗 EGFR 突变阳性的晚期 NSCLC 的疗效及患者的耐受性[40]。该试验设计与 EURTAC 类似，并纳入了 165 例亚洲患者。厄洛替尼较化疗显著延长了无进展生存期（主要研究终点）[13.1 个月 vs 4.6 个月；HR=0.16；95% CI（0.1，0.26）；P<0.000 1]。厄洛替尼组也表现出较好的有效率（83% vs 36%）。

总之，上述研究结果显示检测 EGFR 突变状态是判断肺癌患者能否从 EGFR-TKI 一线治疗中获益的最好方法。多项研究均显示吉非替尼或厄洛替尼较化疗能有效提高无进展生存期、治疗有效率及生活质量。尚无一项研究显示总生存期的获益，很可能是由于各治疗组在发生疾病进展后各种治疗方法的高交叉率。依据这些数据，目前在既往未治疗的复发或转移患者中检测 EGFR 突变状态已相当普遍；EGFR 突变阳性的患者更倾向应用 EGFR-TKIs；EGFR 野生型肿瘤不推荐一线应用 EGFR-TKIs。

在既往未接受治疗的不吸烟或少量吸烟患者中一线应用卡铂-紫杉醇联合厄洛替尼也在相关临床试验中得到了研究[41]。81 例应用单药厄洛替尼的患者及 100 例应用化疗+厄洛替尼的患者在主要终点——无进展生存期上结果相似（5.0 个月 vs 6.6 个月；P=0.198 8）。EGFR 突变阳性患者在两组中的治疗效果均优于突变阴性者。鉴于此，在根据人群及突变状态选择的患者中，在 EGFR-TKIs 一线治疗的基础上增加化疗并无额外获益。

维持治疗

双盲、随机对照Ⅲ期临床试验 SATURN 评估了晚期 NSCLC 患者接受一线铂类方案化疗后继续应用厄洛替尼作为维持治疗的疗效[42]。患者结束 4 个周期化疗后且无证据显示进展或转移的状态下，随机接受 150mg/d 的厄洛替尼或安慰剂，直至进展或不可耐受的毒性。主要研究终点是无进展生存期，次要研究终点是 EGFR 突变阳性患者的无进展生存期。两组间腺癌或鳞癌所占比例类似。该研究达到了两个主要研究终点。厄洛替尼组相较安慰剂组无进展生存期显著延长 [HR=0.71；95% CI（0.62，0.82）；P<0.000 1]。EGFR 突变阳性患者无进展生存期也显著延长 [HR=0.10；95% CI（0.04，0.25）；P<0.000 1]，EGFR 突变阴性患者也得出类似结果 [HR=0.78；95% CI（0.63，0.96）；P=0.018 5]。

表 26.1 EGFR-TKIs 与化疗一线治疗含 EGFR 突变的 NSCLC Ⅲ 期临床试验比较

试验	区域	EGFR-TKIs	化疗	病例数	中位 PFS(月)	HR	有效率
IPASS (Mok,2009)	东亚	吉非替尼	卡铂-紫杉醇	261	9.5 vs 6.3	0.48 (0.36,0.64) $P<0.0001$	71.2% vs 47.3%
First-SIGNAL (Lee,2009)	韩国	吉非替尼	顺铂-吉西他滨	42	8.4 vs 6.7	0.61 (0.31,1.22) $P=0.084$	84.6% vs 37.5%
NEJ002 (Maemondo,2010)	日本	吉非替尼	卡铂-紫杉醇	230	10.8 vs 5.4	0.30 (0.22,0.41) $P<0.001$	73.7% vs 30.7%
WJTOG3405 (Mitsudomi,2010)	日本	吉非替尼	顺铂-多西他赛	177	9.2 vs 6.3	0.49 (0.34,0.71) $P<0.0001$	62.1% vs 32.2%
EURTAC (Rosell,2012)	西班牙,法国,意大利	厄洛替尼	顺铂-多西他赛 顺铂-吉西他滨 卡铂-多西他赛 卡铂-吉西他滨	173	9.7 vs 5.2	0.37 (0.25,0.54) $P<0.0001$	58% vs 15%
OPTIMAL (Zhou,2011)	中国	厄洛替尼	卡铂-吉西他滨	165	13.1 vs 4.6	0.16 (0.1,0.26) $P<0.0001$	83% vs 36%

ATLAS 作为一项双盲、随机对照ⅢB期临床试验，在含铂双药化疗+贝伐单抗治疗结束的患者中，比较了应用贝伐单抗单药或联用厄洛替尼作为维持治疗的疗效[43]。该试验于第二次计划中期分析后关闭，并已达到了无进展生存期的最终目标。贝伐单抗+厄洛替尼组的中位无进展生存期为4.8个月，贝伐单抗单药治疗组为3.7个月[HR=0.722；95% CI（0.592，0.881）；P=0.0012]。因此，ATLAS试验的结论是一线应用化疗联合贝伐单抗的晚期NSCLC患者，维持治疗选用贝伐单抗联合厄洛替尼能显著延长无进展生存期且副反应较典型，但在预期范围。

在美国，厄洛替尼已被监管机构批准用于一线治疗后疗效评价为CR、PR或SD患者的维持治疗，而在欧洲则是适用于一线治疗后SD的患者。

挽救治疗

名为NCIC CTG BR.21的随机对照Ⅲ期临床试验比较了厄洛替尼与安慰剂在一线或二线化疗失败的晚期NSCLC中的疗效[27]。731例患者按2∶1的比例随机分配接受150mg/d剂量的厄洛替尼或安慰剂。厄洛替尼组的客观缓解率为8.9%，显著高于安慰剂组（1%），P<0.001。中位治疗反应维持时间分别为7.9个月与3.7个月；无进展生存期分别为2.2个月与1.8个月（HR=0.61；P<0.001）。总生存期上也是厄洛替尼组占优势（6.7个月 vs 4.7个月；HR=0.70；P<0.001）。亚组分析显示女性、不吸烟者、亚裔及腺癌患者对厄洛替尼反应性更佳。最常见的毒副反应包括皮疹和腹泻，总体易控制，尤其在肿瘤症状及生活质量上，厄洛替尼组较安慰剂控制得更好[27]。

由于 IDEAL-1、IDEAL-2两项Ⅱ期临床试验取得了不错的结果[44-45]，后续开展了ISEL临床试验。ISEL是一项随机对照Ⅲ期临床试验，观察吉非替尼二线或三线治疗晚期NSCLC对患者生存期的影响[30]。按照原计划的2∶1分配比例，1129例患者随机接受250mg/d剂量的吉非替尼，另外563例患者接受安慰剂。主要终点是总治疗人群及肺腺癌患者的生存时间。中位随访时间为7.2个月，两种治疗方案下所有患者的总生存期无显著差异[5.6个月 vs 5.1个月；HR=0.89；95% CI（0.77，1.02）；P=0.087]，对812例肺腺癌患者的中位总生存期也无显著差异[6.3个月 vs 5.4个月；HR=0.84；95% CI（0.68，1.03）；P=0.089]。在预先计划的亚组分析中，不吸烟亚裔患者的生存期显著延长[30,46]。

我们同时回顾了BR.21和ISEL临床试验的结果，发现吉非替尼和厄洛替尼有相似的有效率（8% vs 9%）。但厄洛替尼对所有入组患者均有生存获益，而吉非替尼仅对腺癌或不吸烟患者有生存获益。有趣的是，在ISEL研究中，45%接受吉非替尼治疗的患者发生疾病进展并有18%最近一次化疗有效，但28%接受厄洛替尼治疗的患者疾病进展，有38%最近一次化疗有效。这引起一些疑问，即这些差异是否会影响ISEL和BR.21试验中吉非替尼和厄洛替尼的疗效[47]。

INTEREST临床试验在既往接受过铂类化疗的晚期NSCLC患者中直接比较了吉非替尼与多西他赛的疗效。对1433例患者的研究结果显示，吉非替尼对中位总生存期的延长效果不亚于多西他赛[7.6个月 vs 8.0个月；HR=1.020；95% CI（0.905，1.150）][8]。作为预先计划分析的一部分，研究进行了肿瘤活检来分析生物标志物与临床结果的关系。EGFR阳性突变患者接受吉非替尼治疗后在无进展生存期及客观缓解率方面显著优于多西他赛组。EGFR阳性突变患者吉非替尼治疗组的中位无进展生存期为7.0个月，而多西他赛组为4.1个月[HR=0.16；95% CI（0.05，0.49）；P=0.001]。吉非替尼组的有效率为42.1%，多西他赛组为21.1%（P=0.04）[48]。

TITAN试验同样也比较了厄洛替尼与化疗二线治疗的疗效差异。TITAN试验主要招募了那些接受维持治疗临床试验SATURN筛查，并在完成4个周期一线铂类双药化疗后疾病进展的患者。患者随机接受化疗（多西他赛或培美曲塞）或厄洛替尼[49]。主要观察终点是意向治疗人群的总生存期。然而由于该研究招募患者速度过慢，导致其比事先计划更早关闭。424例患者的最终入组使得该研究结果说服力不强。但该研究仍然显示厄洛替尼组在中位总生存期上与化疗组相差不大（厄洛替尼组5.3个月 vs 化疗组5.5个月）。因为肺鳞癌不应使用培美曲塞，该研究在剔除30例接受培美曲塞治疗的肺鳞癌患者后又进行了单独分析。

但这并未显著改变最终的研究结果。TITAN 研究的结果进一步巩固了 INTEREST 试验的结论,支持了 EGFR 抑制剂作为一种二线治疗方案对提高特定人群总生存期（overall survival，OS）的效果并不亚于化疗的观点。

基于 EGFR-TKIs 对 EGFR 阳性突变患者的疗效更为突出的事实,研究人员开展了一项新的Ⅲ期临床试验,以比较厄洛替尼与多西他赛在既往接受过化疗的 EGFR 野生型 NSCLC 患者中的疗效（TAILOR 研究）。TAILOR 研究尚未得到其主要终点－总生存期,但中期分析显示,作为次级终点的无进展生存期在化疗组要显著高于厄洛替尼组 [HR = 0.70；95% CI（0.53，0.94）；P = 0.016]。该结果提示化疗可能更适用于 EGFR 野生型 NSCLC 患者的挽救治疗[50]。

SELECT 试验评估了西妥昔单抗联合化疗在既往接受过治疗的患者中的疗效。这项多中心、开放、随机对照Ⅲ期临床试验,将培美曲塞或多西他赛分别联用西妥昔单抗,主要目的是观察西妥昔单抗－培美曲塞组对比培美曲塞单药组的无进展生存期。意向治疗人群由 938 例患者构成,其中 605 例纳入培美曲塞组（301 例应用西妥昔单抗－培美曲塞联合治疗；304 例应用培美曲塞单药）。西妥昔单抗－培美曲塞的中位无进展生存期为 2.9 个月,培美曲塞组为 2.8 个月 [HR = 1.03；95% CI（0.87，1.21）；P = 0.76]。两组的中位总生存期分别为 6.9 个月与 7.8 个月 [HR = 1.01；95% CI（0.86，1.20）；P = 0.86],客观缓解率分别为 6.6% 和 4.3% [OR = 1.59；95% CI（0.78，3.26）；P = 0.20]。按病理类型、EGFR 免疫组化染色强度或病理学评分（H-score）分组比较,各组间疗效无显著差异。西妥昔单抗－培美曲塞治疗组的毒副反应更大,主要包括皮肤毒性、胃肠道症状（腹泻、腹痛）及低镁血症。联用多西他赛时也有类似结果。所以在该人群中联合应用培美曲塞和西妥昔单抗并不能提高疗效[51]。

其他酪氨酸激酶抑制剂及单克隆抗体

目前关于 EGFR-TKIs 耐药机制的研究热点主要集中在 MET 癌基因复制及 EGFR 的二次突变。T790M 突变是发生获得性耐药的主要机制,占所有病例的 50% 以上。不可逆的 EGFR 抑制剂、针对 MET 的靶向治疗及双通路阻断等正在研究中。

达可替尼（PF - 00299804）是一种广泛的 HER 抑制剂,通过不可逆结合 EGFR 中的 ATP 域、HER2 及 HER4 发挥作用,而厄洛替尼则通过竞争性、可逆性结合 EGFR 酪氨酸激酶域来阻断信号通路。达可替尼在表达 L858R 及 T790M 突变的细胞系中仍能阻断 EGFR[52-53]。在一项国际间、多中心、开放性随机对照Ⅱ期临床试验中,188 例化疗失败患者随机接受达可替尼（45mg/d）或厄洛替尼（150mg/d）。达可替尼延长了无进展生存期（主要终点）[2.86 个月 vs 1.91 个月；HR = 0.66；95% CI（0.47，0.91）；P = 0.012][54]。这是在既往未接受过 TKIs 治疗患者中首次获得的关于不可逆 EGFR-TKIs 的随机临床数据。该结果为晚期 NSCLC 患者提供了另一个更完全抑制 HER 信号通路的潜在治疗选择。

D019/XL647 是一种以 EGFR、VEGFR - 2、HER2 及 Ephrin type B 受体 4 为靶点的小分子酪氨酸激酶抑制剂。在一项评估两种给药方案的Ⅱ期临床试验中,有效率达到 20%,无进展生存期为 9.3 个月[55]。这是一种仍需继续临床观察的化合物。

阿法替尼（BIBW 2992）是一种不可逆 ErbB 家族抑制剂。它与吉非替尼及厄洛替尼这类可逆性 EGFR-TKIs 的不同之处在于,其进入细胞后与 EGFR 半胱氨酸残基共价结合从而达到 EGFR 信号的持续抑制。阿法替尼同时对 HER2、HER3、HER4 及 EGFR 耐药 T790M 突变均有抑制活性。

在日本开展了一项在既往接受过厄洛替尼或吉非替尼治疗的晚期 NSCLC 患者中应用阿法替尼的Ⅱ期临床试验。主要观察终点是客观缓解率。阿法替尼可达到 69% 的 8 周以上疾病控制率及 4.4 个月的中位无进展生存期,因此被认定为有效[56]。

在另一项临床试验中,厄洛替尼治疗后进展的患者接受了阿法替尼－西妥昔单抗联合治疗。40mg 剂量的阿法替尼可使所有 22 例患者达到疾病控制,使肿瘤体积缩小达 76%[57]。

LUX-Lung 2 是一项在 EGFR 突变阳性肺腺癌患者中确定阿法替尼疗效的临床试验。接受阿法替尼作为一线治疗的 61 例患者中，无进展生存期为 12 个月。在表达 19 外显子缺失及 *L858R* 突变的患者中，无进展生存期可延长至 13.7 个月[58]。

基于这些结果，LUX-Lung 3 作为一项开放性、随机对照Ⅲ期临床试验，比较了阿法替尼与有效性、耐受性均较好的化疗方案顺铂 - 培美曲塞在 *EGFR* 突变阳性的晚期 NSCLC 患者中作为一线治疗的疗效。该研究达到了主要研究终点（独立观察组），显示阿法替尼组有效延长了无进展生存期（中位无进展生存期 11.1 个月 *vs* 6.9 个月；HR = 0.58；$P = 0.0004$）[59]。按包括性别、年龄、人种、*EGFR* 突变情况、ECOG 评分及吸烟史划分的各亚组危险比均小于 1（正在吸烟者或既往吸烟者的危险比为 1.04）。对 308 例表达 *EGFR* 突变（Del19 或 L858R）患者的预先计划分析显示，阿法替尼组的中位无进展生存期为 13.6 个月，顺铂 - 培美曲塞组为 6.9 个月。阿法替尼组的客观缓解率也显著较高（在所有患者中为 56.1% *vs* 22.6%；$P < 0.001$。在突变阳性患者中为 60.8% *vs* 22.1%；$P < 0.0001$）。同时，疾病控制率也有所提高：有 47% 的阿法替尼组患者在 12 个月随访期时尚未发生进展，而在化疗组这一比例仅为 22%。亚洲患者的无进展生存期显著较长。最常见的药品不良反应是腹泻和皮疹，但无患者因皮疹而中断阿法替尼治疗。有 3 例患者发生了间质性肺病样不良反应。非亚洲患者的耐受性总体较差。依据患者的症状及调查问卷，阿法替尼能显著延缓癌症相关症状的发生并提高患者的生活质量。

Necitumumab（IMC - 11F8）是另一种经过临床试验测试的针对性抑制 *EGFR* 的完全人源化单克隆抗体。2011 年 2 月，在一项比较 necitumumab 联合顺铂 - 培美曲塞方案化疗或单独化疗一线治疗转移性肺鳞癌患者的Ⅲ期临床试验——INSPIRE 中，necitumumab 组的血栓栓塞发生率过高导致其被迫终止[60]。此前，Ⅰ期和Ⅱ期临床试验并未报道有血栓栓塞的发生[61]。

靶向抑制 *EGFR* 平行或下游通路来治疗 NSCLC 的一些药物也正在研制中。MET 抑制剂是其中正在发展的一类药物。对 EGFR 和 MET 通路双重抑制的理论依据是 MET 通路与厄洛替尼、吉非替尼耐药相关；临床前及临床试验结果显示两药的协同作用或能克服耐药性[62-64]。

Tivantinib（ARQ 197）是一种 MET 受体酪氨酸激酶非 ATP 竞争、选择性口服抑制剂。一项全球性、随机双盲Ⅱ期临床试验在既往未使用 EGFR 抑制剂的晚期 NSCLC 患者中比较了厄洛替尼 + ARQ 197 与厄洛替尼 + 安慰剂的疗效。该研究纳入了 167 例患者，结果显示联合治疗能显著延长无进展生存期（主要终点）［16.1 周 *vs* 9.7 周；HR = 0.81；95% CI（0.57，1.15）；$P = 0.23$］。在非鳞癌、*KRAS* 突变、*EGFR* 野生型患者中，无进展生存期延长尤为明显[65]。基于这些令人鼓舞的试验结果，又开展了一项新的双盲、随机对照Ⅲ期临床试验以比较 ARQ 197 + 厄洛替尼与安慰剂 + 厄洛替尼在治疗晚期非鳞状细胞 NSCLC 患者的疗效差异。主要研究目的是评价意向治疗人群的总生存期[66]。

Onartuzumab（OAM4558）是一种特异性结合 MET 细胞外域的重组单价人单克隆抗体。一项国际间、随机双盲Ⅱ期临床试验比较了厄洛替尼 + Onartuzumab 及厄洛替尼 + 安慰剂用于二线或三线治疗晚期 NSCLC 的疗效差异。在肿瘤组织表达高水平 MET 的患者中联用 MET 单克隆抗体与厄洛替尼能显著提高无进展生存期及总生存期，并使疾病进展风险下降近 2 倍，死亡风险下降 3 倍[67]。而紧接着该研究的是一项名为 Met Lung 的多中心、随机对照Ⅲ期临床试验，该试验将在既往至少 1 个但不超过 2 个铂类化疗方案治疗失败的晚期 NSCLC 患者中进行，主要观察终点是总生存期[68]。

拉帕替尼是一种口服 EGFR、HER - 2 双通路可逆性抑制剂。EGFR 能同 HER2 形成二聚体及异二聚体进而传导信号，同时抑制两种受体相对于单独抑制 EGFR 或许能带来更大的临床获益。一项多中心、开放性、随机对照Ⅱ期临床试验评估了拉帕替尼作为一线或二线方案治疗晚期 NSCLC 患者的疗效。尽管耐受性良好，但拉帕替尼并没有在意向治疗人群中达到预先计划的有效率。一部分患者能维持肿瘤稳定状态 24 周或更少。在这种情况下，该剂量的单药拉帕替尼有效率较低[69]。

总 结

调控 EGFR 通路已发展为 NSCLC 治疗手段之一。可逆性 EGFR-TKIs—厄洛替尼、吉非替尼已被证实对晚期 NSCLC，特别是 EGFR 阳性突变患者有效。但原发及获得性耐药则是另一个值得持续关注的问题。包括不可逆性 EGFR-TKIs 及单克隆抗体在内的一些新的治疗手段正在研发和评估中。这一变革定义了 NSCLC 治疗中分子分型的标准。

（倪 阳 邹知耕 译）

参考文献

[1] Cohen S. Isolation of a mouse submaxillary gland protein accelerating incisor eruption and eyelid opening in the new born animal. J Biol Chem, 1962, 237: 1555-1562.

[2] Herbst RS, Prager D, Hermann R, et al. TRIBUTE: a phase Ⅲ trial of erlotinib hydrochloride (OSI-774) combined with carboplatin and paclitaxel chemotherapy in advanced non-small-cell lung cancer. J Clin Oncol, 2005, 23: 5892-5899.

[3] Gatzemerier U, Pluzanska A, Szczesna A, et al. Phase Ⅲ study of erlotinib in combination with cisplatin and gemcitabine in advanced non-small-cell lung cancer: the Tarceva Lung Cancer Investigation Trial. J Clin Oncol, 2007, 25: 1545-1552.

[4] Giaccone G, Herbst RS, Manegold C, et al. Gefitinib in combination with gemcitabine and cisplatin in advanced non-small-cell lung cancer: A phase Ⅲ trial-INTACT 1. J Clin Oncol, 2004, 22: 777-784.

[5] Herbst RS, Giaccone G, Schiller JH, et al. Gefitinib in combination with paclitaxel and carboplatin in advanced non-small-cell lung cancer: A phase Ⅲ trial-INTACT 2. J Clin Oncol, 2004, 22: 785-794.

[6] Pirker R, Pereira JR, Szczesna A, et al. Cetuximab plus chemotherapy in patients with advanced non-small-cell lung cancer (FLEX): An open-label randomized phase Ⅲ trial. Lancet, 2009, 373: 1525-1531.

[7] Lynch TJ, Patel T, Dreisbach L, et al. Cetuximab and first-line taxane/carboplatin chemotherapy in advanced non-small-cell lung cancer: results of the randomized multicenter phase Ⅲ trial BMS099. J Clin Oncol, 2010, 28: 911-917.

[8] Kim E, Herbst RS, Moon J, et al. SWOG 0536: Phase Ⅱ trial of carboplatin, paclitaxel, cetuximab and bevacizumab followed by cetuximab and bevacizumab in advanced non-small cell lung cancer. J Thor Oncol, 2008, 3: S266.

[9] Tracy S, Mukohara T, Hansen M, et al. Gefitinib induces apoptosis in the EGFRL858R non-smallcell lung cancer cell line H3255. Cancer Res, 2004, 64: 7241-7244.

[10] Gumerlock PH, Pryde BJ, Kimura T, et al. Enhanced cytotoxicity of docetaxel OSI-774 combination in non-small cell lung carcinoma (NSCLC). Proc Am Soc Clin Oncol, 2003, 662 (abstr 2661).

[11] Solit DB, She Y, Lobo J, et al. Pulsatile administration of the epidermal growth factor receptor inhibitor gefitinib is significantly more effective than continuous dosing for sensitizing tumors to paclitaxel. Clin Cancer Res, 2005, 11: 1983-1989.

[12] Mok TS, Wu YL, Yu CJ, et al. Randomized, placebo-controlled, phase Ⅱ study of sequential erlotinib and chemotherapy as first-line treatment for advanced non-small-cell lung cancer. J Clin Oncol, 2009, 27: 5080-5087.

[13] Mok TS, Wu YL, Thongprasert S, et al. A randomized placebo-controlled phase Ⅲ study of intercalated erlotinib with gemcitabine-platinum in firstline advanced non-small cell lung cancer (NSCLC): FASTACT-Ⅱ. J Clin Oncol, 2012, 30 (suppl): Abstr 7519.

[14] Mok TS, Lee JS, Zhang L, et al. Biomarker analyses and overall survival (OS) from the randomized, placebo-controlled, phase 3, FASTACT-2 study of intercalated erlotinib with first-line chemotherapy in advanced non-small-cell lung cancer. ESMO, 2012: Abstr 1023.

[15] Hirsch FR, Kabbinavar F, Eisen T, et al. A randomized, phase Ⅱ, biomarker-selected study comparing erlotinib to erlotinib intercalated with chemotherapy in first-line therapy for advanced non-small cell lung cancer. J Clin Oncol, 2011, 29: 3567-3573.

[16] Reck M, Buchholz E, Romer KS, et al. Gefitinib monotherapy in chemotherapy-naive patients with inoperable stage Ⅲ/Ⅳ non-small-cell lung cancer. Clin Lung Cancer, 2006, 7: 406-411.

[17] Niho S, Kubota K, Goto K, et al. First-line single agent treatment with gefitinib in patients with advanced non-small-cell lung cancer: A phase Ⅱ study. J Clin Oncol, 2006, 24: 64-69.

[18] Giaccone G, Gallegos RM, Le Chevalier T, et al. Erlo-

tinib for frontline treatment of advanced nonsmall cell lung cancer: a phase Ⅱ study. Clin Cancer Res, 2006, 12: 6049 – 6055.

[19] Lee DH, Kim SW, Suh C, et al. Phase Ⅱ study of erlotinib for chemotherapy-naïve patients with advanced or metastatic non-small cell lung cancer who are ineligible for platinum doublets. Cancer Chemother Pharmacol, 2011, 67: 35 – 39.

[20] Yang CH, Yu CJ, Shih JY, et al. Specific EGFR mutations predict treatment outcome of stage ⅢB/Ⅳ patients with chemotherapy-naive non-smallcell lung cancer receiving first-line gefitinib monotherapy. J Clin Oncol, 2008, 26: 2745 – 2753.

[21] Hesketh PJ, Chansky K, Wozniak AJ, et al. Southwest Oncology Group phase Ⅱ trial (S0341) of erlotinib (OSI-774) in patients with advanced nonsmall cell lung cancer and a performance status of 2. J Thorac Oncol, 2008, 3: 1026 – 1031.

[22] Goss G, Ferry D, Wierzbicki R, et al. Randomized phase Ⅱ study of gefitinib compared with placebo in chemotherapy-naïve patients with advanced nonsmall-cell lung cancer and poor performance status. J Clin Oncol, 2009, 27: 2253 – 2260.

[23] Lee SM, Khan I, Upadhyay S, et al. Firstline erlotinib in patients with advanced non-smallcell lung cancer unsuitable for chemotherapy (TOPICAL): A double-blind, placebo-controlled, phase 3 trial. Lancet Oncol, 2012, 13 (11): 1161 – 1170.

[24] Jackman DM, Yeap BY, Linderman NI, et al. Phase Ⅱ clinical trial of chemotherapy-naïve patients ≥ 70 years of age treated with erlotinib for advanced non-small cell lung cancer. J Clin Oncol, 2007, 25: 760 – 766.

[25] Crino L, Cappuzzo F, Zatloukal P, et al. Gefitinib versus vinorelbine in chemotherapy-naive elderly patients with advanced non-small-cell lung cancer (INVITE): A randomized, phase Ⅱ study. J Clin Oncol, 2008, 26: 4253 – 4260.

[26] Gridelli C, Ciardiello F, Gallo C, et al. First-line erlotinib followed by second-line cisplatingemcitabine chemotherapy in advanced non-small cell lung cancer: the TORCH randomized trial. J Clin Oncol, 2012, 30: 3002 – 3011.

[27] Shepherd FA, Pereira J, Ciuleanu TE, et al. A randomized placebo-controlled trial of erlotinib in patients with advanced non-small cell lung cancer (NSCLC) following failure of 1st line or 2nd line chemotherapy. A National Cancer Institute of Canada Clinical Trials Group (NCIC CTG) trial. J Clin Oncol, 2004, 22: 622s.

[28] Shepherd FA, Rodrigues PJ, Cieleanu TE, et al. Erlotinib in previously treated non-small-cell lung cancer. N Engl J Med, 2005, 353: 123 – 132.

[29] Kim ES, Hirsh V, Mok T, et al. Gefitinib versus docetaxel in previously treated non-small-cell lung cancer (INTEREST): A randomised phase Ⅲ trial. Lancet, 2008, 372: 1809 – 1818.

[30] Thatcher N, Chang A, Parikh P, et al. Gefitinib plus best supportive care in previously treated patients with refractory advanced non-small cell lung cancer: results from a randomised, placebo-controlled, multicentre study (Iressa Survival Evaluation in Lung Cancer). Lancet, 2005, 366: 1527 – 1537.

[31] Inoue A, Suzuki T, Fukuhara T, et al. Prospective phase Ⅱ study of gefitinib for chemotherapy naive patients with advanced non-small-cell lung cancer with epidermal growth factor receptor gene mutations. J Clin Oncol, 2006, 24: 3340 – 3346.

[32] Sequist LV, Martins RG, Spigel D, et al. Firstline gefitinib in patients with advanced non-small cell lung cancer harboring somatic EGFR mutations. J Clin Oncol, 2008, 26: 2442 – 2449

[33] Mok TS, Wu YL, Thongprasert S, et al. Gefitinib or carboplatin-paclitaxel in pulmonary adenocarcinoma. N Engl J Med, 2009, 361: 947 – 957.

[34] Lee JS, Park K, Kim SW, et al. Presented at World Conference on Lung Cancer. A randomized phase Ⅲ study of gefitinib (IRESSA) versus standard chemotherapy (gemcitabine plus cisplatin) as a first-line treatment for never-smokers with advanced or metastatic adenocarcinoma of the lung, 2009.

[35] Mitsudomi T, Morita S, Yatabe Y, et al. Gefitinib versus cisplatin plus docetaxel in patients with non-small-cell lung cancer harbouring mutations of the epidermal growth factor receptor (WJTOG3405): An open label, randomized phase 3 trial. Lancet Oncol, 2010, 11: 121 – 128.

[36] Maemondo M, Inoue A, Kobayashi K, et al. Gefitinib or chemotherapy for non-small-cell lung cancer with mutated EGFR. N Engl J Med, 2010, 362: 2380 – 2388.

[37] Han JY, Park K, Kim SW, et al. First-SIGNAL: first-line single-agent iressa versus gemcitabine and cisplatin trial in never-smokers with adenocarcinoma of the lung. J Clin Oncol, 2012, 30: 1122 – 1128.

[38] Inoue A, Kobayashi K, Maemondo M, et al. Updated o-

verall survival results from a randomized phase III trial comparing gefitinib with carboplatinpaclitaxel for chemonaïve non-small cell lung cancer with sensitive EGFR gene mutations (NEJ002). Ann Oncol, 2013, 24 (1): 54–59.

[39] Rosell R, Carcereny E, Gervais R, et al. Erlotinib versus standard chemotherapy as first-line treatment for European patients with advanced EGFR mutationpositive non-small-cell lung cancer (EURTAC): A multicenter, open-label-randomised phase 3 trial. Lancet Oncol, 2012, 13: 239–246.

[40] Zhou C, Wu YL, Chen G, et al. Erlotinib versus chemotherapy as first-line treatment for patients with advanced EGFR mutation-positive non-small-cell lung cancer (OPTIMAL, CTONG-0802): A multicenter, open-label, randomized, phase 3 study. Lancet Oncol, 2011, 12: 735–742.

[41] Jäanne PA, Wang X, Socinski MA, et al. Randomized phase II trial of erlotinib alone or with carboplatin and paclitaxel in patients who were never or light former smokers with advanced lung adenocarcinoma: CALGB 30406 trial. J Clin Oncol, 2012, 30 (17): 2063–2069.

[42] Cappuzzo, F, Ciuleanu T, Stelmakh L, et al. Erlotinib as maintenance treatment in advanced nonsmall- cell lung cancer: a multicentre, randomised, placebo-controlled phase 3 study. Lancet Oncol, 2010, 11: 521–529.

[43] Miller VA, O'Connor P, Soh C, et al. A randomized, double-blind, placebo-controlled, phase IIIb trial (ATLAS) comparing bevacizumab (B) therapy with or without erlotinib (E) after completion of chemotherapy with B for first-line treatment of locally advanced, recurrent, or metastatic non-small cell lung cancer (NSCLC). J Clin Oncol, 2009, 27: 18s, LBA8002.

[44] Fukuoka M, Yano S, Giaccone G, et al. Multiinstitutional randomized phase II trial of gefinitib for previously treated patients with advanced nonsmall-cell lung cancer. J Clin Oncol, 2003, 21: 2237–2246.

[45] Kris MG, Natale RB, Herbst RS, et al. Efficacy of gefitinib, an inhibitor of the epidermal growth factor receptor tyrosine kinase, in symptomatic patients with non-small cell lung cancer: A randomized trial. JAMA, 2003, 290: 2149–2158.

[46] Hirsch FR, Varella-Garcia M, Bunn PA, Jr., et al. Molecular predictors of outcome with gefitinib in a phase III placebo-controlled study in advanced nonsmall cell lung cancer. J Clin Oncol, 2006, 24: 5034–5042.

[47] Wang Y, Schmid-Bindert, Zhou C. Erlotinib in the treatment of advanced non-small cell lung cancer: An update for clinicians. Ther Adv Med Oncol, 2011, 4: 19–29.

[48] Douillard JY, Shepherd FA, Hirsh V, et al. Molecular predictors of outcome with gefitinib and docetaxel in previously treated non-small-cell lung cancer: data from the randomized phase III INTEREST trial. J Clin Oncol, 2010, 28: 744–752.

[49] Ciuleanu T, Stelmakh L, Cicenas S, et al. Efficacy and safety of erlotinib versus chemotherapy in second-line treatment of patients with advanced, nonsmall-cell lung cancer with poor prognosis (TITAN): A randomised multicentre, open-label, phase 3 study. Lancet Oncol, 2012, 13: 300–308.

[50] Garassino MC, Martelli O, Bettini A, et al. TAILOR: A phase III trial comparing erlotinib with docetaxel as the second-line treatment of NSCLC patients with wild-type (wt) EGFR. J Clin Oncol, 2012, 30 (suppl): Abstr LBA7501.

[51] Kim ES, Neubauer MA, Cohn AL, et al. SELECT: Randomized phase III study of docetaxel (D) or pemetrexed (P) with or without cetuximab (C) in recurrent or progressive non-small cell lung cancer (NSCLC) after platinum-based therapy. J Clin Oncol, 2012, 30 (suppl): Abstr 7502.

[52] Engelman JA, Zejnullahu K, Gale CM, et al. PF00299804, an irreversible pan-ERBB inhibitor, is effective in lung cancer models with EGFR and ERBB2 mutations that are resistant to gefitinib. Cancer Res, 2007, 67: 11924–11932.

[53] Gonzales AJ, Hook KE, Althaus IW, et al. Antitumor activity and pharmacokinetic properties of PF-00299804, a second-generation irreversible pan-erbB receptor tyroside kinase inhibitor. Mol Cancer Ther, 2008, 7: 1880–1889.

[54] Ramalingam SS, Blackhall F, Krzakowski M, et al. Randomized phase II study of dacomitinib (PF-00299804), an irreversible pan-human epidermal growth factor receptor inhibitor, versus erlotinib in patients with advanced non-small cell lung cancer. J Clin Oncol, 2012, 30: 3337–3344.

[55] Pietanza MC, Gadgeel SM, Dowlati A, et al. Phase II study of the multitargeted tyroside kinase inhibitor XL647 in patients with non-small-cell lung cancer. J Thorac Oncol, 2012, 7: 856–865.

[56] Yamamoto N, Katakami N, Atagi S, et al. A phase II

trial of afatinib (BIBW 2992) in patients (pts) with advanced non-small cell lung cancer previously treated with erlotinib (E) or gefitinib (G). J Clin Oncol, 2011, 29 (suppl): Abstr 7524.

[57] Janijigian YY, Groen HJ, Horn L, et al. Activity and tolerability of afatinib (BIBW 2992) and cetuximab in NSCLC patients with acquired resistance to erlotinib or gefitinib. J Clin Oncol, 2011, 29 (suppl): Abstr7525.

[58] Yang JC, Shih JY, S WC, et al. Afatinib for patients with lung adenocarcinoma and epidermal growth factor receptor mutations (LUX-Lung 2): A phase 2 trial. Lancet Oncol, 2012, 13: 539-548.

[59] Yang JC, Schuler MH, Yamamoto N, et al. LUXLung 3: A randomized, open-label, phase III study of afatinib versus pemetrexed and cisplatin as first-line treatment for patients with advanced adenocarcinoma of the lung harboring EGFR-activating mutations. J Clin Oncol, 2012, 30 (suppl): Abstr LBA7500.

[60] Lilly, Bristol-Myers Squibb stop enrollment in one of two phase III lung cancer trials of necitumumab. Bristol-Myers Squibb website, 2012. http://bms.newshq.businesswire.com/pressrelease/rd-news/lilly-bristol-myers-squibb-stop-enroll ment-one-two-phase-iii-lung-cancer-trial.

[61] Tabernero J, Cervantes A, Delaunoit T, et al. A phase 2 study of IMC-11F8, a monoclonal antibody directed against the EGFR, in combination with mFOLFOX-6 chemotherapy in the first-line treatment of advanced or metastatic colorectal carcinoma. Ann Oncol, 2009, 20: 18-19.

[62] Merchant M, Zhang YW, Su Y, et al. Combination efficacy with MetMAb and erlotinib in a NSCLC tumor model highlight therapeutic opportunities for c-Met inhibitors in combination with EGFR inhibitors. Proceedings of the 99th Annual Meeting of the American Association for Cancer Research. San Diego, CA, USA, 2008: Abstract 1336.

[63] Janne PA, Wax M, Leach JW, et al. Targeting MET with XL184 to reverse EGFR tyrosine kinase inhibitor (TKI) resistance in NSCLC: Impact of preclinical studies on clinical trial design. EJC, 2008, 6 (Suppl): Abstr174.

[64] Wakelee HA, Gettinger SN, Engelman JA, et al. A phase Ib/II study of XL184 (BMS 907351) with and without erlotinib (E) in patients (pts) with non-small cell lung cancer (NSCLC). J Clin Oncol, 2010, 28 (suppl): Abstr 3017.

[65] Schiller JH, Akerley WL, Brugger W, et al. Results from ARQ 197-209: A global randomized placebo-controlled phase II clinical trial of erlotinib plus ARQ 197 versus erlotinib plus placebo in previously treated EGFR inhibitor-naive patients with locally advanced or metastatic non-small cell lung cancer (NSCLC). J Clin Oncol, 2010, 28 (suppl): Abstr LBA7502.

[66] Scagliotti GV, Novello S, Schiller JH, et al. Rationale and design of MARQUEE: A phase III, randomized, double-blind study of tivantinib plus erlotinib versus placebo plus erlotinib in previously treated patients with locally advanced or metastatic, nonsquamous, non-small-cell lung cancer. Clin Lung Cancer, 2012, 13: 391-395.

[67] Spigel DR, Ervin TJ, Ramlau R, et al. Final efficacy results from OAM4558g, a randomized phase II study evaluating MetMAb or placebo in combination with erlotinib in advanced NSCLC. J Clin Oncol, 2011, 29 (suppl): Abstr 7505.

[68] Spigel DR, Edelman MJ, Mok T, et al. The MetLUNG study: A randomized, double-blind, phase III study of onartuzumab (MetMAb) plus erlotinib versus placebo plus erlotinib in patients with advanced, MET-positive non-small cell lung cancer (NSCLC). J Clin Oncol, 2012, 30 (suppl): Abstr TPS7616.

[69] Ross HJ, Blumenschein GR, Aisner J, et al. Randomized phase II multicenter trial of two schedules of lapatinib as first-or second-line monotherapy in patients with advanced or metastatic non-small cell lung cancer. Clin Cancer Res, 2010, 16: 1938-1949.

第27章
非小细胞肺癌中表皮生长因子受体耐药机制

Erminia Massarelli
Department of Thoracic Head and Neck Medical Oncology, The University of Texas MD Anderson Cancer Center, Houston, TX, USA

引 言

肺癌是造成美国癌症患者死亡的首要原因[1]。对高危人群进行肺癌筛查最近已被批准[2],但不幸的是仍有大部分非小细胞肺癌(NSCLC)患者确诊时已属晚期。作为针对表皮生长因子受体(*EGFR*)阳性突变的靶向药物,表皮生长因子受体酪氨酸激酶抑制剂(EGFR-tyrosine kinase inhibitors,EGFR-TKIs)——厄洛替尼、吉非替尼的问世及临床成功应用,改变了 NSCLC 的治疗模式[3-5]。目前,这类药物已获得美国 FDA 批准用于晚期 NSCLC 的一线治疗。

EGFR 家族包括4个成员:EGFR、人类表皮生长因子受体2(HER2)、HER3 及 HER4。相关活性配体通过与受体的细胞外结构域特异性结合诱发受体的(同)异二聚体化,进而激活胞质酪氨酸激酶,刺激包括 Ras/细胞外信号调节激酶通路,磷脂酰肌醇-3激酶(PI3K)/v-AKT 小鼠胸腺瘤病毒癌基因(AKT)通路,信号转导和转录激活因子通路以及细胞内信号转导通路在内的多条细胞内信号通路[6]。*EGFR* 基因编码酪氨酸激酶区的突变与 EGFR-TKIs 疗效的提高密切相关,而这种认识更好地表征突变类型及它们的功能意义。

EGFR 突变在高加索 NSCLC 患者中的发生率约为15%,在亚洲患者中约为30%,基因突变通常与腺癌、女性、不吸烟等特征密切相关[7]。最常见的 *EGFR* 激活突变包括18外显子点突变(6%)、19外显子插入或缺失(6%)、20外显子的插入或重复和点突变(9%)以及21外显子的点突变(39%)[7]。这些突变打破了 EGFR 激酶激活及抑制状态的平衡,促进了激酶活性的释放,最终导致对 EGFR 的"癌基因依赖"及肿瘤生长存活优势的建立[7-8]。赋予 EGFR-TKI 治疗敏感性最典型的突变位于19外显子(缺失,尤其是 E746-A750del 缺失)和21外显子上(L858R)。表达这些突变的患者对 EGFR-TKIs 治疗有效率高(高达70%),且较 *EGFR* 野生型患者中位生存期显著延长(达27个月)[9-10]。

EGFR-TKIs 原发性耐药通常是由于 EGFR 基因突变致第一代 EGFR-TKIs 无效,如20外显子插入突变或其他影响 EGFR 信号通路的体细胞突变,如 KRAS[11-12]。原发性耐药也可能由于 EGFR-TKI 耐药的从头显现或 *EGFR* 基因的失活突变。在表达 *EGFR* 有效突变的患者中应用厄洛替尼或吉非替尼的临床数据显示,这些患者最终会发展为可逆性 EGFR-TKIs 耐药,一般认为发生这种耐药的原因可能是 *EGFR* 基因发生获得性突变或其他 *EGFR* 基因型之外的相关机制,例如旁路信号通路的激活。

旁路信号通路的激活参与了 EGFR-TKIs 的原发和获得性耐药。主要的旁路信号包括 PI3K/AKT 通路[13],胰岛素样生长因子1受体[14]以及间质表皮转化因子(c-MET)[15-16]。MET 基因扩增能同时介导原发和获得性耐药的发生。另外,由于肿瘤异质性,多重耐药机制可在同一患者中同时存在。

本章将具体阐述 NSCLC 患者发生 EGFR-TKIs 原发和获得性耐药的已知相关机制。

EGFR-TKIs 原发性耐药

图27.1 阐述了 *EGFR* 突变的 NSCLC 患者发生

原发性耐药的机制及发生频率，这些机制主要包括发生 EGFR 耐药突变、ErbB 家族其他成员受体发生突变或扩增以及其他激活逃逸途径相关基因的突变，如 v-Ki-ras2 Kirsten 大鼠肉瘤病毒癌基因同源物，KRAS，原癌基因 B-Raf（BRAF），磷脂酰肌醇 -4，5-二磷酸激酶催化亚基（PIK3CA），磷酸酶和张力蛋白同源物（PTEN）缺失[7, 10, 11,13, 17-23]。

EGFR 耐药突变

EGFR 基因 20 外显子插入突变占整个 EGFR 突变的 1%～10%，而大多数该类突变与 EGFR-TKIs 的耐药有关[12]。表 27.1 综合了原发性耐药的突变类型。20 外显子插入突变在 N 端或在其相反的 C 端位置插入残基。尽管尚未报道有晶体结构形成，但其可能会影响激酶结构域的功能[24]。插入突变主要限制在 EGFR 基因 C 端之后的 N 端半段结构（M766 到 C775）及紧随 C 端的喜好位置（A767～C775），对调控 EGFR 酪氨酸激酶活性起关键作用[25]。该关键区域调控激酶状态，使其控制腺苷-5′-三磷酸与 EGFR-TKI 结合并事实上推动 C 端结构的行程，最终形成并激活激酶结构域[26]。据报道，有一些 C 端 20 外显子插入突变影响了 E762～Y764 残基及 EGFR 活性[7, 13, 27-28]，其中一项研究显示 2 例表达 Y764_V765insHH 或 M766_A767insA 突变的患者应用 EGFR-TKIs 后疾病控制时间延长，说明了这些突变能介导至少中等水平的药物敏感性[29]。

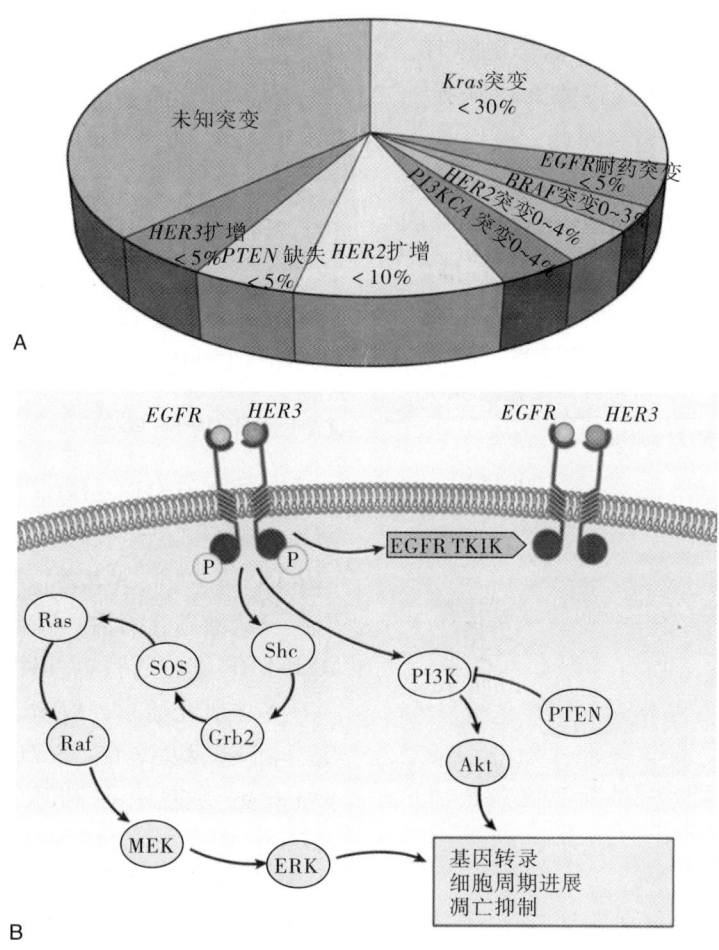

图 27.1 EGFR-TKIs 原发性耐药机制。A. 肺癌 EGFR 抑制治疗原发性耐药中已知驱动癌基因范围及相对发生频率。B. EGFR 下游分子激活以及其他 ErbB 酪氨酸激酶家族成员绕过 EGFR-TKIs 抑制的 EGFR 信号通路诱导 EGFR-TKIs 原发性耐药

诸如D770_N771（insNPG）、D770_（insSVQ）、D770_（insG）、N771T-（30）及H773_V774insH[31]在内的插入突变介导了对厄洛替尼和吉非替尼从原发到临床的耐药。一项美国亚裔NSCLC患者EGFR突变特点的研究[32]，确定了两种提高激酶活性并介导厄洛替尼耐药的20外显子突变类型（N771GY_delN771insGY和A767_V769dup）。其他两项研究也证实了A767_V769dupASV为耐药突变[31,33]。Q787R转染相比L858R转染能降低吉非替尼的体外敏感性，Q787R与L858R共转染显示敏感性居中[17]。

口服非可逆性EGFR、HER2抑制剂［来那替尼（HKI-272），阿法替尼（BIBW2992）］及达可替尼（PF00299804）的研究结果显示，表达A767_V769dupASV、D770_N771insNPG、delN771insGY和H773_V774insH突变细胞同转染经典耐药基因T790M的肿瘤细胞模型对上述化合物的IC$_{50}$基本相似，相较L858R经典突变转染和19外显子缺失型的灵敏度减少约100倍。因此，可以预见阿法替尼和PF00299804对这类肿瘤比对EGFR敏感的突变肿瘤（L858R和19外显子缺失）的临床效果差。

表27.1　EGFR原发性耐药20外显子突变

插入及缺失	点突变
D770_N771 ins NPG/D770 N771insNPG	A763V
N771GY delN771insGY	K806E
N771dupN	
A767_V769dupASV	L777G
H773 V774insH/M/dup H	P772R
DelA767 V769	S784F
770_771ins VDSVDNP	V769L/M
S768 V769EinsVAS	V774M
V769D770delinsGI	Y801C
V768D770dupSVD	
M766V769insWPA	
S768D770dupSVD	
A767S768insSVR	

来源：摘自Massarelli E, Johnson FM, Erickson HS, et al. Uncommon Epidermal Growth Factor Receptor mutations in non-small cell lung cancer and their mechanisms of EGFR tyrosine kinase inhibitors sensitivity and resistance. Lung Cancer, 2013

在一项关于来那替尼的Ⅱ期临床试验中，3例20外显子突变（S768_D770dupSVD、H773_V774dupHV、delN771insGF）的NSCLC患者对治疗没有反应[34]。一项PF00299804的Ⅰ期临床试验显示，6例表达EGFR20外显子插入突变的患者中仅有1例（表达delA770insGY突变）对治疗有效[35]。在一项纳入11例表达EGFR 20外显子插入突变患者应用阿法替尼（BIBW2992）的Ⅱ期临床试验中，只有1例疗效为部分有效，而这些患者的无进展生存期均较短[36-37]。热休克蛋白90抑制剂已在EGFR突变阳性的晚期NSCLC患者中进行了研究，包括EGFR在内的突变癌基因合成蛋白更需要热休克蛋白90作为分子伴侣进而发挥作用[38]。而一项在76例晚期NSCLC患者中进行的关于热休克蛋白90抑制剂——IPI-504的Ⅱ期临床试验显示，其在EGFR突变患者中的有效率极低（4%）[39]。

在表达多种EGFR突变的患者中，EGFR-TKIs的疗效尚不确定，并取决于参与的突变种类是否与发生单个突变的患者相似[40-41]。然而，同时表达G719S和L858R的患者对吉非替尼的疗效不佳[40,42-45]，但L858R+D761Y，L858R+L747S和L858R+T854A这几种混合突变的耐药性低于L858R+T790M突变[48]。

KRAS 和 BRAF 突变

RAS基因编码21kDa膜结合鸟苷酸结合蛋白家族，调控细胞生长、分化和凋亡。3个RAS基因（HRAS、K-RAS、N-RAS）中任一基因的点突变会引起三磷酸鸟苷酶活性降低，进而诱导RAS-RAF-MEK-ERK细胞质激酶级联激活。

多项研究显示，KRAS与EGFR突变为互斥突变[7,11,49]。KRAS在NSCLC中的突变率为20%~30%，主要集中在肺腺癌（30%）和吸烟者（17%）中[50]。KRAS突变最常见的类型为密码子12中胸腺嘧啶鸟嘌呤残基替换，引起KRAS的持续激活。关于KRAS突变对NSCLC患者生存的影响尚存在争议，但是越来越多的证据显示KRAS突变与EGFR-TKIs的有效率低有关[11,17,51-53]。

BRAF突变仅在2%~3%的NSCLC患者中出现，通常与RAS和EGFR突变互斥，主要在现时及曾经吸烟的患者中表达[21]。相比于其他肿瘤（如恶性黑色素瘤），BRAF 突变而非 V600E 替换在肺癌中的发生率更高[21]。含有 BRAF 突变的患者预后更差[22]。

PIK3CA 突变和 PTEN 缺失

PI3K/Akt 级联信号通路是另一条由 EGFR 激活并对细胞生长存活起关键作用的通路[54-55]。PIK3CA 基因（编码 PI3K 激酶 p110 亚基）的激活突变及抑癌基因 PTEN 表达缺失导致了这条癌基因通路的异常激活。PTEN 缺失牵涉到多重机制，包括体细胞突变（如常染色体显性 Cowden 综合征）[56]，引起位于染色体 10q 的 Cowden 等位基因缺失的零星突变[57]，启动子甲基化引起的基因沉默[58]以及促进基因沉默的特定微小 RNA（microRNA）的上调[59]。这些基因沉默和蛋白失活的机制最终导致肿瘤中 PTEN 表达缺失。而在临床前模型中，PI3K 和 PTEN 的表达与 EGFR-TKIs 的耐药相关[60-62]。

PIK3CA 基因编码 PI3K 激酶的主要催化亚基——p110α 异构体，其突变率为 3%~4%，并在 12%~20% 的肺鳞癌中有扩增[63-65]。PIK3CA 突变与 EGFR 和 KRAS 突变并不相互排斥[64-66]。在既往未接受 EGFR-TKIs 治疗的 EGFR 突变阳性患者中也可以检测到 PIK3CA 突变[64,67]。在一项研究中，所有表达 PIK3CA 突变的患者均同时存在 EGFR 突变，PIK3CA 突变存在于 9 和 20 外显子中[67]。然而，体外研究显示，PI3K 主催化亚基（PIK3CA）突变同样也被视为 EGFR-TKIs 获得性耐药的一种机制[68]，该机制在 2 例 EGFR 突变阳性并在 EGFR-TKIs 治疗过程中发生疾病进展的患者中也得到验证[69]。

研究表明，PTEN 缺失也是 EGFR 阳性突变患者发生 TKIs 耐药的潜在机制[13]，与吉非替尼治疗人群的总生存期预后不良相关[70]。在 EGFR 野生型肿瘤中，同时出现 PTEN 缺失和 PIK3CA 突变往往预示吉非替尼治疗预后较差[18]。

ErbB 家族成员：突变和扩增

包括 HER2、HER3 和 HER4 在内的其他 ErbB 家族成员在 EGFR-TKIs 耐药中发挥了关键作用，因为在与配体结合后 EGFR 会与其他 ErbB 家族成员形成同（异）二聚体。HER2 基因突变，往往与 EGFR 突变互斥，在肺腺癌中表达率较低（4%）[7,19,71]，且大部分发生于女性、不吸烟、亚裔及肺腺癌患者。HER2 突变的最常见类型是引起 HER2 激酶持续激活的 20 外显子框内插入[7,19,71]。

最近的研究发现，在不表达 EGFR-T790M 突变的 EGFR-TKI 耐药肺癌中存在 HER2 扩增的表达[20]。但 HER2 扩增与 EGFR-TKIs 治疗敏感性之间的相关性尚存在争议[72-75]。

EGFR-TKIs 的获得性耐药

EGFR-TKIs 的获得性耐药可以由 EGFR 基因的二次突变引起，最常见的是 20 外显子 T790M 突变，或引起其他旁路信号通路激活，使肿瘤摆脱"癌基因依赖"状态。MET 扩增、肝细胞生长因子（hepatocyte growth factor，HGF）过表达及胰岛素样生长因子-1 受体通路是与 EGFR 通路激活间接相关的最常见的逃逸机制。另一个新近发现的耐药机制是组织学转变，通常是转变为小细胞肺癌[69]。图 27.2 总结了 EGFR-TKI 获得性耐药的发生频率和发生机制[20, 69, 76-77]。

EGFR 获得性突变

T790M 是最常见的获得性耐药突变[78-80]。T790M 位于 EGFR 催化区内结合 EGFR-TKIs 的腺苷三磷酸结合口袋结构中，而该位点对腺苷三磷酸的亲和性高于 EGFR-TKIs[25]。

EGFR-T790M 突变位置与介导伊马替尼耐药的 BCR-ABL1、KIT 和 PDGFRA 等基因催化区突变类似[ABL1 基因 T315 突变为异亮氨酸（I），KIT 基因 T670I 突变及 PDGFRA 基因 T764I 突变][81-82]。

激酶活性位点附近的苏氨酸残基的突变会稳定 EGFR 酪氨酸激酶活性构象[83]。对 EGFR-TKIs 获得性耐药患者的临床组织切片研究显示，T790M 突变出现在约 50% 的肺腺癌患者中[84]。部分患者初诊时即有部分肿瘤细胞表达 T790M 突变[13]，而在第一代 EGFR-TKIs 治疗过程中，不断的克隆选择导致 T790M 肿瘤细胞持续扩增，最终在整个肿块中占主导地位[85-86]。

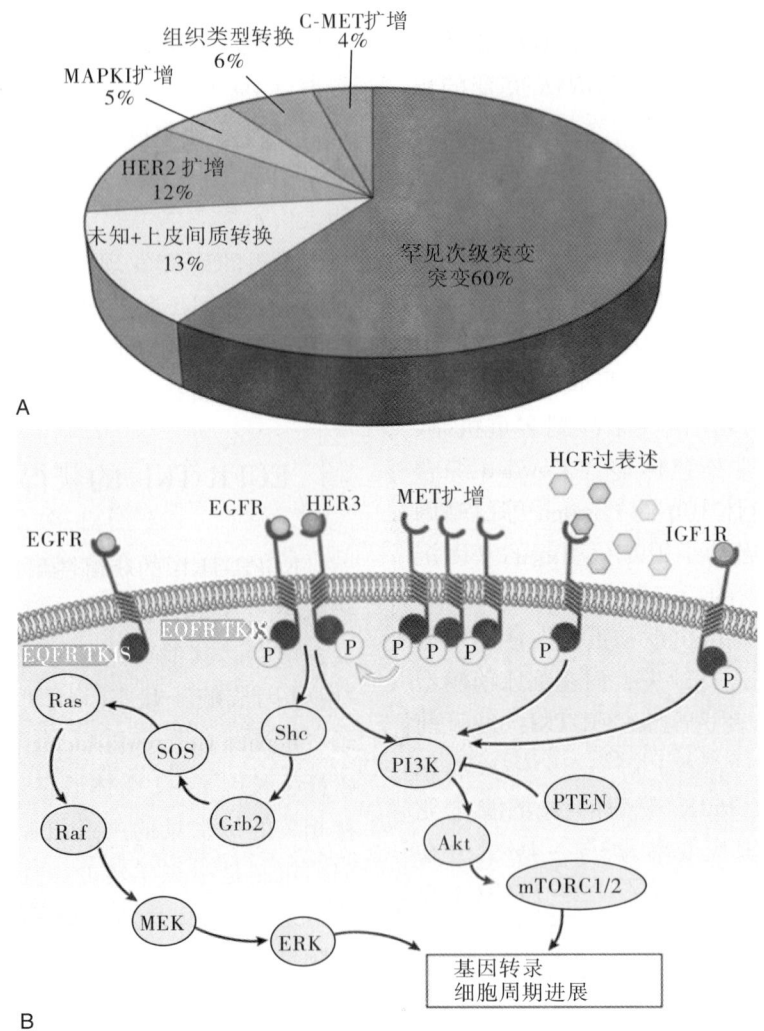

图27.2 EGFR-TKIs获得性耐药机制。A. 肺癌 EGFR 抑制治疗获得性耐药中已知驱动癌基因范围及相对发生频率。B. EGFR 抑制剂获得性耐药信号通路示意图。EGFR 继发性 T790M 突变导致其对 EGFR-TKIs 亲和性降低。MET 或 IGFR 激活诱导 PI3K/Akt 通路活性升高，该效应不依赖于 EGFR 活性

体外研究显示，T790M 突变细胞相较于其 EGFR-TKI 敏感的未突变细胞，其在厄洛替尼和非可逆性 EGFR 抑制剂 BIBW2992 作用下生长不占优势[87]。文献报道这种生长动力学的差异与部分获得性耐药患者的"突然紧张"和"再反应"现象有一定相关性，说明耐药肿瘤细胞很可能是由 TKI、敏感细胞和 TKI 耐药细胞构成的混合体[80]。当撤除选择性压力（TKI）后，之前细胞周期停滞的 TKI 敏感细胞比耐药细胞生长更快，肿瘤也重新对 EGFR-TKIs 敏感。在获得性耐药患者中，T790M 也和惰性表型相关。对 93 例 EGFR 突变及 TKI 获得性耐药肺癌患者的活检标本检测显示，T790M 介导耐药患者的预后更好[88]。T790M 介导耐药的惰性表型意味着这些患者即使在疾病进展后继续服用单药 TKI，有时也能获得数月的生存期[89]；最终发展为恶性程度更高的表型往往意味着分子机制上的"第三重打击"，而其中的具体机制有待进一步研究。T790M 突变与更佳预后的相关性显示了活检在评估患者疗效中的重要临床价值。

其他一些对 EGFR-TKIs 非敏感的不常见获得性突变有 L747S、D761Y 和 T854A[16,46,48]。对一例脑转移患者的研究表明，外显子 19 的 D761Y 突变降低了 EGFR-L858R 突变对 EGFR-TKIs 的敏感性[46]。L747S 二次突变影响 EGFR 催化裂口；一例肺癌患者对单药吉非替尼长时间有效并最终发生了该等位基因突变[6,30]。L747S 耐药模式不及 L858R-T790M 明显。最近，在一例长期接受吉非

替尼和厄洛替尼治疗的患者中发现了 T854A 突变。该位点突变为疏水丙氨酸残基后可能增加选择性口袋结构的大小，最终下调其与 TKI 的结合力；该发现有体外和体内试验数据的支持[16,90]。

HER2 扩增

最近，研究人员用荧光免疫杂交技术显示 HER2 扩增在 12% 的获得性耐药肿瘤中表达而且在未治疗肺腺癌患者中的表达率仅为 1%[20]。值得注意的是，HER2 扩增与 EGFR-T790M 突变相互排斥。该结果揭示了一项之前未知的 EGFR-TKIs 耐药机制，并为在发生获得性耐药的 EGFR 突变患者中检测 HER2 基因状态并使之成为潜在治疗靶点提供了理论基础。

MAPK1 扩增

一例接受厄洛替尼治疗并发生耐药患者的活检切片显示发生了 MAPK1 基因扩增，而在治疗前的组织切片中并没有该扩增出现[76]。耐药肿瘤也没有表达 EGFR-T790M 或 MET 扩增等更常见的耐药机制[76]。

MET 扩增

c-MET 约占所有 EGFR 突变、并发生 EGFR-TKIs 获得性耐药机制的 20%，但其在未治 EGFR 突变阳性的患者中的表达率仅为 3%[15-16]。在 MET 基因扩增的肿瘤，通过共受体 HER3 刺激细胞引起 PI3K 通路激活，从而抑制 EGFR-TKIs 的效果[15]。约有 50% 表达 MET 扩增的患者同时表达 T790M 突变，但尚不清楚吉非替尼或厄洛替尼治疗是否优先选择 c-MET 扩增克隆。在最近的两项研究中，荧光原位杂交显示，在所报道病例中有 3%[77] 和 5%[69] 高表达 MET 扩增。最近的研究中 MET 扩增表达率偏低可能是因为在临床样本中检测该基因突变尚存在难度。而最初的两项研究则运用了多种检测方法，包括阵列式基因体杂交比较法、实时定量 PCR 法及荧光原位杂交等来综合评估 MET 的扩增量[15-16]。

对 16 份获得性耐药的 NSCLC 患者的标本进行分析显示，25%（4/16）的患者标本中检测到了 MET 扩增，但这 4 份标本在吉非替尼治疗前 MET 扩增的表达率极低（<1%）。并且，在这 4 份标本中，吉非替尼治疗后 HGF 表达量较治疗前显著升高。该结果表明 HGF 与 MET 扩增共同加速了肿瘤生长。

HGF 过表达

在无 MET 扩增的情况下 HGF 过表达是 EGFR-TKI 耐药的机制之一[91]。对吉非替尼耐药的肺腺癌患者的组织标本研究显示，不表达 T790M 突变或 MET 扩增的肺癌细胞中 HGF 表达水平较高。HGF 过表达能诱导含有 EGFR-TKIs 敏感突变的肺腺癌细胞对吉非替尼或厄洛替尼耐药[91]。HGF 过表达不需要 ErbB3 磷酸化，而是通过 MET 磷酸化来刺激 PI3K/AKT 通路激活。体外实验显示当把吉非替尼敏感的肺癌细胞与产生 HGF 的成纤维细胞共培养时，原本敏感的肺癌细胞会对吉非替尼产生耐药[92]。此外，HGF 抗体或 HGF 拮抗剂 - NK4 可以消除成纤维细胞分泌 HGF 诱导的耐药[92]，提示 HGF 抑制剂可以用来逆转 EGFR-TKIs 耐药。

IGF-1R 信号通路和其他通路

其他并行信号通路可能也构成了 EGFR-TKIs 的耐药机制，如血管内皮生长因子受体（VEGFR）和 IGF-1R。将 NSCLC 细胞系暴露于抗 EGFR 抗体时会引起血管内皮生长因子（VEGF）上调 4 倍[93]。VEGF 通路的激活能共刺激肿瘤细胞。相似的是，IGF-1R 能激活 EGFR 通路下游靶点，从而绕过细胞对 EGFR 的依赖性[14]。在持续接触第一代 TKI 的 NSCLC 细胞中，IGF-1R 活性的提高能引起细胞增殖[94]。

组织学类型转换

Sequist 等[69] 最近报道了一项 37 例 EGFR-TKI 治疗后进展并再次活检的晚期 NSCLC 病例的研究。37 例患者中有 5 例的肿瘤组织学类型转变为小细胞肺癌（SCLC）。这些转化肿瘤患者对治疗 SCLC 的经典化疗方案有效。

表皮-间质转化（EMT）

包括 NSCLC 在内的多种上皮癌症都有表皮-间质转化（epithelial-mesenchymal transition, EMT）

的发生。EMT 与细胞黏附蛋白如 E - 钙黏蛋白的缺失相关,并增加细胞浸润、迁移和增殖能力[95]。相关基础和临床试验的结果提示 EMT 标志蛋白与 EGFR 抑制剂效果受限有关,而即便患者不表达 *EGFR* 突变,上皮表型也意味着其对 TKI 治疗有较好的反应[96]。在与 EMT 相关的几个分子标志中,受体酪氨酸激酶 Axl 有望成为判定 EGFR-TKI 耐药的潜在靶点[97]。

药物相互作用

药物相互作用也能影响 EGFR-TKI 的血浆浓度。厄洛替尼与细胞色素 P450 - 3A4(CYP3A4)诱导剂间的药物相互作用能引起次优药物暴露,同时可能降低抗肿瘤作用[98]。吸烟能降低血浆 EGFR-TKIs 浓度。在一项Ⅲ期临床试验中,吸烟的 NSCLC 患者中厄洛替尼稳定血浆浓度约比已戒烟或不吸烟患者低 2 倍[99]。该效应同时伴随吸烟诱导细胞色素 P450(CYP)1A 异构体的增加,致使厄洛替尼血浆清除率提高 24%[99]。一项在健康志愿者中进行的评估厄洛替尼单剂量药代动力学的研究中,吸烟者的药物清除速度要显著快于已戒烟或不吸烟者[100]。吸烟者的 AUC 曲线下 0 至无穷大面积分别是不吸烟者和已戒烟者的 1/3 ~ 1/2。在另一项对 35 例吸烟肺癌患者进行的研究中,稳定状态的药代动力学分析显示,当厄洛替尼剂量从 150mg 增至 300mg 时,患者的血药浓度成比例升高,但是吸烟患者推荐使用的具体药物剂量尚不清楚。

肿瘤异质性

肿瘤异质性或许在 EGFR-TKI 耐药中起重要作用[101]。事实上,在最近的一项研究中,30% 参与研究的患者有肿瘤异质性,*EGFR* 突变的含量与 EGFR-TKIs 的有效性和患者的预后相关[101]。

研究 EGFR-TKIs 获得性耐药的另一个挑战是不能持续获得肿瘤组织以用于确定 *EGFR* 突变。目前的一些临床试验考虑到了肿瘤的异质性,并正在测试治疗的最佳时间和策略,预防或延缓耐药的发生。

总 结

总之,*EGFR* 突变明确了一类 NSCLC 患者可从 EGFR-TKIs 在内的靶向治疗中获益。然而,最大的挑战在于克服 EGFR-TKIs 的原发和获得性耐药。在更换治疗方案前确定 EGFR-TKIs 耐药是有必要的,优先推荐对耐药肿瘤进行活检来指导下一步的治疗。

(倪 阳 韩 玥译)

参考文献

[1] Siegel R, Naishadham D, Jemal A. Cancer statistics, 2013. CA Cancer J Clin, 2013, 63(1): 11 - 30.
[2] Aberle DR, Adams AM, Berg CD, et al. Reduced lung-cancer mortality with low-dose computed tomographic screening. N Engl J Med, 2011, 365(5): 395 - 409.
[3] Lynch TJ, Bell DW, Sordella R, et al. Activating mutations in the epidermal growth factor receptor underlying responsiveness of non-small-cell lung cancer to gefitinib. N Engl J Med, 2004, 350(21): 2129 - 2139.
[4] Paez JG, Janne PA, Lee JC, et al. EGFR mutations in lung cancer: correlation with clinical response to gefitinib therapy. Science, 2004, 304(5676): 1497 - 1500.
[5] Pao W, Miller V, Zakowski M, et al. EGF receptor gene mutations are common in lung cancers from "never smokers" and are associated with sensitivity of tumors to gefitinib and erlotinib. Proc Natl Acad Sci USA, 2004, 101(36): 13306 - 13311.
[6] Kumar A, Petri ET, Halmos B, et al. Structure and clinical relevance of the epidermal growth factor receptor in human cancer. J Clin Oncol, 2008, 26(10): 1742 - 1751.
[7] Shigematsu H, Lin L, Takahashi T, et al. Clinical and biological features associated with epidermal growth factor receptor gene mutations in lung cancers. J Natl Cancer Inst, 2005, 97(5): 339 - 346.
[8] Gazdar AF, Minna JD. Deregulated EGFR signaling during lung cancer progression: mutations, amplicons, and autocrine loops. Cancer Prev Res(Phila), 2008, 1(3): 156 - 160.
[9] Costa DB, Kobayashi S, Tenen DG, et al. Pooled analysis of the prospective trials of gefitinib monotherapy for EGFR-mutant non-small cell lung cancers. Lung Cancer, 2007, 58(1): 95 - 103.
[10] Sequist LV, Martins RG, Spigel D, et al. First-line gefitinib in patients with advanced non-small-cell lung cancer harboring somatic EGFR mutations. J Clin Oncol,

2008, 26 (15): 2442-2449.

[11] Pao W, Wang TY, Riely GJ, et al. KRAS mutations and primary resistance of lung adenocarcinomas to gefitinib or erlotinib. PLoS Med, 2005, 2 (1): e17.

[12] Yasuda H, Kobayashi S, Costa DB. EGFR exon 20 insertion mutations in non-small-cell lung cancer: preclinical data and clinical implications. Lancet Oncol, 13 (1): e23-31.

[13] Sos ML, Koker M, Weir BA, et al. PTEN loss contributes to erlotinib resistance in EGFR-mutant lung cancer by activation of Akt and EGFR. Cancer Res, 2009, 69 (8): 3256-3261.

[14] Guix M, Faber AC, Wang SE, et al. Acquired resistance to EGFR tyrosine kinase inhibitors in cancer cells is mediated by loss of IGF-binding proteins. J Clin Invest, 2008, 118 (7): 2609-2619.

[15] Engelman JA, Zejnullahu K, Mitsudomi T, et al. MET amplification leads to gefitinib resistance in lung cancer by activating ERBB3 signaling. Science, 2007, 316 (5827): 1039-1043.

[16] Bean J, Riely GJ, Balak M, et al. Acquired resistance to epidermal growth factor receptor kinase inhibitors associated with a novel T854A mutation in a patient with EGFR-mutant lung adenocarcinoma. Clin Cancer Res, 2008, 14 (22): 7519-7525.

[17] Tam IY, Chung LP, Suen WS, et al. Distinct epidermal growth factor receptor and KRAS mutation patterns in non-small cell lung cancer patients with different tobacco exposure and clinicopathologic features. Clin Cancer Res, 2006, 12 (5): 1647-1653.

[18] Fidler MJ, Morrison LE, Basu S, et al. PTEN and PIK3CA gene copy numbers and poor outcomes in non-small cell lung cancer patients with gefitinib therapy. Br J Cancer, 2011, 105 (12): 1920-1926.

[19] Sasaki H, Shimizu S, Endo K, et al. EGFR and erbB2 mutation status in Japanese lung cancer patients. Int J Cancer, 2006, 118 (1): 180-184.

[20] Takezawa K, Pirazzoli V, Arcila ME, et al. HER2 amplification: a potential mechanism of acquired resistance to EGFR inhibition in EGFR-mutant lung cancers that lack the second-site EGFRT790M mutation. Cancer Discov, 2012, 2 (10): 922-933.

[21] Paik PK, Arcila ME, Fara M, et al. Clinical characteristics of patients with lung adenocarcinomas harboring BRAF mutations. J Clin Oncol, 2011, 29 (15): 2046-2051.

[22] Marchetti A, Felicioni L, Malatesta S, et al. Clinical features and outcome of patients with non-small-cell lung cancer harboring BRAF mutations. J Clin Oncol, 2011, 29 (26): 3574-3579.

[23] Cappuzzo F, Toschi L, Domenichini I, et al. HER3 genomic gain and sensitivity to gefitinib in advanced non-smallcell lung cancer patients. Br J Cancer, 2005, 93 (12): 1334-1340.

[24] Pao W, Chmielecki J. Rational, biologically based treatment of EGFR-mutant non-small-cell lung cancer. Nat Rev Cancer, 2010, 10 (11): 760-774.

[25] Yun CH, Mengwasser KE, Toms AV, et al. The T790M mutation in EGFR kinase causes drug resistance by increasing the affinity for ATP. Proc Natl Acad Sci USA, 2008, 105 (6): 2070-2075.

[26] Eck MJ, Yun CH. Structural and mechanistic underpinnings of the differential drug sensitivity of EGFR mutations in non-small cell lung cancer. Biochim Biophys Acta, 2010, 1804 (3): 559-566.

[27] Linardou H, Dahabreh IJ, Bafaloukos D, et al. Somatic EGFR mutations and efficacy of tyrosine kinase inhibitors in NSCLC. Nat Rev Clin Oncol, 2009, 6 (6): 352-366.

[28] Murray S, Dahabreh IJ, Linardou H, et al. Somatic mutations of the tyrosine kinase domain of epidermal growth factor receptor and tyrosine kinase inhibitor response to TKIs in non-small cell lung cancer: an analytical database. J Thorac Oncol, 2008, 3 (8): 832-839.

[29] Yasuda H, Kobayashi S, Costa DB. EGFR exon 20 insertion mutations in non-small-cell lung cancer: preclinical data and clinical implications. Lancet Oncol, 2012, 13 (1): e23-e31.

[30] Greulich H, Chen TH, Feng W, et al. Oncogenic transformation by inhibitor-sensitive and-resistant EGFR mutants. PLoS Med, 2005, 2 (11): e313.

[31] Yuza Y, Glatt KA, Jiang J, et al. Allele-dependent variation in the relative cellular potency of distinct EGFR inhibitors. Cancer Biol Ther, 2007, 6 (5): 661-667.

[32] Harada T, Lopez-Chavez A, Xi L, et al. Characterization of epidermal growth factor receptor mutations in non-small-cell lung cancer patients of African-American ancestry. Oncogene, 2011, 30 (15): 1744-1752.

[33] Engelman JA, Zejnullahu K, Gale CM, et al. PF00299804, an irreversible pan-ERBB inhibitor, is effective in lung cancer models with EGFR and ERBB2 mutations that are resistant to gefitinib. Cancer Res, 2007, 67 (24): 11924-11932.

[34] Sequist LV, Besse B, Lynch TJ, et al. Neratinib, an ir-

[34] reversible pan- ErbB receptor tyrosine kinase inhibitor: results of a phase II trial in patients with advanced non-small-cell lung cancer. J Clin Oncol, 2010, 28 (18): 3076-3083.

[35] Janne PA, Boss DS, Camidge DR, et al. Phase I doseescalation study of the pan-HER inhibitor, PF299804, in patients with advanced malignant solid tumors. Clin Cancer Res, 2011, 17 (5): 1131-1139.

[36] Shih J, Yu CJ, Su W. Activity of BIBW 2992, an irreversible EGFR/HER1 TKI, in lung adenocarcinoma patients harboring less common EGFR mutations. Ann Oncol, 2011, 21 (Suppl 8): 415.

[37] Yang CH, Shih J, Chao T. Use of BIBW 2992, a novel irreversible EGFR/HER2 TKI to induce regression in patients with adenocarcinoma of the lung and activating EGFR mutations preliminary results of a single-arm phase II clinical trial. Proc Am Soc Clin Oncol, 2008, 26 (15S) (May 20 Supplement): 8026.

[38] Shimamura T, Lowell AM, Engelman JA, et al. Epidermal growth factor receptors harboring kinase domain mutations associate with the heat shock protein 90 chaperone and are destabilized following exposure to geldanamycins. Cancer Res, 2005, 65 (14): 6401-6408.

[39] Sequist LV, Gettinger S, Senzer NN, et al. Activity of IPI-504, a novel heat-shock protein 90 inhibitor, in patients with molecularly defined non-small-cell lung cancer. J Clin Oncol, 2010, 28 (33): 4953-4960.

[40] Wu SG, Chang YL, Hsu YC, et al. Good response to gefitinib in lung adenocarcinoma of complex epidermal growth factor receptor (EGFR) mutations with the classical mutation pattern. Oncologist, 2008, 13 (12): 1276-1284.

[41] Zhang GC, Lin JY, Wang Z, et al. Epidermal growth factor receptor double activating mutations involving both exons 19 and 21 exist in Chinese non-small cell lung cancer patients. Clin Oncol (R Coll Radiol), 2007, 19 (7): 499-506.

[42] Chou TY, Chiu CH, Li LH, et al. Mutation in the tyrosine kinase domain of epidermal growth factor receptor is a predictive and prognostic factor for gefitinib treatment in patients with non-small cell lung cancer. Clin Cancer Res, 2005, 11 (10): 3750-3757.

[43] Hata A, Yoshioka H, Fujita S, et al. Complex mutations in the epidermal growth factor receptor gene in non-small cell lung cancer. J Thorac Oncol, 2010, 5 (10): 1524-1528.

[44] Jiang J, Greulich H, Janne PA, et al. Epidermal growth factorindependent transformation of Ba/F3 cells with cancer-derived epidermal growth factor receptor mutants induces gefitinib-sensitive cell cycle progression. Cancer Res, 2005, 65 (19): 8968-8974.

[45] Mitsudomi T, Yatabe Y. Mutations of the epidermal growth factor receptor gene and related genes as determinants of epidermal growth factor receptor tyrosine kinase inhibitors sensitivity in lung cancer. Cancer Sci, 2007, 98 (12): 1817-1824.

[46] Balak MN, Gong Y, Riely GJ, et al. Novel D761Y and common secondary T790M mutations in epidermal growth factor receptor-mutant lung adenocarcinomas with acquired resistance to kinase inhibitors. Clin Cancer Res, 2006, 12 (21): 6494-6501.

[47] Costa DB, Schumer ST, Tenen DG, et al. Differential responses to erlotinib in epidermal growth factor receptor (EGFR) -mutated lung cancers with acquired resistance to gefitinib carrying the L747S or T790M secondary mutations. J Clin Oncol, 2008, 26 (7): 1182-1184; author reply 4-6.

[48] Costa DB, Halmos B, Kumar A, et al. BIM mediates EGFR tyrosine kinase inhibitor-induced apoptosis in lung cancers with oncogenic EGFR mutations. PLoS Med, 2007, 4 (10): 1669-1679; discussion 80.

[49] Janne PA, Engelman JA, Johnson BE. Epidermal growth factor receptor mutations in nonsmall-cell lung cancer: Implications for treatment and tumor biology. J Clin Oncol, 2005, 23 (14): 3227-3234.

[50] Graziano SL, Gamble GP, Newman NB, et al. Prognostic significance of K-ras codon 12 mutations in patients with resected stage I and II non-small-cell lung cancer. J Clin Oncol, 1999, 17 (2): 668-675.

[51] Eberhard DA, Johnson BE, Amler LC, et al. Mutations in the epidermal growth factor receptor and in KRAS are predictive and prognostic indicators in patients with non-small-cell lung cancer treated with chemotherapy alone and in combination with erlotinib. J Clin Oncol, 2005, 23 (25): 5900-5909.

[52] Massarelli E, Varella-Garcia M, Tang X, et al. KRAS mutation is an important predictor of resistance to therapy with epidermal growth factor receptor tyrosine kinase inhibitors in non-small-cell lung cancer. Clin Cancer Res, 2007, 13 (10): 2890-2896.

[53] Zhu CQ, da Cunha Santos G, Ding K, et al. Role of KRAS and EGFR as biomarkers of response to erlotinib in National Cancer Institute of Canada Clinical Trials Group Study

BR.21. J Clin Oncol, 2008, 26 (26): 4268-4275.

[54] Cantley LC. The phosphoinositide 3-kinase pathway. Science, 2002, 296 (5573): 1655-1657.

[55] Osaki M, Oshimura M, Ito H. PI3K-Akt pathway: Its functions and alterations in human cancer. Apoptosis, 2004, 9 (6): 667-676.

[56] Di Cristofano A, Pesce B, Cordon-Cardo C, et al. Pten is essential for embryonic development and tumour suppression. Nat Genet, 1998, 19 (4): 348-355.

[57] Frayling IM, Bodmer WF, Tomlinson IP. Allele loss in colorectal cancer at the Cowden disease/juvenile polyposis locus on 10q. Cancer Genet Cytogenet, 1997, 97 (1): 64-69.

[58] Goel A, Arnold CN, Niedzwiecki D, et al. Frequent inactivation of PTEN by promoter hypermethylation in microsatellite instability-high sporadic colorectal cancers. Cancer Res, 2004, 64 (9): 3014-3021.

[59] Meng F, Henson R, Wehbe-Janek H, et al. MicroRNA-21 regulates expression of the PTEN tumor suppressor gene in human hepatocellular cancer. Gastroenterology, 2007, 133 (2): 647-658.

[60] Janmaat ML, Kruyt FA, Rodriguez JA, et al. Response to epidermal growth factor receptor inhibitors in non-small cell lung cancer cells: limited antiproliferative effects and absence of apoptosis associated with persistent activity of extracellular signal-regulated kinase or Akt kinase pathways. Clin Cancer Res, 2003, 9 (6): 2316-2326.

[61] Engelman JA, Janne PA, Mermel C, et al. ErbB-3 mediates phosphoinositide 3-kinase activity in gefitinibsensitive non-small cell lung cancer cell lines. Proc Natl Acad Sci USA, 2005, 102 (10): 3788-3793.

[62] Yamasaki F, Johansen MJ, Zhang D, et al. Acquired resistance to erlotinib in A-431 epidermoid cancer cells requires down-regulation of MMAC1/PTEN and up-regulation of phosphorylated Akt. Cancer Res, 2007, 67 (12): 5779-5788.

[63] Hiles ID, Otsu M, Volinia S, et al. Phosphatidylinositol 3-kinase: structure and expression of the 110 kd catalytic subunit. Cell, 1992, 70 (3): 419-429.

[64] Kawano O, Sasaki H, Endo K, et al. PIK3CA mutation status in Japanese lung cancer patients. Lung Cancer, 2006, 54 (2): 209-215.

[65] Kawano O, Sasaki H, Okuda K, et al. PIK3CA gene amplification in Japanese non-small cell lung cancer. Lung Cancer, 2007, 58 (1): 159-160.

[66] Okudela K, Suzuki M, Kageyama S, et al. PIK3CA mutation and amplification in human lung cancer. Pathol Int, 2007, 57 (10): 664-671.

[67] Sun Y, Ren Y, Fang Z, et al. Lung adenocarcinoma from East Asian neversmokers is a disease largely defined by targetable oncogenic mutant kinases. J Clin Oncol, 2010, 28 (30): 4616-4620.

[68] Engelman JA, Mukohara T, Zejnullahu K, et al. Allelic dilution obscures detection of a biologically significant resistance mutation in EGFR-amplified lung cancer. J Clin Invest, 2006, 116 (10): 2695-2706.

[69] Sequist LV, Waltman BA, Dias-Santagata D, et al. Genotypic and histological evolution of lung cancers acquiring resistance to EGFR inhibitors. Sci Transl Med, 2011, 3 (75): 75ra26.

[70] Buckingham LE, Coon JS, Morrison LE, et al. The prognostic value of chromosome 7 polysomy in non-small cell lung cancer patients treated with gefitinib. J Thorac Oncol, 2007, 2 (5): 414-422.

[71] Stephens P, Hunter C, Bignell G, et al. Lung cancer: intragenic ERBB2 kinase mutations in tumours. Nature, 2004, 431 (7008): 525-526.

[72] Cappuzzo F, Varella-Garcia M, Shigematsu H, et al. Increased HER2 gene copy number is associated with response to gefitinib therapy in epidermal growth factor receptor-positive non-small-cell lung cancer patients. J Clin Oncol, 2005, 23 (22): 5007-5018.

[73] Cappuzzo F, Bemis L, Varella-Garcia M. HER2 mutation and response to trastuzumab therapy in non-small-cell lung cancer. N Engl J Med, 2006, 354 (24): 2619-2621.

[74] Cappuzzo F, Ligorio C, Toschi L, et al. EGFR and HER2 gene copy number and response to first-line chemotherapy in patients with advanced non-small cell lung cancer (NSCLC). J Thorac Oncol, 2007, 2 (5): 423-429.

[75] Daniele L, Macri L, Schena M, et al. Predicting gefitinib responsiveness in lung cancer by fluorescence in situ hybridization/chromogenic in situ hybridization analysis of EGFR and HER2 in biopsy and cytology specimens. Mol Cancer Ther, 2007, 6 (4): 1223-1229.

[76] Ercan D, Xu C, Yanagita M, et al. Reactivation of ERK signaling causes resistance to EGFR kinase inhibitors. Cancer Discov, 2012, 2 (10): 934-947.

[77] Arcila ME, Oxnard GR, Nafa K, et al. Rebiopsy of lung cancer patients with acquired resistance to EGFR inhibitors and enhanced detection of the T790M mutation using a locked nucleic acid-based assay. Clin Cancer Res, 2011, 17 (5): 1169-1180.

[78] Pao W, Miller VA, Politi KA, et al. Acquired resistance

[79] Kobayashi S, Boggon TJ, Dayaram T, et al. EGFR mutation and resistance of non-small-cell lung cancer to gefitinib. N Engl J Med, 2005, 352 (8): 786-792.

[80] Kosaka T, Yatabe Y, Endoh H, et al. Analysis of epidermal growth factor receptor gene mutation in patients with nonsmall cell lung cancer and acquired resistance to gefitinib. Clin Cancer Res, 2006, 12 (19): 5764-5769.

[81] Azam M, Seeliger MA, Gray NS, et al. Activation of tyrosine kinases by mutation of the gatekeeper threonine. Nat Struct Mol Biol, 2008, 15 (10): 1109-1118.

[82] Carter TA, Wodicka LM, Shah NP, et al. Inhibition of drug-resistant mutants of ABL, KIT, and EGF receptor kinases. Proc Natl Acad Sci USA, 2005, 102 (31): 11011-11016.

[83] Raben D, Helfrich B, Chan DC, et al. The effects of cetuximab alone and in combination with radiation and/or chemotherapy in lung cancer. Clin Cancer Res, 2005, 11 (2 Pt 1): 795-805.

[84] Suda K, Onozato R, Yatabe Y, et al. EGFR T790M mutation: A double role in lung cancer cell survival. J Thorac Oncol, 2009, 4 (1): 1-4.

[85] Inukai M, Toyooka S, Ito S, et al. Presence of epidermal growth factor receptor gene T790M mutation as a minor clone in non-small cell lung cancer. Cancer Res, 2006, 66 (16): 7854-7858.

[86] Maheswaran S, Sequist LV, Nagrath S, et al. Detection of mutations in EGFR in circulating lung-cancer cells. N Engl J Med, 2008, 359 (4): 366-377.

[87] Chmielecki J, Foo J, Oxnard GR, et al. Optimization of dosing for EGFR-mutant non-small cell lung cancer with evolutionary cancer modeling. Sci Transl Med, 2011, 3 (90): 90ra59.

[88] Oxnard GR, Arcila ME, Sima CS, et al. Acquired resistance to EGFR tyrosine kinase inhibitors in EGFR-mutant lung cancer: distinct natural history of patients with tumors harboring the T790M mutation. Clin Cancer Res, 2011, 17 (6): 1616-1622.

[89] Mok TS. Living with imperfection. J Clin Oncol, 2010, 28 (2): 191-192.

[90] Avizienyte E, Ward RA, Garner AP. Comparison of the EGFR resistance mutation profiles generated by EGFR-targeted tyrosine kinase inhibitors and the impact of drug combinations. Biochem J, 2008, 415 (2): 197-206.

[91] Yano S, Wang W, Li Q, et al. Hepatocyte growth factor induces gefitinib resistance of lung adenocarcinoma with epidermal growth factor receptoractivating mutations. Cancer Res, 2008, 68 (22): 9479-9487.

[92] Wang W, Li Q, Yamada T, et al. Crosstalk to stromal fibroblasts induces resistance of lung cancer to epidermal growth factor receptor tyrosine kinase inhibitors. Clin Cancer Res, 2009, 15 (21): 6630-6638.

[93] Viloria-Petit A, Crombet T, Jothy S, et al. Acquired resistance to the antitumor effect of epidermal growth factor receptor-blocking antibodies in vivo: a role for altered tumor angiogenesis. Cancer Res, 2001, 61 (13): 5090-6101.

[94] Nguyen KS, Kobayashi S, Costa DB. Acquired resistance to epidermal growth factor receptor tyrosine kinase inhibitors in non-small-cell lung cancers dependent on the epidermal growth factor receptor pathway. Clin Lung Cancer, 2009, 10 (4): 281-289.

[95] Thiery JP, Acloque H, Huang RY, et al. Epithelialmesenchymal transitions in development and disease. Cell, 2009, 139 (5): 871-890.

[96] Yauch RL, Januario T, Eberhard DA, et al. Epithelial versus mesenchymal phenotype determines in vitro sensitivity and predicts clinical activity of erlotinib in lung cancer patients. Clin Cancer Res, 2005, 11 (24 Pt 1): 8686-8698.

[97] Zhang Z, Lee JC, Lin L, et al. Activation of the AXL kinase causes resistance to EGFR-targeted therapy in lung cancer. Nat Genet, 2012, 44 (8): 852-860.

[98] Mir O, Blanchet B, Goldwasser F. Druginduced effects on erlotinib metabolism. N Engl J Med, 2011, 365 (4): 379-380.

[99] Hamilton M, Wolf JL, Rusk J, et al. Effects of smoking on the pharmacokinetics of erlotinib. Clin Cancer Res, 2006, 12 (7Pt 1): 2166-2171.

[100] Clark GM, Zborowski DM, Santabarbara P, et al. Smoking history and epidermal growth factor receptor expression as predictors of survival benefit from erlotinib for patients with non-small-cell lung cancer in the National Cancer Institute of Canada Clinical Trials Group study BR.21. Clin Lung Cancer, 2006, 7 (6): 389-394.

[101] Bai H, Wang Z, Wang Y, et al. Detection and clinical significance of intratumoral EGFR mutational heterogeneity in Chinese patients with advanced non-small cell lung cancer. PLoS One, 2013, 8 (2): e54170.

第28章
EGFR 抑制剂的预测性肿瘤生物标志物

Lucia Kim[1], Geoffrey Liu[2], Ming-Sound Tsao[3]
1. Department of Pathology, Inha University School of Medicine, Incheon, South Korea
2. Department of Medicine, Medical Biophysics, and Epidemiology, University of Toronto, Toronto, ON, Canada
3. Department of Laboratory Medicine and Pathobiology, University of Toronto, Toronto, ON, Canada

肿瘤的发生牵涉到癌基因逐步激活及抑癌基因的失活。在多种类型的癌症中，肿瘤细胞"依赖"于特定的癌基因突变（驱动基因），并需要这些基因的持续作用来维持其恶性表型。因此，抑制这些突变基因能显著诱导肿瘤细胞凋亡和减少其对正常细胞的不良影响[1]。"癌基因依赖"的概念将肿瘤治疗的理念由化疗转向靶向抑制特异驱动癌基因产物的个体化治疗。

表皮生长因子受体（EGFR）在包括非小细胞肺癌（NSCLC）在内的多种上皮来源癌症中普遍高表达。*EGFR* 酪氨酸激酶（TK）区突变几乎特定地出现于 NSCLC 特别是肺腺癌中[2-5]。*EGFR* 基因通常也会大量扩增[6-7]。靶向抑制 EGFR 通路能引起大量癌细胞死亡从而获得显著的临床疗效[3,8]。EGFR 是 NSCLC 治疗的分子靶点，其中两类主要的靶向药物是以吉非替尼、厄洛替尼为代表的 EGFR 酪氨酸激酶小分子抑制剂（TKIs）和以西妥昔单抗为代表的 EGFR 特异性单克隆抗体，对它们的临床疗效已有了深入研究。但在未选择的 NSCLC 患者中，EGFR 抑制剂的有效性并不优于化疗药物[9-10]，仅有某一亚类患者表现出显著疗效。女性、不吸烟、东亚及肺腺癌患者对 EGFR 靶向治疗的有效率更高[11-12]。尽管 *EGFR* 突变是预测患者对 EGFR 抑制剂敏感性最有效的指标[3,8,13]，但患者对治疗的反应仍有很大不同。一小部分表达 *EGFR* 突变的患者对 EGFR 抑制剂原发耐药，而临床上也确定了一些 *EGFR* 突变非依赖性的治疗有效患者。为了成功应用 EGFR 抑制剂治疗 NSCLC，判断哪些患者会对治疗有效显得尤为关键。因此，了解与药物敏感性相关的生物学过程并找到预测 EGFR 抑制剂疗效的标志物对患者以及治疗方法的选择都非常重要。这里我们将回顾 NSCLC 中 EGFR 通路相关分子生物学异常及它们与 EGFR 抑制剂的临床相关性，并探讨可以指导 EGFR 抑制剂临床用药的预测性生物标志物。

EGFR

EGFR 是酪氨酸激酶受体（receptor tyrosine kinase，RTK）家族成员之一，该家族包括 EGFR（ERBB1/HER1）、HER2（ERBB2）、HER3（ERBB3）和 HER4（ERBB4）。*EGFR* 基因位于 7 号染色体短臂上（7p11.2）。EGFR 蛋白由 4 个功能区组成：细胞外配体结合区、跨膜区、细胞内酪氨酸激酶区以及 C 端调控区。酪氨酸激酶区含有 1 个位于 C 端与 N 端之间的 ATP 结合口袋结构。表皮生长因子（EGF）、转化生长因子-α（transforming growth factor，TGF-α）、双向调节因子等配体与 EGFR 的胞外区特异性结合后能引起两个 EGFR 之间二聚体化或 EGFR 与另一个其他家族受体间的异二聚体化。二聚体化的受体通过结合 ATP 激活了内在的酪氨酸激酶并促进胞质区酪氨酸残基的自磷酸化。磷酸化的酪氨酸残基作为多种连接分子的结合点，随之激活下游信号，包括 RAS/RAF/MAPK、PI3K/AKT 和 STAT 通路，进而调控细胞增殖、凋亡、运动、分化和黏附。越来越多的证据表明选择性阻断 EGFR 或其下游通路是治疗癌症的有效手段。肿瘤对 TKIs 的反应性或耐药性受多种因素影响，包括 *EGFR* 基因突变类型、*EGFR* 基因拷贝数目、*KRAS* 突变及其他因素（图 28.1）。

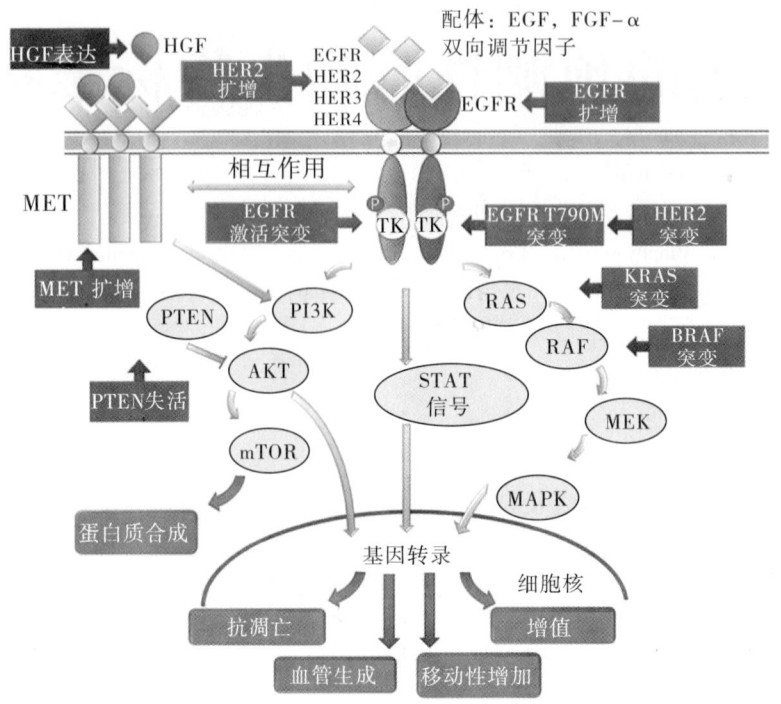

图 28.1（见彩插） EGFR 及相关分子信号通路。EGFR 与相应配体结合诱导受体形成同（异）二聚体，进而通过酪氨酸残基自磷酸化激活细胞内酪氨酸激酶。EGFR 激活引起下游信号级联放大，主要包括 RAS、PI3K/AKT 和 STAT 通路，并最终导致增殖、抗凋亡、移动性增加及血管生成等一系列细胞反应。MET 扩增引起 HER3 依赖的 PI3K/Akt 通路激活，并导致 *EGFR* 突变肿瘤的获得性耐药。图中显示了针对 EGFR 及与药敏（蓝盒）或耐药（红盒）相关下游分子的遗传及表观遗传学改变

EGFR 突变

EGFR 突变分布于 18～21 外显子间，特别是在 ATP 结合口袋区域附近[3,8]。ATP 结合口袋参与受体激活的同时也是 ATP 的竞争结合物 EGFR-TKIs 的结合位点。*EGFR* 突变使其惰性构象不稳定，并促进激酶激活[14]，诱导受体胞质区酪氨酸残基的受体非依赖性激活及自磷酸化[15-16]，从而引起了下游 AKT 和 STAT 通路的选择性激活，促进细胞存活[17]；它还能增强肿瘤细胞的成瘤能力和转化能力[15-16]。NSCLC 对 *EGFR* 突变的依赖在肿瘤表型的起始及维持上起到关键作用[1]。*EGFR* 突变肿瘤对 EGFR-TKIs 的亲和力提升高[15]，而 EGFR-TKIs 治疗诱导的生存和凋亡信号的临时不平衡最终引起细胞死亡[18]。

EGFR 敏感突变

NSCLC 中最常见的敏感突变是 19 外显子缺失和 20 外显子点突变（L858R）[3,8,19]。746～750 密码子周边的 19 外显子缺失及密码子 858（L858R）处亮氨酸-精氨酸的替换突变约占所有敏感（经典）*EGFR* 突变的 85%～90%[3,8,20-21]。在对 EGFR-TKIs 治疗有效的 NSCLC 患者中 *EGFR* 突变发生率非常高，大多数研究报告数据均 > 70%，而对 EGFR-TKIs 耐药的患者中突变率不足 10%[22]。在多项临床试验中，60%～80% 的未接受过化疗且表达敏感突变的患者对 EGFR-TKIs 治疗有效，而仅有约 10% 的 *EGFR* 野生型患者对治疗有反应（表 28.1）[4,5,7,21-28]。

EGFR 突变肿瘤与 EGFR-TKIs 治疗有效的 NSCLC 患者类似，表现出一些独特的临床病理特征。*EGFR* 突变倾向于但并不仅限于女性、不吸烟、东亚及肺腺癌患者[3-4,21]。*EGFR* 突变在女性及不吸烟患者中的高发生率提示 *EGFR* 突变的发生牵涉到一些与吸烟无关的其他致癌机制。在亚洲人群中，约 30%～50% 的患者表达 *EGFR* 突变，而在高加索患者中突变率仅为 10%～20%[4,24,29]。然而，亚洲患者与其他地区患者（主要为高加索人）*EGFR* 突变类型和突变位置的差异不大[30]。根据肿瘤的病理类型，*EGFR* 突变与乳头状、腺泡样及贴壁样腺癌

相关[2]，且大部分表达甲状腺转录因子－1（TTF－1）。后一种关联引发了如下假说，即 *EGFR* 突变肿瘤代表了终末呼吸单元型腺癌[31]。

在东亚人群中，*EGFR* 突变阳性的鳞癌所占比例不低[32-34]，且免疫组化分子标记物研究显示部分 *EGFR* 阳性突变的鳞癌表现出局灶性腺癌样分化[34-35]。由于一些通过穿刺活检确诊的 *EGFR* 突变阳性肺鳞癌代表采样不完全的腺鳞癌或与鳞癌表型类似的低分化腺癌，因此在单纯鳞癌中，*EGFR* 的真实突变率可能很低[35-36]。然而，最近日本的一项研究发现，应用一种突变高敏检测方法，249 例患者中 *EGFR* 突变率达到 13%[34]。癌症基因图谱计划也在 176 例肺鳞癌患者中确定了 2 例 *EGFR* 突变肿瘤，且这 2 例都是较罕见的 *L861Q* 突变[36-37]。EGFR-TKIs 在 *EGFR* 突变的肺鳞癌患者中的疗效似乎比其在突变肺腺癌中的有效性低[34,37]。小细胞肺癌（SCLC）发生 *EGFR* 突变非常罕见，绝大多数这类患者既往不吸烟但含有一定的腺癌成分。EGFR-TKIs 在这类患者中的疗效也不好[38-39]。

EGFR 耐药突变

所有初始对 TKIs 治疗有效的 NSCLC 患者均含有 *EGFR* 突变，但由于药物耐药最终均导致疾病进展。20 外显子内 790 密码子（T790M）苏氨酸替换为蛋氨酸的突变类型，出现在了约 50% 的服用 EGFR-TKIs 并出现疾病进展的 *EGFR* 突变阳性患者中[40-41]。*T790M* 突变通常与 *EGFR* 敏感突变呈顺式排列[40]，并在出现时表现出协同激酶活性及转化潜能[15,42]。*T790M* 突变上调了受体亲和力，使 ATP 回调至野生型水平，降低 EGFR-TKIs 效力从而引起耐药[41,43-44]。然而矛盾的是，患者因发生 *T790M* 突变而获得的耐药相比其他耐药突变的患者预后可能更好[41]。新一代 EGFR-TKIs 正在着力克服这种药物耐药性，研究结果尚未公布。

表 28.1 未接受化疗或既往接受治疗的患者对 EGFR-TKIs 的有效率

试验	患者种族	EGFR-TKI	TKI 治疗有效的 EGFR 敏感突变患者数	TKI 治疗有效*的 EGFR 敏感突变患者比例	TKI 治疗有效的野生型 EGFR 患者数	TKI 治疗有效的野生型 EGFR 患者比例
一种或多种既往化疗（二线或以上）						
IDEAL（Bellet 等，2005）[5]	混合	吉非替尼	13	46%	61	10%
BR.21（Zhuet 等，2008）[23]	混合	吉非替尼	15	27%	101	7%
ISEL（Hirschet 等，2006）[7]	混合	吉非替尼	16	38%	116	3%
INTEREST（Douillardet 等，2010）[4]	混合	吉非替尼	19	42%	106	7%
未接受化疗（一线）						
IPASS（Moket 等，2009）[24]	东亚	吉非替尼	132	71%	91	1%
WJTOG3405（Mitsudomi 等，2010）[25]	日本人	吉非替尼	58	62%	NA	NA
NEJ002（Maemondo 等，2010）[26]	日本人	吉非替尼	114	74%	NA	NA
OPTIMAL（Zhou 等，2011）[27]	中国人	厄洛替尼	82	83%	NA	NA
EURTARC（Rosell 等，2012）[28]	欧美白人	厄洛替尼	77	64%	NA	NA

*有效：完全缓解或部分缓解；NA：数据不可用

用直接测序法很少能在未接受 EGFR-TKI 治疗的患者中检测到 T790M 突变[40]。但如果应用高敏检测手段，其在表达 EGFR 敏感突变的 NSCLC 患者中表达率可达 38%[45-48]，提示小部分 T790M 突变已存在于接受 TKI 治疗的原发肿瘤中，而在 TKI 的淘汰压力下 T790M 突变细胞选择性富集并最终产生耐药性（图 28.2）[45-46]。治疗前 T790M 突变表达水平与 EGFR-TKIs 治疗患者无进展生存期的缩短密切相关，且为 EGFR-TKI 治疗有效性的负相关因子[45,47]。但在 EGFR 突变阳性的早期 NSCLC 患者中，T790M 突变常与 EGFR-TKI 治疗预后良好有关[48]。

其他罕见突变

G719X 和 L861Q 突变在 NSCLC 患者中较少见，约占所有突变类型的 3%~5%。它们或独立存在或与其他 EGFR 突变共表达从而形成复合突变[20]。G719 与 L861 突变相比于经典突变对 EGFR-TKIs 的敏感性稍低[14,16,20]。表现为 18 碱基对 EGFR 19 外显子的插入突变是最近报道的一种肺腺癌 EGFR-TKIs 敏感突变[49]。20 外显子 A767~C775 区小范围的插入或复制突变占所有 EGFR 酪氨酸激酶区突变的 3%~4%，并与 TKI 原发性耐药相关[16,50]。L747S、D761Y 及 T854A 等二次突变极少发生在 EGFR-TKIs 获得性耐药中[51-53]。其他罕见突变可能单独或与 L858R、G719X 及 L861Q 等敏感突变同时发生[54,55]，这些复合突变相较于 G719X 或 L858R 突变能减弱 EGFR 抑制剂的作用[20,52-55]。

EGFR 突变在临床中的作用

EGFR-TKIs 的总有效率在不同种族 EGFR 突变患者中没有差异，但可能受患者之前接受过的化疗的影响（表 28.1），但该数据需考虑的偏倚因素是未接受化疗的患者大部分来自于亚洲，而之前接受过化疗的患者主要来自于多种族西方人群（表 28.1）[4,5,7,23-28]。在东亚及高加索人群中进行的比较 EGFR-TKIs 与传统化疗作为一线治疗的 III 期临床试验显示，EGFR 突变阳性患者如果首先应用 TKIs 能显著延长无进展生存期（表 28.2）[24-28,56]。更重要的是，野生型 EGFR 患者如果首先接受化疗会比其首先接受 TKIs 时无进展生存期更长，该结果在一系列包括 EGFR 野生型和 EGFR 突变型的东亚及高加索肺癌患者中都得到了验证[24,57]。但在所有 EGFR 突变阳性占比例较高的 III 期临床研究中，不同用药次序导致的总生存期差异不大，可能原因是疾病进展后多种替代疗法的交叉应用（表 28.2）[13,25,27-28,58]。这些研究结果明确了 EGFR 突变状态是 EGFR-TKIs 治疗的预测指标，特别是当其作为一线治疗时。对 EGFR 突变阳性患者，TKIs 应作为一线治疗选择。而如果患者的 EGFR 突变为阴性，则推荐传统化疗[13,57]。一线化疗后维持应用厄洛替尼或吉非替尼也能带来无进展生存期的显著获益[59-60]。SATURN 试验还发现了 TKI 维持治疗能带来总生存获益，且与肿瘤的组织学类型或 EGFR 突变状态无关，但该 INFORM 试验未获得相似结果[59,61]。不同于 EGFR-TKIs，EGFR 突变状态不是西妥昔单抗疗效的一个预测指标[62]。

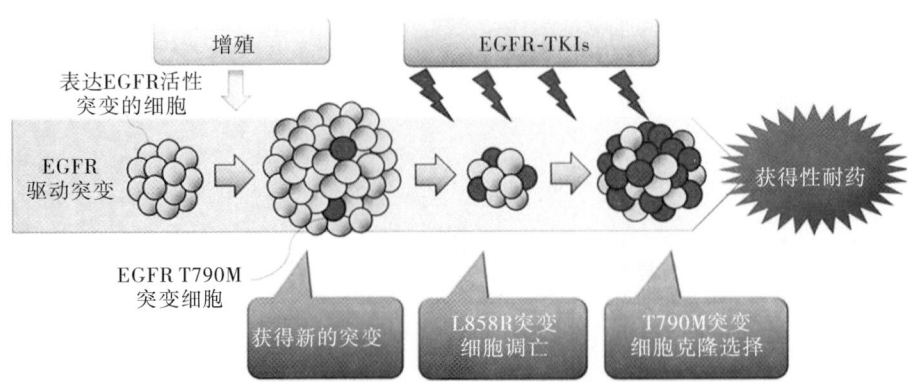

图 28.2　EGFR T790M 突变介导的获得性耐药机制概述。肿瘤细胞增殖诱导多种遗传异常的细胞混合克隆，其中小部分肿瘤细胞含有 T790M 突变。在 EGFR-TKIs 作用下，含有 EGFR 敏感突变的肿瘤细胞发生凋亡，但 T790M 突变细胞继续增殖，进而引起耐药

表28.2 EGFR-TKIs Ⅲ期临床试验生存结果

试验	病例数	治疗分组	患者选择	无进展生存期 HR(95%CI)	无进展生存期 P	总生存期 HR(95%CI)	总生存期 P
既往至少接受一次化疗（二线或以上）							
BR.21 (Shepherd等,2005)[11]	731	厄洛替尼 vs 安慰剂	无	0.61 (0.51,0.74)	<0.001	0.70 (0.58,0.85)	<0.001
ISEL (Hirsch等,2006)[7]	1 692	吉非替尼 vs 安慰剂	无	NA	NA	0.89 (0.77,1.02)	0.087
INTEREST (Douillard等,2010)[4]	1 433	吉非替尼 vs 多西他赛	无	1.04 (0.93,1.18)	0.47	1.02 (0.91,1.15)	NS
LUX-Lung1 (Miller等,2012)[119]	585	阿法替尼 vs 安慰剂	E/G治疗后进展	0.38 (0.31,0.48)	<0.000 1	1.08 (0.86,1.35)	0.74
既往未接受化疗（一线治疗）							
IPASS (Mok等,2009; Fukuoka等,2011)[13, 24]	1 217	吉非替尼 vs 卡铂/紫杉醇	ADC;非吸烟者	0.74 (0.65,0.85)	<0.001	0.90 (0.79,1.02)	0.11
WJTOG3405 (Mitsudomi等,2010)[25]	175	吉非替尼 vs 顺铂/多西他赛	EGFR突变	0.49 (0.34,0.71)	<0.000 1	1.64 (0.75,3.58)	0.211
NEJ002 (Inoue等,2013)[58]	224	吉非替尼 vs 卡铂/紫杉醇	EGFR突变	0.32 (0.24,0.44)	<0.001	0.89 (0.63,1.24)	0.483
EURTARC (Rosell等,2012)[28]	173	厄洛替尼 vs 铂类双药化疗	EGFR突变	0.37 (0.25,0.54)	<0.000 1	1.04 (0.65,1.68)	0.87
OPTIMAL (Zhou等,2011)[27]	165	厄洛替尼 vs 卡铂/吉西他滨	EGFR突变	0.16 (0.10,0.26)	<0.000 1	1.04 (0.69,1.58)	0.69
LUX-Lung3 (Yang等,2012)[56]	345	阿法替尼 vs 顺铂/培美曲塞	EGFR突变	0.58 (0.43,0.78)	0.000 4	NA	NA
TORCH (Gridelli等,2012)*[57]	760	厄洛替尼 vs 顺铂/吉西他滨	无	1.21 (1.04,1.42)	NS	1.24 (1.04,1.47)*	NS
化疗后给予TKI（维持治疗）							
SATURN (Cappuzzo等,2010)[59]	884	厄洛替尼 vs 安慰剂	CTx后未进展	0.71 (0.62,0.82)	<0.000 1	0.81 (0.70,0.95)	0.009
INFORM (Zhang,2012)[60]	296	吉非替尼 vs 安慰剂	无	0.42 (0.33,0.55)	<0.000 1	0.86 (0.62,1.14)	0.26

* 这项试验是评价一线化疗后予以二线厄洛替尼维持治疗及相反顺序的交叉研究。ADC：腺癌；CTx：化疗；E/G：厄洛替尼或吉非替尼；NA：在行文时数据尚不可用；NS：不显著

EGFR 突变类型决定了肿瘤对 EGFR-TKIs 敏感性的差异。19 外显子缺失突变对 EGFR-TKIs 治疗的有效性（63%～100%）高于 21 外显子突变（50%～67%）[63-65]，但患者的生存期没有显著差异。目前比较厄洛替尼和吉非替尼有效性的数据相对有限[63,66-67]。尽管表达 *EGFR* 突变的患者在应用这两种药物时生存期没有显著差异，但对于 *EGFR* 野生型患者，厄洛替尼较吉非替尼的临床获益更大[23,59,66-67]。另外，厄洛替尼对吉非替尼治疗失败的患者可能可提供一些获益[68]。

虽然获得性耐药通常发生在表达敏感突变并起初对 EGFR-TKIs 治疗有效的 NSCLC 患者中，但有一部分患者在终止 TKI 治疗后会出现爆发式进展[69-70]。停用 TKIs 后疾病复发的患者通常不含有 *T790M* 突变并可能仍对 TKI 治疗有效。因此，对 *EGFR* 突变阳性、停用 TKI 后复发的肺癌患者，重新启用 EGFR-TKIs 是一种可供选择的治疗方法[71]。

突变检测方法

多项临床试验报道了一小部分未检出 *EGFR* 突变的患者仍对 EGFR-TKIs 治疗有效，其中一种解释是尽管排除了其他作为病因的遗传突变，但检测方法的灵敏度仍较低。*EGFR* 突变检测的标准方法是直接测序法（图 28.3A），能检测所有类型的突变，相对精确且经济。但由于大多数 NSCLC 组织被炎症细胞、基质成纤维细胞、内皮细胞等非肿瘤组织浸润，致其灵敏度较低。直接测序法要求用不少于 40% 的突变肿瘤细胞来完成检测[72]。晚期肺癌患者的诊断主要靠小样本活检或细胞学，由于混杂有较多非肿瘤细胞，样本中肿瘤细胞数不一定能达到 *EGFR* 基因测序标准。因此具有更高灵敏度的可检测 1%～5% 肿瘤细胞的检测方法已经开发出来，如蝎形探针扩增阻滞突变系统法（amplification refractory mutation system, ARMS）[45,73]，基于实时荧光定量聚合酶链反应（PCR）的片段长度分析法[74]，限制性片段长度多态性分析[40,75]、高分辨熔化曲线分析[76]、突变富集 PCR[46]、变性高效液相色谱技术[77]等。每种方法各有优缺点，因此可检测所有潜在突变且灵敏度高、成本低廉的相关技术仍在努力开发中。

最近，突变特异性单克隆抗体的免疫组化被用于检测 *EGFR* 突变蛋白（图 28.3B）[78]。这些抗体能分别识别具有共同 15bp 缺失的 *L858R* 突变和 19 外显子突变。不同于 15bp 缺失，尽管 *EGFR* 19 外显子突变特异性抗体对 19 外显子突变敏感性稍低[79]，但其可以直接在肿瘤细胞中评估 *EGFR* 突变状态，往往这些肿瘤细胞数目不足以行 DNA 提取以供分子检测[78]。因此，突变特异 *EGFR* 免疫组化分析可用于初筛或不能行分子检测的患者。

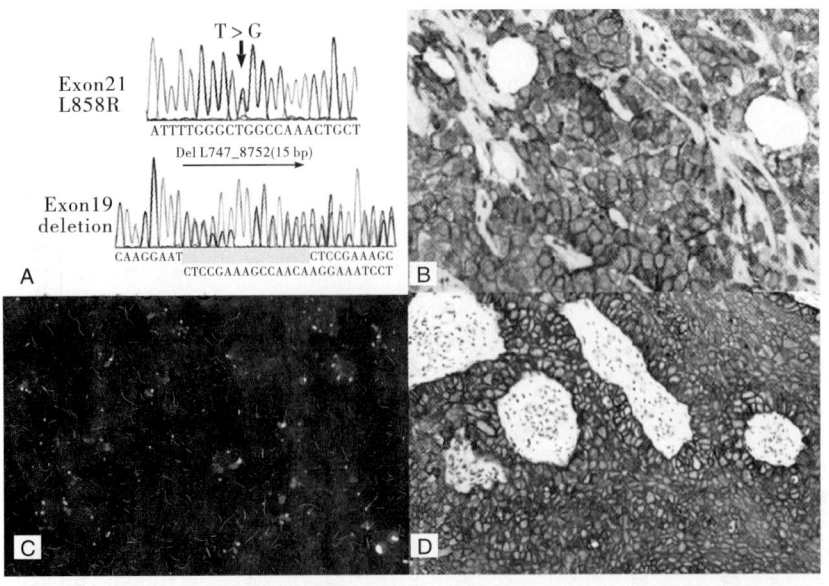

图 28.3（见彩插） 检测 *EGFR* 突变，基因拷贝数及蛋白表达的通常检测手段。A. *EGFR* L858R 点突变及 19 外显子缺失突变的直接测序结果。B. *EGFR* L858R 突变特异性抗体的免疫组化显示了其在 *EGFR* 突变肿瘤细胞膜及胞质内的染色模式。C. 荧光原位杂交检测到的 *EGFR* 扩增（红色信号，*EGFR* 基因探针；绿色信号，7 号染色体着丝粒探针）。D. 免疫组化法检测的 *EGFR* 蛋白表达显示其在肺鳞癌细胞膜上特定的染色特点

EGFR 基因拷贝数

检测 EGFR 基因拷贝数（gene copy number, GCN）变化及剂量的方法主要包括荧光原位杂交（fluorescent in situ hybridization, FISH）、银染原位杂交（silver in situ hybridization, SISH）及实时定量 PCR。FISH 是常用的检测方法，且 FISH 法检测 EGFR 基因数被科罗拉多大学分类系统研究最多[80]。当 FISH 结果显示扩增（即 EGFR 基因簇紧凑且 EGFR 基因/7 号染色体比值≥2 或在≥10% 的分析细胞中每个细胞 EGFR 拷贝数≥15）或多染色体（有≥40% 的细胞基因拷贝数≥4）时，被定义为 EGFR 基因拷贝升高（图 28.3C）。EGFR GCN 在 NSCLC 患者中表达率变化较大，一般在 22%～70%，主要取决于试验设计和纳入人群[7]。在亚洲以外人群中，22%～48% 的患者高表达 GCN，而东亚患者的表达率为 42%～70%[6,13,61]。肺腺癌中 EGFR 扩增与 EGFR 突变密切相关，在 EGFR GCN 高表达患者中有 80% 同时表达 EGFR 突变[7,13,23,81]。GCN 升高理论上会引起突变等位基因的转录和基因活性的升高[81-82]。通过该机制，EGFR 突变及高 GCN 的肿瘤可能更依赖 EGFR 信号并对靶向治疗反应性越好[83]。EGFR 突变参与肺癌起始阶段，并在癌前病变或早期肺腺癌中高表达，而 EGFR 扩增参与腺癌进展后期并在肿瘤细胞中呈异质性分布[82,84]。

关于 EGFR 高 GCN 在 NSCLC 患者中的临床意义相关的试验结果尚存在争议。以安慰剂为主的对照组的多项研究显示高 EGFR GCN 与 EGFR-TKI 治疗有效率高及总生存期显著延长相关[7,23]，但如果将经典化疗作为研究对照，相关试验结果则不具有可重复性[4,13]。另外，高 EGFR GCN 在 EGFR-TKI 治疗中的有利作用可能仅局限于高加索人群，而在东亚患者中不明显[6,85]。目前，EGFR GCN 分析不推荐作为 EGFR-TKIs 治疗患者的常规方法。

EGFR 蛋白表达

EGFR 蛋白表达易于用免疫组化法检测到（图 28.3D），在 NSCLC 患者中表达率为 60%～80%[4,7,61,86]。免疫组化检测到的 EGFR 蛋白表达与 EGFR 敏感突变、高 EGFR GCN 及患者的临床特征均无显著相关性[88]。多数研究的检测方法、检测抗体及评分体系均不尽相同，从而造成各个研究间试验结果的差异[85]。而多项临床试验关于 EGFR 蛋白表达在 EGFR-TKIs 治疗中的预测作用也不一致[4,13,29,59,61]。FLEX 研究显示在一线化疗联用西妥昔单抗治疗的晚期 NSCLC 中，EGFR 高表达（IHC 评分≥200 分）可有效预测生存期的延长[87]。该研究中，免疫组化评分系统被用于评价肿瘤细胞膜染色强度（0～3 级）和每个染色强度的染色细胞比例。尽管免疫组化检测 EGFR 蛋白表达并不是筛选对 EGFR-TKI 治疗有效患者的最佳方法，但其可作为预测化疗联合西妥昔单抗治疗效果的指标，且有待进一步的前瞻性研究证实。

EGFR 基因多态性

患者的基因多态性差异会造成 EGFR 抑制治疗效果的不同。EGFR 基因的第一个内含子中含有一个临近下游增强序列的高度多态的 CA 双核苷酸简单重复序列，且该重复序列数量的增多与转录活性的降低和 EGFR 低表达相关[89]。EGFR 短 CA 重复序列相较于长序列的患者对 EGFR-TKIs 的有效性更好、生存期更长[90-92]，但相关临床试验的结果并不支持这一结论[61,93]。因此，有待进一步研究来明确基因多态性是否为 EGFR-TKIs 治疗的独立预测因子，或者仅与其他分子或临床因素耦合发生[85]。

KRAS 突变

KRAS 基因编码产物是 EGFR 下游 RAS/RAF/MAPK 通路中的 GTP 结合蛋白成员之一。在 NSCLC 中，KRAS 突变包括 12、13 密码子或罕见的 61 密码子突变[94]，最常见的突变类型是 G12C 突变（43%）[95]。突变的 RAS 蛋白对抑制 RAS-GTP 活性的 GTP 酶激活蛋白不敏感，从而导致 RAS 在不依赖上游配体激酶的情况下持续激活。KRAS 突变见于 10%～30% 的 NSCLC 患者，特别在高加索黏液腺癌患者中多见[96-97]。KRAS 突变于吸烟患者中发生率更高并有多种突变类型。KRAS 转换突变（G→A）在非吸烟患者中多见而颠换突变（G→T 或 G→C）在吸烟患者中多见。

突变型 KRAS 及野生型 KRAS 患者对 EGFR-TKIs

的有效率分别是 3% 和 26%[97]。尽管 KRAS 突变状态可能作为一个 EGFR-TKIs 治疗有效率的不良预测因子[94]，但其对生存差异的预测作用尚未明确[4,9,23,61]。KRAS 和 EGFR 突变通常为互斥突变[7,94]，KRAS 野生型患者中存在较大比例的治疗无效者，而 KRAS 突变型/EGFR 野生型患者及 KRAS 野生型/EGFR 野生型肺癌患者的生存期无显著差异[64,97]。目前，尽管 KRAS 突变一定程度上可确定 EGFR-TKIs 治疗无效的亚组患者，但不推荐其作为判定患者是否对 EGFR-TKIs 治疗有效的筛选方法。

最近的研究显示，不同 KRAS 突变状态与细胞内不同信号通路的激活[98]以及患者接受 EGFR-TKIs 治疗[99]、其他靶向治疗[98]及辅助化疗[100]的预后相关。接受 EGFR-TKIs 治疗的 G12C KRAS 突变患者的无进展生存期比非 G21C 突变组显著缩短，但两组间的总生存期无差异[99]。在评价厄洛替尼、凡德他尼、贝沙罗汀联合厄洛替尼或索拉非尼的 BATTLE 临床试验中，表达 G12C 或 G12V KRAS 突变患者的无进展生存期显著短于其他类型 KRAS 突变或野生型 KRAS 患者[98]。KRAS 13 密码子突变的 NSCLC 患者辅助化疗后的生存期显著较差[100]。尽管纳入该研究的 KRAS 突变患者数目较少，但该结果仍令人振奋。KRAS 突变类型作为预测因子的作用有待进一步确定。

其他生物标志物

HER2 通常与 EGFR 形成二聚体，一对 HER2 聚合产生的信号强度显著高于其他二聚体[101]。FISH 法检测 2%～23% 的 NSCLC 高表达 HER2 GCN，这些患者通常为女性、肺腺癌、不吸烟患者[101-102]。高 HER2 GCN 增加了 EGFR 突变阳性患者对吉非替尼的敏感性，但该效应仅局限于 EGFR/HER2 均为阳性的患者[102]。HER2 突变极少作为 NSCLC 的驱动突变，通常见于不吸烟的肺腺癌患者[101,103]。大多数 HER2 突变是酪氨酸激酶域的 20 外显子插入突变[103]。相较于野生型 HER2，突变 HER2 的催化转换能力更强，可显著抑制细胞凋亡。另外，大多数含有 HER2 突变的肿瘤对 EGFR-TKIs 耐药但对能同时抑制 HER2 及 EGFR 的新靶向药物敏感[104]。因此，共同抑制 EGFR 和 HER2 或许将成为 NSCLC 治疗的新靶点。然而，由于 NSCLC HER2 突变率很低，因此其在临床试验中的预测作用较难确定。

研究人员还试图确定相关血清蛋白表达谱来预测 EGFR-TKIs 治疗的有效率。Taguchi 等运用基质辅助激光解吸电离（matrix-assisted laser desorption ionization，MALDI）质谱分析开发了一套预测方法，并根据 8 种蛋白的表达谱确定了 EGFR-TKIs 治疗获益的一群 NSCLC 患者亚组[105]。这种血清蛋白质组分析"VeriStrat®"能将 EGFR-TKIs 治疗或 EGFR、VEGF 抑制剂联合治疗的患者分为预后好及预后差两组[105-107]。然而，其临床预测作用并未在 BR. 21 试验中得到确认[108]。因此，仍有必要进行前瞻性随机对照试验来确定其临床预测作用。

EGFR 检测的临床应用

目前多项临床试验[13,24-26]显示晚期 NSCLC 通常需要行基因检测来明确哪些患者最有可能从 EGFR-TKIs 一线治疗中获益[109-110]，诸如性别、种族、吸烟史等临床指标并不能单独作为 EGFR-TKIs 治疗的选择指标[24]。FISH 法检测 EGFR GCN 及免疫组化检测 EGFR 蛋白表达等方法并不推荐用于指导治疗[109-110]。KRAS 检测也并不推荐作为常规检测，因为其结果对于临床决策意义不大。但随着新的 MEK 抑制剂在 KRAS 突变患者中取得的初步疗效，这种情况将很快得到改变[111]。

EGFR 突变应在所有含腺癌成分的晚期 NSCLC，而不应只在单纯鳞癌、SCLC 或神经内分泌癌中进行检测[112-113]。在病理组织类型难以确定的情况下，如 TTF-1、p63 或 p40、CK5/6 及黏液素等免疫指标的应用将有助于明确腺癌的特征。对于病理类型不是腺癌但临床特征高度倾向 EGFR 突变的患者（如不吸烟者），也有必要进行 EGFR 突变检测（图 28.4）[112]。

由于 EGFR-TKIs 敏感突变 90% 为 19 外显子及 21 外显子 L858R 突变，因此常规检测中至少要包含这两种突变。在肿瘤标本足够的情况下，L861Q、G719X 及 E709X 等少见突变的检测也是有益的。T790M 在原发肿瘤中不常见且其表达并不能排除厄洛替尼、吉非替尼等一代 TKIs 的临床应用，故其检测为可选项。但检测 T790M 突变可为将针对该突变有效的不可逆抑制剂作为首选治疗提供理论依据（表28.3）。

EGFR 突变检测确立了一种新的临床模式，即获取足够的肿瘤组织样本，用于明确诊断和病理亚型并进行分子检测。组织切片及帮助鉴别诊断的免疫组化结果需妥善保存，从而有剩余足够的样本来进行分子分析[113]。尽管组织样本要优于细胞学样本[110,114]，但有些情况下细胞学样本或许是唯一可用的材料。肿瘤细胞数量、保存状态及 DNA 质量是细胞学样本的主要考虑因素。所有在组化样本中检测到的突变也能在细胞学样本中得到确认，细胞学组织块是一个绝佳的替代，因为显微镜检和癌细胞百分计数技术即将实现[115]。在活检及细胞学样本均难以获得的情况下，外周血血清或许是另外一个选择。尽管外周血检测的敏感性仍待提高，但最近的一项研究显示，利用高通量技术分离外周血循环肿瘤细胞可以将检测灵敏度提高至临床可接受水平[45]，但运用外周血清及循环肿瘤细胞检测 EGFR 突变结果的重要性需要进一步研究确定[45,116]。

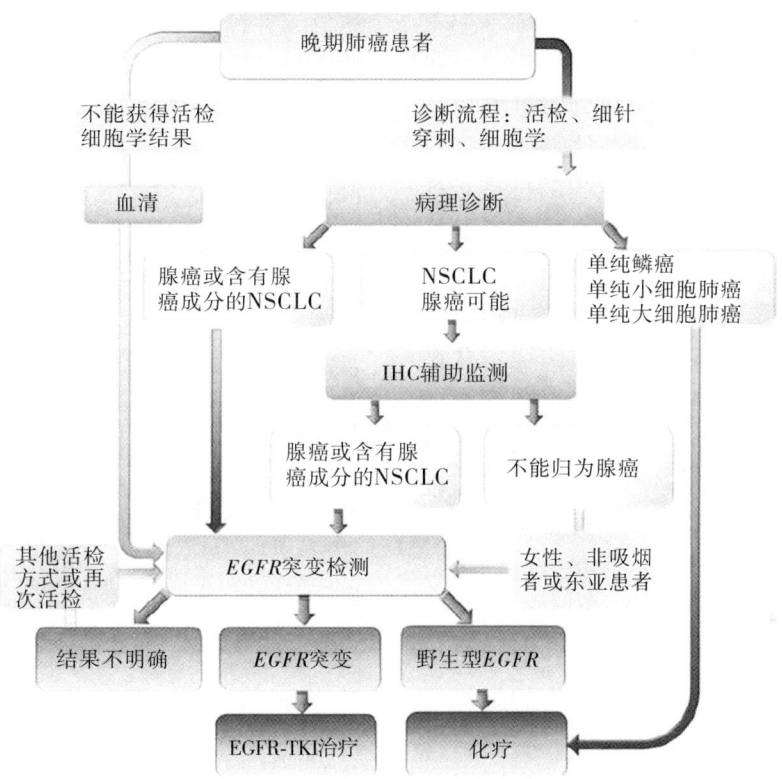

图 28.4 新确诊的晚期 NSCLC 患者对于指导一线 EGFR-TKIs 治疗 EGFR 突变检测的决策流程

表 28.3 NSCLC 患者 EGFR-TKIs 治疗预测生物标志物

生物标志物	发生频率	密切相关人群亚组	EGFR-TKIs 疗效	常规临床实践效果观察
EGFR 敏感突变	东亚人群 30%～50%/非亚洲人群 10%～20%	东亚人，女性，非吸烟者，ADC	敏感	推荐 EGFR-TKIs 一线治疗
EGFR T790M 突变	获得性耐药患者中 50%	含有 EGFR 敏感突变患者	耐药	获得性耐药患者
高基因拷贝数 EGFR	东亚人 42%～70%/非亚洲人群 22%～48%	与 EGFR 突变密切相关	敏感	不推荐
EGFR 蛋白表达量	60%～80%	SqCC 中更多见	不明确	不推荐
KRAS 突变	10%～30%	ADC，吸烟者，欧美白人	耐药	支持
HER2 扩增	2%～23%	女性，非吸烟者，ADC	敏感	需进一步验证
HER2 突变	约 2%	非吸烟者，ADC	耐药	需进一步验证

ADC：腺癌；SqCC：鳞癌

肺癌基因组异质性的临床意义有待充分阐明。转移灶的基因特性可以与原发灶或其他转移灶类似或不同[113]。选择分子病理组织样本的重要临床因素包括组织易于获取，可迅速固定并有足够数量的肿瘤细胞[114,117]。符合肿瘤细胞数量和质量相关要求的任何标本都可用于检测，相关决策应由经验丰富的病理科医生制订。样本在获取后立即进行固定对DNA的保存十分关键。新鲜冰冻、甲醛固定石蜡包埋及乙醇固定的组织均适用于分子检测。由于可能会引起DNA降解，应避免使用酸性或重金属固定剂及脱钙溶剂。理想的样本应含有较大比例的肿瘤细胞，而坏死及黏液成分尽可能少。通常在含有至少50%肿瘤成分时推荐应用直接测序法[114]，组织学上超过40%肿瘤成分即有可能被检测到[72]。对于肿瘤成分较少的标本，推荐显微分离法富集肿瘤细胞以提高异质性组织检测的准确性。

对于晚期患者，及时快速诊断非常重要。完成时间（turn-around time，TAT）指组织样本从被分子病理实验室接收到最终形成正式诊断报告的时间。5个工作日是EGFR突变检测的一个理想完成时间，而最长不应超过10个工作日[112,114]。推荐在获得结果3d之内即给予EGFR-TKIs治疗[112]。为避免TAT延长，一些研究中心在初诊时即进行"习惯性"的分子检测。而随着可同时检测多种突变的高通量复合检测方法的发展，这种应用趋势也越来越明显。对于肿瘤细胞成分较少的组织切片，以往只提供直接测序检测方法的实验室需进行灵敏度更高的检测。我们需综合考虑灵敏度、特异度、可检测的突变谱及TAT等因素来选择合适的检测方法。符合各个机构要求的检测方法都可选用并执行该方法的验证。

未来生物标志物的发展和展望

自发现EGFR突变作为EGFR-TKIs治疗的有效预测指标以来，EGFR即成为研究最为深入的分子之一。小部分EGFR突变患者对EGFR抑制剂不敏感以及部分EGFR野生型患者对其敏感的相关分子机制尚在研究中，新的生物标志物的临床应用也仍在探索中。进一步寻找其他驱动突变及新的生物标志物以选择对其他靶向治疗有效的患者的研究仍在继续。另外，研发一种快速且低价的突变检测方法以有效的灵敏度检测所有可能的EGFR突变是有必要的。对个性化治疗而言，能够同时检测包括EGFR基因在内的多个突变的高级筛查系统正在持续研发中，并将很快应用于临床[118]。简单快速分离肺癌患者外周血循环肿瘤细胞的技术能监测生物标志物状态并相应地调整治疗方案[45]。

治疗过程中出现的获得性耐药是个性化治疗的一大障碍。大量研究结果揭示了耐药的生物学机制，并提出一些遗传及表观遗传过程（见第27章，NSCLC的EGFR耐药机制）。肺癌是一种组织学及遗传学异质性肿瘤，由多种药物敏感性不同的细胞混合组成。正如由EGFR T790M突变介导的获得性耐药（图28.2），药物治疗筛选出罕见的、介导耐药的遗传学异常或许将成为一个主要障碍。与药物疗效及耐药相关的肿瘤异质性的临床应用需要进一步阐明，如何调控遗传异质性以克服靶向药物耐药是一个亟待解决的问题。

（韩 玥 倪 阳 译）

参考文献

[1] Weinstein I. Addiction to oncogenes-the Achilles heel of cancer. Science, 2002, 297: 63-64.

[2] Yatabe Y. EGFR mutations and the terminal respiratory unit. Cancer Metastasis Rev, 2010, 29: 23-36.

[3] Paez JG, Janne PA, Lee JC, et al. EGFR mutations in lung cancer: correlation with clinical response to gefitinib therapy. Science, 2004, 304: 1497-1500.

[4] Douillard JY, Shepherd FA, Hirsh V, et al. Molecular predictors of outcome with gefitinib and docetaxel in previously treated non-small-cell lung cancer: data from the randomized phase Ⅲ INTEREST trial. J Clin Oncol, 2010, 28: 744-752.

[5] Bell DW, Lynch TJ, Haserlat SM, et al. Epidermal growth factor receptor mutations and gene amplification in non-small-cell lung cancer: molecular analysis of the IDEAL/INTACT gefitinib trials. J Clin Oncol, 2005, 23: 8081-8092.

[6] Dahabreh IJ, Linardou H, Kosmidis P, et al. EGFR gene copy number as a predictive biomarker for patients receiving tyrosine kinase inhibitor treatment: a systematic review

and meta-analysis in non-small-cell lung cancer. Ann Oncol, 2011, 22: 545-552.

[7] Hirsch FR, Varella-Garcia M, Bunn PA, Jr., et al. Molecular predictors of outcome with gefitinib in a phase Ⅲ placebo-controlled study in advanced non-small-cell lung cancer. J Clin Oncol, 2006, 24: 5034-5042.

[8] Lynch TJ, Bell DW, Sordella R, et al. Activating mutations in the epidermal growth factor receptor underlying responsiveness of non-small-cell lung cancer to gefitinib. N Engl J Med, 2004, 350: 2129-2139.

[9] Kim ES, Hirsh V, Mok T, et al. Gefitinib versus docetaxel in previously treated non-small-cell lung cancer (INTEREST): A randomised phase Ⅲ trial. Lancet, 2008, 372: 1809-1818.

[10] Giaccone G, Herbst RS, Manegold C, et al. Gefitinib in combination with gemcitabine and cisplatin in advanced non-small-cell lung cancer: a phase Ⅲ trial-INTACT 1. J Clin Oncol, 2004, 22: 777-784.

[11] Shepherd FA, Rodrigues Pereira J, Ciuleanu T, et al. Erlotinib in previously treated non-small-cell lung cancer. N Engl J Med, 2005, 353: 123-132.

[12] Vincent MD, Kuruvilla MS, Leighl NB, et al. Biomarkers that currently affect clinical practice: EGFR, ALK, MET, KRAS. Curr Oncol, 2012, 19: S33-44.

[13] Fukuoka M, Wu YL, Thongprasert S, et al. Biomarker analyses and final overall survival results from a phase Ⅲ, randomized, open-label, first-line study of gefitinib versus carboplatin/paclitaxel in clinically selected patients with advanced non-smallcell lung cancer in Asia (IPASS). J Clin Oncol, 2011, 29: 2866-2874.

[14] Yun CH, Boggon TJ, Li Y, et al. Structures of lung cancer-derived EGFR mutants and inhibitor complexes: Mechanism of activation and insights into differential inhibitor sensitivity. Cancer Cell, 2007, 11: 217-227.

[15] Mulloy R, Ferrand A, Kim Y, et al. Epidermal growth factor receptor mutants from human lung cancers exhibit enhanced catalytic activity and increased sensitivity to gefitinib. Cancer Res, 2007, 67: 2325-2330.

[16] Greulich H, Chen TH, Feng W, et al. Oncogenic transformation by inhibitor-sensitive and -resistant EGFR mutants. PLoS Med, 2005, 2: e313.

[17] Sordella R, Bell DW, Haber DA, et al. Gefitinibsensitizing EGFR mutations in lung cancer activate anti-apoptotic pathways. Science, 2004, 305: 1163-1167.

[18] Sharma SV, Gajowniczek P, Way IP, et al. A common signaling cascade may underlie "addiction" to the Src, BCR-ABL, and EGF receptor oncogenes. Cancer Cell, 2006, 10: 425-435.

[19] Gazdar AF. Activating and resistance mutations of EGFR in non-small-cell lung cancer: role in clinical response to EGFR tyrosine kinase inhibitors. Oncogene, 2009, 28 (Suppl 1): S24-31.

[20] Wu JY, Yu CJ, Chang YC, et al. Effectiveness of tyrosine kinase inhibitors on "uncommon" epidermal growth factor receptor mutations of unknown clinical significance in non-small cell lung cancer. Clin Cancer Res, 2011, 17: 3812-3821.

[21] Riely GJ, Politi KA, Miller VA, et al. Update on epidermal growth factor receptor mutations in non-small cell lung cancer. Clin Cancer Res, 2006, 12: 7232-7241.

[22] Sequist LV, Bell DW, Lynch TJ, et al. Molecular predictors of response to epidermal growth factor receptor antagonists in non-small-cell lung cancer. J Clin Oncol, 2007, 25: 587-595.

[23] Zhu CQ, da Cunha Santos G, Ding K, et al. Role of KRAS and EGFR as biomarkers of response to erlotinib in National Cancer Institute of Canada Clinical Trials Group Study BR. 21. J Clin Oncol, 2008, 26: 4268-4275.

[24] Mok TS, Wu YL, Thongprasert S, et al. Gefitinib or carboplatin-paclitaxel in pulmonary adenocarcinoma. N Engl J Med, 2009, 361: 947-957.

[25] Mitsudomi T, Morita S, Yatabe Y, et al. Gefitinib versus cisplatin plus docetaxel in patients with non-small-cell lung cancer harbouring mutations of the epidermal growth factor receptor (WJTOG3405): an open label, randomised phase 3 trial. Lancet Oncol, 2010, 11: 121-128.

[26] Maemondo M, Inoue A, Kobayashi K, et al. Gefitinib or chemotherapy for non-small-cell lung cancer with mutated EGFR. NEngl J Med, 2010, 362: 2380-2382.

[27] Zhou C, Wu YL, Chen G, et al. Erlotinib versus chemotherapy as first-line treatment for patients with advanced EGFR mutation-positive non-smallcell lung cancer (OPTIMAL, CTONG-0802): A multicentre, open-label, randomised, phase 3 study. Lancet Oncol, 2011, 12: 735-742.

[28] Rosell R, Carcereny E, Gervais R, et al. Erlotinib versus standard chemotherapy as firstline treatment for European patients with advanced EGFR mutation-positive non-small-cell lung cancer (EURTAC): A multicentre, open-label, randomized phase 3 trial. Lancet Oncol, 2012, 13: 239-246.

[29] Tsao MS, Sakurada A, Cutz JC, et al. Erlotinib in lung

[30] Pao W, Chmielecki J. Rational, biologically based treatment of EGFR-mutant non-small-cell lung cancer. Nat Rev Cancer, 2010, 10: 760–774.

[31] Yatabe Y, Kosaka T, Takahashi T, et al. EGFR mutation is specific for terminal respiratory unit type adenocarcinoma. Am J Surg Pathol, 2005, 29: 633–639.

[32] Park SH, Ha SY, Lee JI, et al. Epidermal growth factor receptor mutations and the clinical outcome in male smokers with squamous cell carcinoma of lung. J Korean Med Sci, 2009, 24: 448–452.

[33] An SJ, Chen ZH, Su J, et al. Identification of enriched driver gene alterations in subgroups of nonsmall cell lung cancer patients based on histology and smoking status. PLoS ONE, 2012, 7: e40109.

[34] Hata A, Katakami N, Yoshioka H, et al. How sensitive are epidermal growth factor receptortyrosine kinase inhibitors for squamous cell carcinoma of the lung harboring EGFR gene-sensitive mutations? J Thorac Oncol, 2013, 8: 89–95.

[35] Rekhtman N, Paik PK, Arcila ME, et al. Clarifying the spectrum of driver oncogene mutations in biomarker-verified squamous carcinoma of lung: lack of EGFR/KRAS and presence of PIK3CA/AKT1 mutations. Clin Cancer Res, 2012, 18: 1167–1176.

[36] Hammerman PS, Sos ML, Ramos AH, et al. Comprehensive genomic characterization of squamous cell lung cancers. Nature, 2012, 489: 519–525.

[37] Shukuya T, Takahashi T, Kaira R, et al. Efficacy of gefitinib for non-adenocarcinoma non-smallcell lung cancer patients harboring epidermal growth factor receptor mutations: a pooled analysis of published reports. Cancer Sci, 2011, 102: 1032–1037.

[38] Shiao TH, Chang YL, Yu CJ, et al. Epidermal growth factor receptor mutations in small cell lung cancer: a brief report. J Thorac Oncol, 2011, 6: 195–198.

[39] Tatematsu A, Shimizu J, Murakami Y, et al. Epidermal growth factor receptor mutations in small cell lung cancer. Clin Cancer Res, 2008, 14: 6092–6096.

[40] Pao W, Miller VA, Politi KA, et al. Acquired resistance of lung adenocarcinomas to gefitinib or erlotinib is associated with a second mutation in the EGFR kinase domain. PLoS Med, 2005, 2: e73.

[41] Oxnard GR, Arcila ME, Sima CS, et al. Acquired resistance to EGFR tyrosine kinase inhibitors in EGFR-mutant lung cancer: distinct natural history of patients with tumors harboring the T790M mutation. Clin Cancer Res, 2011, 17: 1616–1622.

[42] Godin-Heymann N, Bryant I, Rivera MN, et al. Oncogenic activity of epidermal growth factor receptor kinase mutant alleles is enhanced by the T790M drug resistance mutation. Cancer Res, 2007, 67: 7319–7326.

[43] Yoshikawa S, Kukimoto-Niino M, Parker L, et al. Structural basis for the altered drug sensitivities of non-small cell lung cancer-associated mutants of human epidermal growth factor receptor. Oncogene, 2013, 32 (1): 27–38.

[44] Yun CH, Mengwasser KE, Toms AV, et al. The T790M mutation in EGFR kinase causes drug resistance by increasing the affinity for ATP. Proc Natl Acad Sci USA, 2008, 105: 2070–2075.

[45] Maheswaran S, Sequist LV, Nagrath S, et al. Detection of mutations in EGFR in circulating lungcancer cells. N Engl J Med, 2008, 359: 366–377.

[46] Inukai M, Toyooka S, Ito S, et al. Presence of epidermal growth factor receptor gene T790M mutation as a minor clone in non-small cell lung cancer. Cancer Res, 2006, 66: 7854–7858.

[47] Rosell R, Molina MA, Costa C, et al. Pretreatment EGFR T790M mutation and BRCA1 mRNA expression in erlotinib-treated advanced non-smallcell lung cancer patients with EGFR mutations. Clin Cancer Res, 2011, 17: 1160–1168.

[48] Fujita Y, Suda K, Kimura H, et al. Highly sensitive detection of EGFR T790M mutation using colony hybridization predicts favorable prognosis of patients with lung cancer harboring activating EGFR mutation. J Thorac Oncol, 2012, 7: 1640–1644.

[49] He M, Capelletti M, Nafa K, et al. EGFR exon 19 insertions: a new family of sensitizing EGFR mutations in lung adenocarcinoma. Clin Cancer Res, 2012, 18: 1790–1797.

[50] Yasuda H, Kobayashi S, Costa DB. EGFR exon 20 insertion mutations in non-small-cell lung cancer: preclinical data and clinical implications. Lancet Oncol, 2012, 13: e23–31.

[51] Bean J, Riely GJ, Balak M, et al. Acquired resistance to epidermal growth factor receptor kinase inhibitors associated with a novel T854A mutation in a patient with EGFR-mutant lung adenocarcinoma. Clin Cancer Res, 2008, 14: 7519–7525.

[52] Balak MN, Gong Y, Riely GJ, et al. Novel D761Y and common secondary T790M mutations in epidermal growth factor receptor-mutant lung adenocarcinomas with acquired resistance to kinase inhibitors. Clin Cancer Res, 2006, 12: 6494-6501.

[53] Massarelli E, Johnson FM, Erickson HS, et al. Uncommon Epidermal Growth Factor Receptor mutations in non-small cell lung cancer and their mechanisms of EGFR tyrosine kinase inhibitors sensitivity and resistance. Lung Cancer, 2013, 80: 235-241.

[54] Tam IY, Leung EL, Tin VP, et al. Double EGFR mutants containing rare EGFR mutant types show reduced in vitro response to gefitinib compared with common activating missense mutations. Mol Cancer Ther, 2009, 8: 2142-2151.

[55] Kancha RK, von Bubnoff N, Peschel C, et al. Functional analysis of epidermal growth factor receptor (EGFR) mutations and potential implications for EGFR targeted therapy. Clin Cancer Res, 2009, 15: 460-467.

[56] Yang JC, Shih JY, Su WC, et al. Afatinib for patients with lung adenocarcinoma and epidermal growth factor receptor mutations (LUX-Lung 2): A phase 2 trial. Lancet Oncol, 2012, 13: 539-548.

[57] Gridelli C, Ciardiello F, Gallo C, et al. First-line erlotinib followed by second-line cisplatingemcitabine chemotherapy in advanced non-smallcell lung cancer: the TORCH randomized trial. J Clin Oncol, 2012, 30: 3002-3011.

[58] Tsao MS, Sakurada A, Ding K, et al. Prognostic and predictive value of epidermal growth factor receptor tyrosine kinase domain mutation status and gene copy number for adjuvant chemotherapy in non-small cell lung cancer. J Thorac Oncol, 2011, 6: 139-147.

[59] Cappuzzo F, Ciuleanu T, Stelmakh L, et al. Erlotinib as maintenance treatment in advanced nonsmall-cell lung cancer: a multicentre, randomised, placebo-controlled phase 3 study. Lancet Oncol, 2010, 11: 521-529.

[60] Zhang L, Ma S, Song X, et al. Gefitinib versus placebo as maintenance therapy in patients with locally advanced or metastatic non-small-cell lung cancer (INFORM; C-TONG 0804): A multicentre, double-blind randomised phase 3 trial. Lancet Oncol, 2012, 13: 466-475.

[61] Brugger W, Triller N, Blasinska-Morawiec M, et al. Prospective molecular marker analyses of EGFR and KRAS from a randomized, placebocontrolled study of erlotinib maintenance therapy in advanced non-small-cell lung cancer. J Clin Oncol, 2011, 29: 4113-4120.

[62] Khambata-Ford S, Harbison CT, Hart LL, et al. Analysis of potential predictive markers of cetuximab benefit in BMS099, a phase Ⅲ study of cetuximab and first-line taxane/carboplatin in advanced nonsmall-cell lung cancer. J Clin Oncol, 2010, 28: 918-927.

[63] Jackman DM, Yeap BY, Sequist LV, et al. Exon 19 deletion mutations of epidermal growth factor receptor are associated with prolonged survival in non-small cell lung cancer patients treated with gefitinib or erlotinib. Clin Cancer Res, 2006, 12: 3908-3914.

[64] Jackman DM, Miller VA, Cioffredi LA, et al. Impact of epidermal growth factor receptor and KRAS mutations on clinical outcomes in previously untreated non-small cell lung cancer patients: Results of an online tumor registry of clinical trials. Clin Cancer Res, 2009, 15: 5267-5273.

[65] Mitsudomi T, Kosaka T, Endoh H, et al. Mutations of the epidermal growth factor receptor gene predict prolonged survival after gefitinib treatment in patients with non-small-cell lung cancer with postoperative recurrence. J Clin Oncol, 2005, 23: 2513-2520.

[66] Cho BC, Im CK, Park MS, et al. Phase Ⅱ study of erlotinib in advanced non-small-cell lung cancer after failure of gefitinib. J Clin Oncol, 2007, 25: 2528-2533.

[67] Wu WS, Chen YM, Tsai CM, et al. Erlotinib has better efficacy than gefitinib in adenocarcinoma patients without EGFR-activating mutations, but similar efficacy in patients with EGFR-activating mutations. Exp Ther Med, 2012, 3: 207-213.

[68] Vasile E, Tibaldi C, Chella A, et al. Erlotinib after failure of gefitinib in patients with advanced non-small cell lung cancer previously responding to gefitinib. J Thorac Oncol, 2008, 3: 912-914.

[69] Riely GJ, Kris MG, Zhao B, et al. Prospective assessment of discontinuation and reinitiation of erlotinib or gefitinib in patients with acquired resistance to erlotinib or gefitinib followed by the addition of everolimus. Clin Cancer Res, 2007, 13: 5150-5155.

[70] Chaft JE, Oxnard GR, Sima CS, et al. Disease flare after tyrosine kinase inhibitor discontinuation in patients with EGFR-mutant lung cancer and acquired resistance to erlotinib or gefitinib: implications for clinical trial design. Clin Cancer Res, 2011, 17: 6298-6303.

[71] Oxnard GR, Janjigian YY, Arcila ME, et al. Maintained sensitivity to EGFR tyrosine kinase inhibitors in EGFR-

[72] Warth A, Penzel R, Brandt R, et al. Optimized algorithm for Sanger sequencing-based EGFR mutation analyses in NSCLC biopsies. Virchows Arch, 2012, 460: 407-414.

[73] Newton CR, Graham A, Heptinstall LE, et al. Analysis of any point mutation in DNA: The amplification refractory mutation system (ARMS). Nucleic Acids Res, 1989, 17: 2503-2516.

[74] Molina-Vila MA, Bertran-Alamillo J, Reguart N, et al. A sensitive method for detecting EGFR mutations in non-small cell lung cancer samples with few tumor cells. J Thorac Oncol, 2008, 3: 1224-1235.

[75] Kawada I, Soejima K, Watanabe H, et al. An alternative method for screening EGFR mutation using RFLP in non-small cell lung cancer patients. J Thorac Oncol, 2008, 3: 1096-1103.

[76] Do H, Dobrovic A. Limited copy number-high resolution melting (LCN-HRM) enables the detection and identification by sequencing of low level mutations in cancer biopsies. Mol Cancer, 2009, 8: 82.

[77] Chin TM, Anuar D, Soo R, et al. Detection of epidermal growth factor receptor variations by partially denaturing HPLC. Clin Chem, 2007, 53: 62-70.

[78] Yu J, Kane S, Wu J, et al. Mutation-specific antibodies for the detection of EGFR mutations in non-small-cell lung cancer. Clin Cancer Res, 2009, 15: 3023-3028.

[79] Brevet M, Arcila M, Ladanyi M. Assessment of EGFR mutation status in lung adenocarcinoma by immunohistochemistry using antibodies specific to the two major forms of mutant EGFR. J Mol Diagn, 2010, 12: 169-176.

[80] Cappuzzo F, Hirsch FR, Rossi E, et al. Epidermal growth factor receptor gene and protein and gefitinib sensitivity in non-small-cell lung cancer. J Natl Cancer Inst, 2005, 97: 643-655.

[81] Soh J, Okumura N, Lockwood WW, et al. Oncogene mutations, copy number gains and mutant allele specific imbalance (MASI) frequently occur together in tumor cells. PLoS ONE, 4: e7464.

[82] Sholl LM, Yeap BY, Iafrate AJ, et al. Lung adenocarcinoma with EGFR amplification has distinct clinicopathologic and molecular features in neversmokers. Cancer Res, 2009, 69: 8341-8348.

[83] Gazdar AF, Minna JD. Deregulated EGFR signaling during lung cancer progression: Mutations, amplicons, and autocrine loops. Cancer Prev Res (Phila), 2008, 1: 156-160.

[84] Yatabe Y, Takahashi T, Mitsudomi T. Epidermal growth factor receptor gene amplification is acquired in association with tumor progression of EGFR-mutated lung cancer. Cancer Res, 2008, 68: 2106-2111.

[85] John T, Liu G, Tsao MS. Overview of molecular testing in non-small-cell lung cancer: Mutational analysis, gene copy number, protein expression and other biomarkers of EGFR for the prediction of response to tyrosine kinase inhibitors. Oncogene, 2009, 28 (Suppl 1): S14-23.

[86] Hirsch FR, Varella-Garcia M, Bunn PA, Jr., et al. Epidermal growth factor receptor in non-small-cell lung carcinomas: Correlation between gene copy number and protein expression and impact on prognosis. J Clin Oncol, 2003, 21: 3798-3807.

[87] Pirker R, Pereira JR, von Pawel J, et al. EGFR expression as a predictor of survival for firstline chemotherapy plus cetuximab in patients with advanced non-small-cell lung cancer: analysis of data from the phase 3 FLEX study. Lancet Oncol, 2012, 13: 33-42.

[88] Pinter F, Papay J, Almasi A, et al. Epidermal growth factor receptor (EGFR) high gene copy number and activating mutations in lung adenocarcinomas are not consistently accompanied by positivity for EGFR protein by standard immunohistochemistry. J Mol Diagn, 2008, 10: 160-168.

[89] Gebhardt F, Burger H, Brandt B. Modulation of EGFR gene transcription by secondary structures, a polymorphic repetitive sequence and mutations-a link between genetics and epigenetics. Histol Histopathol, 2000, 15: 929-936.

[90] Nie Q, Wang Z, Zhang GC, et al. The epidermal growth factor receptor intron1 (CA) n microsatellite polymorphism is a potential predictor of treatment outcome in patients with advanced lung cancer treated with Gefitinib. Eur J Pharmacol, 2007, 570: 175-181.

[91] Han SW, Jeon YK, Lee KH, et al. Intron 1 CA dinucleotide repeat polymorphism and mutations of epidermal growth factor receptor and gefitinib responsiveness in non-small-cell lung cancer. Pharmacogenet Genomics, 2007, 17: 313-319.

[92] Liu G, Gurubhagavatula S, Zhou W, et al. Epidermal growth factor receptor polymorphisms and clinical outcomes in non-small-cell lung cancer patients treated with gefitinib. Pharmacogenomics J, 2008, 8: 129-138.

[93] Liu G, Cheng D, Ding K, et al. Pharmacogenetic analysis of BR. 21, a placebo-controlled randomized phase III clinical trial of erlotinib in advanced non-small cell lung cancer. J Thorac Oncol, 2012, 7: 316-322.

[94] Riely GJ, Marks J, Pao W. KRAS mutations in non-small cell lung cancer. Proc Am Thorac Soc, 2009, 6: 201-205.

[95] Roberts PJ, Stinchcombe TE. KRAS mutation: Should we test for it, and does it matter? J Clin Oncol, 2013, 31: 1112-1121.

[96] Finberg KE, Sequist LV, Joshi VA, et al. Mucinous differentiation correlates with absence of EGFR mutation and presence of KRAS mutation in lung adenocarcinomas with bronchioloalveolar features. J Mol Diagn, 2007, 9: 320-326.

[97] Mao C, Qiu LX, Liao RY, et al. KRAS mutations and resistance to EGFR-TKIs treatment in patients with non-small cell lung cancer: a meta-analysis of 22 studies. Lung Cancer, 2010, 69: 272-278.

[98] Ihle NT, Byers LA, Kim ES, et al. Effect of KRAS oncogene substitutions on protein behavior: Implications for signaling and clinical outcome. J Natl Cancer Inst, 2012, 104: 228-239.

[99] Fiala O, Pesek M, Finek J, et al. The dominant role of G12C over other KRAS mutation types in the negative prediction of efficacy of epidermal growth factor receptor tyrosine kinase inhibitors in non-small cell lung cancer. Cancer Genet, 2013, 206: 26-31.

[100] Shepherd FA, Domerg C, Hainaut P, et al. Pooled analysis of the prognostic and predictive effects of KRAS mutation status and KRAS mutation subtype in early-stage resected non-small-cell lung cancer in four trials of adjuvant chemotherapy. J Clin Oncol, 2013, 31 (17): 2173-2181.

[101] Swanton C, Futreal A, Eisen T. Her2-targeted therapies in non-small cell lung cancer. Clin Cancer Res, 2006, 12: 4377s-4383s.

[102] Cappuzzo F, Varella-Garcia M, Shigematsu H, et al. Increased HER2 gene copy number is associated with response to gefitinib therapy in epidermal growth factor receptor-positive non-small-cell lung cancer patients. J Clin Oncol, 2005, 23: 5007-5018.

[103] Arcila ME, Chaft JE, Nafa K, et al. Prevalence, clinicopathologic associations, and molecular spectrum of ERBB2 (HER2) tyrosine kinase mutations in lung adenocarcinomas. Clin Cancer Res, 2012, 18: 4910-4918.

[104] Wang SE, Narasanna A, Perez-Torres M, et al. HER2 kinase domain mutation results in constitutive phosphorylation and activation of HER2 and EGFR and resistance to EGFR tyrosine kinase inhibitors. Cancer Cell, 2006, 10: 25-38.

[105] Taguchi F, Solomon B, Gregorc V, et al. Mass spectrometry to classify non-small-cell lung cancer patients for clinical outcome after treatment with epidermal growth factor receptor tyrosine kinase inhibitors: A multicohort cross-institutional study. J Natl Cancer Inst, 2007, 99: 838-846.

[106] Kuiper JL, Lind JS, Groen HJ, et al. VeriStrat ((R)) has prognostic value in advanced stage NSCLC patients treated with erlotinib and sorafenib. Br J Cancer, 2012, 107 (11): 1820-1825.

[107] Akerley W, Boucher K, Rich N, et al. A phase II study of bevacizumab and erlotinib as initial treatment for metastatic non-squamous, non-small cell lung cancer with serum proteomic evaluation. Lung Cancer, 2012, 79 (3): 307-311.

[108] Carbone DP, Ding K, Roder H, et al. Prognostic and predictive role of the VeriStrat plasma test in patients with advanced non-small-cell lung cancer treated with erlotinib or placebo in the NCIC Clinical Trials Group BR. 21 trial. J Thorac Oncol, 2012, 7: 1653-1660.

[109] Keedy VL, Temin S, Somerfield MR, et al. American Society of Clinical Oncology provisional clinical opinion: epidermal growth factor receptor (EGFR) Mutation testing for patients with advanced non-small-cell lung cancer considering first-line EGFR tyrosine kinase inhibitor therapy. J Clin Oncol, 2011, 29: 2121-2127.

[110] Ellis PM, Blais N, Soulieres D, et al. A systematic review and Canadian consensus recommendations on the use of biomarkers in the treatment of non-small cell lung cancer. J Thorac Oncol, 2011, 6: 1379-1391.

[111] Janne PA, Shaw AT, Pereira JR, et al. Selumetinib plus docetaxel for KRAS-mutant advanced nonsmall-cell lung cancer: A randomised, multicentre, placebo-controlled, phase 2 study. Lancet Oncol, 2013, 14: 38-47.

[112] Salto-Tellez M, Tsao MS, Shih JY, et al. Clinical and testing protocols for the analysis of epidermal growth factor receptor mutations in East Asian patients with non-small cell lung cancer: A combined clinical-molecular pathological approach. J Thorac Oncol, 2011, 6: 1663-

1669.

[113] Travis WD, Brambilla E, Noguchi M, et al. International Association for the Study of Lung Cancer/American Thoracic Society/European Respiratory Society international multidisciplinary classification of lung adenocarcinoma. J Thorac Oncol, 2011, 6: 244-285.

[114] Pirker R, Herth FJ, Kerr KM, et al. Consensus for EGFR mutation testing in non-small cell lung cancer: results from a European workshop. J Thorac Oncol, 2010, 5: 1706-1713.

[115] da Cunha Santos G, Saieg MA, Geddie W, et al. EGFR gene status in cytological samples of nonsmall cell lung carcinoma: Controversies and opportunities. Cancer Cytopathol, 2011, 119: 80-91.

[116] Brevet M, Johnson ML, Azzoli CG, et al. Detection of EGFR mutations in plasma DNA from lung cancer patients by mass spectrometry genotyping is predictive of tumor EGFR status and response to EGFR inhibitors. Lung Cancer, 2011, 73: 96-102.

[117] Gately K, O' Flaherty J, Cappuzzo F, et al. The role of the molecular footprint of EGFR in tailoring treatment decisions in NSCLC. J Clin Pathol, 2012, 65: 1-7.

[118] Su Z, Dias-Santagata D, Duke M, et al. A platform for rapid detection of multiple oncogenic mutations with relevance to targeted therapy in nonsmall-cell lung cancer. J Mol Diagn, 2011, 13: 74-84.

[119] Miller VA, Hirsh V, Cadranel J, et al. Afatinib versus placebo for patients with advanced, metastatic non-small-cell lung cancer after failure of erlotinib, gefitinib, or both, and one or two lines of chemotherapy (LUX-Lung 1): A phase 2b/3 randomised trial. Lancet Oncol, 2012, 13: 528-538.

第29章
肺癌的免疫治疗

Jay M. Lee[1], Steven M. Dubinett[2], Sherven Sharma[2]
1. Division of Thoracic Surgery, Jonsson Comprehensive Cancer Center, David Geffen School of Medicine at UCLA, Los Angeles, CA
2. Division of Pulmonary and Critical Care Medicine, Department of Medicine, UCLA Lung Cancer Research Program, David Geffen School of Medicine at UCLA, Los Angeles, CA, USA

肿瘤的免疫治疗

目前尽管有多种免疫刺激方法治疗胸部恶性肿瘤，但仍没有一种被证实是切实有效的。然而这种基于免疫的方法在治疗黑色素瘤和肾癌方面比较有效，说明胸部恶性肿瘤是非免疫原性的，所以也就不能用免疫学方法进行干预治疗。然而，随着肿瘤相关抗原（tumor associated antigens，TAA）的发现，细胞及分子免疫学的发展，以及对肿瘤免疫新的认识，促进了免疫治疗这一前景广阔的治疗策略的发展。现在有很多关于肺癌免疫学方面的研究，而临床试验主要集中于诱导产生特异性的抗肿瘤免疫反应，可以分为以下几大类：①阻断免疫抑制节点的单克隆抗体；②肿瘤蛋白及肽疫苗；③树突状细胞疫苗；④修饰的肿瘤细胞疫苗；⑤免疫佐剂疫苗；⑥基因载体疫苗。在本章节中，我们将讨论免疫治疗方法的发展，尤其是在非小细胞肺癌（NSCLC）中的临床应用，并总结对这些免疫治疗方法所进行的临床研究的最新数据。

肺癌治疗的靶向免疫调控

肿瘤依靠免疫抑制机制逃避免疫系统，其中一条免疫抑制途径是靠肿瘤表达程序性死亡配体-1（PD-L1）介导的，通过与T细胞表面的程序性死亡受体1（PD-1）结合，从而阻止对肿瘤的免疫监视，且阻止免疫系统攻击肿瘤功能的激活。单克隆抗体阻断了癌症患者体内的PD-L1或PD-1，导致了肿瘤的消减，改善患者的长期生存[1]。

虽然在所有癌症患者中，肿瘤基因突变或表观基因突变诱导产生的肿瘤抗体是大量存在的，但是肿瘤通过诱导对肿瘤特异性T细胞产生耐受来逃避免疫攻击，还可以通过表达配体与抑制受体结合并抑制肿瘤微环境中T细胞的功能来逃避免疫攻击。调节T细胞及负调控分子治疗的实际目的即清除免疫耐受。在临床前期研究及早期临床试验中，针对B7家族复合物的抑制性抗体，包括负调节受体、细胞毒T淋巴细胞相关抗原4（CTLA-4）以及PD-1，他们均表达于激活的T细胞上，已经证明是免疫治疗有价值的目标。PD-1是一种T细胞共抑制受体，它有一个结构与CTLA-4相似，但是却有不同的生物学功能及配体特异性[2]。PD-1有2个已知的配体，程序性死亡配体-1（PD-L1，B7-H1）及程序性死亡配体-2（PD-L2，B7-DC）[4-5]，与CTLA-4的配体——CD80（B7-1）及CD86（B7-2）不同，PD-L1选择性表达于许多肿瘤组织，并且表达于肿瘤微环境中对炎性刺激应答的细胞上。PD-1及PD-L1的相互作用加强了体外试验中的免疫应答，介导了临床前期的抗肿瘤活性[7-8]。PD-L1是原发性PD-1的配体，在实体瘤中其表达上调，可抑制细胞因子的产生，且抑制PD-1$^+$、肿瘤浸润相关CD4$^+$及CD8$^+$ T淋巴细胞的细胞毒作用[7,9-10]，这种特性使得PD-L1成为一种可能有价值的癌症免疫治疗靶点。

BMS-936559是一种具有高度亲和力、全人源化、PD-L1特异性的IgG4（S228P）单克隆抗体，它同时抑制PD-L1与PD-1及CD80的结合。曾有一项多中心I期临床试验评估过这一抗体，它是通过血管内给药用于所选择的进展期癌症患者。抗PD-L1抗体每14d给药一次，共6周的疗程，可以延长到16个疗程，甚至可延长至患者完全缓解或者证实疾病进展。这项研究结果证明，抗体介导的PD-L1阻断可诱导肿瘤的持续退缩（ORR 6%~17%），延长疾病稳定期（24周12%~41%），是在进展期癌症患者中进行的，包括NSCLC、黑色素瘤及肾细胞癌[1]。在进展期NSCLC接受抗PD-L1治疗的患者中，49例中有5例客观有效（10%），这个结果出乎意料。虽然黑色素瘤及肾癌对免疫治疗是有效的（例如IL-2及抗CTLA-4），但是NSCLC曾被认为是非免疫原性，对以免疫为基础的治疗收效甚微。抗PD-L1的另一项重要特征是其在多种肿瘤中的持续性作用，尤其在进展期肿瘤患者及研究中前期接受其他治疗的患者中，这种特征尤为显著，其持续性作用貌似强于多数接受化疗或酶抑制剂治疗的患者，虽然以前并未进行直接对照试验[11]。进行抗PD-L1试验的肺癌患者，76例中14例有效。NSCLC各种病理学类型的客观有效率如下：18例鳞癌患者中6例有效（33%），56例非鳞癌患者中7例有效（12%），2例未知病理类型患者中1例有效。该治疗最常见的副作用为乏力、皮疹和腹泻，其他少见的副作用为发热，与免疫系统激活相一致。在PD-1的靶向治疗临床试验中，有5%的患者终止治疗，在PD-L1的靶向治疗中，有6%的患者终止治疗，均归因于严重副作用，并且有3例接受PD-1靶向治疗的患者因无法控制的肺部浸润而死亡，其肺部浸润是PD-1靶向药物引起的[1]。这些抑制途径在治疗上的潜力已被研究者注意到，其可阻断肿瘤被免疫系统识别。另外，关于PD-1靶向药物的II期临床试验正在进行中，III期临床试验包括黑色素瘤、NSCLC及肾癌患者，正在计划中。PD-1途径靶向药物也是作为临床试验最优先使用的药物，该临床试验由美国国家癌症研究所（NCI）的免疫治疗临床试验网进行。

肿瘤蛋白和肽疫苗

激活的原癌基因、失活的肿瘤抑制基因和基因突变是肺癌发生相关的分子事件，同时也是疫苗策略中理想的肿瘤抗原。蛋白和肽经过加工以后经MHC分子被APC细胞提呈给T细胞，从而诱导产生一系列特异的免疫反应[12]。肿瘤蛋白中只有一小段肽序列是有免疫原性的，这些肽被称为抗原表位，根据细胞规则的复杂设定，它们被MHC分子提呈在细胞表面[12]。肽比蛋白小，更容易生产，并可以产生现有技术容易检测到的免疫反应。但是，肽只能被特异的HLA分子提呈，这种限制性可能使其不能被广泛应用于所有患者[12]。治疗用的肽癌症疫苗，目的是诱导强大的CD8和CD4 T细胞反应，需要宿主的抗原提呈细胞（antigen presenting cells，APC）的参与，以更有效地提呈肽抗原，从而激活各自的T细胞亚型。肽疫苗的合理应用是基于大量的临床前期研究，这些临床研究证实，实体瘤的根治需要T淋巴细胞。细胞毒性T淋巴细胞（cytotoxic T-lymphocytes，CTLs），或称之为CD8 T细胞，为代表性的原发性效应细胞，它参与了肿瘤特异性免疫介导的肿瘤细胞的杀伤。CTL识别、结合并杀伤靶细胞，是通过3个分子的相互作用，包括抗原特异性受体（antigen-specific receptor，TCR）及多肽，后者是通过靶细胞提呈给CTL，需要以I级主要组织相容性复合体抗原（major histocompatibility complex antigens，MHC）的存在为前提（MHC又被称为人类白细胞抗原或缩写为HLA）。所有体细胞表面都表达人类白细胞抗原（human lymphocyte antigen，HLA）分子，并通过他们把抗原提呈给T细胞。细胞内的整个蛋白被加工成小的肽片段（长度为8~10个氨基酸），并排布于含HLA分子的细胞表面。HLA-肽复合物促使CTLs识别肿瘤相关抗原，因此，对表达此抗原的癌细胞起到靶向杀伤作用。许多原发肿瘤表达特异性HLA分子，从而能被肿瘤相关抗原特异性CTLs识别并杀伤。通过疫苗识别及再引入肿瘤相关特异性多肽，提高了其浓度，对免疫系统来说，可激活及募集足够的CTLs杀伤癌细胞。治疗性肿瘤疫苗所用的单一肽抗原或少量多肽抗原是有迹可循的，它是基于一种假设，这种假设就是，最初被诱导的针对单一或少量抗原的抗肿瘤反应，经过宿主的抗原提呈细胞（antigen presenting cell，APC）摄入及提呈死亡的肿瘤细胞，演变为对大量肿瘤相关抗原广泛的免疫反应。

除了干细胞，一般的正常细胞中黑色素瘤的相关抗原（melanoma-associated antigen，MAGE）是不表达的[13]。迄今为止，有超过50个MAGE基因被确定，这些基因在胚胎发育、生殖细胞发展、细胞周期以及凋亡过程中发挥着重要的生理学和病理学作用[13]。几乎超过75%的小细胞肺癌（SCLC）和接近40%的NSCLC患者中都表达MAGE基因，因此这种睾丸癌抗原开始被人们作为免疫治疗的靶点。Atanackovic等报道了一项利用MAGE-3蛋白疫苗成功地在早期NSCLC（Ⅰ期及Ⅱ期）患者中诱导特异性的体液和细胞免疫的试验[14]。17例表达MAGE-3的NSCLC患者被分为两组，一组仅接受MAGE-3蛋白免疫，而另外一组接受MAGE-3蛋白和AS02B佐剂的联合免疫。在第1组的9例患者中，1例患者有低水平的抗体滴度，另外7例患者有HLA-A2限制的针对MAGE-3 271-279位的肽的CD8$^+$T细胞反应[14]。相反，另外一组的8例患者中，有7例患者诱导出很高的抗体滴度并4例同时伴有HLA-DP4限制的针对MAGE-3 243-258位肽的CD4$^+$T细胞反应[14]。1例患者同时还存在HLA-A1限制的针对MAGE-3 168-176位肽的CD8$^+$T细胞反应。虽然这些免疫反应与临床的相关性还不清楚，但这也说明除了传统上理解的CD8$^+$T细胞免疫反应，CD4$^+$T细胞介导的免疫以及抗体的产生也是很重要的。另外，这项研究也给人们提供了进一步研究联合体液免疫和细胞免疫的疫苗研究策略的基础，以研究这种方法的临床效果。GlaxoSmithKline的特异性疫苗针对表达MAGE-3的NSCLC，它包含提纯的MAGE-3重组蛋白，在含AS02B免疫佐剂系统的脂质体制剂中。基于此疫苗在NSCLC患者中的早期研究，一项检测此疫苗的大型临床试验正在筹备中（被称为MAGRIT Ⅲ期临床试验）。全世界许多研究中心此刻正在参与这项临床试验，管理全世界术后患者。这项研究的主要研究重点为无病生存期，包括在全部人群中及未进行术后化疗的队列中的无病生存期[15]。

经过一个阶段的长期发展，在Ⅱ期临床试验中，MUC1肽疫苗在NSCLC受试者中延长其生存期，这也为更多大规模的肺癌Ⅲ期临床试验提供了理论依据[16-17]。此疫苗的靶点是黏蛋白1（mucin 1，MUC1），MUC1是一种在肺癌中广泛表达的抗原。BLP25脂质体疫苗是治疗肺癌患者的一种方法，它的靶点是肺癌患者中MUC1相关抗原暴露出的肽核心。MUC1是一种细胞膜糖蛋白，它在许多癌症中过表达，例如NSCLC、乳腺癌、结直肠癌、前列腺癌、胰腺癌、卵巢癌和多发性骨髓瘤。MUC1促进肿瘤的生长及存活，并与疾病的进展及预后差相关。MUC1作为抗肿瘤的靶点，是基于许多临床前期研究及临床研究。MUC1在肿瘤细胞中的表达方式与在正常细胞中是不同的。超过80%的肿瘤细胞表达MUC1，而超过60%的NSCLC细胞表达MUC1[18]。BLP25脂蛋白疫苗由含25个氨基酸的MUC1序列构成（STAPPAHGVTSAPDTRPAPGSTAPP），它保持了MUC1的特异性，比一串MUC1拷贝数要大一点，其碳端为棕榈酸根结合赖氨酸，促使脂肽合并为脂质体微粒。这种疫苗是一种冻干制剂，它包含BLP25脂肽，免疫佐剂磷酰脂A及3种脂质：胆固醇，[1-（2,3-二羟基丙氧基羟基磷酰）氧基-3-十四酰氧基丙-2-基]十四酸酯，二棕榈酰磷脂酰胆碱。这些脂质的作用是佐剂，以增强MUC1肽疫苗的免疫原性。单磷酰脂质A是一种toll样受体4（TLR4）拮抗剂，可激活树突状细胞及巨噬细胞。脂质体转运系统便于抗原提呈细胞的摄取，以利于脂肽运送到细胞内环境，被MHC分子提呈，激活特异性T细胞，从而识别及把表达MUC1的癌细胞作为靶点。令人鼓舞的是，L-BLP25癌疫苗目前在一项Ⅲ期临床试验中被评估，以治疗不可切除的、Ⅲ期NSCLC（用于NSCLC的药物称为emepepimut-S）。令人乐观的有两点：一是这种疫苗在应用的患者身上体现出有利的毒性研究进展；另一点是患有局部Ⅲ期NSCLC的患者生存期延长。目前为止，在针对L-BLP25癌疫苗的研究中，尚无对疫苗接种反应的足够免疫监控。这些研究缺乏关于疫苗复合物的免疫反应的资料，如通过对MUC1特异性的细胞毒性T淋巴细胞在免疫接种前后的量化，以及它如何与患者的全部临床表现相关联。令人振奋的是，关于免疫反应量化的遗漏将随着研究的进展而得到完善。

树突状细胞疫苗

抗肿瘤免疫的主要机制是 T 淋巴细胞介导的对肿瘤细胞的杀伤，特别是扩增能够识别 MHC 分子提呈的癌细胞抗原的细胞毒性 T 淋巴细胞，这正是大多数免疫治疗策略想要达到的目的。APC 在 T 细胞活化过程中起着重要作用，它能够提呈肿瘤抗原，提供 CTL 反应所必需的共刺激信号。在适宜的条件下，APC 能够迁移到肿瘤的微环境中，克服肿瘤的阻碍而发挥作用。T 细胞活化引起 CTL 反应，进而识别并杀伤肿瘤细胞，而且能产生细胞因子，如 IFN-γ 和 TNF-α，抑制肿瘤细胞的增殖及血管生成。CTL 也能利用穿孔素和 Fas 裂解肿瘤细胞。因此，目前治疗方案致力于寻找肿瘤抗原，提供具有免疫原性的抗原，调节 T 细胞反应以增加 CTL 的数量，从而增强反应效应。

DC（dendritic cells）细胞是功能非常强的 APC 细胞，能够提呈肿瘤相关抗原到 T 细胞，因此能启动肿瘤特异的免疫反应[22-24]。DC 细胞起源于骨髓的白细胞，能高表达 MHC 和共刺激分子[25]。因此，它们能捕获抗原，形成大量能引起免疫反应的 MHC-肽复合物[25]，它们转移到次级淋巴器官，选择抗原特异的 T 细胞并刺激使其活化。使用合适的细胞因子，能够得到大量的 DC 细胞。增殖的 $CD34^+$ 细胞和非增殖的 $CD14^+$ 祖细胞都能产生 DC 细胞，$CD34^+$ 细胞需要 GM-CSF 和肿瘤坏死因子 TNF-α，而 $CD14^+$ 细胞需要 GM-CSF 和 IL-4。

由于 DC 细胞在肿瘤免疫中的重要性，有多种将活化的 DC 细胞应用于肿瘤免疫治疗中的方法[26-27]，很多临床试验探索基于 DC 治疗策略的可行性和安全性[28-32]。有报道将 DC 作为肿瘤相关抗原的载体，负载整个细胞和肽片段的研究。Hirschowitz 等将自体同源的 DC 负载异源 NSCLC 细胞系的凋亡小体，这种细胞系高表达 5 种已知抗原：Her2/neu、CEA、WT1、Mage2 和 survivin[31]。Kontani 等研究将局部晚期或转移性肺癌患者 8 例或 6 例乳腺癌患者的自体 DC 用 MUC1 阳性肿瘤患者（9 例）的 MUC1 肽片段或 MUC1 阴性肿瘤患者（5 例）的自体肿瘤裂解产物负载[32]。Antonia 等报道了一种疫苗策略，即使用带有野生型 P53 的腺病毒感染的自体 DC[30]。

对引起免疫细胞募集和活化的细胞和分子事件的考察表明可以越过肿瘤部位的阻碍，利用细胞因子和趋化因子在实体瘤位点引起肿瘤免疫。研究已经发现，在临床前小鼠肿瘤模型中，瘤内接种基因改造的 DC 能表达次级淋巴组织因子等，具有抗肿瘤的作用[33-35]。基于这种临床试验模型，一项进展期 NSCLC 的临床试验在洛杉矶加利福尼亚大学被启动（与美国癌症中心合作，称为干预进展的捷径项目）。这项临床试验是对晚期 NSCLC 患者以剂量递增的方式瘤内注射 DC-AdCCL21。符合产品生产质量管理规范（good manufacturing practice，GMP）认证的 DC-AdCCL21 拷贝缺陷的病毒[36]，通过 RAID 项目被研制出来，以用于临床 I 期试验。人 DC 细胞通过腺病毒 CCL21 转导，产生 CCL21，从而吸引 T 细胞及 DC 细胞。通过 IFN-γ 的酶联免疫斑点法的评估，初步发现阐释了肿瘤特异性系统免疫反应。在患者中，对治疗前后浆细胞细胞因子多重方法的估测，揭示了 IL-2、IFN-γ、IL-12 以及 CXCL10 的诱导。通过肿瘤活检后免疫组化分析，揭示了表达 CD4 的肿瘤浸润性淋巴细胞的汇集。

修饰的肿瘤细胞疫苗

肿瘤和正常细胞在抗原组成和生物学行为上具有本质的不同，并且遗传不稳定是肿瘤形成的一个关键因素[37]。在肿瘤的发生发展过程中，肿瘤细胞中的基因突变最终会导致新的抗原形成[37]。因此，自体和异体肿瘤可以作为疫苗试验中丰富的肿瘤抗原库。

自体肿瘤疫苗的优势是能够产生针对患者特异性的免疫反应，避免了肿瘤细胞抗原表型的确定过程。但是，患者自己所能提供的肿瘤细胞数量有限，这是限制这种疫苗可推广性的一个因素，而以此理论为基础的疫苗试验也只限于招募经手术切除肿瘤的患者。基因修饰疫苗已经在几个临床前肿瘤模型中得到了很好的应用。细胞因子 GM-CSF 可以推动记忆性免疫，阻止肿瘤的复发和转移。GM-CSF 能够调节 DC 细胞的增殖、成熟和迁移，从而增强抗肿瘤免疫。经过基因工程修饰能够分泌 GM-CSF 的 NSCLC 细胞，经过放射处理做成自体肿瘤疫苗，已经于临床 I 期试验中在 NSCLC 转移患者中进行了测试[38]。为了去除自体肿瘤对病毒转染的需要，包含自体肿瘤细胞和分泌 GM-CSF 的异体肿瘤细胞系的联合疫苗 GVAX 被用于临床试验[39-40]。因为 GVAX 疫苗对晚期 NSCLC 患者无效，人们开始在其他恶性肿瘤上验证其效果。

异源抗原消除了对于患者自身肿瘤的需求，成为疫苗试验中吸引人的肿瘤抗原来源。肿瘤细胞系可用来作为异源全细胞疫苗。恶性肿瘤常常通过缺失共刺激分子改变细胞表面表型，这些共刺激分子是形成有效抗肿瘤免疫所必需的[41]，其中最关键的共刺激分子包括 CD80、CD86 和 CD40L[41]。研究表明，肺癌细胞能够下调细胞表面的 MHC 分子的表达。所以一些研究从肿瘤细胞系的基因改造着手以使其表达必需的共刺激分子和 MHC 分子，从而诱导抗肿瘤免疫[42-43]。Raez 等人将 B7.1（CD80）和 HLA A1 或者 A2（MHC I 期分子）转入人肺腺癌细胞系，以此疫苗为基础对 II B 和 IV 期的 NSCLC 患者进行了 I 期临床试验[43]。虽然相对于自体肿瘤疫苗，异体疫苗展现出了很多方面的优势，但是其主要问题是这种策略所基于的假设的局限性，它认为细胞系表达的肺癌抗原与患者独特的肿瘤抗原是一致的，并且这种抗原表型在不同的患者中是共有的。

免疫佐剂疫苗

转化生长因子 TGF-β 是一种能够在正常细胞和肿瘤细胞中抑制细胞增殖和诱导凋亡的蛋白，是一种肿瘤抑制基因，并能调节血管生成[44-46]。TGF-β 受体或者 Smad 的基因突变会导致 TGF-β 受体-Smad 通路的抑制，从而促进肿瘤的发生[44-45]。所有的人类肿瘤都会过表达 TGF-β，这可以促进肿瘤细胞侵袭转移，从而诱发 EMT[44]。它还能抑制包括细胞毒性 T 细胞、自然杀伤细胞、巨噬细胞和树突状细胞在内的淋巴细胞的增殖和分化，从而提供肿瘤介导的一种免疫逃避机制。TGF-β_2 水平也与肿瘤患者的免疫抑制呈正相关，与 NSCLC 患者的预后呈负相关。

Nemunaitis 等的最近报告将 belagenpumatucel-L——一种 TGF-β_2 反义基因修饰的异源细胞系瘤苗应用于 II～IV 期患者的临床 II 期研究[47]。如果免疫反应的提高与良好的临床结果相关，这个试验证明，如果能找到一种能提供具有免疫优势的肿瘤抗原的同种异源肿瘤细胞系作为瘤苗，就能起到很好的抗肿瘤作用。将这种方法与靶向 TGF 通路的治疗结合起来能起到更好的效果。

抗独特型的单克隆抗体能模拟蛋白和非蛋白的抗原表位，可以诱导产生针对肿瘤抗原的免疫反应。当这个抗原不是蛋白或不能轻易获得足够的量时，抗独特型抗体疫苗就非常理想。SCLC 源于神经外胚层，因此有一些特异的分化抗原，可以作为潜在的靶点[48]。Bec2 就是一个模拟 GD3 的抗独特型单克隆抗体，GD3 是一种来源于神经外胚层、表达于肿瘤细胞表面的神经节苷脂抗原，参与很多细胞功能，包括细胞与细胞识别、细胞基质间接触以及细胞分化[48-49]。Giaccone 等进行了 Bec2 与 BCG 联合免疫的临床 III 期试验，患者之前经过化疗和胸部放疗并产生了很好的效果，患者身上的 SCLC 被限制[49]。515 例患者在 10 周多的时间内接种 Bec2/BCG 疫苗，共接种 5 次，免疫毒性表现为皮肤溃疡和轻度流感样症状[49]。但是接种了疫苗的患者，生存期和无进展存活期并没有延长，生活质量也没有明显提高[49]。观察组和免疫组的中位生存期分别为 16.4 个月和 14.3 个月[49]。总之，这个研究表明，Bec2/BCG 疫苗对经过化疗和胸部放疗的限制性 SCLC 患者没有临床意义。抗独特型抗体疫苗仅在肺癌治疗上进入临床 III 期。其他一系列的研究确定了几种钥孔血蓝蛋白结合的 SCLC 相关疫苗具有免疫原性，包括 GM2、Globo H、fucosyl GM1 以及聚唾液酸等[48]。

基因载体疫苗

基因运输载体被用来作为药物的运输系统，可以高效表达胞内或分泌到肿瘤环境中的目的蛋白[50-51]。MUC-1 是一种糖蛋白，通常情况下位于分泌黏液素的上皮细胞表面，高表达于乳腺癌、卵巢癌及结肠癌，这说明 MUC-1 的异常表达常见于腺癌。NSCLC 患者中能检测到这种蛋白的体液反应具有诊断意义[52]。Mennecier 等在晚期 NSCLC 患者身上进行了 TG4010 的临床Ⅱ期试验，这是一种带有 MUC-1 抗原及 IL-2 的重组 NDA 疫苗载体[53]。一项多种心随机试验纳入了 65 例ⅢB 和Ⅳ期 NSCLC 患者，给予 TG4010 及顺铂和长春瑞滨联合治疗，或单用 TG4010，病情发展后再联合两药物化疗[53]。第一组中，有 68%（24/35）的患者部分缓解[53]；第二组中，2 例患者病情稳定，随后联合治疗后，14 例患者中有 3 例出现部分缓解，患者能够很好地耐受 TG4010 注射位点常见的不良反应[53]。该研究初步表明，TG4010 联合常规化疗治疗 NSCLC 取得了振奋人心的结果。

总　结

免疫疗法的挑战是如何利用细胞和分子免疫的优势来达到有效安全地增强抗肿瘤免疫应答的目的。当我们能很好地了解围绕肿瘤免疫监视、肿瘤免疫编辑、肺癌形成中宿主细胞网络的协同作用、肿瘤介导的免疫抑制以及调节 T 细胞活性的免疫调控节点等一系列复杂的问题后，这一目标才有可能实现。导致疫苗效能低下的几个难题包括：①最佳抗原和免疫佐剂的合理选择；②如何确定产生了适当的免疫反应；③诱导长期免疫记忆；④肿瘤诱导的免疫抑制和免疫逃逸。一个完整的疫苗策略必须包括：①免疫细胞的活化、归巢以及在肿瘤部位的积聚；②中断限制免疫反应的调节机制；③同时还必须具备指导多个免疫成分对肿瘤进行协调有效的攻击的能力。目前很清楚的是一个有效的抗肿瘤免疫反应需要 APC、淋巴细胞和 NK 细胞之间复杂的相互作用，需要下调免疫抑制剂活性及免疫调控节点。当阐明了抑制抗肿瘤免疫的机制时，我们将可以为有效治疗肺癌开发免疫靶点，从而发现更多的治疗机会。

（王　娇　译）

参考文献

[1] Brahmer JR, Tykodi SS, Chow LQ, et al. Safety and activity of antiPD-L1 antibody in patients with advanced cancer. New England Journal of Medicine, 2012, 366（26）：2455-2465. PubMed PMID：22658128. Pubmed Central PMCID：3563263.

[2] Okazaki T, Honjo T. PD-1 and PD-1 ligands：From discovery to clinical application. International Immunology, 2007, 19（7）：813-824. PubMed PMID：17606980.

[3] Freeman GJ, Long AJ, Iwai Y, et al. Engagement of the PD-1 immunoinhibitory receptor by a novel B7 family member leads to negative regulation of lymphocyte activation. Journal of Experimental Medicine, 2000, 192（7）：1027-1034. PubMed PMID：11015443. Pubmed Central PMCID：2193311.

[4] TsengSY, OtsujiM, GorskiK, et al. B7-DC, a new dendritic cell molecule with potent costimulatory properties for T cells. Journal of Experimental Medicine, 2001, 193（7）：839-846. PubMed PMID：11283156. Pubmed Central PMCID：2193370.

[5] Latchman Y, Wood CR, Chernova T, et al. PD-L2 is a second ligand for PD-1 and inhibits T cell activation. Nature Immunology, 2001, 2（3）：261-268. PubMed PMID：11224527.

[6] Fife BT, Pauken KE, Eagar TN, et al. Interactions between PD-1 and PDL1 promote tolerance by blocking the TCR-induced stop signal. Nature Immunology, 2009, 10（11）：1185-1192. PubMed PMID：19783989. Pubmed Central PMCID：2778301.

[7] Dong H, Strome SE, Salomao DR, et al. Tumor-associated B7-H1 promotes T-cell apoptosis：A potential mechanism of immune evasion. Nature Medicine, 2002, 8（8）：793-800. PubMed PMID：12091876.

[8] Iwai Y, Ishida M, Tanaka Y, et al. Involvementof PD-L1 ontumorcells in the escape from host immune system and tumor immunotherapy by PD-L1 blockade. Proceedings of the National Academy of Sciences of the United States of America, Pubmed Central PMCID：129438, 2002.

[9] Hino R, Kabashima K, Kato Y, et al. Tumor cell expression of programmed cell death-1 ligand 1 is a prognostic factor for malignant melanoma. Cancer, 2010, 116（7）：1757-1766. PubMed PMID：20143437.

[10] Taube JM, Anders RA, Young GD, et al. Colocalization of inflammatory response with B7-h1 expression in human melanocytic lesions supports an adaptive resistance mechanism of immune escape. Science Translational Medicine, 2012, 4（127）：127ra37. PubMed PMID：22461641.

[11] Holt GE, Podack ER, Raez LE. Immunotherapy as a strategy for the treatment of non-small-cell lung cancer. Therapy, 2011, 8（1）：43-54. PubMed PMID：

[12] Ribas A, Butterfield LH, Glaspy JA, et al. Current developments in cancer vaccines and cellular immunotherapy. Journal of Clinical Oncology, 2003, 21 (12): 2415-2432. PubMed PMID: 12805342.

[13] Tsai JR, Chong IW, Chen YH, et al. Differential expression profile of MAGE family in non-small-cell lung cancer. Lung Cancer, 2007, 56 (2): 185-192. PubMed PMID: 17208331.

[14] Atanackovic D, Altorki NK, Stockert E, et al. Vaccine-induced CD4 + T cell responses to MAGE-3 protein in lung cancer patients. Journal of Immunology, 2004, 172 (5): 3289-3296. PubMed PMID: 14978137.

[15] GSK1572932A Antigen-specific cancer immunotherapeutic as adjuvant therapy in patients with non-small cell lung cancer [Internet]. 2013 [cited March 24, 2011]. Available from: http://www.clinicaltrials.gov/ct2/show/NCT00480025 term = MAGE – A3&rank =8.

[16] Butts C, Murray N, Maksymiuk A, et al. Randomized phase ⅡB trial of BLP25 liposome vaccine in stage ⅢB and Ⅳ nonsmall-cell lung cancer. J Clin Oncol, 2005, 23 (27): 6674-6681.

[17] Sangha R, Butts C. L-BLP25: a peptide vaccine strategy in non small cell lung cancer. Clin Cancer Res, 2007, 13 (15 Pt 2): s4652-4654.

[18] Vlad AM, Kettel JC, Alajez NM, et al. MUC1 immunobiology: Fromdiscoverytoclinical applications. Adv Immunol, 2004, 82: 249-293.

[19] Peng L, Krauss JC, Plautz GE, et al. T cell-mediated tumor rejection displays diverse dependence upon perforin and IFN-gamma mechanisms that cannot be predicted from in vitro T cell characteristics. Journal of Immunology, 2000, 165 (12): 7116-7124. PubMed PMID: 11120842.

[20] Poehlein CH, Hu HM, Yamada J, et al. TNF plays an essential role in tumor regression after adoptive transfer of perforin/IFN-gamma double knockout effector T cells. Journal of Immunology, 2003, 170 (4): 2004-2013. PubMed PMID: 12574370.

[21] Seki N, Brooks AD, Carter CR, et al. Tumor-specific CTL kill murine renal cancer cells using both perforin and Fas ligand-mediated lysis in vitro, but cause tumor regression in vivo in the absence of perforin. Journal of Immunology, 2002, 168 (7): 3484-3492. PubMed PMID: 11907109.

[22] Aragoneses-Fenoll L, Corbi AL. Dendritic cells: still a promising tool for cancer immunotherapy. Clinical & Translational Oncology, 2007, 9 (2): 77-82. PubMed PMID: 17329218.

[23] Fong L, Engleman EG. Dendritic cells in cancer immunotherapy. Annual Review of Immunology, 2000, 18: 245-273. PubMed PMID: 10837059.

[24] Banchereau J, Palucka AK. Dendritic cells as therapeutic vaccines against cancer. Nature Reviews Immunology, 2005, 5 (4): 296-306. PubMed PMID: 15803149.

[25] Pardoll DM. Spinning molecular immunology into successful immunotherapy. Nature Reviews Immunology, 2002, 2 (4): 227-238. PubMed PMID: 12001994.

[26] Banchereau J, Steinman RM. Dendritic cells and the control of immunity. Nature, 1998, 392 (6673): 245-252. PubMed PMID: 9521319.

[27] Timmerman JM, Levy R. Dendritic cell vaccines for cancer immunotherapy. Annual Review of Medicine, 1999, 50: 507-529. PubMed PMID: 10073291.

[28] Nair SK, Hull S, Coleman D, et al. Induction of carcinoembryonic antigen (CEA)-specific cytotoxic T-lymphocyte responses in vitro using autologous dendritic cells loaded with CEA peptide or CEA RNA in patients with metastatic malignancies expressing CEA. International Journal of Cancer, 1999, 82 (1): 121-124. PubMed PMID: 10360830.

[29] Sharma S, Miller P, Stolina M, et al. Multi-component gene therapy vaccines for lung cancer: Effective eradication of established murine tumors in vivo with Interleukin 7/Herpes Simplex Thymidine Kinase-transduced autologous tumor and ex vivo-activated dendritic cells. Gene Therapy, 1997, 4: 1361-1370.

[30] Antonia SJ, Mirza N, Fricke I, et al. Combination of p53 cancer vaccine with chemotherapy in patients with extensive stagesmallcelllungcancer. Clinical Cancer Research, 2006, 12 (3 Pt 1): 878-887. PubMed PMID: 16467102.

[31] Hirschowitz EA, Foody T, KryscioR, et al. Autologous dendritic cell vaccines for non-small-cell lung cancer. Journal of Clinical Oncology, 2004, 22 (14): 2808-2815. PubMed PMID: 15254048.

[32] Kontani K, Taguchi O, Ozaki Y, et al. Dendritic cell vaccine immunotherapy of cancer targeting MUC1 mucin. International Journal of Molecular Medicine, 2003, 12 (4): 493-502. PubMed PMID: 12964025.

[33] Yang SC, Hillinger S, Riedl K, et al. Intratumoral administration of dendritic cells overexpressing CCL21 generates systemic antitumor responses and confers tumor im-

munity. Clinical Cancer Research, 2004, 10 (8): 2891-2901. PubMed PMID: 15102698.

[34] Yang SC, Batra RK, Hillinger S, et al. Intrapulmonary administration of CCL21 gene-modified dendritic cells reduces tumor burden in spontaneous murine bronchoalveolar cell carcinoma. Cancer Research, 2006, 15, 66 (6): 3205-3213. PubMed PMID: 16540672.

[35] Sharma S, Stolina M, Luo J, et al. Secondary lymphoid tissue chemokine mediates T cell-dependent antitumor responses in vivo. Journal of Immunology, 2000, 164 (9): 4558-4563. PubMed PMID: 10779757.

[36] Baratelli F, Takedatsu H, Hazra S, et al. Preclinical characterization of GMP grade CCL21-gene modified dendritic cells for application in a phase I trial in non-small cell lung cancer. J Transl Med, 2008, 6 (1): 38. PubMed PMID: 18644162.

[37] Pardoll D. Does the immune system see tumors as foreign or self? Annual Review of Immunology, 2003, 21: 807-839. PubMed PMID: 12615893.

[38] Salgia R, Lynch T, Skarin A, et al. Vaccination with irradiated autologous tumor cells engineered to secrete granulocytemacrophage colony-stimulating factor augments antitumor immunity in some patients with metastatic non-small-cell lung carcinoma. Journal of Clinical Oncology, 2003, 21 (4): 624-630. PubMed PMID: 12586798.

[39] Nemunaitis J, Sterman D, Jablons D, et al. Granulocyte macrophage colony-stimulating factor gene-modified autologous tumor vaccines in non-small-cell lung cancer. Journal of the National Cancer Institute, 2004, 96 (4): 326-331. PubMed PMID: 14970281.

[40] NemunaitisJ, JahanT, RossH, et al. Phase 1/2trial of autologoustumor mixed with an allogeneic GVAX vaccine in advancedstage non-small-cell lung cancer. Cancer Gene Therapy, 2006, 13 (6): 555-562. PubMed PMID: 16410826.

[41] Singh NP, Yolcu ES, Taylor DD, et al. Anovelapproach to cancer immunotherapy: tumor cells decorated with CD80 generate effective antitumor immunity. Cancer Research, 2003, 63 (14): 4067-4073. PubMed PMID: 12874008.

[42] Raez LE, Cassileth PA, Schlesselman JJ, et al. Induction of CD8 T-cell-Ifn-gamma response and positive clinical outcome after immunization with gene-modified allogeneic tumor cells in advanced non-small-cell lung carcinoma. Cancer Gene Therapy, 2003, 10 (11): 850-858. PubMed PMID: 14605671.

[43] Raez LE, Cassileth PA, Schlesselman JJ, et al. Allogeneic vaccination with a B7.1 HLA-A gene-modified adenocarcinoma cell line in patients with advanced nonsmall-cell lung cancer. Journal of Clinical Oncology, 2004, 22 (14): 2800-2807. PubMed PMID: 15254047.

[44] Pardali K, Moustakas A. Actions of TGF-beta as tumor suppressor and pro-metastatic factor in human cancer. Biochimica et biophysicaacta, 2007, 1775 (1): 21-62. PubMed PMID: 16904831.

[45] Levy L, Hill CS. Alterations in components of the TGF-beta superfamily signaling pathways in human cancer. Cytokine & Growth Factor Reviews, 2006, 17 (1-2): 41-58. PubMed PMID: 16310402.

[46] Gajewski TF, Meng Y, Harlin H. Immune suppression in the tumor microenvironment. Journal of Immunotherapy, 2006, 29 (3): 233-240. PubMed PMID: 16699366.

[47] Nemunaitis J, Dillman RO, Schwarzenberger PO, et al. Phase II study of belagenpumatucel-L, a transforming growth factor beta-2 antisense gene-modified allogeneic tumor cell vaccine in non-small-cell lung cancer. Journal of Clinical Oncology, 2006, 24 (29): 4721-4730. PubMed PMID: 16966690.

[48] Krug LM. Vaccine therapy for small cell lung cancer. Seminars in Oncology, 2004, 31 (1 Suppl 1): 112-116. PubMed PMID: 14981589.

[49] Giaccone G, Debruyne C, Felip E, et al. Phase III study of adjuvant vaccination with Bec2/bacille Calmette-Guerin in responding patients with limited-disease small-cell lung cancer (European Organisation for Research and Treatment of Cancer 08971-08971B; Silva Study). Journal of Clinical Oncology, 2005, 23 (28): 6854-6864. PubMed PMID: 16192577.

[50] Toloza EM, Morse MA, Lyerly HK. Gene therapy for lung cancer. Journal of Cellular Biochemistry, 2006, 99 (1): 1-22. PubMed PMID: 16767697.

[51] Hege KM, Carbone DP. Lung cancer vaccines and gene therapy. Lung Cancer, 2003, 41 (Suppl 1): S103-113. PubMed PMID: 12867069.

[52] Hirasawa Y, Kohno N, Yokoyama A, et al. Natural autoantibody to MUC1 is a prognostic indicator for non-small cell lung cancer. American Journal of Respiratory and Critical Care Medicine, 2000, 161 (2 Pt 1): 589-594. PubMed PMID: 10673204.

[53] Mennecier B, Ramlau R, Rolski J. Phase II study evaluating clinical efficacy of TG 4010 (MVA-MUC1 IL2) in association with cisplatin and binorelbine in a patient with non small cell lung cancer//Roth JA, Cox JD, Hong WK (eds). Lung Cancer: Chichester. UK: John Wiley & Sons, Ltd, 2006.

第 30 章
非小细胞肺癌治疗中的新型及新兴药物

Anne S. Tsao[1], Jack A. Roth[2]
Department of Thoracic/Head and Neck Medical Oncology, The University of Texas MD Anderson Cancer Center, Houston, TX, USA
Department of Thoracic and Cardiovascular Surgery, The University of Texas MD Anderson Cancer Center, Houston, TX, USA

引 言

快速 DNA 测序技术的出现，导致了肿瘤学模式的转变。基因治疗与新型靶向药物的研发均在肿瘤学领域得到发展。本章节将从新型靶向药物及基因治疗两方面讲述他们对非小细胞肺癌（NSCLC）治疗的影响。在靶向治疗部分，将从 HSP90、MET/HCF、MEK、PI3K/AKT/mTOR、PARP、NOTCH/Hedgehog 通路及有丝分裂等分子或通路为靶点进行阐述，并研究每类药物背后的原理，同时提供临床药物发展的最新情况。基因治疗部分则集中在 p53 基因的替代研究，阐述迄今为止所完成的临床试验，并探讨 FUS1 替代 DOTAP 的临床试验结果。

新型靶向药物

HSP 90 抑制剂

热休克蛋白 90（heat-shock protein 90，HSP90）是 ATP 依赖的分子伴侣。据推测它在癌细胞中过表达，并通过多种分子伴侣复合物来稳定蛋白并促进其活化。假设 HSP90 可能优先作用于突变蛋白，尤其是来源于癌基因扩增的蛋白。那么可以据此推测，抑制 HSP90 可致潜在多个癌蛋白和多条信号通路的降解。目前，一些 HSP90 仍在研究中。

从已公布的Ⅱ期临床试验数据来看，IPI - 504（瑞他霉素盐酸盐，Infinity Pharmaceuticals 制药公司）在前期未接受过化疗的 76 例 NSCLC 患者中，尤其在 EML4 ALK 阳性易位者中发挥着重要作用，其中共有 3 例 ALK 易位者，有 2 例为部分缓解，1 例肿瘤缩小约 24%，临床评效为稳定。治疗耐受性良好，最常见副作用为 1~2 级乏力、恶心和腹泻。3 级及以上肝功能异常发生率为 11.8%[1]。在临床研究中，Retaspimycin HCl 与多西紫杉醇联合不仅仅用于试验组，也用于 ALK 阳性易位者。

Ganetespib（STA - 9090）是第二代 HSP90 抑制剂，与第一代安莎霉素类药物相比具有不同的结构。Ganetespib 在某些肿瘤的Ⅰ期试验中表明其具有单剂活性，最常见的不良反应为轻中度腹泻。最重要的是，在其他已报道的 HSP90 抑制剂试验中表明，它不存在肝脏剂量限制性或眼毒性。Ganetespib 的Ⅱ期临床试验报告[2]显示，它在 ALK 阳性患者中存在活性，4 例有效者（n = 72）均为 ALK 阳性患者。8 例 ALK 阳性患者中有 6 例肿瘤缩小。目前正在对 ganetespib 与多西他赛联合（GALAXY 试验）以及作为单药用于 ALK 阳性患者进行试验研究。

MET 抑制剂或 HCF 抑制剂

MET（N - 对甲基 1 - N′- 硝基 - N - 亚硝基胍）基因位于 7 号染色体，用于编码跨膜受体。肝细胞生长因子（hepatocyte growth factor，HGF）是 c-MET 受体的唯一配体，它可导致下游信号传导途径的二聚化及后续活化，并在伤口愈合和胚胎发育中发挥重要作用。在异常表型中可通过一些机制，包括 MET 突变，通过基因扩增或拷贝数增益使蛋白质过度表达，以及减少受体降解使 c-MET 激活。MET 基因扩增提示 NSCLC 的预后不良，而且与 EGFR 酪氨酸激酶抑制剂耐药相关[3]。

已经有一些方法可靶向作用于 MET 和 HGF 通路。Onartuzumab（OAM4558g，MetMAb；Genentech，Inc. San Francisco，California），一种抗 MET 单臂人源性 5D5 抗体。在先前的 II 期临床试验中，它被用来评估厄洛替尼联合或不联合 onartuzumab 对 NSCLC 患者的治疗效果，数据显示两组间无统计学差异。然而，在 MET 阳性的患者中，厄洛替尼与 onartuzumab 联合用药可导致无疾病进展时间和总生存的获益[4]。MET 阳性的定义为：通过免疫组化染色，具有中等或较强染色强度的肿瘤细胞占 50%。与厄洛替尼单药治疗相比，联合用药的 MET 阴性患者具有更差的无疾病进展时间和总生存时间。而 MET 阳性患者的这一阳性结果并没有受 EGFR 突变或荧光原位杂交（fluorescent in situ hybridization，FISH）结果的影响。厄洛替尼与 onartuzumab 联合用药最常见的不良反应包括皮疹、腹泻、乏力、恶心、食欲减退、血管神经性水肿及贫血。其他正在进行的一项 onartuzumab II 期试验，正在对该药一线治疗非鳞状细胞 NSCLC 和鳞状细胞 NSCLC 进行研究。1 项随机 III 期临床试验正在对 MET 阳性的 NSCLC 患者（二线或三线治疗）给予厄洛替尼（150mg/d），联合或不联合 onartuzumab（为 15mg/kg，静脉滴注，每 3 周 1 次）进行研究。

Tivantinib（ARQ197，ArQule and Daiichi Sankyo，Woburn，MA）是一种口服的非 ATP 竞争性小分子抑制剂，靶向作用于 c-MET 受体酪氨酸激酶。一项 III 期临床试验正在对既往未接受过 2 线以上治疗方案（MARQUEE，NCT01377376）的非鳞状细胞 NSCLC 患者，应用厄洛替尼联合或不联合 tivantinib 进行治疗。厄洛替尼联合或不联合 tivantinib（720mg/d）的现有 II 期临床试验数据显示，在改善 167 例未经治疗的 NSCLC 患者的生存方面无统计学差异[5]。联合用药的中位 PFS 为 3.8 个月，单药厄洛替尼为 2.3 个月 [HR = 0.81；95% CI（0.57，1.16）；P = 0.24]。中位总生存期方面，联合用药组为 8.5 个月，单药组为 6.9 个月 [HR = 0.87；95% CI（0.44，1.27）；P = 0.47]。在亚组分析中，对 KRAS 突变患者（n = 15）联合应用 tivantinib 和厄洛替尼可显著改善其 PFS [HR = 0.18；95% CI（0.05，0.70）；P < 0.01] 及 OS [HR = 0.43；95% CI（0.12，1.5）；P = 0.17]。该试验中联合用药的常见不良反应为皮疹、贫血和腹泻。一项 II 期临床试验正在对 KRAS 阳性突变的 NSCLC 患者联合应用厄洛替尼及 tivantinib 进行调查研究（NCT01395758）。

Carbozantinib（XL184，Exelixis，Inc. San Francisco，CA）是一种 c-MET、RET 和 VEGFR2 的小分子酪氨酸激酶抑制剂。Carbozantinib 已于 2012 年 11 月获得 FDA 批准用于甲状腺髓样癌的治疗。一项 IB/II 期临床试验正在对 NSCLC 患者进行 carbozanitinib 与厄洛替尼的预处理研究。Ficlatuzumab（AV-299，AVEO，Cambridge，MA）是一种人源化抗 HGF IgG1 单克隆抗体，可抑制配体与受体的结合。一项 II 期随机临床试验，对亚洲不吸烟或很少量吸烟的 NSCLC 患者应用吉非替尼联合或不联合 ficlatuzumab（20mg/kg）进行治疗，公布的初步结果表明，EGFR 突变患者可从治疗获益，此类患者低表达 c-MET，而高表达间质肝细胞生长因子[6]。

MEK 抑制剂

丝裂原活化蛋白（mitogen-activated protein，MAPK）/细胞外信号调节激酶（extracellular signal-regulated kinase，ERK）通路通过生长因子进行信号传导。MAPK 激酶或 MEK 可迅速下调 RAS，引起 RAS/RAF/MEK/ERK 通路的信号异常、失调以及肿瘤的发生。直接抑制 MEK 可降低 MAPK/ERK 信号，并影响随后的细胞生长。最近，对接受前期临床研究的 MEK 抑制剂进行严格审查，结果表明 BRAF 或 RAS 基因突变细胞系对 MEK 抑制剂敏感[7]。一项 II 期随机临床试验对未经治疗过的 NSCLC 患者口服司美替尼（AZD6244，ARRY-142886，AstraZeneca/Array BioPharma）治疗，与培美曲塞治疗相比，两者在生存方面无显著差异[8]。该试验和临床前期研究提示司美替尼药物研究将集中在 RAS 和 RAF 变异的人群。司美替尼可阻断 MEK1 及 MEK2 酶的亚型。

后续的 II 期临床试验证实，对前期确诊为 KRAS 突变的 NSCLC 患者口服司美替尼治疗，效果显著[9]。该试验将多西他赛联合司美替尼（75mg，每天 2 次）与单药多西他赛治疗进行对比，结果显示联合用药组有效率显著（35% vs 0；

$P < 0.001$），PFS 为 6 个月（$P = 0.0158$）。司美替尼与多西他赛联合用药的主要副反应为皮疹、乏力、中性粒细胞减少和发热性中性粒细胞减少症[9]。目前，一项 I 期临床试验正在对 BRAF 突变患者应用司美替尼做进一步的研究。许多变构酶抑制剂和 MEK2 或小分子抑制剂也正在研发中，其中包括 trametinib（GSK1120212，Glaxo Smith Kline）、PD325901（Pfizer）、MEK162（Novartis）和 GDC-0973/XL518（Genentech）。

PI3K/AKT/mTOR 通路抑制剂

基于磷酸肌醇 3-激酶（PI3K）/蛋白激酶 B（AKT）/哺乳动物雷帕霉素靶蛋白（mTOR）通路在调节细胞凋亡中的作用，它已被广泛用于 NSCLC 治疗的研究。在肿瘤学中，它是实体肿瘤最常见的失调通路[10]。PI3K/AKT/mTOR 通路是由胞外生长因子与多个跨膜受体激酶结合，从而激活细胞内信号传导途径。上游基因突变或扩增（例如 RAS 突变、ErbB2 过表达）可致异常信号的产生，基因突变也可导致通路调节剂或抑制剂的缺乏（例如 PTEN 缺失）或 PI3K、AKT 基因的扩增或突变[10-12]。

PI3K 家族由 3 种类别的脂质激酶组成，它们具有不同的脂质产物和靶向特异性。脂质产物可作为第二信使，激活细胞的增殖、分化、凋亡以及葡萄糖稳态[12]。最常见的变异发生在 IA 类 PI3Ks，它是异源二聚体蛋白与 P110 催化发生脂质底物磷酸化而成的亚基[10,12]。一些 PI3K 的小分子抑制剂（聚丙胺 PI3K 或亚型特异性）正在进行 I 期和 II 期 NSCLC 临床试验，同时双 PI3K-mTOR 抑制剂的 I 期试验也在研究中。

BKM120（诺华）是一种口服的聚丙胺 I 类 PI3K 抑制剂，一些 I 期临床试验正在对其进行研究，它可能在抗肿瘤 PI3KCA 基因突变方面起作用[13]。PI3KCA 编码人类 P110 蛋白，是 I 类 PI3K 的催化亚基。与 BKM-120 相关的主要不良反应为瘙痒、皮疹、黏膜炎、恶心、厌食、腹泻、乏力、高血糖和情绪改变[14]。BKM-120 正在联合卡铂与培美曲塞用于非鳞状细胞 NSCLC 患者，以及联合厄洛替尼用于 EGFR 突变，且以前接受过 EGFR 酪氨酸激酶抑制剂治疗的 NSCLC 患者。

GDC-0941（Genentech 公司）是一种 ATP 竞争性抑制剂，选择性地结合 PI3K 亚型 p100α 和 p100δ。对卡铂-紫杉醇-GDC-0941+/-贝伐单抗进行 I 期临床试验研究，初步显示其毒性为：1~2 级脱发、乏力、恶心、口腔炎、厌食、白细胞减少、感觉异常、鼻出血、关节痛、周围神经病变及皮疹[15]；也有 III 级和 IV 级中性粒细胞减少，但这并不会导致剂量限制。在亚组分析中，鳞癌患者的总反应率比非鳞癌高（71% vs 38%）。卡铂-紫杉醇-GDC0941 的一项 II 期试验正在对鳞癌的 NSCLC 患者进行研究。

PX-866（Oncothyreon）是一种口服的不可逆性聚丙胺 I 类 PI3K 抑制剂，与 PI3K 亚型共价结合。实体瘤的一项 I 期临床试验指出，其最常见的副作用为恶心、呕吐、腹泻以及可逆性转氨酶升高[16]。虽然没有统计学差异，但在该试验中，PIKCA 突变患者的疾病稳定性持续时间较长。一项将 PX-866 和多西他赛联合用于转移性 NSCLC 患者或头颈部鳞癌患者的 II 期临床试验正在进行中。

AKT，也被称为蛋白激酶 B，是一种丝-苏氨酸特异性蛋白激酶。存在 3 种亚型，但 AKT1 和 AKT2 与肿瘤形成相关。AKT1 在细胞存活中发挥重要作用，而 AKT2 在胰岛素信号传导途径的葡萄糖转运中发挥作用。AKT 抑制剂包括 ATP 类似物和非催化位点抑制剂。变构抑制剂结合在 PH（pleckstrin-homology）结构域的 AKT 蛋白，从而诱导构象变化，并防止 AKT 定位于质膜而被激活。MK-2206（Merck）是第一个可口服的 $AKT_{1,2,3}$ 变构抑制剂，因此存在时间最长。MK-2206 的前期临床试验已经表明，它可以增加 EGFR 酪氨酸激酶抑制剂的活性，并且使 MET 难治表型的 NSCLC 细胞系再度敏化。一项 I 期临床试验[17]研究显示，其剂量限制性毒性为广义的非泡性斑丘疹。主要不良反应包括皮疹、恶心、呕吐、腹泻和高血糖。该试验中，一例同时存在 PTEN 丢失和 KRAS G12D 突变的患者，24 周时肿瘤显著缩小。另外 2 例神经内分泌患者，肿瘤缩小持续时间为 32 周[17]。一些 MK-2206 的 II 期临床试验正在进行中，包括 MK-2206 与 AZD6244（MEK 抑制剂）联合用于 KRAS 基因突变的患者，以及 MK-2206 与厄洛替尼联合用于厄洛替尼难治性 NSCLC 患者。其他 AKT 抑制剂也在研究中，包括 GSK2141795

和 GSK2110183（Glaxo Smith Kline）、GDC-0068（Genentech）及 LY2780301（Eli Lilly）。

哺乳动物雷帕霉素靶蛋白（mTOR）是一种由 FRAP1 基因编码的丝（苏）氨酸蛋白激酶，它在细胞增殖、运动和凋亡中发挥调节作用。mTOR 蛋白可形成 mTOR 复合物 1（mTORC1），它可以调控蛋白合成并靶向作用于 p70-S6 激酶 1（S6K1）和 4E-BP1（真核起始因子 4E 结合蛋白 1）。S6K1 同时提供一个正反馈循环给 mTORC1。mTOR 的络合物也形成 mTORC2（包括 mTOR、Rictor、GBL、mSIN1），并通过 F-肌动蛋白应力纤维、桩蛋白、CDC42 和蛋白激酶 C，在丝氨酸残基 S473 及细胞骨架上调节 AKT 磷酸化。

目前已有一些 mTOR 抑制剂被开发，其中依维莫司和西罗莫司已被 FDA 批准用于某些肿瘤类型，但不包括 NSCLC。迄今为止，依维莫司在 NSCLC 患者中，无论是作为单药或与化疗或新剂型联合用药，均没有表现出显著的临床获益[18-22]。坦西莫司单药用于 NSCLC 患者的[23]疗效有限，西罗莫司也被作为维持治疗用于广泛期 NSCLC，但没有表现出临床获益[24]。Ridaforolimus（MK-8669，Merck）是一种小分子抑制剂，与西妥昔单抗联合用于 NSCLC 患者的治疗正在研究中，且在一项 II 期临床试验中，用于所有 KRAS 突变的 NSCLC 患者。

BEZ235（Novartis）是一种口服咪唑喹啉衍生物，聚丙胺 PI3K 抑制剂可抑制 mTORC1 与 mTORC2[25]。在第一个 I 期临床试验中，遇到的主要不良反应为恶心、呕吐、腹泻、乏力、贫血、厌食[26]。正在研究的其他 I 期临床试验（NCT01343498）正在评估每天两次的给药方案[27]。一项独立的实体瘤 I 期临床试验正在根据前期临床试验所证实的协同作用，来评估 BEZ235 与依维莫司的联合用药情况[28]。其他的一些 mTORC1/2 抑制剂还包括 INK128（Intellikine）、OSI-027（OSI 制药）和 AZD8055（Astra Zeneca）。

PARP 抑制剂

聚腺苷二磷酸核糖聚合酶（poly-adenosine diphosphate-ribose polymerase，PARP）由几种调节 DNA 修复和细胞凋亡的蛋白组成。该 PARP 酶的主要作用是通过 DNA 连接酶Ⅲ、DNA 聚合酶 β 以及支架蛋白的 X 射线交叉互补基因 1（XRCC1）来识别单链 DNA 断裂和启动碱基剪切修复机制。在有明显 DNA 损伤的细胞中，PARP 可以消耗细胞的 ATP，以努力修复 DNA，并由此诱导细胞裂解和死亡。PARP 也参与程序性细胞死亡[29]。

当 PARP 被抑制，细胞的单链 DNA 缺口出现，最终导致细胞复制过程中双链断裂。在基因突变（BRCA1 或 BRCA2）的肿瘤细胞中，PARP 抑制剂可诱发多种 DNA 链断裂，并最终导致细胞死亡。此外，PARP 抑制剂将 PARP 结合在 DNA 上，该复合物会妨碍复制，从而对细胞产生毒性[30]。

一些 PARP 抑制剂正在作为单药以及与其他剂型联合用于 NSCLC 患者。目前进行的一项 II 期临床试验正在对 veliparib（ABT-888，Abbott，Abbott Park，IL）联合或不联合卡铂-紫杉醇治疗 NSCLC 患者进行评价。而 veliparib 与细胞周期蛋白依赖性激酶抑制剂 SCH727965 联合用于 BRCA 突变肿瘤正在进行 I 期临床试验。SWOG 的 I 期临床试验（NCI8811），将卡铂-紫杉醇-veliparib 与放疗联合用于 III 期 NSCLC 的治疗也在研究中。Olaparib（AZD2281，Astra Zeneca，London，England）作为一种口服剂型，已在 BRCA 突变的乳腺癌和卵巢癌（BRCA1/2 突变或野生型）中广泛研究[31-32]。在这些试验中，患者应用 olaparib 最常见的副作用有恶心、呕吐、乏力、贫血。此外，西班牙的 Lung Group 正在进行一项 IB/II 期临床试验，将吉非替尼联合或不联合 olaparib 应用于 EGFR 突变的 NSCLC 患者的治疗。

Notch 与 hedgehog 抑制剂

肿瘤干细胞具有多能性并可自我更新，而且被认为与有效治疗后的肿瘤复发或疾病进展密切相关。Notch 和 Hedgehog 是参与肿瘤干细胞持续增殖的重要信号通路[33]。Notch 受体（1~4）是一种单次跨膜受体，它可被位于邻近细胞上的 5 种配体 [Delta-like 1（DLL1）、DLL3、DLL4、Jagged 1 和 Jagged 2] 所激活[34-35]。Notch 信号转导通路是多细胞生物中高度保守的通路之一[36]。一旦 Notch 受体和配体结合，其胞外域就会被 ADAM 家族的金属蛋白酶 TACE（TNF-α 转化酶）从膜上切割。随后，该受体的 γ 分泌酶裂解细胞膜受体，使 Notch 横移至细胞核，从而激活转录因子 CSL 并调节基因表达[34-36]。

迄今为止，多数 Notch 信号传导途径的抑制剂为 γ-分泌酶抑制剂，其中 REGN421（Regeneron）作为一种人类单克隆抗体 Delta 4-配体正在进行一项 I 期临床试验。γ-分泌酶抑制剂可增加聚腺苷二磷酸核糖聚合酶抑制剂的裂解，并诱导细胞凋亡。目前进行的一项 I/II 期试验正在对 NSCLC 患者进行 RO4929097 联合厄洛替尼治疗。RO4929097 同时也正接受一线治疗后的维持治疗研究。另外一个 γ-分泌酶抑制剂 PF-03084014 正在一项实体瘤的 I 期临床试验中进行评估[37]。

Hedgehog 通路是哺乳动物发育的主要调节剂，并参与调节成熟干细胞。有 2 个跨膜受体启动 hedgehog 信号传导途径：Patched homologue-1（PTCH1）与 Patched homologue-2（PTCH2）。Hedgehog 蛋白由细胞分泌，并附着于邻近细胞的 PTCH1 和（或）PTCH2 上。PTCH1 可抑制 7 次跨膜蛋白 Smoothened 同源物（SMO），以防止 glioma 相关癌基因同源物（glioma-associated oncogene homologue，GLI）活化。GLI 活化可诱发 hedgehog 靶基因的转录调控，以及随后的细胞增殖与存活[38]。在基底细胞癌中，可识别出 PTCH1 或 SMO 基因的突变[39,40]。Vismodegib（GDC-0449，Genentech，South San Francisco，CA）于 2012 年 1 月获得 FDA 批准用于基底细胞癌的治疗。与 vismodegib 相关的主要副作用是味觉减退、脱发与肌肉痉挛[40]。ECOG1508 的一项随机 II 期临床研究正在对 vismodegib 进行调查研究，该研究应用顺铂-依托泊苷联合或不联合 vismodegib 或 IMG-A12（胰岛素样生长因子受体）对广泛期 SCLC 患者进行化疗。

有丝分裂抑制剂

有几种不同的方法可以对有丝分裂进行抑制，其中有 4 种方法正在进行积极的药物研发：微管蛋白结合剂、微管蛋白酶抑制剂、有丝分裂酶抑制剂以及有丝分裂检查点抑制剂。微管蛋白结合剂能稳定微管，并通过连接至 α-微管蛋白异源二聚体亚基来防止解离。微管蛋白酶抑制剂或有丝分裂驱动蛋白可阻碍纺锤体功能，从而引起有丝分裂停滞及细胞死亡。有丝分裂酶抑制剂属于丝-苏氨酸激酶，它靶向作用于 aurora 激酶和 polo 样激酶（polo-like kinase，PLK）调节细胞分裂。有丝分裂检查点抑制剂是 DNA 损伤敏化剂，在正常细胞中，检查点 1（Chk1）的活化会导致细胞周期停滞，而且它是充分修复 DNA 的关键。大多数检查点抑制剂是通过静脉注射给药，但口服剂型也正在研发中。

有些微管蛋白结合剂已经被 FDA 批准用于乳腺癌和肺癌。一些常见的微管蛋白结合剂有紫杉醇（批准用于肺癌和乳腺癌）、埃博霉素、abraxane（用于肺癌和乳腺癌）、艾日布林（用于乳腺癌）和伊沙匹隆（用于乳腺癌）。艾日布林是软海绵素 B 的合成类似物，它可以抑制微管聚合，并将微管蛋白螯合成非功能性集合体。在实体瘤中应用 eribulin 与卡铂的 IB 期临床试验显示，其主要不良反应为中性粒细胞减少、血小板减少、疲乏、恶心。目前一些研究正在对艾日布林联合标准化疗和厄洛替尼治疗 NSCLC 进行研究。伊沙匹隆是一种微管稳定埃坡霉素 B 类似物，它对表达 β3-微管蛋白（β3T）且对紫杉耐药的转移性乳腺癌具有抗肿瘤活性。在 NSCLC 中，对于应用紫杉类药物治疗的晚期 NSCLC 患者而言，高 β3T 水平是一个预后不良因素[41]。但是，一项 II 期随机临床试验对伊沙匹隆或紫杉醇联合卡铂进行研究表明，β3T 表达不同并不能显示出生存差异[42]。Abraxane 是一种纳米颗粒的白蛋白结合紫杉醇（NAB 紫杉醇），是紫杉醇与白蛋白相结合的剂型。一项 III 期临床试验研究[43]表明，与卡铂-紫杉醇相比，在 NSCLC 患者尤其是鳞癌患者中应用 abraxane 和卡铂进行化疗表现出显著的有效性。Abraxane 已于 2012 年 10 月被 FDA 批准用于 NSCLC 的治疗。

极光激酶有 3 种亚型（A、B、C），但只有极光激酶 A 和 B 是潜在的治疗靶标。抑制极光激酶 A 可使有丝分裂延迟、单极纺锤体和染色体分离失误，而抑制极光激酶 B 会导致细胞分裂异常、多倍体和细胞凋亡。目前一些极光激酶抑制剂正在研究中，极光激酶 A 抑制剂 ENMD-0276（Entremed）和 MLN8237（Millenium）正在进行 I 期和 II 期临床试验。初步研究结果表明，其剂量限制性毒性是骨髓抑制和黏膜炎。极光激酶 B 抑制剂 GSK1070916A（Glaxo Smith Kline）和 AZD1152（Astra Zeneca）也在实体瘤及白血病患者中进行Ⅰ期和Ⅱ期临床试验。另外还有几个panaurora激酶抑制剂正在进行Ⅰ期和Ⅱ期临床试验。迄今为止，还没有极光激酶抑制剂对 NSCLC 进行特殊研究试验的，它们在 NSCLC 治疗中的作用仍然未知。

Polo 样激酶（polo-like kinase，PLK）参与细胞周期的所有阶段，但主要作用于 M 期。PLK-1 在具有较高组织学分级的高分期 NSCLC 中过表达，而且与染色体不稳定和异倍体有关。前期临床对 NSCLC 的鼠异种移植物模型进行研究表明，通过 siRNA 对 PLK-1 进行抑制可降低肝转移及肿瘤细胞的生长[44]。BI6727（Boehringer Ingelhcim）靶向作用于 PLK-1 ATP 结合部，可破坏纺锤体组装从而导致细胞周期停滞和细胞凋亡。BI6727 的实体肿瘤Ⅰ期临床试验（n=65）所报道的剂量限制性毒性为骨髓抑制。一项 3 组Ⅱ期临床试验中，对 NSCLC 患者随机应用单药 BI6727、单药培美曲塞或两药联合进行治疗，目前正在加拿大进行研究（计划 n=150，主要终点为 PFS）。

驱动蛋白抑制剂正处于发展初期。作为一类剂型，它们可引起中性粒细胞减少、乏力、贫血、恶心、皮疹和低钠血症。Ispinesib（SB-715992，Glaxo Smith Kline）作用于有丝分裂纺锤体驱动蛋白（kinesin spindle protein，KSP）Eg5，额外毒性为高血糖，但没有神经毒性。LY-2523355（Eli Lilly）是 Eg5 的变构抑制剂，目前正在 SCLC 中进行Ⅱ期临床试验。SB-743921（Glaxo Smith Kline）作用于 KSP Eg5，目前也在 SCLC 和 NSCLC 中进行Ⅱ期临床试验。

大多数检查点抑制剂都推测与 DNA 损伤剂（如化疗）联用可更好地发挥作用。在前期临床模型中，对检查点激酶 1 抑制剂 LY2603618（Eli Lilly/ Array Biopharma）进行的研究显示，它与培美曲塞有协同活性，尤其是在 p53 突变的肿瘤细胞。国际上一项单组Ⅱ期临床试验正在对 LY2603618-培美曲塞联合治疗转移性 NSCLC 患者进行研究，并包括了药物的基因组学分析。一项Ⅰ/Ⅱ期临床试验正在对 LY2603618 联合顺铂与培美曲塞进行研究，主要集中在非鳞状 NSCLC 的第二阶段部分（主要目标为 PFS）。AZD7762（Astra Zeneca）为检查点 1/2 的 ATP 竞争性抑制剂，一项Ⅰ期临床试验正在对该试剂进行研究。

总结及新型靶向药物的未来走向

本节所讨论的靶向治疗并不包括所有的新药或正在研发中的某些药物。所选择的通路和剂型，重点是因为它们最大限度地跟随临床发展，而且在 NSCLC 治疗领域有更多的发展潜力。可以预料，随着对肿瘤细胞生物学更深层次的理解，新药开发也将有更光明的未来。最终可以预料，NSCLC 患者将被识别驱动突变，从而决定它们的初始治疗计划。随后，在疾病进展期，肿瘤将被重新活检，从而发现额外突变或通路失调，并直接进行靶向治疗。这一个性化用药的新模式已经在其他章节针对 NSCLC 的 EGFR 突变、EML-4ALK 易位和 BRAF 突变阐述过了。

肺癌靶向基因治疗

过去 20 年的研究已经建立了肺癌的遗传学基础。烟草烟雾中所含的 100 多种致癌物可使肿瘤抑制基因以及 DNA 修复基因灭活，并且激活肿瘤生长调节基因[45]。从组织学上来讲，有吸烟史的人，他的正常支气管黏膜可见多种基因损伤。大约 15% 的肺癌病例发生在从不吸烟的个体，这些病例的肿瘤遗传信息也是不同的[46]。在这本书其他部分所讨论的全基因组测序已经发现驱动突变将导致许多癌基因的持续活化。小分子药物可阻断癌基因的激活，从而导致短暂但具有戏剧性的应答，然而，仅有少于 10% 的肺癌患者检测出存在个体基因突变[47]。最近全基因组测序检测出肿瘤抑制基因中最常见的基因突变[48]。在肺癌中最常发生突变的基因是肿瘤抑制基因 p53，它最先应用于肺癌基因治疗。

p53 蛋白监测细胞应激和 DNA 损伤，它既可以在 DNA 广泛损伤时使生长停滞以促进 DNA 修复，也可以诱导细胞程序性死亡（细胞凋亡）[49]。当细胞受到癌基因活化、缺氧或 DNA 损伤刺激时，完整的 p53 通路可决定该细胞是否将接收的信号用于阻止其停滞在细胞周期的 G1 期，是否尝试 DNA 修复，或细胞是否通过凋亡进行自毁。以前，人们认为基因疗法不能替代所有癌细胞中的受损基因，因此也不会有显著疗效。当癌细胞触发细胞凋亡时对野生型 p53 基因的表达进行研究，为基因疗法提供了理论依据[50]。事实上，仅修复一个缺陷基因就足以触发细胞凋亡，这表明目前癌细胞中 DNA 损伤会使癌细胞准备好通过一个单一通路诱导凋亡事件。

P53 基因替代

上述研究表明，在 p53 功能缺陷的肿瘤细胞中野生型 p53 基因的表达即可介导细胞凋亡，也可使细胞生长停滞，这两者对癌症患者而言都具有治疗益处。初始研究表明，用逆转录病毒载体修复功能性 p53 基因，可以抑制某些人肺癌细胞系的生长，但不是全部。第一个进行 p53 基因治疗的研究表明，在原位人肺癌模型中用反转录病毒的表达载体对该基因进行治疗，可抑制肿瘤生长[51]。这项研究首次证明，修复单个肿瘤抑制基因的功能可使人类癌细胞在体内消退。由于使用逆转录病毒的固有局限性，包括基因组整合和不可靠的转基因表达，使得后续肺癌 p53 基因替代研究使用腺病毒载体（Ad-P53）[52]。原始的腺病毒载体是删除 E1 区的血清型 5 复制 – 缺陷载体。随后的研究表明，在人原位肺癌的小鼠模型中 Ad-p53 可抑制肿瘤的生长[53]，而且在各种其他肿瘤细胞系及小鼠体内异种移植肿瘤模型中，其诱导细胞凋亡并抑制细胞增殖[54-56]。旁观者杀伤效应（通过转基因细胞杀伤非转基因细胞）是非常必要的，因为病毒载体并不转导所有的癌细胞，该效应将涉及血管生成的调节[57-58]、免疫上调[59-61]，并且分泌可溶性促凋亡蛋白[62]。

P53 基因替代的临床试验

首个 p53 基因替代临床试验方案，使用复制缺陷型逆转录病毒载体，通过 β 肌动蛋白启动子驱动野生型 p53 的表达[63]。将基因或载体的构建体注射到 59 例不能手术切除，且常规治疗后进展的 NSCLC 肿瘤患者体内，9 例患者中有 3 例表现出肿瘤消退的证据，且没有载体相关毒性，这表明了 p53 基因治疗的可行性和安全性。

随后的 P53 临床试验采用人腺病毒 p53 表达载体。一项 I 期临床试验纳入 28 例对常规治疗无效的 NSCLC 患者，该试验证实，80% 的可评估患者成功进行了基因转染[64]；46% 的患者可检测到 p53 表达，表达该基因的患者除 1 例外，其他均发生细胞凋亡，更重要的是，没有观察到显著毒性。有 2 例患者的肿瘤体积缩小超过 50%，其中 1 例在最终治疗后无肿瘤复发时间超过 1 年；另外一例对放化疗耐受的上叶支气管肿瘤几乎完全消退。其他对头颈部肿瘤患者的研究也为 Ad-p53 基因转染作为一种可行的临床策略提供了有利证据，研究表明它可以使基因转录和基因表达获得成功，具有低毒性，可消退肿瘤，而且可以显示 p53 生物标记物的预反应能力[65-67]。

基因替代与放化疗联合

对培养的 NSCLC 细胞及裸鼠的人异种移植物应用 P53 基因疗法联合顺铂进行治疗显示，顺铂与 p53 基因治疗的顺序给药可增强 p53 基因产物的表达[68-69]。对 Ad-p53 基因转染联合放疗进行研究表明，导入 p53 腺病毒可增加 p53 缺陷肿瘤细胞对体外射线的敏感性[56]。

24 例对先前常规治疗无效的 NSCLC 患者应用 Ad-p53 和顺铂进行治疗[70]。75% 的患者应用含顺铂或卡铂的方案会发生肿瘤进展。静脉应用顺铂达 6 个月，随后 3d 通过瘤体内注射 Ad-p53 基因，结果显示 17 例患者的病情稳定至少 2 个月，2 例患者达到部分缓解；79% 的肿瘤活检显示凋亡细胞的数量明显增加。

一项 II 期临床试验对每一例参加试验的 NSCLC 患者评价两个可比较的转移灶[71]。所有患者均接受化疗，用卡铂联合紫杉醇治疗 3 个周期，或用顺铂加长春瑞滨治疗 3 个周期，之后将 p53 腺病毒直接注射到一个病灶内。接受卡铂联合紫杉醇化疗并从中获益的患者，并没有发现 Ad-p53 基因转染所带来的额外益处。然而，顺铂和长春瑞滨方案治疗失败的患者，通过测定肿瘤大小显示，与对照组病灶相比，接受 p53 腺病毒局部注射的病变明显消退。

前期临床研究表明，对某些肿瘤而言，p53 基因替代可能增强放疗敏感性[56,72-75]，基于此结论，一项临床试验正在对 p53 基因转染结合外照射放疗[76]进行研究。一般因状态差而无法接受外科手术的患者，在接受化疗联合 60Gy 放疗超过 6 周，并在第 1、18、32 天应用 Ad-p53 基因注射治疗时存在高风险。19 例患者接受局部 NSCLC 治疗，1 例完全缓解（5%），11 例部分缓解（58%），3 例病灶稳定（16%）。在完成治疗后3个月，活检显示12例患者无肿瘤存活（63%），3例（16%）存在肿瘤存活，4例患者（21%）由于肿瘤进展、早期死亡或体力差没有进行活检；1年的无疾病进展生存率为45.5%；1年后13例可评价的患者中，5例（39%）完全缓解，3例（23%）部分缓解或病情稳定。大部分治疗失败是由于无局部进展的转移性疾病所引起。

在这项研究中，治疗前后进行肿瘤活检，就可以详细地研究基因表达。12例患者中对9例进行配对活检，其组织标本中检测到p53腺病毒载体特异性的DNA。对11例有充足样本的患者进行载体DNA和mRNA分析，8例显示注射后增加了可检测载体DNA相关的mRNA表达。在Ad-p53注射后24h，12个配对活检组织中有11个检测到注射后增加了p53 mRNA的表达，11个中有10个增加了3倍以上。对注射前的活检标本进行免疫组化染色表明，p53蛋白的表达为阴性；Ad-p53注射后p53蛋白表达呈阳性。染色结果证实了p53蛋白表达于治疗后样本的癌细胞核中。与治疗前活检相比，p53腺病毒注射24h后及治疗期间显示p21（CDKN1A）mRNA的增加有统计学差异。治疗期间较治疗前相比，MDM2 mRNA表达水平较高。FAS mRNA水平在治疗期间无明显变化。注射p53腺病毒24h后BAK mRNA表达显著增加，这似乎是由于p53腺病毒注射导致标志物的急性上调。

瘤体内注射p53腺病毒的安全性良好。进行p53腺病毒注射治疗，最常见的不良反应为发热和寒战、乏力、注射部位疼痛、恶心、呕吐。这些副反应大部分为轻度至中度。迄今为止，还没有明确p53腺病毒注射的最大耐受剂量。基于Ad-p53联合放疗治疗头颈部肿瘤患者的完全缓解数量在增加，Ad-p53在中国已被批准应用于人体，成为首个获得指定和认可的基因治疗试剂[22]。

转移灶的系统基因治疗

肺癌的局部控制非常重要，但多数肺癌患者因全身转移而死亡。肿瘤疫苗可以增强全身免疫反应，从而作用于癌细胞异常表达蛋白，如突变的p53。肿瘤细胞中突变的p53会发生构象改变，并且半衰期长，这表明p53基因可以作为肿瘤抗原和疫苗靶点[77-80]。一项临床试验将最有效的抗原呈递细胞——树突状细胞导入Ad-p53，对广泛期SCLC进行治疗[81]。广泛期SCLC患者未经治疗的中位生存期为2~4个月，而化疗后可达6~8个月。患者首先接受常规化疗，其自体树突状细胞在体外经Ad-p53处理，可激活细胞并导致p53蛋白的高表达。对那些化疗后至少达到稳定的患者应用疫苗注射治疗，每周2次，共3~6次。如果患者病情发生进展，则进行化疗。29例治疗者中，有1例部分缓解，7例稳定，21例进展。发生进展的患者接受二线化疗，并完成了临床随访。21例接受二线化疗的患者，完全或部分缓解率为61.9%。11例患者在首次疫苗治疗后存活时间达1年。临床反应与疫苗诱导的免疫反应相关。已公布的广泛期SCLC患者二线化疗的客观缓解率为5%~30%。

全基因组测序已确定的驱动子突变，是小分子靶向药物研发的依据。目前的临床试验中，许多小分子药物靶向作用于肿瘤存活的关键通路。目前3大主要挑战已显现出来：首先，人类肿瘤中所检测到的驱动突变频率小于10%；其次，尽管开始反应剧烈，但这种反应是暂时性的，一般为6个月或更少；最后，在肿瘤抑制基因中发现最常见的突变为p53突变，但迄今为止，小分子一直无法恢复肿瘤抑制基因的功能。如果基因转染至肿瘤的远隔部位是可行的，成功恢复抑癌基因的功能才能得以完成。最近，随着纳米合成囊泡的发展，有报道指出它可以封装质粒DNA，经静脉注射后可转染细胞[82-83]。这已被用于人弥散性肺癌的小鼠异种移植模型研究。除p53外，其他肿瘤抑制基因也可使用这种技术进行转染。在多种人类肿瘤的体外试验及临床前期动物模型中，3p21.3的多个基因表现出不同程度的肿瘤抑制活性。该位点上其中一个肿瘤抑制基因TUSC2（也称FUS1）在多数肺癌中并不表达。当野生型TUSC2在肺癌细胞中表达，细胞凋亡途径将被激活并发生细胞死亡。为了将这些研究成果转化为临床应用中的肿瘤分子治疗，研制了一个系统治疗策略，将新型TUSC2表达质粒载体与N-[1-(2,3-二油氧基)丙基]-N,N,N-三甲基氯化铵（DOTAP）：胆固醇（DOTAP：Chol）纳米囊泡整合，称为TUSC2纳米囊泡，用于肺癌和肺转移的治疗[82,83]。将 TUSC2 纳米囊泡静脉注射到老鼠体内来承载 A549 肺转移试验,可显著降低转移灶的数量;而且承受肺癌的动物在接受 TUSC2 纳米囊泡处理后,与对照动物相比,其生存时间显著延长。这些研究为Ⅳ期肺癌患者静脉应用 TUSC2 介导的分子治疗的临床试验提供了合理性[84]。对先前接受过铂类基础方案化疗的肺癌复发或转移患者,每 3 周静脉应用 N-[1-(2,3-二油氧基)丙基]-N,N,N-三甲基氯化铵(DOTAP):胆固醇纳米囊泡封装的 FUS-1 表达质粒(DOTAP:chol-FUS-1),按逐渐增加的剂量进行治疗。31 例患者接受了 6 种剂量水平的治疗(0.01~0.09mg/kg)。MTD 被最终确定为 0.06mg/kg。有 5 例患者达到病情稳定(2.6~10.8 个月,其中包括两个弱效)。1 例患者在 PET 成像中呈完整代谢反应。RT-PCR 分析显示,8 个治疗后的肿瘤组织标本中有 7 个检测到 FUS-1 质粒表达,但预处理标本及外周血淋巴细胞在对照组中均无表达。对 3 例患者的配对活检标本进行近似结扎法免疫组织化学染色,证实预处理组织中低背景 FUS-1 蛋白染色,但在治疗后的组织中 FUS-1 蛋白强染色(10~25 倍)。对治疗后高表达 FUS-1 mRNA 和蛋白的 2 例患者进行 RT-PCR 基因表达谱分析显示,其内在凋亡通路在治疗后发生了显著变化。2 例治疗后的患者,其细胞凋亡阵列中 S2 有 29 个基因被修改。该研究表明 DOTAP:chol-FUS-1 可以安全地经静脉给药途径应用于肺癌患者,它可以使人原发和转移性肿瘤摄取该基因,导致转基因及基因产物表达,在 FUS-1 调控通路上发生特异性改变以及发挥抗肿瘤效应;这在已有的研究中是第一次对系统性 DOTAP:胆固醇纳米囊泡基因治疗进行报道。未来还计划将基因治疗与其他靶向治疗药物进行联合。

基因治疗的未来展望

本章中所总结的临床试验表明,与最初基因治疗不适用于肿瘤的预测相反,基因替代疗法靶向作用于肿瘤抑制基因可以通过激活已知通路的方式使肿瘤消退,且毒副作用小。

随着肿瘤基因治疗日渐成熟,有一些问题仍需要解决,包括:更有效的全身基因转染载体的开发、最佳基因靶点的鉴定、联合治疗的优化、更灵敏的用于监测肿瘤细胞基因摄取和表达的预测技术以及克服治疗耐药的策略。

大量的靶向基因治疗方法正在 NSCLC 中进行积极的临床研发。与此同时,定量蛋白质组学及基因组技术变得更加容易,这促使个体化治疗试图通过唯一的肿瘤特异性分子信号来匹配特定的靶向基因治疗。

(孟 敏 叶 欣 译)

参考文献

[1] Sequist LV, Gettinger S, Senzer NN, et al. Activity of IPI-504, a novel heat-shock protein 90 inhibitor, in patients with molecularly defined non-small-cell lung cancer. J Clin Oncol, 2010, 28: 4953-4960.

[2] Wong K, Koczywas M, Goldman J, et al. An open-label phase Ⅱ study of the HSP90 inhibitor ganetespib (STA-9090) as monotherapy in patients with advanced NSCLC [abstract 7500]. J Clin Oncol, 2011, 29: 7500.

[3] Engelman JA, Zejnullahu K, Mitsudomi T, et al. MET amplification leads to gefitinib resistance in lung cancer by activating ERBB3 signaling. Science, 2007, 316: 1039-1043.

[4] Spigel D, Ervin T, Ramlau R, et al. Final efficacy results from OAM4558g, a randomized phase Ⅱ study evaluating MetMAb or placebo in combination with erltoinib in advanced NSCLC [Abstract 7505]. J Clin Oncol, 2011, 29: 7505.

[5] Sequist LV, von Pawel J, Garmey EG, et al. Randomized phase Ⅱ study of erlotinib plus tivantinib versus erlotinib plus placebo in previously treated non-small-cell lung cancer. J Clin Oncol, 2011, 29: 3307-3315.

[6] Mok T, Park K, Jac J, et al. Randomized phase Ⅱ study of ficlatuzumab (formerly AV-299), an anti-hepatocyte growth factor (HGF) monoclonal antibody (MAb) in combination with gefitinib (G) in Asian patients (pts) with NSCLC. J Clin Oncol, 2011, 29: TPS213.

[7] Davies BR, Logie A, McKay JS, et al. AZD6244 (ARRY-142886), a potent inhibitor of mitogen-activated protein kinase/extracellular signal-regulated kinase kinase 1/2 kinases: mechanism of action in vivo, pharmacokinetic/pharmacodynamic relationship, and potential for combination in preclinical models. Mol Cancer Ther, 2007, 6:

[8] Hainsworth JD, Cebotaru CL, Kanarev V, et al. A phase II, open-label, randomized study to assess the efficacy and safety of AZD6244 (ARRY-142886) versus pemetrexed in patients with non-small cell lung cancer who have failed one or two prior chemotherapeutic regimens. J Thorac Oncol, 2010, 5: 1630 – 1636.

[9] Pasi A, Janne ATS, Pereira JR, et al. Phase II double-blind, randomized study of selumetinib (SEL) plus docetaxel (DOC) versus DOC plus placebo as second-line treatment for advanced KRAS mutant non-small cell lung cancer (NSCLC). J Clin Oncol, 2012, 30: 7503.

[10] Engelman JA. Targeting PI3K signalling in cancer: opportunities, challenges and limitations. Nat Rev Cancer, 2009, 9: 550 – 562.

[11] Sansal I, Sellers WR. The biology and clinical relevance of the PTEN tumor suppressor pathway. J Clin Oncol, 2004, 22: 2954 – 2963.

[12] Katso R, Okkenhaug K, Ahmadi K, et al. Cellular function of phosphoinositide 3-kinases: Implications for development, homeostasis, and cancer. Annu Rev Cell Dev Biol, 2001, 17: 615 – 675.

[13] Maira SM, Pecchi S, Huang A, et al. Identification and characterization of NVP-BKM120, an orally available pan-class I PI3-kinase inhibitor. Mol Cancer Ther, 2012, 11: 317 – 328.

[14] Bendell JC, Rodon J, Burris HA, et al. Phase I, dose-escalation study of BKM120, an oral pan-Class I PI3K inhibitor, in patients with advanced solid tumors. J Clin Oncol, 2012, 30: 282 – 290.

[15] Besse B, Gomez-Roca C, Ware JA, et al. A phase Ib study to evaluate the PI3-kinase inhibitor GDC-0941 with paclitaxel (P) and carboplatin (C), with and without bevacizumab (BEV), in patients with advanced non-small cell lung cancer (NSCLC). J Clin Oncol, 2011, 29: 3044.

[16] Hong DS, Bowles DW, Falchook GS, et al. A multicenter phase I trial of PX-866, an oral irreversible phosphatidylinositol 3-kinase inhibitor, in patients with advanced solid tumors. Clin Cancer Res, 2012, 18: 4173 – 4182.

[17] Yap TA, Yan L, Patnaik A, et al. First-in-man clinical trial of the oral pan-AKT inhibitor MK-2206 in patients with advanced solid tumors. J Clin Oncol, 2011, 29: 4688 – 4695.

[18] Price KA, Azzoli CG, Krug LM, et al. Phase II trial of gefitinib and everolimus in advanced non-small cell lung cancer. J Thorac Oncol, 2010, 5: 1623 – 1629.

[19] Gridelli C, Rossi A, Morgillo F, et al. A ran-domized phase II study of pemetrexed or RAD001 as second-line treatment of advanced non-small-cell lung cancer in elderly patients: treatment rationale and protocol dynamics. Clin Lung Cancer, 2007, 8: 568 – 571.

[20] Papadimitrakopoulou VA, Soria JC, Jappe A, et al. Everolimus and erlotinib as second-or third-line therapy in patients with advanced non-small-cell lung cancer. J Thorac Oncol, 2012, 7: 1594 – 1601.

[21] Soria JC, Shepherd FA, Douillard JY, et al. Efficacy of everolimus (RAD001) in patients with advanced NSCLC previously treated with chemotherapy alone or with chemotherapy and EGFR inhibitors. Ann Oncol, 2009, 20: 1674 – 1681.

[22] Vansteenkiste J, Solomon B, Boyer M, et al. Everolimus in combination with pemetrexed in patients with advanced non-small cell lung cancer previously treated with chemotherapy: a phase I study using a novel, adaptive Bayesian dose-escalation model. J Thorac Oncol, 2011, 6: 2120 – 2129.

[23] Hidalgo M, Buckner JC, Erlichman C, et al. A phase I and pharmacokinetic study of temsirolimus (CCI – 779) administered intravenously daily for 5 days every 2 weeks to patients with advanced cancer. Clin Cancer Res, 2006, 12: 5755 – 5763.

[24] Pandya KJ, Dahlberg S, Hidalgo M, et al. A randomized, phase II trial of two dose levels of tem-sirolimus (CCI – 779) in patients with extensive-stage small-cell lung cancer who have responding or stable disease after induction chemotherapy: A trial of the Eastern Cooperative Oncology Group (E1500). J Thorac Oncol, 2007, 2: 1036 – 1041.

[25] Maira SM, Stauffer F, Brueggen J, et al. Identification and characterization of NVP-BEZ235, a new orally available dual phosphatidylinositol 3-kinase/mammalian target of rapamycin inhibitor with potent in vivo antitumor activity. Mol Cancer Ther, 2008, 7: 1851 – 1863.

[26] Burris H, Sharma S, Herbst RS, et al. First-in-human phase I study of the oral PI3K inhibitor BEZ235 in patients (pts) with advanced solid tumors. J Clin Oncol, 2010, 28: 3005.

[27] NCI: http: //clinicaltrials. gov/show/NCT01343498.

[28] Xu CX, Li Y, Yue P, et al. The combination of RAD001 and NVP – BEZ235 exerts synergistic anti-cancer activity

[29] Annunziata CM, O'Shaughnessy J. Poly (ADP-ribose) polymerase as a novel therapeutic target in cancer. Clin Cancer Res, 2010, 16: 4517-4526.

[30] Helleday T. The underlying mechanism for the PARP and BRCA synthetic lethality: Clearing up the misunderstandings. Mol Oncol 2011, 5: 387-393.

[31] Fong PC, Boss DS, Yap TA, et al. Inhibition of poly (ADP-ribose) polymerase in tumors from BRCA mutation carriers. N Engl J Med, 2009, 361: 123-134.

[32] Ledermann J, Harter P, Gourley C, et al. Olaparib maintenance therapy in platinum-sensitive relapsed ovarian cancer. N Engl J Med, 2012, 366: 1382-1392.

[33] Alison MR, Lin WR, Lim SM, et al. Cancer stem cells: In the line of fire. Cancer Treat Rev, 2012, 38: 589-598.

[34] Guruharsha KG, Kankel MW, Artavanis-Tsakonas S. The Notch signalling system: recent insights into the complexity of a conserved pathway. Nat Rev Genet, 2012, 13: 654-666.

[35] Kopan R, Ilagan MX. The canonical Notch signaling pathway: unfolding the activation mechanism. Cell, 2009, 137: 216-233.

[36] Artavanis-Tsakonas S, Rand MD, Lake RJ. Notch signaling: Cell fate control and signal integration in development. Science, 1999, 284: 770-776.

[37] Weiss GJ. Doubling down with inhibitors of Notch and Hedgehog signaling pathways. J Thorac Oncol, 2012, 7: S409-410.

[38] Rahnama F, Shimokawa T, Lauth M, et al. Inhibition of GLI1 gene activation by Patched1. Biochem J, 2006, 394: 19-26.

[39] Tang JY, Mackay-Wiggan JM, Aszterbaum M, et al. Inhibiting the hedgehog pathway in patients with the basal-cell nevus syndrome. N Engl J Med, 2012, 366: 2180-2188.

[40] Von Hoff DD, LoRusso PM, Rudin CM, et al. Inhibition of the hedgehog pathway in advanced basal-cell carcinoma. N Engl J Med, 2009, 361: 1164-1172.

[41] Seve P, Mackey J, Isaac S, et al. Class III beta-tubulin expression in tumor cells predicts response and outcome in patients with non-small cell lung cancer receiving paclitaxel. Mol Cancer Ther, 2005, 4: 2001-2007.

[42] Dumontet C, Jordan MA, Lee FF. Ixabepilone: Targeting beta III-tubulin expression in taxane-resistant malignancies. Mol Cancer Ther, 2009, 8: 17-25.

[43] Socinski MA, Bondarenko I, Karaseva NA, et al. Weekly nab-paclitaxel in combination with carboplatin versus solvent-based paclitaxel plus carboplatin as first-line therapy in patients with advanced non-small-cell lung cancer: final results of a phase III trial. J Clin Oncol, 2012, 30: 2055-2062.

[44] Kawata E, Ashihara E, Kimura S, et al. Admin-istration of PLK-1 small interfering RNA with atelocollagen prevents the growth of liver metastases of lung cancer. Mol Cancer Ther, 2008, 7: 2904-2912.

[45] Denissenko MF, Pao A, Tang M, et al. Prefer-ential formation of benzo pyrene adducts at lung cancer mutational hotspots in p53. Science, 1996, 274: 430-432.

[46] Thu KL, Vucic EA, Chari R, et al. Lung adenocarcinoma of never smokers and smokers harbor differential regions of genetic alteration and exhibit different levels of genomic instability. PLoS ONE, 2012, 7: e33003.

[47] Pal SK, Figlin RA, Reckamp K. Targeted therapies for non-small cell lung cancer: An evolving land-scape. Mol Cancer Ther, 2010, 9: 1931-1944.

[48] Hammerman PS, Hayes DN, Wilkerson MD, et al. Comprehensive genomic characterization of squamous cell lung cancers. Nature, 2012, 489: 519-525.

[49] Burns TF, El-Deiry WS. The p53 pathway and apoptosis. J Cell Physiol, 1999, 181: 231-239.

[50] Fujiwara T, Grimm EA, Mukhopadhyay T, et al. A retroviral wild-type p53 expression vector penetrates human lung cancer spheroids and inhibits growth by inducing apoptosis. Cancer Res, 1993, 53: 4129-4133.

[51] Fujiwara T, Cai DW, Georges RN, et al. Therapeutic effect of a retroviral wild-type p53 expression vector in an orthotopic lung cancer model. J Natl Cancer Inst, 1994, 86: 1458-1462.

[52] Zhang WW, Fang X, Mazur W, et al. High-efficiency gene transfer and high-level expression of wild-type p53 in human lung cancer cells mediated by recombinant adenovirus. Cancer Gene Ther, 1994, 1: 5-13.

[53] Georges RN, Mukhopadhyay T, Zhang Y, et al. Prevention of orthotopic human lung cancer growth by intratracheal instillation of a retroviral antisense Kras construct. Cancer Res, 1993, 53: 1743-1746.

[54] Bouvet M, Fang B, Ekmekcioglu S, et al. Suppression of the immune response to an adenovirus vector and enhancement of intratumoral transgene expression by low-dose etoposide. Gene Ther, 1998, 5: 189-195.

[55] Nielsen LL, Dell J, Maxwell E, et al. Efficacy of p53 adenovirus-mediated gene therapy against human breast cancer xenografts. Cancer Gene Ther, 1997, 4: 129-138.

[56] Spitz FR, Nguyen D, Skibber JM, et al. Adenoviral-mediated wild-type p53 gene expression sensitizes colorectal cancer cells to ionizing radiation. Clin Cancer Res, 1996, 2: 1665-1671.

[57] Dameron KM, Volpert OV, Tainsky MA, et al. Control of angiogenesis in fibroblasts by p53 regulation of thrombospondin-1. Science, 1994, 265: 1582-1584.

[58] Miyashita T, Reed JC. Tumor suppressor p53 is a direct transcriptional activator of the human bax gene. Cell, 1995, 80: 293-299.

[59] Carroll JL, Nielsen LL, Pruett SB, et al. The role of natural killer cells in adenovirus-mediated p53 gene therapy. Mol Cancer Ther, 2001, 1: 49-60.

[60] Molinier-Frenkel V, Le Boulaire C, Le Gal FA, et al. Longitudinal follow-up of cellular and humoral immunity induced by recombinant adenovirus-mediated gene therapy in cancer patients. Hum Gene Ther, 2000, 11: 1911-1920.

[61] Yen N, Ioannides CG, Xu K, et al. Cellular and humoral immune responses to adenovirus and p53 protein antigens in patients following intratumoral injection of an adenovirus vector expressing wild-type. P53 (Ad-p53). Cancer Gene Ther, 2000, 7: 530-536.

[62] Owen-Schaub LB, Zhang W, Cusack JC, et al. Wild-type human p53 and a temperature-sensitive mutant induce Fas/APO-1 expression. Mol Cell Biol, 1995, 15: 3032-3040.

[63] Roth JA, Nguyen D, Lawrence DD, et al. Retrovirus-mediated wild-type p53 gene transfer to tumors of patients with lung cancer. Nat Med, 1996, 2: 985-991.

[64] Swisher SG, Roth JA, Nemunaitis J, et al. Adenovirus-mediated p53 gene transfer in advanced non-small-cell lung cancer. J Natl Cancer Inst, 1999, 91: 763-771.

[65] Clayman GL, El-Naggar AK, Lippman SM, et al. Adenovirus-mediated p53 gene transfer in patients with advanced recurrent head and neck squamous cell carcinoma. Journal of Clinical Oncology, 1998, 16: 2221-2232.

[66] Peng Z. Current status of gendicine in China: Recombinant human Ad-p53 agent for treatment of cancers. Human Gene Therapy, 2005, 16: 1016-1027.

[67] Nemunaitis J, Clayman G, Agarwala SS, et al. Biomarkers predict p53 gene therapy efficacy in recur-rent squamous cell carcinoma of the head and neck. Clin Cancer Res, 2009, 15: 7719-7725.

[68] Fujiwara T, Grimm EA, Mukhopadhyay T, et al. Induction of chemosensitivity in human lung cancer cells in vivo by adenovirus-mediated transfer of the wild-type p53 gene. Cancer Res, 1994, 54: 2287-2291.

[69] Nguyen DM, Spitz FR, Yen N, et al. Gene therapy for lung cancer: enhancement of tumor suppression by a combination of sequential systemic cisplatin and adenovirus-mediated p53 gene transfer. J Thorac Cardiovasc Surg, 1996, 112: 1372-1376; discussion 1376-1377.

[70] Nemunaitis J, Swisher SG, Timmons T, et al. Adenovirus-mediated p53 gene transfer in sequence with cisplatin to tumors of patients with non-small-cell lung cancer. J Clin Oncol, 2000, 18: 609-622.

[71] Schuler M, Herrmann R, De Greve JL, et al. Adenovirus-mediated wild-type p53 gene transfer in patients receiving chemotherapy for advanced non-small-cell lung cancer: results of a multicenter phase II study. J Clin Oncol, 2001, 19: 1750-1758.

[72] Broaddus WC, Liu Y, Steele LL, et al. Enhanced radiosensitivity of malignant glioma cells after adenoviral p53 transduction. J Neurosurg, 1999, 91: 997-1004.

[73] Feinmesser M, Halpern M, Fenig E, et al. Expression of the apoptosis-related oncogenes bcl-2, bax, and p53 in Merkel cell carcinoma: can they predict treatment response and clinical outcome? Hum Pathol, 1999, 30: 1367-1372.

[74] Jasty R, Lu J, Irwin T, et al. Role of p53 in the regulation of irradiation-induced apoptosis in neuroblastoma cells. Mol Genet Metab, 1998, 65: 155-164.

[75] Sakakura C, Sweeney EA, Shirahama T, et al. Overexpression of bax sensitizes human breast cancer MCF-7 cells to radiation-induced apoptosis. Int J Cancer, 1996, 67: 101-105.

[76] Swisher S, Roth JA, Komaki R, et al. A phase II trial of adenoviral mediated p53 gene transfer (RPR/INGN 201) in conjunction with radiation therapy in patients with localized non-small cell lung cancer (NSCLC). Amer Soc Clin Oncol, 2000, 19: 461a.

[77] Chada S, Mhashilkar A, Roth JA, et al. Development of vaccines against self-antigens: The p53 paradigm. Curr Opin Drug Discov Devel, 2003, 6: 169-173.

[78] Ishida T, Chada S, Stipanov M, et al. Dendritic cells transduced with wild-type p53 gene elicit potent anti-

tumour immune responses. Clin Exp Immunol, 1999, 117: 244-251.

[79] Mayordomo JI, Loftus DJ, Sakamoto H, et al. Therapy of murine tumors with p53 wild-type and mutant sequence peptide-based vaccines. J Exp Med, 1996, 183: 1357-1365.

[80] Nikitina EY, Clark JI, Van Beynen J, et al. Dendritic cells transduced with full-length wild-type p53 generate antitumor cytotoxic T lymphocytes from peripheral blood of cancer patients. Clin Cancer Res, 2001, 7: 127-135.

[81] Antonia SJ, Mirza N, Fricke I, et al. Combination of p53 cancer vaccine with chemotherapy in patients with extensive stage small cell lung cancer. Clin Cancer Res, 2006, 12: 878-887.

[82] Ito I, Ji L, Tanaka F, et al. Liposomal vector potent antitumor activity against human lung cancer in vivo. Cancer Gene Ther, 2004, 11: 733-739.

[83] Uno F, Sasaki J, Nishizaki M, et al. Myristoylation of the fus1 protein is required for tumor suppression in human lung cancer cells. Cancer Res, 2004, 64: 2969-2976.

[84] Lu C, Stewart DJ, Lee JJ, et al. Phase I clinical trial of systemically administered TUSC2（FUS1）-nanoparticles mediating functional gene transfer in humans. PLoS ONE, 2012, 7: e34833.

第31章
转移性肺癌的新临床试验设计

Vassiliki A. Papadimitrakopoulou
Department of Thoracic/Head and Neck Medical Oncology, The University of Texas MD Anderson Cancer Center, Houston, TX, USA

引 言

肺癌是一种可导致器官功能衰竭的疾病，在所有恶性肿瘤中死亡率很高[1]，由于确诊时通常已处于晚期，故不适合行根治性手术治疗[2]。虽然化疗在治疗肿瘤中应用十分广泛，但从目前已报道的临床结果来看，在非选择患者中更换化疗药物以及联合用药均没有显著的疗效[3]。

分子生物学和基因谱的最新研究进展促使许多新型抗癌药物的研发，这些药物在肿瘤细胞中可特异性地靶向作用于异常通路和（或）基因及蛋白质。新药的广泛应用表明，需要有一套更有效的系统来快速、准确识别有效药物用于Ⅲ期试验。美国FDA有两套机制分别对药物及生物制品进行正常审批和快速审批[4]。正常审批需要证明临床获益，例如生存期延长、生活质量提高或者有其他益处。快速审批则专门针对那些治疗严重或危及生命疾病出现的新药或生物制剂进行审批，要求替代性终点疗效良好，这也被认为是"非常有可能预知的临床获益"，并需要在随后的试验中确认该临床获益。虽然第二种类型的审批可以使新药更早地进入临床，但在替代药物选择及最终药物审批的不确定性上仍存在疑虑。在转移性非小细胞肺癌（NSCLC），合适的终点与特定患者群体的获益相关联，包括总生存期（OS）和无疾病进展生存期（PFS）。而关键的新方法及其他感兴趣的潜在替代终点（如反应率、8周疾病控制率）目前正在积极的发展和讨论。除了识别良好的替代物之外，可能的影像生物标记物或生化、遗传、分子生物学生物标记物，都需要进行新的Ⅱ期研究设计。

临床试验中的替代终点

目前对晚期NSCLC中RR和OS之间的关联进行系统回顾发现，一线抗肿瘤治疗可以改善OS（$P<0.0001$），但这与RR存在很大差异，需要进一步做获益检测[5]。对晚期NSCLC单独应用药物吉非替尼或厄洛替尼治疗的Ⅱ、Ⅲ期临床试验进行系统回顾发现，RR和中位OS之间存在很强的相关性，也被认定为疾病控制率（disease control rate，DCR）和中位OS之间存在正向但较弱的关联。在应用EGFR-TKI治疗的人群中，RR可能逐步替代OS[6]；与DCR相比，RR是一个更好的替代指标，因为DCR即包括了*EGFR*突变治疗有效患者，也包括了那些惰性病灶的患者，但RR只包括EGFR突变治疗有效的患者。早期临床试验中疾病稳定（stable disease，SD）有助于长期获益[7]，但它可能不是惰性肿瘤的有效终点。在靶向治疗随机试验研究中SD就作为终止研究的终点[8]。在安慰剂对照的随机Ⅱ期终止试验中，对预处理的转移性NSCLC应用索拉非尼单药治疗，存在显著PFS获益，并显著提高SD率[9]。RR的使用通常基于传统影像终点，将肿瘤负荷分为反应或不反应，这常常不能捕捉到患者获益。因为他们可能会错过一个事实，即治疗后残存肿瘤的残留影像可能主要由坏死组织组成。使用总生存率作为临床试验终点的主要优势在于它是一个临床相关结果，但需要一个对照队列，受交叉设计及随后治疗的影响，需要较长时间的随访。相比之下，肿瘤缓解率很容易标准化，它是一个早期

结果，但容易受测量不准的影响，尽管 PFS 没有被挽救疗法混淆，但易受调查者的偏见影响而且仅部分被认定为可替代生存获益。

BATTLE 试验使用 8 周 DCR［实体瘤疗效评价标准（RECIST 标准）中的完全缓解、部分缓解或 SD］作为主要终点，因为这一终点需要更短的时间，而且被认为可以预测 OS。104 例患者 8 周疾病控制的中位 OS 为 11.3 个月，而 8 周无疾病控制的中位 OS 为 7.5 个月（$P=0.002$）[10]，详细内容我们将在本章节的后续部分继续讨论。

其他新的终点包括分子及成像生物标志物。分子生物标记物被证实可能具有预测性，其作为替代终点使用可探寻耐药机制，但在早期临床药物研发期间通常不进行对应验证。如果药物靶点非普遍存在，则需要根据特定的肿瘤相关分子标记物存在与否来选择患者，以提高临床获益[11]。然而，通常情况下肿瘤药物的真正靶点是未知的，甚至当它已经被认为具有靶向抑制时，也并不足以使肿瘤缩小或患者获益[12-13]。成像花费昂贵，而且几乎不增加反应评估，新的正电子发射断层显像剂和其他新型成像方法仍在研究中。

新试验设计的需求

随着 II 期及 III 期临床试验中关键部分的成本逐渐升高，药物创新的风险越来越大，这使得药品创新的效率降低[14-15]。尽管行业研发的投入在增加，但获得上市许可的新分子药物数量却没有增加。传统药品研发的做法是将临床研发分成几个连续的阶段，在分离事件中监测其发展。新型临床研发及试验设计中提高效率及降低损耗的方式在克服一些挑战中起着关键作用。在过去的 20 年间越来越多的随机 II 期研究设计采用检测试剂或在 II 期研究中设置联合 PFS 作为主要终点[16-17]。随机终止设计[18]已经被许多研究者用于分子靶向药物研究。在这种设计中所有患者最初都需在规定的时间接受研究试剂的治疗，然后病情稳定的患者在规定的时间随机继续或终止，从而在假定反应人群中评估药物的疗效。上述类型的设计就索拉非尼[9]而言非常有用，尤其在药品初始反应时或病情稳定后将预期提供一些其他额外益处。这种设计的缺点是大量患者需要进行初始治疗，为了定义一个较小亚组，将使他们过多暴露于无效治疗中，因此该设计的益处可能不易实现。即便如此，如果获得益处的亚组不是由分子构成或其他确定的方式分类，那么这些药物的进一步测试可能存在困难。

新型药物研发的核心是新工具，包括模拟与仿真、贝叶斯（Bayesian）方法论以及适应性设计。

分子靶向药物在试验设计中的影响

对疾病发病机制的分子解析[19]促使我们将患者的分子标志物与靶向治疗选择进行配对，这彻底改变了该领域的治疗方式，其中 EGFR-TKI 对治疗 *EGFR* 突变肿瘤，以及 ALK-TKI 治疗 EML-ALK 易位肿瘤[20-21]存在确切获益。NSCLC 患者在确诊肿瘤时检测这些和其他生物标志物，逐渐成为一种可以被接受的方法，因为它会影响治疗决策以及患者的疗效[22]。对高表达棘皮动物微管相关蛋白样-4 或间变性淋巴瘤激酶（EML4－ALK）的晚期 NSCLC 患者（主要是腺癌及非吸烟者）应用克唑替尼进行靶向治疗，表现出一定疗效[23]，克唑替尼已于 2011 年 8 月通过美国 FDA 批准[24]。I 期临床试验中可见其在生物标志物阳性者中存在活性，且 RR 与中位生存均未达到 61%[20,25-26]。为弥补克唑替尼对照组数据的缺乏，82 例未经克唑替尼处理或 ALK 阳性疾病、ALK 阴性或 EGFR 阴性的患者被用于做对照数据分析证实，克唑替尼在 OS 上显著获益[26]。克唑替尼的批准不同于目前的常规抗癌药物，因为它基于 RR 而不是 PFS 或 OS 获益。

然而，大部分临床试验设计在传统上都不是基于相关研究进展，而是以组织学为基础；这种 I 期和 II 期试验设计将导致 III 期研究的失败或出现患者群体临床获益的可疑边缘统计。事实上，目前只有两个靶向信号通路药物被美国 FDA 批准用于未经选择的 NSCLC 患者：EGFR-TKI 厄洛替尼和贝伐单抗［单克隆抗体靶向血管内皮细胞生长因子（vascular endothelial growth factor, VEGF）］。

在靶向治疗的早期临床试验中，探索生物标

志物被一个事实阻碍，即 NSCLC 临床试验中，多数新型靶向治疗不用于初始治疗，而是作为二线、三线或更后续的治疗方案；而且对分子进行分析所得出的临床试验结论通常在病例亚组中完成[27-28]，并基于存档的诊断标本。因此，这对复发和难治性肿瘤而言，可能丢失生物学及突变的演变数据。另一个原因是在早期临床试验中，选择诊断性检测以确认应答患者亚组很困难，因为肿瘤通路并不是简单的被治疗药物干预，从而导致反馈机制及其他并行信号通路的活化。前期临床系统所衍生的分子预测信号的应用，在临床上通常不可靠[29-30]，临床预测信号的研发需要大量的临床数据对早期临床试验中的无效信号进行验证。抗癌药物中只有少部分生物标记物可作为一种诊断手段来选择应答的患者亚组，其中包括雌激素受体 IHC、HER-2 IHC/DNA 杂交检测、EGFR IHC、C-KIT IHC、BCR-ABL 染色体、PML-RAR 染色体、5 号染色体和 RAS 突变，它们中只有 3 个获得了 FDA 批准（HER-2 IHC/DNA 杂交检测、EGFR IHC 和 C-KIT IHC）。

BATTLE 试验

设想并努力捕获所有参与者给药时的生物标志物状态，已在里程碑式的 BATTLE 试验中得到实现[10]。

NSCLC 中的 4 个独立治疗性临床试验（即厄洛替尼、凡德他尼、厄洛替尼+贝沙罗汀、索拉非尼）具有伞形结构（图 31.1）。对所有患者，包括至少一线治疗失败的患者进行肿瘤针吸活检，其目的是获得最新生物标记物状态，然后将其随机分到 4 个治疗组中。研究者发现，根据活检标本的多种检测结果进行治疗分配是可行的，并且安全风险最小。生物标志物分析是实时完成的，包含大量的基因突变、基因拷贝数，并对每一个样品进行免疫组织化学分析。根据这些研究结果将患者分成预定义的生物标记物特征组，然后可以用来评价治疗型生物标记物的相互作用。最初的 97 例患者被随机分到 4 个不同的治疗组，被分到每个治疗组的机会均为 25%，然后对这 97 例患者的结果进行评估，对感兴趣的数据——8 周疾病控制率与每个治疗组中生物标志物的状态进行比较。

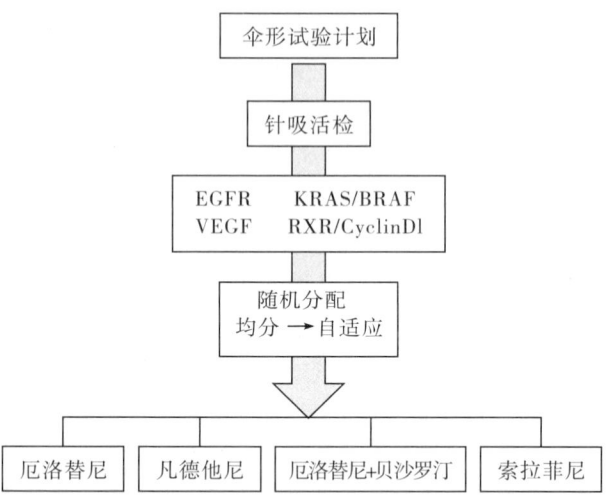

图 31.1 BATTLE 试验图解。患者最初被随机均分为 4 个组，随后进行自适应随机化

在此至前这一研究终点是总生存时间的一个合理替代指标[31]；对于此类需要一个快速结果以促进贝叶斯自适应的方法而言，该终点并不常见，但却十分必要。

对 20 种生物标志物治疗组进行分析，获得的 8 周疾病控制率（4 种治疗，每组 5 个生物标志物，产生 20 种组合）是研究中治疗分配所用的自适应随机化设计的基础。有了这个信息，将来随机概率的调整会使用贝叶斯模型。此调整意味着如果发现患者活检中有一个特定生物标记物，根据之前治疗的 8 周 DCR 数据，他（她）将有 >25% 的概率被随机给予之前具有相同生物标记物的患者已经进行的较好治疗。积累的数据越多且自适应存在时，则越多具有特定标记的患者将得到特定治疗，后续类似患者分配到该疗法的概率也较高。该创新的适应性随机化设计，旨在提高每例患者接受最有效试验性治疗的机会，既往类似患者的 8 周 DCR 基准为 30%，且没有一项设计能确定生物标志物和治疗之间是否存在显著相关性。实际上 20 种生物标记物与治疗配对中，有 8 种达到有效标准，有 >80% 的概率实现 30% 的 8 周 DCR，其中一些配对与我们目前所认识的药效标志物预测一致，例如 *KRAS/BRAF* 突变将响应索拉非尼[32]。这一观察报告为继续在这些 *KRAS* 突变的肿瘤患者中研究 RAF-MEK-ERK 信号传导轴更有效的抑制剂提供了帮助。用于生物标记物分组的技术资格检测可能会影响到这些强调关于生物标志物与治疗匹配需要明确证据的结果。这项

Ⅱ期研究设计并没有直接比较平均随机组与自适应随机组，这种比较可以提供一个最终证据，即自适应将导致更好的结果。

尽管这些优势对患者及肿瘤学专家都非常有吸引力，但引入并实现某种程度上"个体化用药"的想法由于受到非均等分组的影响使得贝叶斯设计对治疗效果的精确估计变小[33]。

该研究的主要成就是使科学界认可了一个事实，即对难治性肺癌治疗前进行重复活检是有价值并且可行的。这些操作程序实际上被证明是安全的（接受肺活检的患者发生严重并发症的概率<1%），而且实时生物标志物评估在治疗分配之前进行是可行的。

最近，在此创新设计的基础上一项类似研究[BATTLE-2（NCT01248247）]已经开始。BATTLE-2涉及之前治疗的肺癌患者，并包括厄洛替尼和索拉非尼治疗组，以及其他两个研究性治疗：AKT抑制剂MK-2206与MEK抑制剂AZD6244组合，以及MK-2206与厄洛替尼的组合（图31.2）。该研究对生物标志物进行选择的方法以及对肿瘤进行分类的方式与BATTLE试验不同。

该研究的前半部分，利用临床验证的生物标志物（如KRAS突变）来定义生物标志物组，并用于适应性治疗分配。一组有限、需预先指定的生物标志物将在肿瘤活检组织中进行评估。对结果进行分析后，生物标志物被认为可以潜在预测每个试验治疗的反应，这将在第二部分的研究中被用于治疗分配决策。需注意的是，最初的BATTLE试验，生物标志物群的预指定及固有属性不允许进行多个生物标志物治疗的配对确认，这种情况可通过采用更多探索性的方法来避免。该研究还允许在研究的第二部分灵敏性自适应生物标志物的选择，以便形成生物标记物和治疗的配对，并要求在这样的数据出现时需对试验进行修改。如以上所述的影像及分子分析2（I-SPY2）研究，除临床验证的生物标记物之外，一组候选及探索性的生物标志物也正在研究中，它试图定义一组生物标记物，在第二部分临床试验中可以使4组中的每个个体都更好地适应其随机性。

BATTLE研究设计在新药的靶点生物学特征不确定或尚未明确其作用机制的情况下更具有显著优势。在某些情况下，实时、复杂的生物标志物分析可加速鉴定及进一步测试潜在生物标志物与治疗的关系。相反，在更好地理解药物靶点假说及其生物学特征以后，与具有成熟假说的任何潜在生物标志物试验或在限制较少患者人群中进行的、将定义明确的生物标志物纳入回顾性分析的传统靶向治疗研究相比，适应性随机策略可能效率较低。BATTLE方法代表了一种新的疗法，它与配对的预测生物标志物进行联合研发将更有效。BATTLE试验的创新点在于，它在基于预处理活检组织分配的单一研究中将4个不同的治疗组与5种生物标志物分类进行结合。在影像及分子分析2（I-SPY 2）试验中，类似的方法采用的是一系列研究调查来预测治疗反应，这涉及在刚诊断为乳腺癌并符合条件的患者中应用紫杉醇进行新辅助治疗[34]。I-SPY 2代表了一种探索生物标记物的独特方法，除了病理完全缓解这一主要终点外，它还测试、解析验证标志物，并使合格的标志物作为新药被检测，采用适应性设计研究每种药物的生物标志物特性，并利用组织管理原则及复杂生物信息学，来消除临床试验中的低效率。其目标基于疾病的分子特性（生物标志物特性）来进一步明确患者亚群的改进治疗方案。该方案比标准疗法具有更有效的贝叶斯预测率。如果有任何生物标记物特性显示出低改善率，该方案将会被舍弃。

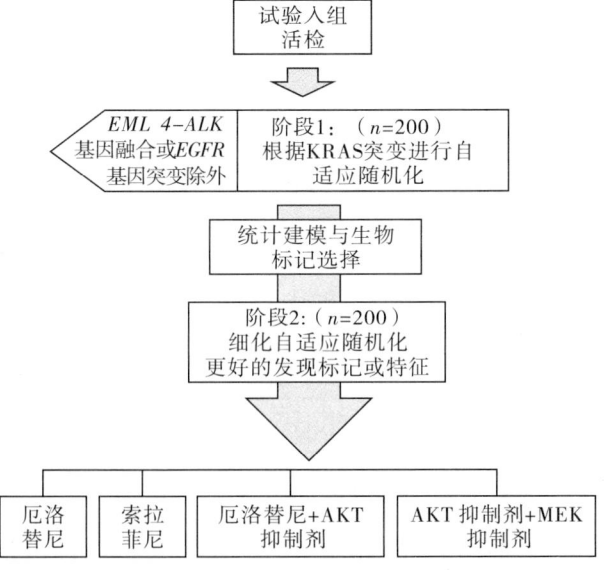

图31.2 BATTLE-2试验图解。研究之初便应用自适应随机化将患者分为4个组。具有 EGFR 敏感突变或 EML4/ALK 基因融合的肿瘤患者被排除在外

I-SPY 2 中的生物标志物被分为 3 种不同类型，即美国 FDA 批准的标准生物标记物、尚未被 FDA 批准合格但有望决定试验资格或测量肿瘤反应的标志物和探索性生物标记物。

统计设计与 BATTLE 和 I-SPY 2 不同，已经提出了随机试验，其中包括预测生物标志物的假设[35-36]。这些设计不要求将预先规定的生物标记物检测用于治疗分配，从而避免了筛选失败的问题。不必预先指定一组生物标记物在入组前进行测试，其主要优点是解决了在关键性试验开始时我们对哪些亚组可以从新治疗方案中获益知之甚少的问题。

创新临床试验设计的未来展望

就抗肿瘤药物的监管批准而言，尽管 OS 是肿瘤试验的传统终点，但是考虑到后续治疗的混杂影响，OS 获益可能会造成靶向治疗时代不可克服的挑战。与此同时，延长 PFS 的幅度不仅必须有统计学差异而且要有临床意义。临床研发有效性的提高可以通过采用更加综合的模式得到改善，提高灵活性并最大限度地利用积累的知识。药物研发模式的核心是新工具，包括建模和模拟、贝叶斯方法和适应性设计，例如无缝自适应设计和样本量再评估方法。这些新试验设计要求统计分析有显著差异，模拟并协调运筹以验证自己的操作特色，因此往往需要更多的时间规划并拟订发展计划。监管机构和机构审查委员会还需要分析批准设计的形式，而这些讨论有时可能需要相当长的时间。将这些方法应用于药物研发，虽然带来了益处，但也带来了挑战并为它的实现设置了障碍。BATTLE 试验提供了证据证明我们能够成功地提高肺癌临床试验的研究门槛，包括为所有参与者进行全面的预处理活检和基因分型。我们认为这样的努力有很大的潜力，将成倍增加我们对靶向治疗获益患者的理解，并有可能加速及提高药物研发的进程。新标准已对获取组织进行设定，并实时执行综合性生物标志物的评价，这将允许对目前不同靶点的新药物研究情况进行调查，并将加快调查进程。实际上，目前正在探讨创建这些设计去替代传统的药物研发和设计。

这种研发战略是 III 期注册试验的主方案，该试验对特定疾病同时运用多种新治疗方案进行测试。但是，这种试验并不像 I-SPY 2 和 BATTLE II 期适应性筛选试验那样，而是一个多组、多标记或药物的 III 期试验，以促使新治疗方案被 FDA 批准。与适应性筛选试验对标记物和药物之间的未知关联进行分析不同，多药注册试验中的筛选是专门用来治疗组分配和验证临床应用的。多药注册试验中的每个生物标记物都将有相应的处理，治疗的分配将基于验证的诊断鉴定结果。这种类型的试验中，对患者进行入组筛选是一种全民参与，将指导他们如何根据筛查诊断测试的结果分配入组。

多组注册研究与传统替代多个两组注册研究相比有许多优点。首先，就药物而言，它在生物标记物与选择患者群体方面已显示出希望，它在独立试验下将这些研究进行分组，并具有一个共同的对照组，这降低了总体筛选的失败率。其次，通过单一的主方案获得操作效率，可以根据研究需要来修改药物的选入和剔除。治疗疾病的每种药物将用相同的方法进行测试，主方案也将提供一致性。如果能满足预先指定的有效性和安全性标准，赞助商可能会鼓励在主注册试验中应用他们的药物，药物和相应的诊断也将被批准。最后，通过提高一些特定疾病的药物研发效率，该试验有可能比其他可行的方法更快地提供安全、有效的药物给患者。可以通过克服内部阻碍的方法使新型试验设计和方法进入临床研发。监管机构和赞助商也已经意识到创新设计的独特优势，最重要的是增加这些现代化工具。

（孟 敏 叶 欣 译）

参考文献

[1] Siegel R, Naishadham D, Jemal A. Cancer statistics, 2012. CA Cancer J Clin, 2012, 62: 10-29.

[2] NCCN. Clinical Practice Guidelines in Oncology, National Comprehensive Cancer Network. Non-small cell lung cancer, 2012.

[3] Schiller JH, Harrington D, Belani CP, et al. Comparison of four chemotherapy regimens for advanced non-small-cell lung cancer. N Engl J Med, 2002, 346: 92-98.

[4] Johnson JR, Ning YM, Farrell A, et al. Accelerated ap-

[5] Johnson KR, Ringland C, Stokes BJ, et al. Response rate or time to progression as predictors of survival in trials of metastatic colorectal cancer or non-small-cell lung cancer: A meta-analysis. Lancet Oncol, 2006, 7: 741-746.

[6] Tsujino K, Kawaguchi T, Kubo A, et al. Response rate is associated with prolonged survival in patients with advanced non-small cell lung cancer treated with gefitinib or erlotinib. J Thorac Oncol, 2009, 4: 994-1001.

[7] Tolcher AW. Stable disease is a valid end point in clinical trials. Cancer J, 2009, 15: 374-378.

[8] Hales RK, Banchereau J, Ribas A, et al. Assessing oncologic benefit in clinical trials of immunotherapy agents. Ann Oncol, 2010, 21: 1944-1951.

[9] Wakelee HA, et al. A double-blind randomized discontinuation phase-II study of sorafenib (BAY 43-9006) in previously treated non-small-cell lung cancer patients: Eastern cooperative oncology group study E2501. J Thorac Oncol, 2012, 7 (10): 1574-1582.

[10] Kim ES, Herbst RS, Wistuba, et al. The BAT-TLE trial: personalizing therapy for lung cancer. Cancer Discov, 2011, 1: 44-53.

[11] Dy GK, Adjei A. Patient selection for rational development of novel anticancer agents//Kaufman H, Wadler S, Antman K (eds), Cancer Drug Discovery and Development Molecular Targeting in Oncology. Totowa: NJ, Humana Press, Inc., 2007: 639-646.

[12] Adjei AA, Cohen RB, Franklin W, et al. Phase I pharmacokinetic and pharmacodynamic study of the oral, small-molecule mitogen-activated protein kinase kinase 1/2 inhibitor AZD6244 (ARRY-142886) in patients with advanced cancers. J ClinOncol, 2008, 26: 2139-2146.

[13] Friday BB, YuC, Dy GK, et al. BRAF V600E disrupts AZD6244-induced abrogation of negative feedback pathways between extracellular signal-regulated kinase and Raf proteins. Cancer Res, 2008, 68: 6145-6153.

[14] Adams CP, Brantner VV. Spendingonnewdrug development. Health Econ, 2010, 19 (2): 130-141.

[15] Adams CP, Brantner VV. Estimating the cost of new drug development: Is it really 802 million dollars? Health Aff (Millwood), 2006, 25: 420-428.

[16] Phase II trials in the EORTC. The Protocol Review Committee, the Data Center, the Research and Treatment Division, and the New Drug Development Office. European Organization for Research and Treatment of Cancer. Eur J Cancer, 1997, 33: 1361-1363.

[17] Van Glabbeke M, Steward W, Armand JP. Non-randomised phase II trials of drug combinations: Often meaningless, sometimes misleading. Are there alternative strategies? Eur J Cancer, 2002, 38: 635-638.

[18] Rosner GL, Stadler W, Ratain MJ. Randomized discontinuation design: Application to cytostatic anti-neoplastic agents. J Clin Oncol, 2002, 20: 4478-4484.

[19] Kris MG, Johnson BE, Kwiatkowski DJ, et al. Identification of driver mutations in tumor specimens from 1000 patient with lung adenocarcinoma: The NCI's Lung Cancer Mutation Consortium (LCMC). J Clin Oncol, 2011, 29 (Suppl).

[20] Kwak EL, Bang YJ, Camidge DR, et al. Anaplastic lymphoma kinase inhibition in non-small-cell lung cancer. N Engl J Med, 2010, 363: 1693-1703.

[21] Mok TS, Wu YL, Thongprasert S, et al. Gefitinib or carboplatin-paclitaxel in pulmonary adenocarcinoma. N Engl J Med, 2009, 361: 947-957.

[22] Azzoli CG, Baker S, Jr., Temin S, et al. American Society of Clinical Oncology Clinical Practice Guideline update on chemotherapy for stage IV non-small-cell lung cancer. J Clin Oncol, 2009, 27: 6251-6266.

[23] Horn L, Pao W. EML4-ALK: Honinginonanew target in non-small-cell lung cancer. J Clin Oncol, 2009, 27: 4232-4235.

[24] XALKORI (Crizotinib) capsules, oral (package insert) New York, Pfizer Labs.

[25] Camidge DR, Bang YJ, Kwak EL, et al. Progression-free survival (PFS) from a phase I study of crizotinib (PF-02341066) in patients with ALK-positive non-small cell lung cancer (NSCLC). J Clin Oncol, 2011, 29: 15S.

[26] Shaw AT, Yeap B, Solomon B, et al. Impact of crizotinb on survival in patients with advanced ALK-positive NSCLC compared with historical controls. J Clin Oncol, 2011, 29: 15S.

[27] Eberhard DA, Johnson BE, Amler LC, et al. Mutations in the epidermal growth factor receptor and in KRAS are predictive and prognostic indicators in patients with non-small-cell lung cancer treated with chemotherapy alone and in combination with erlotinib. J Clin Oncol, 2005, 23: 5900-5909.

[28] Tsao MS, Sakurada A, Cutz JC, et al. Erlotinib in lung cancer-molecular and clinical predictors of outcome. N

Engl J Med, 2005, 353: 133 - 144.

[29] Baggerly K, Coombes K. Deriving chemosensitivity from cell lines: Forensic bioinformatics and reproducible research in highthroughput biology. Ann Appl Stat, 2009, 3: 1309 - 1334.

[30] Potti A, Dressman HK, Bild A, et al. Genomic signatures to guide the use of chemotherapeutics. Nat Med, 2006, 12: 1294 - 1300.

[31] Lara PN, Jr., Redman MW, kelly k, et al. Disease control rate at 8 weeks predicts clinical benefit in advanced non-small-cell lung cancer: Results from Southwest Oncology Group randomized trials. J Clin Oncol, 2008, 26: 463 - 467.

[32] Massarelli E, Varella-Garcia M, Tang X, et al. KRAS mutation is an important predictor of resistance to therapy with epidermal growth factor receptor tyro-sine kinase inhibitors in non-small-cell lung cancer. Clin Cancer Res, 2007, 13: 2890 - 2896.

[33] Thall PF, Wathen JK. Practical Bayesian adaptive randomisation in clinical trials. Eur J Cancer, 2007, 43: 859 - 866.

[34] Barker AD, Sigman CC, Kelloff GJ, et al. I-SPY 2: An adaptive breast cancer trial design in the setting of neoadjuvant chemotherapy. Clin Pharmacol Ther, 2009, 86: 97 - 100.

[35] Baker SG, Sargent DJ. Designing a randomized clinical trial to evaluate personalized medicine: A new approach based on risk prediction. J Natl Cancer Inst, 2010, 102: 1756 - 1759.

[36] Freidlin B, Jiang W, Simon R. The cross-validated adaptive signature design. Clin Cancer Res, 2010, 16: 691 - 698.

第 32 章
非小细胞肺癌临床试验的新统计学模型

J. Jack Lee, *Caleb T. Chu*

Department of Biostatistics, the University of Texas MD Anderson Cancer Center, Houston, TX, USA

引 言

近年来，肿瘤生物学的快速发展使我们对于肺癌分子及基因组机制有了更深刻的研究，也为更新更有效治疗方法的出现提供了肥沃的土壤。例如，图 32.1A[1]展示了肺癌组织病理学的传统分型，包括腺癌、鳞癌及大细胞癌。1987 年，KRAS 基因突变被确认，继而，2004 年激活的 EGFR 突变被发现。2009 年及以后，大量的罕见突变，如 EML4-ALK 重排也在肺癌中被发现。随着个体化突变的涌现，许多突变被发现是互相重叠的，而且在分子学结构上形成了有趣的交叉（图 32.1B）[2]。尽管突变是普遍存在的，但特殊类型的激活突变在患者中还是罕见的。如果所有已知的突变都被考虑到，那么超过 50% 的患者都存在分子学变异。这表明，针对分子靶点的治疗是肿瘤治疗中有前景的一种方法。

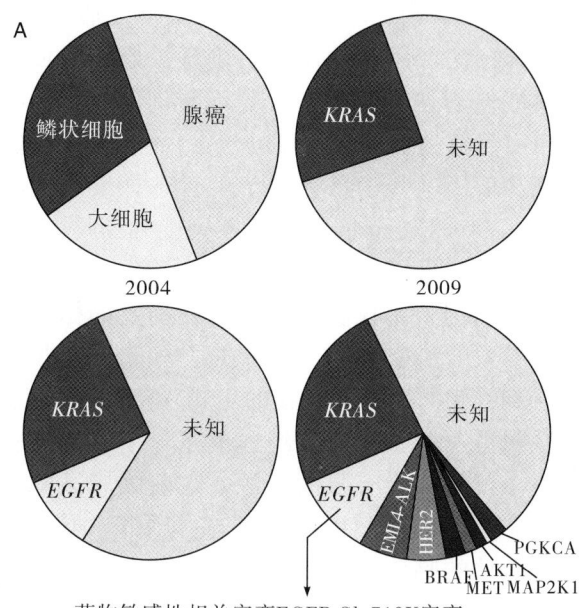

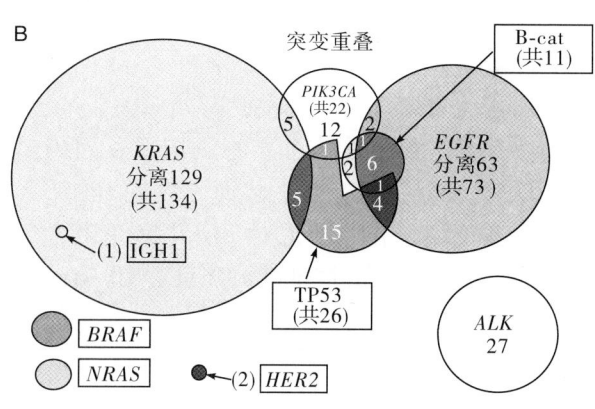

图 32.1 NSCLC 分类的演变。A. 有史以来的传统认识；1987 年发现 KRAS 突变；2004 年发现 EGFR 突变；2009 年许多新的突变确定。B. 常见、罕见及重叠的突变

来源：[1] Pao W, Girard N. New driver mutations in non-small-cell lung cancer. Lancet Oncology, 2011, 12（2）：175-180. 经许可，摘自 Elsevier. [2] Sequist LV, Heist RS, Shaw AT, et al. Implementing multiplexed genotyping of non-small-cell lung cancers into routine clinical practice. Ann Oncol, 2011, 22（12）：2616-2624. 经许可，摘自牛津大学出版社

过去的20年里，突变这一生物学发现为肿瘤靶向药物的出现铺平了道路，最著名的例子是伊马替尼。在1960年，慢性淋巴细胞白血病中，费城染色体被首次报道。然而，直到30年后，*BCR-ABL* 的功能及其在肿瘤发生中的作用才被阐明。它为后来高活性的 BCR-ABL 蛋白抑制剂，即 ST1571（伊马替尼）的出现，提供了重要的功能学解释。在确凿的证据出现后，即在体外及动物实验中，伊马替尼可有效抑制表达 BCR-ABL 的细胞。1998年，开始在患者体内进行新药物试验。Ⅰ期研究的结果令人鼓舞，从而有了1999年的Ⅱ期临床试验。令人惊讶的是，31例患者全部持续每天口服伊马替尼至少300mg，血细胞恢复到正常；在20例患者中，有9例治疗5个月或更长时间后，未发现携带费城染色体的细胞。这一结果导致了2000年的Ⅲ期临床试验，并且这种药物在2001年及2002年分别被FDA批准用于治疗慢性淋巴细胞白血病及胃肠间质瘤[3]。

1994年EGFR酪氨酸激酶抑制剂被首次发现。1997年吉非替尼进行了Ⅰ期临床试验，验证了它的耐受性，并阐述它的作用机理。2000年，Ⅱ期临床试验证明，在非小细胞肺癌（NSCLC）中，250mg/d 吉非替尼具有临床意义的活性。2003年，FDA同意了尽快将吉非替尼作为三线治疗方案来治疗标准化疗失败的进展期NSCLC患者。然而，接下来的Ⅲ期临床试验证明，在NSCLC一线标准化疗中，加用吉非替尼并未提高疗效。2005年，FDA撤销了在新发肺癌中吉非替尼的应用，因为它未被证实对总生存期有益。然而，最近IPASS临床试验重新证实，吉非替尼对 *EGFR* 突变患者有特殊疗效[4]。吉非替尼被批准，并且近10年已被除美国等60多个国家应用。相反，另一种相似的 EGFR TKI，厄洛替尼，于2004年被FDA批准应用于一线化疗方案失败的局部进展期及转移的NSCLC患者。即使市场上有活性药物，临床试验设计及策略仍然很重要，它为药物的成功发展起到重要作用[5]。

另一个吸引人的事情是克唑替尼的发展，它的主要复合物于2005年被发现。在NSCLC中的临床检测始于2006年，EML4 - ALK 易位于2007年被发现并报道。2008年发现了第1例携带EML4 - ALK 易位的肿瘤患者对克唑替尼有治疗效应。截至2009年，一项关于肺癌的Ⅲ期临床试验被发起，克唑替尼于2011年被FDA批准用于 *EML4 - ALK* 易位的患者[6]。

靶向药物的发展，与 *EGFR* 突变及 *EML4 - ALK* 易位的发现是同步的，它改变了肺癌的临床诊断及治疗。在许多大型医学中心，新诊断的肺癌患者，通过针吸活组织检查取得诊断标本，并进行基因组分析。这种实践也被扩展到小的诊所。随着更廉价及更有效的基因检测技术以前所未有的速度出现，我们期待这种发展潮流能够持续。在不久的将来，新诊断的肺癌患者一旦在诊所预约诊疗，他们会立即拥有他们所患肿瘤的基因学图谱。并且，复发的肺癌患者，可以再次活检取新鲜的组织进行进一步的分子及基因学检测，确定其最有效的二线或三线治疗方案。

特异性分子匹配使靶向治疗应运而生，然而，显而易见的是，靶向药物不是对所有患者都有效。肺癌是癌症中排名第一位的死亡原因，但从整体来看是持续降低的，NSCLC的5年生存率一直徘徊在15%左右。已知的敏感突变非常稀少，接受靶向治疗一段时间的患者，可能会发展为耐药。诊断和预测标志物的出现及确认，是一项长期且有挑战性的任务。我们需要不断询问自己：我们是否有足够的信息为肺癌的治疗做出合理的选择？我们如何用这些信息为每个患者选择最有效的治疗方式？对部分有匹配的敏感突变和药物的病例，有效的治疗方案可以使患者得到相应的治疗。但在其他病例中，我们仍缺乏足够确定的标志物来选择有效的治疗方案。然而在过去的10年里，我们看到，靶向药物及潜在的生物学标志物被发现，其数量迅速增长。这已经远远超过了临床试验的数量，仅仅因为有限的资源，这些临床试验可以在一个给定的时间内同时进行。因此，发展高效及创新性的临床试验，用于检测新药及收集关于生物学标志物的预后和预测能力的资料，变得尤为重要。在这一章中，我们将首先提供一个概述，阐明标准及新颖的临床试验如何用于寻找NSCLC的新药。相关有效的统计学问题、伦理问题及新颖的临床试验设计将被讨论。

临床试验是药物开发这一领域的基石。在寻找安全有效的治疗方法的同时，临床试验是十分必要的，这也为循证医学奠定了基础。缺乏合理严格的临床试验，临床药物的发展将会被严重限制。随着知识的进步及疾病治疗方法的改善，临床试验及临床实践的协作变得尤为重要[7-10]。

随着药物的发展，当一个突变的分子被分离出来，相关的靶向药物也应运而生，有可能为患者提供更有效的治疗方法。然而，靶向药物的有效性因人而异，对许多药物来说，可能根本没有作用。研发新药具有挑战性的环节在于评估治疗的有效性，以及明确预后及预测的标记物。此外，检测到每个患者的标记物，可以为患者提供相对更有效的治疗方法。因此，一个好的临床试验需具备以下几点：①测试治疗的有效性；②明确预后及预测的标志物；③为参加临床试验的患者提供最好的治疗。

尽管临床试验已经有50多年历史了，但标准的临床试验设计是严格的，需要很长的研究时间。最近的研究提出了应用新方法以提高试验效率，以便能使患者得到更有效的治疗。满足这种需求的一个主要统计学创新是在自适应设计里应用贝叶斯方法（Bayesian）。在接下来的两个小节中，我们将介绍贝叶斯统计学和自适应设计。随后，我们将阐述贝叶斯自适应设计如何应用于一项有创意的临床试验，为进展期肺癌研究设计的 BATTLE 试验就是个例子。最后，我们将会给其他新的设计进行概述，并用一章总结。

贝叶斯统计学和其相关的临床试验

统计学是一门定量推理科学，它提供了一个框架来评估信息中包含的数据的不确定性。统计数据用来量化事件的可能性，以便正确地推理。统计数据还可以应用于设计更有效率的临床试验，从而及时准确地推断，以推动临床研究。

有两种主要方法进行统计推理：主要频率论的方法和贝叶斯方法。虽然著名的贝叶斯定理由牧师托马斯·贝叶斯提出，在他去世后的1763年出版，远远早于主要频率论的成名，但是与频率论相比，贝叶斯方法历来未被充分利用，也被低估了。贝叶斯方法对待未知参数（如新药在未经治疗的Ⅳ期NSCLC中的有效率）是随机的，对待已知的数据是固定的。贝叶斯方法是计算所给数据中参数的概率；而频率论的方法则是计算所给参数的数据的概率。因此，这两种方法是互补的。

如何使用贝叶斯方法？简单来说，贝叶斯方法有以下几步：①获得感兴趣的参数的先验分布（一个对已知或从过去的数据估计的预定义的测量）；②计算数据的可能性（研究期间收集的数据）；③综合这两方面的信息形成后验分布。后验分布就变成了先验分布的后续评估。贝叶斯方法的一些独特优点为：①与频率论的方法相比，贝叶斯方法更直观和直接解决手头的问题。例如，它可以直接计算的概率零假设是正确，而频率论方法计算的概率数据的零假设是正确的（例如 P 值）——提供了一种间接的评估零假设是否是正确的方法。②贝叶斯方法可模拟未知参数的分布及正确定位不同程度的不确定性。例如，在亚组的患者和（或）多中心试验中，可以构造一个层次的贝叶斯模型来评估药物的反应率。③试验期间，贝叶斯方法提供更频繁的监测和制订临时决策，因此，它提供了一个连续学习的平台。大多数临床试验进行了一段时间。因此，需要经常监视中期结果，可以早期判断是否积累了足够的资料。④贝叶斯方法采用的是在学习中前进的方法，其潜在的学习特性使得贝叶斯方法容易被掌握。可根据目前观测到的数据获取的知识来引导临床试验的进行。例如，一项临床试验设计，将与结果匹配的随机化合并，随着临床试验的进行，从而使得更多患者能接受更好的治疗。并且，根据观测到的结果，一种自适应样本量估计过程可以估算试验规模。⑤贝叶斯方法可为正在制订的知情决策提供有用的信息。利用贝叶斯决策理论方法，临床试验研究人员可以指定"效用"或"损失"的各种事件。例如，"对于被治愈的癌症患者，何谓效用（或重要性）；对于由治疗引起长期毒性的患者，何谓损失？"贝叶斯方法制订的主观偏好结果明确并定量地帮助调查人员或患者做出明智的决定。最大化有效作用或最小化损失作用决定了试验的最优决策行为。

然而，贝叶斯方法有其局限性，因为它需要规范的先验分布。正式加入之前收集的信息前、期间和以外的试验可以提高临床试验效率，但基于之前的选择，可增加结果的敏感性。缘于更好计算算法的发展及更快的电脑发展，贝叶斯方法在计算机算法上被加强了，这种挑战被减轻了。为了实现贝叶斯设计临床试验，额外的基础设施往往是必要的。专业软件程序是需要的，用来研究设计、模拟、行为准则，并分析数据。基于网络的应用程序，尤其对于数据的及时输入，临时分析和报告是有用的。临床试验的成功，不仅需要恰当工具的发展，也需要及时、准确地执行结果评价、自适应随机化、数据分析和推理。

贝叶斯方法蕴含着巨大的前景，提高临床试验的效率和灵活性，非常适合学习。贝叶斯方法提供优秀的工具，以寻找有效的治疗方法和具有预测功能的生物标记物，寻求生物标志物个性化治疗——所有都是为了在试验内外以更有效的治疗方法治疗更多患者这个目标。不久的将来，BATTLE 临床试验的例子，如 BATTLE-2 将会被阐明。贝叶斯的相对优点和频率论的方法仍然是在统计数据里争论的主题。更好的统计方法对患者参与试验可能导致更有效的临床试验设计，降低样本大小，得到更准确的结论和更好的结果。贝叶斯方法提供了一个更好的有吸引力的替代试验。这些类型的试验应该被更多设计并实施，从而证明其是真正受益的[11]。

自适应设计

在肿瘤学领域，临床药物的研发是一个漫长又昂贵的过程，成功率仅为 5%[12-13]。自适应设计允许研究者基于中期分析数据对试验进行调整，从而使临床试验更加适合于药物研发。在药物研发的早期阶段，新药和（或）药物之间联合作用的效果和毒性通常是未知的。随着试验的持续进行，自适应设计可以使用观察获取的信息来指导研究的实施。通过动态调整将患者转移到更安全、疗效更好的治疗方案中，这样的设计通常效率更高，仅需要较少的患者即可达到研究目的，并且也符合临床试验受试者伦理诉求[12-16]。文献中已提及许多自适应设计[17-21]。用于早期药物研发的自适应设计的大多数相关特征为：①动态调整剂量水平；②将患者动态分组或动态随机化到不同的剂量水平或治疗方案中；③允许基于中期分析结果来增加、减少或分等级给予治疗方案或剂量；④随着试验进展，动态调整样本量。许多自适应设计都是在贝叶斯框架下构建的，但并非所有设计都是这样。由于推论不受抽样方案的限制，即便研究的实施偏离了原始设计，贝叶斯方法本质上也更具灵活性和动态调整性[22-23]。对于所有的自适应设计，应当谨慎选择设计参数，并且提前进行模拟研究，从而校准研究设计，使其达到理想的工作特性。

本书选择了几个自适应设计来说明它们如何应用于药物研发。

连续性重新评估设计（CRM）

连续性重新评估设计（continual reassessment methed, CRM）是一种基于模型的方法，用于评估剂量-毒性曲线，并随后确定最大耐受剂量（maximum tolerated dose, MTD）。试验开始前，需提前指定一个单参数剂量-毒性曲线模型，如双曲正切函数模型、逻辑回归模型或功效模型。在明确模型参数的先验分布后，将最接近目标毒性水平的剂量用于治疗下一个患者。CRM 允许研究者根据当前数据，以最接近估计的 MTD 水平的剂量治疗患者。后来对 CRM 提出的修正意见补充了一些安全规程，如从最低剂量开始，不跨越剂量水平等[25]。CRM 的结果是剂量快速升级，并且利用所有可获得的信息来确定 MTD。在 Garrett-Mayer 的一篇论文中可以找到关于 CRM 的一个很好的教程[26]。最近的几篇论文从不同方面扩展了原始的 CRM，以提高其实用性和准确性，包括时间事件 CRM（TITE-CRM）、控制过量用药的剂量递增方法（escalation with over-dose control, EWOC）和贝叶斯模型平均 CRM（BMA-CRM）等[27-29]。

预测概率设计（PPD）

两阶段或三阶段设计通常用于评估新药的初始疗效[30]。尽管这些设计控制了假阳性和假阴性错误率，并且允许基于中期数据分析结果的早期无效停止，但是这种严格的研究设计可能很难遵循，因为必须在预先指定的固定数量的患者中评价药物反应。预测概率设计（predictive probability design, PPD）是一种基于贝叶斯预测概率的高效灵活的设计方式[31]。基于中期观察数据，假设当前趋势稳定，并且试验持续进行到纳入预计的最大样本量，由此计算某种阳性结论（拒绝无效假设）的概率来获得预测概率。可以根据预测概率的强度做出继续或终止试验的决定。该设计允许对试验结果进行持续监测。因此，当新的治疗方案无效时，PPD 能够很有效地在纳入样本量较小的早期终止试验。在试验实施偏离原始设计的情况下，PPD 在控制错误率方面仍然能够保持稳定。在评价研究结果方面，它比传统的多阶段设计更具可修改性，因而更易于实施。

生物标记物分层贝叶斯动态随机设计（BSBARD）

肿瘤的分子标记可用于鉴定预测标记物，从而寻找针对患者个体的最适合的靶向治疗。生物标记物分层贝叶斯动态随机设计（biomarker stratified bayesian adaptive randomization design，BSBARD）采用基于结果的动态调整的随机化方法将患者特征与靶向药物进行匹配。所有患者在随机化之前取活检标本进行生物标记物评估。通常采用一个短期的研究终点指标，例如在预定时间内（8周）的反应率或疾病控制率。贝叶斯概率模型或贝叶斯逻辑模型可用于分析结局指标的特征。根据试验累积数据计算最新的反应率，按照随机化率，将患者动态地随机分配到不同的治疗方案中。对于每一种生物标记物谱，高效能组的随机化率也高，反之亦然。可以增加早期终止规则，这样，低效能组可以暂停随机化。研究者提出的设计应当具备以下预期的工作特征：①识别有效药物的概率高；②暂停无效药物；③利用与其生物标记物谱相对应的有效药物治疗更多的患者。随着试验的进行，试验设计持续动态调整，包括改进参数估计值，并据此将患者分配到效能更高的一组。

标准设计方法与创新设计方法的比较

在这样的背景下，文献中已经提出了几种评价靶向药物的研究设计[32]。在此，我们比较了最近提出的 5 种设计方法的工作特性，这 5 种设计分别是：简单随机设计、标记物分层设计、标记物策略设计[33]、高效靶向设计[34-35]和生物标记物分层贝叶斯动态随机设计（BSBARD）。图 32.2 展示了这些设计的原理。在简单随机设计中，患者在标记物未知的情况下，被平均分配到标准治疗组或靶向治疗组。简单随机设计可以用于检测药物在整个患者群体中的总体治疗效果。根据患者标记物状态的析因分析，也可分别对标记物阴性和阳性患者的治疗效果进行检验。然而，对于样本量较小的研究来说，两个治疗组的患者中标记物状态的分布可能并不均衡。如果回顾性检测标记物，缺失率可能会很高。另一方面，根据标记物状态分层设计的方法也要求标记物检测结果在基线时已知。根据标记物状态分层之后，患者也被平均分配到标准治疗组或靶向治疗组。标记物的预测效果可以通过 A 组和 C 组的比较进行检验。A 组和 B 组，C 组和 D 组的比较分析可以分别用于标记物阴性或阳性组内治疗效果的评估。预测效果可以通过标记物阴性和标记物阳性组治疗反应的比值进行检验。在标记物策略设计中，患者首先根据策略进行随机化。随机分入非策略组的患者，既可以接受标准治疗（图 32.2 未展示），也可再次接受随机化，平均分配到标准治疗组或靶向治疗组。对于随机分入基于标记物策略组的患者，他们治疗方案的分配是确定的。标记物阴性者接受标准治疗，而标记物阳性者接受靶向治疗。两种策略治疗结果的差异可以通过 A+B 组和 C+D 组的比较进行检验。A 和 B 两组之间的比较可以检验未经筛选的患者群体的治疗效果。同样，经过筛选的患者群体的治疗效果可以通过 C 和 D 两组的比较来检验。然而，标记物策略设计是非常低效的，在比较不同策略治疗结果时需要较大的样本量，因为相似的患者类型的重叠特性可能将他们置于不同策略的相同治疗组中。在基于标记物策略的一组中，标记物效果和治疗方案效果无法区分，因为它们在设计上是完全混杂的。高效靶向设计是一种浓缩的设计类型，试验仅针对标记物阳性患者进行治疗。标记物阴性的患者脱离研究方案。该设计能够回答靶向治疗是否对于标记物阳性患者有效这一问题，但是无法评估靶向治疗对于标记物阴性患者的效力。

BSBARD 是一种基于模型的方法，逐步评估不同标记物状态两组的疗效。该设计与标记物分层设计类似，不同之处在于根据标记物状态有条件地实施随机化。该设计并非使用均等随机化方法，而是采用标记物协变量调整的动态随机化方法，以将更多的患者分配到更优越的治疗组。这种设计可以回答治疗方案效果、标记物效果、治疗和标记物的交互作用，以及利用试验期间收集的

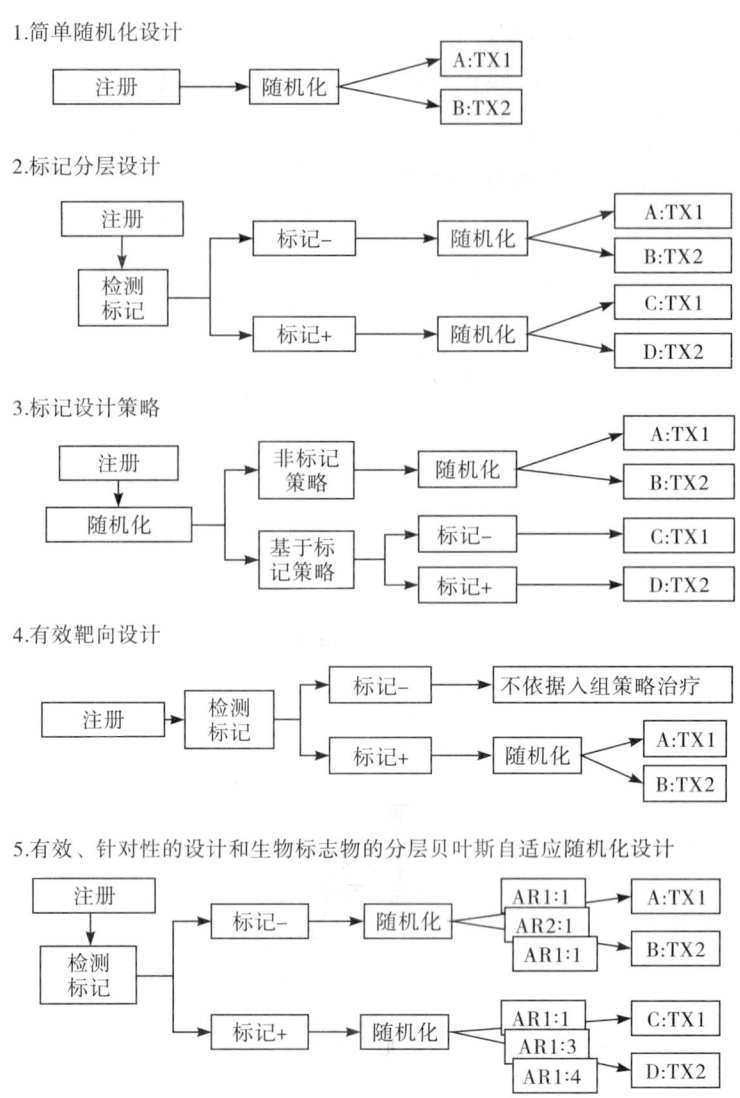

图32.2 简单随机设计、标记物分层设计、标记物策略设计、高效靶向设计和生物标记物分层贝叶斯动态随机设计（BSBARD）原理图。AR：动态随机化；TX1：标准治疗；TX2：靶向治疗

可用数据为患者提供更有效的治疗。

自适应设计面临的挑战

自适应设计提供了一种合理的、灵活的方法可供学习。为了根据中期数据对研究进行调整，研究终点指标需要在一个合理的短时间内进行客观地测量和观察。入组患者例数的增长不能比研究数据的累积更快。该设计还需要额外的基础工作支持，包括试验开展期间稳健的终点指标评价机制，及时将试验数据输入中央数据库，以及用于患者分组的专用软件地开发。可以从网址 http://biostatistics.mdanderson.org/SoftwareDownload 下载许多有用的工具。

BATTLE 试验：案例研究

生物标记物整合的靶向治疗方法消除肺癌（BATTLE）试验是在难治性的经治肺癌患者中开展的第一个前瞻性的、强制性活检的、基于生物标记物的动态调整的随机化研究[36-37]。从 2006 年到 2009 年，BATTLE 试验纳入了 341 例患者，其中有 255 例进行了随机分组。活检后的组织标本进行生物标记物谱分析。根据估计的预测值的等级顺序，将患者分配到 5 个生物标记物组中的一个：①EGFR 突变、扩增或多倍体；②KRAS 或 BRAF 突变；③ VEGF 和 VEGFR－2 的表达；

④RXR α、β 或 γ 过表达和（或）细胞周期蛋白 D1 过表达或扩增；⑤没有上述生物标记物。在初始将 97 例患者均等随机化分组之后，其余 158 例患者根据其各自的相关分子标记物情况，通过动态调整随机化分配到 4 个研究组之一：厄洛替尼、凡德他尼、厄洛替尼加贝沙罗汀、索拉非尼。

研究的主要终点指标是 8 周疾病控制率，对于本研究患者群体来说，DCR 已被证实是总生存的一个很好的替代指标[38]。基于数据的初步分析，本研究的无效假设是 DCR 为 30%，备择假设是 DCR 为 50%。统计学设计是基于贝叶斯分级模型的动态随机化，这种设计通过基于患者个体生物标记物谱得到随机化概率，随机化概率与观察功效成比例，从而将更多的患者分配到更有效的治疗组中。在动态随机化之前，患者通过均等随机化的方式分到 4 个治疗组中，对模型进行修整，从而计算随机化概率。试验设计同时允许，如果某一标记物组患者 DCR>50% 的概率小于 0.1，那么将暂停该组效果不佳的治疗。试验结束时，某一标记物组患者 8 周 DCR>30% 的后验概率大于 0.8 时，治疗才被视为有效。本研究设计概要详见图 32.3A。

研究的结论是，8 周的总体 DCR 为 46%。这项研究证实了几个预先指定的假设，例如厄洛替尼在 EGFR 突变患者中效果好，凡德他尼在 VEGFR-2 表达的患者中效果好，厄洛替尼加贝沙罗汀在细胞周期蛋白 D1 高表达的患者中效果好。这项研究也产生了一些有趣的假设。例如，索拉非尼在 KRAS 突变的患者中表现出疗效，这有待未来的试验研究进一步证实。图 32.4B 给出了编号 1、2、3 和 5 这 4 个生物标记物组分配到 4 个治疗组的最终的随机化概率分布（值得注意的是，编号 4 的生物标记物组只有 6 例患者，因此该组未在图中展示）。

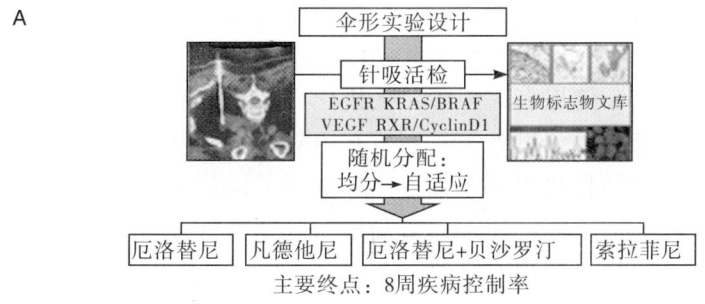

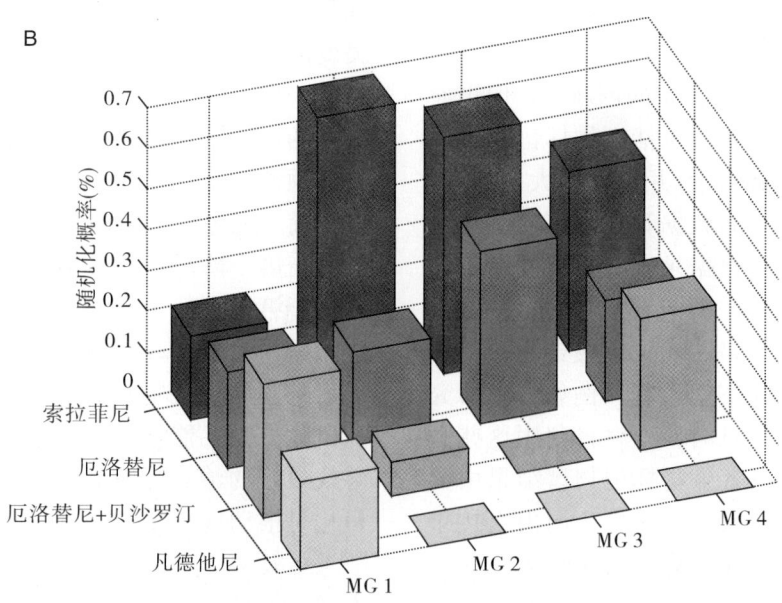

图 32.3（见彩插） BATTLE 试验。A. BATTLE 试验设计图。B. BATTLE 试验结束时不同治疗组和标记物组的动态随机化概率

BATTLE 试验动态调整特征之一就是低效能的治疗方案/标记物配对组暂停随机化。例如，BATTLE 试验结束时，分析数据提示，凡德他尼对 KRAS/BRAF 突变组无效，凡德他尼以及厄洛替尼加贝沙罗汀都对 VEGF/VEGFR-2 过表达组无效。因此，随机化概率被设置为 0（图 32.3B）。这种暂停或早期停止的规则能够避免将患者分配到无效治疗组，而将他们重新分配到更有效的治疗组中。贝叶斯框架允许试验过程中不断更新信息。不断更新的后验分布可用于指导研究的实施，如根据结果动态调整随机化概率，由于治疗无效或功效原因的早期终止等。

BATTLE 试验为个体化治疗肺癌建立了一个新的范本[39-40]。我们可以从这一开创性的试验中学到很多宝贵的经验。该试验证实，在复发性肺癌患者中获取新鲜活检组织不仅可行，而且在复发时确定肿瘤的标记物谱方面也是非常重要的[41]。这使得研究可以为每一例患者寻找最有效的治疗方案。前瞻性地收集患者的组织标本并进行生物标记物分析可以为未来工作的重大发现提供宝贵的信息。该试验平均每月招募 9.5 例患者，患者数量的增加保持稳定，说明临床团队和患者都很好地执行了根据结果动态调整的随机化设计。在贝叶斯分级模型下，治疗效果和预测标记物都得到了有效评估。这种"边走边学"的方法非常具有吸引力，因为随着试验的向前推进，这种方式能够最大限度地利用累积的患者数据来改善治疗效果。

BATTLE 试验尽管具有一定的创新性，但也面临许多挑战。为了实时获取包括生物标记物、患者资格、治疗效果以及毒副作用在内的大量信息，我们必须开发基于网络的数据管理系统。基于网络的应用程序允许远程数据录入，并通过内置数据类型、值以及范围核查来进行数据的质量控制。它还具有自动发送电子邮件或生成报告和数据下载功能，以利于对研究实施监督。例如，当研究护士录入患者的基线信息时，程序将利用这些数据来核查患者资格。患者生物标记物谱结果由分子病理学实验室的工作人员在活检 2 周内直接录入基于网络的系统。在完成患者资格核查，并完成生物标记物谱分析后，研究护士可以通过点击应用程序中的随机化按钮来执行随机化。这将通过网络服务调用 R 编写的动态随机化代码。R 代码将读取当前数据，执行贝叶斯计算，并相应地随机化患者。然后，随机化结果被发送到药房，药房配送合适的药物。除了满足一般的数据库安全性要求之外，这一系统还具备基于角色的安全控制功能，这样每个研究协作者对于相关的数据都有他/她自己的读/写权限。这样一个数据库对于 BATTLE 试验以及之后类似的动态随机化试验的实施来说是非常必要的。因此，高质量的数据通过一种更准确、完整和及时的方式被收集起来。

在我们的研究中，38% 的患者通过均等随机化分组，而其余 62% 的患者接受了动态随机化分组。回顾研究设计，我们认为动态随机化过程应该更早开始启动。我们的试验设计要求是，每个治疗/标记物组至少招募到一例患者才启动动态随机化。事实上，由于标记物组 4 的患者非常少，导致动态随机化过程的启动被延迟。最初的均等随机化方法是可以被替代的，可以事先选取一个适当的有效样本量来控制均等随机化的百分比。Lee 等的研究可以看到关于根据结果动态调整的随机化方法的讨论[42]。设计的另一个缺点是，我们在 BATTLE 试验设计中预先指定了生物标记物，并进行了标记物的组合分组。事实证明，某些标记物（如 RXR 相关的标记物）根本无法预测治疗效果。此外，将标记物进行降维分组并不是一个好主意，因为同一组中的标记物其预测强度是不同的。例如，预测厄洛替尼治疗组的 DCR、EGFR 突变的预测效果最强，其次是 EGFR 基因扩增。EGFR 蛋白表达几乎没有预测价值。因此，标记物分组的设计方式最终削弱了某些更为重要的标记物的预测强度。从 BATTLE 试验总结经验后，我们目前正在进行一个两阶段的 BATTLE-2 试验的设计。第一阶段识别预测标记物，将识别的标记物用于第二阶段（图 32.4）。我们得到的一个重要经验是，当确实存在有效的治疗方案，并且治疗方案与预测标记物相关时，根据结果动态调整的随机化方法，能够将患者获益最大化。我们正在寻找最好的治疗方案和预测标记物。动态调整随机化是推动这一过程的非常明智的选择。

尽管多年来，临床试验中开发了很多贝叶斯方法，但是真正付诸实践的方法少之又少。然而，近年来，贝叶斯方法在临床试验中的应用大幅度增长[11]。由于其不断更新信息的固有特性，贝叶斯框架是动态调整的临床试验设计的理想选择。可以通过校准设计参数来控制频率论上的Ⅰ类和Ⅱ类错误。

总之，BATTLE试验是肺癌领域首个已经完成的、基于生物标记物的动态调整的随机化研究。它也激励着类似动态调整试验研究的发展[43-49]。实时活检、生物标记物分析以及动态调整的随机化，这些举措使得我们向实现个体化治疗肺癌迈出了实质性的一步。我们应该进行更多像BATTLE一样的试验，来改进动态调整试验的设计和实施。这将进一步提高癌症有效疗法研发的效率。

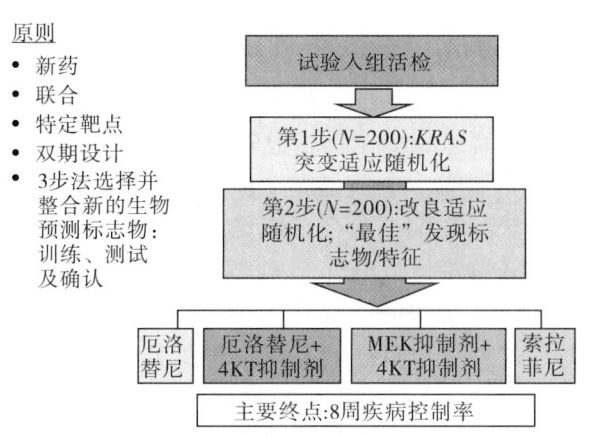

图32.4 BATTLE-2试验原则和设计图

其他创新性设计

文献中提到许多关于靶向药物研发的其他创新性设计方案。下面我们列出其中一些，并对每种设计进行简要的讨论。

1. 动态序列设计（adaptive signature design, ASD）[50]：这是一种将基因序列作为预测标记物来确定有效治疗方案的设计。这种设计可以分辨出某种治疗方案是广泛有效，还是仅对一部分患者有效。这是一种两阶段设计。第一阶段的主要工作是开发"分类器"。例如，鉴定一组高表达或者低表达并且与药物的敏感性和抵抗性相关的基因。第二阶段是进行两个步骤的假设检验。首先，在所有受试者中检验治疗效果，检验水准为α_1。如果检验结果有统计学意义，那么我们可以认为这种治疗方案对所有患者都是有效的。如果结果没有统计学意义，那么继续在"敏感"的亚组（第一阶段鉴定）中检验治疗效果，检验水准为α_2。如果这时候检验结果有统计学意义，那么我们可以认为这种治疗方案仅对敏感的亚组有效。整体的检验水准控制在α水平，$\alpha = \alpha_1 + \alpha_2$。例如，我们可以设置$\alpha_1 = 0.04$，$\alpha_2 = 0.01$，$\alpha = 0.05$。

2. 动态阈值设计（adaptive threshold design, ATD）[51]：在确定了基因序列之后，阈值选择的问题依然存在。ATD将所有患者总体治疗效果的检验与在敏感亚组中预先指定的标记物切点的建立和验证相结合。当新的治疗方案广泛有效时，ATD也保留了检验整体效果的能力。与不进行人群选择的研究设计相比，当敏感患者的比例较低时，这种设计能够明显提高效率。最近的一篇文章增加了交叉验证来提高预测的准确性[52]。

3. 随机化中止设计（randomized discontinuation design, RDD）[53-54]：在一项随机化研究中，必然有一部分患者被随机分配到"标准治疗"组或对照组，而其他患者将被随机分配到"新疗法"组或试验组。这样，将有部分患者无法享受新疗法，为解决这方面的顾虑，RDD预先为所有患者提供新疗法。对于新疗法有效的患者，治疗方案将持续至病情进展。对于使用新疗法出现病情进展的患者，新疗法将停止，并给予下一线治疗。而对于病情稳定的患者，将其均等随机化分配到对照组和试验组。这种设计不要求研究具有已知的预测标记物，并且可允许所有患者都享受新的治疗方案。它也可以筛选出一个更同质的研究人群来评价其停止新疗法后的治疗效果。然而，与简单随机化研究相比，这种设计可能研究效率较低。而且对于随机分组到停止新疗法组的患者，停止了潜在有效的治疗方案也存在伦理学问题[55-57]。

4. Ⅱ/Ⅲ无缝连接设计（seamless phase Ⅱ/Ⅲ designs, SP23D）[58-60]：该设计始于一个随机化的Ⅱ期试验，设有一个阳性对照组（标准治疗）和几个不同治疗方案和（或）剂量的试验组。它使用Ⅱ期试验的一个短期终点指标（例如2周期治疗后的客观反应率）来替代长期终点指标［例如总生存（OS）］。在进行试验中期分析后，弃掉无效组或高毒性组。如果至少有一个试验组有希望，那么研究将进入Ⅲ设计，设有一个标准治疗组和一个或多个选定治疗方案的试验组。通常使用长期终点指标（例如OS）作为Ⅲ期试验的主要终点。Ⅱ期试验阶段收集的信息，将用于Ⅲ期阶段以提高效率。此外，SP23D也消除了Ⅱ期和Ⅲ期试验之间的"空隙"，并节省了试验实施时间。

5. 个体化设计[61-64]：随着基因检测在覆盖范围和深度方面的全方位发展，可以预见，没有任何两个患者具有完全相同的基因图谱。当每一例患者个体的标记物谱都被独特地鉴定出来，那么如何针对每例患者开发最有效的治疗方案将是我们面临的挑战。个体化设计允许在单个患者中进行多周期交叉试验来比较多种治疗方案的效果。在癌症领域，随着时间的推移，患者的病情会逐渐恶化。因此，时间趋势需要随着时间的推移进行修正。例如，当根据不同治疗进展时间的比较决定给予何种治疗方案时，治疗线应该适当模型化。此外，贝叶斯分级模型可用于多个个体化试验的信息汇总。

6. 篮子研究：篮子研究是基于基因型的临床试验设计。这种研究对所有参与者，不论疾病部位或组织学特点，都进行全面的基因检测。根据突变类型、分子变异或通路异常，将患者归类到"篮子"中去。然后确定匹配的靶向治疗，并将治疗分配到"篮子"中，从而"篮子"中的患者能够得到相应的治疗。目标是每个"篮子"每种肿瘤类型至少纳入10~15例受试者[65]。例如，将患者分组到EGFR、EML4-ALK、HER-2、BRAF、AKT/MTOR、KRAS等几个"篮子"中，然后针对不同的篮子给予匹配的靶向治疗。随后可以确定不同分子图谱和不同部位肿瘤的治疗效果。如果药物对某个特定疾病部位的特定亚组有效，那么可以设计进一步的研究来丰富该亚组队列。如果药物效果具有压倒性优势，在药物批准之前，仅需要治疗少数患者来验证结果。该设计在罕见的基因组畸变研究方面非常有效。

7. 动态治疗方案（dynamic treatment regimen, DTR）[66-67]：大多数临床试验的目的都是在静态环境中寻找最佳治疗方案，而DTR的不同之处在于，它寻求最佳的治疗顺序，从而达到最佳治疗效果，如延长总体生存期。例如，治疗方案A可能是获得最高反应率的最佳初始治疗方案。当疾病出现进展，最佳的解救治疗是方案B，然而该方案可能在延长总生存期方面不是特别有效。另一个选择是治疗方案C，它作为一线治疗时，效果可能略逊于方案A。但是当疾病出现进展，继续方案D治疗在控制疾病和延长总生存期方面非常有效。在这种情况下，DTR提示，C-D的治疗顺序优于A-B的治疗顺序。DTR要求在一个复杂的环境下，运用一种复杂的动态程序算法来明确定义进程，只有这样，DTR设计才会有效。无论是方法学的发展，还是临床应用，这都是一个激动人心的课题。不过，该领域尚处于起步阶段。

8. 平台设计：众所周知，只有极小部分的癌症患者能够参与到临床试验中。尽管研究者已经尽力提高入组率，临床试验的参与率预计仅有3%~5%[68-69]。与传统的临床试验"以试验为中心"的方式相反，平台设计采用"以患者为中心"的方法。平台设计的主题是，每例患者都有一些信息，所有患者的全部信息被持续不断地收集起来，统一形成一个信息库，从而使以后的患者获益。传统的临床试验都有明确的、通常是非常严格的纳入标准，以确保纳入一组同质的患者，从而减少患者之间的变异性。这样做是为了使不同治疗组之间可以进行比较，而不受其他不适当因素的影响。对于具有特定选择性入组标准的试验，我们可能需要筛选大量的患者才能招募到试验要求的样本量，例如通过鉴定EML4-ALK易位来招募患者。整个过程漫长而低效。在平台设计中，所有患者都接受基因组分析。根据基因分析结果，不同的患者被引导进入不同的试验环境，不丢弃任何一例患者。例如，对于有实际价值突变的患者，当具备分子谱与靶向治疗匹配的1级证据时，患者将接受相应的治疗。包括利用EGFR抑制剂，如吉非替尼和厄洛替尼治疗具有EGFR突变的患者。另一个例子是利用克唑替尼治疗EML4-ALK易位的患者。

不具备有实际价值突变，但是推测正在研发中的靶向药物可能对其携带的异常分子谱有效，这类患者视为具有2级证据。这样的患者可以入组相应的试验，并通过动态调整的随机化分配到最有效的治疗组。例如，AKT抑制剂和MEK抑制剂都有积极的发展。类似于"篮子"试验的概念，具有AKT或MEK突变的患者可以进入AKT或MEK相关的试验。如果没有合适的试验，患者可能会根据医生选择的药物进行治疗。治疗结果可以作为个体化试验的一部分,并且随后通过个体患者的 meta 分析进行整合。

3 级证据的定义是,靶向治疗效果与某个预测标记物的相关性信息较弱或缺乏。对于那些不具备实际价值突变或推定治疗方案的患者,可以将其纳入未经选择的患者群体进行试验,从而筛查有效药物。一旦发现不同寻常的反应,将信息汇总并检验,从而形成新的假设,用于设计新的试验。在平台设计下,每个临床试验都可视为一个模块,可以根据需要插入平台或从中取出。所有的患者都被引导进入最好的治疗方案和(或)试验。所有收集到的信息均可用于目前以及未来的药物研发,从而大力提高临床研究的效率。

总 结

总而言之,自适应设计是药物研发领域非常明智又符合伦理学要求的方法。它可用于高效鉴别有效药物、淘汰无效药物、检测和验证预后及预测标记物,并将有效治疗与患者的生物标记物谱相匹配。自适应设计适合于靶向治疗药物的发展,并且为个体化医疗目标的实现提供了一个合理的途径。其他创新性设计包括个体化设计、篮子试验、Ⅱ/Ⅲ期无缝连接设计、动态治疗方案、平台设计等,为传统研究设计提供了具有吸引力的替代方案,这些创新性设计允许任何患者入组试验,并且基于患者的标记物谱、可获得的治疗方案、医生的选择或统计学算法等因素选择治疗方案。这些设计允许以统一的方式收集信息,然后将其汇总形成知识数据库,以促进科学发展并使以后的患者获益。应该继续开发和落实更多新颖的试验设计,让梦想变成现实。

(吕艳丽 王 娇 译)

参考文献

[1] Pao W, Girard N. New driver mutations in non-small-cell lung cancer. Lancet Oncology, 2011, 12 (2): 175-180.

[2] Sequist LV, Heist RS, Shaw AT, et al. Implementing multiplexed genotyping of non-small-cell lung cancers into routine clinical practice. Ann Oncol, 2011, 22 (12): 2616-2624.

[3] Capdeville R, Buchdunger E, Zimmermann J, et al. Glivec (STI571, imatinib), a rationally developed, targeted anticancer drug. Nat Rev Drug Discov, 2002, 1 (7): 493-502.

[4] Mok TS, Wu YL, Thongprasert S, et al. Gefitinib or carboplatin-paclitaxel in pulmonary adenocarcinoma. New England Journal of Medicine, 2009, 361 (10): 947-957.

[5] Herbst RS, Fukuoka M, Baselga J. Gefitinib-a novel targeted approach to treating cancer. Nat Rev Cancer, 2004, 4 (12): 956-965.

[6] Shaw AT, Yasothan U, Kirkpatrick P. Crizotinib. Nat Rev Drug Discov, 2011, 10 (12): 897-898.

[7] Rosenberg WM, Sackett DL. On the need for evidence-based medicine. Therapie, 1996, 51 (3): 212-217.

[8] Sackett DL, Rosenberg WM, Gray JA, et al. Evidence based medicine: what it is and what it isn't. BMJ, 1996, 312 (7023): 71-72.

[9] Guyatt G. Users' Guides to the Medical Literature: Essentials of Evidence-based Clinical Practice, 2nd edn. New York: McGraw-Hill Medical, xxii, 2008, 359 pp.

[10] Montori VM, Guyatt GH. Progress in evidence-based medicine. JAMA, 2008, 300 (15): 1814-1816.

[11] Lee JJ, Chu CT. Bayesian clinical trials in action. Stat Med, 2012, 31 (25): 2955-2972.

[12] Chen EX, Siu LL. Development of molecular targeted anticancer agents: Successes, failures and future directions. Curr Pharm Des, 2005, 11 (2): 265-272.

[13] Schmidt C. Adaptive design may hasten clinical trials. J Natl Cancer Inst, 2007, 99 (2): 108-109.

[14] Bauer P, Brannath W. The advantages and disadvantages of adaptive designs for clinical trials. Drug Discov Today, 2004, 9 (8): 351-357.

[15] Booth CM, Calvert AH, Giaccone G, et al. Design and conduct of phase Ⅱ studies of targeted anticancer therapy: Recommendations from the task force on methodology for the development of innovative cancer therapies (MDICT). Eur J Cancer, 2008, 44 (1): 25-29.

[16] Chang M, Chow SC, Pong A. Adaptive design in clinical research: issues, opportunities, and recommendations. J Biopharm Stat, 2006, 16 (3): 299-309; discussion 11-12.

[17] Cheung YK, Inoue LY, Wathen JK, et al. Continuous Bayesian adaptive randomization based on event times

with covariates. Stat Med, 2006, 25 (1): 55-70.

[18] Jones CL, Holmgren E. An adaptive Simon Two Stage Design for Phase 2 studies of targeted therapies. Contemp ClinTrials, 2007, 28 (5): 654-661.

[19] Smith MK, Jones I, Morris MF, et al. Implementation of a Bayesian adaptive design in a proof of concept study. Pharm Stat, 2006, 5 (1): 39-50.

[20] Yin G, Li Y, Ji Y. Bayesian dose-finding in phase I/II clinical trials using toxicity and efficacy odds ratios. Biometrics, 2006, 62 (3): 777-784.

[21] Zohar S, Chevret S. Recent developments in adaptive designs for Phase I/II dose-finding studies. J Biopharm Stat, 2007, 17 (6): 1071-1083.

[22] Berry DA. Introduction to Bayesian methods III: use and interpretation of Bayesian tools in design and analysis. Clin Trials, 2005, 2 (4): 295-300; discussion 1-4, 64-78.

[23] Berry DA. Bayesian clinical trials. Nat Rev Drug Discov, 2006, 5 (1): 27-36.

[24] O'Quigley J, Pepe M, Fisher L. Continual reassessment method: a practical design for phase 1 clinical trials in cancer. Biometrics, 1990, 46 (1): 33-48.

[25] Goodman SN, Zahurak ML, Piantadosi S. Some practical improvements in the continual reassessment method for phase I studies. Stat Med, 1995, 14 (11): 1149-1161.

[26] Garrett-Mayer E. The continual reassessment method for dose-finding studies: A tutorial. Clin Trials, 2006, 3 (1): 57-71.

[27] Ying Kuen Cheung, Chappell R. Sequential designs for phase I clinical trials with late-onset toxicities. Biometrics, 2000, 56 (4): 1177-1182.

[28] Babb J, Rogatko A, Zacks S. Cancer phase I clinical trials: Efficient dose escalation with overdose control. Statistics in Medicine, 1998, 17 (10): 1103-1120.

[29] Yin G, Yuan Y. Bayesian model averaging continual reassessment method in phase I clinical trials. Journal of the American Statistical Association, 2009, 104 (487): 954-968.

[30] Simon R. Optimal two-stage designs for phase II clinical trials. Control Clin Trials, Mar, 1989, 10 (1): 1-10.

[31] Lee JJ, Liu DD. A predictive probability design for phase II cancer clinical trials. Clin Trials, 2008, 5 (2): 93-106.

[32] Sargent DJ, Conley BA, Allegra C, et al. Clinical trial designs for predictive marker validation in cancer treatment trials. J Clin Oncol, 2005, 23 (9): 2020-2027.

[33] Lee JJ, Xuemin G, Suyu L. Bayesian adaptive randomization designs for targeted agent development. Clin Trials, 2010, 7 (5): 584-596.

[34] Maitournam A, Simon R. On the efficiency of targeted clinical trials. Stat Med, 2005, 24 (3): 329-339.

[35] Simon R, Maitournam A. Evaluating the efficiency of targeted designs for randomized clinical trials. Clin Cancer Res, 2004, 10 (20): 6759-6763.

[36] Zhou X, Liu S, Kim ES, et al. Bayesian adaptive design for targeted therapy development in lung cancer: A step toward personalized medicine. Clin Trials, 2008, 5 (3): 181-193.

[37] Kim ES, Herbst RS, Wistuba, et al. The BATTLE trial: personalizing therapy for lung cancer. Cancer Discov, 2011, 1 (1): 44-53.

[38] Lara PN, Jr., Redman MW, kelly K, et al. Disease control rate at 8 weeks predicts clinical benefit in advanced non-small-cell lung cancer: Results from Southwest Oncology Group randomized trials. J Clin Oncol, 2008, 26 (3): 463-467.

[39] Rubin EH, Anderson KM, Gause CK. The BATTLE trial: A bold step toward improving the efficiency of biomarker-based drug development. Cancer Discov, 2011, 1 (1): 17-20.

[40] Sequist LV, Muzikansky A, Engelman JA. A new BATTLE in the evolving war on cancer. Cancer Discov, 2011, 1 (1): 14-16.

[41] Tam AL, Kim ES, Lee JJ, et al. Feasibility of image-guided transthoracic core-needle biopsy in the BATTLE lung trial. J Thorac Oncol, 2013, 8 (4): 436-442.

[42] Lee JJ, Chen N, Yin G. Worth adapting? Revisiting the usefulness of outcome-adaptive randomization. Clin CancerRes, 2012, 18 (17): 4498-4507.

[43] Allison M. Reinventing clinical trials. Nat Biotechnol, 2012, 30 (1): 41-49.

[44] Berry DA, Herbst RS, Rubin EH. Reports from the 2010 Clinical and Translational Cancer Research Think Tank meeting: design strategies forpersonalized therapy trials. Clin Cancer Res, 2012, 18 (3): 638-644.

[45] Gold KA, Kim ES, Lee JJ, et al. The BATTLE to personalize lung cancer prevention through reverse migration. Cancer Prev Res (Phila), 2011, 4 (7): 962-972.

[46] Kelloff GJ, Sigman CC. Cancer biomarkers: Selecting the

[47] Lai TL, Lavori PW, Shih MC, et al. Clinical trial designs for testing biomarker-based personalized therapies. Clin Trials, 2012, 9 (2): 141-154.

[48] Printz C. BATTLE to personalize lung cancer treatment. Novel clinical trial design and tissue gathering procedures drive biomarker discovery. Cancer, 2010, 116 (14): 3307-3308.

[49] Rubin EH, Gilliland DG. Drug development and clinical trials: The path to an approved cancer drug. Nat Rev Clin Oncol, 2012, 9 (4): 215-222.

[50] Freidlin B, Simon R. Adaptive signature design: an adaptive clinical trial design for generating and prospectively testing a gene expression signature for sensitive patients. Clin Cancer Res, 2005, 11 (21): 7872-7878.

[51] Jiang W, Freidlin B, Simon R. Biomarker adaptive threshold design: A procedure for evaluating treatment with possible biomarker-defined subset effect. J Natl Cancer Inst, 2007, 99 (13): 1036-1043.

[52] Freidlin B, Jiang W, Simon R. The crossvalidated adaptive signature design. Clin Cancer Res, 2010, 16 (2): 691-698.

[53] Ratain MJ, Eisen T, Stadler WM, et al. Phase II placebo-controlled randomized discontinuation trial of sorafenib in patients with metastatic renal cell carcinoma. J Clin Oncol, 2006, 24 (16): 2505-2512.

[54] Rosner GL, Stadler W, Ratain MJ. Randomized discontinuation design: application to cytostatic antineoplastic agents. J Clin Oncol, 2002, 20 (22): 4478-4484.

[55] Capra WB. Comparing the power of the discontinuation design to that of the classic randomized design on time-to-event endpoints. Control Clin Trials, 2004, 25 (2): 168-177.

[56] Stadler WM, Rosner G, Small E, et al. Successful implementation of the randomized discontinuation trial design: An application to the study of the putative antiangiogenic agent carboxyaminoimidazole in renal cell carcinoma-CALGB 69901. J Clin Oncol, 2005, 23 (16): 3726-3732.

[57] Pacey S, Ratain MJ, Flaherty KT, et al. Efficacy and safety of sorafenib in a subset of patients with advanced soft tissue sarcoma from a Phase II randomized discontinuation trial. Invest New Drugs, 2011, 29 (3): 481-488.

[58] Bretz F, Schmidli H, Konig F, et al. Confirmatory seamless phase II/III clinical trials with hypotheses selection at interim: General concepts. Biom J, 2006, 48 (4): 623-634.

[59] Inoue LY, Thall PF, Berry DA. Seamlessly expanding a randomized phase II trial to phase III. Biometrics, 2002, 58 (4): 823-831.

[60] Stallard N. A confirmatory seamless phase II/III clinical trial design incorporating short-term endpoint information. Stat Med, 2010, 29 (9): 959-971.

[61] Gabler NB, Duan N, Vohra S, et al. N-of-1 trials in the medical literature: a systematic review. Med Care, 2011, 49 (8): 761-768.

[62] Lillie EO, Patay B, Diamant J, et al. The n-of-1 clinical trial: the ultimate strategy for individualizing medicine? Per Med, 2011, 8 (2): 161-173.

[63] Zucker DR, Ruthazer R, Schmid CH. Individual (N-of-1) trials can be combined to give population comparative treatment effect estimates: methodologic considerations. J Clin Epidemiol, 2010, 63 (12): 1312-1323.

[64] Zucker DR, Schmid CH, McIntosh MW, et al. Combining single patient (N-of-1) trials to estimate population treatment effects and to evaluate individual patient responses to treatment. J Clin Epidemiol, 1997, 50 (4): 401-410.

[65] Willyard C. 'Basket studies' will hold intricate data for cancer drug approvals. Nature medicine, 2013, 19 (6): 655.

[66] Murphy SA. Optimal dynamic treatment regimes. Journal of the Royal Statistical Society: Series B (Statistical Methodology), 2003, 65 (2): 331-355.

[67] Wang L, Rotnitzky A, Lin X, et al. Evaluation of viable dynamic treatment regimes in a sequentially randomized trial of advanced prostate cancer. J Am Stat Assoc, 2012, 107 (498): 493-508.

[68] Murthy VH, Krumholz HM, Gross CP. Participation in cancer clinical trials: race-, sex-, and age-based disparities. JAMA, 2004, 291 (22): 2720-2726.

[69] Nass SJ, Balogh E, Mendelsohn J. A National Cancer Clinical Trials Network: Recommendations from the Institute of Medicine. Am J Ther, 2011, 18 (5): 382-391.

第33章
肿瘤的微环境、血管生成及靶向治疗

John V. Heymach[1], Tina Cascone[2]

1. Department of Thoracic/Head and Neck Medical Oncology, the University of Texas MD Anderson Cancer Center, Houston, TX, USA
2. Department of Medicine, Division of Medical Education, Barnes-Jewish Hospital/Washington University School of Medicine in St. Louis, St. Louis, MO, USA

肿瘤的血管生成

实体肿瘤的生长及扩散有赖于血液供应[1-2]。事实上，肿瘤直径生长到超过数毫米后即可出现局部氧分压下降和营养匮乏，由此可引发新生血管的生成，以便满足肿瘤进一步生长的需要[3]。血管生成包括从已有的血管发展形成新的血管和为满足组织不断增长的需要而进行的血管重建。在伤口愈合、生殖周期等生理情况下，这一过程受到严格的促血管生成及抗血管生成因素之间复杂平衡的调控。在癌症等病理状态下，对失控刺激的持续应答最终导致了病理性的血管生成[4]。通过旁分泌及自分泌的方式，肿瘤微环境中富集了多种与体细胞及肿瘤细胞上的相应受体相结合的生长因子，处于活化状态的肿瘤相关血管内皮细胞经历了一系列的细胞病理生理过程（例如细胞迁移、蛋白酶合成、细胞分裂）并最终导致了新生血管网络的形成。然而，部分血管由于缺乏周细胞（壁细胞）的包绕从而导致了肿瘤血管不同于正常器官固有的高渗透性[5]，这也造成了肿瘤组织间液体压力升高并超过了正常器官[6]，从而限制了肿瘤细胞对抗肿瘤药物的摄取，给肿瘤的治疗带来了负面影响[6]。另外，肿瘤血管周细胞的丢失还促进了转移的发生[7]。

通过抑制肿瘤血管生成来限制肿瘤生长和预防癌细胞转移的研究目前很活跃。在接下来的部分中，我们将讨论肺癌中调节血管生成的因素、抗肿瘤血管生成治疗肺癌出现耐药的分子机制和血管生成抑制剂治疗肺癌的临床进展。

肿瘤血管生成的调控

血管生成的发生被认为是促血管生成因子及抗血管生成因子失衡的结果[8]。刺激促血管生成蛋白合成的最重要因素之一是组织中正常氧气张力水平的下降[9]。缺氧通过转录的低氧诱导因子-1α（HIF-1α），从而导致调节血管生成及糖酵解基因上调[10]。HIF-1α在包括肺癌的多种人类恶性肿瘤及相应的转移组织中存在过表达[11]。对早期非小细胞肺癌（NSCLC）患者进行术中肺癌组织氧分压测量证实了缺氧的存在[12]。NSCLC细胞中由缺氧诱发的HIF-1α上调与临床的相关性在于它能够引发肿瘤对化疗[13]和放疗的抵抗。

癌基因激活及抑癌基因的突变也能引发肿瘤的血管生成开关。例如，p53的缺失[14]或Ras的激活[15]与促血管生成蛋白血管内皮生长因子（VEGF）水平升高相关。通过突变或配体结合实现的EGFR受体的激活能够导致HIF-1α的上调及VEGF和其他促血管生成分子的分泌增多。抑癌基因LKB1的丢失也能够引起HIF-1α上调及肿瘤侵袭性增加[16-18]。有报道显示肿瘤相关的间质细胞可能是NSCLC中生成促血管生成蛋白的主要细胞来源[19]。肿瘤相关的巨噬细胞表达大量的血管生成因子[20]，人类肺部恶性肿瘤组织中巨噬细胞的明显增多与血管生成及不良预后相关[21]。

有报道显示，不同类型的肿瘤血管生成应答的程度不同，其中肺癌拥有的正在分裂的内皮细胞的数量最少[22]。事实上，一项纳入了500例Ⅰ期NSCLC患者的研究发现，有16%的研究对象未发现新生血管生成的组织学依据[23]。部分肺癌中缺乏活跃的血管生成可能是由于正常肺组织本身含有丰富的毛细血管，这一点可能对该部分肺癌患者的抗血管生成治疗提供重要启示。不依赖新生血管生成的肿瘤是通过增殖以接近之前存在的血管来实现继续生长的，这一过程被称为"血管拉拢"[24]。在接下来的部分，我们将对几种促血管生成蛋白进行讨论并对它们在肺癌中发挥作用的证据进行综述。

VEGF因子受体信号通路

VEGF是关键的血管生成调节因子之一，这一细胞因子能够刺激新生血管形成所需要的全部过程[5,25]。VEGF属于生长因子家族，包含5种VEGF配体（VEGFs A~E）及胎盘生长因子（placental growth factor, PLGF）。这些配体通过与3种不同的VEGF受体（VEGFR1-VEGFR3）结合来发挥效应[26]。VEGF-A被认为是VEGF配体中与血管生成相关的最重要的一种，它通过与主要分布在内皮细胞表面的VEGF-R2结合来介导效应[27]。VEGF-R2信号传导的激活刺激了受体的自体磷酸化和二聚体化，进而引发一系列内皮细胞活动，包括迁移、蛋白酶合成、细胞分裂及存活[28]。VEGFC和VEGFD配体与淋巴管内皮细胞的VEGFR3结合后可以发出促进淋巴管生成的信号[29]。

VEGF-A的表达从很大程度上受到HIF1-α和组织氧合状态的调节。在正常肺组织中，VEGF在Ⅱ型肺泡上皮细胞、细支气管Clara细胞、平滑肌细胞和肺泡成肌纤维细胞中均有表达[30]。在Ⅰ期NSCLC中，VEGF的表达和微血管密度之间存在相关性，这与不良的预后有关[31]。小细胞肺癌（SCLC）中也存在着高度的血管化，但这一特点似乎并不依赖于VEGF的表达[32]。曾有报道显示，VEGF在NSCLC原发灶及相对应的脑转移灶中均有表达，然而，与脑转移相关的血管中，成熟的、有周细胞覆盖的血管占60%，这一比例高于原发灶[33]。磷酸化的VEGFR2在试验性的NSCLC异种移植物的肿瘤相关性内皮细胞上表达，对它进行抑制在某些肿瘤模型中可以改善患者的生存期[19]。VEGFR3信号转导的确切作用和肺癌中淋巴管的生成尚不明确。

成纤维细胞生长因子受体信号通路

成纤维细胞生长因子（fibroblast growth factors, FGFs）是一个肝素结合蛋白大家族，在新生血管形成、伤口愈合、生长发育及癌症中起作用[34]。癌症中研究最多的FGFs是酸性FGF（FGF1）和碱性FGF（FGF2）。FGF2是最早从癌细胞中获得并被分离和克隆的促血管生成蛋白中的一员[35]。FGFs通过与4个高亲和性的受体（FGFR1~4）之一结合发挥作用[36]。FGFs及其受体在多种不同类型的细胞表面均有表达，包括内皮细胞、平滑肌细胞、胶质细胞、成纤维细胞及巨噬细胞。

从非血管化的纤维瘤到高度血行转移的纤维肉瘤均发现了FGF的输出是激发血管生成的开关[37]。肺鳞癌中经常出现FGF、FGFR1和FGFR2的过表达[38]，并且观察到了FGFR1的扩增[39]。在包括肺癌在内的多种恶性肿瘤患者的血清和尿液里均发现了FGF2水平的上升[40]。事实上，在NSCLC中，血清FGF2水平与肿瘤的体积、高复发率及较差的生存相关[41]。最新的证据提示在接受放疗的Ⅱ~Ⅲ期NSCLC患者中，肿瘤细胞FGF的表达在局部控制、无远处转移及总生存方面是一个独立的负向预测因子[42]。在NSCLC的试验模型中，对VEGFR途径的抑制产生获得性耐药的肿瘤与FGFR家族成员的上调有关[19]。

表皮生长因子受体信号通路

EGFR属于ErbB家族受体中的一员，这一家族也包括HER2（ErbB2）、HER3（ErbB3）及Her4（ErbB4）。EGF或转化生长因子α（TGFα）配体与EGFR结合导致后者激活，进而刺激同源二聚体和异二聚体的形成，最终导致细胞内效应蛋白丝裂原活化蛋白（mitogen-activated protein, MAP）激酶、磷酸肌醇化3-激酶/Akt以及信号转导和转录活化蛋白的激活。EGFR信号转导的激活通过刺激癌细胞分裂、侵袭、存活及转移来促进肿瘤进展[43-44]。EGFR及其配体在NSCLC的发展过程中往往是过表达的[45]。最近的研究显示EGFR在刺激新生毛细血管形成中发挥作用，同时发现从试验用的肿瘤中分离出的内皮细胞由于表达EGFR且能够对EGF配体做出应答而与正常器官中分离出的内皮细胞不同[46]。另外，应用EGFR和VEGFR信号通路小分子TKIs治疗表达TGFα的试验用NSCLC可以产生明显的抗血管生成作用，并能降低转移频率、改善生存[47]。

血小板源性生长因子信号途径

血小板源性生长因子及受体（the platelet derived growth factors and receptors，PDGF/Rs）能够将周细胞募集并维持在血管网络的生发部位，因此被广泛认为是血管成熟的关键调节因子[48]。PDGF配体家族包括4个结构相关的可溶性多肽，以同源或异源二聚体的形式存在，可以同两种酪氨酸激酶受体PDGFR-α和PDGFR-β结合[49]。大多数实体肿瘤在内皮细胞或血管周细胞上表达PDGFR[50]，该受体过表达与多种肿瘤的预后差有关[51-52]。PDGFs在体内也表现出刺激血管生成的作用[53-54]，提示一些内皮细胞存在高亲和力的PDGF受体。PDGF信号通路通过促进周细胞募集及血管成熟发挥促进肿瘤血管生成的作用[55]。事实上，只有成熟、有壁细胞覆盖的血管才能正常发挥作用。为了稳定内皮细胞通道，促血管生成的内皮细胞释放PDGF-B以吸引PDGF-β阳性的周细胞[56-57]。一项小鼠胶质瘤模型的实验研究支持了该观点，该研究发现了PDGF依赖性的周细胞向肿瘤血管的募集[58]。已经在小鼠前列腺癌骨转移的模型中发现了PDGF-β受体在骨转移瘤内皮细胞中的表达，但正常骨组织或周围肌肉转移瘤中分布的内皮细胞未发现该受体的表达[59]。PDGF-β缺失导致周细胞缺乏，最终引起血管渗漏、迂曲、微血管瘤形成及出血，抑制PDGFR可以通过周细胞脱落使得血管不成熟、易于退变而削弱肿瘤的生长[60]。由于内皮细胞的存活依赖周细胞VEGF的合成，所以周细胞能够保护内皮细胞免于VEGF的撤退并使其对VEGF阻滞剂耐药[61]。数个多靶点受体酪氨酸激酶抑制剂已经被开发出来，初始研究显示PDGF信号途径的阻断可以通过消耗周细胞提高成熟、正常化的血管对VEGF抑制的灵敏度[4]。

抑制肺癌血管生成的治疗策略

针对肿瘤相关内皮细胞的靶向治疗作为控制肿瘤生长的一种方法因几个原因被认为相当具有吸引力。例如，内皮细胞具有遗传稳定性，因此不易对治疗产生耐药[62]；另外，抗肿瘤血管生成的治疗为靶向治疗，所以很少会产生类似化疗的全身毒性。

多数抑制肿瘤新生血管生成应答的努力集中在VEGF/R信号途径。验证抗VEGF治疗效果的实验发现这些药物可以通过缩小血管直径、减少血管迂曲及通过积极的动员周细胞至血管壁及使基底膜正常化来提高血管成熟度等最终使肿瘤血管正常化[63]。总的来说，这些效应最终导致了微血管密度的暂时性降低和肿瘤组织间液体压力的下降，进而改善氧气和药物的传递[64]。临床前研究令人振奋的结果激发了人们测试多种抑制肿瘤血管生成药物在不同肿瘤治疗中效果的热情。

VEGF靶向治疗：美国FDA批准的药物

抗VEGF单克隆抗体贝伐珠单抗与人类VEGF结合并抑制VEGF的功能[65]。贝伐珠单抗是首个获得美国FDA批准的抗血管生成药物。这一决定主要是基于一项Ⅲ期临床试验的结果。该临床试验发现接受贝伐珠单抗联合标准化疗治疗的结肠癌及NSCLC患者在无进展生存期（PFS）和（或）总生存期（OS）以及客观反应率方面均有改善[66-67]。贝伐珠单抗单药治疗NSCLC被证实无效[68]，不过，与单纯化疗相比，它与标准一线化疗联合治疗晚期非鳞状NSCLC能够延长PFS和OS[67]。

目前，贝伐珠单抗联合化疗用于Ⅰ~Ⅲ期NSCLC的辅助治疗或新辅助治疗的效果正接受评估。纪念斯隆·凯瑟琳癌症中心近期已完成了名为BEACON（Bevacizumab and Chemotherapy for Operable NSCLC，贝伐珠单抗联合化疗治疗可切除的NSCLC）的一项单中心Ⅱ期临床试验（NCT00130780），这项研究纳入了一批存在可切除病灶的临床分期为ⅠB～ⅢA（T1-3N0-2M0）的NSCLC患者，研究的主要目标是观察含铂化疗联合贝伐珠单抗方案用于非鳞状NSCLC的新辅助治疗能否提高病理降期率，即与诱导治疗前的临床分期相比最终病理分期任何程度的降低。一项被称为ECOG的Ⅲ期随机临床试验（E1505）正在招募患者，旨在比较ⅠB（>4cm）～ⅢA期包括鳞癌在内获得完全切除的NSCLC患者接受联合或不联合贝伐珠单抗辅助化疗的效果，目前该研究结果尚未公布（NCT00324805）。

由于会显著提高食管气管瘘的发生率，故在不能手术的ⅢB期NSCLC中不推荐进行贝伐珠单抗联合同步放化疗[70]。VEGF途径的抑制不仅影响肿瘤相关血管的生长，也会对正常器官的血管造成一些影响。这就可以解释为什么贝伐珠单抗的毒性包括血栓栓塞事件、出血、伤口愈合困难、高血压及蛋白尿[71]。另外，鳞癌通常属于贝伐珠单抗的使用禁忌证，因为该类患者相对容易出现咯血。

VEGF/R及EGFR靶向治疗的联合应用

针对促使肿瘤生长、进展及转移的多种关键途径进行的靶向治疗已经改善了多种恶性肿瘤的临床结局。这一做法可以通过一种复合制剂或多种制剂的联用来实现。在NSCLC的异体移植模型中进行的临床前试验发现VEGF/R联合EGFR途径的治疗方式是合理的。事实上，与单独应用贝伐珠单抗或抗EGFR-TKI厄洛替尼（Tarceva）相比，二者联用能起到更强的肿瘤抑制作用[72]。SWOG（Southwest Oncology Growp）研究作为一项Ⅱ期临床试验对抗EGFR单克隆抗体西妥昔单抗（Erbitux®）与贝伐珠单抗及化疗联用进行了评估，并为我们展示了一种具有前景、毒性可耐受的抗肿瘤治疗模式[73]。一项Ⅰ、Ⅱ期研究测试了在既往接受过治疗的晚期非鳞状NSCLC患者中联合应用厄洛替尼及贝伐珠单抗的效果，显示出12.6个月的中位OS和6.2个月的中位PFS[74]。另外一项Ⅱ期临床试验纳入了相似数量的患者，发现贝伐珠单抗联合厄洛替尼获得了能与贝伐珠单抗联合化疗相媲美的疗效，二者的中位OS分别为13.7个月及12.6个月[75]。最终，BeTa Ⅲ期试验对这种联合用药在接受过治疗的晚期NSCLC患者中的应用进行了研究，尽管并未达到与厄洛替尼单药相比延长总生存期的主要终点（中位OS：9.3个月 vs 9.2个月；$P=0.75$），但却获得了PFS的显著延长[76]。ATLAS Ⅲ期试验将贝伐珠单抗联合厄洛替尼与贝伐珠单抗联合安慰剂用于一线治疗后的维持治疗进行了比较，因中期分析发现前组PFS较后组显著延长而提前终止了研究[77]。

VEGFR途径的酪氨酸激酶抑制剂

针对肿瘤血管生成所涉及的几个关键信号通路（如VEGFR、PDGFR、FGFR、Raf及c-KIT）所研制的小分子酪氨酸激酶抑制剂已经展示出了比单靶点药物更强的抗肿瘤作用，目前正在临床开发阶段。另外，这些药物可以口服给药，因此患者应用时更加方便。相反，非目标激酶的抑制导致了更广的毒性谱，尤其是当这些复合物与化疗联合应用时可能会出现额外的毒副作用。已经被美国FDA批准的多靶点抗血管生成药物包括舒尼替尼（肾细胞癌、肝细胞癌、胰腺神经内分泌肿瘤）、索拉非尼（肾细胞癌、肝细胞癌）、凡德他尼（甲状腺髓样癌）、帕生帕尼以及阿西替尼（肾细胞癌）。然而，这些药物并不能使NSCLC患者取得生存获益。

舒尼替尼（Sutent®，SU11248）是一种口服的小分子酪氨酸激酶抑制剂，以VEGFR-1、VEGFR-2、VEGFR-3、PDGFR、KIT、FLT3、RET及CSF-1R为靶点，已经在美国及欧洲被批准用于晚期肾细胞癌的治疗及伊马替尼抵抗或耐药的胃肠间质瘤（gastrointestinal stromal tumor, GIST）。对多种异种移植物模型进行的临床前研究发现舒尼替尼对包括NSCLC在内的多种肿瘤具有抑制作用[78]。事实上，与单独应用相比，舒尼替尼与多西他赛、培美曲塞、吉西他滨或顺铂等化疗药物联用的肿瘤抑制作用更强[79-80]。Ⅱ期试验评估了舒尼替尼单药持续或间歇给药治疗接受过治疗的NSCLC患者的效果，发现该药能够起效且患者耐受良好[81]。另外，一项Ⅰ期临床研究发现舒尼替尼与吉西他滨和铂类联用可以获得有前景的肿瘤反应率[82]。Ⅱ期临床试验 SUN1058 和Ⅲ期试验 SUN1087 正在评估厄洛替尼单药或与舒尼替尼联合用于晚期 NSCLC 患者的效果，旨在研究 EGFR 和 VEGF/R 双信号通路的阻断作用。在最近报道的一项Ⅲ期临床试验中，Scagliotti 等发现在难治性 NSCLC 中舒尼替尼联合厄洛替尼与厄洛替尼单药相比并不能改善总生存情况[83]，然而，前者获得了 PFS 的延长、客观缓解率（ORR）的改善以及更高的 3 级不良反应发生率。

索拉非尼（Nexavar®）以 Raf、VEGFR-2 和 VEGFR-3、PDGFR 和 KIT 为靶点，获准用于晚期肾细胞癌及肝细胞癌[84]。以细胞系及异种移植物模型为研究对象的临床前试验发现，索拉非尼与 EGFR 抑制剂、威罗菲尼、顺铂或吉非替尼联用能够显著推迟肿瘤生长[85-87]。来自一些Ⅱ期临床试验的数据显示，索拉非尼单独用于既往接受过多次治疗的转移性 NSCLC 患者在疾病稳定时间、总生存期及中位无进展生存期方面均有显著延长，分别为 2 个月[88]、6.8 个月及 2.8 个月[89]。近期的Ⅱ期临床试验——BATTLE 试验发现带有 KRAS 突变的既往接受过治疗的肺癌患者能够从索拉非尼的治疗中获益，强调了用于识别靶向获益人群的生物标志物的重要性[90]。亦有研究对比了索拉非尼联合培美曲塞与培美曲塞单药用于肺癌二线治疗。Ⅱ期研究 NCCTG N0626 在非鳞状 NSCLC 患者中发现这两种治疗具有相似的中位 PFS（3.4 个月 vs 4.1 个月；$P = 0.22$）和 OS（9.4 个月 vs 9.7 个月；$P = 0.49$）[91]。针对既往接受过治疗的 168 例晚期 NSCLC 的一项研究显示，索拉非尼联合厄洛替尼并未显著改善缓解率（remission rate，RR）、PFS 或 OS[92]。在另外一项Ⅱ期试验中，50 例未行化疗的晚期 NSCLC 患者也接受了这种联合治疗并获得了类似的结果[93]。Gridelli 等评估了索拉非尼联合吉西他滨或厄洛替尼用于既往未接受过治疗的老年晚期 NSCLC 患者，在 RR 和 OS 方面并未获得明显改善（索拉非尼+吉西他滨组与索拉非尼+厄洛替尼组 6.5% ~ 10.3%；6.5 个月 vs 12.6 个月）[94]。一项Ⅲ期临床研究 ESCAPE 比较了卡铂+紫杉醇联合或不联合索拉非尼的疗效，亚组分析发现在非鳞状 NSCLC 中联合索拉非尼并未获得显著的总生存期改善，而在鳞癌患者中甚至表现出了有害作用[95]。另外一项设计类似的Ⅲ期研究 NExUS（NCT00449033）比较了顺铂+吉西他滨方案联合与不联合索拉非尼的治疗效果，并最终因未能达到它的主要终点 OS 而提前终止。

凡德他尼（Zactima®，ZD6474）是以 RET、VEGFR2-3 和 EGFR 为靶点的口服 TKI，是首个获得美国 FDA 认证的用于有症状或进展的晚期甲状腺髓样癌的全身治疗药物[96]。体外试验及临床前研究发现在浓度较低时，凡德他尼对 VEGFR2 的抑制作用要强于 EGFR[97]。相比于单独用药，凡德他尼与标准的含铂化疗方案联用治疗未经化疗的 NSCLC 患者能够带来更高的反应率和更长的 PFS[98]。在一项Ⅱ期临床试验中，凡德他尼联合多西他赛比多西他赛单药治疗以往化疗失败的 NSCLC 更有优势[99]，作为二线用药，与吉非替尼相比能够显著延长 PFS[100]。ZEAL Ⅲ期临床研究发现凡德他尼联合培美曲塞并未获得生存改善，然而，这种联合治疗改善了 ORR，同时能够延长症状恶化的时间[101]。ZODIAC Ⅲ期临床试验比较了凡德他尼联合多西他赛和安慰剂联合多西他赛一线治疗后进展的晚期 NSCLC，在凡德他尼组获得了主要终点 PFS 的延长（PFS：HR = 0.79；$P <0.001$），但是这一延长的 PFS 并未最终转化为总生存的显著改善[102]。最常见的严重不良反应是粒细胞减少性发热，凡德他尼组的发生率为 7%，安慰剂组为 6%。Ⅲ期临床试验 ZEST 在未经选择的既往接受过至少一线化疗失败的晚期 NSCLC 患者中比较了凡德他尼与标准二线治疗厄洛替尼的作用[103]。与厄洛替尼相比，在 PFS 方面凡德他尼组并未显出显著改善（凡德他尼组中位 PFS 为 2.6 个月，厄洛替尼组为 2.0 个月）。另外，在次要终点 OS（HR = 1.01；$P = 0.83$）、ORR（均为 12%）及至疼痛症状恶化的时间（HR = 0.92；$P = 0.28$）方面二者无统计学差异。在非劣效性研究中这两种药物在 PFS 和 OS 方面表现相当；在毒副作用方面，凡德他尼要比厄洛替尼更为严重，发生 3 级以上不良反应的概率要高于后者（50% vs 40%）。ZEPHYR 是一项以安慰剂为对照的随机双盲Ⅲ期临床试验，研究发现凡德他尼联合最佳支持治疗用于 EGFR-TKI 治疗或者一线或二线化疗失败的晚期 NSCLC 与单纯最佳支持治疗相比无明显总生存获益（HR = 0.95；$P = 0.52$；试验组中位 OS 为

8.5 个月，对照组为 7.8 个月）。然而，凡德他尼组在 PFS（HR = 0.63；$P < 0.001$）及 ORR（2.6% vs 0.7%；$P = 0.028$）方面表现出了显著优势[104]。

西地尼布（Recentin®，AZD2171）是以 VEGFR-1、VEGFR-2、VEGFR-3、PDGFR 及 KIT 为靶点的口服酪氨酸激酶抑制剂[105]。目前人们主要研究它与化疗联用的效果。Ⅰ期试验发现这种药物与标准化疗联合应用有望带来较好的抗肿瘤效果[106]。基于这些令人鼓舞的结果，Ⅱ、Ⅲ期临床试验 BR.24 对卡铂 + 紫杉醇联合西地尼布或安慰剂一线治疗晚期 NSCLC 进行了比较。尽管Ⅱ期试验显示西地尼布与安慰剂相比具有更高的 RR（38% vs 16%；$P < 0.0001$）及更长的 PFS（HR = 0.77），但这项试验因为毒性增加而提前停止（尽管已将西地尼布的剂量降至 30mg）[107]。考虑到毒性反应，Ⅲ期试验 NCIC BR29 采用了相似的设计以进一步研究西地尼布 20mg 联合卡铂及多西他赛的治疗效果，然而由于中期分析效果欠佳，该试验已于近期停止[108]。Ⅱ期试验 N0528 在类似的患者群体中研究了吉西他滨/卡铂联合或不联合西地尼布（45mg/d，口服）的安全性及有效性。尽管试验组的中位 PFS（6.3 个月 vs 4.5 个月；HR = 0.69；$P = 0.15$）、中位 OS（11.8 个月 vs 9.9 个月；HR = 0.66；$P = 0.16$）以及 3 级及更高级别的毒性发生率（71% vs 45%；$P = 0.01$）有轻度升高，但二者的客观反应率并无显著差异（20% vs 18%；$P = 1.0$）[109]。

帕唑帕尼（GW786034，Glaxo Smith Kline）是具有抗 VEGFR-1、VEGFR-2、VEGFR-3、PDGFR-α/β，FGFR-1 及 FGFR-3 活性的小分子酪氨酸激酶抑制剂[110]。在非转移性 NSCLC 患者中，帕唑帕尼单药作为新辅助治疗手段在Ⅰ、Ⅱ期患者中取得了令人鼓舞的治疗效果[111]，出现的不良反应以 1~2 级为主，包括高血压、腹泻及疲乏。该药物在辅助治疗及晚期治疗方面的安全性及有效性正在进一步研究中[112]。

新 药

以 VEGFR、PDGFR 或 FGFR 信号途径为作用靶点的更新的抗血管生成药物正在以临床前试验的形式被研究，并显示出了具有前景的抗肿瘤作用。目前有进行到不同阶段的临床试验正在对该药物进行评估。

阿西替尼（AG-013736，Pfizer）是一种以 VEGFR-1、VEGFR-2、VEGFR-3、PDGFR-β 和 c-KIT 为靶点的口服酪氨酸激酶抑制剂，对多种实体肿瘤有中度抗肿瘤作用[113]。在一项Ⅱ期临床研究中，晚期 NSCLC 患者应用单药阿西替尼获得了 14.6 个月的中位 OS，这远远超出了人们对这一人群生存的预期，其毒性也在可接受范围内[114]。另外一些评估阿西替尼与标准化疗联合用于一线治疗的Ⅱ期临床试验正在进行，其中 AGILE1030 试验对阿西替尼联合紫杉醇-卡铂及贝伐珠单抗联合紫杉醇或卡铂进行了比较，AGILE1039 对阿西替尼联合培美曲塞-顺铂与仅用两联化疗相比的获益情况进行了评估。Ⅱ期临床试验 AGILE1038 正在研究阿西替尼联合顺铂-吉西他滨治疗肺鳞癌。

莫特塞尼靶向作用于所有的 VEGFRs 以及 PDGFR、c-kit 和 RET[115]。近期的结果显示莫特塞尼每天用药联合卡铂-紫杉醇与贝伐珠单抗联合卡铂-紫杉醇一线治疗晚期 NSCLC 疗效相当[116]。由于鳞癌患者死亡率及咯血的发生率更高，对莫特塞尼联合卡铂-紫杉醇进行研究的Ⅲ期临床试验 MONET1 目前正在招募晚期非鳞状 NSCLC 患者。2011 年 ASCO 上研究人员公布了该试验的初步结果：联合治疗组的中位 PFS（5.6 个月 vs 5.4 个月；HR = 0.78；$P = 0.0006$）和 RR（40% vs 26%；$P < 0.0001$）的改善有统计学意义，但中位 OS 并无显著差异（13.0 个月 vs 11.0 个月；HR = 0.89；$P = 0.13$）。

尼达尼布 BIBF 1120 是一种针对所有 VEGFRs、PDGFR-α/β、FGFR1、FGFR-2、FGFR-3、Src 家族成员和 flt-3 的口服小分子抑制剂[117]。一项Ⅱ期临床试验发现 BIBF 1120 单药用于经过治疗的 NSCLC 可以使 48% 的患者获得病情稳定[118]，中位 PFS 及 OS 分别为 6.9 周和 21.9 周。目前，一些Ⅲ期临床试验正在评估 BIBF 1120 与化疗联用的有效性（LUME-Lung 2、

NCT00806819 以及 LUME-Lung 1、NCT00805194）。

血管阻断剂（VDAs）

血管生成抑制剂阻止了来自原有血管系统的新生血管的形成，而血管阻断剂（vascular disrupting agents，VDAs）则靶向作用于已形成的肿瘤血管的内皮细胞，最终导致肿瘤血管系统的瓦解并剥夺了肿瘤的氧气和营养供应[119]。

Vadimezan（ASA404）是一种黄酮乙酸类似物，在一项Ⅱ期临床试验中与化疗联用治疗 NSCLC 初步显示出了令人鼓舞的结果[120]；然而这些发现在Ⅲ期临床试验中并未得到证实。事实上，一项关于 vadimezan 联合卡铂或紫杉醇一线治疗 NSCLC 的Ⅲ期临床试验因试验组和安慰剂组的 OS 无统计学差异（中位 OS 分别为 13.4 个月 vs 12.7 个月；HR = 1.01；P = 0.535）而未达到它的主要研究终点[121]。基于这些结果以及二线治疗的失败，诺华公司已经终止了 vadimezan 在肺癌中的研究。

ABT-751 是另外一种在临床前实验中显示出强有力抗肿瘤活性的 VDAs。已经有Ⅰ/Ⅱ期临床试验对该药物与多西他赛联合用于 NSCLC 的二线治疗进行了评估[122]。不幸的是，这项试验并未表现出主要终点 PFS 的改善（ABT-751 组和安慰剂组的中位 PFS 分别为 2.3 个月和 1.9 个月；P = 0.82）。然而，一项亚组分析显示 ABT-751 能延长肺鳞癌的 OS（P = 0.034；中位生存期为 3.3 个月 vs 8.1 个月）。

SCLC 的抗血管生成治疗

抗肿瘤血管生成药物在 SCLC 中的临床应用较少被深入研究。一项随机、双盲、与安慰剂对照的Ⅲ期临床试验 IFTC0001 比较了多药联合化疗（顺铂、依托泊苷、表柔比星及环磷酰胺）联合或不联合沙利度胺（400mg）用于初治的广泛期 SCLC 患者[123]，结果显示经过最初两个周期的 PC-DE 方案治疗后，ORR 为 81.5%，92 例患者被随机分配到安慰剂组（n = 43）或沙利度胺组（n = 49）。在随访时间至少为 3 年的前提下，尽管沙利度胺组患者的中位生存时间与安慰剂组相比有所延长，但并无统计学差异（HR = 0.74；11.7 个月 vs 8.7 个月；P = 0.16）。一项探索性研究发现体力状况 PS（performance status）评分 1~2 分的患者接受沙利度胺治疗后可以获得生存期的显著延长（HR = 0.59；P = 0.02）和更缓慢的疾病进展（HR = 0.54；P = 0.02）。应用沙利度胺与神经毒性、便秘和需要输注红细胞的发生率提高有关，约有 1/3 的患者因为副作用停用了沙利度胺。不幸的是，这些试验结果是否能被推广到支持抗血管生成药物用于 SCLC 的治疗尚存在争议，一方面是由于纳入的研究对象较少，另一方面是由于沙利度胺除抗血管生成作用外尚存在调节免疫等其他作用机制。

几项Ⅱ期临床试验研究了抗 VEGFR 治疗用于初治的广泛期 SCLC。Horn 等近期发表了Ⅱ期临床试验 E3501 的最终结果，这项试验研究了贝伐珠单抗联合顺铂 + 依托泊苷一线治疗广泛期 SCLC 的有效性和安全性[124]。共有 63 例患者接受了贝伐珠单抗 + 顺铂 + 依托泊苷治疗，并以贝伐珠单抗单药作为后续治疗直到死亡或疾病进展。6 个月 PFS 率为 30.2%，中位 PFS 为 4.7 个月，OS 为 10.9 个月，反应率为 63.5%。试验组的治疗方案在毒性方面耐受良好，比单纯化疗组仅增加了轻微的副作用。生物标志物分析显示较高的 VCAM 基线水平预示显著升高的进展或死亡风险，但是并未发现治疗、生物标志物及结局三者之间的其他关系。

一项多中心Ⅱ期临床试验研究了贝伐珠单抗联合伊立替康 + 卡铂一线治疗体力状况 ECOG 评分 0~1 分的广泛期 SCLC，并在既定化疗计划完成后在疾病无进展的前提下给予贝伐珠单抗维持治疗[125]。共纳入 51 例患者，据报道 ORR 为 84%，包括 1 例完全缓解和 42 例部分缓解。中位 TTP 和 OS 分别为 9.13 个月和 12.1 个月。最常见的严重副作用为粒细胞减少、血小板减少、胃肠道反应和乏力（20%），并未出现明显出血事件。近期发表的一项类似的Ⅱ期试验 CALGB30306 报道了 72 例广泛期 SCLC 初治患者应用顺铂 + 伊立替康联合贝伐珠单抗的有效性[126]，结果显示中位 PFS 和 OS 均有延长，分别为 7.0 个月和 11.6 个月，ORR 为 75%。然而，研究的主要终点即 1 年生存率为 50%~65% 并未达到。3 例患者在治疗期间因肺炎、卒中和心力衰竭死亡。在调整了年龄和 PS 评分的影响之后，研究者发现高血压与生存改善相关（$P = 0.04$），较低的基线 VEGF 水平预示着更差的 PFS（$P = 0.03$）。

鉴于抗 VEGF 治疗在"单臂研究"中具有前景的表现，以安慰剂为对照的双盲随机 Ⅱ 期试验 SALUTE 纳入了 52 例广泛期 SCLC 患者，研究贝伐珠单抗对比安慰剂联合顺铂或卡铂+依托泊苷一线化疗 4 个周期序贯单药贝伐珠单抗或安慰剂治疗直至病情进展或毒性不能耐受的有效性及安全性[127]。贝伐珠单抗组中位 PFS 高于安慰剂组（5.5 个月 vs 4.4 个月），但 OS 并无显著差异（贝伐珠单抗组和安慰剂组分别为 9.4 个月和 10.9 个月）。ORR 分别为 58% 和 48%，中位反应持续时间分别为 4.7 个月和 3.2 个月。贝伐珠单抗治疗组出现 3 级或以上不良反应的频率更高，然而并未出现新的或意料之外的安全信号。Hellenic 肿瘤研究协作组在一项 Ⅱ 期临床试验中评估了紫杉醇联合贝伐珠单抗治疗复发的化疗耐药的 SCLC[128]。试验共纳入了 30 例一线化疗完成后 3 个月内复发的 PS 评分 0～2 分的 SCLC 患者。整体 ORR 为 20%，疾病控制率（DCR）为 36.7%，中位 PFS 和 OS 分别为 2.7 个月和 6.3 个月。3、4 级及以上的毒性仅限于粒细胞减少、腹泻和乏力，另包括 1 例非致死性肺栓塞。Hoosier 肿瘤协作组的 LUN06-113 研究是一项正在进行中的随机、双盲 Ⅱ 期临床试验，目的是观察顺铂+依托泊苷联合或不联合凡德他尼用于初治的广泛期 SCLC，目前正在招募患者，初始结果尚未报道（NCT00613626）。韩国国家癌症中心目前与 Bayer 公司合作进行了一项随机 Ⅱ 期临床试验，目的是评估索拉非尼作为维持治疗用于接受铂类为基础的诱导化疗并获得 CR 或 PR 的广泛期 SCLC 患者能否延长 PFS 和 OS（NCT01159327）。

也有一些临床试验正在研究将抗血管生成药物纳入局限期 SCLC 治疗计划的获益情况。首个研究纳入了 60 例局限期 SCLC 患者，评估了放化疗后（4 个周期的伊立替康+卡铂联合同步放疗）获得病情缓解或稳定的患者接受贝伐珠单抗单药维持治疗（10mg/kg，每 2 周给药 1 次，共 10 次）的效果[129]。完全缓解及部分缓解率分别为 27% 和 53%；中位随访时间为 24 个月的前提下未能达到中位 PFS，中位 OS 为 17.5 个月；1 年和 2 年生存率分别为 70% 和 29%。在一项 Ⅱ 期临床试验中，局限期 SCLC 患者接受了 4 个周期贝伐珠单抗+伊立替康联合卡铂方案化疗同步放疗[70]。4 个周期全身治疗后病情稳定或缓解的患者接受了单药贝伐珠单抗作为维持治疗直到疾病进展或持续了 6 个月。这项试验的中位随访时间为 14 个月，然而，由于安全性方面的问题，该试验于 2007 年 3 月被提前终止，其主要终点 PFS 并未达到。8 例患者因为试验提前终止未完成放化疗而未能参与疗效评估；21 例患者按计划完成了全部诱导治疗，8 例患者完成了 25 次贝伐珠单抗维持治疗。ORR 为 88%，4 例患者达到完全缓解（CR），11 例患者达到部分缓解（PR），1 例患者评效为疾病稳定（SD）。总生存因试验终止未能被评估。3～4 级不良反应包括腹泻（21%）、食管炎（14%）、乏力（17%）、疼痛（14%）、中性粒细胞减少（18%）、白细胞减少（10%）和血小板减少（28%），1 例患者死于治疗相关的肠穿孔。

对抗血管生成治疗起效的生物标记物

受治疗调节的生物标记物的发现将极大地有利于抗血管生成治疗的临床应用。事实上，活性生物标记有利于决定抗肿瘤的合适剂量[130]、选择哪些患者能从某个特定药物中获益从而避免其他患者承担毒性风险及监测治疗反应，也有利于我们深入了解血管生成抑制剂耐药的机制。因此，人们对识别能够预测治疗结局及有助于抗血管生成治疗个体化的生物标记物投入了大量的精力。迄今为止，已经有多个能够预测治疗结局的生物标志物被发现，但尚未发现可以作为可靠的常规预测工具用来识别哪些患者能够从血管生成抑制剂治疗中获益最多的标志物。

高血压

高血压是抗血管生成治疗最常见的 3 级或以上的不良反应[131-132]。贝伐珠单抗通过降低一氧化氮的合成导致高血压，这与血管系统中 VEGF 的有效阻断相关。Dahlberg 等近期报道了 Ⅲ 期临床试验 ECOG4599D 的亚组分析结果，发现 NSCLC 患者应用贝伐珠单抗后发生高血压（>150/

100mmHg或舒张压至少比基线水平高出20mmHg）与更好的临床结局呈正相关[133]。实际上，该研究观察到紫杉醇＋卡铂＋贝伐珠单抗治疗组（PCB组）的高血压患者与单纯化疗组（PC组）高血压患者相比，具有显著延长的OS（HR＝0.60；P＝0.001），校正后的PFS HR为0.54（P＜0.0001）。当把PCB组的非高血压患者与PC组的非高血压患者相比较时，发现OS HR为0.86（P＝0.05），PFS HR为0.72（P＜0.0001）。总之，这些数据表明，接受贝伐珠单抗联合标准化疗过程中出现高血压与更好的临床结局相关。6项关于阿西替尼的Ⅱ期临床试验共纳入了230例不同肿瘤类型的患者，其中包括30例NSCLC患者，最终数据分析显示了类似于ECOG4599的结果，即舒张压大于90mmHg可以作为潜在的预示更长OS的生物标记[134]。有必要开展一些前瞻性的研究，以验证高血压是否能够作为临床实践中预测治疗反应的可靠生物标记。

循环中的细胞因子

VEGF是研究最为广泛的预测性生物标记之一。循环中VEGF水平的升高及可溶性VEGFR2浓度的下降已经在评估VEGFR酪氨酸激酶抑制剂安全性和抗肿瘤活性的Ⅰ期和Ⅱ期研究中反复报道过，提示这些变化可能表示这类药物的一类特殊效应[135-137]。然而，只有部分研究发现这些变化和临床结局改善之间存在关联。最近，Ebos等发现，荷瘤小鼠和非荷瘤小鼠体内VEGF和VEGFR-2水平的变化可能代表了一种全身性的与肿瘤无关且为剂量依赖性的宿主来源应答的结果，并可能与舒尼替尼的最佳抗肿瘤剂量相关[135]。利用多路复用微球阵列技术及ELISA法，Hanrahan等进行了一项探索性的回顾性分析，旨在研究凡德他尼治疗NSCLC的3项Ⅱ期临床试验中基线循环VEGF水平与PFS间的相关性，发现较低的基线循环VEGF水平可能预示着接受凡德他尼治疗的晚期NSCLC患者与吉非替尼治疗组相比，或者凡德他尼＋多西他赛组与多西他赛单药治疗组相比有PFS优势。一项纳入了123例NSCLC患者的Ⅱ期临床试验按一线治疗方案不同将患者随机分成3组，分别为凡德他尼单药（V）、卡铂联合紫杉醇（CP）及三药联合治疗组（VCP），关于基线和治疗过程中细胞因子和血管生成因子（cytokine and angiogenic factors，CAFs）水平的分析显示，在治疗第43天时，仅在V组观察到了VEGF的上升和可溶性VEGFR2（sVEGFR2）的下降，而在该组患者中VEGF的上升与疾病进展风险增加有关[138]。在同一项研究中，较高的HGF基线水平与V组患者中较差的PFS显著相关，但在VCP组患者中未发现该关联[139]。这些发现与我们最近报道的一项临床前实验结果相一致，即在接受凡德他尼治疗直到进展的NSCLC异种移植物模型中，HGF/c-MET途径的表达上升与活化和治疗抵抗的发生相关。对接受帕唑帕尼治疗的早期NSCLC患者的血浆样本进行分析发现，治疗后血浆sVEGFR2和IL-4水平的变化与肿瘤缩小显著相关，基线HGF和IL-12水平与肿瘤对帕唑帕尼的治疗反应有关，暗示了CAF谱或许能够用于判断患者是否能从VEGFR-TKIs治疗中获益[137]。然而，也有人报道了关于将治疗前VEGF水平作为临床结局预测性生物标记的有效性的相反数据。例如，一项评估晚期NSCLC患者应用化疗联合贝伐珠单抗治疗的Ⅱ、Ⅲ期临床试验发现治疗前血浆中较高的循环VEGF水平尽管与ORR改善显著相关，但尚不能够作为生存（PFS和OS）的预测性标记物[141]。基于以上这些发现我们可以明白把循环VEGF作为预测NSCLC生存获益的生物标记尚需进一步的研究。

VEGF的单核苷酸多态性（SNPs）

探究VEGF的基因型及单核苷多态性（single nucleotide polymorphisms，SNPs）是目前一项新兴的研究领域。现已表明，SNPs可能会影响药物代谢和排泄的效率，通过基因表达的改变或转录后修饰影响治疗反应。携带变异的C等位基因的 $VEGF$ +405G＞C多态性与早期NSCLC的生存改善有显著相关[142]。纳入了133例晚期NSCLC患者的ECOG4599试验显示VEGFA-634GG、ICAM1 469T/C及IL-8 -251T/A的SNP特征是OS和PFS的最佳预测因子[143]，提示了血管生成通路上涉及的分子遗传学变异与临床结局之间存在重要的相关性。E2501是一项已停止的随机Ⅱ期临床试验[144]，对索拉非尼对比安慰剂治疗二线化疗失败的转移性NSCLC进行了研究，该试验的一项相关研究对 SNP 作为索拉非尼的生物标记进行了评估。来自 88 份血浆样本的 DNA 分析显示 VEGFA - 1498CC 和 VEGFA - 634CC 基因型与改善的 PFS 相关[145]。

其他生物标记物

研究者发现较高的微血管密度（microvascular density，MVD）能够反映供应肿瘤的血管数量和 NSCLC 患者较差的生存、肿瘤进展和转移之间存在显著相关性[146]。鉴于这一相关性，人们假设 MVD 与抗血管生成治疗的反应和获益间存在关联。然而，尽管在临床前模型中证实了 MVD 预测治疗反应的标志物作用，但这一点却未在临床试验阶段得以验证[147]。

循环内皮细胞（circulating endothelial cells，CECs）来自血管壁并表达成熟内皮细胞的表型。大量的证据表明 CECs 在肿瘤患者中是增多的[148]。抗血管生成治疗可以诱导内皮细胞脱离肿瘤血管系统，这会导致那些对治疗有反应的患者血流中的 CECs 增加[149-150]。这些发现使 CECs 作为一种可以预测肿瘤血管生成抑制剂治疗反应的新的生物标志物得以识别[151]，也就是说，具有高水平的 CECs 的患者可能对该治疗有反应。一些评估抗肿瘤血管生成治疗的临床试验测量了 CEC 水平，发现治疗过程中该水平的下降与 PFS 改善之间呈正相关[152]。另外，较高的基线 CECs 水平与较高的治疗反应率相关，然而，在疾病出现进展时可以检测到 CEC 水平的显著升高[153]。总而言之，这些数据提示，尽管人们正在努力寻找能够预测更好的临床结局和抗血管治疗耐药的生物标志物，但迄今为止，尚未出现一种标记物已经被批准进入临床作为常规应用。

肿瘤对抗血管生成治疗的耐药

尽管抗血管生成药物临床应用的最初结果较好，但是无论是临床治疗反应的强度还是生存获益均远低于临床前实验的预期。事实上，并非所有肿瘤都能对该治疗有反应，而那些最初有反应的肿瘤最终也会出现复发和进展。在本小节，我们将回顾目前已知的使肿瘤开始对抗抗 VEGF 治疗的细胞学和分子学机制。

近期的临床前研究提出了肿瘤避开 VEGFR 信号途径阻滞的一种可能方式，即通过开发血管生成的替代信号途径。事实上，进一步的研究发现，在临床前癌症模型中，尽管抗 VEGFR 治疗最初阻断了新生血管生成和肿瘤生长，血管生成和肿瘤进展最终还是通过癌细胞合成 FGF 家族相关分子的增加得以恢复[154]。一些常见的癌细胞遗传学改变也被证实能够允许肿瘤生长减少对血管生成的依赖。$p53$ 抑癌基因失活的癌细胞能够更好地耐受低氧环境[155]，$p53$ 缺失型肿瘤对抗血管生成治疗明显不敏感[156]。也有证据表明一些癌细胞为了应对抗血管生成治疗可以改变它们的生长方式。在恶性黑色素瘤脑转移的实验模型中，恶性黑色素瘤细胞在接受抗 VEGF 治疗的同时通过"拉拢"原有的脑血管而继续生长[157]。

大量的证据提示，除了癌细胞本身，存在于肿瘤微环境中的间充质细胞在介导肿瘤对抗血管生成治疗的抵抗中也扮演着重要的角色。在一些肿瘤实验模型中，VEGF/R 抑制剂耐药有赖于肿瘤募集 CD11b$^+$ Gr-1$^+$ 粒细胞的能力[158]。CD11b$^+$ Gr-1$^+$ 髓细胞由数个细胞亚群组成，包括中性粒细胞、巨噬细胞及树突状细胞，定位至恶性肿瘤并对癌细胞产生的细胞因子做出应答（例如粒细胞-巨噬细胞集落刺激因子）。CD11b$^+$ Gr-1$^+$ 细胞是促血管生成蛋白的重要来源，也能产生数种免疫抑制分子[159]，这两点均能支持肿瘤进展。另有研究提示肿瘤相关成纤维细胞在介导肿瘤对抗 VEGF 药物耐药的过程中也起到了一定作用。在小鼠淋巴瘤模型中用抗体中和 VEGF 导致了来自肿瘤相关成纤维细胞的血小板源性生长因子（platelet-derived growth factor，PDGF-C）的上调，这足以维持血管生成并保证肿瘤发展[160]。

癌细胞和间充质细胞在抗血管生成治疗耐药中的相对贡献在不同癌症亚型中有一定差异[161-162]。我们的团队近期报道了在人类 NSCLC 的小鼠模型中发现的一种以前未知的一系列间充质适应，包括间充质 EGFR 和 FGFR 家族成员的上调，以及 EGFR 驱动的周细胞募集和促进 VEGF 抑制耐药的血管重塑。此外，我们的研究结果还表明，VEGFR 和 EGFR 双途径靶向治疗可以显著延长患者的生存期，推迟耐药的发生，这一点与研究晚期 NSCLC 治疗策略的临床试验的发现部分一致[19,163]。

总 结

尽管在近几十年中人们在抗血管生成治疗领域开展了广泛的研究并将其上升为一种抗肿瘤治疗策略，但时至今日，只有贝伐珠单抗被批准与标准含铂两联方案联合用于晚期或转移性 NSCLC 的临床治疗。这一成功使抗血管生成药物种类迅速增多，包括单克隆抗体、受体酪氨酸激酶抑制剂和 VDAs，目前正处于临床前和临床开发的不同阶段。抗血管生成治疗在早期 NSCLC 中的应用尚无定论。目前人们正致力于更好地了解与 NSCLC 生长和增殖相关的分子异常以及这些异常对治疗的反应及临床结局的影响。这将指导人们进一步发现和验证用于识别肿瘤血管靶向治疗最佳获益人群的活性生物标记物。

贝伐珠单抗在 NSCLC 中增加的获益是有限的，并且所有患者均出现了耐药。因此，未来的研究也包括了进一步了解介导肺癌对这些药物固有性或获得性耐药产生的细胞学和分子学机制，以改善患者的临床结局。

（韩晓颖　叶　欣　译）

参考文献

[1] Folkman J. Role of angiogenesis in tumor growth and metastasis. Semin Oncol, 2002, 29: 15-18.

[2] Folkman J. What is the evidence that tumors are angiogenesis dependent? J Natl Cancer Inst, 1990, 82: 4-6.

[3] Weis SM, Cheresh DA. Tumor angiogenesis: molecular pathways and therapeutic targets. Nat Med, 2011, 17: 1359-1370.

[4] Carmeliet P, Jain RK. Molecular mechanisms and clinical applications of angiogenesis. Nature, 2011, 473: 298-307.

[5] Dvorak HF, Brown LF, Detmar M, et al. Vascular permeability factor/vascular endothelial growth factor, microvascular hyperpermeability, and angiogenesis. Am J Pathol, 1995, 146: 1029-1039.

[6] Jain RK. Vascular and interstitial barriers to delivery of therapeutic agents in tumors. Cancer Metastasis Rev, 1990, 9: 253-266.

[7] Xian X, Hakansson J, Stahlberg A, et al. Pericyteslimit tumor cell metastasis. J Clin Invest, 2006, 116: 642-651.

[8] Carmeliet P, Jain RK. Angiogenesis in cancer and other diseases. Nature, 2000, 407: 249-257.

[9] Harris AL. Hypoxia—a key regulatory factor in tumour growth. Nat Rev Cancer, 2002, 2: 38-47.

[10] Semenza GL. Regulation of mammalian O2 homeostasis by hypoxia-inducible factor 1. Annu Rev Cell Dev Biol, 1999, 15: 551-578.

[11] Zhong H, De Marzo AM, Laughner E, et al. Overexpression of hypoxiainducible factor 1alpha in common human cancers and their metastases. Cancer Res, 1999, 59: 5830-5835.

[12] Le QT, Chen E, Salim A, et al. An evaluation of tumor oxygenation and gene expression in patients with early stage non-small cell lung cancers. Clin Cancer Res, 2006, 12: 1507-1514.

[13] Song X, Liu X, Chi W, et al. Hypoxia-induced resistance to cisplatin and doxorubicin in non-small cell lung cancer is inhibited by silencing of HIF-1alpha gene. Cancer Chemother Pharmacol, 2006, 58: 776-784.

[14] Niklinska W, Burzykowski T, Chyczewski L, et al. Expression of vascular endothelial growth factor (VEGF) in non-small cell lung cancer (NSCLC): Association with p53 gene mutation and prognosis. Lung Cancer, 2001, 34 (Suppl 2): S59-64.

[15] Rak J, Mitsuhashi Y, Bayko L, et al. Mutant ras oncogenes upregulate VEGF/VPF expression: implications for induction and inhibition of tumor angiogenesis. Cancer Res, 1995, 55: 4575-4580.

[16] Ji H, Ramsey MR, Hayes DN, et al. LKB1 modulates lung cancer differentiation and metastasis. Nature, 2007, 448: 807-810.

[17] Gao Y, XiaoQ, Ma H, et al. LKB1 inhibits lung cancer progression through lysyl oxidase and extracellular matrix remodeling. Proceedings of the National Academy of Sciences of the United States of America, 2010, 107: 18892-18897.

[18] Marcus AI, Zhou W. LKB1 regulatedpathways in lung cancer invasion and metastasis. Journal of Thoracic Oncology, 2010, 5: 1883-1886.

[19] Cascone T, Herynk MH, Xu L, et al. Upregulated stromal EGFR and vascular remodeling in mouse xenograft models of angiogenesis inhibitor-resistant human lung ad-

enocarcinoma. J Clin Invest, 2011, 121: 1313-1328.
[20] Sica A, Allavena P, Mantovani A. Cancer related inflammation: the macrophage connection. Cancer Lett, 2008, 267: 204-215.
[21] Takanami I, Takeuchi K, Kodaira S. Tumorassociated macrophage infiltration in pulmonary adenocarcinoma: Association with angiogenesis and poor prognosis. Oncology, 1999, 57: 138-142.
[22] Eberhard A, Kahlert S, Goede V, et al. Heterogeneity of angiogenesis and blood vessel maturation in human tumors: Implications for antiangiogenic tumor therapies. Cancer Res, 2000, 60: 1388-1393.
[23] Pezzella F, Pastorino U, Tagliabue E, et al. Non-small-cell lung carcinoma tumor growth without morphological evidence of neo-angiogenesis. Am J Pathol, 1997, 151: 1417-1423.
[24] Ribatti D, Vacca A, Dammacco F. New non-angiogenesis dependent pathways for tumour growth. Eur J Cancer, 2003, 39: 1835-1841.
[25] Ferrara N. Vascular endothelial growth factor: basic science and clinical progress. Endocr Rev, 2004, 25: 581-611.
[26] Nilsson M, Heymach JV. Vascular endothelial growth factor (VEGF) pathway. J Thorac Oncol, 2006, 1: 768-770.
[27] Ferrara N, Davis-Smyth T. The biology of vascular endothelial growth factor. Endocr Rev, 1997, 18: 4-25.
[28] Hicklin DJ, Ellis LM. Role of the vascular endothelial growth factor pathway in tumor growth and angiogenesis. J Clin Oncol, 2005, 23: 1011-1027.
[29] He Y, Karpanen T, Alitalo K. Role of lymphangiogenic factors in tumor metastasis. Biochim Biophys Acta, 2004, 1654: 3-12.
[30] Fehrenbach H, Kasper M, Haase M, et al. Differential immunolocalization of VEGF in rat and human adult lung, and in experimental rat lung fibrosis: light, fluorescence, and electron microscopy. Anat Rec, 1999, 254: 61-73.
[31] Han H, Silverman JF, Santucci TS, et al. Vascular endothelial growth factor expression in stage I non-small cell lung cancer correlates with neoangiogenesis and a poor prognosis. Ann Surg Oncol, 2001, 8: 72-79.
[32] Stefanou D, Batistatou A, Arkoumani E, et al. Expression of vascular endothelial growth factor (VEGF) and association with microvessel density in small-cell and non-small-cell lung carcinomas. Histol Histopathol, 2004, 19: 37-42.
[33] Jubb AM, Cesario A, Ferguson M, et al. Vascular phenotypes in primary non-small cell lung carcinomas and matched brain metastases. Br J Cancer, 2011, 104: 1877-1881.
[34] Beenken A, Mohammadi M. The FGF family: Biology, pathophysiology and therapy. Nat Rev Drug Discov, 2009, 8: 235-253.
[35] Shing Y, Folkman J, Sullivan R, et al. Heparin affinity: purification of a tumor-derived capillary endothelial cell growth factor. Science, 1984, 223: 1296-1299.
[36] Eswarakumar VP, Lax I, Schlessinger J. Cellular signaling by fibroblast growth factor receptors. Cytokine Growth Factor Rev, 2005, 16: 139-149.
[37] Kandel J, Bossy-Wetzel E, Radvanyi F, et al. Neovascularization is associated with a switch to the export of bFGF in the multistep development of fibrosarcoma. Cell, 1991, 66: 1095-1104.
[38] Behrens C, Lin HY, Lee JJ, et al. Immunohistochemical expression of basic fibroblastgrowth factor and fibroblast growth factor receptors 1 and 2 in the pathogenesis of lung cancer. Clin Cancer Res, 2008, 14: 6014-6022.
[39] Weiss J, Sos ML, Seidel D, et al. Frequent and focal FGFR1 amplification associates with therapeutically tractable FGFR1 dependency in squamous cell lung cancer. Sci Transl Med, 2010, 2: 62ra93.
[40] Nguyen M, Watanabe H, Budson AE, et al. Elevated levels of an angiogenic peptide, basic fibroblast growth factor, in the urine of patients with a wide spectrum of cancers. J Natl Cancer Inst, 1994, 86: 356-361.
[41] Brattstrom D, Bergqvist M, Hesselius P, et al. Elevated preoperative serum levels of angiogenic cytokines correlate to larger primary tumours and poorer survival in non-small cell lung cancer patients. Lung Cancer, 2002, 37: 57-63.
[42] Rades D, Setter C, Dahl O, et al. Fibroblast growth factor 2—a predictor of outcome for patients irradiated for stage Ⅱ-Ⅲ non-small-cell lung cancer. Int J Radiat Oncol Biol Phys, 2012, 82: 442-447.
[43] Hynes NE, Lane HA. ERBB receptors and cancer: The complexity of targeted inhibitors. Nat Rev Cancer, 2005, 5: 341-354.
[44] Ciardiello F, Tortora G. EGFR antagonists in cancer treatment. New England Journal of Medicine, 2008, 358: 1160-1174.
[45] Herbst RS, Heymach JV, Lippman SM. Lung cancer. N

Engl J Med, 2008, 359: 1367 - 1380.

[46] Amin DN, Hida K, Bielenberg DR, et al. Tumor endothelial cells express epidermal growth factor receptor (EGFR) but not ErbB3 and are responsive to EGF and to EGFR kinase inhibitors. Cancer Res, 2006, 66: 2173 - 2180.

[47] Wu W, Onn A, Isobe T, et al. Targeted therapy of orthotopic human lung cancer by combined vascular endothelial growth factor and epidermal growth factor receptor signaling blockade. Mol Cancer Ther, 2007, 6: 471 - 483.

[48] Lindahl P, Johansson BR, Leveen P, et al. Pericyte loss and microaneurysm formation in PDGF-B-deficient mice. Science, 1997, 277: 242 - 245.

[49] Cao Y, Cao R, Hedlund EM. Regulation of tumor angiogenesis and metastasis by FGF and PDGF signaling pathways. J Mol Med (Berl), 2008, 86: 785 - 789.

[50] Pietras K, Sjoblom T, Rubin K, et al. PDGF receptors as cancer drug targets. Cancer Cell, 2003, 3: 439 - 443.

[51] Hermanson M, Funa K, Hartman M, et al. Platelet-derived growth factor and its receptors in human glioma tissue: expression of messenger RNA and protein suggests the presence of autocrine and paracrine loops. Cancer Res, 1992, 52: 3213 - 3219.

[52] Nister M, Libermann TA, Betsholtz C, et al. Expression of messenger RNAs for platelet-derived growth factor and transforming growth factor-alpha and their receptors in human malignant glioma cell lines. Cancer Res, 1988, 48: 3910 - 3918.

[53] Oikawa T, Onozawa C, Sakaguchi M, et al. Three isoforms of plateletderived growth factors all have the capability to induce angiogenesis in vivo. Biol Pharm Bull, 1994, 17: 1686 - 1688.

[54] Risau W, Drexler H, Mironov V, et al. Platelet-derived growth factor is angiogenic in vivo. Growth Factors, 1992, 7: 261 - 266.

[55] Hellstrom M, Kalen M, Lindahl P, et al. Role of PDGF-B and PDGFR-beta in recruitment of vascular smooth muscle cells and pericytes during embryonic blood vessel formation in the mouse. Development, 1999, 126: 3047 - 3055.

[56] Hellberg C, Ostman A, Heldin CH. PDGF and vessel maturation. Recent Results Cancer Res, 2010, 180: 103 - 114.

[57] Gaengel K, Genove G, Armulik A, et al. Endothelial-mural cell signaling in vascular development and angiogenesis. Arterioscler Thromb Vasc Biol, 2009, 29: 630 - 638.

[58] Guo P, Hu B, Gu W, et al. Platelet-derived growth factor-B enhances glioma angiogenesis by stimulating vascular endothelial growth factor expression in tumor endothelia and by promoting pericyte recruitment. Am J Pathol, 2003, 162: 1083 - 1093.

[59] Uehara H, Kim SJ, Karashima T, et al. Effects of blocking platelet-derived growth factor-receptor signaling in a mouse model of experimental prostate cancer bone metastases. J Natl Cancer Inst, 2003, 95: 458 - 470.

[60] Bergers G, Song S, Meyer-Morse N, et al. Benefits of targeting both pericytes and endothelial cells in the tumor vasculature with kinase inhibitors. J Clin Invest, 2003, 111: 1287 - 1295.

[61] Bergers G, Hanahan D. Modes of resistance to anti-angiogenic therapy. Nat Rev Cancer, 2008, 8: 592 - 603.

[62] Kerbel RS. Inhibition of tumor angiogenesis as a strategy to circumvent acquired resistance to anticancer therapeutic agents. Bioessays, 1991, 13: 31 - 36.

[63] Jain RK. Molecular regulation of vessel maturation. Nat Med, 2003, 9: 685 - 693.

[64] Jain RK, Duda DG, Clark JW, et al. Lessons from phase Ⅲ clinical trials on anti-VEGF therapy for cancer. Nat Clin Pract Oncol, 2006, 3: 24 - 40.

[65] Ferrara N, Hillan KJ, Gerber HP, et al. Discovery and development of bevacizumab, an anti-VEGF antibody for treating cancer. Nat Rev Drug Discov, 2004, 3: 391 - 400.

[66] Hurwitz H, Fehrenbacher L, Novotny W, et al. Bevacizumab plus irinotecan, fluorouracil, and leucovorin for metastatic colorectal cancer. N Engl J Med, 2004, 350: 2335 - 2342.

[67] Sandler A, Gray R, Perry MC, et al. Paclitaxel-carboplatin alone or with bevacizumab for non-small-cell lung cancer. N Engl J Med, 2006, 355: 2542 - 250.

[68] Johnson DH, Fehrenbacher L, Novotny WF, et al. Randomized phase Ⅱ trial comparing bevacizumab plus carboplatin and paclitaxel with carboplatin and paclitaxel alone in previously untreated locally advanced or metastatic non-small-cell lung cancer. J Clin Oncol, 2004, 22: 2184 - 2191.

[69] Reck M, von Pawel J, Zatloukal P, et al. Phase Ⅲ trial of cisplatin plus gemcitabine with either placebo or bevacizumab as first-line therapy for nonsquamous non-small-cell lung cancer: AVAil. Journal of Clinical Oncology,

[70] Spigel DR, Hainsworth JD, Yardley DA, et al. Tracheo-esophageal fistula formation in patients with lung cancer treated with chemoradiation and bevacizumab. Journal of Clinical Oncology, 2010, 28: 43-48.

[71] Kamba T, McDonald DM. Mechanisms of adverse effects of anti-VEGF therapy for cancer. British Journal of Cancer, 2007, 96: 1788-1795.

[72] Sandler A, Herbst R. Combining targeted agents: Blocking the epidermal growth factor and vascular endothelial growth factor pathways. Clinical Cancer Research, 2006, 12: 4421s-4425s.

[73] Gandara D, Kim ES, Herbst RS, et al. S0536: Carboplatin, paclitaxel, cetuximab and bevacizumab followed by cetuximab and bevacizumab maintenance in advanced NSCLC: A SWOG phase II study. J Clin Oncol, 2009, 27: 15s (suppl; abstr 8015).

[74] Herbst RS, Johnson DH, Mininberg E, et al. Phase I/II trial evaluating the anti-vascular endothelial growth factor monoclonal antibody bevacizumab in combination with the HER-1/epidermal growth factor receptor tyrosine kinase inhibitor erlotinib for patients with recurrent non-small-cell lung cancer. J Clin Oncol, 2005, 23 (11): 2544-2555.

[75] Herbst RS, O'Neill VJ, Fehrenbacher L, et al. Phase II study of efficacy and safety of bevacizumab in combination with chemotherapy or erlotinib compared with chemotherapy alone for treatment of recurrent or refractory non small-cell lung cancer. J Clin Oncol, 2007, 25: 4743-4750.

[76] Herbst RS, Ansari R, Bustin F, et al. Efficacy of bevacizumab plus erlotinib versus erlotinib alone in advanced non-small-cell lung cancer after failure of standard first-line chemotherapy (BeTa): A doubleblind, placebo-controlled, phase 3 trial. Lancet, 2011, 377: 1846-1854.

[77] Miller VA, O'Connor P, Soh C, et al. A randomized, double-blind, placebo-controlled, phase IIIb trial (ATLAS) comparing bevacizumab (B) therapy with or without erlotinib (E) after completion of chemotherapy with B for first-line treatment of locally advanced, recurrent, or metastatic non-small cell lung cancer (NSCLC). ASCO Annual Meeting Proceedings. J Clin Oncol, 2009, 27: abstr LBA8002..

[78] Christensen JG. A preclinical review of sunitinib, a multitargeted receptor tyrosine kinase inhibitor with anti-angiogenic and antitumour activities. Annals of Oncology, 2007, 18 (Suppl 10): x3-10.

[79] Wang D, Jiang Z, Zhang L. Concurrent and sequential administration of sunitinib malate and docetaxel in human non-small cell lung cancer cells and xenografts. Medical Oncology, 2012, 29: 600-606.

[80] Christensen J, Hall C, Hollister B. Antitumor efficacy of sunitinib malate in concurrent and sequential combinations with standard chemotherapeutic agents in non-small cell lung cancer (NSCLC) nonclinical models//99th Annual Meeting of the American Association for Cancer Research. San Diego, California, 2008.

[81] Socinski MA, Novello S, Brahmer JR, et al. Multicenter, phase II trial of sunitinib in previously treated, advanced non-small-cell lung cancer. J Clin Oncol, 2008, 26: 650-656.

[82] Reck M, Frickhofen N, Cedres S, et al. Sunitinib in combination with gemcitabine plus cisplatin for advanced non-small cell lung cancer: a phase I dose-escalation study. Lung Cancer, 2010, 70: 180-187.

[83] Scagliotti GV, Krzakowski M, Szczesna A, et al. Sunitinib plus erlotinib versus placebo plus erlotinib in patients with previously treated advanced non-small-cell lung cancer: a phase III trial. Journal of Clinical Oncology, 2012, 30: 2070-2078.

[84] Escudier B, Eisen T, Stadler WM, et al. Sorafenib in advanced clear-cell renal-cell carcinoma. N Engl J Med, 2007, 356: 125-134.

[85] Morgillo F, Martinelli E, Troiani T, et al. Antitumor activity of sorafenib in human cancer cell lines with acquired resistance to EGFR and VEGFR tyrosine kinase inhibitors. PloS One, 2011, 6: e28841.

[86] Martinelli E, Troiani T, Morgillo F, et al. Synergistic antitumor activity of sorafenib in combination with epidermal growth factor receptor inhibitors in colorectal and lung cancer cells. Clinical Cancer Research, 2010, 16: 4990-5001.

[87] Carter CA, Chen C, Brink C, et al. Sorafenib is efficacious and tolerated in combination with cytotoxic or cytostatic agents in preclinical models of human non-small cell lung carcinoma. Cancer Chemotherapy and Pharmacology, 2007, 59: 183-195.

[88] Schiller J, Lee J, Hanna N, et al. A randomized discontinuation phase II study of sorafenib versus placebo in patients with nonsmall cell lung cancer who have failed at least two prior chemotherapy regimens: E2501. J Clin Oncol, 2008, 26: abstr 8014.

[89] Blumenschein GR, Jr, Gatzemeier U, et al. Phase Ⅱ, multicenter, uncontrolled trial of single-agent sorafenib in patients with relapsed or refractory, advanced non-small-cell lung cancer. J Clin Oncol, 2009, 27: 4274-4280.

[90] Kim E, Herbst R, Wistuba I, et al. The BATTLE trial (Biomarker-integrated Approaches of Targeted Therapy for Lung Cancer Elimination): Personalizing therapy for lung cancer. Cancer Discovery, 2011, 1: 43-51.

[91] Molina J, Dy G, Foster N, et al. A randomized phase Ⅱ study of pemetrexed (PEM) with or without sorafenib (S) as second-line therapy in advanced non-small cell lung cancer (NSCLC) of nonsquamous histology: NCCTG N0626 study. J Clin Oncol, 2011, 29 (suppl): abstr 7513.

[92] Spigel DR, Burris HA, 3rd, et al. Randomized, double-blind, placebo-controlled, phase Ⅱ trial of sorafenib and erlotinib or erlotinib alone in previously treated advanced non-small-cell lung cancer. Journal of Clinical Oncology, 2011, 29: 2582-2589.

[93] Lind JS, Dingemans AM, Groen HJ, et al. A multicenter phase Ⅱ study of erlotinib and sorafenib in chemotherapy-naive patients with advanced non small cell lung cancer. Clinical Cancer Research, 2010, 16: 3078-3087.

[94] Gridelli C, Morgillo F, Favaretto A, et al. Sorafenib in combination with erlotinib or with gemcitabine in elderly patients with advanced non-small-cell lung cancer: a randomized phase Ⅱ study. Annals of Oncology, 2011, 22: 1528-1534.

[95] Scagliotti GV, Parikh P, von Pawel J, et al. Phase Ⅲ study comparing cisplatin plus gemcitabine with cisplatin plus pemetrexed in chemotherapy-naive patients with advanced-stage non-small-cell lung cancer. J Clin Oncol, 2008, 26: 3543-3551.

[96] Wells SA, Jr, Gosnell JE, et al. Vandetanib for the treatment of patients with locally advanced or metastatic hereditary medullary thyroid cancer. Journal of Clinical Oncology, 2010, 28: 767-772.

[97] Wedge SR, Ogilvie DJ, Dukes M, et al. ZD6474 inhibits vascular endothelial growth factor signaling, angiogenesis, and tumor growth following oral administration. Cancer Research, 2002, 62: 4645-4655.

[98] Heymach JV, Paz-Ares L, De Braud F, et al. Randomized phase Ⅱ study of vandetanib alone or with paclitaxel and carboplatin as first-line treatment for advanced non-small-cell lung cancer. J Clin Oncol, 2008, 26: 5407-5415.

[99] Heymach JV, Johnson BE, Prager D, et al. Randomized, placebo-controlled phase Ⅱ study of vandetanib plus docetaxel in previously treated non small-cell lung cancer. J Clin Oncol, 2007, 25: 4270-4277.

[100] Natale RB, Bodkin D, Govindan R, et al. Vandetanib versus gefitinib in patients with advanced non-small cell lung cancer: Results from a two-part, doubleblind, randomized phase Ⅱ Study. J Clin Oncol, 2009, 27: 2523-2529.

[101] de Boer RH, Arrieta O, Yang CH, et al. Vandetanib plus pemetrexed for the second-line treatment of advanced non-small cell lung cancer: A randomized, double-blind phase Ⅲ trial. Journal of Clinical Oncology, 2011, 29: 1067-1074.

[102] Herbst RS, Sun Y, Eberhardt WE, et al. Vandetanib plus docetaxel versus docetaxel as second-line treatment for patients with advanced non-small-cell lung cancer (ZODIAC): A double-blind, randomised, phase 3 trial. Lancet Oncol, 2010, 11: 619-626.

[103] Natale RB, Thongprasert S, Greco FA, et al. Phase Ⅲ trial of vandetanib compared with erlotinib in patients with previously treated advanced non-small-cell lung cancer. J Clin Oncol, 2011, 29: 1059-1066.

[104] Lee JS, Hirsh V, Park K, et al. Vandetanib versus placebo in patients with advanced non-small-cell lung cancer after prior therapy with an epidermal growth factor receptor tyrosine kinase inhibitor: a randomized, double-blind phase Ⅲ trial (ZEPHYR). Journal of Clinical Oncology, 2012, 30: 1114-1121.

[105] Wedge SR, Kendrew J, Hennequin LF, et al. AZD2171: A highly potent, orally bioavailable, vascular endothelial growth factor receptor-2 tyrosine kinase inhibitor for the treatment of cancer. Cancer Res, 2005, 65: 4389-4400.

[106] Laurie SA, Gauthier I, Arnold A, et al. Phase I and pharmacokinetic study of daily oral AZD2171, an inhibitor of vascular endothelial growth factor tyrosine kinases, in combination with carboplatin and paclitaxel in patients with advancednon-small-cell lung cancer: the National Cancer Institute of Canada clinical trials group. Journal of Clinical Oncology, 2008, 26: 1871-1878.

[107] Goss GD, Arnold A, Shepherd FA, et al. Randomized, double-blind trial of carboplatin and paclitaxel with either daily oral cediranib or placebo in advanced non-small-cell lung cancer: NCIC clinical trials group BR24 study. J Clin Oncol, 2010, 28: 49-55.

[108] Laurie S, Solomon B, SeymourL, et al. A randomized double-blind trial of carboplatin plus paclitaxel (CP) with daily oral cediranib (CED), an inhibitor of vascular endothelial growth factor receptors, or placebo (PLA) in patients (pts) with previously untreated advanced non-small cell lung cancer (NSCLC): NCIC Clinical Trials Group study BR29. ASCO Annual Meeting Proceedings. Journal of Clinical Oncology, 2012.

[109] Dy GK, Mandrekar SJ, Nelson GD, et al. A randomized phase II Study of gemcitabine and carboplatin with or without cediranib as first-line therapy in advanced non-small-cell lung cancer: North Central Cancer Treatment Group Study N0528. Journal of Thoracic Oncology, 2013, 8: 79-88.

[110] Kumar R, Knick VB, Rudolph SK, et al. Pharmacokinetic-pharmacodynamic correlation from mouse to human with pazopanib, a multikinase angiogenesis inhibitor with potent antitumor and antiangiogenic activity. Molecular Cancer Therapeutics, 2007, 6: 2012-2021.

[111] Altorki N, Lane ME, Bauer T, et al. Phase II proof-of-concept study of pazopanib monotherapy in treatment-naive patients with stage I/II resectable non-small-cell lung cancer. Journal of Clinical Oncology, 2010, 28: 3131-3137.

[112] Ellis PM, Al-Saleh K. Multitargeted antiangiogenic agents and NSCLC: Clinical update and future directions. Critical Reviews in Oncology/Hematology, 2012, 84: 47-58.

[113] Choueiri TK. Axitinib, a novel anti-angiogenic drug with promising activity in various solid tumors. Current Opinion in Investigational Drugs, 2008, 9: 658-671.

[114] Schiller JH, Larson T, Ou SH, et al. Efficacy and safety of axitinib in patients with advanced non-small-cell lung cancer: Results from a phase II study. Journal of Clinical Oncology, 2009, 27: 3836-3841.

[115] Polverino A, Coxon A, Starnes C, et al. AMG 706, an oral, multikinase inhibitor that selectively targets vascular endothelial growth factor, platelet-derived growth factor, and kit receptors, potently inhibits angiogenesis and induces regression in tumor xenografts. Cancer Research, 2006, 66: 8715-8721.

[116] Blumenschein GR, Jr, Reckamp K, et al. Phase 1b study of motesanib, an oral angiogenesis inhibitor, in combination with carboplatin/paclitaxel and/or panitumumab for the treatment of advanced non-small cell lung cancer. Clinical Cancer Research, 2010, 16: 279-290.

[117] Hilberg F, Roth GJ, Krssak M, et al. BIBF 1120: Triple angiokinase inhibitor with sustained receptor blockade and good antitumor efficacy. Cancer Research, 2008, 68: 4774-4782.

[118] Reck M, Kaiser R, Eschbach C, et al. A phase II double-blind study to investigate efficacy and safety of two doses of the triple angiokinase inhibitor BIBF 1120 in patients with relapsed advanced non-small-cell lung cancer. Annals of Oncology, 2011, 22: 1374-1381.

[119] Thorpe PE. Vascular targeting agents as cancer therapeutics. Clinical Cancer Research, 2004, 10: 415-427.

[120] McKeage MJ, Von Pawel J, Reck M, et al. Randomised phase II study of ASA404 combined with carboplatin and paclitaxel in previously untreated advanced non small cell lung cancer. British Journal of Cancer, 2008, 99: 2006-2012.

[121] Lara PN, Jr, Douillard JY, Nakagawa K, et al. Randomized phase III placebocontrolled trial of carboplatin and paclitaxel with or without the vascular disrupting agent vadimezan (ASA404) in advanced non-small-cell lung cancer. Journal of Clinical Oncology, 2011, 29: 2965-2971.

[122] Rudin CM, Mauer A, Smakal M, et al. Phase I/II study of pemetrexed with or without ABT-751 in advanced or metastatic non-small-cell lung cancer. Journal of Clinical Oncology, 2011, 29: 1075-1082.

[123] Pujol JL, Breton JL, Gervais R, et al. Phase III double-blind, placebo-controlled study of thalidomide in extensive disease small-cell lung cancer after response to chemotherapy: An intergroup study FNCLCC cleo04 IFCT 00-01. Journal of Clinical Oncology, 2007, 25: 3945-3951.

[124] Horn L, Dahlberg SE, Sandler AB, et al. Phase II study of cisplatin plus etoposide and bevacizumab for previously untreated, extensive-stage small-cell lung cancer: Eastern Cooperative Oncology Group Study E3501. Journal of Clinical Oncology, 2009, 27: 6006-6011.

[125] Spigel DR, Hainsworth JD, Simons L, et al. Irinotecan, carboplatin, and imatinib in untreated extensive-stage small-cell lung cancer: A phase II trial of the Minnie Pearl Cancer Research Network. J Thorac Oncol, 2007, 2: 854-861.

[126] Ready NE, Dudek AZ, Pang HH, et al. Cisplatin, iri-

notecan, and bevacizumab for untreated extensive-stage small-cell lung cancer: CALGB 30306, a phase II study. Journal of Clinical Oncology, 2011, 29: 4436-4441.

[127] Spigel DR, Townley PM, Waterhouse DM, et al. Randomized phase II study of bevacizumab in combination with chemotherapy in previously untreated extensive-stage small cell lung cancer: results from the SALUTE trial. Journal of Clinical Oncology, 2011, 29: 2215-2222.

[128] Mountzios G, Emmanouilidis C, Vardakis N, et al. Paclitaxel plus bevacizumab in patients with chemoresistant relapsed small cell lung cancer as salvage treatment: a phase II multicenter study of the Hellenic Oncology Research Group. Lung Cancer, 2012, 77: 146-150.

[129] Patton J, Spigel D, Greco F, et al. Irinotecan (I), carboplatin (C), and radiotherapy (RT) followed by maintenance bevacizumab (B) in the treatment (tx) of limitedstage small cell lung cancer (LS-SCLC): Update of a phase II trial of the Minnie Pearl Cancer Research Network. 2006 ASCO Annual Meeting Proceedings. J Clin Oncol, 2006, 24: 7085.

[130] Norden-Zfoni A, Desai J, Manola J, et al. Blood-based biomarkers of SU11248 activity and clinical outcome in patients with metastatic imatinib-resistant gastrointestinal stromal tumor. Clin Cancer Res, 2007, 13: 2643-2650.

[131] Launay-Vacher V, Deray G. Hypertension and proteinuria: a class-effect of antiangiogenic therapies. Anti-Cancer Drugs, 2009, 20: 81-82.

[132] Izzedine H, Ederhy S, Goldwasser F, et al. Management of hypertension in angiogenesis inhibitortreated patients. Annals of Oncology, 2009, 20: 807-815.

[133] Dahlberg SE, Sandler AB, Brahmer JR. Clinical course of advanced non-small-cell lung cancer patients experiencing hypertension during treatment with bevacizumab in combination with carboplatin and paclitaxel on ECOG 4599. Journal of Clinical Oncology, 2010, 28: 949-954.

[134] Rini BI, Schiller JH, Fruehauf JP, et al. Diastolic blood pressure as a biomarker of axitinib efficacy in solid tumors. Clinical Cancer Research, 2011, 17: 3841-3849.

[135] Ebos JM, Lee CR, Christensen JG, et al. Multiple circulating proangiogenic factors induced by sunitinib malate are tumor independent and correlate with antitumor efficacy. Proc Natl Acad Sci USA, 2007, 104: 17069-17074.

[136] Batchelor TT, Sorensen AG, di Tomaso E, et al. AZD2171, a pan-VEGF receptor tyrosine kinase inhibitor, normalizes tumor vasculature and alleviates edema in glioblastoma patients. Cancer Cell, 2007, 11: 83-95.

[137] Nikolinakos PG, Altorki N, Yankelevitz D, et al. Plasma cytokine and angiogenic factor profiling identifies markers associated with tumor shrinkage in early-stage non-small cell lung cancer patients treated with pazopanib. Cancer Res, 2010, 70: 2171-2179.

[138] Hanrahan EO, Lin HY, Kim ES, et al. Distinct patterns of cytokine and angiogenic factor modulation and markers of benefit for vandetanib and/or chemotherapy in patients with non-small-cell lung cancer. Journal of Clinical Oncology, 2010, 28: 193-201.

[139] Hanrahan E, Lin H, Du D, et al. Correlative analyses of plasma cytokine/angiogenic factor (C/AF) profile, gender and outcome in a randomized, three-arm, phase II trial of 1st-line vandetanib (VAN) and/or carboplatin plus paclitaxel (CP) for advanced non small cell lung cancer (NSCLC) 2007 ASCO Annual Meeting Proocedings. J Clin Oncol, 2007, 25: 7593.

[140] Cascone T, Herynk MH, Xu L, et al. Increased HGF is associated with resistance to VEGFR tyrosine kinase inhibitors (TKIs) in nonsmall cell lung cancer (NSCLC). AACR Annual Meeting#376, 2010.

[141] Dowlati A, Gray R, Sandler AB, et al. Cell adhesion molecules, vascular endothelial growth factor, and basic fibroblast growth factor in patients with non-small cell lung cancer treated with chemotherapy with or without bevacizumab—an Eastern Cooperative Oncology Group Study. Clin Cancer Res, 2008, 14: 1407-1412.

[142] Heist RS, Zhai R, Liu G, et al. VEGF polymorphisms and survival in early stage non-small-cell lung cancer. Journal of Clinical Oncology, 2008, 26: 856-862.

[143] Zhang W, Dahlberg S, Yang D, et al. Genetic variants in angiogenesis pathway associated with clinical outcome in NSCLC patients (pts) treated with bevacizumab in combination with carboplatin and paclitaxel: Subset pharmacogenetic analysis of ECOG 4599. J Clin Oncol, 2009, 27: abstr 8032.

[144] Wakelee HA, Lee JW, Hanna NH, et al. A double-blind randomized discontinuation phase-II study of sorafenib (BAY 43-9006) in previously treated non-small-cell lung cancer patients: Eastern cooperative on-

cology group study E2501. Journal of Thoracic Oncology, 2012, 7: 1574-1582.

[145] Zhang W, Lee J, Schiller J, et al. Use of germline polymorphisms in VEGF to predict tumor response and progression-free survival in non-small cell lung cancer (NSCLC) patients treated with sorafenib: subset pharmacogenetic analysis of Eastern Cooperative Oncology Group (ECOG) trial E2501// ProcAmSoc Clin Oncol, 2010, 28 (suppl): abstr7607.

[146] Trivella M, Pezzella F, Pastorino U, et al. Microvessel density as a prognostic factor in non-small-cell lung carcinoma: a meta-analysis of individual patient data. Lancet Oncol, 2007, 8: 488-499.

[147] Sessa C, Guibal A, Del Conte G, et al. Biomarkers of angiogenesis for the development of antiangiogenic therapies in oncology: tools or decorations? Nat Clin Pract Oncol, 2008, 5: 378-391.

[148] Mancuso P, Burlini A, Pruneri G, et al. Resting and activated endothelial cells are increased in the peripheral blood of cancer patients. Blood, 2001, 97: 3658-3661.

[149] Goon PK, Lip GY, Stonelake PS, et al. Circulating endothelial cells and circulating progenitor cells in breast cancer: relationship to endothelial damage/dysfunction/apoptosis, clinicopathologic factors, and the Nottingham Prognostic Index. Neoplasia, 2009, 11: 771-779.

[150] Bertolini F, Shaked Y, MancusoP, et al. The multifaceted circulating endothelial cell in cancer: towards marker and target identification. Nat Rev Cancer, 2006, 6: 835-845.

[151] Mancuso P, Calleri A, Cassi C, et al. Circulating endothelial cells as a novel marker of angiogenesis. Adv Exp Med Biol, 2003, 522: 83-97.

[152] Ronzoni M, Manzoni M, Mariucci S, et al. Circulating endothelial cells and endothelial progenitors as predictive markers of clinical response to bevacizumab-based first-line treatment in advanced colorectal cancer patients. Annals of Oncology, 2010, 21: 2382-2389.

[153] Dellapasqua S, Bertolini F, Bagnardi V, et al. Metronomic cyclophosphamide and capecitabine combined with bevacizumab in advanced breast cancer. Journal of Clinical Oncology, 2008, 26: 4899-4905.

[154] Casanovas O, Hicklin DJ, Bergers G, et al. Drug resistance by evasion of antiangiogenic targeting of VEGF signaling in late-stage pancreatic islet tumors. Cancer Cell, 2005, 8: 299-309.

[155] Graeber TG, Osmanian C, Jacks T, et al. Hypoxiamediated selection of cells with diminished apoptotic potential in solid tumours. Nature, 1996, 379: 88-91.

[156] Yu JL, Rak JW, Coomber BL, et al. Effect of p53 status on tumor response to antiangiogenic therapy. Science, 2002, 295: 1526-1528.

[157] Leenders WP, Kusters B, Verrijp K, et al. Antiangiogenic therapy of cerebral melanoma metastases results in sustained tumor progression via vessel cooption. Clin Cancer Res, 2004, 10: 6222-6230.

[158] Shojaei F, Wu X, Malik AK, et al. Tumor refractoriness to anti-VEGF treatment is mediated by CD11b + Gr1 + myeloid cells. Nat Biotechnol, 2007, 25: 911-920.

[159] Ferrara N. Role of myeloid cells in vascular endothelial growth factor-independent tumor angiogenesis. Curr Opin Hematol, 2010, 17: 219-224.

[160] Crawford Y, Kasman I, Yu L, et al. PDGF-C mediates the angiogenic and tumorigenic properties of fibroblasts associated with tumors refractory to anti-VEGF treatment. Cancer Cell, 2009, 15: 21-34.

[161] Ebos JM, Kerbel RS. Antiangiogenic therapy: impact on invasion, disease progression, and metastasis. Nat Rev Clin Oncol, 2011, 8: 210-221.

[162] Weis SM, Cheresh DA. Tumor angiogenesis: Molecular pathways and therapeutic targets. Nature Medicine, 2011, 17: 1359-1370.

[163] Casanovas O. The adaptive stroma joining the antiangiogenic resistance front. J Clin Invest, 2011, 121: 1244-1247.

第34章
转移性非小细胞肺癌的抗肿瘤血管生成药物

Millie Das[1,2], Heather Wakelee[2]
1. VA Palo Alto Heath Care System, Palo Alto, CA, USA
2. Division of Oncology, Stanford University/Stanford Cancer Institute, Stanford, CA, USA

引言

自从发现血管生成在肿瘤的生长和发展中起着至关重要的作用以来,开展抗血管生成药物治疗各种恶性肿瘤,包括非小细胞肺癌(NSCLC)引起了医学界很大的兴趣[1]。血管内皮生长因子(VEGF)是一种血管生成的关键介质,已成为一个重要的NSCLC治疗靶点。VEGF家族包含5种糖蛋白(VEGF-A、VEGF-B、VEGF-C、VEGF-D、胎盘生长因子),结合3种酪氨酸激酶受体:VEGF受体1(VEGFR-1)/fms样酪氨酸激酶I(flt1)、VEGFR-2/激酶插入域受体(kinase insert domain receptor,KDR)和VEGFR-3/flt4。配体受体结合激活下游信号传导,诱发内皮细胞增殖和迁移,以及增加现有的血管渗透性[2]。NSCLC抗血管生成药物研究包括针对VEGF单克隆抗体、VEGF受体酪氨酸激酶抑制剂(TKIs)以及不涉及抑制VEGF的血管破坏药物(vascular disrupting agents,VDAs),见表34.1。本章回顾了这些抗血管生成药物治疗NSCLC的数据。

表34.1 抗血管生成药物研究的特异性靶点

肿瘤细胞	VEGF配体	血管内皮细胞
TKIs	雷莫芦单抗	VDAs
贝伐珠单抗	可溶性血管内皮生长因子受体融合蛋白	TKIs

TKI:酪氨酸激酶抑制剂;VDA:血管破坏剂;VEGF:血管内皮生长因子

单克隆抗体VEGF/VEGFR

贝伐珠单抗

贝伐珠单抗是一种针对VEGF-A的人源化单克隆抗体,目前仍然是唯一已通过美国FDA认证的治疗NSCLC的抗血管生成药物。认证基于许多重要的研究结果。在最初的Ⅱ期临床研究中,99例患者被随机分配为3组:单纯化疗组(卡铂/紫杉醇)、化疗加贝伐珠单抗7.5mg/kg体重组和化疗加贝伐珠单抗15mg/kg体重组。接受贝伐珠单抗联合化疗组的患者在完成化疗后允许继续贝伐珠单抗单药治疗达18个周期。重要的是,单纯化疗组患者进展后可转为接受贝伐珠单抗治疗。结果表明,高剂量贝伐珠单抗组和单独化疗组的客观缓解率(ORR为31.5% vs 18.8%)和无进展生存期(PFS为7.4个月 vs 4.2个月,$P=0.023$),前者优于后者,但两组的总生存期(overall survival,OS)无显著差异(17.7个月 vs 14.9个月,$P=0.63$)。此外,低剂量贝伐珠单抗较单独化疗似乎没有任何优势。OS没有受益的可能原因为相对较少的患者数量以及能转为贝伐珠单抗维持治疗的患者数量也较少。在这项研究中观察到9.0%的患者出现肺出血,其中4例为倾向于低剂量贝伐珠单抗治疗的鳞癌患者的主要死亡原因[3]。鉴于该试验观察到肺出血可能与鳞癌相关,后续的Ⅲ期临床试验排除了接受贝伐珠单抗治疗的鳞癌患者。基于令人鼓舞的Ⅱ期研究数据,许多不同的Ⅲ期研究已经开始评估一线应用贝伐珠单抗为基础的治疗方案(表34.2)。

东方肿瘤协作组（Eastern Cooperative Group，ECOG）4599 是具有里程碑意义的Ⅲ期临床研究，878 例复发或进展的 NSCLC 患者随机分组接受一线卡铂/紫杉醇方案化疗加或不加贝伐珠单抗 15mg/kg 体重的 3 周治疗方案，排除了合并或病理类型为鳞癌、有严重咯血史和发生脑转移的患者。与单纯接受化疗组相比，联合贝伐珠单抗组患者的 ORR（35% vs 15%，$P < 0.001$）及 PFS［6.2月 vs 4.5 个月；HR = 0.66；95% CI（0.57，0.77）；$P < 0.001$］均得到提高。而且，主要研究终点 OS 显著改善［12.3 个月 vs 10.3 个月；HR = 10.3；95% CI（0.67，0.92）；$P = 0.003$］。然而，贝伐珠单抗也与毒性增加有关，包括增加出血、粒细胞减少性发热及死亡（联合组 15 例，单纯化疗组为 2 例）的风险[4]。特别是那些年龄超过 70 岁接受贝伐珠单抗治疗的患者 3~5 级的毒性反应明显增加（87% vs 61%；$P < 0.001$），但 ORR 和 PFS 仍受益，主张该亚组患者应慎用贝伐珠单抗[5]。尽管存在这些限制，但 ECOG 4599 是第一个证明贝伐珠单抗在晚期 NSCLC 治疗中能使患者生存受益的抗血管生成药物，对贝伐珠单抗被批准应用于 NSCLC 的治疗起到了重要作用。

AVAiLⅢ期试验将 1 043 例复发或进展的 NSCLC 患者随机分为顺铂/吉西他滨加或不加贝伐珠单抗（7.5mg/kg 或 15mg/kg 体重）。3 种药物均为每 3 周的第 1 天给药，另外第 8 天给予吉西他滨。虽然相比仅接受化疗患者的主要研究终点 PFS（6.1 个月），低剂量贝伐珠单抗组的 PFS（6.7 个月；HR = 0.75；$P = 0.003$）及高剂量贝伐珠单抗组（6.5 个月；HR = 0.82；$P = 0.03$）均得到了明显改善；贝伐珠单抗组（低剂量：13.6 个月，HR = 13.6，$P = 0.420$；高剂量：13.4 个月，HR = 1.03，$P = 0.761$）和单纯化疗组（13.1 个月）的 OS 并没有显著延长[6-7]。大部分患者（61%~65%）继续接受其他后续治疗可以解释该试验 OS 为何并不受益[8]。重要的是，这项研究也表明，贝伐珠单抗可以安全地应用于服用足量抗凝药物的患者，因为 9% 的入组患者接受抗凝治疗与华法林或低分子量肝素后开始试验，没有患者出现肺出血。

为了进一步评估贝伐珠单抗治疗 NSCLC 的安全性和有效性，许多研究已经完成或正在进行。PASSPORT 研究显示，贝伐珠单抗可安全地应用于已治疗过的脑转移患者[9]。为了评价贝伐珠单抗联合多种不同化疗方案治疗的安全性进行了Ⅳ期临床试验（SAiL）。在这项研究中，患者接受含顺

表 34.2 NSCLC Ⅲ期研究中贝伐珠单抗为基础的一线治疗结果

试验	方案	PFS（月）	OS（月）
ECOG 4599[4]	卡铂/紫杉醇	4.5	10.3
	卡铂/紫杉醇/贝伐珠单抗	6.2	12.3
		HR = 0.66，$P < 0.001$	HR = 0.79，$P = 0.003$
AVAiL[6-7]	顺铂/吉西他滨	6.1	13.1
	顺铂/吉西他滨/贝伐珠单抗	6.5	13.4
		HR = 0.82，$P = 0.03$	HR = 1.03，$P = 0.761$
POINT-BREAK[12]	卡铂/紫杉醇/贝伐珠单抗→贝伐珠单抗维持	6.0	12.6
	卡铂/培美曲塞/贝伐珠单抗→培美曲塞/贝伐珠单抗维持	5.6	13.4
		HR = 0.83，$P = 0.012$	HR：1.00，$P = 0.949$
AVAPERL[13]	顺铂/培美曲塞/贝伐珠单抗→贝伐珠单抗维持	6.6	15.7
	顺铂/培美曲塞/贝伐珠单抗→贝伐珠单抗/培美曲塞维持	10.2	未达到
		HR = 0.50，$P < 0.001$	HR = 0.75，$P = 0.23$
ATLAS[14-15]	铂类为基础的化疗→贝伐珠单抗维持	3.7	14.4
	铂类为基础的化疗→贝伐珠单抗/厄罗替尼维持	4.8	13.3
		HR = 0.72，$P = 0.001\ 2$	HR = 0.92，$P = 0.56$

铂方案化疗联合贝伐珠单抗 OS（14.7个月），患者接受含卡铂方案化疗联合贝伐珠单抗的 OS 为 14.3 个月，不含铂类方案化疗联合贝伐珠单抗（OS 为 8.1 个月），单药化疗联合贝伐珠单抗（OS 为 9.4 个月）。1% 的患者出现≥3 级肺出血，3% 的患者出现 3~5 级出血（不包括肺出血）[10]。另一项研究发现，贝伐珠单抗联合其他常用的含铂类方案化疗也是有效的，包括卡铂/培美曲塞[11]。最近完成的 III 期 POINT-BREAK 试验比较了两组进展期非鳞癌 NSCLC 患者：卡铂/培美曲塞/贝伐珠单抗诱导治疗之后，培美曲塞/贝伐珠单抗维持（A 组）和卡铂/紫杉醇/贝伐珠单抗诱导治疗之后贝伐珠单抗维持（B 组）。结果表明，主要终点 OS 并没有显著差异（A 组 12.6 个月，B 组 13.4 个月；HR=1.00；P=0.949），次要终点（ORR：A 组 34.1%，B 组 33.0%）和疾病控制率（DCR：A 组 65.9%，B 组 69.8%）也没有显著差异[12]。AVAPERL 试验是另一项最近完成的研究，在患者完成了 4 个周期的顺铂/培美曲塞/贝伐珠单抗治疗后，比较贝伐珠单抗维持和贝伐珠单抗/培美曲塞维持治疗。接受贝伐珠单抗/培美曲塞维持治疗组的 PFS 显著优于单药贝伐珠单抗维持治疗组（10.2 个月 vs 6.6 个月；P<0.001），接下来 11 个月的随访显示贝伐珠单抗/培美曲塞组的 OS 无统计学差异（HR=0.75；P=0.23）[13]。ECOG 5508 试验正在研究贝伐珠单抗维持治疗晚期 NSCLC 患者的效果。患者接受 4 个周期的 E4599 方案治疗，那些病情稳定的患者随机进行单药贝伐珠单抗、培美曲塞（每 3 周 500mg/m²）或两药联合直到疾病进展或出现难以耐受的毒性。目前进行中的 III 期 ECOG 1505 研究正在评估贝伐珠单抗应用于早期治疗的地位，I~III 期已手术切除的 NSCLC 患者随机接受 4 个周期以铂类为基础的术后辅助化疗加或不加贝伐珠单抗，现在已经完成收益和暂时性安全分析，并未发现存在预料之外的毒性[14]。

已有热衷于贝伐珠单抗结合其他靶向治疗药物在维持治疗和二线治疗方面的研究，包括厄罗替尼，一种口服型表皮生长因子受体（EGFR）抑制剂。在 III 期 ATLAS 研究中，晚期 NSCLC 患者在完成 4 个周期的以铂类为基础的化疗后被随机分组接受贝伐珠单抗（15mg/kg 体重）+ 厄罗替尼（150mg/d）维持与贝伐珠单抗维持联合安慰剂治疗。尽管主要终点 PFS 贝伐珠单抗/厄罗替尼相比贝伐珠单抗维持/安慰剂有所改善（4.8 个月 vs 3.7 个月；HR=3.7；P=0.001 2）[15]，次要终点 OS 却并没有显著改善 [14.4 个月 vs 13.3 个月；95% CI（0.70，1.21）；P=0.56][16]。II 期二线试验随机将患者分为 3 组：厄罗替尼+贝伐珠单抗、化疗（多烯紫杉醇或培美曲塞）+贝伐珠单抗及单独化疗组。中位 PFS 在贝伐珠单抗联合化疗（4.8 个月）或联合厄罗替尼（4.4 个月）相较于单纯化疗（3 个月）是改善的[17]。III 期β试验将 636 例一线化疗后疾病进展的患者随机分组接受厄罗替尼加（或）不加贝伐珠单抗。尽管联合治疗组的 PFS 显著延长（3.4 个月 vs 1.7 个月；HR=0.62；P<0.62），主要终点 OS 在两组却无不同（9.3 个月 vs 9.2 个月；HR=0.97；P=0.75）[18]。最终，从贝伐珠单抗联合厄罗替尼治疗 III 期 NSCLC 的 I、II 期研究结果发现 45 例患者中有 29% 发生 3~4 级食管炎，包括食管气管瘘，但并没有显著改善有效性[19]。

雷莫芦单抗

雷莫芦单抗（IMC-1121B）是一种针对 VEGFR-2 的单克隆抗体，早期多种恶性肿瘤临床试验已研究过，包括 NSCLC。涉及晚期 NSCLC 患者应用雷莫芦单抗联合卡铂/紫杉醇作为一线治疗的试验评估发现 59% 的 OR 和 97% 的 DCR 与雷莫芦单抗相关[20]。这些令人振奋的结果催生了其他有关雷莫芦单抗在转移性 NSCLC 治疗中的研究，包括一个根据组织学随机分组的 II 期临床试验：非鳞癌组患者接受铂类/培美曲塞加（或）不加雷莫芦单抗×（4~6）周期，随后是两组均接受培美曲塞维持，鳞癌组接受铂类/吉西他滨加（或）不加雷莫芦单抗×（4~6）周期，随后是雷莫芦单抗组接受雷莫芦单抗维持治疗。非鳞癌组登记已完成，鳞癌组登记正在进行（临床试验，官方 ID：NCT 01160744）。RECEL III 期临床研究也正在进行中，将进展的转移性 NSCLC 患者在接受前期以铂为基础的治疗后随机分组，多西他赛加（或）不加雷莫芦单抗（临床试验，官方 ID：NCT 01168973）。

小分子酪氨酸激酶抑制剂

当前 NSCLC 的治疗进展中已有数种抗血管生成小分子酪氨酸激酶抑制剂（tyrosine kinase inhibitors，TKIs）。TKIs 的优势包括可同时抑制多个受体，从而提供单药活性的可能性；通常是口服制剂，患者使用更方便。尽管有这些优点，但当这些药物与化疗联合时，其多靶点激酶抑制作用和潜在的添加剂所致的毒性反应令人担忧。下面我们回顾包括将 VEGF 作为靶点的治疗 NSCLC 的选择性小分子 TKIs 药物（表 34.3）。

索拉非尼

索拉非尼是一种口服的针对 VEGFR-2 和 VEGFR-3、血小板源生长因子（platelet-derived growth factor receptor，PDGFR）β 受体、RAF 激酶、c-kit 受体、Ret 和 fms 样酪氨酸激酶受体 3（Flt3）的多种激酶抑制剂，基于 III 期临床研究显示其可延长 PFS[21-22]，被 FDA 批准用于治疗转移性肾细胞癌（renal cell carcinoma，RCC）和进展期肝细胞癌（hepatocellwlar carcinoma，HCC）。索拉非尼治疗 NSCLC 的评估是在 II 期 ECOG 2501 试验中进行的，342 例晚期 NSCLC 患者在前期至少行 2 种化疗方案失败后，口服 2 个周期索拉非尼 400mg，每天 2 次。2 个周期治疗后病情稳定的患者（$n=97$）被随机分配接受继续索拉非尼或安慰剂治疗。索拉非尼组与安慰剂组相比，PFS 延长（3.6 个月 vs 1.9 个月；$P=0.01$）[23]。另一项涉及 52 例患者的 II 期试验发现：复发或难治性晚期 NSCLC 患者行单药索拉非尼 400mg，每天 2 次不间断治疗，59% 的可评价患者达疾病稳定（stable disease，SD），PFS 为 5.5 个月。治疗相关毒性是可控的，且与之前的试验相似，其中 10% 的患者出现手足反应[24]。

有希望的 II 期临床试验结果引导两大 III 期试验对索拉非尼联合化疗的评估。III 期 ESCAPE 试验采取随机双盲、安慰剂对照方法将晚期 NSCLC 患者随机分为接受卡铂和紫杉醇一线治疗加或不加索拉非尼 2 组。一个临时分析显示鳞癌患者的毒性增加且主要研究终点 OS 可能无法达成，故研究早期即终止[25]。NEXUS III 期试验研究索拉非尼联合顺铂/吉西他滨，显示 PFS 受益而主要研究终点 OS 没有改善[26]。在 II 期研究设计中，索拉非尼联合厄洛替尼取得了令人鼓舞的结果，需要进一步评估[27-28]。最近，BATTLE 研究是第一次完成的前瞻性、基于生物标志物的自适应随机研究，根据从不同患者的生物标志物分析得到的结果将中、晚期 NSCLC 患者随机分为 4 组：厄洛替尼、凡德他尼、厄洛替尼联合蓓萨罗丁或索拉非尼组。自适应随机分组相较平均随机分组中，K-ras 突变者应用索拉非尼治疗被发现存在无显著统计学意义的 DCR 改善倾向（61% vs 32%；$P=0.11$）。这表明 K-ras 基因突变的患者可能从索拉非尼治疗中获益，尽管这相关性需要进一步的额外临床试验证实[29]。

舒尼替尼

舒尼替尼是一种 TKI 口服制剂，抑制 VEGFR-1、VEGFR-2，VEGFR-3，PDGFRα/β、c-kit、Flt-3 和 RET，被美国 FDA 批准用于治疗晚期 RCC 和伊马替尼耐药的胃肠道间质瘤。舒尼替尼在 NSCLC 治疗中的评价在两个单独的第二阶段试验取得了令人鼓舞的结果[30-31]。随后的第三阶段

表 34.3　抗血管小分子酪氨酸激酶抑制剂及其靶点

靶点	索拉非尼	舒尼替尼	帕唑帕尼	凡德他尼	西地尼布	莫特塞尼	阿昔替尼	BIBF1120	卡博替尼
VEGFR-1	x	x	x		x	x	x		
VEGFR-2	x	x	x	×	x	x	x		
VEGFR-3	x	x	x	x	x	x	x		
PDGFR	x	x	x	x		x	x	x	
c-kit	x	x	x	x					x
EGFR				×					
其他	Raf、Flt 3	Ret、Flt 3				Ret		FGFR	MET、Ret、Flt 3

的研究比较了舒尼替尼/厄洛替尼以及安慰剂/厄洛替尼，结果显示既往治疗晚期 NSCLC 患者 OR（10.6% vs 6.9%；P = 0.047 1）和 PFS 提高（3.6 个月 vs 2.0 个月；P = 0.002 3），但 OS 没有改善（9.0 个月 vs 8.5 个月；P = 0.138 8）[32]。目前正在研究 NSCLC 患者应用舒尼替尼治疗，包括 II 期 CALGB 30704 试验评价舒尼替尼作为二线治疗（临床试验，官方 ID：NCT00698815）和 III 期 CALGB 30607 舒尼替尼作为维持治疗的研究（临床试验，官方 ID：NCT00693992）。

帕唑帕尼

帕唑帕尼是一种针对 VEGFR-1、VEGFR-2、VEGFR-3 和 PDGFR-β、c-kit 的口服抑制剂，2009 年被美国 FDA 批准用于治疗晚期 RCC。在 NSCLC 中，帕唑帕尼被证明疗效是在一个小的 II 期试验中，I、II 期 NSCLC 患者接受帕唑帕尼 800mg/d×（2~6）周（中位数 16d）术前新辅助治疗，30 例（86%）的肿瘤体积缩小，最常见的不良事件是 2 级高血压、疲劳和腹泻[33]。这些令人鼓舞的初步结果使帕唑帕尼在更多的治疗 NSCLC 的试验中得以进行，包括最近完成的 II 期开放标签的多中心随机对照研究，比较了帕唑帕尼/培美曲塞与顺铂/培美曲塞作为一线治疗转移性 NSCLC 患者（临床试验，官方 ID：NCT00871403）。其他研究已经完成了预期收益，包括 II 期随机、安慰剂对照研究厄洛替尼联合帕唑帕尼治疗以前曾接受过治疗的 NSCLC 患者（临床试验，官方 ID：NCT01027598）和 II 期研究比较了帕唑帕尼/紫杉醇与卡铂/紫杉醇作为一线方案治疗晚期 NSCLC（临床试验，官方 ID：NCT00866528）。

凡德他尼

凡德他尼是一种口服给药的血管内皮生长因子受体抑制剂（VEGFR-2、VEGFR-3）、RET、和表皮生长因子受体（EGFR）。凡德他尼联合化疗的 II 期临床研究取得了令人鼓舞的结果，促成了进一步评估 4 个单独的凡德他尼的 III 期临床研究中治疗转移性 NSCLC[34]。III 期 ZODIAC 试验随机分配晚期 NSCLC 患者接受多西他赛/凡德他尼或多西他赛/安慰剂作为二线治疗。虽然加用凡德他尼改进了 ORR（17% vs 10%；P = 0.000 1）和 PFS（HR = 0.79；P < 0.000 1），但主要研究终点 OS 并未改善（HR = 0.91；P = 0.196）[35]。III 期 ZEAL 试验中，患者被随机分配二线接受凡德他尼/培美曲塞或安慰剂/培美曲塞。结果表明，ORR（19% 培美曲塞/凡德他尼 vs 8% 培美曲塞/安慰剂组；P < 0.001）和肺癌症状恶化延迟时间（18.1 周培美曲塞/凡德他尼 vs 12.1 周培美曲塞/安慰剂组；P = 0.005 2）延长更青睐那些接受凡德他尼治疗的患者，虽然这项研究并没有达到主要研究终点 PFS（HR = 0.86；P = 0.108）[36]。III 期 ZEST 随机将以前接受凡德他尼或厄洛替尼治疗的患者分组，并没有发现显著的 PFS 改善［HR = 0.98；95% CI（0.87，1.10）；P = 0.721］[37]。最后，在 III 期 ZEPHYR 研究中，晚期进展的 NSCLC 患者经过化疗和厄洛替尼治疗后，随机接受凡德他尼单药与安慰剂治疗。接受凡德他尼治疗的患者的 PFS 改善（HR = 0.63；P < 0.000 1），但主要研究终点 OS 不符合（HR = 0.95；P = 0.527）[38]。总之，这些研究令人失望的结果使凡德他尼对 NSCLC 的进一步研究已被暂停。

西地尼布

西地尼布（AZD2171）抑制 VEGFR-1 和 VEGFR-2，PDGFR-β 和 c-kit，其与化疗联合已经在一些单独的试验中研究用于晚期 NSCLC。在 BR24 II、III 期试验中，296 例晚期 NSCLC 患者随机接受卡铂/紫杉醇加（或）不加西地尼布作为一线治疗。虽然中期研究结果表明联用西地尼布可有较高的 ORR 和 PFS，但研究被提前中止，因为西地尼布在 30mg 剂量下产生过度的毒性，包括严重的高血压、胃肠道毒性及发热性嗜中性粒细胞减少症[39]。随后的 BR29 II/III 期试验将西地尼布减量为 20mg/d 并联合卡铂/紫杉醇，但该研究因中期研究分析提示西地尼布没有达到预先指定的 PFS 疗效标准而中止（临床试验，官方 ID：NCT00795340）。在西地尼布联合培美曲塞治疗复发性 NSCLC 的 II 期临床研究已经完成，结果令人期待（临床试验，官方 ID：NCT00410904）。

莫特赛尼

莫特赛尼（AMG 706）是一种选择性的 VEG-

FR-1、VEGFR-2 和 VEGFR-3，PDGFR-β、c-kit 和 RET 的抑制剂，已被研究作为各种恶性肿瘤中单药治疗或联合化疗[40-41]。在一项 NSCLC 的 Ⅱ 期临床研究中，非鳞癌患者应用莫特赛尼或者贝伐珠单抗联合卡铂/紫杉醇化疗作为一线治疗，莫特赛尼给药剂量为 125mg/d 组与贝伐珠单抗组疗效相仿，中位 PFS 为 7.7 个月（贝伐珠单抗 8.3 个月）和中位 OS 为 14 个月（贝伐珠单抗 14 个月）[8]。然而，双盲、安慰剂对照的 MONET1 Ⅲ 期研究，莫特赛尼联合卡铂/紫杉醇在非鳞癌晚期患者没有达到其主要研究终点 OS（HR=0.89；P=0.137），导致对该药物进一步研究的热情减退[42]。

阿西替尼

阿西替尼（AG-013736）是一种靶点为 VEGFR-1、VEGFR-2、VEGFR-3、PDGFR-β 和 c-kit 的口服 TKI 药物。一项包含 32 例晚期 NSCLC 患者的 Ⅱ 期临床试验对阿西替尼单药治疗给予了评估。在这项试验中，28% 的患者之前未接受化疗。ORR 为 9%，中位 PFS 为 4.9 个月 [95% CI（3.6，7.0）]，中位 OS 为 14.8 个月 [95% CI（10.7，无法估计）]。阿西替尼的一般耐受性可，有 3 级毒性疲劳（22%）、高血压（9%）及低钠血症（9%）[43]。总体而言，鉴于治疗 NSCLC 良好的单药疗效，关于阿西替尼治疗鳞癌和非鳞癌患者的 Ⅱ 期临床试验正在开展。在非鳞状 NSCLC 患者，有两个研究：AGILE 1030 对比阿西替尼/卡铂/紫杉醇与贝伐珠单抗/卡铂/紫杉醇（临床试验，官方 ID：NCT00600821），AGILE 1039 对比阿西替尼/顺铂/培美曲塞与顺铂/培美曲塞（临床试验，官方 ID：NCT007687855）。在鳞状 NSCLC，AGILE1038 试验随机分配患者接受阿西替尼/顺铂/吉西他滨或顺铂/吉西他滨（临床试验，官方 ID：NCT00735904）。

BIBF 1120

BIBF 1120 是一种针对 VEGFR-1、VEGFR-2、VEGFR-3、PDGFR-α/β 和成纤维细胞生长因子受体（fibroblast growth factor receprors，FGFR）1~3 的口服抑制剂，有研究其作为单药或联合化疗在 NSCLC 中的疗效。73 例复发性晚期 NSCLC 患者的 Ⅱ 期临床研究显示：BIBF1120 作为一种单药治疗方案，患者耐受性良好，中位 PFS 为 11.6 周，中位 OS 为 37.7 周，DCR（CR、PR 或 SD）为 46%。最常见的 3 级或 4 级毒副反应为恶心、呕吐、腹泻和肝功能检查值升高[44]。另有一项 BIBF 1120 剂量逐增的 Ⅰ 期临床试验研究了其与卡铂/紫杉醇联合作为晚期 NSCLC 患者的一线治疗。这项研究结果表明，当 BIBF 1120 与卡铂/紫杉醇联合治疗时，最大耐受剂量为 200mg，每天 2 次[45]。有两项 Ⅲ 期研究在 BIBF 1120 联合化疗二线治疗 NSCLC 已完成应计项目，结果令人期待：LUME-Lung1（组合多西他赛）和 LUME-Lung2（联合培美曲塞；临床试验，官方 ID：分别为 NCT00805194 和 NCT00806819）。

卡博替尼

卡博替尼（XL-184）是针对 VEGFR-2、MET、RET、Kit 和 Flt3 的 TKI 类药物，在亚临床阶段肺肿瘤模型中可抑制肿瘤生长和内皮细胞的增殖[46]。在一项卡博替尼 ⅠB/Ⅱ 期研究中，之前用或不用厄罗替尼治疗的晚期 NSCLC 患者，临床证据支持厄罗替尼进行预处理的患者采用卡博替尼与厄罗替尼联合治疗的耐受性良好，其中包括 EGFR T790M 和 MET 扩增者，而且额外的结果可被预期[47]。单药或者联合厄罗替尼的其他靶向药物治疗 NSCLC 的临床试验正在进行中。

血管阻断剂

血管阻断剂（VDAs）靶向作用于已形成的肿瘤血管，导致血流阻断与肿瘤中心坏死。研究发现，NSCLC 中的 VDAs 包括 ASA-404、fosbretabulin、bavituximab 和 omrabulin。在 ATTRACT-1 Ⅲ 期卡铂/紫杉醇加（或）不加 ASA-404 的研究中，ASA-404 的加入没有导致 OS 的改善[48]，随后的 ATTRACT-2 Ⅲ 期研究二线多西他赛加（或）不加 ASA-404 早期即停止，因为中期研究结果显示，主要研究终点 OS 不可能达成，导致该药物的进一步研究停止。FALCON Ⅱ 期临床试验随机分组转移性非鳞癌的患者接受卡铂/紫杉醇/贝伐珠单抗加（或）不加 fosbretabulin。令人鼓舞的是，最初的数据显示接受 fosbretabulin 者的 ORR 达 56%

（仅接受卡铂/紫杉醇/贝伐珠单抗者为36%），肿瘤总径>10cm者的OS亦改善[14.2个月 vs 11个月，HR=0.67；95% CI（0.26,0.7）][49]。巴维昔单抗是一种单克隆VDA抗体，靶向作用于磷脂酰丝氨酸/β₂糖蛋白1复合物，与卡铂/紫杉醇联合治疗NSCLC单组的Ⅱ期研究[50]。2012年发表了两项Ⅱ期随机临床研究，包括单抗巴维昔一线（在与卡铂/紫杉醇联合）和二线（联合多西他赛）治疗NSCLC（临床试验，官方ID：NCT01160601和NCT01138163）。然而，初步数据随后由于与编码和分布的差异被撤回，该药的未来尚不清楚。最后，ombrabulin是一种新的VDA，是考布他汀A4类似物和模拟微管蛋白结合剂，在一项跨国、安慰剂对照、Ⅱ期DISRUPT试验中，将转移性NSCLC患者随机分配接受紫杉类和铂类一线治疗加（或）不加ombrabulin（临床试验，官方ID：NCT01293630）。研究已经完成权责发生制，结果正在等待。

其他抗肿瘤血管生成药物

阿柏西普

阿柏西普（VEGF-Trap, ZALTRAP）是一种重组融合蛋白，结合VEGFR-1、VEGFR-2、胎盘生长因子（placental growth factor, PLGF），被美国FDA批准用于治疗黄斑变性。最近，阿柏西普也获得了FDA批准用于治疗转移性结直肠癌，基于Ⅲ期VELOUR研究发现阿柏西普联合FOLFIRI方案化疗可以改善PFS（HR=0.758；P=0.000 07）和OS（HR=0.817；P=0.003 2）[51]。一项对NSCLC的Ⅱ期临床研究使之前经过严格预处理的晚期患者接受阿柏西普单药治疗，静脉注射剂量为4.0mg/kg体重，每2周1次，提示ORR为2%［95% CI（0.002,0.072%）］，PFS为2.7个月，OS为6.2个月[52]。随后的Ⅲ期VITAL试验比较阿柏西普/多西他赛和安慰剂/多烯紫杉醇治疗局部晚期或转移性铂类药物化疗失败的NSCLC患者。尽管加用阿柏西普，ORR（23.3% vs 8.9%）和PFS［HR=0.82；95% CI（0.716,0.937）］有所改善，但主要研究终点OS［HR=1.01；95% CI（0.868,1.174）］在两组之间无统计学差异，导致该药在NSCLC治疗中的进一步发展充满不确定性[53]。此外，一项阿柏西普单组Ⅱ期临床研究提示与顺铂/培美曲塞联合治疗初治的晚期或转移性NSCLC患者，ORR为26.3%［95% CI（12.3,40.3）］和PFS为5个月［95% CI（4.3,7.1）］，然而这项试验提前停止了，因为在42例登记入组的患者中出现高于预期的可逆性后部白质脑病综合征（reversible posterior leukoencephalopathy syndrome, RPLS）发生率（3例确诊）。有趣的是，涉及3个大型安慰剂对照的阿柏西普联合化疗试验都没有RPLS安全的meta分析报道[54]。

抗血管生成治疗的生物标记物

寻找抗血管生成药物治疗的预测性生物标志物仍然是一个还未实现的重要目标。缺乏可靠的生物标志物阻碍了贝伐珠单抗和其他抗血管生成疗法的发展，在没有发现更好的生物标志物之前，这些药物真正的潜力将无法实现。高血压是临床上对应于血管内皮生长因子靶向治疗中有用的生物标志物，最初是在舒尼替尼治疗RCC试验中发现[55]。在NSCLC中，ECOG 4599分析了应用贝伐珠单抗导致高血压与临床获益的关系[56]。更重要的是，这种反应只能在开始治疗后进行评估，导致建立替代标记的努力方向尚未确定。血管生成的血清和血浆候选生物标志物已被广泛研究。第一个被研究的生物标志物是血管内皮生长因子的血浆浓度。在ECOG 4599研究中，高基线血浆血管内皮生长因子水平与贝伐珠单抗的高反应性相关，但没有预测生存受益[57]。最近，血液循环中血管内皮生长因子基线水平在预测贝伐珠单抗治疗包括胃癌在内的其他恶性肿瘤中的作用好像更有前途。Ⅲ期AVAGAST试验中，血浆VEGF-A高基线水平的胃癌患者的总体预后较差，尽管他们倾向于应用贝伐珠单抗治疗反应率高和生存延长[58]。在肾脏和胰腺癌患者，类似的生存受益差异也能观察到[59]。

除了血管内皮生长因子，各种其他生物标志物在抗血管生成治疗的试验中也被探讨。ECOG 4599试验中也测量过血浆中纤维母细胞生长因子（basic fibroblast growth factor, bFGF）、可溶性细胞间黏附分子（intercellular adhesion molecule, ICAM）、E-选择素的基线和治疗期水平。基线

ICAM 水平被证明是预后因素而不是预测因子，因为两组低基线 ICAM 水平患者相比高 ICAM 都有更高的反应率和更好的整体存活率（$P=0.00005$）[57]。有关血管生成的基因变异，如单核苷酸多态性（single nucleotide polymorphisms，SNPs），也被研究作为潜在的预测生物标志物。尽管血管内皮生长因子的多态性似乎与生存相关，但通过 E4599、VEGF、VEGFR1、ICAM-1 和表皮生长因子的单核苷酸多态性分析却没有一个确定的结果[60]。胰腺癌或 RCC 患者参加了2个独立的贝伐珠单抗Ⅲ期临床试验，其对 SNP 的分析表明，两组试验中接受贝伐珠单抗治疗的一个 VEGFR-1 单核苷酸多态性与 PFS 明显相关，另外在胰腺癌组与 OS 相关。此外血管内皮生长因子单核苷酸多态性的研究仍在继续[59]。

也有研究分析多种血浆标记物以识别 VEGFR-TKI 反应相关的特征性标记。细胞因子和血管生成因子（cytokines and angiogenic factors，CAFs）的变化与 VEGFR 酪氨酸激酶抑制剂治疗肺癌患者的临床预后相关，但令人感兴趣的细胞因子在研究中是可变的[61-62]。研究人员也在评估接受血管内皮生长因子抑制剂治疗的其他方法，如检测循环内皮细胞（circulating endothelial cells，CECs），但是将这些生物标志物纳入大试验存在重要的方法论问题需要去克服。最后，利用最新进展的基因表达分析和蛋白质组学，研究人员已经能够将高水平的促血管生成细胞因子，如白细胞介素-6（IL-6）与各种恶性肿瘤患者较差的预后相关联[63-64]，也发现高 IL-6 水平可预测卵巢透明细胞癌舒尼替尼治疗的反应[65]。随着临床上对有效的抗血管生成治疗的生物标志物的研究，未来涉及这些药物的试验应该包含探索性和验证性生物标志物分析，以帮助我们更好地理解。

总　结

抗血管生成药物在 NSCLC 的治疗中表现出了良好的效果，包括 FDA 批准的治疗晚期非鳞 NSCLC 的单克隆抗体贝伐珠单抗。在具有里程碑意义的 ECOG 4599 研究中，贝伐珠单抗联合卡铂/紫杉醇作为一线治疗晚期 NSCLC，PFS 和 OS 均获得了改善，另外的研究扩展了贝伐珠单抗联合其他化疗方案以及治疗脑转移瘤。其他抗血管生成疗法，如小分子酪氨酸激酶抑制剂，包括以 VEGFR 为靶点的药物，虽仍在不同临床开发阶段，但从正在进行的研究来看是值得期待的 VDAs 药物。可靠的抗血管生成治疗预测生物标志物的发现是一个关键的问题，只有解决了这个问题才能建立这些药物治疗肺癌的确切地位。最终，根据临床试验确定最佳治疗组合和剂量时间表对改善患者的疗效至关重要，也许更重要的是提前识别最有可能使患者从可用的抗血管生成疗法中获益的生物标志物。

（李文红　叶　欣　译）

参考文献

[1] Folkman J. Tumor angiogenesis: therapeutic implications. N Engl J Med, 1971, 285（21）: 1182-1186. PubMed PMID: 4938153.

[2] Ferrara N, Gerber HP, LeCouter J. The biology of VEGF and its receptors. Nat Med, 2003, 9（6）: 669-676. PubMed PMID: 12778165.

[3] Johnson DH, Fehrenbacher L, Novotny WF, et al. Randomized phase Ⅱ trial comparing bevacizumab plus carboplatin and paclitaxel with carboplatin and paclitaxel alone in previously untreated locally advanced or metastatic non-small-cell lung cancer. J Clin Oncol, 2004, 22（11）: 2184-2191. PubMed PMID: 15169807.

[4] Sandler A, Gray R, Perry MC, et al. Paclitaxel-carboplatin alone or with bevacizumab for non-small-cell lung cancer. NEngl J Med, 2006, 355（24）: 2542-2550. PubMed PMID: 17167137.

[5] Hanna N, Shepherd FA, Fossella FV, et al. Randomized phase Ⅲ trial of pemetrexed versus docetaxel in patients with non-small-cell lung cancer previously treated with chemotherapy. J Clin Oncol, 2004, 22（9）: 1589-1597. PubMed PMID: 15117980.

[6] Reck M, von Pawel J, Zatlouka P, et al. Phase Ⅲ trial of cisplatin plus gemcitabine with either placebo or bevacizumab as first-line therapy for nonsquamous non small-cell lung cancer: AVAiL. J Clin Oncol, 2009, 27（8）: 1227-1234. PubMed PMID: 19188680.

[7] Reck M, von Pawel J, Zatloukal P, et al. Overall survival with cisplatin-gemcitabine and bevacizumab or placeboas first-line therapy for nonsquamous non-small-cell lung canc-

er: results from a randomised phase Ⅲ trial (AVAiL). Ann Oncol, 2010, 21 (9): 1804-1809. PubMedPMID: 20150572. Pubmed Central PMCID: 2924992.

[8] Blumenschein GR, Jr., Kabbinavar F, Menon H, et al. A phase Ⅱ, multicenter, open-label randomized study of motesanibor bevacizumab in combination with paclitaxel and carboplatin for advanced nonsquamous non-small-cell lung cancer. Ann Oncol, 2011, 22 (9): 2057-2067. PubMed PMID: 21321086.

[9] Socinski MA, Langer CJ, Huang JE, et al. Safety of bevacizumabin patients with non-small-cell lung cancer and brain metastases. J Clin Oncol, 2009, 27 (31): 5255-5261. PubMed PMID: 19738122.

[10] Crino L, Dansin E, Garrido P, et al. Safety and efficacy of first-line bevacizumab-based therapy in advanced non-squamous non-small-cell lung cancer (SAiL, MO19390): a phase 4 study. Lancet Oncol, 2010, 11 (8): 733-740. PubMed PMID: 20650686.

[11] Patel JD, Hensing TA, Rademaker A, et al. Phase Ⅱ study of pemetrexed and carboplatin plus bevacizumab with maintenance pemetrexed and bevacizumab as first-line therapy for nonsquamous non-small-cell lung cancer. JClin Oncol, 2009, 27 (20): 3284-3289. PubMed PMID: 19433684.

[12] Patel J, Socinski M, Garon EB, et al. A randomized, open-label, phase 3, superiority study of Pemetrexed (Pem) + Carboplatin (Cb) + Bevacizumab (B) followed by maintenance Pem + B versus Paclitaxel (Pac) + Cb + B followed by maintenance B in patients (pts) with stage Ⅲ B or Ⅳ nonsquamous non-small cell lung cancer (NS-NSCLC). 2012 Chicago Multidisciplinary Symposium in Thoracic Oncology. Chicago, IL, 2012.

[13] Barlesi F, de Castro J, Dvornichenko V, et al. Final efficacy outcomes for patients (pts) with advanced non-squamousnon-small cell lung cancer (NSCLC) randomised to continuation maintenance (mtc) with Bevacizumab (bev) or Bev + Pemetrexed (pem) after first-line (1L) Bev-cisplatin (cis) -pem treatment (Tx). Eur J Cancer, 2011, 47 (Suppl 2): 16.

[14] Wakelee HA, Dahlberg SE, Keller SM, et al. Interim report of on-study demographics and toxicity from E1505, a phase Ⅲ randomized trial of adjuvant (adj) chemotherapy (chemo) with or without bevacizumab (B) for completely resected early-stage non-small cell lung cancer (NSCLC). J Clin Oncol, 2011, 29 (Suppl): Abstract7013.

[15] Miller MJ, Lindsay H, Valverde-Ventura R, et al. Evaluation of the BioVigilant IMD-A, a novel optical spectroscopy technology for the continuous and real-time environmental monitoring of viable and nonviable particles. Part I. Review of the technology and comparative studies with conventional methods. PDA J Pharm Sci Technol, 2009, 63 (3): 245-258. PubMed PMID: 20069798.

[16] Kabbinavar FF, Miller VA, Johnson BE, et al. Overall survival (OS) in ATLAS, a Phase Ⅲb trial comparing bevacizumab (B) therapy with or without erlotnib (E) after completion of chemotherapy (chemo) with B for first-line treatment of locally advanced, recurrent, or metastatic non-small-cell lung cancer (NSCLC). J Clin Oncol, 2010, 28 (15S): Abstract 7526.

[17] Herbst RS, Prager D, Hermann R, et al. TRIBUTE: a phase Ⅲ trial of erlotinib hydrochloride (OSI-774) combined with carboplatin and paclitaxel chemotherapy in advanced non-small-cell lung cancer. J Clin Oncol, 2005, 23 (25): 5892-5899. PubMed PMID: 16043829.

[18] Herbst RS, Ansari R, Bustin F, et al. Efficacy of bevacizumab plus erlotinib versus erlotinib alone in advanced non-small-cell lung cancer after failure of standard first-line chemotherapy (BeTa): a double-blind, placebo-controlled, phase3 trial. Lancet, 2011, 377 (9780): 1846-1854. PubMed PMID: 21621716.

[19] Socinski MA, Stinchcombe TE, Moore DT, et al. Incorporating bevacizumab and erlotinib in the combined-modality treatment of stage Ⅲ non-small-cell lung cancer: Results of a phase Ⅰ/Ⅱ trial. J Clin Oncol, 2012, 30 (32): 3953-3959. PubMed PMID: 23045594.

[20] Camidge DR, Ballas MS, Dubey S, et al. A phase Ⅱ, open-label study of ramucirumab (IMC-1121B), an IgG1 fully human monoclonal antibody (MAb) targeting VEGFR-2, in combination with paclitaxel and carboplatin as firstline therapy in patients (pts) with stage Ⅲb/Ⅳ non small cell lung cancer (NSCLC). J Clin Oncol, 2010, 28 (15s): Abstract 7588.

[21] Escudier B, Eisen T, Stadler WM, et al. Sorafenib in advanced clear cell renal-cell carcinoma. N Engl J Med, 2007, 356 (2): 125-134. PubMed PMID: 17215530.

[22] Llovet JM, Ricci S, Mazzaferro V, et al. Sorafenib in advanced hepatocellular carcinoma. N Engl J Med, 2008, 359 (4): 378-390. PubMed PMID: 18650514.

[23] Schiller J, Lee JW, Hanna H, et al. A randomized discontinuation phase Ⅱ study of sorafenib versus placebo in patients with non-small cell lung cancer who have failed at

least two prior chemotherapy regimens: E2501. J Clin Oncol, 2008, 26 (May20 suppl): Abstract 8014.

[24] Blumenschein GR, Jr., Gatzemeier U, Fossella F, et al. Phase II, multicenter, uncontrolled trial of single-agent sorafenib in patients with relapsed or refractory, advanced non-small-cell lung cancer. J Clin Oncol, 2009, 27 (26): 4274-4280. PubMed PMID: 19652055.

[25] Scagliotti G, von Pawel J, Reck M, et al. Sorafenib plus carboplatin/paclitaxel in chemonaiive patients with stage ⅢB-Ⅳ non-small cell lung cancer: interim analysis results from the phase Ⅲ, randomized, double-blind, placebo-controlled, ESCAPE (Evaluation of Sorafenib, Carboplaitn and Paclitaxel Efficacy in NSCLC) trial. J Thorac Oncol, 2008, 4 (S97).

[26] Paz-Ares LG, Biesma B, Heigener D, et al. Phase Ⅲ, randomized, double-blind, placebo-controlled trial of Gemcitabine/Cisplatin alone or with Sorafenib for the firstline treatment of advanced, nonsquamous non-small cell lung cancer. J Clin Oncol, 2012, 30 (25): 3084-3092. PubMed PMID: 22851564.

[27] Spigel DR, Burris HA, 3rd, Greco FA, et al. Randomized, double-blind, placebo-controlled, phase Ⅱ trial of sorafenib and erlotinib or erlotinib alone in previously treated advanced non-small-cell lung cancer. J Clin Oncol, 2011, 29 (18): 258-2589. PubMed PMID: 21576636.

[28] Gridelli C, Morgillo F, Favaretto A, et al. Sorafenib in combination with erlotinib or with gemcitabine in elderly patients with advanced non-small-cell lung cancer: A randomized phase Ⅱ study. Ann Oncol, 2011, 22 (7): 1528-1534. PubMedPMID: 21212155.

[29] Kim ES, Herbst RS, Wistuba II, et al. The BATTLE Trial: Personalizing therapy for lung cancer. Cancer Discov, 2011, 1 (1): 44-53.

[30] Socinski MA, Novello S, Brahmer JR, et al. Multicenter, phase Ⅱ trial of sunitinib in previously treated, advanced non-small-cell lung cancer. J Clin Oncol, 2008, 26 (4): 650-656. PubMed PMID: 18235126.

[31] Novello S, Scagliotti GV, Rosell R, et al. Phase Ⅱ study of continuous daily sunitinib dosing in patients with previously treated advanced non-small cell lung cancer. Br J Cancer, 2009, 101 (9): 1543-1548. PubMed PMID: 19826424. Pubmed Central PMCID: 2778527.

[32] Scagliotti GV, Krzakowski M, Szczesna A, et al. Sunitinib plus erlotinib versus placebo plus erlotinib in patients with previously treated advanced non-small-cell lung cancer: a phase Ⅲ trial. J Clin Oncol, 2012, 30 (17): 2070-2078. PubMed PMID: 22564989.

[33] Altorki N, Lane ME, Bauer T, et al. Phase Ⅱ proof-of-concept study of pazopanib monotherapy in treatment-naive patients with stage Ⅰ/Ⅱ resectable non-small-cell lung cancer. J Clin Oncol, 2010, 28 (19): 3131-3137. PubMed PMID: 20516450.

[34] Heymach JV, Paz-Ares L, De Braud F, et al. Randomized phase Ⅱ study of vandetanib alone or with paclitaxel and carboplatin as first-line treatment for advanced non-small-cell lung cancer. J Clin Oncol, 2008, 26 (33): 5407-5415. PubMed PMID: 18936474.

[35] Herbst RS, Sun Y, Eberhardt WE, et al. Vandetanib plus docetaxelversus docetaxel as second-line treatment for patients with advanced non-small-cell lung cancer (ZODIAC): A double-blind, randomised, phase 3 trial. Lancet Oncol, 2010, 11 (7): 619-626. PubMed PMID: 20570559. Pubmed Central PMCID: 3225192.

[36] de Boer RH, Arrieta O, Yang CH, et al. Vandetanib plus pemetrexed for the second-line treatment of advanced non-small-cell lung cancer: a randomized, double-blind phase Ⅲ trial. J Clin Oncol, 2011, 29 (8): 1067-1074. PubMed PMID: 21282537.

[37] Natale RB, Thongprasert S, Greco FA, et al. Phase Ⅲ trial of vandetanib compared with erlotinib in patients with previously treated advanced non-small-cell lung cancer. J Clin Oncol, 2011, 29 (8): 1059-1066. PubMed PMID: 21282542.

[38] Lee JS, Hirsh V, Park K, et al. Vandetanib Versus placebo in patients Anti-angiogenic Agents in Metastatic NSCLC 539with advanced non-small-cell lung cancer after prior therapy with an epidermal growth factor receptor tyrosine kinase inhibitor: a randomized, double blind phase Ⅲ trial (ZEPHYR). J Clin Oncol, 2012, 30 (10): 1114-1121. PubMed PMID: 22370318.

[39] Goss GD, Arnold A, Shepherd FA, et al. Randomized, double-blind trial of carboplatin and paclitaxel with either daily oral cediranib or placebo in advanced non-small-cell lung cancer: NCIC clinical trials group BR24 study. J Clin Oncol, 2009, 28 (1): 49-55. PubMed PMID: 19917841.

[40] Sherman SI, Wirth LJ, Droz JP, et al. Motesanib diphosphate in progressive differentiated thyroid cancer. N Engl J Med, 2008, 359 (1): 31-42. PubMed PMID: 18596272.

[41] Rosen LS, Kurzrock R, Mulay M, et al. Safety, phar-

macokinetics, and efficacy of AMG 706, an oral multikinase inhibitor, in patients with advanced solid tumors. J Clin Oncol, 2007, 25 (17): 2369 - 2376. PubMed PMID: 17557949.

[42] Scagliotti GV, Vynnychenko I, Park K, et al. International, randomized, placebo-controlled, double-blind phase III study of motesanib plus carboplatin/paclitaxelin patients with advanced nonsquamous non-small cell lung cancer: MONET1. J Clin Oncol, 2012, 30 (23): 2829 - 2836. PubMed PMID: 22753922.

[43] Schiller JH, Larson T, Ou SH, et al. Efficacy and safety of axitinib in patients with advanced non-small-cell lung cancer: results from a phase II study. J Clin Oncol, 2009, 27 (23): 3836 - 3841. PubMed PMID: 19597027.

[44] Reck M, Kaiser R, Eschbach C, et al. A phase II doubleblind study to investigate efficacy and safety of two doses of the triple angiokinase inhibitor BIBF 1120in patients with relapsed advanced non-small-celllung cancer. Ann Oncol, 2011, 22 (6): 1374 - 1381. PubMed PMID: 21212157.

[45] Doebele RC, Conkling P, Traynor AM, et al. A phase I, openlabel dose-escalation study of continuous treatment with BIBF 1120 in combination with paclitaxel and carboplatin as first-line treatment in patients with advanced non-small-cell lung cancer. Ann Oncol, 2012, 23 (8): 2094 - 2102. PubMed PMID: 22345119.

[46] Yakes FM, Chen J, Tan J, et al. Cabozantinib (XL 184), a novel MET andVEGFR2 inhibitor, simultanously suppresses metastasis, angiogenesis, and tumor growth. Mol Cancer Ther, 2011, 10 (12): 2298 - 2308.

[47] Wakelee HA, Gettinger SN, Engelman JA, et al. A phase IB/II study of XL184 (BMS 907351) with and without erlotinib (E) in ptatients (pts) with non-small cell lung cancer (NSCLC). J Clin Oncol, 2010, 28 (15s): Abstract 3017.

[48] Lara PN, Jr., Douillard JY, Nakagawa K, et al. Randomized phase III placebo-controlled trial of carboplatin and paclitaxel with or without the vascular disrupting agent vadimezan (ASA404) in advanced non-small-cell lung cancer. J Clin Oncol, 2011, 29 (22): 2965 - 2971. PubMed PMID: 21709202.

[49] Garon EB, Kabbinavar FF, Neidhart JA, et al. A randomized phase II trial of a vascular disrupting agent (VDA) fosbretabulin tromethamine (CA4P) with carboplatin (C), paclitaxel (P), and bevacizumab (B) in stage 3B/4nonsquamous non-small cell lung cancer (NSCLC): Analysis of safety and activity of the FALCON trial. J Clin Oncol, 2011, 29 (Suppl.): Abstract 7559.

[50] Digumarti R, Suresh AV, Bhattacharyya GS, et al. Phase II study of bavituximab plus paclitaxel and carboplatin in untreated locally advanced or metastatic non-small cell lung cancer: Interim results. J Clin Oncol, 2010, 28 (15 suppl): Abstract7589.

[51] Van Cutsem E, Tabernero J, Lakomy R, et al. (eds) Intravenous (IV) aflibercept versus placebo in combination with irinotecan/5-FU (FOLFIRI) for second-line treatment of metastatic colorectal cancer (MCRC): Results of a multinational phase 3 trial (EFC10262 - VELOUR). 13th ESMO World Congress on Gastrointestinal Cancer, Abstract 0 - 0024. Barcelona, Spain, 2011, 6: 22 - 25.

[52] Leighl NB, Raez LE, Besse B, et al. A multicenter, phase 2 study of vascular endothelial growth factor trap (Aflibercept) inplatinum and erlotinib-resistant adenocarcinoma ofthe lung. J Thorac Oncol, 2010, 5 (7): 1054 - 1059.

[53] Novello S, Ramlau R, Gorbunova VA, et al. (eds) Afliberceptin combination with docetaxel for second-line treatment of locally advanced or metastatic non-small-cell lung cancer (NSCLC): Final results of a multinational placebo-controlled phase III trial (EFC10261-VITAL). 14th Biennial World Conference on Lung Cancer, Abstract O43.06. Amsterdam, Netherlands, 2011, 7: 3 - 7.

[54] Chen H, Modiano MR, Neal JW, et al. A phase II multicenter study of aflibercept (AFL) in combination with cisplatin (C) and pemetrexed (P) in patients with previously untreated advanced/metastatic nonsquamousnon-small cell lung cancer (NSCLC). J Clin Oncol, 2012, 30 (Suppl): Abstr 7541.

[55] Rini BI, Cohen DP, Lu DR, et al. Hypertension as a biomarker of efficacy in patients with metastatic renal cell carcinoma treated with sunitinib. J Natl Cancer Inst, 2011, 103 (9): 763 - 773. PubMed PMID: 21527770. Pubmed Central PMCID: 3086879.

[56] Dahlberg SE, Sandler AB, Brahmer JR, et al. Clinical course of advanced non small-cell lung cancer patients experiencing hypertension during treatment with bevacizumab in combination with carboplatin and paclitaxel on ECOG 4599. J Clin Oncol, 2010, 28 (6): 949 - 954. PubMed PMID: 20085937. Pubmed Central

PMCID: 2834434.

[57] Dowlati A, Gray R, Sandler AB, et al. Cell adhesion molecules, vascular endothelial growth factor, and basic fibroblast growth factor in patients with non-small cell lung cancer treated with chemotherapy with or without bevacizumab-an Eastern Cooperative Oncology Group Study. Clin Cancer Res, 2008, 14 (5): 1407-1412. PubMed PMID: 18316562.

[58] Van Cutsem E, de Haas S, Kang YK, et al. Bevacizumab in combination with chemotherapy as first-line therapy in advanced gastric cancer: a biomarker evaluation from the AVAGAST randomized phase III trial. J Clin Oncol, 2012, 30 (17): 2119-2127. PubMed PMID: 22565005.

[59] Lambrechts D, Claes B, Delmar P, et al. VEGF pathway genetic variants as biomarkers of treatment outcome with bevacizumab: an analysis of data from the AViTA and AVOREN randomised trials. Lancet Oncol, 2012, 13 (7): 724-733. PubMed PMID: 22608783.

[60] Zhang W, Dahlberg SE, Yang D, et al. Genetic variants in angiogenesis pathway associated with clinical outcome in NSCLC patients (pts) treated with bevacizumab in combination with carboplatin and paclitaxel: Subset pharmacogenetic analysis of ECOG 4599. J Clin Oncol, 2009, 27 (15S): Abstract 8032.

[61] Hanrahan EO, Lin HY, Kim ES, et al. Distinct patterns of cytokine and angiogenic factor modulation and markers of benefit for vandetanib and/or chemotherapy in patients with non-small-cell lung cancer. J Clin Oncol, 2009, 28 (2): 193-201. PubMed PMID: 19949019. Pubmed Central PMCID: 3040010.

[62] Nikolinakos PG, Altorki N, Yankelevitz D, et al. Plasma cytokine and angiogenic factor profiling identifies markers associated with tumor shrinkage in early-stage non-small cell lung cancer patients treated with pazopanib. CancerRes, 2010, 70 (6): 2171-2179. PubMed PMID: 20215520.

[63] Zhu AX, Sahani DV, Duda DG, et al. Efficacy, safety, and potential biomarkers of sunitinib monotherapy in advanced hepatocellular carcinoma: a phase II study. J Clin Oncol, 2009, 27 (18): 3027-3035. PubMed PMID: 19470923. Pubmed Central PMCID: 2702235.

[64] Nilsson MB, Langley RR, Fidler IJ. Interleukin-6, secreted by human ovarian carcinoma cells, is a potent proangiogenic cytokine. Cancer Res, 2005, 65 (23): 10794-10800. PubMed PMID: 16322225. Pubmed Central PMCID: 1534114.

[65] Anglesio MS, George J, Kulbe H, et al. IL6-STAT3-HIF signaling and therapeutic response to the angiogenesis inhibitor sunitinib in ovarian clear cell cancer. Clin Cancer Res, 2011, 17 (8): 2538-2548. PubMed PMID: 21343371.

第35章
靶向淋巴瘤激酶（ALK）重排

Justin F. Gainor, Alice T. Shaw
Department of Medicine, Harcard Medical School, Massachusetts General Hospital, Boston, MA, USA

引 言

全身化疗一直是晚期非小细胞肺癌（NSCLC）患者主要的治疗方式。然而，2004年表皮生长因子受体激活突变的发现成为该病治疗的一个重要转折点[1-3]，这一发现建立了一种新的基于患者肿瘤分子特征的治疗模式。表皮生长因子受体突变患者治疗的成功引领了其他研究寻找新的基因突变或作为药物靶点的"驱动"突变。最终在2007年发现了涉及未分化淋巴瘤激酶（anaplastic lymphoma kinase, ALK）基因的染色体重排。像EGFR突变一样，ALK重排定义为NSCLC一个特定的基因子集。在本章中，我们将：①复习ALK重排的分子机制；②总结ALK阳性患者常见的临床病理学特征；③概述ALK重排检测当前可用的技术；④审查支持ALK靶向治疗的临床试验数据。

天然ALK的分子生物学

ALK基因位于2号染色体，编码1 620个氨基酸受体酪氨酸激酶[4-5]。天然ALK由胞外域、短跨膜区和一个细胞内的酪氨酸激酶结构域构成（图35.1）。作为胰岛素受体超家族中的一员，ALK与白细胞酪氨酸激酶（LTK）、c-ROS癌基因（ROS1）、胰岛素样生长因子-1受体（IGF-1R）和胰岛素受体享有同源性序列。天然ALK在中枢神经系统、睾丸和成人小肠的表达是有限的[6-7]。在小鼠中，ALK仅在胚胎发育和新生神经系统中瞬时表达[8]。这种模式表明ALK的表达对神经系统的发育可能是重要的。然而，在敲除了ALK基因小鼠实验中，小鼠是有活力的，并没有表现出任何明显的发育或形态学异常[9]。另外关于敲除了ALK基因小鼠的分析显示与年龄相关的海马神经前体细胞增加以及行为测试的变化。

目前对天然ALK功能的了解还不完全，通常认为是通过配体诱导的二聚化激活[10]。在果蝇，Jelly Belly（Jeb）已被确定为ALK激活配体和下游信号，而人类同源蛋白目前尚未被确认[11]。在人类，生长因子PTN和MK可能为ALK配体[12-13]。

EML4-ALK在分子发病机制中的地位

ALK致癌基因的活化已在一些恶性肿瘤中确定[14]。在大多数情况下，激活通过染色体易位发生。ALK基因重排首次报道是1994年在间变性大细胞淋巴瘤（anaplastic large cell lymphoma, ALCL）确定的再发的t（2；5）（P23；Q35）易位[7]。这种重排产生嵌合融合蛋白包括核仁磷酸蛋白的氨基末端（NPM1）和羧基末端的ALK。最初的描述ALK重排在其他的恶性肿瘤也被发现，包括炎性肌纤维母细胞瘤、NSCLC、肾细胞癌（renal cell carcinomas, RCC）及其他[15,18]。此外，激活点突变在ALK酪氨酸激酶域已在神经母细胞瘤和间变性甲状腺癌[19-23]中报道。

在NSCLC中ALK基因重排首次被识别是在2007年[17,24]。采用从人肺腺癌组织中制备逆转录cDNA表达文库，Soda及其同事检测到2号染色体上一个小的反转，产生一个包含棘皮动物微管结合样蛋白4（EML4）的1~13号外显子与ALK 20~29外显子的融合基因[17]。这个EML4-ALK嵌

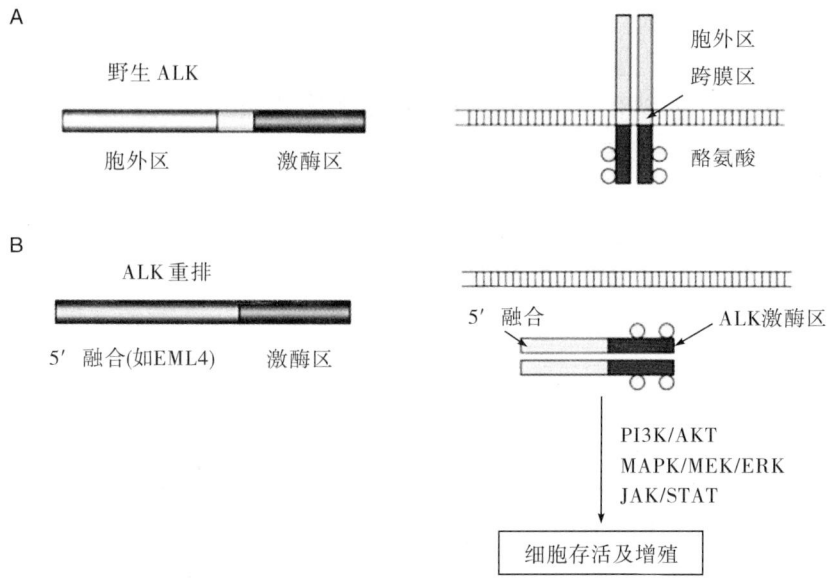

图 35.1 A. 野生 ALK 结构及细胞定位示意图。B. ALK 融合致癌基因示意图。ALK 重排，包含 5′融合受体和大多数通常出现在涉及 2 号染色体倒置的 ALK 酪氨酸激酶域。由此产生的融合蛋白在胞质中异常表达和重新分配

合转录编码 EML4 N-端和 ALK 胞内酪氨酸激酶结酶结构域。结果是，ALK 从细胞膜迁移到胞质中，在这里，EML4 介导 ALK 非配体依赖的二聚化和自动磷酸化[17,25]，反过来导致 ALK 通过 MAPK/MEK/ERK/PI3K/Akt 和 JAK/STAT 信号通路使下游信号激活[26-27]。因此，EML4-ALK 是体外和体内转化[17,28]。事实上，转基因小鼠表达 EML4-ALK 的肺泡 II 型细胞发展为肺多发性腺癌[28]。然而动物在 ALK 抑制剂治疗后，肿瘤又复发了。总之，这些结果表明，EML4-ALK 是一种新型的 NSCLC 的癌驱动因素。

几种不同的 ALK 亲本细胞系已在 NSCLC 中确定，包括驱动蛋白家族成员 5B（KIF5B），驱动蛋白轻链 1（KCL1）和转化生长因子（transforming growth factor，TFG）[24,29-30]。这些重排似乎具有类似的生物学特性[31]。在 NSCLC 中 EML4 是最常见的 ALK 亲本细胞系[32]。此外，EML4-ALK 多变体存在，均含有相同的 ALK 酪氨酸激酶结构域但具有不同的截断 EML4[17,26,33-34]。最常见的是 EML4-ALK 变体 1（49.6%），其次是变体 3a/b（25.6%）以及变体 2（10%）[35]。其他 ALK 变异由少于 15% 的其他情况组成。

ALK 重排患者的临床病理特征

在 NSCLC 的 EML4-ALK 的初步报告中，75 个样本中有 6.7% 发现融合转录[17]。随后的筛选研究估计在未经选择的患者中 ALK 重排的患病率为 3%~5%[26,29,33,36,41]。ALK 重排与独特的临床和病理特征有关，包括年龄小、腺癌组织学及缺乏吸烟史。与 ALK 易位和 EGFR 突变的患者有相似的临床特点。然而，ALK 重排本质上与 EGFR 和 KRAS 基因突变是相互排斥的[36,42]，只有罕见状况下的重叠突变被报告[41,43,51]。关于 ALK 重排的临床病理特征的知识可以指导分子检测和有助于识别这种罕见的患者群体[36]。

ALK 重排与诊断时患者相对年轻有关[36,37,52,54]。中位年龄约为 50 岁，比 ALK 阴性患者年轻 10~15 岁。ALK 重排也明显与有少量吸烟史或不吸烟相关[36,52,53]。从最近克唑替尼的临床试验中建立的数据库来看，约 70% ALK 阳性患者从不吸烟[55-56]。与 EGFR 突变相比，ALK 重排与性别、种族无明显关联。

ALK 阳性肺癌患者也与具有独特的形态特征相关。绝大多数的 ALK 阳性患者（约 97%）为腺癌[55]，也有一个罕见亚组的患者为鳞癌的报道[36,37,55,57-58]。在一个主要以亚洲人群为主的肺癌切除的研究中，ALK 重排也与印戒细胞的存在、一种液腺癌模式和腺泡的生长特性相关[57]。在最近的一个 104 例 ALK 阳性和 215 例 ALK 阴性的肺癌样本分析中，ALK 阳性的原发性肿瘤也与印戒细胞有关[59]。然而，这些相同标本没有表现出较

高的腺泡或黏液生长模式的比例。总的来说，富于印戒细胞和实性优势增长模式已经成为原发性和转移性病变最特异的 ALK 重排的形态学特征。超过 70% 的 ALK 阳性肿瘤显示存在印戒细胞，而同时近一半表现出实性增长模式。尽管如此，这些特征不能作为肿瘤基因分型的替代品；相反，它们可能会预测检测策略的优先次序，特别是在组织有限的情况下。

ALK 重排的预后影响

在之前的描述中，ALK 重排与肿瘤进展期的出现相关[36,52]。此外，我们注意到 ALK 阳性患者具有独特的转移模式。在一份关于晚期患者的报道中，与 ALK 阴性患者相比，ALK 重排与心包、胸膜和肝转移显著相关[60]。多种基因型中，包括有 ALK、EGFR 或 KRAS 改变的患者，脑转移的普遍性没有差异。Choi 等人使用 FDG PET/CT 进行的独立研究中，提出 ALK 重排可能还与侵袭性表型相关[61]。在他们的分析中，与 ALK 阴性的对照组相比，ALK 阳性肿瘤显示出明显较高的最大标准化摄取值及更多的淋巴结和远处转移。

ALK 重排为对 ALK TKI - 克唑替尼响应的预测性标志物，将于下文中更详细地讨论。然而，这些基因改变的预后意义并不明确[62]。在肿瘤早期，已报告了若干相矛盾的研究[47,63-64]。Zhang 等人认定在手术切除后的 ALK 阳性患者中无明显 OS 升高的趋势[47]。与此相反，Yang 等人证实，与 ALK 阴性对照的患者相比，ALK 阳性肿瘤患者病情进展或复发的 5 年风险要高出 2 倍[63]。在一份独立报告中，Kim 及其同事评估了 119 例经过手术切除的患者根据基因型进行无复发存活（recurrence-free survival, RFS）的比较[64]。根据基因分型的 RFS 没有显著差异（EGFR 突变：39.7 个月，ALK 重排：20.0 个月，KRAS 突变：21.4 个月及"三阴性"：26.8 个月；$P = 0.344$）。

在对晚期患者的研究中，ALK 重排的预后意义同样不清楚。早期研究显示 ALK 重排不会使总生存期有所不同[36,65-66]。一项这类研究中，Shaw 等人评估了 36 例克唑替尼 - 野生型 ALK 阳性患者的 OS，与 253 例野生型（WT）对照组相比较，发现两组之间的中位总生存期无显著差异（20 个月 vs 15 个月；$P = 0.244$）[66]。最近，Lee 及其同事报道，ALK 重排与中位总生存期的缩短相关联，虽然统计学差异不显著（ALK 重排：12.2 个月，EGFR 突变：29.6 个月及 WT/WT：19.3 个月；ALK vs WT/WT，$P = 0.127$）[67]。同样，Kimet 等人将涵盖各种基因型的 229 例 NSCLC 患者的中位总生存期进行了对比，发现与 EGFR 阳性或 WT/WT 的患者相比，那些有 ALK 重排的患者统计学意义上的中位总生存期大大缩短了（分别为：14.3 个月 vs 37.2 个月 vs 33.3 个月）[64]。与此相反，Wu 和同事近来报道，39 例有 ALK 重排的患者，与 77 例 WT 对照组相比，OS 升高（14.7 个月 vs 10.3 个月，$P = 0.009$）[68]。总体来说，这些研究受限于回顾性评估、小样本量和测试技术的变异性。然而，总的来说，这些研究显示 ALK 重排不大可能成为有效、明确的预后生物标志物。

ALK 重排的诊断测试

若干不同的技术可用于 ALK 重排的检测。3 种最常被报道的方法包括：ALK 荧光原位杂交（fluorescence in situ hybridization, FISH）、逆转录聚合酶链式反应（reverse transcription-polymerase chain reaction, RT-PCR）和 ALK 免疫组织化学法（immunohistochemistry, IHC）[69]。遗憾的是，没有一种测试完美地适用于所有样本的临床测试。

ALK 荧光原位杂交

ALK FISH 为目前用于诊断 ALK 重排的金标准技术。在克唑替尼的临床试验中，ALK 重排已首先被应用 Vysis ALK Break-Apart FISH 检验分析（雅培分子）进行确认[55-56,70]。测试使用红色和绿色荧光探针，攻击 ALK 内高度保守的断点区域侧面。无 ALK 重排时，两个交叠的探针产生黄色或融合信号。然而，当 ALK 重排存在时，5′绿色探针和 3′红色探针分离，导致典型的"裂隙"信号（图 35.2）。阳性信号定义为由大于两个信号直径的 5′和 3′信号分离。单一孤立的红色 3′探针的存在，可能是通过 5′结合位点的缺失发生的，也被看作是一个阳性信号[71]。如果≥15% 的细胞核具有分离或孤立的红色信号则认为给定的样本存在 ALK 重排。ALK FISH 的主要优点是它是在克唑

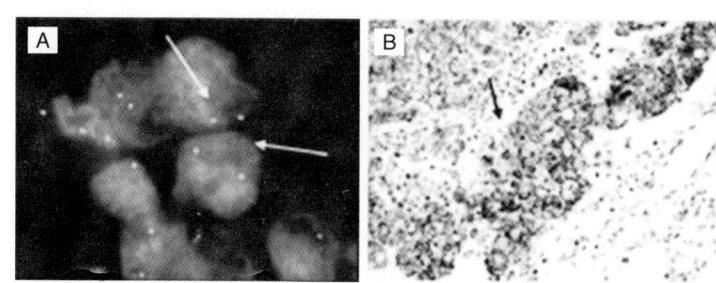

图 35.2（见彩插） A. ALK FISH 揭示了红色和绿色探针分离（箭头），ALK 重排的象征。B. ALK 免疫组化显示 ALK 染色阳性。C. 苏木精和伊红染色显示印戒细胞，一个常见的 ALK 阳性 NSCLC 的形态学特征。摘自 Shaw AT, Yeap BY, Mino-Kenudson M, et al. Clinical features and outcomes of patients with non-small-cell lung cancer who harbor EML4 – ALK, 2009, 27 (26): 4247 – 4253. Reprinted with permission. © (2009) American Society of Clinical Oncology

替尼的临床试验中唯一已通过验证的检验分析技术。ALK FISH 能够在福尔马林固定石蜡包埋的（formalin-fixed paraffin-embedded, FFPE）样本上进行[72]，甚至单个无污染的玻片通常足以做测试。而且，ALK FISH 能检测重排不需要 ALK 5′融合标签或 EML4 – ALK 变异的先备知识。因此，其允许异常 ALK 重排的识别。另一方面，对于例行的临床测试 ALK FISH 还面临若干挑战。特别是，该检验分析需要专业技术和解读经验，因此在日常的病理实验室中也许不能广泛普及。有一点需要注意，ALK FISH 测试比其他技术昂贵。

逆转录聚合酶链式反应（RT-PCR）

对于 ALK 重排的检测，备选的技术为 RT-PCR。此方法使用多路复合引物将框内的 ALK 融合转录子放大[26,33]。而此技术能够获取已知的 ALK 融合变异，RT-PCR 的一个主要的限制是其不能检测涉及异常 5′融合型的 ALK 重排。另外，RT-PCR 结果依赖测试样本的 RNA 的有效性和质量。因为 RNA 在 FFPE 组织中常常退化，早期的对于 ALK 重排的 RT-PCR 筛选工作需要新鲜冷冻的样本[17, 26, 33, 37]。最近，已开发出市场上可行的 RT-PCR 技术，使得 FFPE 样本可以测试[73-75]。虽然如此，作为对克唑替尼的响应预测因素，预期的 RT-PCR 和 ALK FISH 之间还没有进行对比。

免疫组织化学（IHC）

在免疫组织化学（immunohistochemistry, IHC）广泛应用于日常病理实践且正常成人组织中缺乏 ALK 表达的情况下，IHC 已被提议作为 ALK 重排的一种备选检测方法。ALK IHC 现在被用作非霍奇金淋巴瘤的筛选工具。遗憾的是，在 NSCLC 中采用 ALK IHC 出现了较多问题，因为与 ALCL 中所观测到的相比，EML4 – ALK 重排导致 ALK 融合蛋白质表达水平较低[76]。

3 种不同的 ALK IHC 抗体已被研究：ALK1（DAKO, Carpinteria, CA）、D5F3（Cell signaling Technologies, Beverly, MA）和 5A4（Novacastra, Newcastle Cpon Tyne, UK）[52, 59, 76-79]。最初的研究使用的是 ALK1 抗体[52]。而特异性的、于 ALK FISH 阳性样本之中，对 ALK 重排的检测此抗体灵敏度低。随后一系列试验证明此抗体的灵敏度可通过各种信号放大策略而改善[29, 52, 80]。最近，有关两种追加的抗体 D5F3 和 5A4 的数据出现，这两种表现出高灵敏度且其特异度适用于 NSCLC 样本中 ALK 重排的检测[59, 76-79]。ALK IHC 有望成为低成本且快速筛选 ALK 重排的工具。近年来，全自动化及标准化的 ALK IHC 系统已被开发应用于临床实践。一旦这些系统经过检验并经监管机构批准，筛选方法可只包括 ALK IHC 或者与 ALK FISH 相结合。

ALK 抑制剂：克唑替尼

NSCLC 中 ALK 重排的发现立刻引发了研究者对识别此靶点的小分子抑制剂的兴趣。在症状出现之前的测试中，ALK TKI 与 ALK 阳性细胞株和小鼠模型形成鲜明的对比，表现明显活跃，为在临床中追求类似的策略提供了有力的理论依据[17, 26-28, 81]。第一种在 ALK 阳性患者中测试的 ALK 抑制剂即克唑替尼，一种口服小分子酪氨酸激酶。尽管此药物最初是作为间质上皮细胞转化生长因子（c-MET）抑制剂而开发的，很快人们就认识到在细胞株检测分析中克唑替尼以25～50 nmol/L的半极大抑制浓度值有效地抑制了ALK[81-82]。

临床疗效

人体应用克唑替尼研究的第一阶段（PROFILE 1001）于2006年启动，早于NSCLC中的 EML4-ALK（表35.1）的发现[17,70]。这一国际性、多中心临床试验，包括一个剂量递增组群以及一个最大耐受剂量（maximum tolerated dose，MTD）的剂量扩充组群。NSCLC中 EML4-ALK 报道[17]不久之后，两个 ALK 阳性的 NSCLC 患者接受克唑替尼剂量递增试验期间得到了引人瞩目的症状改善[70]。基于这些早期结果，研究点开始预期筛选 ALK 重排的患者。试验还做出了改进，使ALK 阳性 NSCLC 的患者进入到每天 2 次 250mg MTD 的扩大分子组群[70]。在此试验最近更新的结论中，已参加的 NSCLC 的患者总数为 149 例[55]。根据 ALK FISH 测试，所有参与者均为 ALK 重排阳性。在 143 例可评估的患者中，客观有效率（objective response rate，ORR）为 60.8%，包括 3 例 CR 和 84 例 PR。疾病控制率（即 CR、PR 或 SD）第 8 周为 82.5%，第 16 周为 70.6%。总计超过 90% 的 ALK 阳性患者经历了某种程度的肿瘤缩小（图35.3）。重要的是，这些反应似乎是独立且持久的。接受克唑替尼患者的中位无进展生存期（PFS）约为 10 个月。数据截止时中位总生存期还未得出数据[55]。

类似的正在进行的克唑替尼的第二阶段研究始于 2009 年（PROFILE1005；临床试验，官方ID：NCT00932451）。这项单组研究包括晚期、ALK 阳性 NSCLC 已经进行一种或多种治疗后进展的患者。在此次试验的初步报告中，克唑替尼显示出高的 ORR（60%）及近 8 个月的中位 PFS[56]。生活质量和患者症状出现统计学意义上的显著改善（例如咳嗽、呼吸困难、失眠、疲劳）。2011 年 8 月，根据首批参加 PROFILE 1001 试验的 136 例患者和参加 PROFILE 1005 试验的 119 例患者的有效率，克唑替尼获得了美国 FDA 加速批准[83]。此批准条件是正在进行中的将克唑替尼与标准的细胞毒类化疗进行对比的随机试验（PROFILE 1007；临床试验，官方 ID：NCT00932893；PROFILE 1014 报道临床试验，官方 ID：NCT01154140）。其中一个 PROFILE 1007 试验的初步结果近来才被报道[84]。于此第三阶段的随机试验中，之前接受含铂方案治疗的晚期、ALK 阳性 NSCLC 患者，随机分组接受克唑替尼或者培美曲塞、多西他赛两者中的一种作为二线治疗。在初步报告中，克唑替尼治疗在延长主要终点 PFS 上更有优势。未来将克唑替尼与常规化疗进行比较的临床试验可不检测总生存的差别，因为治疗组之间的交叉可能很普遍。在目前缺少随机化数据的情况下，克唑替尼对总生存期的影响是以对参加克唑替尼第一阶段研究的患者进行回顾性分析的方式进行评估[66]。ALK 阳性以克唑替尼二线或三线治疗的患者，与克唑替尼野生型、ALK 阳性控制、施予任何二线疗法的组群相比，1 年和 2 年的总生存期率显著较高（分别为 70% vs 44% 和 55% vs 12%；P = 0.004），这为克唑替尼与提高总生存相关提供了间接证据。

表35.1 克唑替尼在 ALK 阳性 NSCLC 中的选择性临床试验

试验名	分期	描述	客观缓解率	中位PFS
PROFILE 1001（NCT00585195）	I	克唑替尼在晚期 NSCLC 患者中药代动力学和药效学及安全性研究	60%	9.7个月
PROFILE 1005（NCT00932451）	II	克唑替尼在既往接受≥1 种化疗的 ALK 阳性 NSCLC 患者中安全性及有效性研究	60%	8.1个月
PROFILE 1007（NCT00932893）	III	比较 NSCLC 患者中克唑替尼与多西他赛或培美曲塞二线化疗疗效的随机对照试验*	NR	NR
PROFILE 1014	III	比较 ALK 阳性且既往未接受化疗的 NSCLC 中克唑替尼与一线铂类或培美曲塞化疗疗效的随机对照试验	NR	NR

*2012 年 European Society of Medical Oncology 大会的初步试验结果。中位 PFS：中位无进展生存期。ALK：未分化淋巴瘤激酶；NCT：国家临床试验；NR：未报告

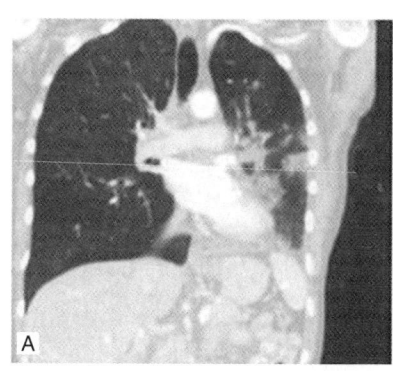 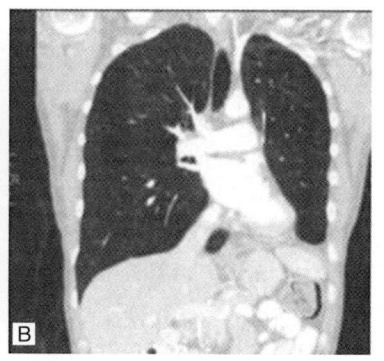

图 35.3　一个晚期 ALK 阳性 NSCLC 患者的显著影像学改变。A. 展示克唑替尼治疗前的影像。B. 表现克唑替尼治疗 8 周后的影像

安全性

总的来说，克唑替尼治疗耐受性良好。常见的治疗相关不良反应事件（treatment-related adverse event，TRAE）包括胃肠道反应，如恶心、呕吐、便秘和腹泻[55-56,70]。大多数患者（50% ~ 64%）也会出现视觉障碍，这通常发生在开始药物治疗的几天之内。这类视觉障碍通常被描述为光线轨迹、闪烁或图像存留，几乎总是与从黑暗到光环境的转换相关。就严重程度而言，目前大多数视觉干扰为 1 级。一部分 PROFILE 1005 患者经眼科详细检查后发现这些视觉障碍并无眼科改变[85]。

接受克唑替尼治疗的一个亚组的患者中观察到周围性水肿[55,70]。在这些患者中，典型周围性水肿通常发生在治疗 2 ~ 3 个月后，考虑可能与克唑替尼抑制了 MET 有关[86]。其他的主要毒性包括肝功能检查指标升高。特别是有 13% 和 9% 的患者的谷丙转氨酶（ALT）和谷草转氨酶（AST）升高[55,83]，常发生在开始治疗后 8 周内，通常是可逆的。亦有报道 7% 和 3% 的患者出现 3 或 4 级 ALT 或 AST 升高。另外，5 例严重潜在的药物相关肝脏毒性已报道（1%），其中 2 例致死[87]。治疗中断后，可能允许继续减少剂量的克唑替尼治疗，但一些患者需要终止治疗。

据报道，1.6% 的患者接受克唑替尼出现罕见的严重或危及生命的不良事件是肺炎[70,83]，导致克唑替尼治疗终止。与克唑替尼相关的其他不良事件包括肾囊肿、QTc 间期延长和无症状的窦性心动过缓[70,83,88]。最后，一个小系列报告显示男子在接受克唑替尼治疗时总睾酮水平迅速减少[89]。这种异常的临床影响和睾酮替代的重要性目前还不清楚。

克唑替尼的获得性耐药

克唑替尼长期治疗的有效性已明显受获得性耐药的限制。获得性耐药的机制大致可概括如下：①靶点的遗传学改变（即 ALK）；②激活替代物或旁路、信号转导通路。获得性耐药最早的报告源自一例 28 岁 ALK 阳性患者经克唑替尼治疗后达 PR，但 5 个月后进展[90]。从这个患者胸腔积液标本的深度测序发现 2 个不重叠的二次突变，L1196M 和 c1156y，位于 ALK 酪氨酸激酶结构域。每个突变都独立赋予体外克唑替尼耐药。值得注意的是，该 *L1196M* 突变发生在保守的 *ALK*"守门"残基，类似于 *EGFR* 的 T790M 和 *ABL* 的 T315I。在随后的克唑替尼获得性耐药报道中，继发的 *ALK* 突变已在大约 30% 的病例中确定[91-93]。这些突变分布在整个激酶和包括错义突变（l1152R、G1202R、S1206Y、G1269Y）和插入（1151Tins）。在体外，这些继发性突变展示对克唑替尼和下一代 ALK 酪氨酸激酶抑制剂灵敏度的差异[91]。

旁路信号是另一个潜在的克唑替尼耐药机制，特别是已经在 ALK 阳性细胞系观察到上调 EGFR 信号增加克唑替尼耐药性[48,91,94]。与这些临床前研究结果一致的是，Katayama 和他的同事们发现，近一半的 ALK 阳性患者观察到克唑替尼耐药的同时 EGFR 活化的免疫组织学证据[91]。在同一研究中，克唑替尼耐药患者中 KIT 基因扩增也被识别，提示异常 KIT 激活也可能介导耐药。其他潜在的目前已报道的克唑替尼耐药机制还包括 *EGFR* 和

KRAS 突变的出现[92]。一个亚组的患者也可出现 ALK 融合基因扩增[91-92]。最后，同一患者出现多种不同的耐药机制[91-92]，这表明，联合治疗对克服耐药可能是必要的。

其他系统疗法

其他系统性治疗 ALK 重排患者的方法的疗效已通过小的回顾性研究得到显著验证[36-67]。在一群 ALK 重排、EGFR 突变或野生型患者中发现，与铂类为基础的化疗患者 ORRs 和 TTP 相似[36]。中位总生存 3 组相似。此外，在一些回顾性研究中，在 ALK 阳性患者中也检测到表皮生长因子受体 TKIs[36,64,67]。同时，这些报告显示接受 EGFR-TKIs 治疗的 ALK 阳性患者的 ORRs 为 0，中位 PFS 为 1.4~1.6 个月。

最近，一些回顾性研究表明，细胞毒性药物培美曲塞可能与增强 ALK 重排患者的反应相关[95-96]。在一份报告中，ALK 阳性接受二线培美曲塞化疗的患者相比表皮生长因子受体突变或野生型患者有较高的反应率和 TTP 延长[96]。在一个单独的研究中，Camidge 等人报道 19 例 ALK 阳性患者接受含培美曲塞方案化疗的中位 PFS 为 9 个月，而 ALK、EGFR 和 KRAS 基因阴性患者的中位 PFS 仅为 4 个月[95]。最近，Shaw 等人报道了培美曲塞治疗 121 例 ALK 阳性和 266 例 ALK 阴性、EGFR 野生型患者的多中心回顾性研究的发现[97]。这项研究表明培美曲塞治疗 ALK 阳性和 ALK 阴性患者，除了培美曲塞联合一线铂类化疗外，PFS 无差异。在后者情况下，中位 PFS 在 ALK 阳性患者为 8.5 个月，而在 ALK、EGFR 和 KRAS 基因阴性患者为 5.4 个月（$P=0.018$）。有趣的是，对没有或有少量吸烟史的患者，ALK 阳性和 ALK 阴性患者的 PFS 相似，这表明吸烟状况可能会混淆培美曲塞的灵敏度和 ALK 重排之间地位的关系。我们期望正在进行的 ALK 阳性患者随机试验的结果可以帮助界定这些关系。

未来发展方向

下一代 ALK 抑制剂

能克服克唑替尼获得性耐药的策略是识别更多有效的新一代 ALK 酪氨酸激酶抑制剂。一批第二代药物目前正在对克唑替尼的敏感性及耐药性进行评估。虽然多个化合物正在临床前试验中，我们将简要回顾一下临床试验中正在审查的药物。

LDK378

LDK378 是一种新颖、高效和选择性的 ALK 抑制剂。在临床前模型中，这种药物已经被证明在体外和体内对 ALK 的高效活性[98]。此外，初步报告，LDK378 首次应用于人类的 I 期研究（临床试验，官方 ID：NCT01283516）显示了其有前景的抗肿瘤活性[99]。基于这些数据，LDK378 由美国 FDA 在 2013 年 3 月授予突破治疗指定状态。

AP26113

AP26113 是一种结构独特、新颖的 ALK 抑制剂，具有相当于克唑替尼约 5~10 倍的效力[100]。在体外，AP26113 已在克唑替尼敏感、含 EML4-ALK 细胞系以及克唑替尼耐药且含 L1196M 把关突变细胞中被证实有活性[100]。AP26113 在 ALK 异种移植模型中还表现出具有抗肿瘤活性。基于这些临床前发现，AP26113 目前正在进行中 I、II 期临床试验（临床试验，官方 ID：NCT01449461）。在这项研究的初步报告中，最常见的不良事件是疲劳和恶心[101]。4 例 ALK 阳性患者中均观察到 PR。LDK378、AP26113 治疗后在中枢神经系统的活性已被观察到，这项研究的剂量探索阶段作为最终的报告正在进行中。

CH5424802

CH5424802 是一种有效、可口服、有独特化工材料的 ALK 抑制剂[102-103]。在最初的临床前研究中，CH5424802 在表达 EML4-ALK 的细胞系和小鼠移植瘤模型中表现出了选择性抗肿瘤活性[102]。此外，CH5424802 诱导异种移植模型中有 EML4-ALK 和随之而来的 L1196M 突变的肿瘤退缩。鉴于这种临床前活性，目前针对 ALK 阳性克唑替尼敏感和耐药的 CH5424802 I、II 期试验正在美国进行（临床试验，官方 ID：NCT01588028）。此外，从一个正在独立进行的针对克唑替尼敏感的 I、II 期试验结果来看，日本 ALK 重排的 NSCLC 呈下降趋势[104,106]。在这项研究的 I 期部分，24 例患者接受 CH5424802 每次 20~300mg，每天 2 次治疗[106]。未观察到剂量限制性毒性，300mg 每天 2 次被认为是 II 期研究的推荐剂量。46 例克唑替尼敏感、ALK 阳性患者在 II 期研究中接受该剂量治疗，43 例患者观察到客观反应（93.5%）。中位治疗时间随访 7.1 个月，中位随访报告时间 7.6 个月的时间。最常见的治疗相关不良事件包括味觉异常、ALT 升高、血清胆红素升高、皮疹和血肌酐升高。与 LDK378 一样，CH5424802 被美国 FDA 授予有突破性进展的治疗方式。

ASP3026

ASP3026 是一种新型选择性的 ALK 抑制剂，已在含 EML4-ALK 细胞系和异种移植模型中证实具有活性[107]。在临床前模型中，ASP3026 也出现积极的反对把关 $L1196M$ 突变。一项 ASP3026 I 期临床试验目前正在进行（临床试验，官方 ID：NCT01401504）。

热休克蛋白 90 抑制剂

获得克唑替尼耐药的另一种方式是针对热休克蛋白 90（HSP90）。HSP90 是一个促进结构折叠和稳定宽范围蛋白质的分子伴侣，包括 EML4-ALK[108-109]。HSP90 抑制剂已在 ALK 阳性细胞系和小鼠模型中表达[109-110]。此外，细胞系的数据表明，尽管克唑替尼获得性耐药，HSP90 仍保持其有效性[100-110]。HSP90 抑制剂在 ALK 阳性 NSCLC 中的临床数据更有限。在一项对 HSP90 的 II 期临床试验，IPI-504 抑制剂对 76 例晚期 NSCLC 的整体反应率为 7%[111]。然而，3 例 ALK 重排患者中，2 例患者出现 PR，1 例有长期 SD。值得一提的是，3 例患者均为克唑替尼敏感。在一项利用 HSP90 抑制剂 AUY922 的 II 期研究初步报告中，21 例（29%）ALK 阳性患者中 6 例为 PR，其中包括 2 例克唑替尼耐药[112]。其他关于克唑替尼耐药 HSP90 抑制剂的研究正在进行。

总 结

总之，目前 ALK 重排是一个代表 NSCLC 的重要分子亚型。像 EGFR 突变，ALK 重排赋予癌基因与 ALK 抑制剂敏感同步状态。克唑替尼的早期成功再次肯定了目前基于肿瘤基因分型的治疗模式。克唑替尼已经是一种对 ALK 阳性的 NSCLC 标准的全身治疗方案。尽管如此，一些重要的挑战仍存在。大多数 ALK 阳性患者应用克唑替尼 1 年后疾病进展。因此，了解克唑替尼的耐药机制和在这些认识基础上识别新的治疗方法以改善 ALK 定向治疗的长期有效性非常有必要。

（李文红　译）

参考文献

[1] Lynch TJ, Bell DW, Sordella R, et al. Activating mutations in the epidermal growth factor receptor underlying responsiveness of non-small-cell lung cancer to gefitinib. N Engl J Med, 2004, 350 (21): 2129-2139.

[2] Paez JG, Janne PA, Lee JC, et al. EGFR mutations in lung cancer: correlation with clinical response to gefitinib therapy. Science, 2004, 304 (5676): 1497-1500.

[3] Pao W, Miller V, Zakowski M, et al. EGF receptor gene mutations are common in lung cancers from "never smokers" and are associated with sensitivity of tumors to gefitinib and erlotinib. Proc Natl Acad Sci USA, 2004, 101 (36): 13306-13311.

[4] Iwahara T, Fujimoto J, Wen D, et al. Molecular characterization of ALK, a receptor tyrosine kinase expressed specifically in the nervous system. Oncogene, 1997, 14 (4): 439-449.

[5] Morris SW, Naeve C, Mathew P, et al. ALK, the chromosome 2gene locus altered by the t (2; 5) in non-Hodgkin's lymphoma, encodes a novel neural receptor tyrosine kinase that is highly related to leukocyte tyrosine kinase (LTK). Oncogene, 1997, 14 (18): 2175-2188.

[6] Pulford K, Lamant L, Morris SW, et al. Detection of anaplastic lymphoma kinase (ALK) and nucleolar protein nucleophosmin (NPM)-ALK proteins in normal and neoplastic cells with the monoclonal antibody ALK1. Blood, 1997, 89 (4): 1394-1404.

[7] Morris SW, Kirstein MN, Valentine MB, et al. Fusion of akinase gene, ALK, to a nucleolar protein gene, NPM, in non-Hodgkin's lymphoma. Science, 1994, 263 (5151): 1281-1284.

[8] Vernersson E, Khoo NK, Henriksson ML, et al. Characterization of the expression of the ALK receptor tyrosine kinase in mice. Gene Expr Patterns, 2006, 6 (5): 448-461.

[9] Bilsland JG, Wheeldon A, Mead A, et al. Behavioral and neurochemical alterations in mice deficient in anaplastic lymphoma kinase suggest therapeutic potential for psychiatric indications. Neuropsychopharmacology, 2008, 33 (3): 685-700.

[10] Chiarle R, Voena C, Ambrogio C, et al. The anaplastic lymphoma kinase in the pathogenesis of cancer. Nat Rev Cancer, 2008, 8 (1): 11-23.

[11] Lee HH, Norris A, Weiss JB, et al. Jelly belly protein activates the receptor tyrosine kinase Alk to specify visceral muscle pioneers. Nature, 2003, 425 (6957): 507-512.

[12] Stoica GE, Kuo A, Aigner A, et al. Identification of anaplastic lymphoma kinase as a receptor for the growth factor pleiotrophin. J Biol Chem, 2001, 276 (20): 16772-16779.

[13] Stoica GE, Kuo A, Powers C, et al. Midkine binds to anaplastic lymphoma kinase (ALK) and acts as a growth factor for different cell types. J Biol Chem, 2002, 277 (39): 35990-35998.

[14] Mano H. ALKoma: a cancer subtype with a shared target. Cancer Discov, 2012, 2 (6): 495-502.

[15] Griffin CA, Hawkins AL, Dvorak C, et al. Recurrent involvement of 2p23 in inflammatory myofibroblastic tumors. Cancer Res, 1999, 59 (12): 2776-2780.

[16] Coffin CM, Patel A, Perkins S, et al. ALK1 and p80 expression and chromosomal rearrangements involving 2p23 in inflammatory myofibroblastic tumor. Mod Pathol, 2001, 14 (6): 569-576.

[17] Soda M, Choi YL, Enomoto M, et al. Identification of the transforming EML4 - ALK fusion gene in non-small-cell lung cancer. Nature, 2007, 448 (7153): 561-566.

[18] Sugawara E, Togashi Y, Kuroda N, et al. Identification of anaplastic lymphoma kinase fusions in renal cancer: largescale immunohistochemical screening by the intercalated antibody-enhanced polymer method. Cancer, 2012, 118 (18): 4427-4436.

[19] Murugan AK, Xing M. Anaplastic thyroid cancers harbor novel oncogenic mutations of the ALK gene. Cancer Res, 2011, 71 (13): 4403-4411.

[20] Mossé YP, Laudenslager M, Longo L, et al. Identification of ALK as552 Lung Cancer a major familial neuroblastoma predisposition gene. Nature, 2008, 455 (7215): 930-935.

[21] Janoueix-Lerosey I, Lequin D, Brugieres L, et al. Somatic and germline activating mutations of the ALK kinase receptor in neuroblastoma. Nature, 2008, 455 (7215): 967-970.

[22] Chen Y, Takita J, Choi YL, et al. Oncogenic mutations of ALK kinase in neuroblastoma. Nature, 2008, 455 (7215): 971-974.

[23] George RE, Sanda T, Hanna M, et al. Activating mutations in ALK provide a therapeutic target in neuroblastoma. Nature, 2008, 455 (7215): 975-978.

[24] Rikova K, Guo A, Zeng Q, et al. Global survey of phosphotyrosine signaling identifies oncogenic kinases in lung cancer. Cell, 2007, 131 (6): 1190-1203.

[25] Webb TR, Slavish J, George RE, et al. Anaplastic lymphoma kinase: Role in cancer pathogenesis and small-molecule inhibitor development for therapy. Expert Rev Anticancer Ther, 2009, 9 (3): 331-356.

[26] Koivunen JP, Mermel C, Zejnullahu K, et al. EML4-ALK fusion gene and efficacy of an ALK kinase inhibitor in lung cancer. Clin Cancer Res, 2008, 14 (13): 4275-4283.

[27] McDermott U, Iafrate AJ, Gray NS, et al. Genomic alterations of anaplastic lymphoma kinase may sensitize tumors to anaplastic lymphoma kinase inhibitors. Cancer Res, 2008, 68 (9): 3389-3395.

[28] Soda M, Takada S, Takeuchi K, et al. A mouse model for EML4 - ALKpositive lung cancer. Proc Natl Acad Sci USA, 2008, 105 (50): 19893-19897.

[29] Takeuchi K, Choi YL, Togashi Y, et al. (2009) KIF5B-ALK, a novel fusion oncokinase identified by an immunohistochemistry-based diagnostic system for ALK-positive lung cancer. Clin Cancer Res, 15 (9): 3143-3149.

[30] Togashi Y, Soda M, Sakata S, et al. KLC1-ALK: A novel fusion in lung cancer identified using a formalinfixed paraffin-embedded tissue only. PLoS One, 2012, 7 (2): e31323.

[31] Pulford K, Lamant L, Espinos E, et al. The emerging normal and disease-related roles of anaplastic lymphoma kinase. Cell Mol Life Sci, 2004, 61 (23): 2939-2953.

[32] Sasaki T, Rodig SJ, Chirieac LR, et al. The biology and treatment of EML4-ALK non-small cell lung cancer. Eur J Cancer, 2010, 46 (10): 1773-1780.

[33] Takeuchi K, Choi YL, Soda M, et al. Multiplex reverse transcription-PCR screening for EML4-ALK fusion transcripts. Clin Cancer Res, 2008, 14 (20): 6618-6624.

[34] Choi YL, Takeuchi K, Soda M, et al. Identification of novel isoforms of the EML4 - ALK transforming gene in non-small cell lung cancer. Cancer Res, 2008, 68 (13): 4971-4976.

[35] Ou SH, Bartlett CH, Mino-Kenudson M, et al. Crizotinib for the treatment of ALK-rearranged non-small cell lung cancer: A success story to usher in the second decade of molecular targeted therapy in oncology. Oncologist, 2012, 17 (11): 1351-1375.

[36] Shaw AT, Yeap BY, Mino-Kenudson M, et al. Clinical features and outcome of patients with non-small-cell lung cancer who harbor EML4 - ALK. J Clin Oncol, 2009, 27 (26): 4247-4253.

[37] Wong DW, Leung EL, So KK, et al. The EML4 - ALK fusion gene is involved in various histologic types of lung cancers from nonsmokers with wild-type EGFR and KRAS. Cancer, 2009, 115 (8): 1723-1733.

[38] Boland JM, Erdogan S, Vasmatzis G, et al. Anaplastic lymphoma kinase immunoreactivity correlates with ALK gene rearrangement and transcriptional up-regulation in non-small cell lung carcinomas. Hum Pathol, 2009, 40 (8): 1152-1158.

[39] Inamura K, Takeuchi K, Togashi Y, et al. EML4 - ALK fusion is linked to histological characteristics in a subset of lung cancers. J Thorac Oncol, 2008, 3 (1): 13-17.

[40] Shinmura K, Kageyama S, Tao H, et al. EML4 - ALK fusion transcripts, but no NPM -, TPM3 -, CLTC -, ATIC -, or TFG-ALK fusion transcripts, in non-small cell lung carcinomas. Lung Cancer, 2008, 61 (2): 163-169.

[41] Martelli MP, Sozzi G, Hernandez L, et al. EML4 - ALK rearrangement in non-small cell lung cancer and non-tumor lung tissues. Am J Pathol, 2009, 174 (2): 661-670.

[42] Takahashi T, Sonobe M, Kobayashi M, et al. Clinicopathologic features of non-small-cell lung cancer with EML4 - ALK fusion gene. Ann Surg Oncol, 2010, 17 (3): 889-897.

[43] Kris M, Johnson B, Kwiatkowski D, et al. Identification of driver mutations in tumor specimens from 1000 patients with lung adenocarcinoma: The NCI's Lung Cancer Mutation Consortium (LCMC). J Clin Oncol, 2011, 29 (suppl): abstr CRA7506.

[44] Popat S, Vieira de Araujo A, Min T, et al. Lung adenocarcinoma with concurrent exon 19 EGFR mutation and ALK rearrangement responding to erlotinib. J Thorac Oncol, 2011, 6 (11): 1962-1963.

[45] Kuo YW, Wu SG, Ho CC, et al. Good response to gefitinib in lung adenocarcinoma harboring coexisting EML4 - ALK fusion gene and EGFR mutation. J Thorac Oncol, 2010, 5 (12): 2039-2040.

[46] Tiseo M, Gelsomino F, Boggiani D, et al. EGFR and EML4 - ALK gene mutations in NSCLC: a case report of erlotinib-resistant patient with both concomitant mutations. Lung Cancer, 2011, 71 (2): 241-243.

[47] Zhang X, Zhang S, Yang X, et al. Fusion of EML4 and ALK is associated with development of lung adenocarcinomas lacking EGFR and KRAS mutations and is correlated with ALK expression. Mol Cancer, 2010, 9: 188.

[48] Sasaki T, Koivunen J, Ogino A, et al. A novel ALK secondary mutation and EGFR signaling cause resistance to ALK kinase inhibitors. Cancer Res, 2011, 71 (18): 6051-6060.

[49] Rimkunas VM, Crosby K, Kelly M, et al. Analysis of receptor tyrosine kinase ROS1 positive tumors in non-small cell lung cancer: Identification of a FIG-ROS1 fusion. Clin Cancer Res, 2012, 18 (16): 4449-4457.

[50] Lee JK, Kim TM, Koh Y, et al. Differential sensitivities to tyrosine kinase inhibitors in NSCLC harboring EGFR mutation and ALK translocation. Lung Cancer, 2012, 77 (2): 460-463.

[51] Yang J, Zhang X, Su J, et al. Concomitant EGFR mutation and EML4 - ALK gene fusion in non-small cell lung cancer. J Clin Oncol, 2011, 29 (suppl): abstr10517.

[52] Rodig SJ, Mino-Kenudson M, Dacic S, et al. Unique clinicopathologic features characterize ALK-rearranged lung adenocarcinoma in the western population. Clin Cancer Res, 2009, 15 (16): 5216-5223.

[53] Shaw AT, Solomon B. Targeting anaplastic lymphoma kinase in lung cancer. Clin Cancer Res, 2011, 17 (8): 2081-2086.

[54] Inamura K, Takeuchi K, Togashi Y, et al. EML4 - ALK lung cancers are characterized by rare other mutations, a TTF-1 cell lineage, an acinar histology, and young onset. Mod Pathol, 2009, 22 (4): 508-515.

[55] Camidge DR, Bang YJ, Kwak EL, et al. Activity and safety of crizotinib in patients with ALK-positive non-small cell lung cancer: updated results from a phase 1 study. Lancet Oncol, 2012, 13 (10): 1011-1019.

[56] Kim D, Ahn M, Shi Y, et al. Results of a global phase II study with crizotinib in advanced ALK-positive non-small cell lung cancer (NSCLC). J Clin Oncol, 2012,

30 (suppl): abstr 7533.

[57] Yoshida A, Tsuta K, Nakamura H, et al. Comprehensive histologic analysis of ALK-rearranged lung carcinomas. Am J Surg Pathol, 2011, 35 (8): 1226-1234.

[58] Yoshida A, Tsuta K, Watanabe S, et al. Frequent ALK rearrangement and TTF-1/p63 co-expression in lung adenocarcinoma with signet-ring cell component. Lung Cancer, 2011, 72 (3): 309-315.

[59] Nishino M, Klepeis VE, Yeap BY, et al. Histologic and cytomorphologic features of ALK rearranged lung adenocarcinomas. Mod Pathol, 2012, 25 (11): 1462-1472.

[60] Doebele RC, Lu X, Sumey C, et al. Oncogene status predicts patterns of metastatic spread in treatment-naive non-small cell lung cancer. Cancer, 2012, 118 (18): 4502-4511.

[61] Choi H, Paeng JC, Kim DW, et al. Metabolic and metastatic characteristics of ALK-rearranged lung adenocarcinoma on FDG PET/CT. Lung Cancer, 2013, 79 (3): 242-247.

[62] Solomon B, Shaw AT. Are anaplastic lymphoma kinase gene rearrangements in non-small celllung cancer prognostic, predictive, or both? J Thorac Oncol, 2012, 7 (1): 5-7.

[63] Yang P, Kulig K, Boland JM, et al. Worse diseasefree survival in never-smokers with ALK+ lung adenocarcinoma. J Thorac Oncol, 2012, 7 (1): 90-97.

[64] Kim HR, Shim HS, Chung JH, et al. Distinct clinical features and outcomes in never-smokers with non-small cell lung cancer who harbor EGFR or KRAS mutations or ALK rearrangement. Cancer, 2012, 118 (3): 729-739.

[65] Varella-Garcia M, Cho Y, Lu X, et al. ALKgene rearrangements in unselected caucasians with non-small cell lung carcinoma (NSCLC). J Clin Oncol, 2010, 28, 15s (suppl): abstr 10533.5

[66] Shaw AT, Yeap BY, Solomon BJ, et al. Effect of crizotinib on overall survival in patients with advanced non-small cell lung cancer harbouring ALK gene rearrangement: A retrospective analysis. Lancet Oncol, 2011, 12 (11): 1004-1012.

[67] Lee JK, Park HS, Kim DW, et al. Comparative analyses of overall survival in patients with anaplastic lymphoma kinase-positive and matched wild-type advanced non-small cell lung cancer. Cancer, 2012, 118 (14): 3579-3586.

[68] Wu SG, Kuo YW, Chang YL, et al. EML4-ALK translocation predicts better outcome in lung adenocarcinoma patients with wild-type EGFR. J Thorac Oncol, 2012, 7 (1): 98-104.

[69] Shaw AT, Solomon B, Kenudson MM. Crizotinib and testing for ALK. J Natl Compr Canc Netw, 2011, 9 (12): 1335-1341.

[70] Kwak EL, Bang YJ, Camidge DR, et al. Anaplastic lymphoma kinase inhibition in non-small-cell lung cancer. N Engl J Med, 2010, 363 (18): 1693-1703.

[71] Camidge DR, Kono SA, Flacco A, et al. Optimizing the detection of lung cancer patients harboring anaplastic lymphoma kinase (ALK) gene rearrangements potentially suitable for ALK inhibitor treatment. Clin Cancer Res, 2010, 16 (22): 5581-5590.

[72] Weickhardt AJ, Aisner DL, Franklin WA, et al. Diagnostic assays for identification of anaplastic lymphoma kinase-positive non-small cell lung cancer. Cancer, 2012, 119 (8): 1467-1477.

[73] Sanders HR, Li HR, Bruey JM, et al. Exon scanning by reverse transcriptase-polymerase chain reaction for detection of known and novel EML4-ALK fusion variants in non-small cell lung cancer. Cancer Genet, 2011, 204 (1): 45-52.

[74] Danenberg P, Stephens C, Cooc J, et al. A novel RT-PCR approach to detecting EML4-ALK fusion genes in archival NSCLC tissue. J Clin Oncol, 2010, 28, 15s (suppl): abstr 10535.

[75] Li T, Mack P, Desai S, et al. Large-scale screening of ALK fusion oncogene transcripts in archival NSCLC tumor specimens using multiplexed RT-PCR assays. J Clin Oncol, 2011, 29 (suppl): abstr 10520.

[76] Mino-Kenudson M, Chirieac LR, Law K, et al. A novel, highly sensitive antibody allows for the routine detection of ALK-rearranged lung adenocarcinomas by standard immunohistochemistry. Clin Cancer Res, 2010, 16 (5): 1561-1571.

[77] McLeer-Florin A, Moro-Sibilot D, Melis A, et al. Dual IHC and FISH testing for ALK gene rearrangement in lung adenocarcinomas in a routine practice: A French study. J Thorac Oncol, 2012, 7 (2): 348-354.

[78] Paik JH, Choe G, Kim H, et al. Screening of anaplastic lymphoma kinase rearrangement by immunohistochemistry in non-small cell lung cancer: correlation with fluorescence in situ hybridization. J Thorac Oncol, 2011, 6 (3): 466-472.

[79] Park HS, Lee JK, Kim DW, et al. Immunohistochemical

screening for anaplastic lymphoma kinase (ALK) rearrangement in advanced non-small cell lung cancer patients. Lung Cancer, 2012, 77 (2): 288-292.

[80] Yi ES, Boland JM, Maleszewski JJ, et al. Correlation of IHC and FISH for ALK gene rearrangement in non-small cell lung carcinoma: IHC score algorithm for FISH. J Thorac Oncol, 2011, 6 (3): 459-465.

[81] Christensen JG, Zou HY, Arango ME, et al. Cytoreductive antitumor activity of PF-2341066, a novel inhibitor of anaplastic lymphoma kinase and c-Met, in experimental models of anaplastic large-cell lymphoma. Mol Cancer Ther, 2007, 6 (12 Pt 1): 3314-3322.

[82] Cui JJ, Tran-Dube M, Shen H, et al. Structure based drug design of crizotinib (PF-02341066), a potent and selective dual inhibitor of mesenchymal-epithelial transition factor (c-MET) kinase and anaplastic lymphoma kinase (ALK). J Med Chem, 2011, 54 (18): 6342-6363.

[83] Food and Drug Administration. Available from: http://www.accessdata.fda.gov/drugsatfda_docs/label/2012/202570s003lbl.pdf.

[84] Shaw A, Kim D, Nakagawa K, et al. Phase III study of crizotinib versus pemetrexed or docetaxel chemotherapy in patients with advanced ALK-positive non-small cell lung cancer. European Society Medical Oncology, abstr LBA1_PR, 2012.

[85] Besse B, Salgia R, Solomon B, et al. Visual disturbances in patients (PTs) with anaplastic lymphoma kinase (ALK)-positive advanced non-small cell lung cancer (NSCLC) treated with crizotinib. Ann Oncol, 2012, 23, 9s (abstr): 1268P.

[86] Spigel D, Ervin T, Ramlau R, et al. Final efficacy results from OAM4558g, a randomized phase II study evaluating MetMab or placebo in combination Targeting ALK Rearrangements 555with erlotinib in advanced NSCLC. J Clin Oncol, 2011, 29 (suppl): abstr 7505.

[87] Schnell P, Safferman A, Barlett C, et al. Clinical presentation of hepatotoxicity-associated crizotinib in ALK-positive (ALK+) advanced non-small cell lung cancer (NSCLC). J Clin Oncol, 2012, 30 (suppl): abstr7598.

[88] Ou SH, Azada M, Dy J, et al. Asymptomatic profound sinus bradycardia (heart rate ≤ 45) in non-small cell lung cancer patients treated with crizotinib. J Thorac Oncol, 2011, 6 (12): 2135-2137.

[89] Weickhardt AJ, Rothman MS, Salian-Mehta S, et al. Rapid-onset hypogonadism secondary tocrizotinib use in men with metastatic non-small celllung cancer. Cancer, 2012, 118 (21): 5302-5309.

[90] Choi YL, Soda M, Yamashita Y, et al. EML4-ALK mutations in lung cancer that confer resistance to ALK inhibitors. N Engl J Med, 2010, 363 (18): 1734-1739.

[91] Katayama R, Shaw AT, Khan TM, et al. Mechanisms of acquired crizotinib resistance in ALK-rearranged lung Cancers. Sci Transl Med, 2012, 4 (120): 120ra17.

[92] Doebele RC, Pilling AB, Aisner DL, et al. Mechanisms of resistance to crizotinib in patients with ALK gene rearranged non-small cell lung cancer. Clin Cancer Res, 2012, 18 (5): 1472-1482.

[93] Lovly CM, Pao W. Escaping ALK inhibition: mechanisms of and strategies to overcome resistance. Sci Transl Med, 2012, 4 (120): 120ps2.

[94] Tanizaki J, Okamoto I, Okabe T, et al. Activation of HER family signaling as a mechanism of acquired resistance to ALK inhibitors in EML4-ALK-positive non-small cell lung cancer. Clin Cancer Res, 2012, 18 (22): 6219-6226.

[95] Camidge DR, Kono SA, Lu X, et al. Anaplastic lymphoma kinase gene rearrangements in non-small cell lung cancer are associated with prolonged progression-free survival on pemetrexed. J Thorac Oncol, 2011, 6 (4): 774-780.

[96] Lee JO, Kim TM, Lee SH, et al. Anaplastic lymphoma kinase translocation: A predictive biomarker of pemetrexed in patients with non-small cell lung cancer. J Thorac Oncol, 2011, 6 (9): 1474-1480.

[97] Shaw AT, Varghese AM, Solomon BJ, et al. Pemetrexed-based chemotherapy in patients with advanced, ALK-positive non-small cell lung cancer. Ann Oncol, 2013, 24 (1): 59-66.

[98] Marsilje TH, Pei W, Chen B, et al. Synthesis, structure-activityrelationship and in vivo efficacy of the novel potentand selective anaplastic lymphoma kinase (ALK) inhibitor5-Chloro-N2-(2-isopropoxy-5-methyl-4-(piperidin-4-yl) phenyl)-N4-(2-(isopropylsulfonyl) phenyl) pyrimidine-2,4-diamine (LDK378) currentlyin phase I and II clinical trials. J Med Chem, 2013, 6.

[99] Shaw A, Camidge R, Felip E, et al. Results of a first-in-human phase I study of the ALK inhibitorLDK378 in advanced solid tumors. Ann Oncol, 2012, 23 (9s): abstr 4400.

[100] Katayama R, Khan TM, Benes C, et al. Therapeutic strategies to overcome crizotinib resistance in non-small cell lung cancers harboring the fusion oncogene EML4-ALK. Proc Natl Acad Sci USA, 2011, 108 (18): 7535-7540.

[101] Gettinger S, Weiss G, Salgia R, et al. A first-in-human dose-finding study of the ALK/EGFR inhibitor AP26113 in patients with advanced malignancies. Ann Oncol, 2012, 23 (9s): abstr 4390.

[102] Sakamoto H, Tsukaguchi T, Hiroshima S, et al. CH5424802, a selective ALK inhibitor capable of blocking the resistant gatekeeper mutant. Cancer Cell, 2011, 19 (5): 679-690.

[103] Kinoshita K, Asoh K, Furuichi N, et al. Design and synthesis of a highly selective, orally active and potent anaplastic lymphoma kinase inhibitor (CH5424802). Bioorg Med Chem, 2012, 20 (3): 1271-1280.

[104] Kiura K, Seto T, Yamamoto N, et al. A first-inhuman phase I/II study of ALK inhibitor CH5424802 in patients with ALK-positive NSCLC. J Clin Oncol, 2012, 30 (suppl): abstr 7602.

[105] Nishio M, Kiura K, Nakagawa K, et al. A phase I/II study of ALK inhibitor CH5424802 in patients with ALK-positive NSCLC; safety and efficacy interim results of the phase II portion. Ann Oncol, 2012, 23 (9s): abstr4410.

[106] Seto T, Kiura K, Nishio M, et al. CH5424802 (RO542802) for patients with ALK-rearranged advanced non-small-cell lung cancer (AF-001JPstudy): A single-arm, open-label, phase 1-2 study. Lancet Oncol, 2013, 4.

[107] Kuromitsu S, Mori M, Shimada I, et al. Antitumor activities of ASP3026 against EML4-ALK-dependent tumor models. Presented at the International Conference of the American Association for Cancer Research-National Cancer Institute-European Organization for Research and Treatment of Cancer. San Francisco: CA, 2011.

[108] Whitesell L, Lindquist SL. HSP90 and the chaperoning of cancer. Nat Rev Cancer, 2005, 5 (10): 761-772.

[109] Chen Z, Sasaki T, Tan X, et al. Inhibition of ALK, PI3K/MEK, and HSP90 in murine lung adenocarcinoma induced by EML4-ALK fusion oncogene. Cancer Res, 2010, 70 (23): 9827-9836.

[110] Normant E, Paez G, West KA, et al. The HSP90 inhibitor IPI-504 rapidly lowers EML4-ALK levels and induces tumor regression in ALK-driven NSCLC models. Oncogene, 2011, 30 (22): 2581-2586.

[111] Sequist LV, Gettinger S, Senzer NN, et al. Activity of IPI-504, a novel heat-shock protein 90 inhibitor, in patients with molecularly defined non-small-cell lung cancer. J Clin Oncol, 2010, 28 (33): 4953-4960.

[112] Felip E, Carcereny E, Barlesi F, et al. Phase II activity of the HSP90 inhibitor AUY922 in patients with ALK-rearranged (ALK+) or EGFR-mutated advanced non-small cell lung cancer (NSCLC). Ann Oncol, 2012, 23 (9s): abstr 4380.

第36章
存在 BRAF 突变的非小细胞肺癌

Renata Ferrarotto, George R. Simon
Department of Thoracic/Head and Neck Medical Oncology, The University of Texas MD Anderson Cancer, Center, Houston, TX, USA

引 言

如今非小细胞肺癌（NSCLC）已经被分为不同的分子实体，而且每一种分子实体都具有其特定的自然病程及相应的靶向治疗。BRAF 是 RAF 家族中的一员，它是由 BRAF 基因编码的一种蛋白激酶。RAF 蛋白家族包含 ARAF、BRAF 及 CRAF 三种同工型。然而，BRAF 是关键下游信号分子 MEK 和 ERK 的主要激活因子。通过 BRAF 突变实现的 RAS-RAF 信号级联的结构性激活会导致肿瘤细胞失控性增殖、生长和转移。一些临床前研究也证明，BRAF 基因突变可以使 BRAF 不依赖上游指令而发出信号[1-2]。识别这些突变能够使我们利用靶向手段特异性地治疗肿瘤。以下是对 BRAF 失调肿瘤的分子发病机制、临床特点及靶向治疗手段的概述。

存在 BRAF 突变的恶性肿瘤的生物学特点

RAF 家族是调节细胞生长、增殖和分化的促分裂素原活化蛋白激酶（mitogen-activated protein kinase, MAPK）信号级联途径中的一组丝氨酸或苏氨酸激酶。这一途径介导了从细胞表面到细胞核内或胞质内靶点的信号转导。它还可以同其他途径发生交互作用，其中最重要的是磷酸肌醇 3-激酶（PI3K/AKT/mTOR）级联途径[3-4]。

如上文所提到的，已被发现的人类 RAF 同源蛋白包括 ARAF、BRAF 及 CRAF，它们具有相同的氨基酸序列并且都包含一个细胞膜募集所必需的 RAS 结合域，一个与活化紧密相关、与调节蛋白相结合的丝氨酸-苏氨酸结构域以及位于羟基端的一个蛋白激酶结构域[5]。然而，BRAF 的基底激酶活性显著高于其他两种 RAF，并且 BRAF 的突变可能性激活关键的下游分子：MEK 及 ERK[1,6-7]。

RAS-GTP 作用于 BRAF 氨基端调节区内的 RAS 结合域，进而通过构象改变促进了 BRAF 磷酸化并进一步引发了 BRAF 的激活。BRAF 的磷酸化激发了其丝氨酸-苏氨酸激酶活性，从而导致了 MEK1/2 及 ERK1/2 的磷酸化和激活，最终引发了可以引发致癌性转化的这一信号途径的活化[7]。

多个单位点的错义突变可以引发 BRAF 的结构性活化。这些突变主要聚集在外显子 11 和 15 的激酶结构域。外显子 15 第 1799 核苷酸上突变（T1799A）是最常见的一种，占人类恶性实体肿瘤的 90%，这一突变可以导致编码产物第 600 位氨基酸的缬氨酸被谷氨酸取代。突变型 BRAF 的激酶活性是野生型 BRAF 的 500 倍[1]。

尽管绝大多数的 BRAF 基因突变会产生激酶激活效应，仍有一些关于 BRAF 基因显性负相关导致激酶活性下降的报道。这些非激活性突变可以反向激活野生型 CRAF 并通过磷酸化激活 ERK[8]。因此，实体恶性肿瘤中的 BRAF 突变可根据激酶活性被描述为高、中间或受损型[7]。

分子致病机制及人类恶性肿瘤中 BRAF 基因突变的发生频率

体细胞的 BRAF 基因突变发生在大约 60% 的

恶性黑色素瘤、36% 的甲状腺乳头状癌及 10% 的结肠癌中[1,9-11]。

BRAF 突变在恶性黑色素瘤及甲状腺癌中的高发促使人们进行了对肺癌中 BRAF 基因 11 和 15 外显子测序的筛选研究。结果在 1.6%~3.0% 的肺腺癌中发现了错义突变[2,11]。近期一些纳入了更多患者并采用了更佳的筛选技术手段的研究在 3%~4.9% 的筛选对象中检出了突变[12-14]。

重要的一点是，在 NSCLC 中发现的 BRAF 突变约有 50% 为 V600E。它们倾向于发生在女性及不吸烟者中。另外 50% 的 BRAF 突变，即通常所指的非 V600E 突变，分布在 15 外显子第 594~606 密码子及 11 外显子第 446~449 密码子之间的狭窄区域，其中最常见的为 11 外显子的 G469A 突变（39%）。非 V600E 突变几乎总是出现在未戒烟者或既往吸烟者中，而很少出现在恶性黑色素瘤中，这一点也许可以反映出烟草相关的致癌作用[12-13]。

尽管有一些个案报道了与 EGFR 突变同时存在的情况，NSCLC 中几乎所有的 BRAF 突变均倾向于独立于 EGFR 和 KRAS 突变以及 EML4-ALK 重排而单独存在。它也几乎只在肺腺癌中被发现，肺鳞癌中非 V600E 突变的发生率仅为 0.2%[13]。

BRAF 突变型恶性黑色素瘤及结直肠癌

为了更好地理解 BRAF 突变型 NSCLC，我们将在本小节介绍关于 BRAF 突变型恶性黑色素瘤及结直肠癌的几个主要临床试验的研究结果。V600E 型突变占 BRAF 突变型恶性黑色素瘤突变类型的 70%~90%，另外 10%~30% 则为 600 密码子赖氨酸被谷氨酸所取代（V600K）[15]。

恶性黑色素瘤中 V600E 突变的高发生率导致了以这一遗传学异常为靶点的药物的开发。威罗菲尼（Zelboraf, Genentech Inc. San Francisco, CA）是 V600E 突变型 BRAF 激酶结构域的第一代抑制剂。一项纳入了 675 例带有 BRAF V600E 突变转移性恶性黑色素瘤患者的关键性 III 期临床试验，对一线治疗采用威罗菲尼与选择达卡巴嗪进行了比较，结果显示二者的反应率（RR）分别为 48% 及 5%，中位无进展生存期（MPFS）分别为 5.3 个月及 1.6 个月（$P<0.001$）。半年总生存率（OS）方面，威罗菲尼组为 84%［95% CI（78%，89%）］，达卡巴嗪组为 64%［95% CI（56%，73%）］[16]。另一项 III 期临床试验比较了第二代 BRAF V600E 突变的激酶抑制剂达拉非尼和达卡巴嗪一线治疗 BRAF V600E 突变阳性的转移性恶性黑色素瘤的效果，结果显示二者的 RR 分别为 50% 及 6%，PFS 分别为 5.1 个月及 2.7 个月，HR 为 0.30［95% CI（0.18，0.51）；$P<0.0001$］。值得注意的是，接受达拉非尼治疗的患者中观察到了脑转移灶的缩小[17]。

然而，BRAF 抑制剂在结直肠癌中的应用目前尚未出现激动人心的效果。在一项评估威罗菲尼治疗带有 BRAF V600E 突变的转移性结直肠癌的 IB 期临床试验中，21 例患者中仅 1 例出现了部分缓解，PFS 为 3.7 个月[18]。BRAF 抑制剂在结直肠癌中作用微弱的一个可能原因在于结直肠癌中 EGFR 的活化，这一活化通过反馈环触发持续的 MAPK 信号传导和（或）抗凋亡的 PI3K/AKT 途径激活，最终导致对 BRAF 抑制剂的原发或获得性耐药[19-21]。

目前，美国 FDA 已批准将威罗菲尼及达拉非尼用于存在 BRAF V600E 突变的转移性恶性黑色素瘤患者。在结直肠癌中，意在评估 BRAF 抑制剂联合 EGFR 或 PI3K 抑制剂治疗效果的研究正在进行中[21]。

BRAF 突变型 SCLC

BRAF 突变的诊断

BRAF 突变往往在采用复合方式进行逆转录酶-聚合酶链反应（reverse transcriptase-polymerase chain reaction, RT-PCR）时被发现。RT-PCR 的一个优势在于可以高度灵敏地鉴别出所有类型的 BRAF 突变基因转录。实际上，那些采用常规 PCR 检测技术的研究机构面临着数个挑战[22]。首先，这项技术的复杂性本身将这一检测形式限制在了较大的癌症中心或商业化的 CLIA（clinical laboratory improvement amendments，临床实验室改进修正体系）认证的实验室；其次，任何以 PCR 为基础的方法必须整合所有已知 BRAF 突变转录物已被验证的引物对；再次，从福尔马林固定组织和石蜡包埋的组织中提取质量合格的 RNA 较困难。考虑到这些条件限制，一个临床诊断实验室将难以完成 BRAF 基因突变的常规检测，故而使得将组织送到专业化中心或实验室进行检测成了惯例[23-24]。

BRAF 突变型 NSCLC 的临床特征

在获得明确的关于人口统计学特征的结论之前，这一独特的分子实体的临床特点有待于进一步的经验积累。从有限的已发表的信息来看，一组具有 BRAF 突变的 NSCLC 患者（n=18）的中位年龄为 64 岁，其中 61% 为女性，所有患者均为白人。这种突变在白人中已属罕见，而在亚洲人中似乎更为罕见。它也几乎不与 EGFR 突变、KRAS 突变及 ALK 重排等更为常见的基因变异类型同时出现。不同于 EGFR 突变和 ALK 重排，BRAF 突变更常见于既往吸烟或尚未戒烟者。实际上，来自 Sloan-Kettering 纪念医院的这 18 例患者均属于有吸烟史或仍未戒烟者。除了这些细节，进一步的临床特征，即这类疾病的自然病史、对化疗的治疗反应、是否易出现脑转移及其他临床特点将随着经验的积累逐渐为人们所知[12]。

BRAF V600E 突变型 NSCLC 的治疗

目前，BRAF 抑制剂治疗肺癌的临床数据是有限的。Gautschi 等报道了首例对威罗菲尼治疗有反应的 V600E 突变型转移性肺腺癌。不幸的是，由于体力评分低下及并发症的作用，该例患者在开始治疗后不久便死亡，故并未从该治疗中取得显著的临床获益[25]。

最近，Peters 等报道了一例从不吸烟的 66 岁男性患者，在同时存在胸膜、淋巴结及肝脏转移的情况下一线应用培美曲塞联合顺铂治疗及培美曲塞维持治疗，之后出现进展。经过分析发现肿瘤存在 BRAF V600E 突变，于是该患者于 2012 年 9 月起开始了威罗菲尼治疗并于治疗 6 周时获得了完全的代谢缓解。直到 2013 年 7 月该报道发出时，该患者仍在接受威罗菲尼治疗且未出现肿瘤相关的任何症状[26]。

肺腺癌中最有力的临床数据来自于一项纳入了 40 例带有 BRAF V600E 突变的转移性肺腺癌患者、意在评估达拉非尼治疗效果的 II 期临床试验，纳入标准为至少一种含铂药物化疗后肿瘤进展。这组患者中从不吸烟者占 32%，≤40 包/年者占 48%，大于 40 包/年者占 20%。在可供进行安全性分析的 25 例患者中仅有 1 例为正在吸烟者。该试验的主要研究终点为 RR，次要研究终点为 PFS、总生存期（overall survival, OS）、安全性、耐受性、药代动力学及有效时间。可供有效性分析的 20 例患者中，有 8 例（40%）获得了部分缓解（partial response, PR），3 例（15%）疗效为稳定。重度吸烟者似乎并未从该治疗中获益。16% 的患者的有效时间在 6~12 个月，另有 2 例患者的有效时间超过了 12 个月（8%）。来自 25 例患者的数据可供安全性分析。44% 的患者出现了 3 级不良反应事件，并导致了 8% 的患者治疗中断。2 例患者（8%）罹患皮肤鳞癌——一项已知的 BRAF V600E 抑制剂的副作用。最常见的不良反应包括疲劳、食欲减退、乏力、皮疹及恶心。最常见的 3 级毒性反应为低磷血症，有 2 例患者（8%）发生低磷血症[27]。

这些令人鼓舞的初步研究结果提示了 BRAF V600E 突变可以作为预测 BRAF V600E 抑制剂治疗敏感性的生物标记。然而，确切的结论还有待于来自该项研究以及将来其他研究的成熟数据的出现。

非 V600E 型 BRAF 突变

在 NSCLC 中，BRAF V600E 型突变大约占 50%。剩余的被归类为非 V600E 型 BRAF 突变者贡献了其他激活性突变的大部分病例，但是也包括了 BRAF 非激活性突变。

威罗菲尼、达拉非尼等 I 型 BRAF 抑制剂特异度地靶向作用于 V600E 突变型激酶。针对其他类型的 BRAF 活化型突变的作用尚属未知。临床前数据提示，非 V600E 型突变对威罗菲尼耐药却对 MEK 抑制剂敏感[28-29]。评估 MEK 抑制剂治疗 BRAF 突变型 NSCLC 的临床研究正在进行（NCT00888134）。

灭活型 BRAF 突变

在一项包括了 32 例接受达沙替尼治疗的 IV 期 NSCLC 患者的 II 期临床研究中（Sprycel, Bristol Myers Squibb, Inc. princeton, NJ），根据最近一次

的随访情况，1例患者获得了完全缓解并在没有任何进一步治疗的情况下无病生存期达4年[30]。Sen等人研究了这例患者的样本，发现了位于11外显子上的激酶灭活型 BRAF 突变——Y472C，它可以通过反向激活 CRAF 来激活 MED 和 ERK[8]。进一步研究表明，带有 G466V BRAF 突变（属另外一种激酶灭活型突变，存在于大约0.87%的肺腺癌中）的细胞系在体外环境中也对达沙替尼敏感，表现为治疗72h后出现不可逆转的细胞老化。这些现象在 BRAF 野生型或激活型突变的细胞系中未能得到复制。达沙替尼作用于存在 BRAF 激酶活性受损的 NSCLC 细胞系后间接抑制了 CRAF 并引发了 BRAF 的二聚体化，最终通过 ERK 活化导致了癌基因诱导的细胞老化[8]。这一机制解释了为何该患者对达沙替尼有如此显著的反应并提示了灭活型 BRAF 突变可以预测患者对这一药物的敏感性[31]。尚需要进一步的临床评估试验来验证这些回顾性的临床及实验室发现。

BRAF 抑制剂的耐药机制

NSCLC 中 BRAF 抑制剂的耐药机制仍有待阐明。不过，人们已经开始尝试模仿 BRAF V600E 阳性恶性黑色素瘤的耐药机制进行研究。在对 BRAF 抑制剂耐药的 bBRAF V600E 突变型恶性黑色素瘤细胞系中尚未发现这一靶向基因的二次突变。通过建立临床前模型，已经有3条可能的途径被确认，包括以下3条途径。

（1）不依赖 BRAF 的 MARK 途径重激活。BRAF 抑制剂敏感型亲代细胞系依靠 BRAF 完成 MAPK 的激活。BRAF 耐药型细胞提高了 CRAF 和 AFAF 的表达，因而能够利用这两种异构体活化 MAPK 的下游信号传导。这或许提示了这一类耐药的细胞系可能会对 RAS 这一下游分子的抑制剂敏感。然而，将多种不同结构的 MEK 抑制剂作用于 BRAF 抑制剂耐药型细胞，结果仅获得了抑制细胞生长的效应，这也暗示可能同时存在额外的旁路机制[32-33]。

（2）酪氨酸激酶替代受体信号（tyrosine kinase replaces the receptor signal, RTK）途径的差异激活。其他的信号途径可能被激活，尤其是 IGF-1R 受体的上调在 BRAF 抑制剂耐药的 BRAF V600E 突变型细胞系中更为显著。虽然亲代黑色素瘤细胞表达 IGF-1R，但是一些 BRAF 抵抗型黑色素瘤细胞的表面表达更高水平的 IGF-1R。有趣的是，已经有报道指出 IGF-1 介导的信号通路的增强并非由于 IGF-1R 基因的扩增或突变。因此，在长期 BRAF 抑制的前提下 IGF-1R 高表达和信号上调的机制尚待进一步阐明。我们有理由假设，BRAF 和 RTKS 之间存在着可能的交联，尤其是 IGF-1R 依赖性的网络[33-35]。

（3）PI3K 的活化和 AKT 的磷酸化。之前已经有研究者阐述了 PI3K/Akt 抗凋亡途径的活化，要么是通过促进 Akt 磷酸化，要么是通过 PTEN 的纯合缺失。IGF/IGF-1R 轴的上调可以诱发 PI3K 信号通路的增强。然而在体外实验中，尽管外源性 IGF-1 增强了 PI3K 的信号转导，但并不足以引发耐药。于是我们有理由相信是 MAPK 和 IGF-1R/PI3K/AKT 信号途径联合起来共同促进了 BRAF 抑制剂抵抗型细胞的存活和增殖[36]。

因此，联合抑制 RAF/MEK 和 PI3K/AKT 途径或许是治疗 BRAF 抑制剂耐药的 BRAF V600E 突变患者的一种手段。在临床前实验中已经观察到了 MEK 和 PI3K 抑制剂联合应用对 BRAF 抑制剂耐药的黑色素瘤细胞系起到的强烈的细胞毒作用。目前，在此类病例中尚有数个以测试 MEK 和 PI3K 抑制剂联合应用的临床试验正在进行。

总 结

BRAF 突变在大约3%的肺腺癌中出现。将近50%的 BRAF 突变为 V600E 型。剩余的突变被归为非 V600E 型，最常见于11和15外显子。BRAF 灭活型突变已有报道但非常罕见。威罗非尼或达拉非尼或许可以治疗存在 BRAF V600E 突变的肺腺癌患者，并有50%的患者被报道获得了至少6个月的持续有效期[27]。针对非 V600E 型 BRAF 突变的临床研究正在进行，类似 MEK 和 PI3K/AKT 抑制剂联合用药的不同靶向治疗联合应用的模式或许可获得临床收益。另有研究报道，1例罕见的灭活型 BRAF 突变患者应用达沙替尼后获得了临床收益[30]。将来随着经验的积累，我们必将对 BRAF 突变的 NSCLC 中这一相对少见的亚群了解更多。

（韩晓颖 译）

参考文献

[1] Davies H, Bignell GR, Cox C, et al. Mutations of the BRAF gene in human cancer. Nature, 2012, 417 (6892): 949-954. Epub 2002/06/18.

[2] Brose MS, Volpe P, Feldman M, et al. BRAF and RAS mutations in human lung cancer and melanoma. Cancer Res, 2002, 62 (23): 6997-7000. Epub 2002/12/04.

[3] Dhillon AS, von Kriegsheim A, Grindlay J, et al. Phosphatase and feedback regulation of Raf-1 signaling. Cell Cycle, 2007, 6 (1): 3-7. Epub 2007/01/16.

[4] Ramjaun AR, Downward J. Ras and phosphoinositide 3-kinase: partners in development and tumorigenesis. Cell Cycle, 2007, 6 (23): 2902-2905. Epub 2007/11/13.

[5] Moelling K, Heimann B, Beimling P, et al. Serine-and threonine-specific protein kinase activities of purified gag-mil and gag-raf proteins. Nature, 1984, 312 (5994): 558-561. Epub 1984/12/06.

[6] Rajagopalan H, Bardelli A, Lengauer C, et al. Tumorigenesis: RAF/RAS oncogenes and mismatch-repair status. Nature, 2002, 418 (6901): 934. Epub 2002/08/29.

[7] Wan PT, Garnett MJ, Roe SM, et al. Mechanism of activation of the RAF-ERK signaling pathway by oncogenic mutations of BRAF. Cell, 2004, 116 (6): 855-867. Epub 2004/03/24.

[8] Sen B, Peng S, Tang X, et al. Kinase-impaired BRAF mutations in lung cancer confer sensitivity to dasatinib. Sci Transl Med, 2012, 4 (136): 136ra70. Epub 2012/06/01.

[9] Kimura ET, Nikiforova MN, Zhu Z, et al. High prevalence of BRAF mutations in thyroid cancer: genetic evidence for constitutive activation of the RET/PTC-RAS-BRAF signaling pathway in papillary thyroid carcinoma. Cancer Res, 2003, 63 (7): 1454-1457. Epub 2003/04/03.

[10] Samowitz WS, Sweeney C, Herrick J, et al. Poor survival associated with the BRAF V600E mutation in microsatellite-stable colon cancers. Cancer Res, 2005, 65 (14): 6063-6069. Epub 2005/07/19.

[11] Naoki K, Chen TH, Richards WG, et al. Missense mutations of the BRAF gene in human lung adenocarcinoma. Cancer Res, 2002, 62 (23): 7001-7003.

[12] Paik PK, Arcila ME, Fara M, et al. Clinical characteristics of patients with lung adenocarcinomas harboring BRAF mutations. J Clin Oncol, 2011, 29 (15): 2046-2051. Epub 2011/04/13.

[13] Marchetti A, Felicioni L, Malatesta S, et al. Clinical features and outcome of patients with non-small-cell lung cancer harboring BRAF mutations. J Clin Oncol, 2011, 29 (26): 3574-3579. Epub 2011/08/10.

[14] Cardarella S, Ogino A, Nishino M, et al. Clinical, pathological and biological features associated with BRAF mutations in non-small cell lung cancer. Clin Cancer Res, 2013, Epub 2013/07/09.

[15] Menzies AM, Haydu LE, Visintin L, et al. Distinguishing clinicopathologic features of patients with V600E and V600K BRAF-mutant metastatic melanoma. Clin Cancer Res, 2012, 18 (12): 3242-3249. Epub 2012/04/27.

[16] Chapman PB, Hauschild A, Robert C, et al. Improved survival with vemurafenib in melanoma with BRAF V600E mutation. N Engl J Med, 2011, 364 (26): 2507-2516. Epub 2011/06/07.

[17] Hauschild A, Grob JJ, Demidov LV, et al. Dabrafenib in BRAFmutated metastatic melanoma: a multicentre, open-label, phase 3 randomised controlled trial. Lancet, 2012, 380 (9839): 358-365. Epub 2012/06/28.

[18] Kopetz S, Hoff PM, Morris JS, et al. Phase Ⅱ trial of infusional fluorouracil, irinotecan, and bevacizumab for metastatic colorectal cancer: efficacy and circulating angiogenic biomarkers associated with therapeutic resistance. J Clin Oncol, 2010, 28 (3): 453-459. Epub 2009/12/17.

[19] Corcoran RB, Ebi H, Turke AB, et al. EGFR-mediated re-activation of MAPK signaling contributes to insensitivity of BRAF mutant colorectal cancers to RAF inhibition with vemurafenib. Cancer Discov, 2012, 2 (3): 227-235. Epub 2012/03/27.

[20] Prahallad A, Sun C, Huang S, et al. Unresponsiveness of colon cancer to BRAF (V600E) inhibition through feedback activation of EGFR. Nature, 2012, 483 (7387): 100-103. Epub 2012/01/28.

[21] Mao M, Tian F, Mariadason JM, et al. Resistance to BRAF inhibition in BRAF-mutant colon cancer can be overcome with PI3K inhibition or demethylating agents. Clin Cancer Res, 2012, 19 (3): 657-667. Epub 2012/12/20.

[22] Szankasi P, Reading NS, Vaughn CP, et al. A quantitative allele-specific PCR test for the BRAF V600E muta-

tion using a single heterozygous control plasmid for quantitation: A model for qPCR testing without standard curves. Journal of Molecular Diagnostics, 2013, 15 (2): 248 – 254. Epub 2013/01/15.

[23] Gonzalez D, Fearfield L, Nathan P, et al. BRAF mutation testing algorithm for vemurafenib treatment in melanoma: recommendations from an expert panel. British Journal of Dermatology, 2013, 168 (4): 700 – 707. Epub 2013/01/31.

[24] Lade-Keller J, Romer KM, Guldberg P, et al. Evaluation of BRAF mutation testing methodologies in formalinfixed, paraffin-embedded cutaneous melanomas. Journal of Molecular Diagnostics, 2013, 15 (1): 70 – 80. Epub 2012/11/20.

[25] Gautschi O, Pauli C, Strobel K, et al. A patient with BRAF V600E lung adenocarcinoma responding to vemurafenib. J Thorac Oncol, 2012, 7 (10): e23 – 24. Epub 2012/06/30.

[26] Peters S, Michielin O, Zimmermann S. Dramatic response induced by vemurafenib in a BRAF V600Emutated lung adenocarcinoma. J Clin Oncol, 2013, 31 (20): e341 – 344. Epub 2013/06/05.

[27] Planchard D, Mazieres J, Riely GJ, et al. Interim results of phase II study BRF113928 of dabrafenib in BRAF V600E mutation-positive non-small cell lung cancer (NSCLC) patients. J Clin Oncol, 2013, 31 (Suppl).

[28] Yang H, Higgins B, Kolinsky K, et al. RG7204 (PLX4032), a selective BRAFV600E inhibitor, displays potent antitumor activity in preclinical melanoma models. Cancer Res, 2010, 70 (13): 5518 – 5527. Epub 2010/06/17.

[29] Trejo CL, Juan J, Vicent S, et al. MEK1/2 inhibition elicits regression of autochthonous lung tumors induced by KRASG12D or BRAFV600E. Cancer Res, 2012, 72 (12): 3048 – 3059. Epub 2012/04/19.

[30] Johnson FM, Bekele BN, Feng L, et al. Phase II study of dasatinib in patients with advanced non-small-cell lung cancer. J Clin Oncol, 2010, 28 (30): 4609 – 4615. Epub 2010/09/22.

[31] Collado M, Serrano M. Senescence in tumours: Evidence from mice and humans. Nat Rev Cancer, 2010, 10 (1): 51 – 57. Epub 2009/12/24.

[32] Alcala AM, Flaherty KT. BRAF inhibitors for the treatment of metastatic melanoma: Clinical trials and mechanisms of resistance. Clin Cancer Res, 2012, 18 (1): 33 – 39. Epub 2012/01/05.

[33] Villanueva J, Vultur A, Lee JT, et al. Acquired resistance to BRAF inhibitors mediated by a RAF kinase switch in melanoma can be overcome by cotargeting MEK and IGF-1R/PI3K. Cancer Cell, 2010, 18 (6): 683 – 695. Epub 2010/12/16.

[34] Villanueva J, Vultur A, Herlyn M. Resistance to BRAF inhibitors: Unraveling mechanisms and future treatment options. Cancer Res, 2011, 71 (23): 7137 – 7140. Epub 2011/12/02.

[35] Girotti MR, Marais R. Deja vu: EGF receptors drive resistance to BRAF inhibitors. Cancer Discov, 2013, 3 (5): 487 – 490. Epub 2013/05/10.

[36] Atefi M, von Euw E, Attar N, Ng C, et al. Reversing melanoma cross-resistance to BRAF and MEK inhibitors by cotargeting the AKT/mTOR pathway. PLoS One, 2011, 6 (12): e28973. Epub 2011/12/24.

第 37 章
肺癌预后及预测的生物标志物特征

Johannes R. Kratz[1], David M. Jablons[2]
1. Departmentof Surgery, Massachusetts General Hospital, Boston, MA, USA
2. Department of Surgery, University of California, San Francisco, CA, USA

引 言

IA 期非小细胞肺癌（NSCLC）的 5 年生存率为 73%，而转移性Ⅳ期患者则只有 17%[1]。手术切除是Ⅰ期、Ⅱ期 NSCLC 的主要治疗手段，也是目前治愈局部病变的唯一希望[2-3]。局限期 NSCLC 完整手术切除后 5 年生存率为 53%[4]，仍低于乳腺癌（98%）[4]和结直肠癌（91%），说明只依据 TNM 分期并不能准确预测肺癌患者的风险和预后[5-6]。

虽然这些患者数据统计的差异在某种程度上可以解释早期肺癌与其他实体瘤的结果差异，但目前普遍认为肺癌相对于其他实体瘤而言具有特殊的侵袭性，在确诊时也更容易发生微转移[7]。该现象已被相关临床试验证实：一项随机前瞻性研究比较了肺叶切除与局限性（段或楔形）切除的Ⅰ期肺癌患者，发现接受肺叶切除的患者局部复发率更低[8]。因此，肺叶切除术被广泛用作Ⅰ期肺癌的标准治疗方法，其既保留了足够的正常肺组织，也更完整的切除隐匿微转移灶。目前所面临的最大挑战之一是：在当前影像学技术和病理学方法都无法检测到的情况下，如何能更准确地预测哪些患者在疾病的早期阶段就已发生亚临床转移。

一旦预测到哪些患者面临亚临床转移及早期死亡风险提高，就应尽可能改变治疗方案。尽管局限性疾病的总体疗效较差，但多个随机对照试验并不支持辅助治疗能给Ⅰ期患者带来显著获益[9]。事实上，如果能确定哪些肿瘤具有高度侵袭性，就可以特异性分选并给予这些患者辅助治疗和（或）扩大根治切除，从而带来最终的临床获益。局部复发及远处转移患者，如被证实是低侵袭性肿瘤，同样也可以从积极的治疗方案中获益。同时，低侵袭性肿瘤患者，也可以减少正常肺组织切除体积并避免化疗毒性反应。通过提供针对性治疗以改善患者预后，已经成为近几年改善乳腺癌和大肠癌患者预后方面的趋势。

TNM 肺癌分期系统是在 2009 年由肺癌国际分期委员会修订并推荐使用的，旨在使目前的分期系统现代化和全球化，以反映最新技术和治疗的进展[10]。尽管对该系统投入了大量精力，但目前的 TNM 分期系统的升级改动仍较少[11]。分子标志物对提高辨别预后水平具有实际意义[12]，因此多名专家推测，肺癌分期系统的下一个重大进展，将由传达肿瘤生物学重要预后信息的生物标志物分类来实现[10,12-13]。

肺癌预后的生物标志物特征

一些研究已经显示了分子生物标志物在细化肺癌预后方面有潜在能力。早在 2001 年，多个研究组报道了肺癌基因表达与正常肺组织相比存在巨大差异。一些研究指出，基因表达模式与患者疗效间存在较强的相关性，这也是有关肺癌预后标志物的首次报道。Bhattacharjee 等报道称，肺腺癌中神经内分泌标志物高表达亚型的预后较差（中位生存期 21 个月，而其他肺腺癌亚类为 41 个月）[14]。但Ⅱ型肺泡标志物高表达的肺腺癌亚型预后较好（中位生存期为 50 个月，其他亚类的为

33 个月)[14]。2002 年，Beer 等报道了 50 个基因标志物与 I 期患者 3 年死亡风险升高相关 (HR = 2.78)[15]。

此后许多其他团队也报道了 NSCLC 预后生物标志物的特征[16-30]。事实上，已公布的多种预后标志物特征，使临床医生不再怀疑其是否有一天能借助于生物标志物的特点去判断 NSCLC 患者的风险。相反，临床医师开始询问标志物中目前有哪些不仅即将应用于临床，且有足够理论依据支持临床日常使用[31]。

事实上，完成这些生物标志物从实验室向临床的转化是相当困难的。大多数预后标志物都基于芯片研究基础[30-31]。微阵列芯片是一个高难度的临床转化平台，通常需要从冷冻组织样本中提取高质量 RNA，但这在社区医院中往往不可行[30]。此外，芯片的数据存在处理、解读及规范化等方面的难题[32]，导致其难以在商业化实验室中推广和迅速普及。各机构的微阵列芯片基因表达结果并不完全一致[33-34]，使得很多实验室将 real-time PCR 作为来确定芯片结果的标准做法。基于基因芯片的这些显著瓶颈，最近已有多篇研究报道了以定量 PCR 为基础的预后标志物[17,19,21-22,25,35]。不同于芯片标志物临床转化方面的多种理论和技术问题，定量 PCR 则应用广泛、价格低廉、易于解读和复制且非常可靠。事实上，专用底物并非必需；福尔马林固定的石蜡包埋组织标本作为测试底物已在肺[35]和其他实体瘤[36-37]有报道。

临床转化的第二个障碍是多数预后生物标志物缺乏临床应用证据。类似于任何临床模型，预后生物标志物在进入临床实践前必须通过验证[38]。与已提出的多种生物标志物相比，其他预后标记的研发不会有质的改变，仅能小幅度提升预后预测水平。尤其是当使用或重复使用公共可用微阵列数据库获取标志物时更是如此[20]。因此，真正的挑战在于在临床工作中严谨的验证预后生物标志物的特性。模型过度拟合是一个常见的统计学研究现象，往往在应用大量预测值及少数观测值建模时发生[38]。较多预测值使得模型中产生大量统计误差，而无法与患者预后相关的真正生物学特性相关联。不幸的是，目前的普遍做法是在相对较小的研究队列中使用芯片去承载成千上万的预测变量，这使得许多 NSCLC 的预后生物标志物特别容易受到这种统计现象的干扰。事实上，根据所试队列的不同，一项随机芯片生物标记的结果可提高 10% ~ 40% 不等的预测效能时间[39]。尽管多种方法可减少统计学中临床模型的过度拟合[38]，但在独立队列研究中进行生物标志物的盲法验证仍是验证过度拟合模型的参考标准。虽然在既往公布的公共芯片数据库中验证相关标志物是目前常用的方法之一，但该技术并不等同于独立盲法验证，因为潜在标志物在正式发布之前，其效能仍要根据验证分析的结果以决定下一步的修改或否决。

迄今为止，只有两个小组报道了独立盲法验证后的预后生物标记结果。2008 年，Shedden 报道了美国国家癌症研究所的一项大型多中心研究结果，即使用独立队列对多个推荐的预后标志物进行盲法验证[20]。442 例 I ~ III 期切除腺癌患者被分为 177 例和 79 例两个治疗队列，以及 82 和 104 例两个验证队列。4 家参与机构获取了相关芯片数据，并各自独立研发了 8 个预后标志物。这些标志物提交给充当裁判的第五机构并重新分配以进行独立盲法验证。不幸的是，这 8 个标志物在不联合其他临床协变量的情况下没有一个能有效地区分 I 期患者。此外，在他们的模型中，该标志物联合临床协变量区分 I 期患者的检测效能甚至劣于单独应用临床协变量建立的预测模型[20]。该结果并非要否认今后高效、独立验证预后标志物的进一步研发。相反，该研究在预后试验研发和验证理想模型方面，强调了预后生物标志物在临床应用之前，需进行独立盲法验证的重要性。

最近，我们团队报道了非鳞状 NSCLC 中通过大规模定量 PCR 法盲法验证的预后生物标志物[35]。这些标志物的特征主要表现在以下方面：①使用福尔马林固定、石蜡包埋（formalin-fixed, paraffin-embedded, FFPE）组织作为底物并用定量 PCR 检测基因表达，从而使其具有高度实用性并可立即应用于临床。②使用了 11 种预测方法，多种统计技术，并拥有 361 例患者的大型队列以减少过度拟合。③使用多个大型独立队列进行国际性盲法验证，其中包括来自北加州 Kaiser Permanente 系统的 433 例于社区医院接受手术切除的 I 期患者，以及来自中国临床试验联盟（China Clinical Trials Consortium，CCTC）的超过 1000 例肿瘤切除患者。

在加州大学旧金山分校开展的 361 例接受外科手术切除的非鳞状 NSCLC 患者队列研究中，通过对已知肺癌通路中密切相关的 11 个基因的检测确定预后生物标记物，依据相关算法及截点将患者分为低、中、高风险类别。Kaplan-Meier 法对不同风险层次肿瘤分析显示，Kdiser Permanente 验证队列中的 I 期肺癌以及 CCTC 验证队列中的各期肺癌患者的预后表现出高度统计学差异[35]。多变量分析也显示，在调整了年龄、性别、吸烟史、组织学和分期后，风险分类是最强的结果预测值，它提高了 I 期患者的风险识别，这超越了国家综合癌症网络（National Comprehensive Cancer Network，NCCN）用来识别高风险 I 期患者（Kaiser 队列）以及分期（CCTC 队列）的标准[40]。该检测方法也成功地对 T1a 淋巴结阴性肿瘤患者进行了危险分层：对于部分亚组，即使完全清扫阴性淋巴结，其 5 年死亡率也高达几乎 50%[41]。随着新的肺癌筛查标准的制定，未来接受手术切除的 T1a 淋巴结阴性肺癌患者数量将会显著增加，因此预后生物标志物在这些特定人群中的作用将显得尤为重要[42]。

肺癌预测的生物标记物特征

预后生物标志物试图提高患者总生存危险分层的识别效能，而预测生物标志物则试图对接受特定治疗的患者进行风险分层，即治疗有效者与无效者。预测标记物的潜在临床价值是显而易见的。对应答患者进行治疗指导，以期显著改善其预后，同时在无应答者中尽量避免这些疗法的毒副作用。理想情况下，多种预测生物标志物的存在将会让每位患者得到最有效的治疗。

文献中描述的分子生物标志物的预测能力，并不像有强大论据支持的单基因预测生物标志物那样，如与表皮生长因子受体通路相关的标志物（见第 29 章）。然而一些研究发现，越来越多的证据显示预后生物标志物也能预测化疗疗效。2010 年，Zhu 等人报道了在 JBR.10 试验中随机接受顺铂/长春瑞滨化疗或临床观察患者的一种预后生物标志物[43]。在先前公开的四个独立芯片数据中，该标志物被作为生存预后指标。此外，该生物标记物可预测随机接受辅助化疗的高危患者而非低危患者的疾病特异性生存期（HR 分别为 0.33 [95% CI（0.17，0.63）] 及 3.67 [95% CI（1.22，11.06）][43]。另一独立研究小组最近利用 Director's Challenge 数据库研发了单独预测化疗反应的标记物，并在 JBR.10 试验的 69 例患者中进行独立验证[44]。肺鳞癌中与培美曲塞有效及耐药相关的预测标记物在最近也有相关报道[45]。

尽管分子生物标志物的预测能力将会在未来的多项前瞻性随机对照试验中得到确切证实，但需注意的是，目前的临床实践指南，如国家综合癌症网络（NCCN）仍推荐 IB 期高危肿瘤患者接受辅助化疗。很多"高危"肿瘤评价标准（分化程度差、血管侵犯、楔形切除、脏层胸膜受累、缺乏足够的淋巴结取样）并没有进行前瞻性研究来证实标准辅助化疗在这些评价标准下所带来的生存获益。然而鉴于"局限性"NSCLC 患者相比其他实体肿瘤预后较差，多数共识团队如 NCCN 建议高危患者行辅助化疗。因此可以预见，如果能够筛选出优于 NCCN 标准的确切的风险识别工具，将会为临床医生在标志物证实的高危患者中进行辅助治疗提供更坚实的依据。

未来展望

提高个体化预后及个体化治疗是目前肺部肿瘤发展趋势。下一个肺癌分期系统的主要版本几乎肯定会包括分子标志物的应用[10,12-13]。一些有前途的新标志物的研发正在起步，包括从痰[46]、血清[47]和胸腔积液标本[48]中研发的预后标志物，从肺癌干细胞中提取的预后标志物[49-50]以及在福尔马林固定的石蜡包埋组织标本中应用芯片技术分析基因表达[51-52]。肺癌中临床验证的预后及预测生物标志正在蓬勃发展，并有望像其在乳腺癌领域一样得到广泛应用[53]。

（孟　敏　叶　欣　译）

参考文献

[1] Mountain CF. Revisions in the international system for

[1] staging lung cancer. Chest, 1997, 111 (6): 1710 – 1717. PubMed PMID: 9187198. Epub 1997/06/01. eng.

[2] Spira A, Ettinger DS. Multidisciplinary management of lung cancer. N Engl J Med, 2004, 350 (4): 379 – 392. PubMed PMID: 14736930. eng.

[3] Spiro SG, Silvestri GA. One hundred years of lung cancer. Am J RespirCrit Care Med, 2005, 172 (5): 523 – 529. PubMed PMID: 15961694. eng.

[4] Jemal A, Siegel R, Xu J, et al. Cancer statistics, 2010. CA Cancer J Clin, 2010, 60 (5): 277 – 300. PubMed PMID: 20610543. Epub 2010/07/09. eng.

[5] Pfannschmidt J, Muley T, Bulzebruck H, et al. Prognostic assessment after surgical resection for non-small cell lung cancer: Experiences in 2083 patients. Lung Cancer, 2007, 55 (3): 371 – 377. PubMed PMID: 17123661. eng.

[6] Fang D, Zhang D, Huang G, et al. Results of surgical resection of patients with primary lung cancer: A retrospective analysis of 1,905 cases. Ann Thorac Surg, 2001, 72 (4): 1155 – 1159. PubMed PMID: 11603429. eng.

[7] Coello MC, Luketich JD, Litle VR, et al. Prognostic significance of micrometastasis in non-small-cell lung cancer. Clin Lung Cancer, 2004, 5 (4): 214 – 225. PubMed PMID: 14967073.

[8] Ginsberg RJ, Rubinstein LV. Randomized trial of lobectomy versus limited resection for T1 N0 non-small cell lung cancer. Lung Cancer Study Group. Ann Thorac Surg, 1995, 60 (3): 615 – 622; discussion 22 – 23. PubMed PMID: 7677489. eng.

[9] Pignon JP, Tribodet H, Scagliotti GV, et al. Lung adjuvant cisplatin evaluation: A pooled analysis by the LACE Collaborative Group. Journal of Clinical Oncology, 2008, 26 (21): 3552 – 3559. PubMed PMID: 18506026. Epub 2008/05/29. eng.

[10] Goldstraw P, Shepherd FA, Pass HI. The Inter-national Staging System for Lung Cancer. Am Soc Clin Oncol, 2009, 29: 462 – 468.

[11] Rami-Porta R, Crowley JJ, Goldstraw P. The revised TNM staging system for lung cancer. Ann Tho-rac Cardiovasc Surg, 2009, 15 (1): 4 – 9. PubMed PMID: 19262443.

[12] Detterbeck FC, Boffa DJ, Tanoue LT. The new lung cancer staging system. Chest, 2009, 136 (1): 260 – 271. PubMed PMID: 19584208. eng N1-Journal Article N1-Review.

[13] D'Amico TA. Molecular biologic staging of lung cancer. Ann Thorac Surg, 2008, 85 (2): S737 – 742. PubMed PMID: 18222207.

[14] Bhattacharjee A, Richards WG, Staunton J, et al. Classification of human lung carcinomas by mRNA expression profiling reveals distinct adenocarcinoma subclasses. Proc Natl Acad Sci USA, 2001, 98 (24): 13 790 – 13 795. PubMed PMID: 11707567. eng.

[15] Beer DG, Kardia SL, Huang CC, et al. Gene-expression profiles predict survival of patients with lung adenocarcinoma. Nat Med, 2002, 8 (8): 816 – 824. PubMed PMID: 12118244. Epub 2002/07/16. eng.

[16] Roepman P, Jassem J, Smit EF, et al. An immune response enriched 72-gene prognostic profile for early-stage non-small-cell lung cancer. Clin Cancer Res, 2009, 15 (1): 284 – 290. PubMed PMID: 19118056. Epub 2009/01/02. eng.

[17] Boutros PC, Lau SK, Pintilie M, et al. Prognostic gene signatures for non-small-cell lung cancer. Proc Natl AcadSci USA, 2009, 106 (8): 2824 – 2828. PubMed PMID: 19196983. Pubmed Central PMCID: 2636731. Epub 2009/02/07. eng.

[18] Sun Z, Wigle DA, Yang P. Non-overlapping and non-cell-type-specific gene expression signatures predict lung cancer survival. J Clin Oncol, 2008, 26 (6): 877 – 883. PubMed PMID: 18281660. Epub 2008/02/19. eng.

[19] Skrzypski M, Jassem E, Taron M, et al. Three-gene expression sig-nature predicts survival in early-stage squamous cell carcinoma of the lung. Clin Cancer Res, 2008, 14 (15): 4794 – 4799. PubMed PMID: 18676750. Epub 2008/08/05. eng.

[20] Shedden K, Taylor JM, Enkemann SA, et al. Gene expression-based survival prediction in lung adenocarcinoma: A multi-site, blinded validation study. Nat Med, 2008, 14 (8): 822 – 827. PubMed PMID: 18641660. Pubmed Central PMCID: 2667337. Epub 2008/07/22. eng.

[21] Raz DJ, Ray MR, Kim JY, et al. A multigene assay is prognostic of survival in patients with early-stage lung adenocarcinoma. Clin Cancer Res, 2008, 14 (17): 5565 – 5570. PubMed PMID: 18765549. Epub 2008/09/04. eng.

[22] Lau SK, Boutros PC, Pintilie M, et al. Three-gene prognostic classifier for early-stage non small-cell lung cancer. J Clin Oncol, 2007, 25 (35): 5562 – 5569. PubMed PMID: 18065728. Epub 2007/12/11. eng.

[23] Larsen JE, Pavey SJ, Passmore LH, et al. Gene expression signature predicts recurrence in lung adenocarcinoma. Clin Cancer Res, 2007, 13（10）：2946－2954. PubMed PMID：17504995. Epub 2007/05/17. eng.

[24] Larsen JE, Pavey SJ, Passmore LH, et al. Expression profiling defines a recurrence signature in lung squamous cell carcinoma. Carcinogenesis, 2007, 28（3）：760－766. PubMed PMID：17082175. Epub 2006/11/04. eng.

[25] Chen HY, Yu SL, Chen CH, et al. A five-gene signature and clinical out-come in non-small-cell lung cancer. N Engl J Med, 2007, 356（1）：11－20. PubMed PMID：17202451. Epub 2007/01/05. eng.

[26] Raponi M, Zhang Y, Yu J, et al. Gene expression signatures for predicting prognosis of squamous cell and adenocarcinomas of the lung. Cancer Res, 2006, 66（15）：7466－7472. PubMed PMID：16885343. Epub 2006/08/04. eng.

[27] Lu Y, Lemon W, Liu PY, et al. A gene expression signature predicts survival of patients with stage I non-small cell lung cancer. PLoS Med, 2006, 3（12）：e467. PubMed PMID：17194181. Pubmed Central PMCID：1716187. Epub 2006/12/30.

[28] Guo L, Ma Y, Ward R, et al. Constructing molecular classifiers for the accurate prognosis of lung adenocarcinoma. Clin Can cer Res, 2006, 12（11 Pt 1）：3344－3354. PubMed PMID：16740756. Epub 2006/06/03. eng.

[29] Tomida S, Koshikawa K, Yatabe Y, et al. Gene expression-based, individualized outcome prediction for surgically treated lung cancer patients. Oncogene, 2004, 23（31）：5360－5370. PubMed PMID：15064725. Epub 2004/04/06. eng.

[30] Kratz JR, Jablons DM. Genomic prognostic models in early-stage lung cancer. Clin Lung Cancer, 2009, 10（3）：151－157. PubMed PMID：19443334. Epub 2009/05/16. eng.

[31] Subramanian J, Simon R. Gene expression-based prognostic signatures in lung cancer：Ready for clinical use？ J Natl Cancer Inst, 2010, 102（7）：464－474. PubMed PMID：20233996. Pubmed Central PMCID：PMC2902824. Epub 2010/03/18. eng.

[32] Michiels S, Koscielny S, Hill C. Interpretation of microarray data in cancer. Br J Cancer, 2007, 96（8）：1155－1158. PubMed PMID：17342085. eng.

[33] Parmigiani G, Garrett-Mayer ES, Anbazhagan R, et al. A cross-study comparison of gene expression studies for the molecular classification of lung cancer. Clin Cancer Res, 2004, 10（9）：2922－2927. PubMed PMID：15131026. eng.

[34] Xu JZ, Wong CW. Hunting for robust gene signature from cancer profiling data：sources of variability, different interpretations, and recent methodological developments. Cancer Lett, 2010, 296（1）：9－16. PubMed PMID：20579805. Epub 2010/06/29. eng.

[35] Kratz JR, He J, Van Den Eeden SK, et al. A practical molecular assay to predict survival in resected non-squamous, non-small-cell lung cancer：Development and international validation studies. Lancet, 2012, 379（9818）：823－832. PubMed PMID：22285053. Pubmed Central PMCID：3294002. Epub 2012/01/31. eng.

[36] Gray RG, Quirke P, Handley K, et al. Validation study of a quantitative multigene reverse transcriptase-polymerase chain reaction assay for assessment of recurrence risk in patients with stage Ⅱ colon cancer. Journal of Clinical Oncology, 2011, 10, 29（35）：4611－4619. PubMed PMID：22067390. Epub 2011/11/10. eng.

[37] Paik S, Shak S, Tang G, et al. A multigene assay to predict recurrence of tamoxifen-treated, node-negative breast cancer. N Engl J Med, 2004, 351（27）：2817－2826. PubMed PMID：15591335. eng N1-Clinical Trial N1-Journal Article N1-Randomized Controlled Trial N1-Research Support, Non-US Gov't.

[38] Steyerberg EW. Clinical Prediction Models：A Practical Approach to Development, Validation, and Updating. New York：Springer, 2009：497 pp.

[39] Starmans MH, Fung G, Steck H, et al. A simple but highly effective approach to evaluate the prognostic performance of gene expression signatures. PLoS ONE, 2011, 6（12）：e28320. PubMed PMID：22163293. Pubmed Central PMCID：PMC3233554. Epub 2011/12/14. eng.

[40] NCCN Clinical Practice Guidelines in Oncology Non-Small Cell Lung Cancer：National Comprehensive Cancer Network, 2012. Available from：http：//www.nccn.org/professionals/physician_ gls/PDF/nscl.pdf.

[41] Kratz JR, Van den Eeden SK, He J, et al. A prognostic assay to identify patients at high risk of mortality despite small, node-negative lung tumors. JAMA, 2012, 308（16）：1629－1631. PubMed PMID：23093159. Epub 2012/10/25. eng.

[42] Bach PB, Mirkin JN, Oliver TK, et al. Benefits and

harms of CT screening for lung cancer: A systematic review of benefits and harms of CT screening for lung cancer. JAMA, 2012: 1-12. PubMed PMID: 22610500. Epub 2012/05/23. Eng.

[43] Zhu CQ, Ding K, Strumpf D, et al. Prognostic and predictive gene signature for adjuvant chemotherapy in resected non-small-cell lung cancer. J ClinOncol, 2010, 28 (29): 4417-4424. PubMed PMID: 20823422. Pubmed Central PMCID: 2988634. Epub 2010/09/09. eng.

[44] Van Laar RK. Genomic signatures for predicting survival and adjuvant chemotherapy benefit in patients with non-small-cell lung cancer. BMC Med Genomics, 2012, 5: 30. PubMed PMID: 22748043. Pubmed Central PMCID: PMC3407714. Epub 2012/07/04. eng.

[45] Hou J, Lambers M, den Hamer B, et al. Expression profiling-based subtyping identifies novel non-small cell lung cancer subgroups and implicates putative resistance to pemetrexed therapy. J Thorac Oncol, 2012, 7 (1): 105-114. PubMed PMID: 22134068. Epub 2011/12/03. eng.

[46] Leng S, Do K, Yingling CM, et al. Defining a gene promoter methylation signature in sputum for lung cancer risk assessment. Clin Cancer Res, 2012, 18 (12): 3387-3395. PubMed PMID: 22510351. Pubmed Central PMCID: PMC3483793. Epub 2012/04/19. eng.

[47] Bianchi F, Nicassio F, Marzi M, et al. A serum circulating miRNA diagnostic test to identify asymptomatic high-risk individuals with early stage lung cancer. EMBO Molecular Medicine, 2011, 3 (8): 495-503. PubMed PMID: 21744498. Pubmed Central PMCID: PMC3377091. Epub 2011/07/12. eng.

[48] Wang T, Lv M, Shen S, et al. Cell-free microRNA expression profiles in malignant effusion associated with patient survival in non-small cell lung cancer. PLoS ONE, 2012, 7 (8): e43268. PubMed PMID: 22937028. Pubmed Central PMCID: PMC3427341. Epub 2012/09/01. eng.

[49] Perumal D, Singh S, Yoder SJ, et al. A novel five gene signature derived from stem-like side population cells predicts overall and recurrence-free survival in NSCLC. PLoS ONE, 2012, 7 (8): e43589. PubMed PMID: 22952714. Pubmed Central PMCID: PMC3430700. Epub 2012/09/07. eng.

[50] Onaitis M, D'Amico TA, Clark CP, et al. A 10-gene progenitor cell signature predicts poor prognosis in lung adenocarcinoma. Ann Thorac Surg, 2011, 91 (4): 1046-1050; discus-sion 50. PubMed PMID: 21353202. Pubmed Central PMCID: PMC3376444. Epub 2011/03/01. eng.

[51] Xie Y, Xiao G, Coombes KR, et al. Robust gene expression signature from formalin-fixed paraffin-embedded samples predicts prognosis of non-small-cell lung cancer patients. Clin Cancer Res, 2011, 17 (17): 5705-5714. PubMed PMID: 21742808. Pubmed Central PMCID: PMC3166982. Epub 2011/07/12. eng.

[52] Jacobson TA, Lundahl J, Mellstedt H, et al. Gene expression analysis using long-term preserved formalin-fixed and paraffin-embedded tissue of non-small cell lung cancer. Int J Oncol, 2011, 38 (4): 1075-1081. PubMed PMID: 21305253. Epub 2011/02/10. eng.

[53] Paik S. Development and clinical utility of a 21-gene recurrence score prognostic assay in patients with early breast cancer treated with tamoxifen. Oncolo-gist, 2007, 12 (6): 631-635. PubMed PMID: 17602054. eng N1-Journal Article N1-Research Support, N. I. H., Extramural.

第 38 章
肺癌脑转移

Ritsuko U. Komaki, Amol J. Ghia
Department of Radiation Oncology, The University of Texas MD Anderson Cancer Center, Houston, TX, USA

引言

肺癌脑转移瘤在脑转移瘤中所占比例较大。10%~25%的肺癌患者确诊时已出现脑转移，40%~50%的肺癌患者有脑转移的趋势[1]。一些研究证明局部进展期肿瘤局控率提高可能导致脑转发移发生率增加。脑转移瘤患者的预后很差，中位生存时间不超过1年。

脑转移的临床表现多种多样，与肿瘤的位置、数目、瘤周水肿程度、出血等因素相关。症状包括头痛、恶心、呕吐、局部肢体无力、癫痫、意识错乱、共济失调、视觉障碍或偶发的颅内神经麻痹。核磁共振成像（MRI）是目前诊断脑转移瘤的金标准，较CT扫描灵敏度高。

对于脑转移瘤最初的治疗包括口服或静脉给予类固醇激素[5]。癫痫患者应给予抗癫痫治疗。由于预防性抗癫痫治疗有相当大的副反应，现临床应用存在很大争议。脑转移瘤的治疗主要根据肿瘤大小、数目、位置、颅外疾病的状况及患者的一般情况来决定。全脑放疗（whole-brain radiation，WBRT）是基本的治疗方式，可作为手术或立体定向放射外科（stereotacic radiosurgery，SRS）后的辅助治疗或局部治疗后的挽救治疗。SRS具有和手术治疗效果一样的局部控制率，并且毒性反应较小，可以作为主要治疗或挽救治疗方式，尤其是对多发或位置较深的病变及无法手术的患者，手术可迅速缓解巨大肿块所引起的症状，对于单发体积较大的脑转移瘤，可作为首选治疗方法。

本章节包括简单地回顾脑转移瘤的病理机制；讨论治疗脑转移瘤的各种方法，包括手术切除、SRS、WBRT和脑预防性照射（prophylactic cranial irradiation，PCI）；还包括脑放疗相关毒性及关于NSCLC和脑转移瘤生物标记物的最新进展。

脑转移瘤的病理改变

肿瘤的转移机制非常复杂，已在其他章节进行了讨论。简单来说，转移的形成需要肿瘤细胞脱离原发病灶到达远离原发病灶的其他特异组织，并且还需要肿瘤细胞适应转移部位的微环境[7-8]。上皮-间叶组织转化被发现参与了转移的过程，其分子机制仍需进一步研究[8]。转移的其他步骤包括血管生成、肿瘤细胞突破基底膜、肿瘤细胞的运输[9]。肿瘤细胞通过动脉循环进入颅内，造成脑转移的高发[9]。脑实质内的转移常位于毛细血管床丰富的灰白质交界区。脑转移瘤的分布大致与脑血流分布一致，符合Ewing提出的"机械假说"[10]。另一个脑转移瘤分布的解释是"种子与土壤"假说，其最初由Paget提出，最新的"种子与土壤"假说认为转移的肿瘤细胞发生基因突变使其适合在宿主的特定微环境中生长[11]，例如前列腺癌易发生骨转移，乳腺癌和黑色素瘤易发生脑转移。这种肿瘤原发与转移灶相关的分子学机制仍需进一步研究[9]。

治疗方式

手术切除

手术切除可作为缓解脑转移瘤症状或明确其病理机制的主要方式，但是，亚组分析提示预后较好的脑转移瘤患者接受手术切除后提高了生存期。在20世纪80年代的一项重要研究中，Patchell等开展的一项随机对照试验研究了手术在48例单发脑转移瘤接受WBRT患者中的作用[12]。特别需要指出的是，将怀疑为脑转移瘤的患者随机分为活检后行WBRT与手术切除后行WBRT两组。WBRT的总剂量为36Gy，分12次。对于接受手术切除的患者，局部复发率（52% vs 20%）与生活质量（2个月 vs 9个月功能独立）明显改善。另外，手术切除组的生存时间（3个月 vs 9个月）与神经性死亡时间（6个月 vs 14个月）亦明显改善，其手术死亡率（4%）与发病率（8%）也是可以接受的。

另外一个荷兰学者主导的Ⅲ期临床试验将患者分为两组，一组接受WBRT（总剂量40Gy，单次2Gy，每天2次），另一组接受上述WBRT及手术切除治疗[13]。结果显示手术切除组的中位生存期（10个月 vs 6个月）提高，尤其是颅外病变稳定的患者。确实，对于身体状态良好、单发脑转移瘤、颅外病变稳定的患者，我们提倡局部治疗。手术后是否给予放射辅助治疗，将在本章节后面部分继续讨论。

立体定向放射外科（SRS）

神经外科医生Lars Leksell 1951年提出了放射外科的概念，17年后第一台γ刀原型机由Karolinska研究所制造出来。立体定向放射外科（stereotactic radiosurgery，SRS）定义为通过立体适形的方式一次给予目标大剂量放疗，同时给予周围正常组织最小的剂量[14]。1987年美国匹兹堡大学医疗中心安装了第一台γ刀[15]。时至今日，SRS仍是脑转移瘤治疗非常重要的治疗方式[16]。SRS可以通过多种放疗技术，包括γ刀、直线加速器或射波刀等实现。

RTOG开展了许多关于SRS治疗脑转移瘤的临床试验。RTOG90-05试验对168例既往接受过SRS治疗的原发或转移性颅内病变的患者进行研究，通过评价最大耐受放疗剂量，探寻针对脑转移瘤的最佳放疗剂量[17]。最大耐受剂量的确定依据肿瘤大小，肿瘤直径≤2cm的最大耐受剂量为24Gy，直径为2.1~3cm的病变最大耐受剂量为18Gy，3.1~4cm的病变最大耐受剂量为15Gy。然而，直径≤2cm的病变真实最大耐受剂量并未确定，因为研究者的限定剂量不超过24Gy。值得注意的是，放射性脑坏死的2年发生率为11%。后续的研究提示针对直径≤2cm的病变，20Gy和24Gy的控制率相同，但前者的相关并发症发生率明显减少[18-19]。

RTOG95-08随机控制试验研究了有1~3个转移瘤的333例患者，分为单纯WBRT治疗组与WBRT+SRS组[20]。WBRT组的总放疗剂量为37.5Gy，分15次，SRS剂量依照ROTG90-05试验剂量。尽管两组间生存无显著差异，但亚组分析显示，对于单发脑转移瘤患者，SRS可以提高其生存率。SRS+WBRT组具有更高的缓解率及1年局部控制率（82% vs 71%）；Cox比例风险回顾模型分析接受SRS是局部控制率的唯一预测因子。WBRT组的局部复发率为43%，较WBRT+SRS组高。另外，WBRT+SRS组患者在治疗6个月后卡氏评分较稳定或得到改善。

目前，尚无随机控制试验研究手术对比SRS。从回顾性研究分析得到的结论往往不够确定，并可能具有选择性偏差[21-23]。SRS的治疗目前还具有争议性，包括转移的数目、患者的身体状态、颅外病变的情况、肿瘤组织类别等因素均影响治疗的选择，因此，需要进一步的临床试验来验证SRS针对脑转移瘤患者的治疗选择。

全脑放疗（WBRT）

早在20世纪初，WBRT已用来治疗脑转移。第一次报道来自于纪念医院，1949—1953年Chao等学者利用分割WBRT治疗38例患者，症状缓解率为63%，推荐剂量为30~40Gy，3~5周完成。后续增加了218例患者，给予30Gy，3周完成，发现接受这一剂量的患者具有较好的治疗反应及生存期[25]，进一步确立了WBRT在治疗颅内转移中的地位。同时，WBRT还可用来快速缓解大的脑转移瘤引起的症状，并作为预防治疗手段防止颅内出现新发转移。我们将在下面的部分进一步讨论。

全脑放疗作为脑转移病灶的基本治疗手段

RTOG主导的多个前瞻性研究用来确定WBRT

的最佳剂量与分割方式。一般来说,针对脑转移瘤患者 WBRT 的剂量为 20~40Gy,1~4 周完成,中位生存期为 4~6 个月(表 38.1)[26],主要对比了各治疗方案下患者的发病率、改善持续时间、进展时间、生存和缓解指数。RTOG7361 研究将 900 例患者随机分为 3 组:20Gy/5f,1 周完成;30Gy/10f,2 周完成;40Gy/15f,3 周完成。3 组的中位生存期相近,20Gy 与 30Gy 组为 15 周,40Gy 组为 18 周。WBRT 被认为可改善大约一半入组患者的神经功能,这与剂量与分割方式有关,但无法提高患者的生存率[27]。另外一项短疗程大分割放疗方案研究(10Gy/1f 或 20Gy/2f)[28]提示中位生存期与 RTOG7361 试验的研究结果差异显著。然而,接受短疗程大分割放疗方案的患者神经毒性明显增加。上述两种治疗方案的快速缓解率相似,但与接受较长疗程的患者(如 30Gy/10f)对比,接受大分割方案患者的症状改善持续时间、神经状态、神经症状完全消失率等均较差。

RTOG 8528 试验研究了加速超分割 WBRT 治疗方案,患者每次接受 1.6Gy,每天 2 次,总剂量分为 48Gy、54.4Gy、64Gy、70.4Gy[29]。尽管中位生存期看似随着剂量的增加在延长(4.8 个月,5.4 个月,7.2 个月,8.2 个月),但各组统计学差异不显著。随后的一项 RTOG 临床Ⅲ期随机试验研究了 445 例卡式评分超过 60 分的患者,分为超分割组(总剂量 54.4Gy,每次 1.2Gy,每天 2 次)和大分割组(总剂量 30Gy,每次 3Gy,每天 1 次)[30]。由于缺少对超分割治疗方式的监督及大分割组神经毒性的分析,目前临床对于 WBRT 治疗大体肿瘤的方案为 30Gy/10f 或 37.5Gy/15f。

表 38.1　RTOG 关于脑转移瘤手后全脑放射治疗的研究

试验名称	研究时间	例数	治疗方案	中位生存期
RTOG 6910	1971—1973	233	30Gy/10f,2 周以上	21 周
Borgelt 等,1980[27]		217	30Gy/15f,3 以上	18 周
		233	40Gy/15f,3 以上	18 周
		227	40Gy/20f,4 以上	16 周
RTOG 7361	1973—1976	447	20Gy/5f,1 周以上	15 周
Borgelt 等,1981[28]		228	30Gy/10F,2 周以上	15 周
		227	40Gy/15f,3 周以上	18 周
RTOG 6901 ultra-rapid Borgel 等,1981[27]	1971—1973	26	10Gy/1f,1d	15 周
RTOG 7361 ultra-rapid Borgelt 等,1981[28]	1973—1976	33	12Gy/2f,2d	13 周
RTOG 7606 favorable pts Kurtz 等,1981[123]	1976—1979	130	30Gy/10f,2 周以上	18 周
		125	50Gy/25f,4 周以上	17 周
RTOG 8528	1986—1989	30	48Gy 1.6Gy/f,每天 2 次	4.8 个月
Accelerated		53	54.5Gy 1.6Gy/f,每天 2 次	5.4 个月
超分割		44	64Gy 1.6Gy/f,每天 2 次	7.2 个月
Sause 等,1993[29]		36	70.4Gy 1.6Gy/f,每天 2 次	8.2 个月
RTOG 9104	1991—1995	213	30Gy/10f	4.5 个月
Murray 等,1997[30]		216	54.4Gy 1.6Gy/f,每天 2 次	4.5 个月
RTOG 7916	1979—1983	193	30Gy/10f,2 周以上	4.5 个月
Misonidazole		200	5Gy/6f,3 周以上	4.1 个月
Phillips 等,1995[32]		196	30Gy/10f,+ Miso	3.1 个月
		190	5Gy/6f,+ Miso	3.9 个月
RTOG 8905	1989—1993	36	37.5Gy/15f,3 周以上	6.1 个月
BrdU		34	37.5Gy/15f,+ BrdUrd	4.3 个月
Komarnicky 等,1991[31]				

BrdU:溴脱氧尿苷;f:分割次数
经 Elsevier 许可,摘自:Sneed PK, Larson DA, Wara WM. Neurosurg Clin N Am, 1996, 7: 505 - 515[26]

部分前瞻性随机临床试验对一些放疗增敏剂进行了研究。RTOG7916 试验评价了放疗增敏剂米索硝唑（misonidazole）对脑转移瘤患者的作用[31]。这项试验共纳入 779 例患者，分为 4 组，分别接受单纯 30Gy/10f（2 周完成）放疗，30Gy/10f 放疗 + 米索硝唑（1g/m²），单纯 30Gy/6f（3 周完成），30Gy/6f + 米索硝唑（2g/m²），患者的中位生存期从 3.1 个月至 4.5 个月，使用米索硝唑与否无显著差异。另一项试验研究了卤代嘧啶溴脱氧尿苷（BrdU）和钆特沙弗林。为了研究 BrdU 作为放疗增敏剂在脑转移瘤中的作用，RTOG89-05 纳入了 72 例患者，接受 WBRT 37.5Gy/15f（3 周完成），同时给予 BrdU（连用 3 周，每周给药 4d，每天 0.8g/m²），其中 5 例接受 BrdU 的患者出现了 4 级、5 级的血液或皮肤毒性反应；接受 BrdU 的患者未显示出生存获益。

另外一项随机试验 RTOG9801 评价了 motaxefin gadolinium（MGd）作为放疗增敏剂在脑转移瘤患者行 WBRT 治疗中的作用[33]。入组 401 例患者，给予单纯 WBRT（30Gy/10f）或 WBRT + MGd［每次照射前 2~5h 给予静脉注射 5mg/（kg·d）］。MGd 的使用并未影响患者的中位生存期，接受 MGd 的患者中位生存期为 5.2 个月，单纯 WBRT 患者的中位生存期为 4.9 个月。回顾分析显示 WBRT 后肿瘤退缩程度与生存时间及神经认知功能的保护相关[34]。神经进展时间在肺癌脑转移瘤患者亚组人群中得到了改善。在随后进行的Ⅲ期临床试验中，对 554 例 NSCLC 脑转移患者随机分组，治疗方案依照 RTOG9801 方案，接受 MGd 组的中位神经进展时间比对照组理想（15.4 个月 vs 10.0 个月），尽管无统计学差异（P=0.11）。

RTOG0118 试验研究了放疗增敏剂沙利度胺（thalidomide）在脑转移患者接受放疗中的作用[36]。患者随机分组为单纯 WBRT（37.5Gy/15f）和 WBRT + 沙利度胺。由于副反应，接近一半的患者未能完成沙利度胺的治疗，因此未显示出生存优势。最新公布的 RTOG0320 放疗增敏剂研究[37]对有 1~3 个脑转移瘤的 NSCLC 患者进行 SBRT 和 SRS，同步给予替莫唑胺或厄洛替尼治疗。结果显示，放疗增敏剂的应用增加了 3~5 级放疗毒性发生率（对照组 11% vs 替莫唑胺 41% vs 厄洛替尼 49%，P<0.001），并且使用放疗增敏剂减少了中位生存期（对照组 13.4 个月 vs 替莫唑胺 6.3 个月 vs 厄洛替尼 6.1 个月）。其他 WBRT 联合放疗增敏剂的效果值得进一步研究探讨。

WBRT 作为局部治疗后的辅助治疗

手术后序贯 WBRT

手术切除脑转移瘤后，WBRT 可防止局部复发。在 Patchell 等报道的前瞻性随机研究中，95 例单发脑转移患者接受了手术完全切除，之后给予观察或 WBRT 放疗（50.4Gy）。接受 WBRT 治疗组较观察组颅内病变复发率（18% vs 70%，P<0.001）明显减少。发生在瘤床的局部复发率（46% vs 10%）与发生在瘤床外的区域复发率（37% vs 14%）明显改善。WBRT 同时减少了因神经原因造成的死亡率（44% vs 14%），但患者的中位生存期并未得到改善。

一系列除 DeAngelis 外的研究关于手术后 WBRT 的研究结果见表 38.2[38-44]。大部分研究显示手术后 WBRT 并未减少颅内复发率[44]。两项回顾性研究显示术后 WBRT 可提高患者的中位生存期（P=0.02）[42-43]。

总之，接受复发后给予 WBRT 的患者死于神经原因的患者数较接受手术切除后给予 WBRT 的患者多，因此，建议手术切除脑转移瘤后即可给予 WBRT。尽管手术切除后常规使用 WBRT 可防止由于神经原因造成的死亡，但也带来了一些争议，包括 WBRT 可以产生长期神经毒性，包括神经认知下降和痴呆。而如果不行术后 WBRT 又会引起肿瘤局部复发造成的神经原因死亡率增加。因此，如果计划术后行 WBRT，应及时开始，即在手术切除后几周内开始，并根据手术侵袭性及患者术后恢复情况调整治疗方案。

SRS 后序贯 WBRT

许多前瞻性试验研究了 SRS 后序贯给予 WBRT。Aoyama 报道了 132 例有 1~4 个直径 <3cm

表 38.2 脑转移瘤切除术后行全脑放疗的研究

研究	原发肿瘤	病例数		肿瘤复发百分率			中位生存期（月）		
		RT	NoRT	RT	NoRT	P	RT	NoRT	P
Doseretz 等，1980[40]	任何	12	21	50%	52%	NS	8	10	NS
Smalley 等，1987[43]	任何	34	51	21%	85%	NA	21	12	0.02
DeAngelis 等，1989[44]	任何	79	19	45%	65%	0.03	21	4	NS
Hagen 等，1990[41]	黑色素瘤	12	21	50%	52%	NS	8	10	NS
Armstrong 等，1994[39]	肺癌	32	32	47%	38%	NS	10	14	NS
Skibber 等，1996[42]	黑色素瘤	22	12	32%	72%	NA	18	6	0.02
Patchell 等，1998[38]	任何	49	46	18%	70%	0.001	11	10	NS

NA：无效；NS：无统计学差异；RT：手术后全脑放疗
来源：经 John Wiley 和 Sons 许可，摘自 Komaki R, Chang E. Whole-brain radiation therapy//Sawaya R (ed.), Intracranial Metastases: Current Management Strategies. MA: Blackwell Publishing, 2004: 126–138[124]

的脑转移瘤患者，随机分为接受 SRS 组和 SRS + WBRT（30Gy/10f）组[45]。接受 WBRT 的患者给予 SRS 时放疗剂量减少 30%。SRS + WBRT 组 1 年局部控制率较单纯 SRS 组提高（89% vs 73%），1 年后新发脑转移发生率降低（42% vs 63.7%）。两组的中位生存期、神经原因死亡、神经功能损伤方面均无显著差异，故作者认为单纯 SRS 可以作为合理的治疗方式，而 WBRT 可作为复发或进展后的补救治疗措施。

相同的一项研究，Chang 等纳入了 58 例肺癌患者，有 1~3 例发生脑转移，根据 RTOG 递归划分分析（recursive partitioning analysis，RPA）进行 1 或 2 级分类后，分为单纯 SRS 组和 SRS + WBRT 组（30Gy/12f）[46]。值得注意的是，在治疗 4 个月后运用霍普金斯言语学习测试法（Hopkins Verbal Learning Test-Revised，HVLT-R）检测上述患者。此项研究开展早期后结束，原因是 SRS + WBRT 明显导致患者出现学习和记忆功能的损伤。加入 WBRT 导致治疗 4 个月后患者的回忆能力明显下降（52% vs 24%）。然而，WBRT 可提高 1 年局部控制率（100% vs 67%）和颅内远处控制率（73% vs 45%）。相反，SRS 组总的中位生存期较高（15 个月 SRS vs 6 个月）。

欧洲癌症治疗研究组织（the Enropean Organization for Research and Treatment of Cancer，EORTC）也进行了类似的研究。359 例研究对象中有 1~3 例脑转移瘤患者，其中 199 例接受 SRS，160 例接受手术治疗，之后随机分为 WBRT 组（30Gy/10 次）与观察组[47]。接受 WBRT 的患者 2 年原位复发率（手术：59% vs 27%；SRS：31% vs 19%）及非原位复发率（手术：42% vs 23%；SRS：48% vs 33%）降低。接受 WBRT 组神经原因相关死亡率较低（28% vs 44%）。在身体状态恶化时间及总生存期方面两组无显著差异。

对于脑转移瘤的初始治疗是否需要行 SRS + WBRT 现仍有争议。不可否认的是加入 WBRT 可以降低颅内远处转移的风险，但缺乏生存获益及增加的毒性又对 SRS 后给予 WBRT 提出了反对意见，对于这类患者，相关临床研究正在开展，以评估患者的生存、生活质量及功能独立。

预防性颅脑照射（prophylactic crania irradiation，PCI）

预防性颅脑照射（prophylactic crania irradiation，PCI）已被证明可以提高患有急性淋巴细胞白血病、累及中枢神经系统的患儿的生存期[48]。随着全身化疗越来越有效，单独累及中枢神经系统的急性淋巴细胞白血病越来越常见，这种现象也在 SCLC 患者中存在[49]。

由于 SCLC 患者脑转移发生率较高，故 20 世纪 70 年代已经开始针对 SCLC 患者进行 PCI 治疗[50]。大约一半的 SCLC 患者如不接受 PCI 治疗，会出现明显的脑转移[51]。然而，由于此类患者生存期较短，故颅内微小转移及颅外中枢神经系统转移发生率被严重低估[52]，而对照针对局限期 SCLC 患者全身治疗的改善及早期应用胸部放疗，PCI 的作用越来越重要[30]。因为 PCI 的神经毒性及不能延长总生存期，尽管能够减少脑转移瘤数目，但 PCI 过去一直不被认为是常规治疗方法，直到对患者治疗前后进行神经心理测试，显示 PCI 不会导致明显的精神退化[53]。

在一项早期的 PCI 研究中，Cox 等发现给予剂量 20Gy/5 次不能减少脑转移瘤的发生率[54]。究其原因可能是总剂量（20Gy）偏低，尽管给予的每次分割剂量大于 2～3Gy。Bieler 等发现接受 PCI 24Gy（每次 3Gy）的患者未出现脑转移瘤的复发，而 54 例未接受 PCI 的患者 16% 出现脑转移瘤的复发（$P<0.05$）[55]。

另外一项 PCI 研究中，Maurer 等将 163 例患者随机分为两组，一组未接受 PCI 治疗，一组接受 PCI 治疗（30Gy/10f）[56]。结果显示，接受 PCI 组较对照组患者出现脑转移瘤的概率降低（4% vs 18%）。其他研究组的结果也显示 PCI 可明显降低脑转移瘤的发生率，但总生存期无明显改善[57-61]。如表 38.3 所示，在较晚的几项研究中，总剂量超过 30Gy 似乎能减少肿瘤复发，这可能与灵敏的脑转移瘤诊断技术的出现、全身化疗有效性的改善、胸部放疗的使用等因素相关[62]。Hirsch 等报道 111 例患者随机分为接受 PCI 组（40Gy）及未接受 PCI 组，发现两组的脑转移瘤发生率无显著差异（PCI 组 9% vs 未接受 PCI 组 13%）[63]。这一结果被认为与 PCI 治疗开始较晚有关，该研究中 PCI 开始于全身治疗结束后 12 周。

上述研究结果发表 20 年后，Auperin 报道的 meta 分析显示，对于 SCLC 治疗后完全缓解的患者，PCI 使这类患者生存获益[64]，其纳入了 987 例患者，分别来自于 1977—1994 年的 7 个临床试验（表 38.4）[65-70]，其中少部分患者（12%～17%）为广泛期病变。结果显示相比对照组，接受 PCI 的患者 3 年存活率明显增高 5.4%（20.7% vs 15.3%），死亡的相对危险度 RR 为 0.84 [95% CI（0.73，0.97）；$P=0.01$]。接受 PCI 的患者 3 年无脑转移瘤存活率亦明显增加（22.3% vs 13.5%；$P<0.001$），3 年累计脑转移发生率从 58.6% 下降到 33.3%（$P<0.001$）。对 4 种放射剂量（8Gy，24～25Gy，30Gy，36～40Gy）分析显示，放疗剂量越大，发生脑转移的概率越小（$P=0.02$），但剂量高低与生存期无相关性。这项 meta 分析还提示，化疗结束后越早介入 PCI 治疗，脑转移发生率越低（小于 4 个月 vs 4～6 个月 vs 大于 6 个月，$P=0.01$）。尽管在大多数随机试验中，PCI 治疗前后未对患者进行神经心理测试，但 meta 分析显示 PCI 治疗后未对患者造成神经心理退化。

表 38.3　关于 SCLC 脑预防照射的早期研究

研究	病例数	放疗方案	脑转移瘤复发率	
			PCI	非 PCI
Cox 等，1978[54]	45	20Gy/5f	17%	20%
Bieler 等，1979[55]	54	24Gy/8f	0	16%
Maurer 等，1980[56]	163	30Gy/10f	4%	18%
Hansen 等，1981[57]	110	40Gy/20f	9%	12%
Eagan 等，1981[57]	30	36Gy/10f	13%	73%
Katensis 等，1982[59]	38	40Gy/10f	12%	44%
Jackson 等，1983[58]	29	30Gy/10f	0	27%
Seydel 等，1985[61]	217	30Gy/10f	5%	22%
Niiranen 等，1989[60]	51	40Gy/20f	0	27%

f：分割次数；PCI：脑预防照射

来源：经 springer science 和 Business Media 许可，摘自 Gregor A, Cull A. Role of prophylactic cranial irradiation: Benefits and late effects//Van Houtte P, Klastersk J, Rocmans P (eds). Progress and Perspectives in the Treatment of Lung Cancer Berlin: Springer-Verlag, 1999: 139 – 149[62]

表 38.4　关于 SCLC 脑预防照射作用的 7 个临床研究及 meta 分析

研究	研究时间	中位随访时间（年）	治疗方式	总剂量/分割次数（单次剂量）	开始治疗至入组中位时间（月）	患者数	生存患者数
U Maryl，Cancer Ctr[65]	1977—1980	18.5	CT	30Gy/10f（3Gy）	3.6	29	2
冈山大学[69]	1981—1986	11.7	CT 或 CT + RT	40Gy/20f（2Gy）	2.5	46	4
PCI-85[66]	1985—1993	8.4	CT 或 CT + RT	24Gy/8f（3Gy）	5.3	300	32
丹麦国家癌症研究所	1985—1991	8.8	CT	24Gy/8（3Gy）	4.4	55	7
UKCCR-EORTC[67]	1987—1995	3.5	CT 或 CT + RT	8~36Gy/（1~18f）*	NA	314	54
PCI-88[68]	1988—1994	5.1	CT 或 CT + RT	24Gy/8f（3Gy）	5.1	211	37
ECOG-RTOG[70]	1991—1994	3.9	CT 或 CT + RT	25Gy/10f（2.5Gy）	NA	32	5

CT：化疗；ECOG-RTOG：RTOG：东部合作组；PCI：脑预防照射；RT：胸部放疗；UKCCR-EORTC：欧洲肿瘤研究治疗组织-英国肿瘤临床研究中心

*第一部分研究包括 3 组治疗组：未行脑预防照射组；24Gy/12f 脑预防照射组；36Gy/18f 脑预防照射组。第二部分研究包括两种治疗组：未行脑预防照射组及脑预防照射组。

来源：经麻省医学协会许可，摘自 Auperin A, Arriagada R, Pigono JP, et al. Prophylactic cranial irradiation for patients with small-cell lung cancer in complete remission. Prophylactic Cranial Irradiation Overview Collaborative Group. N Engl J Med, 1999, 341: 476-484[64]

除了应用于局限期 SCLC，PCI 也应用于广泛期 SCLC 的治疗中。EORTC 主导的一项前瞻性随机试验，入组了 286 例广泛期 SCLC 患者，接受 4~6 个周期化疗后随机分为两组，一组接受 PCI 治疗（20Gy/5f 或 30Gy/12f），一组为观察组[71]。患者接受 PCI 治疗具有较低的有症状脑转移率（15% vs 40%），并且改善了 1 年总生存率（27% vs 13%）。值得注意的是，这项研究在随机分组前，需要经影像学检查确诊无脑转移，同时随访数据提示接受 PCI 的患者生活质量较差[72]。

为了继续探讨 PCI 的最佳放疗剂量，有人开展了一项组间研究，入组的 720 例局限期 SCLC 患者，经化疗与胸部放疗达到完全缓解后，给予 PCI 放疗。一组给予标准剂量（25Gy/10f，每天 1f），一组给予高剂量（36Gy/18f，每天 1 次或 36Gy/24f，每天 2 次）[73]。所有患者均进行颅脑影像学检查。两组的 2 年脑转移发生率无显著差异，标准剂量组有更好的总生存率（42% vs 37%；P = 0.05）。后续的研究显示在 3 年的研究期内，低剂量组与高剂量组在生活质量、神经功能及认知功能方面无显著差异[74]。因此，目前对于 PCI 的标准剂量为 25Gy/10f，每天 1 次。

一些随机试验研究了 PCI 对 NSCLC 患者的作用，其中一项研究是 RTOG 84-03，入组患者为腺癌或大细胞癌，接受 PCI 治疗 30Gy/10f 或观察[75]。1991 年公布的结果显示接受 PCI 的患者较少发生脑转移，但患者的总生存期无明显改善，可能与全身化疗的无效性及 PCI 的开始时间有关。随后来自德国的一项多中心、关于针对可手术 ⅢA 期 NSCLC 患者行新辅助治疗作用的研究，提供了 PCI 在治疗 NSCLC 中的辅助效果信息[76]。在这项研究中，112 例患者被随机分为 2 组，一组为原发病灶手术切除后，给予辅助术后放疗；一组为术前给予化疗，之后给予针对原发病灶的同步放化疗，之后对原发病灶给予根治性切除，该组也接受了术后 PCI（30Gy/10f）治疗。PCI 能够减少 5 年首发脑转移发生率（8% vs 35%），同时是否行 PCI 治疗在神经毒性方面无显著差异。RTOG 0214 Ⅲ期临床试验对比 PCI 在局部进展期 NSCLC 患者治疗中的作用[77]。340 例诊断为 Ⅲ期的 NSCLC 患者接受原发病灶治疗，确定无疾病进展后，随机分为接受 PCI 组（30Gy/15f）或观察组。总生存期及无病生存期两组无显著差异，但 PCI 组的 1 年脑转移发生率明显降低（8% vs 18%）。针对两组患者的神经认知及生活质量的后续研究显示，1 年总认知功能及生活质量两组无显著差异，尽管 PCI 组患者的记忆力（HVLT 测试结果）明显下降[78]。基于上述前瞻性研究，目前不推荐针对

NSCLC 患者行 PCI 治疗。

总之，PCI 治疗可以有效减少脑转移发生率，并且无证据显示 PCI 治疗可出现相关并发症。对于局限性 SCLC 治疗后达到完全缓解的患者及广泛期 SCLC 治疗有效的患者，PCI 均可改善其生存[64,71]。超过 25Gy/10f 的治疗方案对患者无明显获益[73]。PCI 似乎无法对 NSCLC 患者提供生存获益。

颅脑放疗相关毒性

放射治疗相关并发症通常分为急性损伤（发生放射治疗期间）、早期延迟损伤（放疗后 2~4 个月）和晚期损伤（放疗后几个月或几年）。普通的急性损伤包括可逆性脱发、轻度放射性皮炎和轻度乏力。尽管 1970 年曾报道接受单次 10Gy 放疗后，7% 的患者出现致死性放射性脑病[79]，但在如今的放疗分割模式下，放射性脑病极其罕见。嗜睡综合征表现为持续乏力、厌食、易激惹（好发于儿童），常发生于 WBRT 后的 3~10 周，通常在 6 个月内缓解[80-81]。

经 WBRT 治疗获得长期存活，尤其是其中接受多种化疗药物的患者可出现进行性痴呆、共济失调或尿失禁，最终导致伤残或死亡。在一项报道中[44]，12 例患者中有 7 例出现上述情况。进行 CT 扫描发现脑皮质萎缩和脑白质低密度灶。所有 12 例患者接受了单次分割至少 3Gy，每天 1 次的方案照射，其中 9 例在治疗期间接受了单次分割 5Gy 或更大剂量的照射。基于上述发现，为了减轻长期后遗症，作者建议颅脑给予低剂量分割照射，每天 1.8~2Gy，总剂量为 40~45Gy，尤其针对那些预后较好的患者。最近，递归划分分析确定了可获得长期生存的亚组患者。对预后评价的一篇报道中，临床因素如年龄、KPS（karnofsky performance status）评分、中枢神经系统转移灶数目、颅外转移病灶状态等与脑转移瘤患者的预后相关[82]。具有较好预后的亚组患者的中位生存期为 11 个月，预后差的亚组患者的中位生存期为 2.6 个月。对于具有较好预后因子的患者，我们建议单次分割剂量≤3Gy。

WBRT、颅内疾病控制和神经认知功能之间的相互关系十分复杂。简单地说，颅内病灶进展与 WBRT 是出现神经认知功能障碍的一对矛盾风险因子[46,83-85]。相关的进一步研究十分必要，可以筛选确定相对独立的危险因素，指导预后较好患者的 WBRT 治疗。

关于神经心理毒性的研究，不仅针对接受 WBRT 的患者，还有接受全身治疗的患者。Sheline 等诸多学者均研究了电离辐射对中枢神经系统的影响[86-88]。Johnson 等研究了接受治疗后存活 6~13 年的 SCLC 患者，其中 86% 发生了神经心理缺陷，包括定向力、记忆、语言功能等方面[89]。导致上述损伤出现的因素有免疫缺陷、机会性感染、脑微转移灶、大放射野毒性、神经营养化疗药物联合 PCI 的应用及放疗总剂量等。特别需要注意的是，急性淋巴细胞白血病接受 PCI 的同时给予氨甲蝶呤治疗的患儿及 SCLC 接受 PCI 的同时给予洛莫司汀治疗的患者容易发生上述损伤[90-91]。然而，至少一组研究团队发现，在那些接受预防性中枢神经系统照射后出现无法预测的晚期神经后遗症患者中，其一些临床信息与 CT 扫描结果不相符[92]。在我们探讨 PCI 最低有效生物剂量的研究中，发现 25Gy/10f 是有效的，并且比 30Gy/10f 毒性低[93]。在后续的前瞻性研究中，30 例局限期 SCLC 患者同时确诊无脑转移，在接受 PCI 治疗前后进行神经心理测试，研究发现，29 例患者在接受 PCI 治疗前就已经出现轻微认知功能障碍，其中最常见的损伤是言语记忆损伤，之后是前额叶功能障碍和精细运动共济失调。PCI 治疗后无明显的神经功能退化[53]。相似的结果也出现在 2 项后续随机试验中，即前瞻性评估神经认知终点[66-67]，即在 PCI 治疗之前患者已经出现了神经功能损伤，未发现 PCI 有损于神经认知功能。

随着全身治疗作用的提高及患者生存时间的延长，WBRT 造成的晚期损伤越来越受到关注。最近完成的一项 RTOG Ⅲ 期临床试验中，随机分配患者在 WBRT 治疗中使用美金刚胺，该药是在治疗阿尔兹海默病中得到批准使用的一种 N-甲基-D-天门冬氨酸受体激动剂。这项研究的结果待定。适形放射治疗技术可以保护与神经认知功能相关的重要部位，例如照射海马被认为与神经认知功能障碍相关[94-96]。RTOG 目前正在主导 Ⅱ 期临床试验，评估进行海马保护的 WBRT 是否能够帮助保护患者的神经认知功能。

NSCLC 与脑转移的生物标记物

之前的研究已经证实 SCLC、腺癌及大细胞癌患者容易发生脑转移[51,97-99]。在现代分子靶向治疗时代，生物标记物可以指导 NSCLC 患者的治疗。许多研究也已经显示某些基因表达与 NSCLC 患者发生脑转移相关[100-102]，例如 Ki-67、p53、bcl-2、EGFR、Cox-2、BAX 等[101-102]，但其远未达到成为稳定或独立的相关因素。然而，表达模式如多种生物标记物联合表达，有希望准确预测患者是否发生肿瘤脑转移[103]。在一项回顾性研究中，含有 8 种标记物的分子组合能够对 I 期 NSCLC 分组，并能确定其中 37% 的患者可能出现颅脑转移[104]。血清标记物如癌胚抗原，是一种能够预测脑转移发生的危险因子[105-107]。然而，在应用于临床治疗前，任何一个有潜力的生物标记物或生物标记组合都需要前瞻性研究去验证。

EGFR 被报道与脑转移的诊断及治疗相关。现在还不清楚的是，EGFR 的突变或扩增能否预测脑转移瘤的发生[101,108-111]。然而，EGFR 酪氨酸激酶抑制剂吉非替尼和厄洛替尼对 NSCLC 患者的脑转移病灶治疗有效[112-116]，其治疗效果与 EGFR 酪氨酸激酶结构域突变相关[114-116]。EGFR 突变患者较非突变患者对 WBRT 治疗更加敏感，与年龄、功能状态、颅外病变状态、脑转移瘤数目等均为预后的独立预测因子[117-118]。需要注意的是，原发病灶与转移病灶的 EGFR 突变状态可能不一致，如果考虑靶向治疗，原发及转移病灶的 EGFR 状态均应考虑[109,119-121]。

接受传统化疗的 NSCLC 患者发生脑转移瘤的风险较接受分子靶向治疗的 EGFR 突变患者高。在一项报道中，IIIB 或 IV 或复发的合并 EGFR 突变的 NSCLC 患者，接受吉非替尼或厄洛替尼一线治疗，中枢神经系统转移的 1 年发生率为 6%，2 年发生率为 13%[110]。这篇报道的作者提出靶向治疗或许有预防脑转移发生的作用。在后续研究中，EGFR 突变接受分子靶向治疗的患者与接受传统化疗的患者相比[122]，前组可降低 44% 中枢神经系统转移发生率，具有提高吉非替尼或厄洛替尼预防中枢神经系统转移的作用。

但是，这些发现均需要前瞻性试验研究来证实。如前文所提到的，评价替莫唑胺或厄洛替尼同步 SRS + WBRT 作用的 RTOG0320[37]，显示加入厄洛替尼后，3~5 级毒性发生率较单纯 SRS + WBRT 发生率，从 11% 增加到了 49%（P = 0.001），并且缩短了中位生存期（6.1 个月 vs 13.4 个月；P 值无统计学意义）。目前，分子生物特性指导了 NSCLC 的前沿治疗，但是，生物标记物在脑转移瘤应用方面仍未得到确立，值得我们进一步研究。

总 结

总之，WBRT 是一种非常实用的治疗方式，可以用于实体瘤脑转移的治疗，以及局部治疗后的预防复发、预防 SCLC 患者发生脑转移。现已开展了许多前瞻性研究来确定合理的剂量及分割方式、验证同步全身化疗的作用、评估相关毒性。应用于神经影像、神经心理测试、SRS 照射方式、预测脑转移发生的生物标记物检测等方面的诸多新进展，将会更加优化 WBRT 的实施。

（毛 羽 黄 伟 李宝生 译）

参考文献

[1] Yamanaka R. Medical management of brain metastases from lung cancer (Review). Oncology reports, 2009, 22 (6): 1269-1276.

[2] Ceresoli G L, Reni M, Chiesa G, et al. Brain metastases in locally advanced nonsmall cell lung carcinoma after multimodality treatment. Cancer, 2002, 95 (3): 605-612.

[3] Gandara D R, Chansky K, Albain K S, et al. Consolidation docetaxel after concurrent chemoradiotherapy in stage IIIB non-small-cell lung cancer: Phase II Southwest Oncology Group Study S9504. Journal of clinical oncology, 2003, 21 (10): 2004-2010.

[4] Sze G, Milano E, Johnson C, et al. Detection of brain metastases: comparison of contrast-enhanced MR with unenhanced MR and enhanced CT. American Journal of Neuroradiology, 1990, 11 (4): 785-791.

[5] Coia L R, Aaronson N, Linggood R, et al. A report of the consensus workshop panel on the treatment of brain metastases. International Journal of Radiation Oncology Biology

Physics, 1992, 23 (1): 223-227.

[6] Cohen N, Strauss G, Lew R, et al. Should prophylactic anticonvulsants be administered to patients with newly-diagnosed cerebral metastases? A retrospective analysis. Journal of Clinical Oncology, 1988, 6 (10): 1621-1624.

[7] Hanahan D, Weinberg R A. The hallmarks of cancer. Cell, 2000, 100 (1): 57-70.

[8] Hanahan D, Weinberg R A. Hallmarks of cancer: the next generation. Cell, 2011, 144 (5): 646-674.

[9] Gavrilovic I T, Posner J B. Brain metastases: epidemiology and pathophysiology. Journal of neuro-oncology, 2005, 75 (1): 5-14.

[10] Ewing J. Metastasis//Ewing J (ed), Neoplastic Diseases: A Treatise on Tumours. Philadelphia: W. B. Saunders, 1940: 62-74

[11] Paget S. The distribution of secondary growths in cancer of the breast. Cancer metastasis reviews, 1989, 8 (2): 98.

[12] Patchell R A, Tibbs P A, Walsh J W, et al. A randomized trial of surgery in the treatment of single metastases to the brain. New England Journal of Medicine, 1990, 322 (8): 494-500.

[13] Noordijk EM, Vecht CJ, Haaxma-Reiche H, et al. The choice of treatment of single brain metastasis should be based on extracranial tumor activity and age. International Journal of Radiation Oncology Biology Physics, 1994, 29 (4): 711-717.

[14] Leksell L. The stereotaxic method and radiosurgery of the brain. Acta Chir Scand., 1951, 102: 316-319.

[15] Lunsford LD, Maitz A, Lindner G. First United States 201 source cobalt-60 gamma unit for radiosurgery. Stereotactic and Functional Neurosurgery, 1987, 50 (1-6): 253-256.

[16] Jayarao M, Chin L S, Regine W F. Stereotactic Radiosurgery for Brain Metastases. Intracranial Stereotactic Radiosurgery. New York: Thieme Medical Publishers, 2009: 151-62.

[17] Shaw E, Scott C, Souhami L, et al. Single dose radiosurgical treatment of recurrent previously irradiated primary brain tumors and brain metastases: final report of RTOG protocol 90-05. International Journal of Radiation Oncology Biology Physics, 2000, 47 (2): 291-298.

[18] Shehata MK, Young B, Reid B, et al. Stereotatic radiosurgery of 468 brain metastases ≤ 2cm: implications for SRS dose and whole brain radiation therapy. International Journal of Radiation Oncology Biology Physics, 2004, 59 (1): 87-93.

[19] Elliott RE, Rush SC, Morsi A, et al. Local control of newly diagnosed and distally recurrent, low-volume brain metastases with fixed-dose (20Gy) gamma knife radiosurgery. Neurosurgery, 2011, 68 (4): 921-931.

[20] Andrews D W, Scott C B, Sperduto P W, et al. Whole brain radiation therapy with or without stereotactic radiosurgery boost for patients with one to three brain metastases: phase III results of the RTOG 9508 randomised trial. The Lancet, 2004, 363 (9422): 1665-1672.

[21] O'Neill B P, Iturria N J, Link M J, et al. A comparison of surgical resection and stereotactic radiosurgery in the treatment of solitary brain metastases. International Journal of Radiation Oncology Biology Physics, 2003, 55 (5): 1169-1176.

[22] Auchter RM, Lamond JP, Alexander E, et al. A multiinstitutional outcome and prognostic factor analysis of radiosurgery for resectable single brain metastasis. International Journal of Radiation Oncology Biology Physics, 1996, 35 (1): 27-35.

[23] Bindal AK, Bindal RK, Hess KR, et al. Surgery versus radiosurgery in the treatment of brain metastasis. Journal of neurosurgery, 1996, 84 (5): 748-754.

[24] Chao JH, Phillips R, Nickson JJ. Roentgen-ray therapy of cerebral metastases. Cancer, 1954, 7 (4): 682-689.

[25] Chu FC, Hilaris BB. Value of radiation therapy in the management of intracranial metastases. Cancer, 1961, 14 (3): 577-581.

[26] Sneed PK, Larson DA, Wara WM. Radiotherapy for cerebral metastases. Neurosurgery Clinics of North America, 1996, 7 (3): 505-515.

[27] Borgelt B, Gelber R, Kramer S, et al. The palliation of brain metastases: final results of the first two studies by the Radiation Therapy Oncology Group. International Journal of Radiation Oncology Biology Physics, 1980, 6 (1): 1-9.

[28] Borgelt B, Gelber R, Larson M, et al. Ultra-rapid high dose irradiation schedules for the palliation of brain metastases: final results of the first two studies by the Radiation Therapy Oncology Group. International Journal of Radiation Oncology Biology Physics, 1981, 7 (12): 1633-1638.

[29] Sause WT, Scott C, Krisch R, et al. Phase I/II trial of accelerated fractionation in brain metastases RTOG 85-28. International Journal of Radiation Oncology Biology

Physics, 1993, 26 (4): 653 - 657.

[30] Murray KJ, Scott C, Greenberg HM, et al. A randomized phase III study of accelerated hyperfractionation versus standard in patients with unresected brain metastases: a report of the Radiation Therapy Oncology Group (RTOG) 9104. International Journal of Radiation Oncology Biology Physics, 1997, 39 (3): 571 - 574.

[31] Komarnicky LT, Phillips TL, Martz K, et al. A randomized phase III protocol for the evaluation of misonidazole combined with radiation in the treatment of patients with brain metastases (RTOG - 7916). International Journal of Radiation Oncology Biology Physics, 1991, 20 (1): 53 - 58.

[32] Phillips TL, Scott CB, Leibel SA, et al. Results of a randomized comparison of radiotherapy and bromodeoxyuridine with radiotherapy alone for brain metastases: report of RTOG trial 89 - 05. International Journal of Radiation Oncology Biology Physics, 1995, 33 (2): 339 - 348.

[33] Mehta MP, Rodrigus P, Terhaard CH, et al. Survival and neurologic outcomes in a randomized trial of motexafin gadolinium and whole-brain radiation therapy in brain metastases. Journal of Clinical Oncology, 2003, 21 (13): 2529 - 2536.

[34] Li J, Bentzen SM, Renschler M, et al. Regression after whole-brain radiation therapy for brain metastases correlates with survival and improved neurocognitive function. Journal of Clinical Oncology, 2007, 25 (10): 1260 - 1266.

[35] Mehta MP, Shapiro WR, Phan SC, et al. Motexafin gadolinium combined with prompt whole brain radiotherapy prolongs time to neurologic progression in non-small-cell lung cancer patients with brain metastases: Results of a phase III trial. International Journal of Radiation Oncology Biology Physics, 2009, 73 (4): 1069 - 1076.

[36] Knisely JP, Berkey B, Chakravarti A, et al. A phase III study of conventional radiation therapy plus thalidomide versus conventional radiation therapy for multiple brain metastases (RTOG 0118). International Journal of Radiation Oncology Biology Physics, 2008, 71 (1): 79 - 86.

[37] Sperduto PW, Wang M, Robins HI, et al. RTOG 0320: A phase III trial comparing whole brain radiation therapy (WBRT) and stereotactic radiosurgery (SRS) alone versus WBRT with temozolomide (TMZ) or erlotinib for non-small cell lung cancer (NSCLC) and 1 - 3 brain metastases. Cancer Research, 2012, 72 (8 Supplement): 736 - 736.

[38] Patchell RA, Tibbs PA, Regine WF, et al. Postoperative radiotherapy in the treatment of single metastases to the brain: a randomized trial. Jama, 1998, 280 (17): 1485 - 1489.

[39] Armstrong J G, Wronski M, Galicich J, et al. Postoperative radiation for lung cancer metastatic to the brain. Journal of clinical oncology, 1994, 12 (11): 2340 - 2344.

[40] Dosoretz DE, Blitzer PH, Russell AH, et al. Management of solitary metastasis to the brain: the role of elective brain irradiation following complete surgical resection. International Journal of Radiation Oncology Biology Physics, 1980, 6 (12): 1727 - 1730.

[41] Hagen NA, Cirrincione C, Thaler HT, et al. The role of radiation therapy following resection of single brain metastasis from melanoma. Neurology, 1990, 40 (1): 158 - 158.

[42] Skibber JM, Soong S, Austin L, et al. Cranial irradiation after surgical excision of brain metastases in melanoma patients. Annals of Surgical Oncology, 1996, 3 (2): 118 - 123.

[43] Smalley SR, Schray MF, Laws ER, et al. Adjuvant radiation therapy after surgical resection of solitary brain metastasis: association with pattern of failure and survival. International Journal of Radiation Oncology Biology Physics, 1987, 13 (11): 1611 - 1616.

[44] DeAngelis LM, Delattre JY, Posner JB. Radiation-induced dementia in patients cured of brain metastases. Neurology, 1989, 39 (6): 789 - 789.

[45] Aoyama H, Shirato H, Tago M, et al. Stereotactic radiosurgery plus whole-brain radiation therapy vs stereotactic radiosurgery alone for treatment of brain metastases: a randomized controlled trial. Jama, 2006, 295 (21): 2483 - 2491.

[46] Chang EL, Wefel JS, Hess KR, et al. Neurocognition in patients with brain metastases treated with radiosurgery or radiosurgery plus whole-brain irradiation: a randomised controlled trial. The lancet oncology, 2009, 10 (11): 1037 - 1044.

[47] Kocher M, Soffietti R, Abacioglu U, et al. Adjuvant whole-brain radiotherapy versus observation after radiosurgery or surgical resection of one to three cerebral metastases: results of the EORTC 22952 - 26001 study. Journal of Clinical Oncology, 2011, 29 (2): 134 - 141.

[48] Bleyer WA, Poplack DG. Prophylaxis and treatment of

leukemia in the central nervous system and other sanctuaries. Semin Oncol, 1985, 12 (2): 131-48.

[49] Hansen HH, Dombernowsky P, Hirsch F R, et al. Prophylactic irradiation in bronchogenic small cell anaplastic carcinoma. A comparative trial of localized versus extensive radiotherapy including prophylactic brain irradiation in patients receiving combination chemotherapy. Cancer, 1980, 46 (2): 279-284.

[50] Hansen HH. Should initial treatment of small cell carcinoma include systemic chemotherapy and brain irradiation? Cancer chemotherapy Rep, 1973, 3, 4 (2): 239-241.

[51] Komaki R. Prophylactic cranial irradiation for small cell carcinoma of the lung. Cancer Treat Symp. 1985, 2: 35-39.

[52] Nugent JL, Bunn PA, Matthews MJ, et al. CNS metastases in small cell bronchogenic carcinoma. Increasing frequency and changing pattern with lengthening survival. Cancer, 1979, 44 (5): 1885-1893.

[53] Komaki R, Meyers CA, Shin DM, et al. Evaluation of cognitive function in patients with limited small cell lung cancer prior to and shortly following prophylactic cranial irradiation. International Journal of Radiation Oncology Biology Physics, 1995, 33 (1): 179-182.

[54] Cox JD, Petrovich Z, Paig C, et al. Prophylactic cranial irradiation in patients with inoperable carcinoma of the lung. Preliminary report of a cooperative trial. Cancer, 1978, 42 (3): 1135-1140.

[55] Beiler DD, Kane RC, Bernath AM, et al. Low dose elective brain irradiation in small cell carcinoma of the lung. International Journal of Radiation Oncology Biology Physics, 1979, 5 (7): 941-945.

[56] Maurer LH, Tulloh M, Weiss RB, et al. A randomized combinedmodality trial in small cell carcinoma of the lung comparison of combination chemotherapy-radiation therapy versus cyclophosphamide-radiation therapy effects of maintenance chemotherapy and prophylactic whole brain irradiation. Cancer, 1980, 45 (1): 30-39.

[57] Eagan RT, Frytak S, Lee RE, et al. A case for preplanned thoracic and prophylactic whole brain radiation therapy in limited small-cell lung cancer. Cancer clinical trials, 1980, 4 (3): 261-266.

[58] Jackson DV, Richards F, Cooper MR. II, Prophylactic cranial irradiation in small cell lung cancer, 1983, 237: 2730-2733

[59] Katensis AT, Karpasitis N, Giannakakis D. Elective brain irradiation in patients with small cell carcinoma of the lung. Lung cancer: International Congress Series. 1982, 558: 277-284.

[60] Niiranen A, Holsti P, Salmo M. Treatment of small cell lung cancer: two-drug versus four-drug chemotherapy and loco-regional irradiation with or without prophylactic cranial irradiation. Acta Oncologica, 1989, 28 (4): 501-505.

[61] Seydel HG, Creech R, Pagano M, et al. Prophylactic versus no brain irradiation in regional small cell lung carcinoma. American journal of clinical oncology, 1985, 8 (3): 218-223.

[62] Gregor A, Cull A. Role of Prophylactic Cranial Irradiation: Benefits and Late Effects. Progress and Perspective in the Treatment of Lung Cancer. Springer Berlin Heidelberg, 1999: 139-149.

[63] Hirsch FR, Hansen HH, Paulson OB, et al. Development of brain metastases in small cell anaplastic carcinoma of the lung. CNS complications of malignant disease. Macmillan, New York, 1979: 175-184.

[64] Aupérin A, Arriagada R, Pignon JP, et al. Prophylactic cranial irradiation for patients with small-cell lung cancer in complete remission. New England Journal of Medicine, 1999, 341 (7): 476-484.

[65] Aisner J, Wesley MN. The value of prophylactic cranial irradiation given at complete remission in small cell lung cancer. Cancer Treat Rep, 1983, 67: 675-682.

[66] Arriagada R, Le Chevalier T, Borie F, et al. Prophylactic cranial irradiation for patients with small-cell lung cancer in complete remission. Journal of the National Cancer Institute, 1995, 87 (3): 183-190.

[67] Gregor A, Cull A, Stephens RJ, et al. Prophylactic cranial irradiation is indicated following complete response to induction therapy in small cell lung cancer: results of a multicentre randomised trial. European journal of cancer, 1997, 33 (11): 1752-1758.

[68] Laplanche A, Monnet I, Santos-Miranda J A, et al. Controlled clinical trial of prophylactic cranial irradiation for patients with small-cell lung cancer in complete remission. Lung cancer, 1998, 21 (3): 193-201.

[69] Ohonoshi T, Ueoka H, Kawahara S, et al. Comparative study of prophylactic cranial irradiation in patients with small cell lung cancer achieving a complete response: a long-term follow-up result. Lung Cancer, 1993, 10 (1): 47-54.

[70] Wagner H, Kim K, Turrisi A. A randomized phase III

study of prophylactic cranial irradiation versus observation in patients with small cell lung cancer achieving a complete response: final report of an incomplete trial by the Eastern Cooperative Oncology Group and Radiation Therapy Oncology Group (E3589/R92 - 01). Proc Am Soc Clin Oncol. 1996, 15: 376.

[71] Slotman B, Faivre-Finn C, Kramer G, et al. Prophylactic cranial irradiation in extensive small-cell lung cancer. New England Journal of Medicine, 2007, 357 (7): 664 - 672.

[72] Slotman BJ, Mauer ME, Bottomley A, et al. Prophylactic cranial irradiation in extensive disease small-cell lung cancer: short-term health-related quality of life and patient reported symptoms—results of an international phase Ⅲ randomized controlled trial by the EORTC radiation oncology and lung cancer groups. Journal of Clinical Oncology, 2009, 27 (1): 78 - 84.

[73] Le Péchoux C, Dunant A, Senan S, et al. Standard-dose versus higher-dose prophylactic cranial irradiation (PCI) in patients with limited-stage small-cell lung cancer in complete remission after chemotherapy and thoracic radiotherapy (PCI 99 - 01, EORTC 22003 - 08004, RTOG 0212, and IFCT 99 - 01): a randomised clinical trial. The lancet oncology, 2009, 10 (5): 467 - 474.

[74] Le Péchoux C, Laplanche A, Faivre-Finn C, et al. Clinical neurological outcome and quality of life among patients with limited small-cell cancer treated with two different doses of prophylactic cranial irradiation in the intergroup phase Ⅲ trial (PCI99 - 01, EORTC 22003 - 08004, RTOG 0212 and IFCT 99 - 01). Annals of oncology, 2011, 22 (5): 1154 - 1163.

[75] Russell AH, Pajak TE, Selim HM, et al. Prophylactic cranial irradiation for lung cancer patients at high risk for development of cerebral metastasis: results of a prospective randomized trial conducted by the Radiation Therapy Oncology Group. International Journal of Radiation Oncology Biology Physics, 1991, 21 (3): 637 - 643.

[76] Pottgen C, Eberhardt W, Grannass A, et al. Prophylactic cranial irradiation in operable stage Ⅲ A non-small-cell lung cancer treated with neoadjuvant chemoradiotherapy: Results from a German multicenter randomized trial. Journal of Clinical Oncology, 2007, 25 (31): 4987 - 4992.

[77] Gore EM, Bae K, Wong SJ, et al. Phase Ⅲ comparison of prophylactic cranial irradiation versus observation in patients with locally advanced non-small-cell lung cancer: Primary analysis of Radiation Therapy Oncology Group Study RTOG 0214. Journal of Clinical Oncology, 2011, 29 (3): 272 - 278.

[78] Sun A, Bae K, Gore EM, et al. Phase Ⅲ trial of prophylactic cranial irradiation compared with observation in patients with locally advanced non-small-cell lung cancer: neurocognitive and quality-of-life analysis. Journal of Clinical Oncology, 2011, 29 (3): 279 - 286.

[79] Hindo WA, Detrana FA, Lee MS, et al. Large dose increment irradiation in treatment of cerebral metastases. Cancer, 1970, 26 (1): 138 - 141.

[80] Boldrey ES, Heline GE. Delayed transitory clinical manifestations after radiation treatment of intracranial tumors. Acta Radiol: 5 SRC-GoogleScholar, 1996.

[81] Littman P, Rosenstock J, Gale G, et al. The somnolence syndrome in leukemic children following reduced daily dose fractions of cranial radiation. International Journal of Radiation Oncology Biology Physics, 1984, 10 (10): 1851 - 1853.

[82] Sperduto PW, Berkey B, Gaspar LE, et al. A new prognostic index and comparison to three other indices for patients with brain metastases: an analysis of 1,960 patients in the RTOG database. International Journal of Radiation Oncology Biology Physics, 2008, 70 (2): 510 - 514.

[83] Li J, Bentzen SM, Li J, et al. Relationship between neurocognitive function and quality of life after whole-brain radiotherapy in patients with brain metastasis. International Journal of Radiation Oncology Biology Physics, 2008, 71 (1): 64 - 70.

[84] Meyers CA, Smith JA, Bezjak A, et al. Neurocognitive function and progression in patients with brain metastases treated with whole-brain radiation and motexafin gadolinium: results of a randomized phase Ⅲ trial. Journal of clinical oncology, 2004, 22 (1): 157 - 165.

[85] Corn BW, Moughan J, Knisely JP, et al. Prospective evaluation of quality of life and neurocognitive effects in patients with multiple brain metastases receiving whole-brain radiotherapy with or without thalidomide on Radiation Therapy Oncology Group (RTOG) trial 0118. International Journal of Radiation Oncology Biology Physics, 2008, 71 (1): 71 - 78.

[86] Gregor A, Cull A, Traynor E, et al. Neuropsychometric evaluation of long-term survivors of adult brain tumours: relationship with tumour and treatment parameters. Radiotherapy and oncology, 1996, 41 (1): 55 - 59.

[87] Leibel SA, Sheline GE. Tolerance of the central and pe-

ripheral nervous system to therapeutic irradiation. Advances in radiation biology, 2013: 257 – 288.

[88] Sheline GE, Wara WM, Smith V. Therapeutic irradiation and brain injury. International Journal of Radiation Oncology Biology Physics, 1980, 6 (9): 1215 – 1228.

[89] Johnson BE, Patronas N, Hayes W, et al. Neurologic, computed cranial tomographic, and magnetic resonance imaging abnormalities in patients with small-cell lung cancer: further follow-up of 6-to 13-year survivors. Journal of Clinical Oncology, 1990, 8 (1): 48 – 56.

[90] Bleyer WA. Neurologic sequelae of methotrexate and ionizing radiation: a new classification. Cancer treatment reports, 1980, 65: 89 – 98.

[91] Ellison N, Bernath A, Kane R, et al. Disturbing problems of success: Clinical status of long-term survivors of small cell lung cancer//Proc Am Soc Clin Oncol, 1982, 1: 149.

[92] Catane R, Schwade JG, Yarr I, et al. Follow-up neurological evaluation in patients with small cell lung carcinoma treated with prophylactic cranial irradiation and chemotherapy. International Journal of Radiation Oncology Biology Physics, 1981, 7 (1): 105 – 109.

[93] Komaki R, Cox JD, Hartz AJ, et al. Characteristics of long-term survivors after treatment for inoperable carcinoma of the lung. American journal of clinical oncology, 1985, 8 (5): 362 – 370.

[94] Cheung MC, Chan AS. Memory impairment in humans after bilateral damage to lateral temporal neocortex. Neuroreport, 2003, 14 (3): 371 – 374.

[95] Gondi V, Tome WA, Mehta MP. Why avoid the hippocampus? A comprehensive review. Radiotherapy Oncology, 2010, 97 (3): 370 – 376.

[96] Gondi V, Hermann BP, Mehta MP, et al. Hippocampal dosimetry predicts neurocognitive function impairment after fractionated stereotactic radiotherapy for benign or low-grade adult brain tumors. International Journal of Radiation Oncology Biology Physics, 2013, 85 (2): 348 – 354.

[97] Curran WJ, Paulus R, Langer CJ, et al. Sequential vs concurrent chemoradiation for stage III non-small cell lung cancer: randomized Phase III trial RTOG 9410. Journal of the National Cancer Institute, 2011, 103 (19): 1452 – 1460.

[98] Komaki R, Derus SB, Perez-Tamayo C, et al. Brain metastasis in patients with superior sulcus tumors. Cancer, 1987, 59 (9): 1649 – 1653.

[99] Chen AM, Jahan TM, Jablons DM, et al. Risk of cerebral metastases and neurological death after pathological complete response to neoadjuvant therapy for locally advanced nonsmall-cell lung cancer. Cancer, 2007, 109 (8): 1668 – 1675.

[100] Grinberg-Rashi H, Ofek E, Perelman M, et al. The expression of three genes in primary non-small cell lung cancer is associated with metastatic spread to the brain. Clinical cancer research, 2009, 15 (5): 1755 – 1761.

[101] Milas I, Komaki R, Hachiya T, et al. Epidermal growth factor receptor, cyclooxygenase-2, and BAX expression in the primary non-small cell lung cancer and brain metastases. Clinical Cancer Research, 2003, 9 (3): 1070 – 1076.

[102] Bubb RS, Komaki R, Hachiya T, et al. Association of Ki-67, p53, and bcl-2 expression of the primary non-small-cell lung cancer lesion with brain metastatic lesion. International Journal of Radiation Oncology Biology Physics, 2002, 53 (5): 1216 – 1224.

[103] Saad AG, Yeap BY, Thunnissen FB, et al. Immunohistochemical markers associated with brain metastases in patients with nonsmall cell lung carcinoma. Cancer, 2008, 113 (8): 2129 – 2138.

[104] D'Amico T A, Aloia T A, Moore M B H, et al. Predicting the sites of metastases from lung cancer using molecular biologic markers. The Annals of thoracic surgery, 2001, 72 (4): 1144 – 1148.

[105] Arrieta O, Saavedra-Perez D, Kuri R, et al. Brain metastasis development and poor survival associated with carcinoembryonic antigen (CEA) level in advanced non-small cell lung cancer: a prospective analysis. BMC cancer, 2009, 9 (1): 119.

[106] Horinouchi H, Sekine I, Sumi M, et al. Brain metastases after definitive concurrent chemoradiotherapy in patients with stage III lung adenocarcinoma: carcinoembryonic antigen as a potential predictive factor. Cancer science, 2012, 103 (4): 756 – 759.

[107] Lee DS, Kim YS, Jung SL, et al. The relevance of serum carcinoembryonic antigen as an indicator of brain metastasis detection in advanced non-small cell lung cancer. Tumor Biology, 2012, 33 (4): 1065 – 1073.

[108] Matsumoto S, Takahashi K, Iwakawa R, et al. Frequent EGFR mutations in brain metastases of lung adenocarcinoma. International journal of cancer, 2006, 119 (6): 1491 – 1494.

[109] Sun M, Behrens C, Feng L, et al. HER family receptor

abnormalities in lung cancer brain metastases and corresponding primary tumors. Clinical Cancer Research, 2009, 15 (15): 4829-4837.

[110] Heon S, Yeap BY, Britt GJ, et al. Development of Central Nervous System Metastases in Patients with Advanced Non-Small Cell Lung Cancer and Somatic EGFR Mutations Treated with Gefitinib or Erlotinib. Clinical Cancer Research, 2010, 16 (23): 5873-5882.

[111] Lee YJ, Park IK, Park MS, et al. Activating mutations within the EGFR kinase domain: a molecular predictor of disease-free survival in resected pulmonary adenocarcinoma. Journal of cancer research and clinical oncology, 2009, 135 (12): 1647-1654.

[112] Hotta K, Kiura K, Ueoka H, et al. Effect of gefitinib ('Iressa', ZD1839) on brain metastases in patients with advanced non-small-cell lung cancer. Lung Cancer, 2004, 46 (2): 255-261.

[113] Namba Y, Kijima T, Yokota S, et al. Gefitinib in patients with brain metastases from non-small-cell lung cancer: Review of 15 clinical cases. Clinical lung cancer, 2004, 6 (2): 123-128.

[114] Shimato S, Mitsudomi T, Kosaka T, et al. EGFR mutations in patients with brain metastases from lung cancer: association with the efficacy of gefitinib. Neuro-oncology, 2006, 8 (2): 137-144.

[115] Porta R, Sanchez-Torres JM, Paz-Ares L, et al. Brain metastases from lung cancer responding to erloti-nib: the importance of EGFR mutation. European Respiratory Journal, 2011, 37 (3): 624-631.

[116] Bai H, Han B. The effectiveness of erlotinib against brain metastases in non-small cell lung cancer patients. American journal of clinical oncology, 2013, 36 (2): 110-115.

[117] Gow CH, Chien CR, Chang YL, et al. Radiotherapy in lung adenocarcinoma with brain metastases: effects of activating epidermal growth factor receptor mutations on clinical response. Clinical Cancer Research, 2008, 14 (1): 162-168.

[118] Eichler AF, Kahle KT, Wang DL, et al. EGFR mutation status and survival after diagnosis of brain metastasis in nonsmall cell lung cancer. Neuro Oncol, 2010, 12 (11): 1193-1199.

[119] Daniele L, Cassoni P, Bacillo E, et al. Epidermal growth factor receptor gene in primary tumor and metastatic sites from non-small cell lung cancer. Journal of Thoracic Oncology, 2009, 4 (6): 684-688.

[120] Gomez-Roca C, Raynaud CM, Penault-Llorca F, et al. Differential expression of biomarkers in primary non-small cell lung cancer and metastatic sites. Journal of Thoracic Oncology, 2009, 4 (10): 1212-1220.

[121] Han HS, Eom DW, Kim JH, et al. EGFR mutation status in primary lung adenocarcinomas and corresponding metastatic lesions: discordance in pleural metastases. Clinical lung cancer, 2011, 12 (6): 380-386.

[122] Heon S, Yeap BY, Lindeman NI, et al. The impact of initial gefitinib or erlotinib versus chemotherapy on central nervous system progression in advanced non-small cell lung cancer with EGFR mutations. Clinical Cancer Research, 2012, 18 (16): 4406-4414.

[123] Kurtz JM, Gelber R, Brady LW, et al. The palliation of brain metastases in a favorable patient population: a randomized clinical trial by the Radiation Therapy Oncology Group. International Journal of Radiation Oncology Biology Physics, 1981, 7 (7): 891-895.

[124] Komaki R, Chang E. Whole-brain radiation therapy// Sawaya R (ed.), Intracranial Metastases: Current Management Strategies. MA: Blackwell publishing, 2004: 126-138.

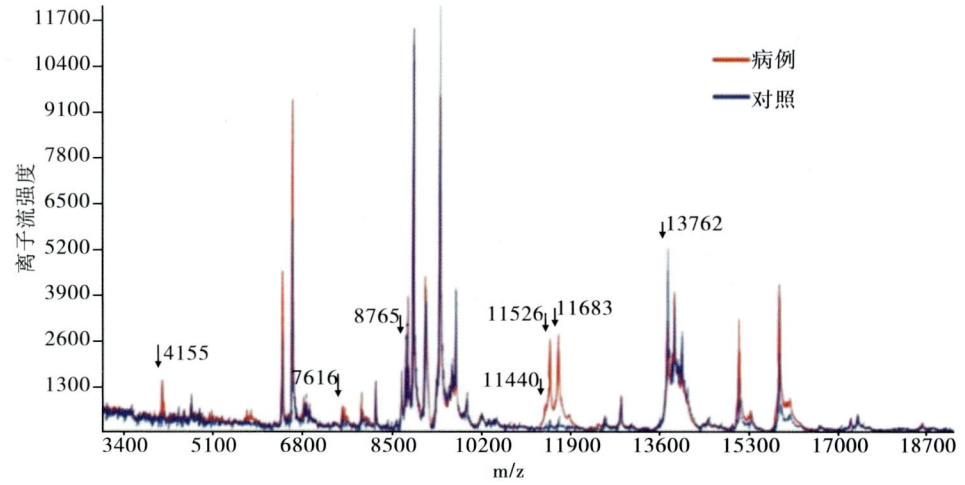

图 5.4 肺癌患者及其对照的 MALDI MS 血清图谱。图中列出了匹配案例（红色，平滑线）和对照（蓝色，点线）的图谱分析的平均强度。箭头代表有差异性的 M/Z 值

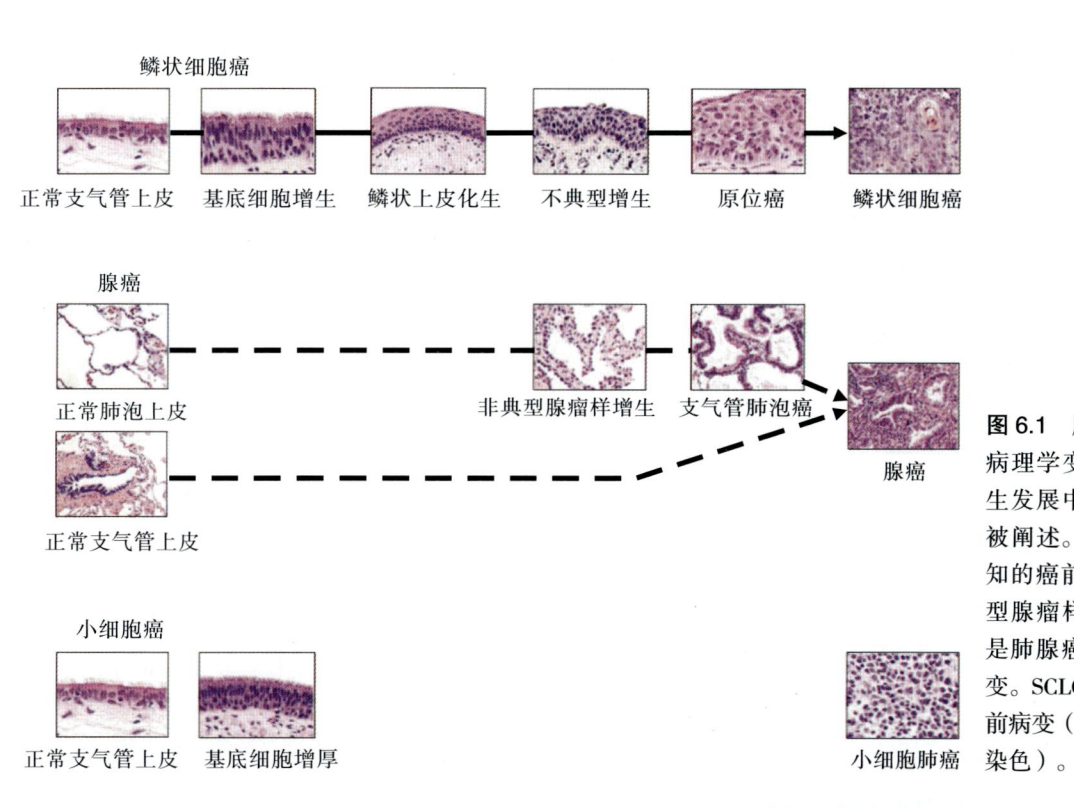

图 6.1 肺癌癌前病变的组织病理学变化总结。肺鳞癌发生发展中癌前病变的次序已被阐述。肺腺癌目前唯一已知的癌前病变是 AAH（非典型腺瘤样增生），其被认为是肺腺癌某一亚型的前驱病变。SCLC 尚未发现明显的癌前病变（经病理组织切片 H-E 染色）。

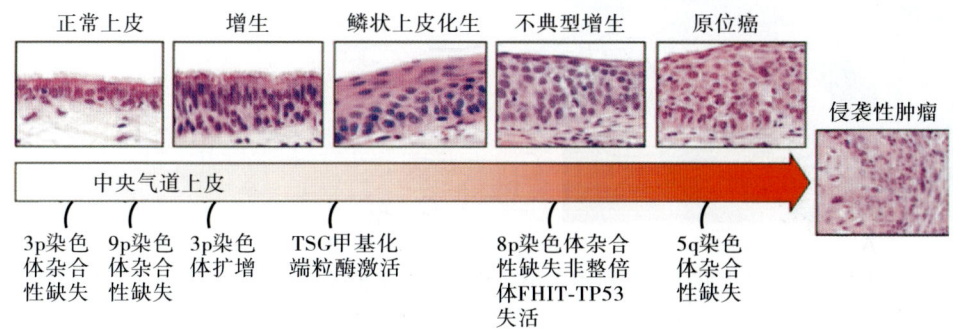

图 6.2 肺鳞癌发病的分子机制。肺鳞癌发病的多步骤中发生一系列分子异常，并可在高危个体中检测到该类异常

1

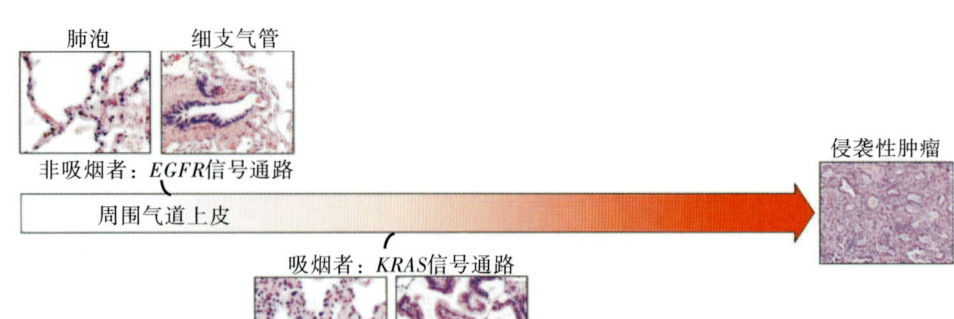

图6.3 肺腺癌的分子学发病机制。吸烟或不吸烟相关性肺腺癌发展中已知至少发生两种病变

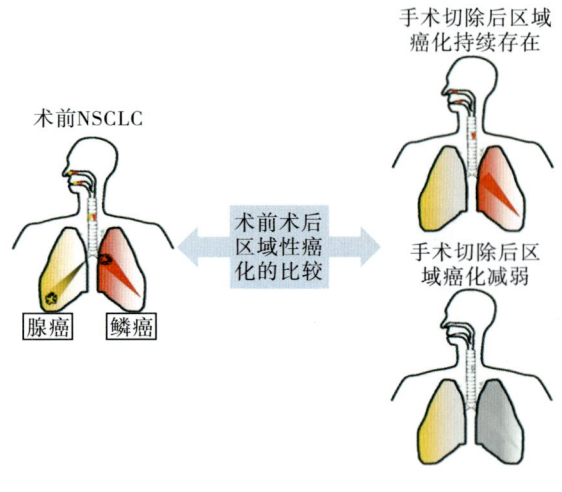

图6.4 早期NSCLC患者中的区域性癌化现象。相较于肺鳞癌，区域性癌化与肺癌的某特定亚型（如肺腺癌）的相关性尚不明确。通过分析肺腺癌（黄色点区）及鳞癌（红色点区）之外多点支气管镜刷检物转录组物来分析局部及远端癌化区域，能为探讨这两种主要病变的分子学发病机制提供线索（左图）。区域性癌化与早期肺癌患者的潜在相关性可通过研究术前及术后分子癌化现象在手术切除后是否持续（右上）或下降（右下）来进行阐明。该类分析将有助于决定肺癌患者术后区域癌化现象与术后复发的相关性。如此，对该效应的分析可能发展为新的预防措施

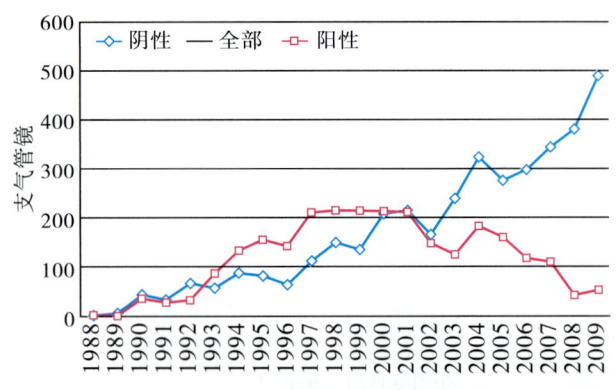

图7.1 1998—2009年加入BCCA肺部健康研究的重度吸烟者的比例。使用自发荧光支气管镜检查及5.8mm的支气管镜活检发现，这些患者存在至少1处以上的支气管异型增生，自2000年开始，支气管异型增生的发病率稳固下降

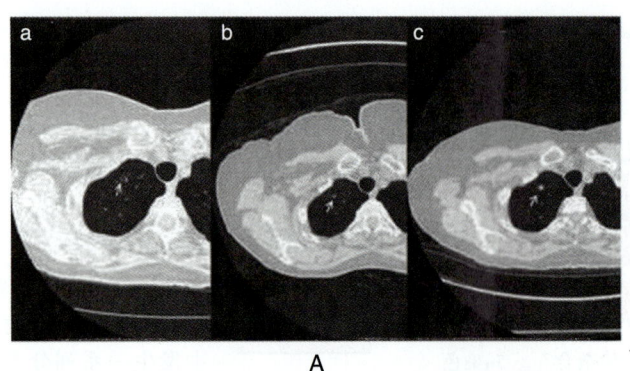
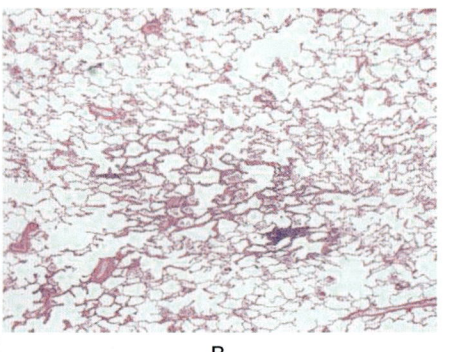

图7.2 A.连续两年的低剂量螺旋CT复查显示右肺上叶（箭头所示）小结节的大小及密度逐渐增加（b、c）。B.肺楔形切除病理检查示AAH

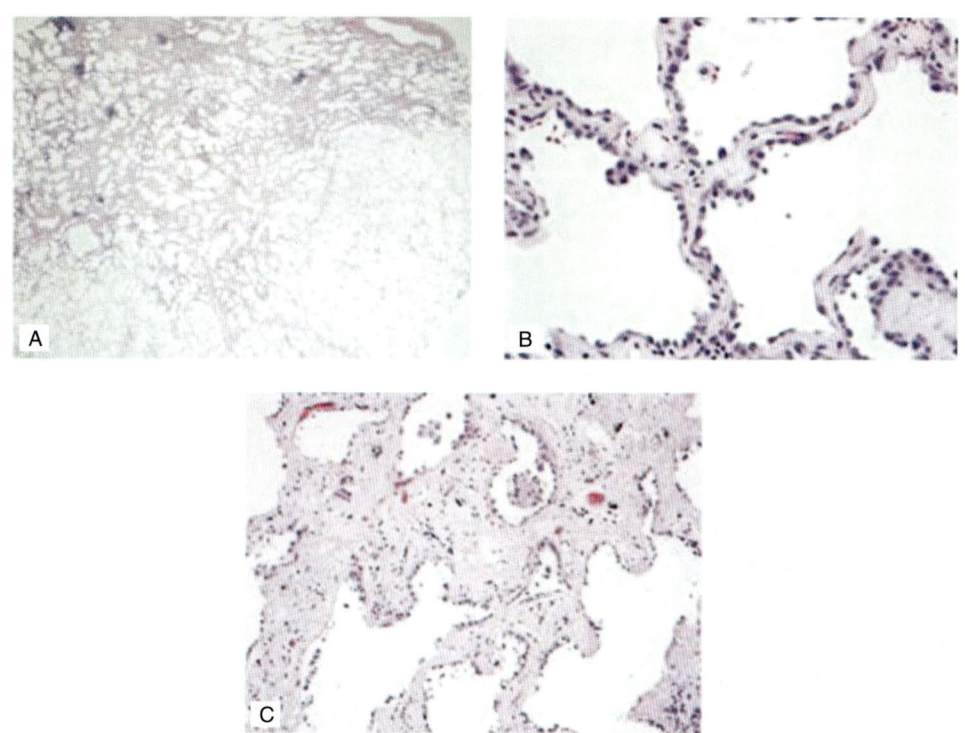

图 8.1 非黏液型 AIS。A. 限制性非黏液型肿瘤单纯鳞屑样生长且无浸润性。苏木精－伊红（H-E）染色 ×1.25。B. 鳞屑样生长或非典型细胞沿肺泡壁薄生长，H-E 染色 ×20；C. 肺泡壁薄纤维化增厚，但没有浸润，只存在鳞屑样生长，H-E 染色 ×20

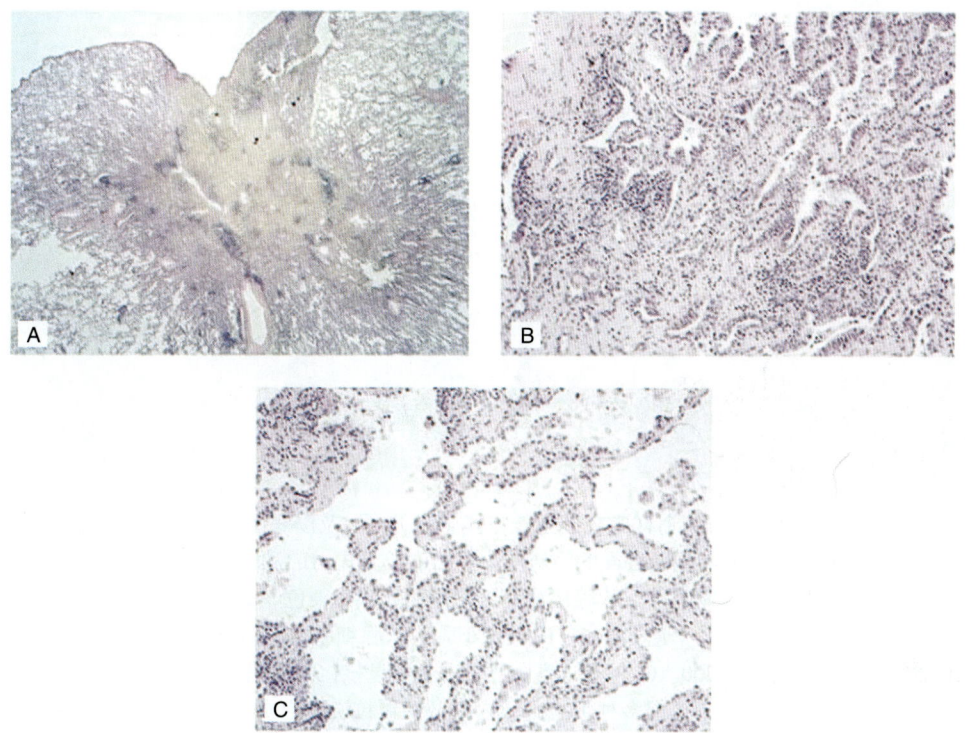

图 8.2 非黏液型 MIA。A. 腺癌鳞屑样生长方式为主且浸润灶小于 5mm，H-E 染色 ×1.25。B. 肿瘤细胞浸润肌纤维母细胞基质，H-E 染色 ×20；C. 其他区域表现为鳞屑样生长，肺泡壁薄生长，H-E 染色 ×20

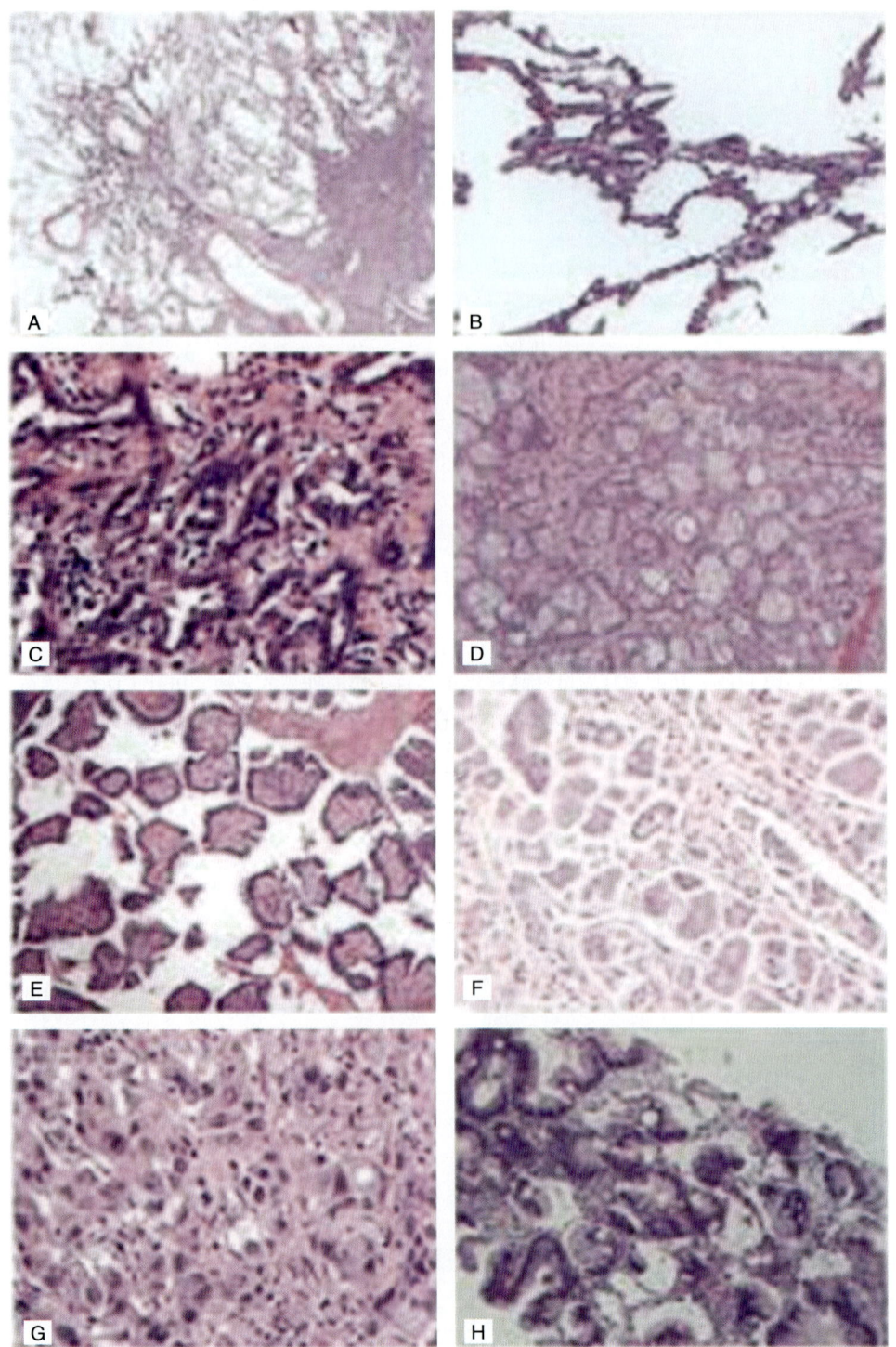

图 8.3 浸润性腺癌的主要组织模式。A. 鳞屑样为主的生长方式（左），以及浸润性腺泡样腺癌（右），H-E 染色 ×100。B. Ⅱ型肺泡上皮细胞和克拉拉细胞沿着肺泡壁表面的鳞屑样为主的生长方式，H-E 染色 ×200。C. 浸润性腺泡样腺癌区，H-E 染色 ×400。D. 包含圆至椭圆形恶性腺体的腺泡状腺癌浸润纤维间质，H-E 染色 ×200。E. 包含恶性立方体柱状肿瘤细胞的乳头状腺癌在纤维芯的表面生长，H-E 染色 ×100。F. 包含小乳头状腺细胞群的微乳头状腺癌在空间上的生长，其中大部分不显示纤维血管轴心，H-E 染色 ×200。G. 带有丰富胞质，以及明显核仁的泡状核的肿瘤细胞构成的实性腺癌被看到，而腺泡样，乳头状以及鳞屑样没有被看到，但多种细胞胞质内嗜碱性颗粒说明胞质内存在黏蛋白。H-E 染色 ×400。H. 浸润性黏液腺癌显示鳞屑样和腺泡样生长。肿瘤由柱状细胞构成，这些柱状细胞的顶端细胞质中被丰富的黏液填充，且能看见小基底核，H-E 染色 ×200

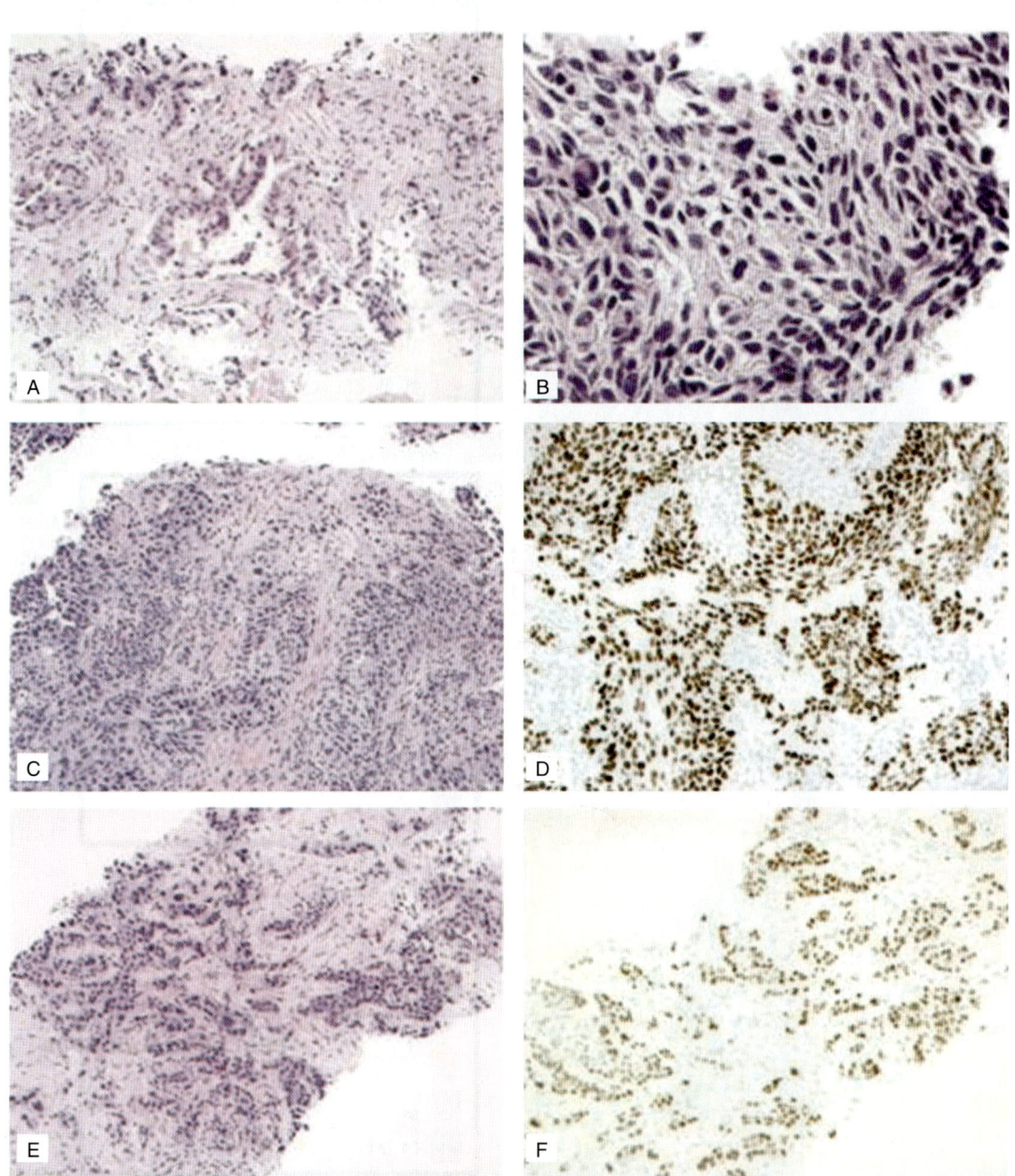

图 8.4 A. 腺癌：肿瘤表现为腺泡样生长模式，苏木精-伊红染色 ×200。B. 鳞状细胞癌：肿瘤表现为角质化。C.NSCLC，良性腺癌：癌细胞没有明显的鳞状或腺状分化，苏木精-伊红染色 ×200。D.TTF-1 染色阳性，从而可以诊断为 NSCLC，良性腺癌，苏木精-伊红染色 ×200。E.NSCLC，良性鳞状细胞癌：癌细胞没有明显的鳞状或腺状分化，苏木精-伊红染色 ×200。F.p63 染色阳性，TTF-1 染色阴性（没显示），从而可以诊断为 NSCLC，良性鳞状细胞癌。p63 免疫组化 ×200

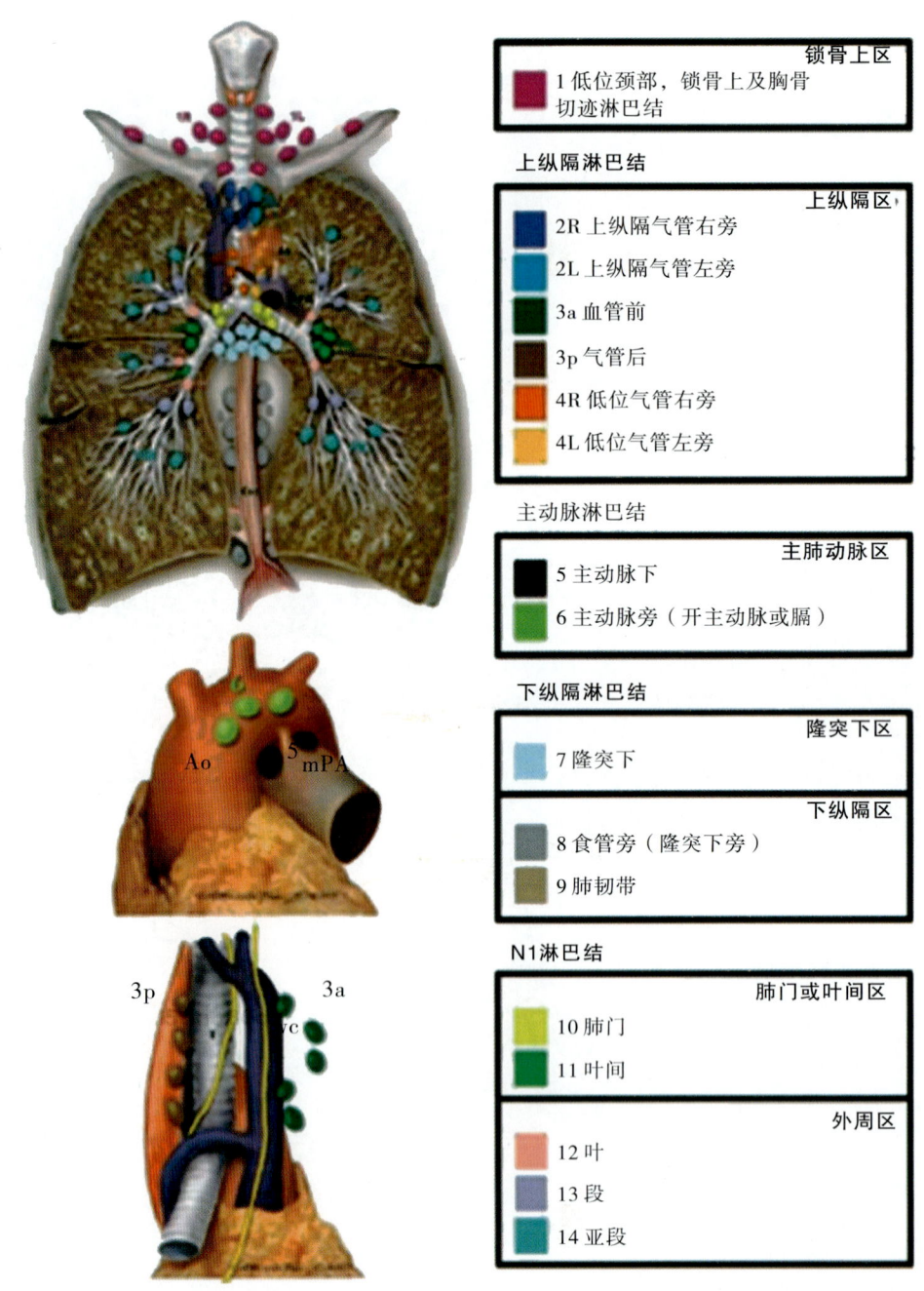

图 12.3 A～F：国际肺癌研究组织 (IASLC) 淋巴结示意图，用于 CT 扫描进行临床分期，横轴位 (A~C)，冠状位 (D)，和矢状位 (E、F) 视野。右和左气管旁区之间的边缘可于 A 和 B 中显示。Ao：主动脉；AV：奇静脉；Br：细支气管；IA：无名动脉；IV：无名静脉；LA：动脉韧带；LIV：左无名静脉；LSA：左锁骨下动脉；PA：肺动脉；PV：肺静脉；RIV：右无名静脉；SVC：上腔静脉[55]。来源：Rusch，2009[55]。经 Lippincott Willams 及 Wilkins 许可出版

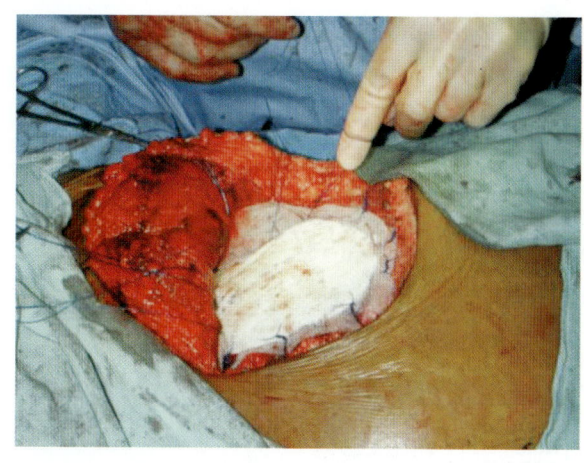

图 15.1 用聚丙烯网和骨水泥重建胸壁

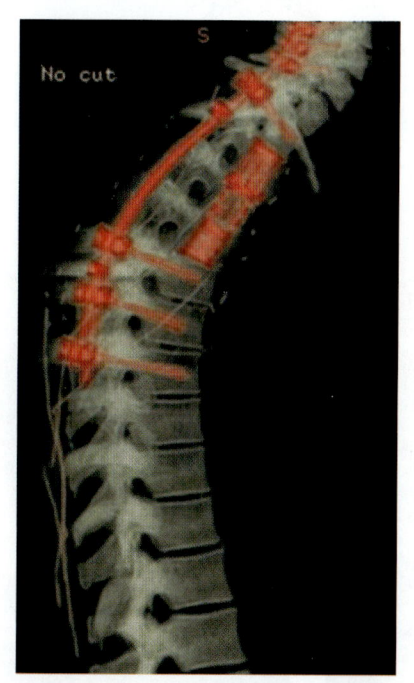

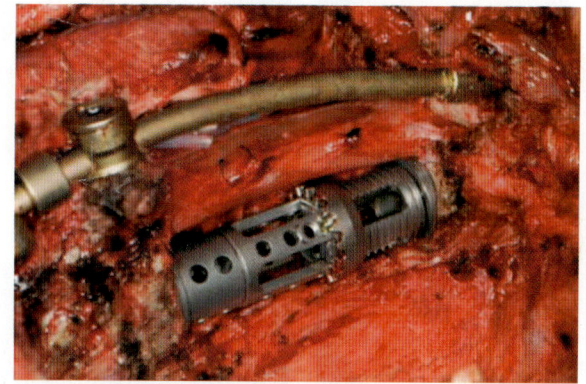

图 15.3 肿瘤侵犯脊柱行扩大切除后重建恢复稳定性。A. 术后影像学。B. 术中照片

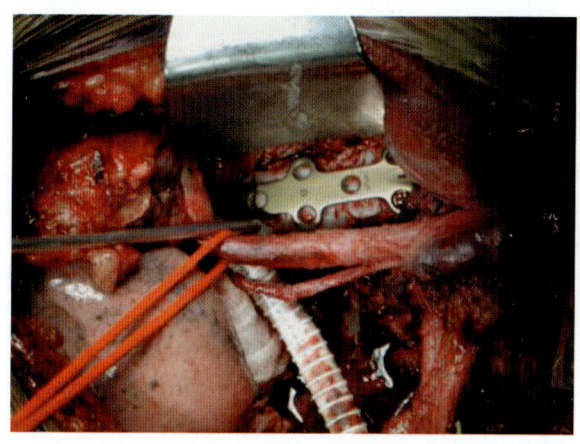

图 15.4 肺上沟瘤联合脊柱（可见固定装置）和锁骨下血管切除（聚四氟乙烯人工血管置换）

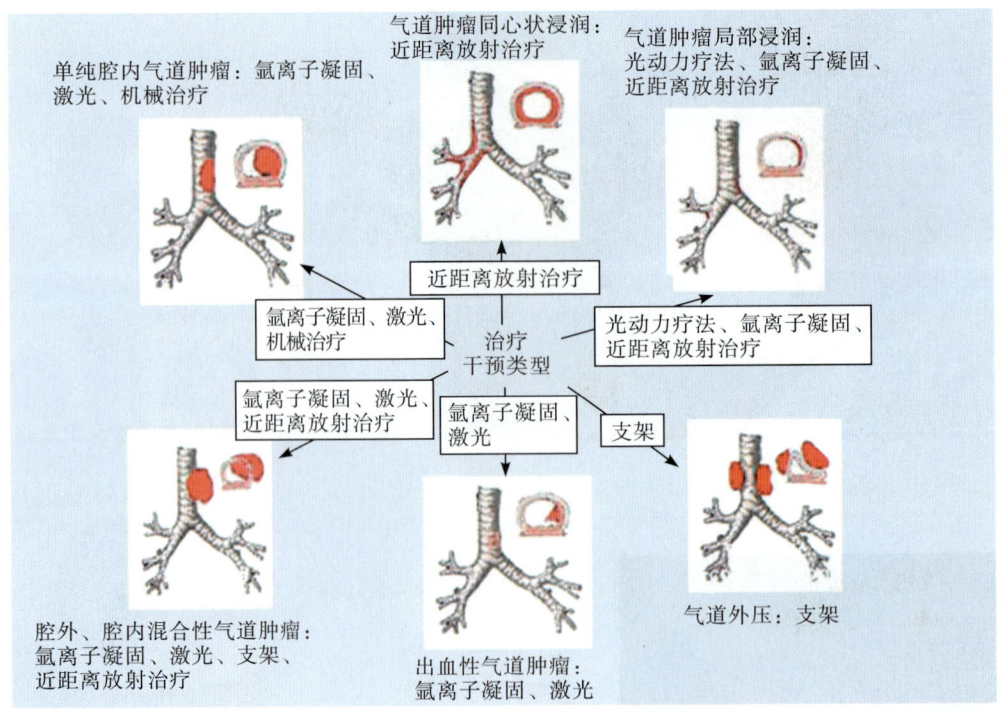

图 16.1 根据位置及病变类型选择适当的内镜治疗方法。经 Dr R. Morice 许可使用

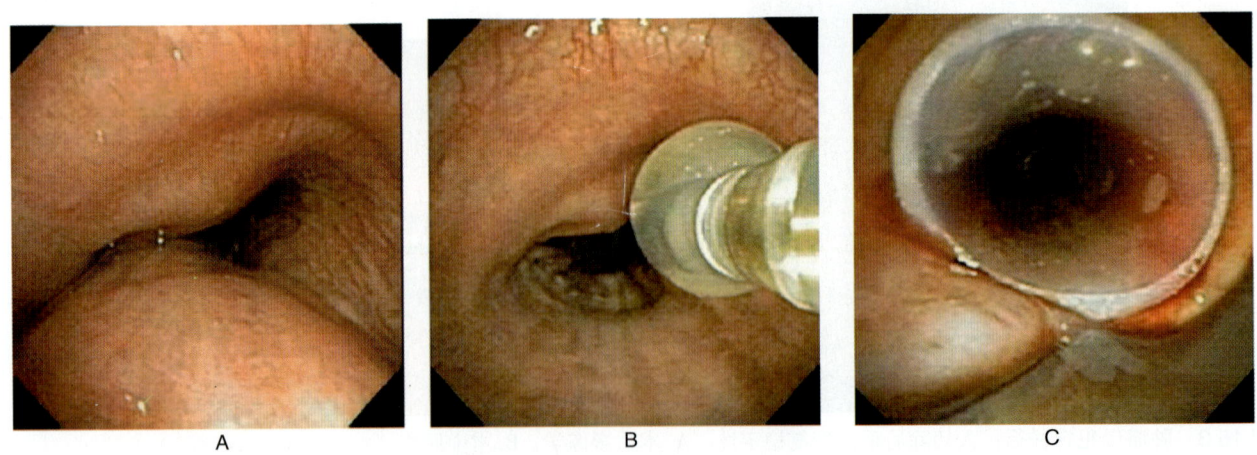

图 16.2 A.69 岁腺样囊性癌女性患者，表现为严重呼吸困难，肿瘤阻塞气管下段及双侧支气管主干。B. 球囊连续扩张气管下段狭窄。C. 球囊连续扩张，植入 Y 形气管支气管硅胶支架之后气道明显恢复

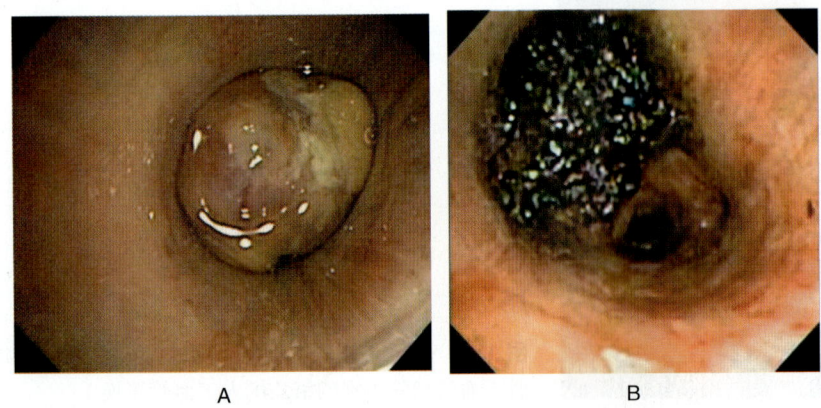

图 16.3 A.49 岁的右肺中叶腺癌女性患者，由于右中间支气管的完全性梗阻出现呼吸困难。B. 右中间支气管经过圈套电灼及氩离子血浆凝固治疗腔内肿瘤后完全再通

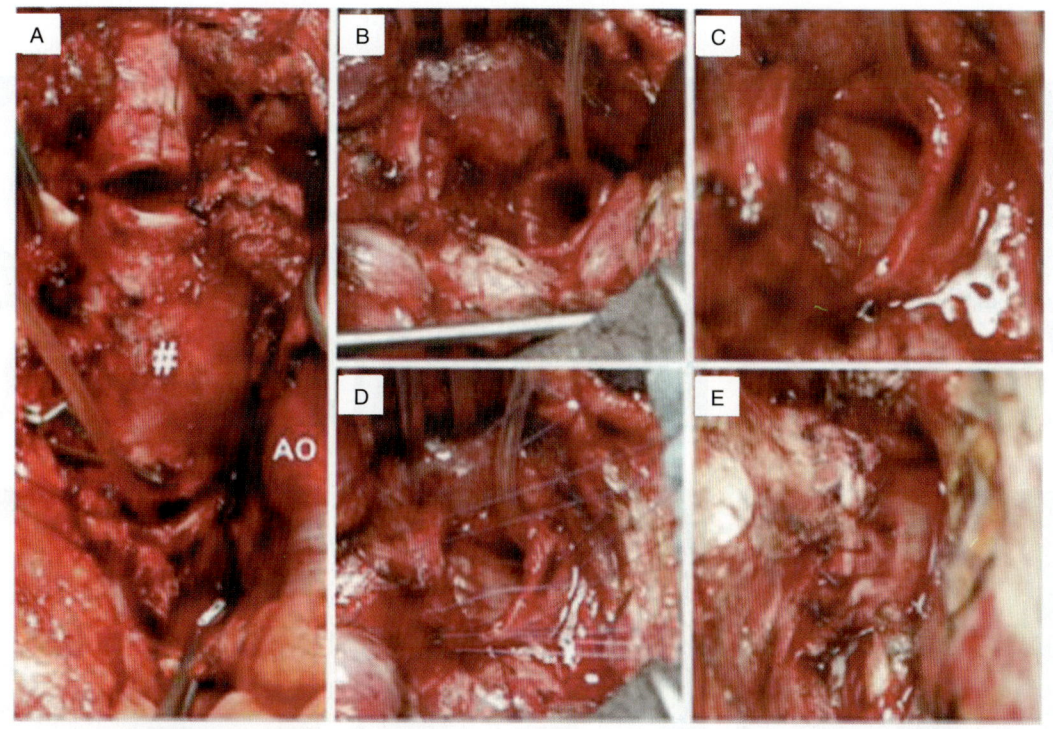

图17.2　A. 正面观：牵拉开主动脉（AO）后，胸腔内中段、远段气管。#：受肿瘤侵犯，需要切除的部分气管。B. 侧面观：切除肿瘤后，气管后壁行连续缝合。C. 收紧连续缝合线。D. 气管前壁间断缝合（7× 缝线）。E. 收紧缝合线，吻合气管

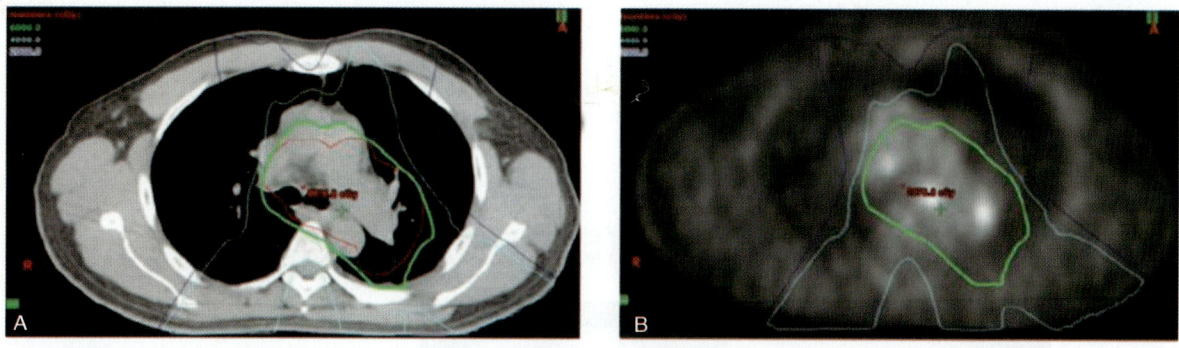

图20.1　一例患有ⅢB期不可手术NSCLC的62岁女性患者。该部位安全地接受了60Gy/30f剂量。治疗计划基于PET-CT融合图像制定。A. 计划CT的一个层面，PTV以红色勾画。B. 相同层面的FDG-PET图像。6 000cGy、4 000cGy、2 000cGy等剂量线分别以绿色、蓝绿色和蓝色标注

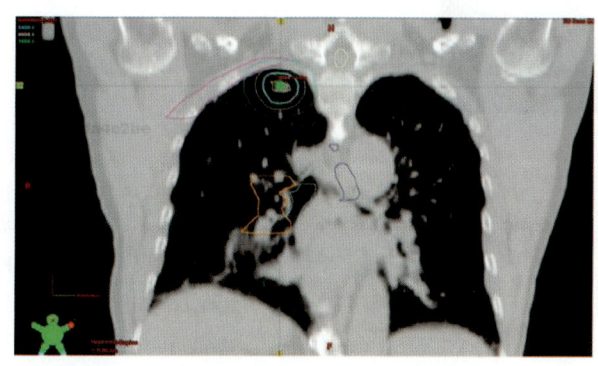

图20.2　一例患有早期不可手术NSCLC的89岁女性患者。该部位安全地接受了54Gy/3f的剂量。黄色勾画线表示大体肿瘤体积（GTV）。绿色、白色和蓝色线分别表示1 000cGy、4 000cGy和5 400cGy等剂量线。需要使其放射剂量最小化的正常结构包括胸壁（品红色）、脊髓（黄色）、食管（蓝色）、支气管树（橙色和蓝色）

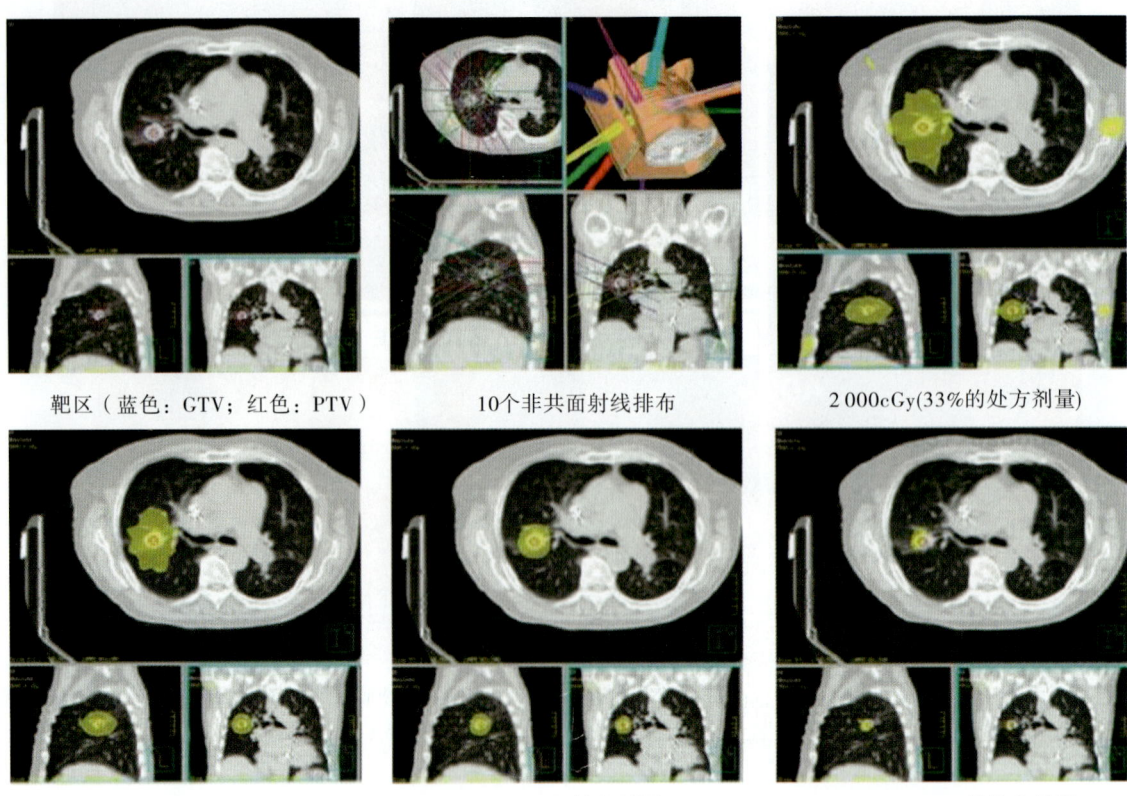

图 21.2 是典型的 SABR 治疗原发性肺癌剂量分布的示例。10 个非共面、非对穿野保证了肿瘤靶区获得高剂量及所有方向上剂量的快速跌落

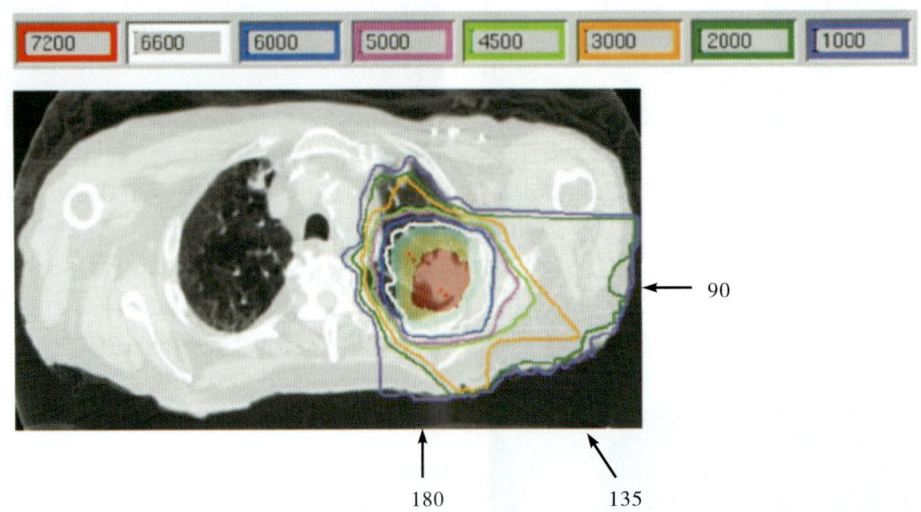

图 22.2 典型被动散射质子放疗计划射束排布。内在肿瘤靶区（internal gross tumor volume, iGTV）标为红褐色；附近临床靶区（CTV）为卡其色（绿）；计划靶区（PTV）为蓝色。箭头指示射束角度。顶部不同颜色数字指示等剂量曲线（cGy）

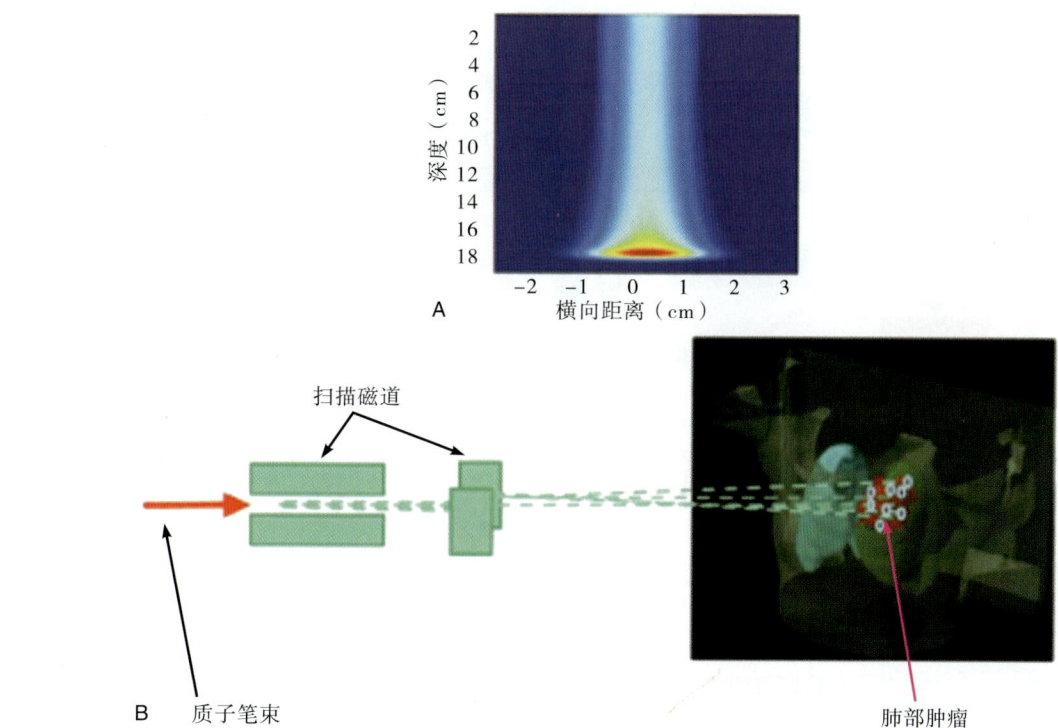

图 22.3　A. 典型动态点扫描。B. 散射束剂量喷涂示意图

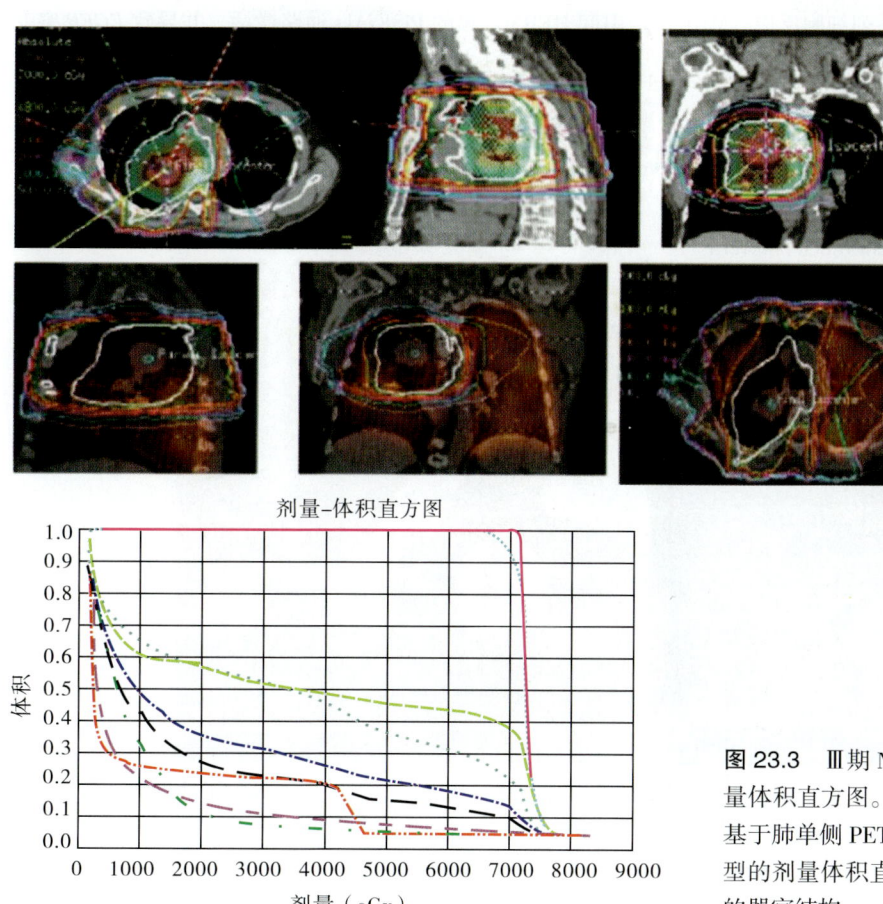

图 23.3　Ⅲ期 NSCLC 放疗计划典型的剂量分布图和剂量体积直方图。上图：基于 CT 图像的 IMRT；中图：基于肺单侧 PET/CT 图像的 IMRT 计划；下图：一个典型的剂量体积直方图。直方图中不同的颜色代表不同的器官结构

11

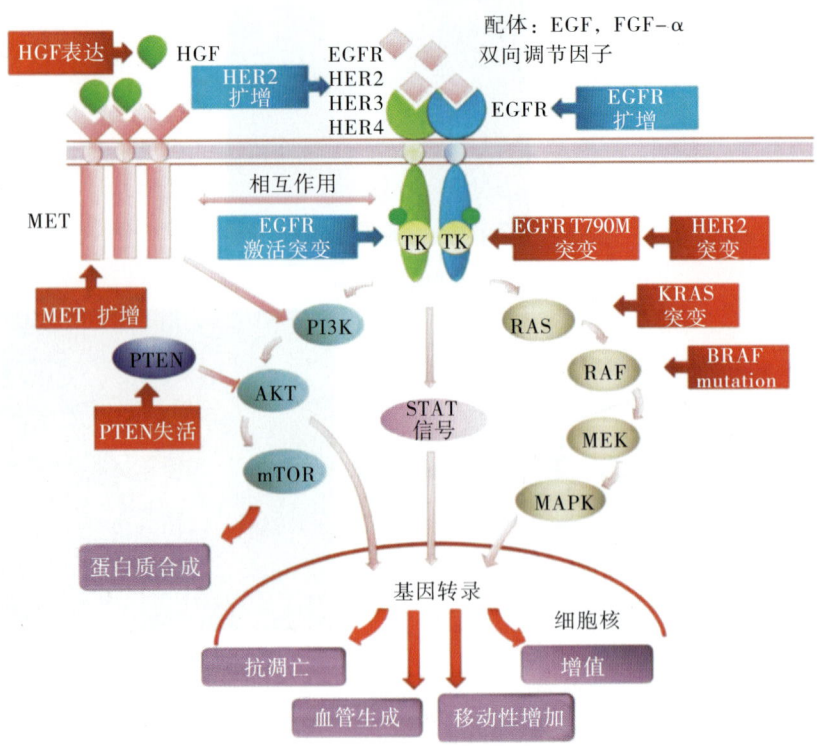

图 28.1 EGFR 及相关分子信号通路。EGFR 与相应配体结合诱导受体形成同（异）二聚体，进而通过酪氨酸残基自磷酸化激活细胞内酪氨酸激酶。EGFR 激活引起下游信号级联放大，主要包括 RAS、PI3K/AKT 和 STAT 通路，并最终导致增殖、抗凋亡、移动性增强及血管生成等一系列细胞反应。MET 扩增引起 HER3 依赖的 PI3K/Akt 通路激活，并导致 *EGFR* 突变肿瘤的获得性耐药。图中显示了针对 EGFR 及与药敏（蓝盒）或耐药（红盒）相关下游分子的遗传及表观遗传学改变

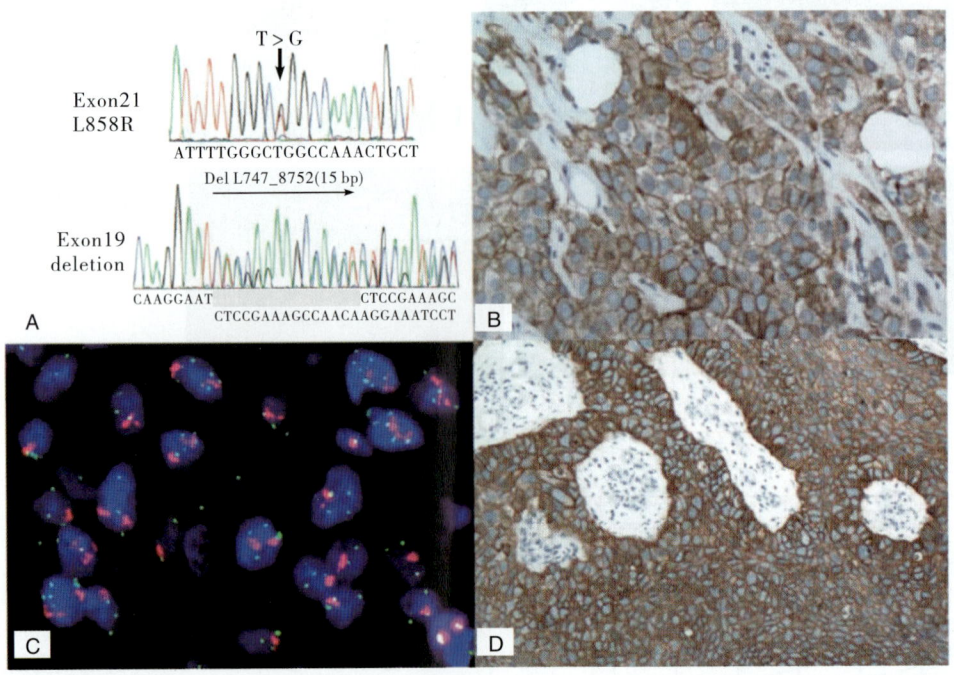

图 28.3 检测 EGFR 突变，基因拷贝数及蛋白表达的通常检测手段。A. *EGFR* L858R 点突变及 19 外显子缺失突变的直接测序结果。B. *EGFR* L858R 突变特异性抗体的免疫组化显示了其在 EGFR 突变肿瘤细胞膜及胞质内的染色模式。C. 荧光原位杂交检测到的 *EGFR* 扩增（红色信号，*EGFR* 基因探针；绿色信号，7 号染色体着丝粒探针）。D. 免疫组化法检测的 *EGFR* 蛋白表达显示其在肺鳞癌细胞膜上特定的染色特点

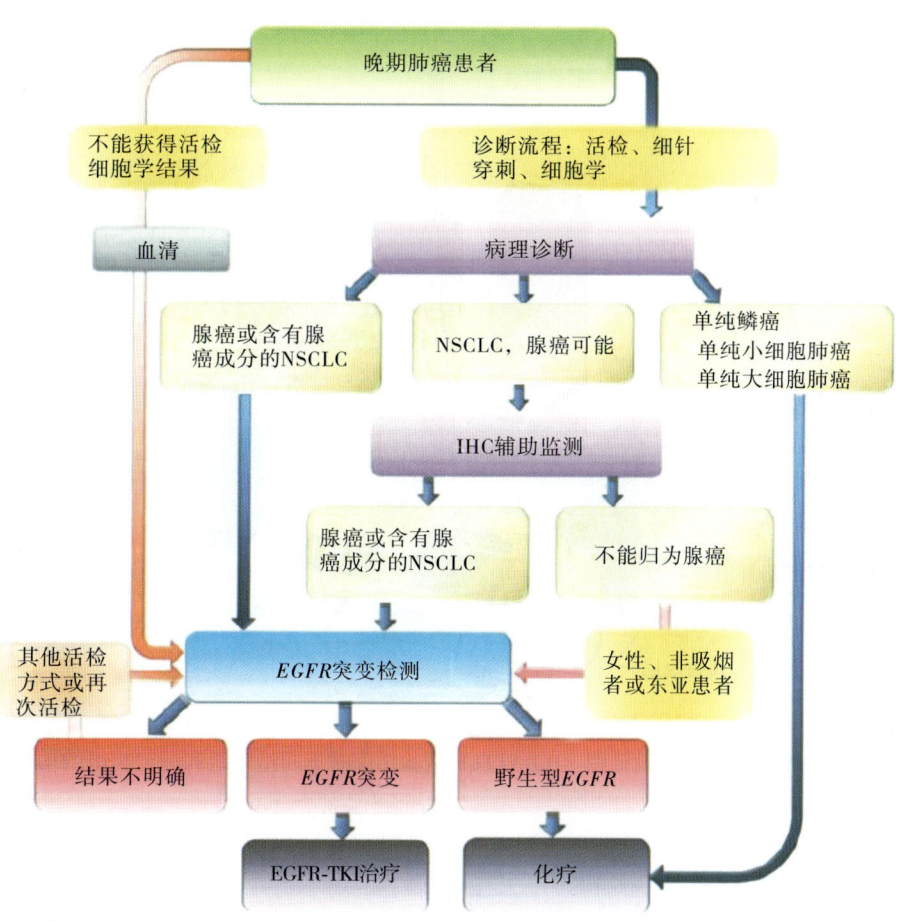

图 28.4 新确诊的晚期 NSCLC 患者对于指导一线 EGFR-TKIs 治疗 *EGFR* 突变检测的决策流程

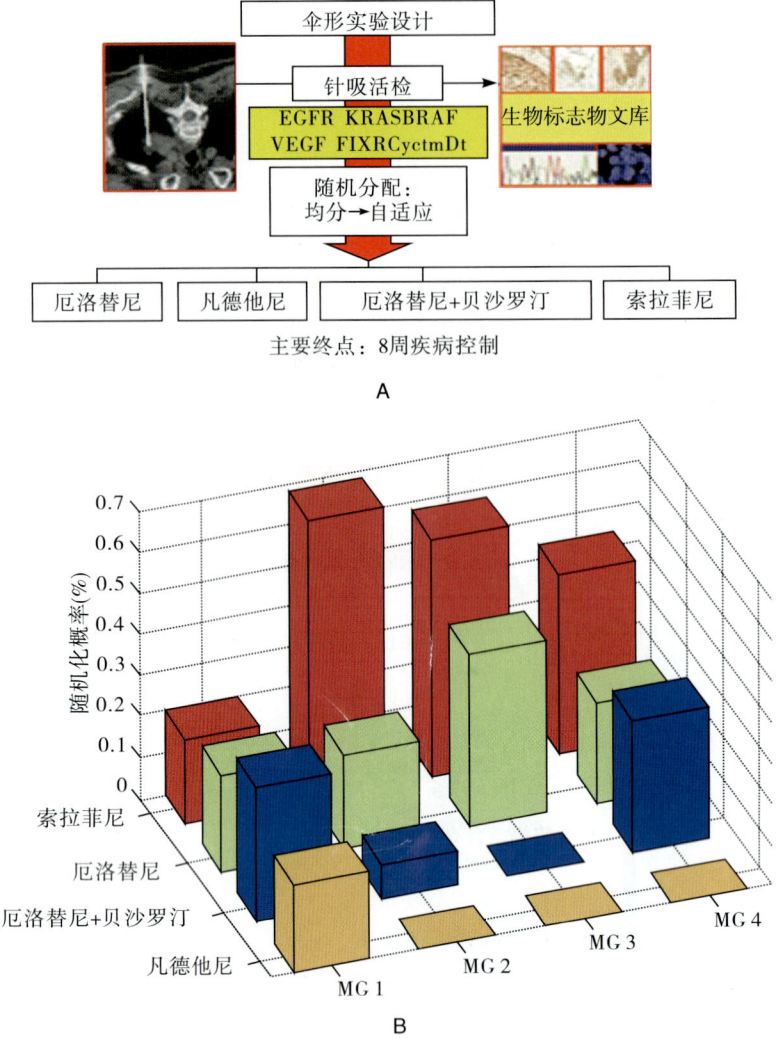

图32.3 BATTLE试验。A.BATTLE试验设计图。B.BATTLE试验结束时不同治疗组和标记物组的动态随机化概率

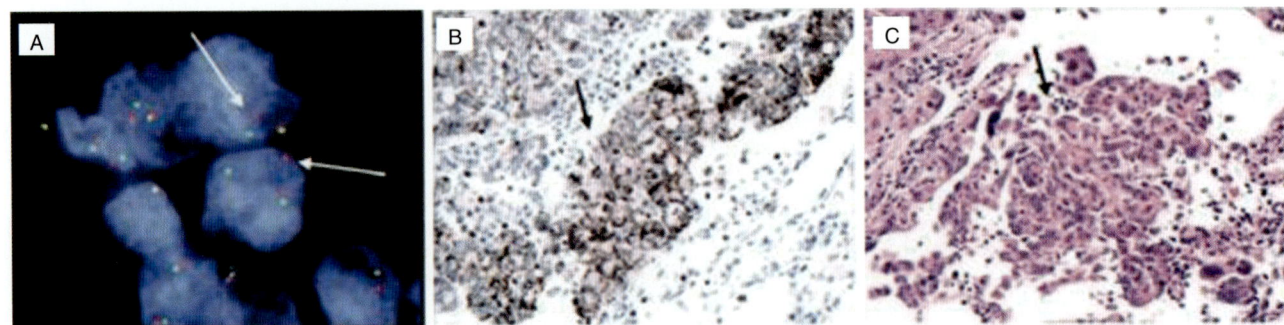

图35.2 A.ALK FISH揭示了红色和绿色探针分离(箭头)，ALK重排的象征。B.ALK免疫组化显示ALK染色阳性。C.H-E染色显示印戒细胞，一个常见的ALK阳性NSCLC的形态学特征。摘自Shaw AT, Yeap BY, Mino-Kenudson M, et al. Clinical features and outcomes of patients with non-small-cell lung cancer who harbor *EML4–ALK*, 2009,27(26): 4247–4253. Reprinted with permission.©(2009) American Society of Clinical Oncology